COMPREHENSIVE MEDICAL TERMINOLOGY

FIFTH EDITION

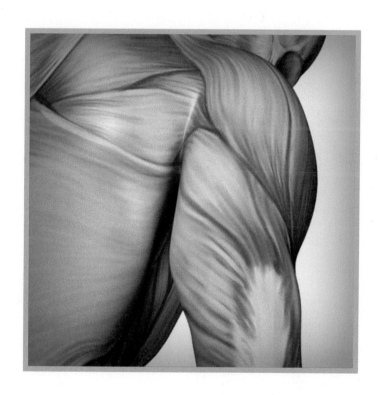

COMPREHENSIVE MEDICAL TERMINOLOGY

FIFTH EDITION

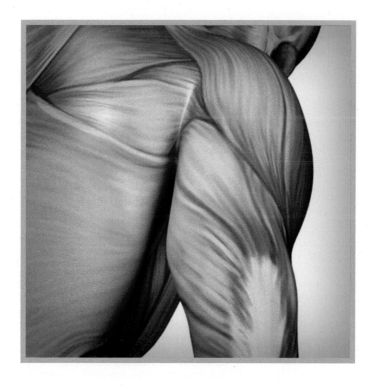

Betty Davis Jones, RN, MA, CMA (AAMA)

Department Chair, Medical Assisting, Phlebotomy, Health Promotions
Gaston College, Dallas, North Carolina

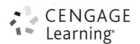

Australia • Brazil • Mexico • Singapore • United Kingdom • United States

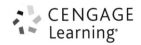

Comprehensive Medical Terminology,
Fifth Edition
Betty Davis Jones

SVP, GM Skills & Global Product Management:
  Dawn Gerrain

Product Director: Matthew Seeley

Senior Director, Development:
  Marah Bellegarde

Product Development Manager: Juliet Steiner

Product Manager: Laura Stewart

Senior Content Developer:
  Debra M. Myette-Flis

Product Assistant: Deborah Handy

Vice President, Marketing Services:
  Jennifer Ann Baker

Marketing Manager: Jonathan Sheehan

Senior Production Director: Wendy Troeger

Production Director: Andrew Crouth

Content Project Manager: Thomas Heffernan

Managing Art Director: Jack Pendleton

Cover image(s): ©iStockPhoto.com/angelhell

For product information and technology assistance, contact us at
Cengage Learning Customer & Sales Support, 1-800-354-9706

For permission to use material from this text or product,
submit all requests online at **www.cengage.com/permissions**
Further permissions questions can be e-mailed to
permissionrequest@cengage.com

Library of Congress Control Number: 2015933403

ISBN: 978-1-285-86954-4

Cengage Learning
20 Channel Center Street
Boston, MA 02210
USA

Cengage Learning is a leading provider of customized learning solutions with employees residing in nearly 40 different countries and sales in more than 125 countries around the world. Find your local representative at
http://www.cengage.com

Cengage Learning products are represented in Canada by Nelson Education, Ltd.

To learn more about Cengage Learning, visit **www.cengage.com**

Purchase any of our products at your local college store or at our preferred online store **www.cengagebrain.com**

Notice to the Reader

Publisher does not warrant or guarantee any of the products described herein or perform any independent analysis in connection with any of the product information contained herein. Publisher does not assume, and expressly disclaims, any obligation to obtain and include information other than that provided to it by the manufacturer. The reader is expressly warned to consider and adopt all safety precautions that might be indicated by the activities described herein and to avoid all potential hazards. By following the instructions contained herein, the reader willingly assumes all risks in connection with such instructions. The publisher makes no representations or warranties of any kind, including but not limited to, the warranties of fitness for particular purpose or merchantability, nor are any such representations implied with respect to the material set forth herein, and the publisher takes no responsibility with respect to such material. The publisher shall not be liable for any special, consequential, or exemplary damages resulting, in whole or in part, from the readers' use of, or reliance upon, this material.

Printed in the United States of America
Print Number: 07   Print Year: 2018

Contents

Chapter 1

Word Building Rules / 1

Chapter 2

Prefixes / 21

Chapter 3

Suffixes / 39

Chapter 4

Whole Body Terminology / 59

Chapter 9

The Blood and Lymphatic Systems / 325

Chapter 10

The Cardiovascular System / 388

Chapter 11

The Respiratory System / 447

Chapter 12

The Digestive System / 491

Chapter 13

The Endocrine System / 554

Chapter 14

The Special Senses / 606

Chapter 15

The Urinary System / 669

Chapter 16

The Male Reproductive System / 719

Chapter 17

The Female Reproductive System / 759

Chapter 18

Obstetrics / 816

Chapter 19

Child Health / 869

Chapter 20

Radiology and Diagnostic Imaging / 917

Dedication

This textbook is dedicated to the many students of medical terminology with whom I have crossed paths. You have challenged my mind to new heights, and your thirst for knowledge makes teaching fun!

Preface

Medical terminology is the key to unlocking a whole new world of knowledge. This knowledge will empower you to communicate on a highly technical level about medical disorders, disease processes, surgical procedures, and treatments. You will learn terms that will allow you to read and interpret medical terms in reports, charts, and other health care environments.

This text has been developed to provide you—the learner—with the skills you need to become an effective communicator in the highly technical world of medicine. Once you understand that medical terms have many interchangeable parts, you will realize that learning medical terms is not as difficult as you might have thought. Couple this with the appropriate word building rules, and you are on your way to expanding your vocabulary by hundreds of new medical words!

Textbook Organization

First, you should familiarize yourself with the organization of this textbook and any supplementary materials that may be available to you. Some of the key points regarding the organization follow.

The textbook begins with Chapter 1, Word Building Rules. It is important that you understand how word elements (parts) are put together to make up medical terms. This knowledge will enable you to build words you have never seen before, simply by knowing the meaning of the word elements and the appropriate way of putting the elements together to form a medical term. Always remember that if you get confused on word building skills, you can return to Chapter 1 for guidance.

Chapters 2 through 4 concentrate on the basics of medical terminology: prefixes, suffixes, and whole body terminology. Chapters 5 through 24 concentrate on body systems and specialty areas of practice. The body systems are arranged in basically the same order as most anatomy and physiology textbooks. This seems to be the most logical approach to keeping the thought processes moving in an orderly pattern, by working from the outside of the body inward.

Chapter Organization

The basic organization for all applicable body systems and specialty chapters includes the following elements: chapter content; objectives; anatomy and physiology; vocabulary; word elements; pathological conditions; diagnostic techniques, treatments, and procedures; common abbreviations; written and audio terminology review; and chapter review exercises.

Chapter content and objectives present learners with a basis for what they are about to learn. They are then grounded with basic information about the specific body system in the anatomy and physiology sections and proceed to the vocabulary and word elements sections to learn specifically the medical terms and word parts appropriate to that chapter. The pathological conditions and diagnostic techniques, treatments, and procedures sections reinforce and elaborate through basic and more extensive definitions many of the terms that have already been introduced in the vocabulary and word part sections.

The abbreviation section presents the most common abbreviations applicable to that chapter. The written and audio terminology review allows learners to write out the definitions and study the pronunciations for the major terms. The chapter review exercises test and assess the learner on the information in the chapter. Additional information on some of these elements is included in the "Pedagogical Features" section following and in the "About the Book" section.

Written and Audio Terminology Review

At the end of each chapter, you will find an alphabetized list of key terms introduced in the chapter. You will write the definition of each term and check it in the glossary. A phonetic pronunciation is included for each term as well as a check box to indicate mastery of the pronunciation.

Chapter Review Exercises

Each chapter has numerous review exercises designed to check your comprehension of the chapter material. You will note that each review activity provides a space for recording your score at the end of the exercise. Ask your instructor for the answers, or check your answers in the chapter. Each exercise question is valued at 5, 10, or 20 points—with the maximum number of points possible being 100. Your goal will be to earn a minimum 80% on each activity. You will be able to gain instant feedback on your level of success by computing your score. Scores lower than 80% indicate a need to go back and review that particular area.

Glossary

A comprehensive glossary has been developed to allow you to check one place for the definition of major terms in the text.

220 CHAPTER 7

polymyositis	Polymyositis is a chronic, progressive disease affecting the skeletal (striated) muscles. It is characterized by muscle weakness of hips and arms and degeneration (atrophy).

(pol-ee-my-oh-SIGH-tis)
poly- = many, much, excessive
myos/o = muscle
-itis = inflammation

The disease is termed *dermatomyositis* when the patient also has a rash on the face, neck, shoulders, chest, and upper extremities. This chronic disease is also characterized by periods of remission ("symptom free") and relapse (symptoms return).

The onset of **polymyositis** is gradual, with patients first experiencing weakness of the hips and shoulders. They may have difficulty getting out of a chair or the bathtub, difficulty climbing stairs, or difficulty reaching for things on the upper shelf of a cabinet or closet. They may experience **arthralgia** (painful joints) accompanied by edema. As the disease progresses, the neck muscles may become so weak that the patient may not be able to raise his or her head from the pillow.

The cause of **polymyositis** is unknown. It is thought to be caused by an autoimmune reaction. It occurs twice as often in women as in men and appears most commonly between the ages of 40 and 60.

Treatment includes high doses of corticosteroids and immunosuppressive drugs, along with reduction of the patient's activities until the inflammation subsides. Response to treatment has resulted in long satisfactory periods of remission in some patients and recovery in others.

rotator cuff tear	A tear in the muscles that form a "cuff" over the upper end of the arm (head of the humerus). See *Figure 7-5.* The rotator cuff helps lift and rotate the arm, and hold the head of the humerus in place during abduction of the arm.

(ROH-tay-tor kuff TAIR)

The individual may experience sudden acute pain, a snapping sensation, and weakness in the arm if a rotator cuff tear develops acutely due to an injury. If the tear has a gradual onset due to repetitive overhead activity or wear and degeneration of the tendon, the pain may be mild at first

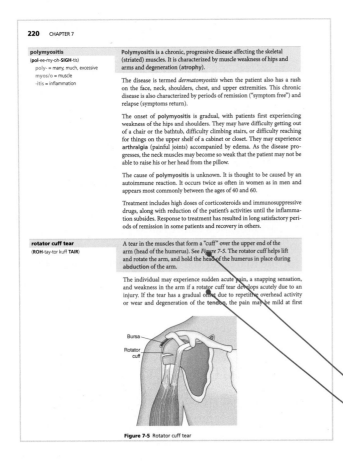

Bursa
Rotator cuff

Figure 7-5 Rotator cuff tear

---

574 CHAPTER 13

Word Element	Pronunciation	"Say It"	Meaning
-tropin gonado**tropin**	**TROH**-pin goh-nad-oh-**TROH**-pin	☐	stimulating effect of a hormone
-uria poly**uria**	**YOO**-ree-ah pol-ee-**YOO**-ree-ah	☐	urine condition

Review Checkpoint

Check your understanding of this section by completing the **Word Elements** exercises in your workbook.

Pathological Conditions

As you study the pathological conditions of the endocrine system, note that the **basic definition** is in a green shaded box followed by a detailed description in regular print. The phonetic pronunciation is directly beneath each term, as well as a breakdown of the component parts of the term where applicable.

The pathological conditions are presented in the same order as the discussion of the endocrine glands, with the exception of the ovaries and testes (which are discussed in detail in the chapters on female and male reproductive systems, respectively). Beneath each **endocrine gland** heading, the pathological conditions are alphabetized for ease of location.

Pituitary Gland

acromegaly	A chronic metabolic condition characterized by the gradual noticeable enlargement and elongation of the bones of the face, jaw, and extremities due to hypersecretion of the human growth hormone after puberty.

(ak-roh-**MEG**-ah-lee)
acr/o = extremities
-megaly = enlarged

The cause of oversecretion of the human growth hormone is most often due to a tumor of the pituitary gland. Treatment for **acromegaly** is aimed at reducing the size of the pituitary gland through surgery or radiation.

diabetes insipidus	A condition caused by a deficiency in the secretion of antidiuretic hormone (ADH) by the posterior pituitary gland, characterized by large amounts of urine and sodium being excreted from the body.

(dye-ah-**BEE**-teez
in-**SIP**-ih-dus)

The person experiencing **diabetes insipidus** will complain of excessive thirst and will drink large volumes of water. The urine is very dilute, with a low specific gravity. ADH (vasopressin) is administered as treatment for **diabetes insipidus**.

Special Features

Simple to Complex Definitions

The presentation of medical terms and conditions in this textbook presents the opportunity to learn a simple, basic definition of a word (along with its component parts) or to learn the basic definition along with a more comprehensive discussion of the disease process, diagnostic techniques and procedures, signs and symptoms, routes of drug administration, and mental disorders. **You will note that the medical term and the basic definition are highlighted in green**. The more comprehensive discussion of the condition follows in regular type. An example follows:

- Basic definition highlighted in green
- More comprehensive discussion

Word Elements Are Reinforced Throughout the Text

The study of word elements is integrated throughout the book. You will note that word elements are repeated in the chapters (to reinforce their meaning again and again) as you expand your studies from basic medical terms to signs and symptoms, disease conditions, and procedures. Note that the medical term will appear in the left-hand column, usually with a phonetic pronunciation immediately beneath the word. The component parts of the medical term (word elements) will be listed directly beneath the phonetic pronunciation. This format will also allow you to see the word in context (as it relates to the particular disease process) while continuing to reinforce the word elements.

- Pronunciation
- Word elements and definition

"Do This" and "Say It" Segments

Where appropriate, we have incorporated "Do This" instructions to involve you actively in the learning process. For example, in the chapter on muscles, the "Do This" instructions are designed to help you learn muscle actions such as extension, flexion, and abduction by having you respond to the directions by actually performing the action. This should reinforce your knowledge of the actions of the various muscles of the body.

The "Say It" segments are designed to have you repeat words and word elements when studying them. Pronouncing the words aloud should help you remember how the words sound, which can also help you spell them correctly when you hear the words pronounced by your instructor or by a physician on a transcription tape. Many times, students misspell words they have not heard before or have not taken the time to familiarize themselves with the sound of the word.

■ "Do This" instructions

■ "Say It" segments

Muscles and Joints **227**

flexion (FLEK-shun)	Flexion is a bending motion. It decreases the angle between two bones. *(Do this: Bend your right elbow and touch the side of your neck with your fingertips. By bending the elbow, you decreased the angle between the lower arm bones and the upper arm bone by bringing them closer together. Keep your arm in this position as you read the next movement description.)*
extension (eks-TEN-shun)	Extension is a straightening motion. It increases the angle between two bones. *(Do this: Remove your fingertips from the side of your neck and straighten your right arm, extending it as if you were going to shake someone's hand. You may now relax your arm. By completing this movement, you increased the angle between the lower arm bones and the upper arm bone by moving them farther apart.)*
abduction (ab-DUCK-shun)	Abduction is the movement of a bone away from the midline of the body. *(Do this: Raise your left arm out from your side until it is almost parallel with your left shoulder. You may now relax your arm. This action moved your arm away from the midline of your body, thus accomplishing the movement of abduction.)*
adduction (ad-DUCK-shun)	Adduction is the movement of a bone toward the midline of the body. *(Do this: First, place both of your hands on top of your head. Now remove your hands from the top of your head and return them to your side. This action moved your arms toward the midline of your body, thus accomplishing the movement of adduction.)*
rotation (roh-TAY-shun)	Rotation is the movement that involves the turning of a bone on its own axis. *(Do this: Turn your head from side to side as if to say "no." This twisting or turning of the head accomplishes the movement of rotation, that is, rotation of the neck.)*
supination (soo-pin-NAY-shun)	Supination is the act of turning the palm up or forward. *(Do this: Place your right hand out, as if to receive change from a cashier. This upward turning of your palm is called supination. Next, place your hands by your side, arms relaxed; turn your palms so they face forward. This forward turning of your palms is also called supination.)*
pronation (proh-NAY-shun)	Pronation is the act of turning the palm down or backward. *(Do this: Place your left hand out, as if to show a ring you are wearing. This downward turning of your palm is called pronation. Next, place your hands by your side, arms relaxed. Turn your palms so that they face backward. This backward turning of your palms is also called pronation.)*

---

218 CHAPTER 7

Word Element	Pronunciation	"Say It"	Meaning
dys- dystonia	DIS dis-TOH-nee-ah	☐	bad, difficult, painful, disordered
electr/o electromyogram	ee-LEK-troh ee-lek-troh-MY-oh-gram	☐	electrical, electricity
fasci/o fasciotomy	FASH-ee-oh fash-ee-OTT-oh-mee	☐	band of fibrous tissue
fibr/o fibroma	FIH-broh fih-BROH-mah	☐	fiber
-graphy electroneuromyography	GRAH-fee ee-lek-troh-noo-roh-my-OG-rah-fee	☐	process of recording
-itis fasciitis	EYE-tis fas-ee-EYE-tis	☐	inflammation
kinesi/o, kines/o kinesiology	kigh-NEE-zee-oh, kigh-NEE-zoh kigh-nee-zee-OL-oh-jee	☐	movement
leiomy/o leiomyofibroma	lye-oh-MY-oh lye-oh-my-oh-fye-BROH-mah	☐	smooth muscle
my/o myalgia	MY-oh my-AL-jee-ah	☐	muscle
myos/o myositis	my-OH-so my-oh-SIGH-tis	☐	muscle
pector/o pectoral	peck-TOR-oh PECK-toh-ral	☐	pertaining to the chest
-plegia hemiplegia	PLEE-jee-ah hem-ee-PLEE-jee-ah	☐	paralysis
rhabdomy/o rhabdomyosarcoma	rab-DOH-my-oh rab-doh-my-oh-sar-KOH-mah	☐	striated muscle; skeletal muscle
tax/o ataxia	TACK-soh ah-TACK-see-ah	☐	coordination, order
tri- triceps	TRY TRY-seps	☐	three
troph/o dystrophy	TROH-foh DIS-troh-fee	☐	development

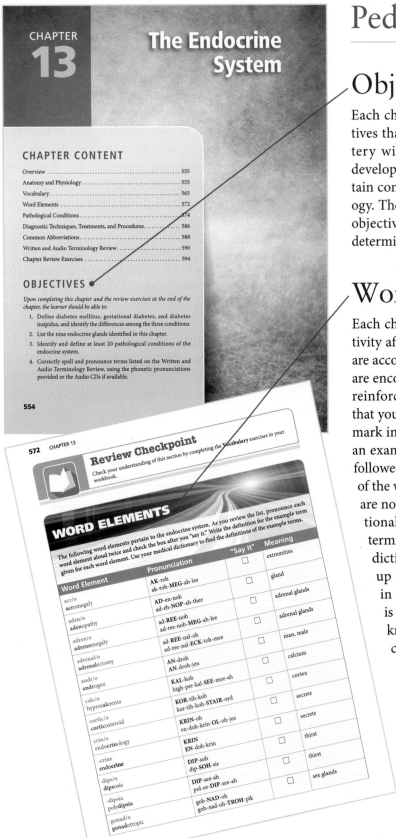

Pedagogical Features

Objectives

Each chapter opens with a list of learning objectives that introduce main areas to target for mastery within the chapter. Objectives have been developed to include standards for learners to attain competency specifically in medical terminology. The review exercises are tied directly to these objectives to help learners assess themselves and determine if they have mastered the content.

Word Elements

Each chapter contains a word element review activity after the vocabulary list. The word elements are accompanied by a phonetic pronunciation. You are encouraged to pronounce these words twice to reinforce your pronunciation skills and indicate that you have achieved success by entering a check mark in the box provided. Each word element has an example term that includes the word element, followed by a space for you to enter the definition of the word. The definitions for the example terms are not included in the text. This was done intentionally because everyone who studies medical terminology needs to know how to use a medical dictionary! These definitions should be looked up in your medical dictionary and recorded in the space provided in your textbook. This is an extra challenge designed to expand your knowledge base. Be careful, though: a medical dictionary is a contagious thing!

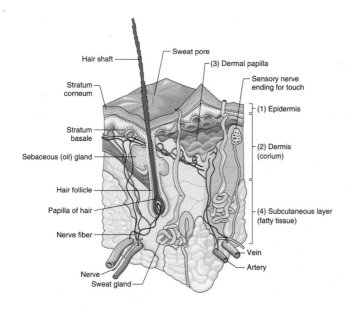

Hair shaft
Sweat pore
(3) Dermal papilla
Stratum corneum
Sensory nerve ending for touch
(1) Epidermis
Stratum basale
(2) Dermis (corium)
Sebaceous (oil) gland
Hair follicle
(4) Subcutaneous layer (fatty tissue)
Papilla of hair
Nerve fiber
Vein
Artery
Nerve
Sweat gland

Color Photos and Illustrations

The body systems and specialty chapters contain more than 400 color photographs and drawings that have been selected to reinforce the specific topics of discussion. Most of the photographs appear beside or immediately following the discussion for immediate reinforcement of your comprehension of the topic. The old saying "A picture is worth a thousand words" is very true in this case. The quality of the photographs and the detail of the artist's illustrations in this textbook will allow you to form a clear mental image of the structure, disease process, or technique being discussed. This will prove particularly helpful when you are reading about a disease or treatment with which you are not familiar.

Changes to the Fifth Edition

Following is a list of major chapter-specific changes for the fifth edition:

- Updated line art and photos have been added to most chapters to enhance learning.

- A new chapter review exercise, a crossword puzzle, has been added to Chapter 1.

- A new photo of ecchymosis has been added to Chapter 5.

- Line art has been replaced with a photo of butterfly rash associated with SLE in Chapter 7.

- A new image for ERCP has been added to Chapter 12.

- A figure has been updated on lateral cross section of the eye in Chapter 14.

- New line art has been added regarding potential sites for ectopic pregnancy in Chapter 18.

- Immunization schedules have been updated, and a new photo added on pediatric urine collection bag in Chapter 19.

- A new image for posteroanterior view has been added to Chapter 20.

- Updates made in Chapter 21 to conform to the changes noted in the *Cancer Facts & Figures*, 2013.

- Two new figures have been added to illustrate placement for sublingual medication and to illustrate placement for buccal medication in Chapter 22.

- Updates have been made to conform to the changes noted in the *DSM-5* and a new chapter review exercise has been added to Chapter 23.

Student Resources

Workbook

The workbook was written to provide you with additional practice to help you learn medical terminology. Assess your mastery of word building; anatomy and physiology; key medical vocabulary; pathological conditions; diagnostic techniques, treatments, and procedures; and common abbreviations by completing the workbook exercises. Review Checkpoint, a feature in the text after major chapter sections, alerts you to go to your workbook and complete the exercises. Multiple exercises have been added to each workbook chapter. These exercises are designed to enhance the learner's ability to define and build medical terms.

Workbook (ISBN: 978-1-3050-7463-7)

Student Companion Website

The Student Companion Website includes animations, slide presentations in PowerPoint®, term-to-definition and definition-to-term quick-access tables for prefixes, suffixes, combining forms, and abbreviations that appear in the textbook. The tables can be used as a quick reference when learners forget the meaning of a word element or when they remember the meaning but forget the particular word element.

Accessing the Student Companion Website:

1. Go to: http://www.CengageBrain.com

2. Register as a new user or log in as an existing user if you already have an account with Cengage Learning or CengageBrain.com.

3. Select **Go to MY Account**.

4. Open the product from the My Account page.

Instructor Companion Site

Resources for instructors include:

- **CogneroTestbank** makes generating tests and quizzes a snap. With over 1,000 questions in a variety of formats to choose from, you can create customized assessments for your students with the click of a button. Add your own unique questions and print tests for easy class preparation.

- Customizable instructor slide presentations created in **PowerPoint**®, including animations, and images, focus on key concepts from each chapter.

- **Electronic Instructor's Manual** includes the following tools:

  - Sample course syllabus

  - Suggested classroom activities

- ❑ Transcription word list exercises
- ❑ Chapter review sheets
- ❑ Sample tests for all chapters
- ❑ Text Answer Keys for chapter review exercises in the text
- ❑ Workbook Answer Keys for exercises in the workbook

The Learning Lab

The Learning Lab is an online homework solution that maps to learning objectives in *Comprehensive Medical Terminology,* Fifth Edition. Interactive, scenario-based activities build students' medical vocabulary, strengthen word building skills, and encourage an understanding of the importance of medical terminology as the basis of communication in the health care workplace, between health care professionals, and with patients. This simulated, immersive environment engages users with its real-life approach. The Learning Lab includes a pre-assessment, learning activities, and a post-assessment organized around the chapters in this text. The post-assessment scores can be posted to the instructor grade book in any learning management system. The amount of time the student spends within the Learning Lab can also be tracked.

IAC Learning Lab to Accompany *Comprehensive Medical Terminology*, 5th Edition, ISBN: 978-1-3050-7517-7

MindTap

MindTap is a fully online, interactive learning experience built upon authoritative Cengage Learning content. By combining readings, multimedia, activities, and assessments into a singular learning path, MindTap elevates learning by providing real-world application to better engage students. Instructors customize the learning path by selecting Cengage Learning resources and adding their own content via apps that integrate into the MindTap framework seamlessly with many learning management systems.

The guided learning path demonstrates the relevance of medical terminology to health care professions through engagement activities, interactive exercises, and procedural videos. Learners apply an understanding of medical terminology through patient education scenarios. These simulations elevate the study of medical terminology by challenging students to apply concepts to practice.

To learn more, visit http://www.cengage.com/mindtap.

About the Author

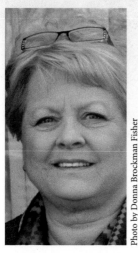

Photo by Donna Brockman Fisher

Betty Davis Jones

Betty Davis Jones, RN, MA, CMA (AAMA), is the department chairperson for medical assisting, phlebotomy, and health promotions at Gaston College, Dallas, North Carolina. She earned her Bachelor of Science degree in Nursing from the University of South Carolina and her Master of Arts degree in Management from Central Michigan University.

Jones, who has taught at Gaston College for more than 30 years, has been instrumental in the development of the medical assisting, phlebotomy, and veterinary medical technology programs at Gaston. She is a member of the American Association of Medical Assistants, the North Carolina Society of Medical Assistants, the Gaston County Chapter of Medical Assistants, and the North Carolina Association of Medical Assisting Educators. Jones has previous credits as a contributing author for several medical assisting textbooks.

Contributor

Dianne Spearman George, RN, BSN, MSN, former department chairperson for the associate degree nursing program at Gaston College, Dallas, North Carolina, has more than 28 years of nursing practice focused on leadership and the needs of the family. Her experience in practicing and teaching health care has been diversified among medical assisting, child health, adult health, mental health, and hospice. As former director of nursing at a local hospice, George was instrumental in opening a new hospice in-patient and residential facility.

Acknowledgments

A textbook is never written solely by one individual. There may be one name on the cover, but there is input from many who support and challenge the author to achieve his or her goal. To the following individuals, I owe a special thanks!

To Deb Myette-Flis a very big thank-you. Thank you again for guiding me and for offering your support throughout this fifth edition. I value your advice and guidance. Your kindness and personalized approach continue to be helpful and most appreciated. You are the best!

Also, my thanks to the staff at Cengage Learning who have worked enthusiastically to see this project through to completion. I never realized just how many individuals were involved in the revision of a textbook!

Product Director: Matthew Seeley

Senior Content Developer: Debra Myette-Flis

Product Assistant: Deborah Handy

Content Project Manager: Thomas Heffernan

Managing Art Director: Jack Pendleton

Thanks to my family for their unending support and enthusiasm for my success in writing. It is much appreciated!

A special thanks to the Gaston College students who have taken medical terminology through our department. Thank you for catching printing errors, for suggesting new ideas, and for sharing such wonderful "teaching" pictures with me of various pathological conditions. I am forever grateful!

Thank you to the members of the Gaston College Medical Assisting Department for your support throughout all of my writing efforts. You are wonderful colleagues and very special friends: Lynn Nichols, MA, CMA (AAMA); Penny Ewing, BS, CMA (AAMA); Dena Bridges AAS, CMA (AAMA); Robin Gun, AAS, CMA (AAMA), and Lythia Bynum, AAS, CMA (AAMA). Thank you to the individuals who have so willingly shared photographs for the fifth edition of this textbook; most of you have been cited with the photograph. These have been wonderful teaching tools, and I appreciate your help. Two individuals, not cited in the text, who served as models are Marla Jones (RN, MSN) and Wendy Altman, CMA (AAMA). Thank you for providing such excellent pictures.

And last but certainly not least, I would like to thank the following Gastonia area physicians and nurses who have so willingly answered my questions, reviewed my chapters, and suggested changes for the fifth edition of this textbook.

List of Physicians and Nurses

Jennifer J. Allran, MSN, PMHCNS/NP-BC
Psychiatry/Mental Health

Costa Andreou, MD, FACC
Cardiology

Todd D. Cohen, MD
Urology

John R. Collier, Jr., MD
Otolaringology – Head and Neck Surgery

Sam Drake, MD
Gastroenterology

Gary L. Dubisky, Jr., DO, FACN
Neurology

Sharon H. Froneberger, RN, BSN
Pediatrics

Dr. Jerry R. Gardner, DC
Chiropractic

Pamela Givens, BSN, CNM, MPH
OB/GYN

Marla Jones Ivester, RN, MSN
Case Management

Dorothy Kodzwa, MD
Endocrinology, Diabetes and Metabolism

Michael Lund, MD
Ophthalmology

Robert Waterhouse, Jr., MD
Urology

Mikell Jarrett, MD
Pulmonology

Reviewers

I am particularly grateful to the reviewers, who have been an invaluable resource in guiding this book as it continues to develop. Their insights, comments, suggestions, and attention to detail were extremely important in updating this textbook.

Jana Allen, MT ASCP
Associate Professor
Volunteer State Community College
Gallatin, Tennessee

Kim Ford
Instructor
Medical Assisting
Catawba Valley Community College
Healthcare Management Technology/
Medical Office Administration
Hickory, North Carolina

Kristin L. Hawthorne
Lead Instructor
Medical Programs
CCI Training Center
Arlington, Texas

Gail P. Orr, RMA (AMT)
Director of Healthcare Education
Governor's Regional Health Science
Academy
Virginia

Karen C. Sansom, MS, RHIA, CPHIMS
Associate Professor
Program Director
Health Information Management
Western Kentucky University
Bowling Green, Kentucky

Tara Weber RN, MSN
Director
Level One Nursing
State Fair Community College
Sedalia, MO

Pi-Ming Yeh, RN, PhD
Assistant Professor
Nursing Department
Missouri Western State University
St. Joseph, Missouri

About the Book and Components

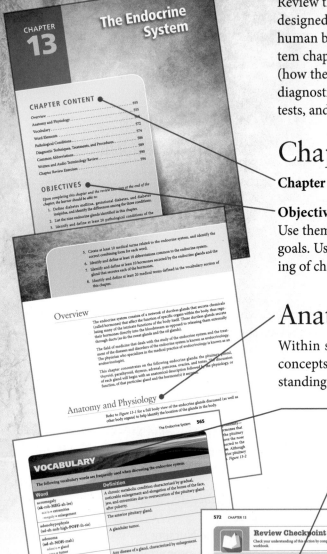

Review these two pages to understand how each chapter has been designed to help you learn medical terminology in the context of human body systems and medical specialties. A typical body system chapter includes anatomy (structure of the body); physiology (how the system works); pathology (conditions and diseases); and diagnostic techniques, treatments, and procedures (examinations, tests, and treatments).

Chapter Opener

Chapter Content provides an outline of major chapter sections.

Objectives identify the key learning objectives for each chapter. Use them before studying the chapter to understand your learning goals. Use them after reading the chapter to test your understanding of chapter content.

Anatomy and Physiology

Within system chapters, these sections introduce you to basic concepts of body structure and function to provide better understanding of medical terms.

Vocabulary and Word Elements

Here is your first practice with medical terms and word parts.

- Study the **Vocabulary** section to learn term definitions plus word part breakdowns and definitions.

- Terms in the Vocabulary section and within the text that are highlighted in **purple** are included in the Written and Audio Terminology Review at the end of the chapter.

- Study and work through the **Word Elements** section to learn more about prefixes, combining forms, and suffixes. It is important to notice how pronunciations differ when the same word part is used in a complete term.

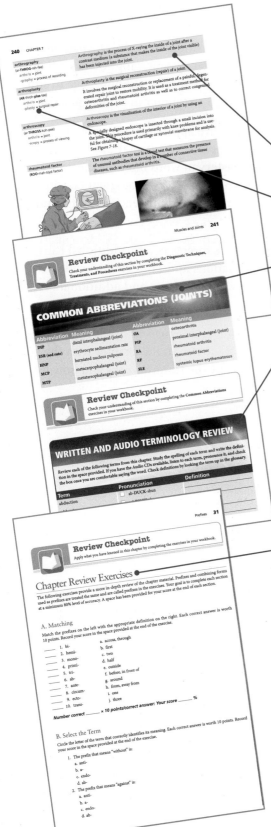

Pathological Conditions and Diagnostic Techniques, Treatments, and Procedures

This book includes comprehensive coverage of major diseases, conditions, treatments, and techniques.

■ Basic definitions are highlighted in green followed by a more comprehensive definition.

■ Terms are broken into word parts to reinforce learning. Word parts appear in blue.

Common Abbreviations

This section presents the most common abbreviations used in today's health care environment.

Written and Audio Terminology Review

This review includes an alphabetical list of medical terms presented in each chapter.

■ Use for review of written definitions; check your definition to those listed in the glossary.

Chapter Review Exercises

Extensive exercises at the end of each chapter help reinforce what you have learned. All exercises include self-assessment scoring to help you immediately determine your competency.

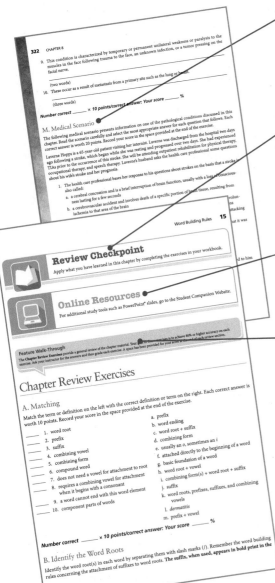

Medical Scenarios

Medical scenarios present information on one of the pathological conditions discussed in the chapter, encouraging you to synthesize information you have learned and apply that knowledge to situations a health care worker might encounter in clinical practice.

The **Review Checkpoint** feature appearing after major chapter sections directs you to complete additional exercises in the workbook to assess your mastery of word building; anatomy and physiology; key medical vocabulary; pathological conditions; diagnostic techniques, treatments, and procedures; and common abbreviations.

The **Online Resources** feature directs you to additional learning opportunities such as animations and PowerPoint® slides available on the Student Companion Website and additional review exercises in the Workbook.

The **Feature Walk-Through** was designed to "walk you through" a feature the first time it is presented in the chapter with the goal of helping you understand how the feature works and how it will help you maximize your learning.

Word Building Rules

CHAPTER CONTENT

OBJECTIVES

Upon completing this chapter and the review exercises at the end of the chapter, the learner should be able to:

1. List the three basic component parts of a word.

2. Correctly state the rule for joining prefixes and suffixes to a word root.

3. Accurately define the terms *word root, suffix, prefix, combining vowel,* and *combining form.*

4. Correctly state the rule for using multiple word roots in a compound word.

5. Demonstrate the ability to apply the word building rules by accurately completing the review exercises located at the end of this chapter.

6. Define an eponym and give an example.

Overview

Studying the language of medicine—that is, medical terminology—is very similar to learning a foreign language. There are rules that must be applied to make the "language" understandable. As a health care professional, you have chosen to learn the language, to master it, and to use it appropriately in the field of medicine. To do this, you must learn the word building rules necessary to expand your knowledge and understanding of medical terminology. Once you have accomplished this, you will possess the power to define words you never thought possible. Sounds exciting, doesn't it? It is! Let's get started.

Word Parts, Combining Forms, and Word Building Rules

Before you begin, remember: **It will be critical for you to learn the word parts, and the rules for combining word parts to create words, to be successful with medical terminology**. It is impossible to memorize thousands of words over the course of one or two quarters or semesters. It *is* possible, however, to memorize the word parts and the rules that will enable you to build the thousands of words you will need to function effectively as a health care professional. As you study this chapter on word building rules, understand that you will probably not master all of the rules in the beginning. This chapter will serve as a reference as you progress through the textbook. When you find that you have difficulty understanding how the words are put together or how to pronounce certain words, return to this chapter and review the word building rules and pronunciation guidelines.

Medical words, like English words, consist of three basic component parts: word roots, prefixes, and suffixes. How you combine the component parts, or word elements, determines the meaning of the word. For example, if one part is changed, the meaning of the word also changes. Review the English word *port* and see the different words you can create by adding to it different prefixes and suffixes. Prefixes appear at the beginning of the word root, whereas suffixes appear at the end of the word root. Notice that the prefixes and the suffixes are bold to emphasize how these word elements can change the meaning of the word root *port*.

port	**re**port	**im**port
support	**ex**port	**trans**port
port**er**	port**able**	

Let's now examine the word parts that we will be using and identifying throughout this text.

Word Root

A word root is the basic foundation of a word, to which component parts are added. By adding other word elements to the root, the meaning of the word changes. A word root is also called the stem or the base of a word and usually has a Greek or Latin origin. All medical words have at least one word root. Some have multiple roots that are joined by a vowel called a combining vowel.

Example: In the word *cardiologist*, the word root is *cardi*, which means "heart." When you see *cardi* (or *card*) as part of a word, you know that the meaning will have something to do with the heart. Another example can be found in *dermatologist*. The root is *dermat*, which means "skin." Anytime you see *dermat* (or *derm*) as part of a word, the meaning will have something to do with the skin.

Word roots keep their same meaning throughout. Adding prefixes and suffixes to the roots, however, changes the meaning of the word. Look at the following words (which contain either the root *cardi*, *card*, *dermat*, or *derm*) and see how the meaning changes by adding word parts. In each word, the root is in color.

Word	Meaning
cardiologist (car-dee-**OL**-oh-jist)	**One who specializes in the study of diseases and disorders of the heart**; *-logist* (one who specializes) is a suffix; *o* is the combining vowel.
cardiology (car-dee-**OL**-oh-gee)	**The study of the heart**; *-logy* (the study of) is a suffix; *o* is the combining vowel.
carditis (car-**DYE**-tis)	**Inflammation of the heart**; *-itis* (inflammation) is a suffix.
cardiac (**CAR**-dee-ak)	**Pertaining to the heart**; *-ac* (pertaining to) is a suffix.
dermatologist (der-mah-**TOL**-oh-jist)	**One who specializes in the study of diseases and disorders of the skin**; *-logist* (one who specializes) is a suffix; *o* is the combining vowel.
dermatology (der-mah-**TOL**-oh-gee)	**The study of the skin**; *-logy* (the study of) is a suffix; *o* is the combining vowel.
dermatitis (der-mah-**TYE**-tis)	**Inflammation of the skin**; *-itis* (inflammation) is a suffix.
dermatosis (der-mah-**TOH**-sis)	**Any condition of the skin**; *-osis* (condition) is a suffix.
acrodermatitis (**ak**-roh-**der**-mah-**TYE**-tis)	**Inflammation of the skin of the extremities**; *-itis* (inflammation) is a suffix; *dermat* is a word root; *acr* (extremities) is a word root; *o* is the combining vowel.
hypodermic (**high**-poh-**DER**-mik)	**Pertaining to under the skin**; *-ic* (pertaining to) is a suffix; *hypo* (under) is a prefix.

Combining Form

A combining form is created when a word root is combined with a vowel. This vowel, known as a combining vowel, is usually an *o*, but occasionally it is an *i*. The combining vowel is used to join the word parts appropriately when creating words. It also helps in pronunciation by allowing the word to flow as opposed to being choppy without the aid of the vowel.

Rule: *Generally, when using more than one word root (as in a compound word), a combining vowel is needed to separate the different word roots regardless of whether the second or third word root begins with a vowel. (There are exceptions to the rule!)*

Example 1:   In the word ***cardiomyopathy***, which means "any disease that affects the structure and function of the heart (i.e., the heart muscle)," there are two word roots: *cardi* (meaning "heart") and *my* (meaning "muscle"). These are followed by the suffix *-pathy*, which means "disease." The best way to determine the number of word roots in a compound word is to look for the combining vowels and divide, or separate, the word into elements. Let's divide the word ***cardiomyopathy*** to illustrate.

cardi	/	*o*	/	***my***	/	*o*	/	*-pathy*
↑		↑		↑		↑		↑
root	+	vowel	+	root	+	vowel	+	suffix

Example 2:   In the word ***myoelectric***, which means "pertaining to the electrical properties of the muscle," there are two word roots: *my* (meaning "muscle") and *electr* (meaning "electric"). These are followed by the suffix *-ic*, which means "pertaining to." The combining vowel is used even though the word root *electr* begins with a vowel.

my	/	*o*	/	***electr***	/	*-ic*
↑		↑		↑		↑
root	+	vowel	+	root	+	suffix

Example 3:   Now comes an exception to the rule. In the word ***lymphadenopathy***, which literally means "any disease of the lymph nodes" (but refers to enlargement of the lymph nodes, by dictionary definition), there are two roots: *lymph* (meaning "lymph") and *aden* (meaning "gland"). These are followed by the suffix *-pathy*, which means "disease." The combining vowel is not used in this word to separate the two roots, as it is in the others. There is not always a clear-cut explanation as to why the vowel is used in combining some roots and not in others, but the rule of using the vowel to separate the word roots in compound words applies more often than not. One might speculate that it is easier to pronounce *lymphadenopathy* without using the *o* than it would be if using the *o* to separate the two roots in this compound word.

lymph	/	***aden***	/	*o*	/	*-pathy*
↑		↑		↑		↑
root	+	root	+	vowel	+	suffix

Rule: *A word cannot end with a combining form (word root + vowel). A suffix is added at the end of the word. A combining vowel will be used if the suffix begins with a consonant. A combining vowel is generally not used if the suffix begins with a vowel. (There are some exceptions to this rule.)*

Example: One word that means "enlargement of the heart" is **megalocardia** (megal/o/card/ia).

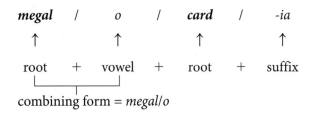

Note that the word root *megal* (enlargement or enlarged) becomes a combining form by adding the vowel *o*. The word root *card* cannot be used as a combining form to end the word because this would create *megalocardo,* which is not a word. These words must use a suffix as an ending. Because the suffix begins with a vowel, the *o* is not used after *card,* and the suffix *-ia* is added to complete the word.

Suffix

A suffix is a word element attached at the end of the word root. Adding a suffix to a word changes the meaning of the word, just as adding different prefixes changes the meaning of the word. Are you beginning to see a pattern here? Just think, a change at the beginning, a change at the end, and you have increased your word building power significantly! All medical words have an ending, or suffix, unless the root is a word itself.

Example: In the word **cardiomegaly**, the suffix is *-megaly* (enlargement or enlarged). When you see the suffix *-megaly* as part of a word, it is referring to something being enlarged.

Note: *-megaly* and *megal/o* are both acceptable word elements; *-megaly* is a suffix and *megal/o* is a combining form. As you continue learning medical terms, you will find other word elements that work as either a suffix or a combining form. Each suffix carries its same meaning regardless of the root to which it is attached.

As you look at the following words using the word root *cardi*, notice how the different suffixes allow you to make several words—all with different meanings but all referring to the heart. The suffix is in color in each word.

Word	Meaning
cardi**algia** (**car**-dee-AL-jee-ah)	**Pain in the heart, heart pain**; *-algia* (pain) is a suffix. Note that a combining vowel was not used with this word because the suffix begins with a vowel.
cardio**centesis** (**car**-dee-oh-sen-TEE-sis)	**Surgical puncture of the heart**; *-centesis* (surgical puncture) is a suffix. The combining vowel was needed with this word because the suffix begins with a consonant.
cardio**megaly** (**car**-dee-oh-MEG-ah-lee)	**Enlargement of the heart**; *o* is the combining vowel, which is needed because the suffix begins with a consonant; *-megaly* (enlargement) is a suffix.

Now that we have explored how changing the suffix also changes the meaning of the word, let's see how a particular suffix dictates whether you use a combining vowel.

Rule: *If the suffix begins with a vowel, the root will attach directly to it. If, however, the suffix begins with a consonant (anything other than a, e, i, o, u, y), the root will need a combining vowel before attaching to the suffix.*

Example: In the word *cardiogram* (cardi/o/gram), which means "a record of the heart's activity," the word root *cardi* (heart) is joined to the suffix *-gram* (record) by the combining vowel *o* because the suffix begins with a consonant.

Now you try the next one! Look at the word **cardialgia**. Identify the word root and the suffix. Was a combining form necessary? Why or why not?

Check your answers in the box immediately following the exercise.

Word root: _____

Suffix: _____

Combining vowel used? _____

If yes, why? _____

If no, why? _____

Answers

Word root: *cardi* _____

Suffix: *-algia* _____

Combining vowel used? <u>No</u> _____

If yes, why? _____

If no, why? <u>The suffix *-algia* begins with a vowel, so the combining vowel is not needed.</u>

_____

How about another one for good measure! Look at the word **carditis**. Identify the word root and the suffix. Was a combining form necessary? Why or why not?

Word root: _____

Suffix: _____

Combining vowel used? _____

If yes, why? _____

If no, why? _____

Answers

Word root: *card* _____

Suffix: *-itis* _____

Combining vowel used? <u>No</u> _____

If yes, why? _____

If no, why? <u>The suffix *-itis* begins with a vowel, so the combining vowel is not needed.</u>

_____

Before we continue with word building rules pertaining to prefixes, it is important to note that Chapters 2 and 3 are devoted to the discussion of prefixes and suffixes, respectively. Word roots, however, are addressed in each "system" chapter throughout the text. Each word, when possible, is separated into its word elements followed by a definition of the element. This appears in the left-hand column next to the medical term.

Prefix

A prefix is a word element added at the beginning of the word. When a prefix is used with a root, it changes (or alters) the meaning of the word. Prefixes are not a part of all medical words.

Rule: *Prefixes are attached directly to the beginning of the word.*

Example: In the word **endocardium**, the prefix is *endo-* (which means "within or inner"). You will always be discussing the inner part, or within, when using the prefix *endo-*. Prefixes keep the same meaning whenever they are attached to a word. What does this mean? If the root doesn't change, and the prefix doesn't change, how does the word change? The same root can change its meaning in a word each time a new prefix is added to it, as we have already seen in the previous example with the word root *port*.

Look at the following words that contain the root *cardi* or *card* and see how using different prefixes makes several words, all with different meanings, but all referring to the heart. In each word, the prefix is in color.

Word	Meaning
endocardium (**en**-doh-**CAR**-dee-um)	**Within the heart, the inner lining of the heart**; *endo-* (within) is a prefix; *-um* (structure, tissue, or thing) is a noun suffix.
intracardiac (**in**-trah-**CAR**-dee-ak)	**Pertaining to within the heart (i.e., pertaining to the interior of the heart chambers)**; *intra-* (within) is a prefix; *-ac* (pertaining to) is an adjective suffix.
pericardial (**pair**-ih-**CAR**-dee-ul)	**Pertaining to around the heart (i.e., pertaining to the pericardium, which is the sac that surrounds the heart)**; *peri-* (around) is a prefix; *-al* (pertaining to) is an adjective suffix. When you first begin to build medical terms, it is important to define each word part (i.e., pertaining to around the heart). Once you become more comfortable, you may give a briefer definition with some of the word endings being understood without actually saying them (i.e., around the heart, instead of pertaining to around the heart).

Now look at the following words containing the word root *men* (which means "menstruation") to see how the different prefixes in these words change the meaning while continuing to refer to menstruation. Again, the prefix is in color in each word.

amenorrhea (ah-**men**-oh-**REE**-ah)	**Absence of menstruation**; *a-* (without or absence of) is a prefix; *-rrhea* (drainage or flow) is a suffix. The *o* is used to combine the word root with the suffix that begins with a consonant.
dysmenorrhea (**dis**-men-oh-**REE**-ah)	**Painful menstrual flow**; *dys-* (bad, difficult, painful, disordered) is a prefix; *-rrhea* (drainage or flow) is a suffix. The *o* is used to combine the word root with the suffix that begins with a consonant.

Word Structure

Generally, words are built using a root and a suffix (or a prefix, word root, and a suffix). As indicated earlier in this chapter, there are exceptions to the rule. You will notice that sometimes a medical term is constructed with only a prefix and a suffix. An example of this is *apnea*, which is composed of the prefix *a-* (without) and the suffix *-pnea* (breathing). One could dissect this word and say that it does have a prefix (*a-*), a root (*pne/o*), and a suffix (*-a*). However, the accepted word element in this word is *-pnea*, which is a suffix. Another example is *analgesia*, which is composed of the prefix *an-* (without) and the suffix *-algesia* (sensitivity to pain).

In the previous pages, we have identified the word elements (word roots, combining forms, prefixes, and suffixes). Now let's see how they fit together to build medical words. There is a logical order to building medical words.

Rule: *A prefix is placed at the beginning of the word. (Applies: always)*

Rule: *A suffix is placed at the end of the word root. (Applies: always)*

Rule: *The use of more than one word root in a word creates the need for combining vowels to connect the roots. This, in turn, creates combining forms used in compound words. (Applies: words that have several components)*

Rule: *A term that comprises multiple word roots (or combining forms) and a suffix is called a compound word.*

Example: *leuk/o* + *cyt* + *-osis* = *leukocytosis*

    word+vowel   word   suffix
    root   root

    combining form

When several combining forms are used, the order is as follows: combining form + combining form + word root + suffix.

Example: *dermat/o + fibr/o + sarc + -oma* = dermatofibrosarcoma

    leuk/o + erythr/o + blast + -osis = leukoerythroblastosis

When defining a medical word, there is also a logical approach.

Rule: *The definition of a medical word usually begins with defining the suffix (the word ending) first and continuing to "read" backward through the word as you define it.*

Example: For the word **carditis**, the definition is: inflammation (*-itis*) of the heart (*card*).

    For the word **cardiomegaly**, the definition is: enlargement (*-megaly*) of the heart (*cardi*). The *o* is a combining vowel.

    For the word *cyanosis*, the definition is: condition (*-osis*) of blueness (*cyan*). A combining vowel is not necessary.

Rule: *When a medical word has a prefix, the definition of the word usually begins with defining the suffix first, the prefix second, and the root(s) last.*

Example: For the word ***intracardiac***, the definition is: pertaining to (*-ac*) within (*intra-*) the heart (*cardi*).

For the word ***pericardial***, the definition is: pertaining to (*-al*) around (*peri-*) the heart (*cardi*).

For the word ***hypoglycemia***, the definition is: blood condition (*-emia*) of low or less than normal (*hypo-*) sugar (*glyc*).

For the word ***hyperhidrosis***, the definition is: condition (*-osis*) of excessive (*hyper-*) sweating (*hidr*).

Rule: *When a medical word identifies body systems or parts, the definition of the word usually begins with defining the suffix first, then defining the organs in the order in which they are studied in the particular body system.*

Example: In the word ***cardiopulmonary***, the definition is: pertaining to (*-ary*) the heart (*cardi*) and lungs (*pulmon*). The *o* is a combining vowel for the two word roots.

In the word ***cardioarterial***, the definition is: pertaining to (*-al*) the heart (*cardi*) and the arteries (*arteri*). The *o* is a combining vowel for the two word roots.

In the word ***hysterosalpingectomy***, the definition is: removal of (*-ectomy*) the uterus (*hyster*) and fallopian tubes (*salping*). The *o* is a combining vowel for the two word roots.

In the word ***nasopharyngitis***, the definition is: inflammation (*-itis*) of the nose (*nas*) and throat (*pharyng*). The *o* is a combining vowel for the two word roots.

Guidelines for Pronunciation

As you continue your study of medical terminology and the word building rules, you must also incorporate a few pronunciation rules or guidelines to help you pronounce the words correctly. Sometimes a medical word is spelled exactly like it sounds; other times it is spelled with a letter, or letters, that produces the same phonetic sound. Let's look at some example words and guidelines for looking up the words in a dictionary.

Note: In the pronunciation of the example words, the part of the word that receives the strongest accent is written in bold uppercase letters. For your convenience, the rules have been simplified in Tables 1-1 and 1-2. These tables can be used as references when a particular word stumps you.

Guidelines for words beginning with the "f" sound: Notice if the word begins with f or with ph.

1. If the word begins with *f*, it will have the "f" sound—as in the word *febrile*, which is pronounced "**FEE**-brill."

2. If the word begins with *ph*, it will also have the "f" sound—as in the word *physiology*, which is pronounced "fizz-ee-**OL**-oh-gee."

Table 1-1 Pronunciation Guideline Chart

"Sounds Like"	Observation	Example Word	Pronunciation
Words beginning with the **"f"** sound	Notice if the word begins with *f*. Notice if the word begins with *ph*.	febrile physiology	"**FEE**-brill" "fiz-ee-**OL**-oh- jee"
Words beginning with the **"j"** sound	Notice if the word begins with *j*. Notice if the word begins with *g* and is followed by an *e*. Notice if the word begins with *g* and is followed by an *i*. Notice if the word begins with *g* and is followed by a *y*.	jejunum genesis gingivitis gyrus	"jee-**JOO**-num" "**JEN**-ee-sis" "jin-jih-**VYE**-tis" "**JYE**-russ"
Words beginning with the **"k"** sound	Notice if the word begins with *k*. Notice if the word begins with *c*. Notice if the word begins with *ch*. Notice if the word begins with *qu*.	kyphosis cornea chorion quadruplet	"kye-**FOH**-sis" "**KOR**-nee-ah" "**KOR**-ree-on" "kwah-**DROOP**-let"
Words beginning with the **"n"** sound	Notice if the word begins with *n*. Notice if the word begins with *pn*. Notice if the word begins with *kn*.	neonatal pneumonia knee	"nee-oh-**NAY**-tal" "new-**MOH**-nee-ah" "**NEE**"
Words beginning with the **"s"** sound	Notice if the word begins with *s*. Notice if the word begins with *c*. Notice if the word begins with *ps*.	sarcoma cervix psychology	"sar-**KOM**-ah" "**SIR**-viks" "sigh-**KOL**-oh-jee"
Words beginning with the **"sk"** sound	Notice if the word begins with *sk*. Notice if the word begins with *sc*. Notice if the word begins with *sch*.	skeleton sclera schizophrenia	"**SKELL**-eh-ton" "**SKLAIR**-ah" "skiz-oh-**FREN**-ee-ah"
Words beginning with the **"z"** sound	Notice if the word begins with *z*. Notice if the word begins with *x*	zygomatic xanthoma	"zeye-go-**MAT**-ik" "zan-**THOH**-mah"

Guidelines for words beginning with the "j" sound: Notice if the word begins with j or with g.

1. If the word begins with *j*, it will have the "j" sound—as in the word *jejunum,* which is pronounced "jee-**JOO**-num."

2. If the word begins with *g* and is followed by the letter *e, i,* or *y*, it will have a "j" sound:

   ■ If the *g* is followed by *e*—as in the word *genesis,* which is pronounced "**JEN**-ee-sis."
   ■ If the *g* is followed by *i*—as in the word *gingivitis,* which is pronounced "**jin**-jih-**VYE**-tis."
   ■ If the *g* is followed by the *y*—as in the word *gyrus,* which is pronounced "**JYE**-russ."

Guidelines for words beginning with the "k" sound: Notice if the word begins with k, c, ch, or qu.

1. If the word begins with *k*, it may have the "k" sound—as in the word *kyphosis,* which is pronounced "kye-**FOH**-sis." However, some words that begin with the

Table 1-2 Additional Rules for Variations in Pronunciations

Beginning/Ending	Rule	Pronunciation	Example Word
Word begins with *c*	If the *c* is followed by *e*	Pronounced as a soft "c" and has a "ss" sound	cervix ("**SIR**-viks")
	If the *c* is followed by *i*	Pronounced as a soft "c" and has a "ss" sound	circumduction ("sir-kum-**DUCK**-shun")
	If the *c* is followed by *y*	Pronounced as a soft "c" and has a "ss" sound	cyst ("**SIST**")
	If the *c* is followed by *a*	Pronounced as a hard "c" and has a "k" sound	cancer ("**CAN**-ser")
	If the *c* is followed by *o*	Pronounced as a hard "c" and has a "k" sound	collagen ("**KOL**-ah-jen")
	If the *c* is followed by *u*	Pronounced as a hard "c" and has a "k" sound	cuticle ("**KEW**-tih-kul")
	If the *c* is followed by a consonant	Pronounced as a hard "c" and has a "k" sound	cheiloplasty ("**KYE**-loh-plas-tee")
Word root ends with *g*	If the *g* is followed by *e*	Pronounced as a soft "g" and has a "j" sound	laryngectomy ("lah-rin-**JEK**-toh-me")
	If the *g* is followed by *i*	Pronounced as a soft "g" and has a "j" sound	pharyngitis ("fair-rin-**JYE**-tiss")
	If the *g* is followed by *a*	Pronounced as a hard "g" and has a "guh" sound	laryngalgia ("lah-rin-**GAL**-jee-ah")
	If the *g* is followed by *o*	Pronounced as a hard "g" and has a "guh" sound	meningocele ("men-**IN**-goh-seel")

letter *k* (as in *knee*) do not have the "k" sound. This variation is discussed in another pronunciation guideline.

2. Some words that begin with the letter *c* will have the "k" sound—as in the word *cornea*, which is pronounced "**KOR**-nee-ah."

3. Some words that begin with the letters *ch* will have the "k" sound—as in the word *chorion*, which is pronounced "**KOR**-ree-on."

4. Words that begin with the letters *qu* will have the "k" sound—as in the word *quadruplet*, which is pronounced "kwah-**DROOP**-let."

***Guidelines for words having the "n" sound: Notice if the word begins with* n, pn, *or* kn.**

1. If the word begins with *n*, it will have the "n" sound—as in the word *neonatal*, which is pronounced "nee-oh-**NAY**-tal."

2. Some words that have the "n" sound begin with *pn*—as in the word *pneumonia*, which is pronounced "new-**MOH**-nee-ah."

3. Some words that have the "n" sound begin with *kn*—as in the word *knee*, which is pronounced "**NEE**."

Guidelines for words beginning with the "s" sound: Notice if the word begins with s, c, *or* ps.

1. If the word begins with *s*, it will have the "s" sound—as in the word *sarcoma*, which is pronounced "sar-**KOM**-ah."

2. Some words that begin with *c* will have the "s" sound—as in the word *cervix*, which is pronounced "**SIR**-viks."

3. Words that begin with *ps* will have the "s" sound because the *p* will be silent—as in the word *psychology*, which is pronounced "sigh-**KOL**-oh-jee."

Guidelines for words beginning with the "sk" sound: Notice if the word begins with sk, sc, *or* sch.

1. Words that begin with *sk* will have the "sk" sound—as in the word *skeleton*, which is pronounced "**SKELL**-eh-ton."

2. Some words that begin with *sc* will have the "sk" sound—as in the word *sclera*, which is pronounced "**SKLAIR**-ah."

3. Some words that begin with *sch* will have the "sk" sound—as in the word *schizophrenia*, which is pronounced "**skiz**-oh-**FREN**-ee-ah."

Guidelines for words having the "z" sound: Notice if the word begins with z *or* x.

1. If the word begins with *z*, it will have the "z" sound—as in the word *zygomatic*, which is pronounced "**zeye**-go-**MAT**-ik."

2. Some words that begin with *x* will have the "z" sound—as in the word *xanthoma*, which is pronounced "zan-**THOH**-mah."

Let's take a look at some additional words and explore the rules for variations in pronunciations.

Rule: *When a word begins with the letter* c, *the rule is as follows: If the* c *is followed by* e, i, *or* y, *the* c *is pronounced as a soft "c" and has an "s" sound.*

Example: In the word *cervix*, the *c* is followed by *e* and the *c* is pronounced as a soft "c." The word is pronounced "**SIR**-viks."

In the word *circumduction*, the *c* is followed by *i* and the *c* is pronounced as a soft "c." The word is pronounced "sir-kum-**DUCK**-shun."

In the word *cyst*, the *c* is followed by *y* and the *c* is pronounced as a soft "c." The word is pronounced "**SIST**."

Rule: *When a word begins with the letter* c, *the rule is as follows: If the* c *is followed by* a, o, u, *or a consonant, the* c *is pronounced as a hard "c" and has a "k" sound.*

Example: In the word *cancer*, the *c* is followed by *a* and the *c* is pronounced as a hard "c." The word is pronounced "**CAN**-ser."

In the word *collagen*, the *c* is followed by *o* and the *c* is pronounced as a hard "c." The word is pronounced "**KOL**-ah-jen."

In the word *cuticle*, the *c* is followed by *u* and the *c* is pronounced as a hard "c." The word is pronounced "**KEW**-tih-kul."

In the word *cheiloplasty*, the *c* is followed by a consonant and the *c* is pronounced as a hard "c." The word is pronounced "**KYE**-loh-plas-tee."

Rule: *When building words with word elements that end in* g *(such as* laryng, pharyng, *and* mening), *the rule is as follows: If the* g *is followed by* e *or* i, *the* g *is pronounced as a soft "g" and has a "j" sound.*

Example: In the word *laryngectomy*, the *g* is followed by *e* and the *g* is pronounced as a soft "g." The word is pronounced "**lah**-rin-**JEK**-toh-me."

In the word *pharyngitis*, the *g* is followed by *i* and the *g* is pronounced as a soft "g." The word is pronounced "**fair**-rin-**JYE**-tiss."

Rule: *When building words with word elements that end in* g *(such as* laryng, pharyng, *and* mening), *the rule is as follows: If the* g *is followed by* a *or* o, *the* g *is pronounced as a hard "g" and has a "guh" sound.*

Example: In the word *laryngalgia*, the *g* is followed by *a* and the *g* is pronounced as a hard "g." The word is pronounced "lah-rin-**GAL**-jee-ah."

In the word *meningocele*, the *g* is followed by *o* and the *g* is pronounced as a hard "g." The word is pronounced "men-**IN**-goh-seel."

Guidelines for Use of Possessive Forms (Eponyms)

As you begin your study of pathological conditions in this textbook, you will note that some diseases are named after individuals and are pronounced and written in the possessive form. These terms are known as eponyms. An eponym (**EP**-oh-nim) is a name for a disease, organ, procedure, or body function that is derived from the name of a person. Three examples of eponyms are Parkinson's disease, named after James *Parkinson*, a British physician; Cushing's syndrome, named after Harvey Williams *Cushing*; and Hodgkin's disease, named after Thomas *Hodgkin*, a British physician.

The decision to express the name of the disease in the possessive form remains an acceptable alternative if dictated and/or if indicated as the preference by the employer or client. Medical journals, dictionaries, and style guides remain divided on this issue—although many have acknowledged the trend away from the possessive form. The learner will notice in this textbook that the author's preference is to use the possessive form of disease names.

WRITTEN AND AUDIO TERMINOLOGY REVIEW

Term	Pronunciation	Definition
acrodermatitis	☐ ak-roh-**der**-mah-**TYE**-tis	_____
amenorrhea	☐ ah-**men**-oh-**REE**-ah	_____
cardiac	☐ **CAR**-dee-ak	_____
cardialgia	☐ **car**-dee-**AL**-jee-ah	_____
cardiocentesis	☐ **car**-dee-oh-sen-**TEE**-sis	_____
cardiologist	☐ **car**-dee-**OL**-oh-jist	_____
cardiology	☐ car-dee-**OL**-oh-gee	_____
cardiomegaly	☐ **car**-dee-oh-**MEG**-ah-lee	_____
carditis	☐ car-**DYE**-tis	_____
dermatitis	☐ **der**-mah-**TYE**-tis	_____
dermatologist	☐ **der**-mah-**TOL**-oh-jist	_____
dermatology	☐ **der**-mah-**TOL**-oh-gee	_____
dermatosis	☐ **der**-mah-**TOH**-sis	_____
dysmenorrhea	☐ **dis**-men-oh-**REE**-ah	_____
endocardium	☐ **en**-doh-**CAR**-dee-um	_____
hypodermic	☐ **high**-poh-**DER**-mik	_____
intracardiac	☐ **in**-trah-**CAR**-dee-ak	_____
pericardial	☐ **pair**-ih-**CAR**-dee-ul	_____
polyuria	☐ **pol**-ee-**YOU**-ree-ah	_____

Review Checkpoint

Apply what you have learned in this chapter by completing the exercises in your workbook.

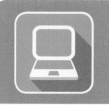

Online Resources

For additional study tools such as PowerPoint® slides, go to the Student Companion Website.

Feature Walk-Through

The **Chapter Review Exercises** provide a general review of the chapter material. Your goal in these exercises is to achieve 80% or higher accuracy on each exercise. Ask your instructor for the answers and then grade each exercise. A space has been provided for your score at the end of each review section.

Chapter Review Exercises

A. Matching

Match the term or definition on the left with the correct definition or term on the right. Each correct answer is worth 10 points. Record your score in the space provided at the end of the exercise.

_____ 1. word root

_____ 2. prefix

_____ 3. suffix

_____ 4. combining vowel

_____ 5. combining form

_____ 6. compound word

_____ 7. does not need a vowel for attachment to root

_____ 8. requires a combining vowel for attachment when it begins with a consonant

_____ 9. a word cannot end with this word element

_____ 10. component parts of words

a. prefix

b. word ending

c. word root + suffix

d. combining form

e. usually an *o*, sometimes an *i*

f. attached directly to the beginning of a word

g. basic foundation of a word

h. word root + vowel

i. combining form(s) + word root + suffix

j. suffix

k. word roots, prefixes, suffixes, and combining vowels

l. *dermatitis*

m. prefix + vowel

Number correct _____ × 10 points/correct answer: Your score _____ %

B. Identify the Word Roots

Identify the word root(s) in each word by separating them with slash marks (/). Remember the word building rules concerning the attachment of suffixes to word roots. **The suffix, when used, appears in bold print in the**

(continued)

first four (4) words. After that, you will have to identify the word root without the help of a bold suffix. All answers appear within this chapter. Each correct answer is worth 10 points. Record your score in the space provided at the end of the exercise.

1. Definition: Enlargement of the heart.

    Root: cardi (the *o* is needed because the suffix *-megaly* begins with a consonant)

    Word: _c a r d i o**m e g a l y**_

2. Definition: Condition in which there is a decrease in the number of white blood cells.

    Root: cyt (the *o* is needed because the suffix *-penia* begins with a consonant)

    Root + vowel: leuk/o (this becomes a combining form due to the compound word)

    Word: _l e u k o c y t o**p e n i a**_

3. Definition: Inflammation of the skin of the extremities.

    Root: dermat (the *o* is not needed because the suffix *-itis* begins with a vowel)

    Root + vowel: acr/o (this becomes a combining form due to the compound word)

    Word: _a c r o d e r m a t**i t i s**_

4. Definition: One who specializes in the study of diseases and disorders of the heart.

    Root: cardi (the *o* is needed because the suffix *-logist* begins with a consonant) (This one may appear to be wrong because *cardi* ends with a vowel. However, remember that it is the beginning of the suffix that determines whether to use the vowel.)

    Word: _c a r d i o**l o g i s t**_

5. Definition: Any condition of the skin.

    Root: _____

    Word: _d e r m a t o s i s_

6. Definition: Painful urination.

    Root: _____

    Word: _d y s u r i a_

7. Definition: Pain in the heart.

    Root: _____

    Word: _c a r d i a l g i a_

8. Definition: One who specializes in the study of diseases and disorders of the skin.

    Root: _____

    Word: _d e r m a t o l o g i s t_

9. Definition: Condition of blueness.

    Root: _____

    Word: _c y a n o s i s_

10. Definition: Inflammation of the heart.

    Root: _____

    Word: _c a r d i t i s_

Number correct _____ *× 10 points/correct answer: Your score* _____ **%**

C. What Is Wrong with This Word?

Each of the following words has been created incorrectly according to the word building rules. Review each word carefully and circle the mistake. Rewrite the word correctly in the space provided, and state your rationale for the change. You may need to refer to the word building rules in the chapter for help. Each correct answer is worth 10 points. Record your score in the space provided at the end of the exercise.

Example:

Wrong:	a men rrhea	
Correct:	amenorrhea	
Rationale:	*The suffix begins with a consonant. Therefore, a combining vowel is needed.*	

1. Wrong: megaly cardio
   Correct: _____
   Rationale: _____

2. Wrong: penia leuko cyto
   Correct: _____
   Rationale: _____

3. Wrong: dermato itis acro
   Correct: _____
   Rationale: _____

4. Wrong: megaly gastro
   Correct: _____
   Rationale: _____

5. Wrong: osis dermato
   Correct: _____
   Rationale: _____

6. Wrong: dys men rrhea
   Correct: _____
   Rationale: _____

7. Wrong: cardio algia
   Correct: _____
   Rationale: _____

8. Wrong: logist dermato
   Correct: _____
   Rationale: _____

9. Wrong: osis cyano
   Correct: _____
   Rationale: _____

(continued)

10. Wrong: <u>itis cardo</u>

    Correct: _____

    Rationale: _____

Number correct _____ **× 10 points/correct answer: Your score** _____ **%**

D. Completion

Read the following statements about word elements, and complete the statement with the correct answer. The spaces provided indicate the number of words in the answer. Each correct answer is worth 10 points. Record your score in the space provided at the end of the exercise.

1. When building a medical word, remember that a word cannot end as a _____. You must drop the vowel and add a _____.

2. The basic foundation of a word is known as the _____ _____.

3. Word roots, prefixes, suffixes, and combining vowels are known as _____ _____ _____.

4. The word element attached directly to the beginning of a word is known as a _____.

5. The word element that requires a combining vowel for attachment when it begins with a consonant is known as a _____.

6. The component part of a word that is usually an *o* but sometimes an *i* is called the _____ _____.

7. The word ending is called a _____.

8. A word root + a vowel is known as a _____ _____.

9. The word element that attaches to the beginning of a word and does not need a vowel for attachment to the root is a _____.

10. A medical word that is made up of a combining form + a word root + a suffix is known as a _____ _____.

Number correct _____ **× 10 points/correct answer: Your score** _____ **%**

E. Review the Rules

Read each statement carefully, and select the correct answer from the options listed. Each correct answer is worth 10 points. Record your score in the space provided at the end of the exercise.

1. When using more than one word root, as in a compound word, a _____ is needed to separate the different word roots. This is done regardless of the second or third word root beginning with a vowel.

   a. prefix

   b. suffix

   c. combining vowel

   d. hyphen

2. If a suffix begins with a vowel, the _____ will attach directly to it.

   a. word root

   b. prefix

c. combining form

d. hyphen

3. If a suffix begins with a consonant (anything other than *a, e, i, o, u, y*), the root will need a(n) _____ before attaching to the suffix.

   a. prefix

   b. hyphen

   c. combining vowel

   d. extra word root

4. A word element added at the beginning of the word is a:

   a. prefix

   b. suffix

   c. combining vowel

   d. hyphen

5. Compound words are usually composed in the following order:

   a. combining form + word root + suffix

   b. combining form + suffix

   c. word root + suffix

   d. prefix + word root

6. The definition of a medical word usually begins with defining the _____ first and continuing to "read" backward through the word as you define it.

   a. prefix

   b. combining form

   c. word root

   d. suffix

7. When a medical word has a prefix, the definition of the word usually begins with defining the suffix first, the prefix _____, and the root(s) last.

   a. third

   b. second

   c. fourth

   d. after the root

8. When a medical word identifies body systems or parts, the definition of the word usually begins with defining the suffix first and then defining the organs _____ in the particular body system.

   a. in the order in which they are studied

   b. in alphabetical order

   c. in reverse order

   d. in any order desired

9. In the medical word *cardiocentesis* (cardi + o + centesis), the word element *-centesis* is a suffix. The combining vowel *o* is used in building this word because:

   a. the suffix always has to have a combining vowel

   b. the suffix begins with a consonant

   c. the root *cardi* ends in a vowel

   d. the vowel is not needed (this word is misspelled)

(*continued*)

10. In the medical word *cardialgia* (cardi + algia), the word element *-algia* is a suffix. The combining vowel *o* is not used in building this word because:

   a. the suffix *-algia* begins with a vowel and a combining vowel is not necessary

   b. the vowel is needed (this word is misspelled)

   c. the root *cardi* ends in a vowel

   d. a suffix never needs a combining vowel

Number correct _____ × *10 points/correct answer: Your score* _____ %

F. Crossword Puzzle

Each crossword answer is worth 10 points. When you have completed the crossword puzzle, total your points and enter your score in the space provided.

Word Building
Rules

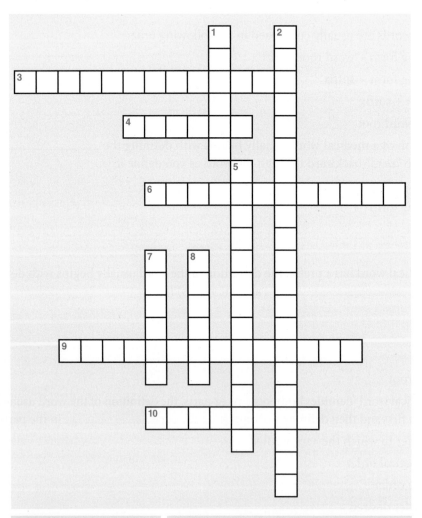

ACROSS

   3 word root + a vowel (2 Words)
   4 word ending
   6 combining form + word root + suffix (2 Words)
   9 usually an "o" but sometimes an "I" (2 Words)
 10 basic foundation of a word (2 Words)

DOWN

   1 requires a combining vowel for attachment when it begins with a consonant
   2 word roots, prefixes, suffixes, and combining vowels (4 Words)
   5 a word cannot end with this word element (2 Words)
   7 does not need a vowel for attachment to the word root
   8 attaches directly to the beginning of a word

Prefixes

CHAPTER CONTENT

OBJECTIVES

Upon completing this chapter and the review exercises at the end of the chapter, the learner should be able to:

1. Define a prefix and state the rule for using prefixes in words.

2. Correctly identify at least 20 prefixes that deal with numbers, colors, measurements, and negatives.

3. Correctly identify at least 10 prefixes that deal with position and direction.

4. Correctly identify at least 30 other prefixes.

5. Demonstrate the ability to create at least 10 new words using prefixes by completing the applicable exercises at the end of the chapter.

Overview

Have you ever drawn a **dia**gram? Have you ever taken a **pre**test? Have you ever taken **anti**biotics? Have you ever received a blood **trans**fusion? Have you ever thought about the many prefixes we use on a daily basis?

While studying this chapter, you will discover many new prefixes. You will also find that some of the prefixes that are part of your regular vocabulary are also used in medical terminology.

Every medical word has a root. Every medical word has an ending, which is either a suffix or a root that is itself a word. Not every medical word, however, has a prefix. When prefixes are used, they are attached directly to the beginning of the word.

The meaning of a prefix will not change from word to word. For example, *hyper-* always means "excessive or more than normal." Any word that has *hyper-* as its prefix will mean "in an excessive or more than normal state." Words with the same root, however, will have different meanings depending on the prefix attached. Look at the following example. Although each word has the same root (*later*, meaning "side"), the addition of different prefixes gives each word a different definition.

Word	Prefix	+	Root	+	Ending		Definition
bilateral	**bi**		later		al	=	pertaining to **two** sides
unilateral	**uni**		later		al	=	pertaining to **one** side
ambilateral	**ambi**		later		al	=	pertaining to **both** sides

Prefixes are attached to words to express numbers, measurements, position, direction, negatives, and color. This chapter concentrates on various categories of prefixes and their meanings. This is not a complete listing of prefixes. Additional prefixes are introduced throughout the text in relevant chapters.

Numbers

Prefixes that express numbers indicate, for example, whether there is one, two, or three, or whether it is single, double, or half. Look at some of the more commonly used prefixes and see how they relate to numbers.

Prefix	Meaning	Example
bi-	two, double	**bi**cuspid (having two cusps or points)
hemi-	half	**hemi**plegia (paralysis of one side [half] of the body)
milli-	one-thousandth	**milli**liter (one-thousandth of a liter)
mono-	one, single	**mono**cyte (a white cell with a singular nucleus)
nulli-	none	**nulli**para (a woman who has borne no children)
primi-	first	**primi**gravida (first pregnancy)

Prefix	Meaning	Example
quadri-	four	**quadri**plegia (paralysis of all four extremities)
semi-	half	**semi**conscious (half conscious)
tetra-	four	**tetra**plegia (paralysis of both arms and both legs; also known as quadriplegia)
tri-	three	**tri**ceps ("a muscle" having three heads)
uni-	one	**uni**nuclear ("a cell" having one nucleus)

Measurement

Prefixes that express measurement indicate quantity such as much, many, or excessive. They often refer to multiples without specifically referring to a number. They also refer to excessive (above normal) conditions. The following prefixes relate to measurements.

Prefix	Meaning	Example
hyper-	excessive	**hyper**lipemia (an excessive or above normal level of blood fats)
hyp-	under, below, beneath, less than normal	**hyp**oxemia (less than normal blood oxygen level)
hypo-	under, below, beneath, less than normal	**hypo**glycemia (less than normal blood sugar)
multi-	many	**multi**para (to bear many "children")
poly-	many, much	**poly**arthritis (inflammation of many joints) **poly**uria (the excretion of large amounts of [much] urine)

Position and/or Direction

Prefixes that express position and/or direction are used to describe a location. The location may be in the middle of, between, under, before, or after a particular body structure, or it may be around, upon, near, or outside an area or structure. The prefixes listed are examples.

Prefix	Meaning	Example
ab-	from, away from	**ab**duct (to move away from the midline of the body)
ad-	toward, increase	**ad**duct (movement toward the midline of the body)
ambi-	both, both sides	**ambi**dextrous (able to use both hands well)

Prefix	Meaning	Example
ante-	before, in front	**ante**cubital ("the space" in front of the elbow)
circum-	around	**circum**oral (around the mouth)
de-	down, from	**de**scend (to come down from)
dia-	through	**dia**gnosis (knowledge through testing)
ecto-	outside	**ecto**pic (outside of its normal location)
endo-	within	**endo**cervical (pertaining to the inner lining of the cervix)
epi-	upon, over	**epi**gastric (upon the stomach)
ex-	out, away from, outside	**ex**tract (to remove a tooth from [away from] the oral cavity)
exo-	outside, outward	**exo**genous (originating outside the body)
extra-	outside, beyond	**extra**hepatic (outside of the liver)
hypo-	under, below, beneath, less than normal	**hypo**glossal (under the tongue)
in-	in, inside, within, not	**in**tubate (to insert a tube inside [into] an organ or body cavity)
infra-	beneath, below, under	**infra**patellar (below the knee)
inter-	between	**inter**costal (between the ribs)
intra-	within	**intra**venous (within a vein)
juxta-	near, beside	**juxta**-articular (pertaining to a location near a joint)
meso-	middle	**meso**derm (the middle of the three layers of the skin)
para-	near, beside, beyond, two like parts	**para**cervical (near, or beside, the cervix)
peri-	around	**peri**anal (around the anus)
pre-	before, in front	**pre**cordial (the region "of the chest wall" in front of the heart)
pro-	in front, before	**pro**gnosis (knowledge before)
re-	back, again	**re**activate (to make active again)
retro-	backward, behind	**retro**flexion (an abnormal position of an organ in which the organ is tilted backward)
sub-	under, below	**sub**lingual (under the tongue)
supra-	above, over	**supra**pubic (above, or over, the pubic area)
trans-	across, through	**trans**urethral (across, or through, the urethra)

Color

Prefixes that express color can, for example, indicate color in reactions, the color of growths or rashes, and the color of body fluids. Some of the following word elements are pure prefixes. Others are combining forms used as prefixes. Most dictionaries identify these forms relating to color as "combining forms," not as prefixes. However, their constant placement at the beginning of the word identifies them more as a prefix than as a combining form, thus the reason for their insertion in this section. The list contains examples of prefixes, and combining forms used as prefixes, that express color. The list is summarized in Table 2-1 for easy reference, listing only the color and the prefix/combining form.

Table 2-1 Prefixes and Combining Forms for Color

Color	Prefix/Combining Form
black	melan/o
blue	cyan/o
gray, silver	glauc/o poli/o
green	chlor/o
purple	purpur/o
red	erythr/o eosin/o rube-
white	alb- albin/o leuk/o
yellow	cirrh/o jaund/o xanth/o

Prefix	Meaning	Example
alb-	white	**alb**ino (person who has a marked deficiency of pigment in the eyes, hair, and skin; has abnormally white skin)
albin/o	white	**albin**ism (condition of abnormally white skin; characterized by absence of pigment in the skin, hair, and eyes)
chlor/o	green	**chlor**ophyll (green pigment in plants that accomplishes photosynthesis)
cirrh/o	yellow, tawny	**cirrh**osis (chronic degenerative disease of the liver with resultant yellowness of the liver and of the skin)
cyan/o	blue	**cyan**oderma (slightly bluish, grayish, slatelike, or dark discoloration of the skin)
eosin/o	red, rosy	**eosin**ophil (bilobed leukocyte that stains a red, rosy color with an acid dye)

Prefix	Meaning	Example
erythr/o	red	**erythr**ocyte (mature red blood cell)
glauc/o	gray, silver	**glauc**oma (disorder of the eye due to an increase in intraocular pressure; creates a dull gray gleam of the affected eye)
jaund/o	yellow	**jaund**ice (yellow discoloration of the skin)
lute/o	yellow	corpus **lute**um (a yellow glandular mass on the surface of the ovary that forms after the ovarian follicle ruptures and releases a mature ovum)
leuk/o	white	**leuk**oplakia (white, hard, thickened patches firmly attached to the mucous membrane in areas such as the mouth, vulva, or penis)
melan/o	black	**melan**oma (darkly pigmented cancerous tumor)
poli/o	gray	**poli**omyelitis (inflammation of the gray matter of the spinal cord)
purpur/o	purple	**purpur**a (collection of blood beneath the skin in the form of pinpoint hemorrhages appearing as red/purple skin discolorations)
rube-	red	**rube**lla (contagious viral disease characterized by fever; coldlike symptoms; and a diffuse, fine, red rash)
xanth/o	yellow	**xanth**oderma (yellow coloration of the skin)

Negatives

Prefixes that express negatives indicate such things as not, without, lack of, and against.

Prefix	Meaning	Example
a-	without, not, no	apnea (without breathing) **Note:** When *a* is used as a prefix, it means "without, not, no"; *a* can also be used as a suffix.
an-	without, not, no	**an**esthesia (without feeling)
ana-	not, without	**ana**plasia (without formation or development)
anti-	against	**anti**dote (a drug or other substance that opposes [works against] the action of a poison)
contra-	against	**contra**ceptive (any device or technique that prevents [works against] conception)
dis-	free of, to undo	**dis**charge (to release a substance or object [to free it from its location])
im-	not	**im**potence (an adult male's inability [not able] to achieve penile erection)
in-	in, inside, within, not	**in**competent (not capable)
non-	not	**non**invasive (pertaining to a diagnostic or therapeutic technique that does not require the skin to be broken [not invaded] or a cavity or organ to be entered)

Common Prefixes

An alphabetical listing of prefixes commonly used in medical terminology is included here for easy reference. As you read the list, note that the prefixes just discussed in the "categories" sections are repeated. In addition, some of the prefixes appear throughout the text as they relate to discussions of specific body systems.

Note: The combining forms used as prefixes to express color have also been included in this list.

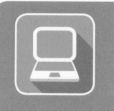

Online Resources

For comprehensive PowerPoint® slides and Quick Access Prefix and Combining Form Tables, go to the Student Companion Website. These tables are a valuable study tool and quick reference for learning prefixes and combining forms. Search by prefix or combining form or by the definition of a prefix or combining form.

Prefix	Meaning	Example
a-	without, not, no	**a**pnea (without breathing)
ab-	from, away from	**ab**errant (wandering away from)
ad-	toward, increase	**ad**duct (movement toward the midline of the body)
alb-	white	**alb**ino (person who has a marked deficiency of pigment in the eyes, hair, and skin; has abnormally white skin)
albin/o	white	**albin**ism (condition of abnormally white skin; characterized by absence of pigment in the skin, hair, and eyes)
ambi-	both, both sides	**ambi**dextrous (able to use both hands well)
an-	without, not, no	**an**esthesia (without feeling)
ante-	before, in front	**ante**cubital ("the space" in front of the elbow)
anti-	against	**anti**dote (a drug or other substance that opposes [works against] the action of a poison)
auto-	self	**auto**graft (a graft transferred from one part of a patient's body to another)
bi-	two, double	**bi**cuspid (having two cusps or points)
bio-	life	**bio**logy (the study of life)
brady-	slow	**brady**cardia (slow heartbeat)
chlor/o	green	**chlor**ophyll (green pigment in plants that accomplishes photosynthesis)

Prefix	Meaning	Example
circum-	around	**circum**duction (movement around in a circle)
cirrh/o	yellow, tawny	**cirrh**osis (chronic degenerative liver disease with resultant yellowness of the liver and skin)
con-	together, with	**con**genital (born with)
contra-	against	**contra**indication (against what is indicated)
cyan/o	blue	**cyan**oderma (slightly bluish, grayish, slatelike, or dark discoloration of the skin)
de-	down, from	**de**scend (to come down from)
dia-	through	**dia**gnosis (knowledge through testing)
dis-	free of, to undo	**dis**location (the displacement [undoing] of any part of the body from its normal position)
dys-	bad, difficult, painful, disordered	**dys**pnea (difficult breathing)
ecto-	outside	**ecto**pic (outside its normal location—as in an ectopic pregnancy, which occurs in the fallopian tubes instead of in the uterus)
endo-	within, inner	**endo**scope (instrument used to look inside the body)
eosin/o	red, rosy	**eosin**ophil (bilobed leukocyte that stains a red, rosy color with an acid dye)
epi-	upon, over	**epi**gastric (pertaining to the region over the stomach)
erythr/o	red	**erythr**ocyte (mature red blood cell)
eu-	well, easily, good, normal	**eu**pnea (normal breathing)
ex-	out, away from, outside	**ex**hale (to breathe out)
exo-	outside, outward	**exo**genous (originating outside the body)
extra-	outside, beyond	**extra**hepatic (outside of the liver)
glauc/o	gray, silver	**glauc**oma (disorder of the eye due to increased intraocular pressure; creates a dull gray gleam of the affected eye)
hemi-	half	**hemi**plegia (paralysis of one side [half] of the body)
hetero-	different	**hetero**geneous (composed of different or unlike substances)
homeo-	likeness, same	**homeo**stasis (a relative constancy [likeness] in the internal environment of the body)
homo-	same	**homo**genesis (having the same origins)

Prefix	Meaning	Example
hydro-	water	**hydro**cephalus (an abnormal accumulation of fluid [water] within the head)
hyp-	under, below, beneath, less than normal	**hyp**oxemia (less than normal blood oxygen level)
hyper-	excessive	**hyper**emesis (excessive vomiting)
hypo-	under, below, beneath, less than normal	**hypo**glycemia (less than normal blood sugar; low blood sugar level)
idio-	individual	**idio**syncrasy (an individual sensitivity to effects of a drug caused by inherited or other bodily constitution factors)
im-	not	**im**potence (an adult male's inability [not able] to achieve penile erection)
in-	in, inside, within, not	**in**competent (not capable) **in**born (acquired during intrauterine life)
infra-	beneath, below, under	**infra**orbital (beneath the bony cavity in which the eyeball is located)
inter-	between	**inter**costal (between the ribs)
intra-	within	**intra**venous (within a vein)
jaund/o	yellow	**jaund**ice (yellow discoloration of the skin)
juxta-	near, beside	**juxta**-articular (pertaining to a location near a joint)
leuk/o	white	**leuk**oplakia (white, hard, thickened patches firmly attached to the mucous membrane in areas such as the mouth, vulva, or penis)
melan/o	black	**melan**oma (a darkly pigmented cancerous tumor)
meso-	middle	**meso**derm (the middle of the three layers of the skin)
meta-	beyond, after	**meta**carpals (pertaining to the bones after the carpal [wrist] bones; i.e., the hand bones)
milli-	one-thousandth	**milli**liter (one-thousandth of a liter)
mono-	one	**mono**cyte (a white cell with a singular nucleus)
multi-	many	**multi**para (to bear many "children")
non-	not	**non**invasive (pertaining to a diagnostic or therapeutic technique that does not require the skin to be broken [not invaded] or a cavity or organ to be entered)
pan-	all	**pan**carditis (inflammation of the entire heart [all])
para-	near, beside, beyond, two like parts	**para**cervical (near, or beside, the cervix)

Prefix	Meaning	Example
per-	through	**per**cussion (striking through)
peri-	around	**peri**anal (around the anus)
poli/o	gray	**poli**omyelitis (inflammation of the gray matter of the spinal cord)
poly-	many, much, excessive	**poly**arthritis (inflammation of many joints) **poly**uria (the excretion of large amounts of [much] urine)
post-	after, behind	**post**cibal (after meals)
pre-	before, in front	**pre**cordial (the region "of the chest wall" in front of the heart)
primi-	first	**primi**gravida (first pregnancy)
pseudo-	false	**pseudo**anorexia ("false anorexia"; a condition in which an individual eats secretly while claiming a lack of appetite and inability to eat)
purpur/o	purple	**purpur**a (collection of blood beneath the skin in the form of pinpoint hemorrhages appearing as red/purple skin discolorations)
quadri-	four	**quadri**plegia (paralysis of all four extremities)
re-	back, again	**re**activate (to make active again)
retro-	backward, behind	**retro**cecal (pertaining to the region behind the cecum)
rube-	red	**rube**lla (a contagious viral disease characterized by fever, coldlike symptoms, and a diffuse, fine red rash [also German measles])
semi-	half	**semi**conscious (half conscious)
sub-	under, below	**sub**cutaneous (under the skin)
supra-	above, over	**supra**pubic (above, or over, the pubic area)
sym-	joined, together	**sym**pathetic (displaying compassion for another's grief; literally, "joined in disease")
syn-	joined, together	**syn**drome (a group of symptoms joined by a common cause; "running together")
tachy-	rapid	**tachy**cardia (rapid heartbeat)
trans-	across, through	**trans**urethral (across, or through, the urethra)
tri-	three	**tri**ceps ("a muscle" having three heads)
ultra-	beyond, excess	**ultra**sound (sound waves at the very high frequency of more than 20,000 vibrations per second)
uni-	one	**uni**nuclear ("a cell" having one nucleus)
xanth/o	yellow	**xanth**oderma (any yellow coloration of the skin)

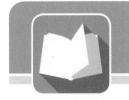

Review Checkpoint

Apply what you have learned in this chapter by completing the exercises in your workbook.

Chapter Review Exercises

The following exercises provide a more in-depth review of the chapter material. Prefixes and combining forms used as prefixes are treated the same and are called prefixes in the exercises. Your goal is to complete each section at a minimum 80% level of accuracy. A space has been provided for your score at the end of each section.

A. Matching

Match the prefixes on the left with the appropriate definition on the right. Each correct answer is worth 10 points. Record your score in the space provided at the end of the exercise.

_____	1. bi-	a. across, through
_____	2. hemi-	b. first
_____	3. mono-	c. two
_____	4. primi-	d. half
_____	5. tri-	e. outside
_____	6. ab-	f. before, in front of
_____	7. ante-	g. around
_____	8. circum-	h. from, away from
_____	9. ecto-	i. one
_____	10. trans-	j. three

_Number correct _____ × 10 points/correct answer: Your score _____ %_

B. Select the Term

Circle the letter of the term that correctly identifies its meaning. Each correct answer is worth 10 points. Record your score in the space provided at the end of the exercise.

1. The prefix that means "without" is:
   a. anti-
   b. a-
   c. endo-
   d. ab-

2. The prefix that means "against" is:
   a. anti-
   b. a-
   c. endo-
   d. ab-

(continued)

3. The prefix that means "not" is:

   a. dys-

   b. ambi-

   c. non-

   d. pan-

4. The prefix that means "bad or difficult" is:

   a. endo-

   b. dys-

   c. non-

   d. post-

5. The prefix that means "both or both sides" is:

   a. ambi-

   b. hemi-

   c. tri-

   d. mono-

6. The prefix that means "between" is:

   a. ecto-

   b. post-

   c. pan-

   d. inter-

7. The prefix that means "false" is:

   a. dys-

   b. pseudo-

   c. endo-

   d. anti-

8. The prefix that means "all" is:

   a. pan-

   b. post-

   c. tri-

   d. hemi-

9. The prefix that means "after or behind" is:

   a. pseudo-

   b. pan-

   c. post-

   d. ante-

10. The prefix that means "within" is:

   a. ecto-

   b. endo-

   c. hemi-

   d. primi-

Number correct _____ × *10 points/correct answer: Your score* _____ %

C. Create a Word

Using the prefixes listed, create a word that best completes each statement dealing with position and direction. If you need assistance, refer to your list of prefixes within the chapter. After you have determined the correct prefix, write the word (without the divisions) in the space provided. Each correct answer is worth 10 points. Record your score in the space provided at the end of the exercise.

inter-	intra-	ambi-	peri-
epi-	dia-	hypo-	supra-
trans-	ab-		

Create a word that means:

1. To move away from the midline of the body

   _____ + duct = _____
   (prefix)   + (root) =   (complete word)

2. Able to use both hands well

   _____ + dextr + ous = _____
   (prefix)   + (root) + (suffix) =   (complete word)

3. Around the mouth

   _____ + or + al = _____
   (prefix)   + (root) + (suffix) =   (complete word)

4. Knowledge through testing

   _____ + gnos + is = _____
   (prefix)   + (root) + (suffix) =   (complete word)

5. Under the tongue

   _____ + gloss + al = _____
   (prefix)   + (root) + (suffix) =   (complete word)

6. Within a vein

   _____ + ven + ous = _____
   (prefix)   + (root) + (suffix) =   (complete word)

7. Above the pubis

   _____ + pub + ic = _____
   (prefix)   + (root) + (suffix) =   (complete word)

8. Across, or through, the urethra

   _____ + urethr + al = _____
   (prefix)   + (root) + (suffix) =   (complete word)

9. Pertaining to the region upon the stomach

   _____ + gastr + ic = _____
   (prefix)   + (root) + (suffix) =   (complete word)

10. Between the ribs

    _____ + cost + al = _____
    (prefix)   + (root) + (suffix) =   (complete word)

Number correct _____ **× 10 points/correct answer: Your score** _____ **%**

D. Crossword Puzzle

Complete the crossword puzzle by entering the applicable prefix for each definition in the spaces provided. Each crossword answer is worth 5 points. When you have completed the puzzle, total your points and enter your score in the space provided.

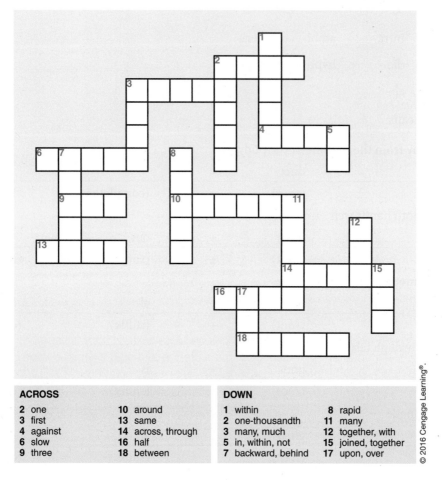

ACROSS

2 one	10 around
3 first	13 same
4 against	14 across, through
6 slow	16 half
9 three	18 between

DOWN

1 within	8 rapid
2 one-thousandth	11 many
3 many, much	12 together, with
5 in, within, not	15 joined, together
7 backward, behind	17 upon, over

© 2016 Cengage Learning®.

Number correct _____ × *5 points/correct answer: Your score* _____ %

E. Proofreading Skills

Read the following Consultation report. For each prefix that appears in bold, define the prefix and indicate if the prefix is spelled correctly. If it is misspelled, provide the correct spelling. Each correct answer is worth 10 points. Record your score in the space provided at the end of the exercise.

Example:

anti- *against* _____

Spelled correctly? ☑ Yes ☐ No _____

1. **epy-** _____

_____

Spelled Correctly? ☐ Yes ☐ No _____

2. **prima-** _____

_____

Spelled Correctly? ☐ Yes ☐ No _____

CONSULTATION

Hillcrest
medical center

PATIENT NAME: Kellie Greene

PATIENT ID: 11049

CONSULTANT:
Paul Bernard, MD, Surgical Services

REQUESTING PHYSICIAN:
George White, MD, Primary Care Physician

DATE OF CONSULTATION:
September 12, 2014

REASON FOR CONSULTATION:
Acute **epy**gastric pain for possible surgical intervention.

HISTORY

This 26-year-old Caucasian female patient was admitted with abdominal pain, nausea, and vomiting. No melena or hematemesis. Pain is in the right epigastrium and right upper quadrant.

She has a prior history of similar bouts but not as bad. She was evaluated in the ER and an obstruction series and abdominal sonogram were ordered by her PCP, Dr. White.

X-rays showed calcification in the right upper quadrant consistent with cholelithiasis. She had a low-grade fever and some chills. No apparent jaundice. She had a uterine and bladder suspension in 1996. She is a **prima**gravida in her second **tri**mester of pregnancy. She had an appendectomy at the age of 18. No history of pancreatitis, alcohol abuse, ulcers, liver disease, or hepatitis. Patient stated that she had **enda**carditis at age 14 following a streptococcal infection. Her recovery was uneventful. She expressed fear that this may be resurfacing. I saw no evidence of this, however.

PHYSICAL EXAMINATION

Physical examination reveals a woman who appears her stated age. She appears to be in considerable discomfort. Temperature 99 degrees Fahrenheit. No apparent jaundice. Neck is normal. Abdomen shows tenderness and guarding in the epigastrium and right upper quadrant. No other mass, hepatosplenomegaly, or hernias noted. Pelvic and rectal are unremarkable.

DIAGNOSTIC DATA

White blood cell count 10.1 with 79% segs. PTT is normal. SMA shows elevated bilirubin at 1.54 with alkaline phosphatase at 442. **Ulter**sound report reveals inflammation of the gallbladder with presence of multiple gallstones. These were reviewed by Dr. Singh, radiologist. Chest x-ray was unremarkable.

IMPRESSION

Cholelithiasis and early obstructive jaundice.

RECOMMENDATION

This patient is currently n.p.o. on IV fluids and **anti**biotics. I talked with the patient about her options: (1) ERCP followed by laparoscopic cholecystectomy, and (2) open cholecystectomy with common duct exploration. She expressed interest in laparoscopic cholecystectomy.

(continued)

CONSULTATION
Patient Name: Kellie Greene
Patient ID: 11049
Date of Consultation: September 12, 2014
Page 2

We plan to do the procedure later today. The nature of the surgery and the possible complications and problems, including stone recurrence, were explained to the patient and her family. Consent for laparoscopic surgery was obtained.

Thank you for allowing me to share in the care of this patient.

_____

Paul Bernard, MD

PB:xx

D: 09/12/2014

T: 09/14/2014

3. **tri-**_____

_____

Spelled Correctly? ☐ Yes ☐ No _____

4. **enda-**_____

_____

Spelled Correctly? ☐ Yes ☐ No _____

5. **ulter-**_____

_____

Spelled Correctly? ☐ Yes ☐ No _____

Number correct _____ *× 20 points/correct answer: Your score* _____ *%*

F. Completion

Complete each statement with the most appropriate prefix. **Note:** Because you are just beginning your study of medical terminology, the meaning of the prefix has been italicized for you. Each correct answer is worth 10 points. Record your score in the space provided at the end of the exercise.

1. A tooth having *two* cusps or points is known as a _____ cuspid tooth.
2. A person who is paralyzed on *one half* (one side) of the body is known to have _____ plegia.
3. A woman who is pregnant for the *first* time is termed a _____ gravida.
4. The excretion of large amounts of urine (*much* urine) is known as _____ uria.
5. The medical term that means "being *without* pain," or refers to an agent that is given to relieve pain, is _____ algesic.
6. A person who is able to use *both* hands well is said to be _____ dextrous.
7. A medication that is placed *under* the tongue is a _____ lingual medication.

8. An _____ venous medication is one that is administered *within* a vein.

9. The term _____ charge means "release of a substance or object in order *to free it from* its location."

10. A diagnostic or therapeutic technique that does not require the skin to be broken (*not* invaded) or a cavity or organ to be entered is said to be a _____ invasive procedure.

Number correct _____ × *10 points/correct answer: Your score* _____ %

G. Word Search

Read each definition carefully, and identify the appropriate word from the list that follows. Enter the word in the space provided; then find it in the puzzle and circle it. The words may be read up, down, diagonally, across, or backward. Each correct answer is worth 10 points. Record your score in the space provided at the end of the exercise.

poly	circum	inter	intra
anti	hyper	hydro	many
first	four	half	

Example: A prefix that means "many, much, excessive."

*poly*_____

1. A prefix that means "around."

_____

2. A prefix that means "between."

_____

3. A prefix that means "within" (other than *endo-*).

_____

4. A prefix that means "against" (other than *contra-*).

_____

5. A prefix that means "excessive."

_____

6. A prefix that means "water."

_____

7. The prefix *multi-* means:

_____

8. The prefix *primi-* means:

_____

9. The prefix *quadri-* means:

_____

10. The prefix *hemi-* means:

_____

Number correct _____ × *10 points/correct answer: Your score* _____ %

Word Search Puzzle

```
P  C  H  C  R  K  F  L  P  A  L  S  Y  I  M
A  O  A  G  E  S  O  I  L  D  U  S  T  U  T
M  I  L  T  M  N  U  E  Z  T  L  N  V  L  D
C  A  F  Y  E  E  R  O  S  H  I  A  C  B  T
I  L  S  S  D  L  N  L  I  E  O  H  I  T  I
R  E  H  E  P  Y  T  T  O  I  E  P  N  L  P
C  R  O  A  I  N  T  E  R  M  A  E  C  O  L
U  R  R  T  N  P  N  E  I  E  R  C  F  E  E
M  A  R  R  P  T  I  G  I  R  E  P  Y  H  S
P  B  V  O  D  A  I  I  N  S  E  R  Y  M  C
E  N  L  C  G  A  S  P  I  N  E  D  S  E  L
N  I  E  H  I  R  C  H  I  S  R  Y  A  I  E
E  A  P  F  I  R  S  T  A  O  D  H  S  G  R
N  L  E  N  N  P  I  L  E  P  S  Y  L  D  O
C  L  A  T  T  L  O  Y  I  U  A  T  C  O  S
E  I  N  E  R  H  C  N  U  T  U  R  E  S  I
F  U  E  R  A  U  R  A  S  M  E  M  N  I  S
P  G  S  I  T  I  L  M  H  P  E  C  N  E  S
```

Suffixes

CHAPTER CONTENT

OBJECTIVES

Upon completing this chapter and the review exercises at the end of the chapter, the learner should be able to:

1. Define a suffix and state the rule for using suffixes in words.

2. Correctly identify at least 10 suffixes that make a word a noun.

3. Correctly identify at least 10 suffixes that make a word an adjective.

4. Correctly identify at least 10 suffixes that deal with instruments and with diagnostic and surgical procedures.

5. Identify and define at least 8 suffixes that deal with specialties and specialists.

Overview

A suffix is the ending of a word. The root to which a suffix is attached may or may not need a combining vowel, depending on whether the suffix begins with a consonant or a vowel.

Example: **Combining Vowel Needed:** *cephal + o + dynia* = **cephalodynia**

Cephal is a word root meaning "head"; *-dynia* is a suffix meaning "pain." Because *-dynia* begins with a consonant (*d*), it is necessary to use the combining vowel *o* to make the word *cephalodynia*—which means "pain in the head."

Rule: *When a suffix begins with a consonant, a combining vowel is used with the word root that attaches to the suffix.*

Example: **Combining Vowel *Not* Needed:** *cephal + algia* = **cephalalgia**

Cephal is a word root meaning "head"; *-algia* is a suffix meaning "pain." Because *-algia* begins with a vowel (*a*), it is not necessary to use a combining vowel to make the word *cephalalgia*—which means "pain in the head."

Rule: *When a suffix begins with a vowel, the word root attaches directly to the suffix without the aid of a combining vowel.*

A suffix makes a word either a noun or an adjective. When the noun ending *-um* is attached to the word root *duoden*, the newly created word *duodenum* is a noun. When the adjective ending *-al* is attached to the same word root, the new word becomes the adjective *duodenal*. In this chapter, we classify the suffixes as either noun endings or adjective endings. Seeing the suffixes in a grouping such as this should help you as you continue to create medical words.

As mentioned in Chapter 2 (on prefixes), the meaning of a particular suffix does not change from word to word. Thus, *-itis* always means "inflammation." Any word that has *-itis* as its suffix denotes inflammation. A word with the same root does change its meaning, however, each time a new suffix is attached. For example, use the word root *gastr* (meaning "stomach") and look at the various definitions that result with the addition of different suffixes. Notice that in each word the suffix is bold, as is the definition of the suffix.

Word	Word Root	+	Suffix		Definition
gastr**algia**	gastr		**-algia**	=	**pain** in the stomach
gastr**itis**	gastr		**-itis**	=	**inflammation** of the stomach
gastr**ic**	gastr		**-ic**	=	**pertaining to** the stomach
gastr**ostomy**	gastr		**-ostomy**	=	**creating a new opening into** the stomach

Suffixes indicate (among other things) surgical procedures, types of surgeries, specialties, specialists, and conditions. Defining medical terms usually begins with the meaning of the suffix. For example, the definition of *gastritis* begins with defining the suffix first, followed by defining the word root. Therefore, the definition of *gastritis* is "**inflammation of** the stomach."

Rule: *When defining a medical term, begin the definition by defining the suffix first, the prefix second, and the root(s) last.*

The remainder of this chapter concentrates on the various categories of suffixes and their meanings. This is not a complete listing of suffixes. Additional suffixes are introduced throughout the text in relevant chapters. The review exercises at the end of the chapter will reinforce your understanding of suffixes and how to use them appropriately in medical terms.

Noun Suffixes

Most of the suffixes in this chapter make a word a noun. Nouns are words used to name a person, place, thing, quality, or action. They can be categorized by their relationship to specialties, surgeries, specialists, conditions, and so on. Some of the basic noun suffixes addressed in this section are used in all categories when building words that have noun endings.

Suffix	Meaning	Example
-a	(*a* is a noun ending)	cyanoder**ma** (skin with a bluish discoloration) **Note:** When *a* is used as a suffix, it is a noun ending; *a* can also be used as a prefix.
-ate	something that . . .	hemolys**ate** (something that results from hemolysis)
-e	(*e* is a noun ending)	dermatom**e** (instrument used to cut the skin; e.g., thin slices of skin for grafting)
-emia	blood condition	hyperglyc**emia** (blood condition in which a greater than normal level of glucose is present in the blood; high blood sugar)
-er	one who	radiograph**er** (one who takes and processes X-rays)
-esis	condition of	enur**esis** (condition of urinary incontinence; bed-wetting)
-ia	condition (*ia* is a noun ending)	parapleg**ia** (condition of paralysis of the lower half of the body)
-iatry	medical treatment, medical profession	pod**iatry** (treatment of diseases and disorders of the foot)
-ion	action, process	conduct**ion** (process in which heat is transferred from one substance to another)
-ism	condition	hirsut**ism** (condition of excessive body hair in a male distribution pattern)
-ist	practitioner	pharmac**ist** (practitioner who prepares/dispenses drugs/medications)
-ole	small or little	arteri**ole** (smallest branch of the arterial circulation; small artery)
-osis	condition	cyan**osis** (condition of blueness)
-tion	process of	relaxa**tion** (the process of reducing tension, as in a muscle when it relaxes after contraction)
-ula	small, little	mac**ula** (small, pigmented spot that appears separate from the surrounding tissue)
-ule	"small one"	ven**ule** (smallest vein that collects blood from a capillary)

Suffix	Meaning	Example
-um	a suffix that identifies singular nouns	duoden**um** (first part of the small intestine)
-us	a suffix that identifies singular nouns	coc**cus** (singular bacterium)
-y	condition; process (noun ending)	myopath**y** (abnormal condition of the muscle)

Plural Words

When a word changes from singular to plural form, the ending of the word also changes. For example, you may have only one cris**is** (singular) or you may have many cris**es** (plural). Use the following rules when changing from singular to plural forms of words.

Rule: *When the singular form of a word ends in -a, change the a to ae to form the plural.*

Example: The singular form *pleura* becomes *pleurae* in the plural form.

Rule: *When the singular form of a word ends in -ax, change the ax to aces to form the plural.*

Example: The singular form *thorax* becomes *thoraces* in the plural form.

Rule: *When the singular form of a word ends in -is, change the is to es to form the plural.*

Example: The singular form *crisis* becomes *crises* in the plural form.

Rule: *When the singular form of a word ends in -ix, -ex, or -yx, change the ix, ex, or yx to ices to form the plural.*

Example: The singular form *appendix* becomes *appendices* in the plural form. The singular form *apex* becomes *apices* in the plural form.

Rule: *When the singular form of a word ends in -on, change the on to a to form the plural.*

Example: The singular form *ganglion* becomes *ganglia* in the plural form.

Rule: *When the singular form of a word ends in -um, change the um to a to form the plural.*

Example: The singular form *bacterium* becomes *bacteria* in the plural form.

Rule: *When the singular form of a word ends in -us, change the us to i to form the plural.*

Example: The singular form *thrombus* becomes *thrombi* in the plural form.

Rule: *When the singular form of a word ends in -ma, change the ma to mata to form the plural.*

Example: The singular form *fibroma* becomes *fibromata* in the plural form.

The rules for changing the singular form to the plural are recapped in the examples in Table 3-1.

Table 3-1 Singular to Plural Suffix Changes

Singular Form		Plural Form
pleura (**PLOO**-rah)	becomes	pleurae (**PLOO**-ree)
thorax (**THOH**-raks)	becomes	thoraces (**THOH**-rah-seez)
diagnosis (**dye**-ag-**NOH**-sis)	becomes	diagnoses (**dye**-ag-**NOH**-seez)
appendix (ah-**PEN**-diks)	becomes	appendices (ah-**PEN**-dih-seez)
apex (**AY**-peks)	becomes	apices (**AY**-pih-seez)
ganglion (**GANG**-glee-on)	becomes	ganglia (**GANG**-glee-ah)
bacterium (back-**TEE**-ree-um)	becomes	bacteria (back-**TEER**-ee-ah)
thrombus (**THROM**-bus)	becomes	thrombi (**THROM**-bye)
fibroma (figh-**BROH**-mah)	becomes	fibromata (figh-**BROH**-mah-tah)

Adjective Suffixes

Adjectives are words that modify nouns by limiting, qualifying, or specifying. Adjective suffixes are normally used to describe the word root to which they are attached. They usually mean "pertaining to," "relating to," "characterized by," or "resembling." There are no specific rules governing which adjective endings go with which words. Sometimes more than one ending will work with the same word root. Understanding the definition and use of a word will help in selecting the most appropriate adjective suffix. The following is a list of some frequently used adjective suffixes.

Suffix	Meaning	Example
ac	pertaining to	cardiac (pertaining to the heart)
-al	pertaining to	duodenal (pertaining to the duodenum)
-ar	pertaining to	ventricular (pertaining to the ventricle)
-ary	pertaining to; relating to	pulmonary (pertaining to the lungs)
-eal	pertaining to	esophageal (pertaining to the esophagus)
-ic	pertaining to	thoracic (pertaining to the thorax)
-ical	pertaining to (-ical is the combination of ic + al)	neurological (pertaining to the study of nerves)
-ile	pertaining to; capable	febrile (pertaining to fever)
-oid	resembling	mucoid (resembling mucus)

Suffix	Meaning	Example
-ory	pertaining to; characterized by	audit**ory** (pertaining to hearing)
-ous	pertaining to	ven**ous** (pertaining to veins)
-tic	pertaining to	cyano**tic** (pertaining to blueness)

Specialties and Specialists

Suffixes that indicate specialties and/or specialists are presented throughout the study of medical terminology, particularly as you learn more about specialties, subspecialties, and the physicians who choose to pursue these specialties as lifelong careers. By the time a physician has earned the title of Board Certified or Diplomate in a particular field of study, this person may have invested as much as three to seven years studying beyond the basic medical degree. The following list identifies the most frequently used suffixes that denote specialties and/or specialists.

Suffix	Meaning	Example
-ician	specialist in a field of study	obstet**rician** (specialist in the field of study of pregnancy and childbirth)
-iatrics	relating to medicine, physicians, or medical treatment	ped**iatrics** (field of medicine that deals with children)
-iatry	medical treatment, medical profession	psych**iatry** (field of medicine that deals with the diagnosis, treatment, and prevention of mental illness)
-iatrist	one who treats; a physician	psych**iatrist** (specialist in the study, treatment, and prevention of mental illness)
-ian	specialist in a field of study	geriatric**ian** (specialist in the field of study of the aging)
-ist	practitioner	pharmac**ist** (one who is licensed to prepare and dispense medications)
-logist	one who specializes in the study of	bio**logist** (one who specializes in the study of living things)
-logy	the study of	bio**logy** (the study of living things)

Instruments, Surgical and Diagnostic Procedures

The following suffixes indicate some type of instrument or a surgical or diagnostic procedure. The procedures vary from those that are performed in a medical office or outpatient setting to those performed in hospital surgery settings. The instruments are used primarily for diagnostic purposes.

Suffix	Meaning	Example
-centesis	surgical puncture	amnio**centesis** (surgical puncture of the amniotic sac to remove fluid for laboratory analysis; an obstetrical procedure)
-clasis	crushing or breaking up	osteo**clasis** (intentional surgical fracture of a bone to correct a deformity)
-desis	binding or surgical fusion	arthro**desis** (fixation of a joint by a procedure designed to accomplish fusion of the joint surfaces)
-ectomy	surgical removal	append**ectomy** (surgical removal of the appendix)
-gram	record or picture	electrocardio**gram** (record of the electrical activity of the heart)
-graph	an instrument used to record	electrocardio**graph** (instrument used to record the electrical activity of the heart)
-graphy	process of recording	electrocardio**graphy** (the process of recording the electrical activity of the heart)
-ize	to make; to treat or combine with	anesthe**tize** (to induce a state of anesthesia; to make one "feelingless")
-lysis	destruction or detachment	dia**lysis** (the removal or detachment of certain elements from the blood or lymph by passing them through a semipermeable membrane)
-meter	an instrument used to measure	pelvi**meter** (instrument used to measure the diameter and capacity of the pelvis)
-metry	the process of measuring	pelvi**metry** (process of measuring the dimensions of the pelvis)
-opsy	process of viewing	bi**opsy** (removal of a small piece of living tissue from an organ or part of the body for "viewing" under a microscope)
-pexy	surgical fixation	colpo**pexy** (surgical fixation of a relaxed vaginal wall)
-plasty	surgical repair	rhino**plasty** (surgical repair of the nose in which the structure of the nose is changed)
-rrhaphy	suturing	nephro**rrhaphy** (the operation of suturing the kidney)
-scope	an instrument used to view	ophthalmo**scope** (instrument used to view the interior of the eye)
-scopy	the process of viewing with a scope	ophthalmo**scopy** (the process of using an ophthalmoscope to view the interior of the eye)
-stomy	the surgical creation of a new opening	colo**stomy** (surgical creation of a new opening between the colon and the surface of the body)
-tomy	incision into	phlebo**tomy** (incision into a vein)
-tripsy	intentional crushing	litho**tripsy** (crushing of a stone in the bladder; may be accomplished by ultrasound or by laser)

Common Suffixes

An alphabetical listing of suffixes commonly used in medical terminology is included here for easy reference. As you read the list, note that the suffixes just discussed in the "categories" section are repeated in this list. Some of the suffixes also appear throughout the text as they relate to discussions of the body.

Suffix	Meaning	Example
-a	(*a* is a noun ending)	cyano**derma** (skin with a bluish discoloration) **Note:** When *a* is used as a suffix, it is a noun ending; *a* can also be used as a prefix.
-ac	pertaining to	cardi**ac** (pertaining to the heart)
-ad	toward, increase	caud**ad** (toward the tail or end of the body)
-al	pertaining to	duoden**al** (pertaining to the duodenum)
-algesia	sensitivity to pain	an**algesia** (without sensitivity to pain)
-algia	pain	cephal**algia** (pain in the head; a headache)
-ar	pertaining to	ventricul**ar** (pertaining to the ventricle)
-ary	pertaining to; relating to	pulmon**ary** (pertaining to the lungs)
-ate	something that . . .	hemolys**ate** (something that results from hemolysis)
-blast	embryonic stage of development	leuko**blast** (immature white blood cell)
-cele	swelling or herniation	cysto**cele** (herniation or protrusion of the urinary bladder through the wall of the vagina)
-centesis	surgical puncture	amnio**centesis** (surgical puncture of the amniotic sac to remove fluid for laboratory analysis; an obstetrical procedure)
-cide	to kill; to destroy	spermi**cide** (chemical substance that kills spermatozoa)
-clasis	crushing or breaking up	osteo**clasis** (the intentional surgical fracture of a bone to correct a deformity)
-cyte	cell	leuko**cyte** (white blood cell)
-desis	binding or surgical fusion	arthro**desis** (fixation of a joint by a procedure designed to accomplish fusion of the joint surfaces)
-dynia	pain	cephalo**dynia** (pain in the head; a headache)
-e	(*e* is a noun ending)	dermato**me** (instrument used to cut the skin; i.e., thin slices of skin for grafting)

Suffix	Meaning	Example
-eal	pertaining to	esophag**eal** (pertaining to the esophagus)
-ectasia	stretching or dilation	gast**rectasia** (stretching or dilation of the stomach)
-ectasis	stretching or dilation	gast**rectasis** (stretching or dilation of the stomach)
-ectomy	surgical removal	append**ectomy** (surgical removal of the appendix)
-emia	blood condition	hyperglyc**emia** (blood condition in which there is a higher than normal level of glucose in the blood; high blood sugar)
-er	one who	radiograph**er** (one who takes and processes X-rays)
-esis	condition of	enur**esis** (condition of urinary incontinence)
-gen	that which generates	glyco**gen** ("that which generates sugar")
-genesis	generating; formation	litho**genesis** (the formation of stones)
-genic	pertaining to formation, producing	litho**genic** (pertaining to the formation of stones)
-gram	record or picture	electrocardio**gram** (record of the electrical activity of the heart)
-graph	an instrument used to record	electrocardio**graph** (instrument used to record the electrical activity of the heart)
-graphy	process of recording	electrocardio**graphy** (the process of recording the electrical activity of the heart)
-gravida	pregnancy	multi**gravida** (a woman who has been pregnant more than once; "many pregnancies")
-ia	condition (*ia* is a noun ending)	parapleg**ia** (condition of paralysis of the lower half of the body)
-ian	specialist in a field of study	geriatric**ian** (specialist in the field of study of the aging)
-iasis	presence of an abnormal condition	cholelith**iasis** (abnormal presence of gallstones in the gallbladder)
-iatric(s)	relating to medicine, physicians, or medical treatment	ped**iatrics** (field of medicine that deals with children)
-iatrician	one who treats; a physician	ped**iatrician** (physician who treats children)
-iatrist	one who treats; a physician	psych**iatrist** (specialist in the study, treatment, and prevention of mental illness)

Suffix	Meaning	Example
-iatry	medical treatment, medical profession	psych**iatry** (field of medicine that deals with the diagnosis, treatment, and prevention of mental illness)
-ic	pertaining to	thorac**ic** (pertaining to the thorax)
-ical	pertaining to (*-ical* is the combination of *ic + al*)	neurolog**ical** (pertaining to the study of nerves)
-ician	specialist in a field of study	obstet**rician** (specialist in the field of study of pregnancy and childbirth)
-ile	pertaining to; capable	feb**rile** (pertaining to fever)
-ion	action; process	conduc**tion** (process in which heat is transferred from one substance to another)
-ism	condition	hirsut**ism** (condition of excessive body hair in a masculine distribution pattern)
-ist	practitioner	pharma**cist** (practitioner who is licensed to prepare and dispense medications)
-itis	inflammation	appendic**itis** (inflammation of the appendix)
-ize	to make; to treat or combine with	anesthet**ize** (to induce a state of anesthesia; to make one "feelingless")
-lepsy	seizure, attack	narco**lepsy** (seizure or sudden attack of sleep)
-lith	stone	rhino**lith** (stone or calculus in the nose)
-lithiasis	presence or formation of stones	chole**lithiasis** (presence of gallstones)
-logy	the study of	bio**logy** (the study of living things)
-logist	one who specializes in the study of	bio**logist** (one who specializes in the study of living things)
-lysis	destruction or detachment	dia**lysis** (removal or detachment of certain elements from the blood or lymph by passing them through a semipermeable membrane)
-lytic	destruction	kerato**lytic** (agent used to destroy hardened skin)
-mania	a mental disorder; a "madness"	megalo**mania** (mental disorder characterized by delusions of grandeur: the patient believes he or she is someone of great importance)
-megaly	enlargement	cardio**megaly** (enlargement of the heart)
-meter	an instrument used to measure	pelvi**meter** (instrument used to measure the diameter and capacity of the pelvis)

Suffix	Meaning	Example
-metry	the process of measuring	pelvi**metry** (the process of measuring the dimensions of the pelvis)
-oid	resembling	muc**oid** (resembling mucus)
-ole	small or little	arteri**ole** (smallest branch of the arterial circulation; a "small" artery)
-oma	tumor	lip**oma** (fatty tumor)
-opia	visual condition	my**opia** (a condition of nearsightedness)
-opsia	visual condition	hemian**opsia** (blindness in one half of the visual field)
-opsy	process of viewing	bi**opsy** (removal of a small piece of living tissue from an organ or part of the body for "viewing" under a microscope)
-ory	pertaining to; characterized by	audit**ory** (pertaining to hearing)
-osis	condition	cyan**osis** (condition of blueness)
-ous	pertaining to	ven**ous** (pertaining to veins)
-pathy	disease	adeno**pathy** (disease of a gland)
-penia	decrease in; deficiency	leukocyto**penia** (decrease in the number of white blood cells)
-pexy	surgical fixation	colpo**pexy** (surgical fixation of a relaxed vaginal wall)
-philia	attraction to	necro**philia** (abnormal attraction to dead bodies)
-phobia	abnormal fear	necro**phobia** (abnormal fear of death and dead bodies)
-plasia	formation or development	hyper**plasia** (excessive formation or development)
-plasty	surgical repair	rhino**plasty** (surgical repair of the nose in which the structure of the nose is changed)
-plegia	paralysis	hemi**plegia** (paralysis of half of the body, of one side of the body)
-pnea	breathing	dys**pnea** (difficult breathing)
-ptosis	drooping or prolapse	colpo**ptosis** (prolapse of the vagina)
-rrhagia	excessive flow or discharge	gastro**rrhagia** (bursting forth of blood from the stomach)
-rrhaphy	suturing	nephro**rrhaphy** (operation of suturing the kidney)
-rrhea	discharge; flow	rhino**rrhea** (flow or drainage from the nose)

Suffix	Meaning	Example
-rrhexis	rupture	arterio**rrhexis** (rupture of an artery)
-scope	an instrument used to view	ophthalmo**scope** (instrument used to view the interior of the eye)
-scopy	the process of viewing with a scope	ophthalmo**scopy** (the process of using an ophthalmoscope to view the interior of the eye)
-stasis	stopping or controlling	hemo**stasis** (stopping or controlling the flow of blood) veno**stasis** (the trapping or "standing still" of blood in an extremity)
-stomy	the surgical creation of a new opening	colo**stomy** (surgical creation of a new opening between the colon and the surface of the body)
-tic	pertaining to	cyano**tic** (pertaining to blueness)
-tion	process of	relaxa**tion** (the process of reducing tension, as when a muscle relaxes after contraction)
-tomy	incision into	phlebo**tomy** (incision into a vein)
-tripsy	intentional crushing	litho**tripsy** (the crushing of a stone in the bladder; may be accomplished by ultrasound or by laser)
-ula	small, little	mac**ula** (small pigmented spot that appears separate from the surrounding tissue)
-ule	"small one"	ven**ule** (smallest vein that collects blood from a capillary)
-um	a suffix that identifies singular nouns	duoden**um** (first part of the small intestines)
-uria	a characteristic of the urine	hemat**uria** (presence of blood in the urine)
-us	a suffix that identifies singular nouns	cocc**us** (singular bacterium)
-y	condition; process (noun ending)	myopath**y** (abnormal condition of the muscles)

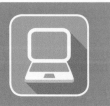

Media Link

To increase your understanding of word structure, go to the Student Companion Website and watch the following animations: **Word Parts Work Together** and **Combining Word Roots**.

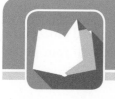

Review Checkpoint

Apply what you have learned in this chapter by completing the exercises in your workbook.

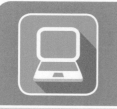

Online Resources

For PowerPoint® slides and comprehensive Quick Access Suffix Tables, go to the Student Companion Website. These tables are a valuable study tool and quick reference for learning suffixes. Search by suffix or by the definition of a suffix.

Chapter Review Exercises

The following exercises provide a more in-depth review of the chapter material. Your goal in these exercises is to complete each section at a minimum 80% level of accuracy. A space has been provided for your score at the end of each section.

A. Replacing

Read each sentence carefully and replace the terms in bold with the applicable noun ending. Each correct answer is worth 10 points. Record your score in the space provided at the end of the exercise.

-algia	-emia	-iatry	-um
-cele	-er	-itis	
-dynia	-genesis	-ole	

1. **One who** takes and processes X-rays is known as a radiograph _____.
2. A **blood condition** in which there is a higher than normal level of glucose in the blood is known as hyperglyc _____.
3. The **treatment** of diseases and disorders of the foot is known as pod _____.
4. The **smallest** branch of the arterial circulation is the arteri _____.
5. To change the word *duodenal* from its adjective form, you would drop the *-al* and add _____ to make the word a noun.
6. **Pain** in the head, or headache, is known as cephal _____.
7. **Herniation** of the bladder through the wall of the vagina is known as a cysto _____.
8. **Pain** in the head can also be called cephalo _____.
9. The **formation of** stones is known as litho _____.
10. **Inflammation** of the appendix is termed appendic _____.

Number correct _____ × *10 points/correct answer: Your score* _____ %

B. Crossword Puzzle

In this puzzle, you will be working with suffixes that indicate instruments and diagnostic or surgical procedures. Each crossword answer is worth 10 points. When you have completed the crossword puzzle, total your points and enter your score in the space provided.

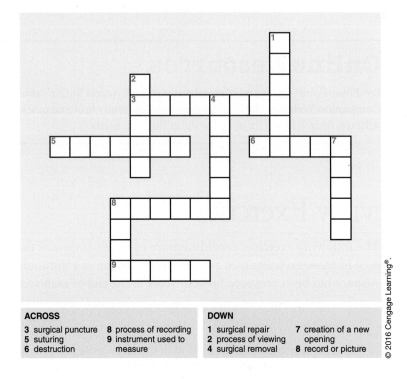

ACROSS

3 surgical puncture
5 suturing
6 destruction
8 process of recording
9 instrument used to measure

DOWN

1 surgical repair
2 process of viewing
4 surgical removal
7 creation of a new opening
8 record or picture

© 2016 Cengage Learning®.

***Number correct* _____ × *10 points/correct answer: Your score* _____ %**

C. Create a Word

Using the suffixes listed, create a word that best completes each statement dealing with specialties, specialists, and specialty instruments. If you need assistance, refer to your list of suffixes within the chapter. After you have determined the correct suffix, write the word (without the divisions) in the space provided. Each correct answer is worth 10 points. Record your score in the space provided at the end of the exercise.

-logist	-scope	-iatrics	-ician
-ist	-logy	-mania	
-iatrist	-iatry	-ian	

Create a word that means:

1. A specialist in the field of study of the aging

   geriatric   +   =

   _____
   (word root)   +   (suffix)   =   (complete word)

2. The study of living things

   bio   +   =

   _____
   (word root)   +   (suffix)   =   (complete word)

3. A specialist in the field of study of pregnancy and childbirth

obstetr	+		=	
(word root)	+	(suffix)	=	(complete word)

4. A pediatrician would use this instrument for viewing the interior of the eye

ophthalm	+	o	+		=	
(root)	+	(vowel)	+	(suffix)	=	(complete word)

5. A specialist in the study, treatment, and prevention of mental illness

psych	+		=	
(word root)	+	(suffix)	=	(complete word)

6. The field of medicine that deals with children

ped	+		=	
(word root)	+	(suffix)	=	(complete word)

7. One who is licensed to prepare and dispense medications

pharmac	+		=	
(word root)	+	(suffix)	=	(complete word)

8. A psychiatrist might treat this mental disorder, which is characterized by delusions of grandeur (the patient believes he or she is someone of great importance)

megal	+	o	+		=	
(root)	+	(vowel)	+	(suffix)	=	(complete word)

9. The field of medicine that deals with the diagnosis, treatment, and prevention of mental illness

psych	+		=	
(word root)	+	(suffix)	=	(complete word)

10. One who specializes in the study of living things

bi	+	o	+		=	
(root)	+	(vowel)	+	(suffix)	=	(complete word)

Number correct _____ **× 10 points/correct answer: Your score** _____ **%**

D. Word Search

Read each definition carefully and identify the applicable word from the list that follows. Enter the word in the space provided and then find it in the puzzle and circle it. The words may be read up, down, diagonally, across, or backward. Each correct answer is worth 10 points. Record your score in the space provided at the end of the exercise.

cardiac	duodenal	ventricular
pulmonary	thoracic	neurological
febrile	mucoid	auditory
venous	cyanotic	

(*continued*)

Example: pertaining to the veins *venous* _____

   1. pertaining to the heart _____

   2. pertaining to the duodenum _____

   3. pertaining to the ventricle _____

   4. pertaining to the lungs _____

   5. pertaining to the thorax _____

   6. pertaining to the nerves _____

   7. pertaining to fever _____

   8. resembling mucus _____

   9. pertaining to hearing _____

  10. pertaining to blueness _____

C	A	R	V	E	N	O	U	S	D	I	A	C	B
A	C	R	F	E	B	R	I	L	E	T	Y	O	R
L	U	E	O	Y	N	T	I	C	H	A	P	Y	I
M	U	C	O	I	D	T	A	O	N	E	B	R	L
N	E	A	U	R	O	L	R	O	T	H	O	O	E
M	U	R	S	C	O	A	T	I	I	D	R	T	F
P	U	D	L	M	C	I	O	N	C	U	A	I	R
F	E	I	B	I	C	R	I	L	E	U	V	D	E
N	O	A	C	U	Y	R	A	N	O	M	L	U	P
S	A	C	U	D	I	D	U	O	D	E	N	A	L
L	A	C	I	G	O	L	O	R	U	E	N	T	R

© 2016 Cengage Learning®.

Number correct _____ × *10 points/correct answer: Your score* _____ %

E. Matching

Match the suffixes on the left with the correct definition on the right. Each correct answer is worth 10 points. Record your score in the space provided at the end of the exercise.

_____	1. -oid	a. discharge; flow
_____	2. -clasis	b. rupture
_____	3. -ectomy	c. instrument used to record
_____	4. -gram	d. surgical fixation
_____	5. -graph	e. surgical removal
_____	6. -pexy	f. record or picture
_____	7. -plasty	g. suturing
_____	8. -rrhaphy	h. surgical repair
_____	9. -rrhea	i. resembling
_____	10. -rrhexis	j. crushing or breaking up

Number correct _____ × *10 points/correct answer: Your score* _____ %

F. Singular to Plural

Look at the singular form of the words following, and change each word ending to the plural form, following the rules presented in this chapter. (HINT: You do not have to change the spelling of the complete word, just the ending to make it a plural form.) The singular ending is printed in bold. Each correct answer is worth 10 points. Record your score in the space provided at the end of the exercise.

SINGULAR FORM	**PLURAL FORM**
Example: cocc**us**	**Example:** cocci
1. pleur**a**	1. _____
2. thor**ax**	2. _____
3. cris**is**	3. _____
4. append**ix**	4. _____
5. ap**ex**	5. _____
6. gangli**on**	6. _____
7. bacteri**um**	7. _____
8. thromb**us**	8. _____
9. fibr**oma**	9. _____
10. diagnos**is**	10. _____

Number correct _____ *× 10 points/correct answer: Your score* _____ *%*

G. Proofreading Skills

Read the following medical report. For each suffix that appears in boldface, define the suffix and indicate if the suffix is spelled correctly. Each correct answer is worth 10 points. Record your score in the space provided at the end of the exercise.

Example Word: *neurologic*

Suffix: _____ *ic* _____

Definition: _____ *pertaining to* _____

HISTORY AND PHYSICAL EXAMINATION

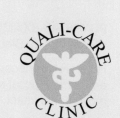

PATIENT NAME: Harold Rivers

PCP: A. Leigh Wells, MD

DATE OF BIRTH: 02/09/1966

AGE: 48

SEX: Male

DATE OF EXAM
06/15/2014

(continued)

HISTORY AND PHYSICAL EXAMINATION
Patient Name: Harold Rivers
PCP: A. Leigh Wells, MD
Date of Exam: 06/15/2014
Page 2

CHIEF COMPLAINT

The patient presents for medical clearance for his scheduled neurologic procedure. Please see Dr. King's detailed note.

PAST HISTORY AND MEDICAL PROBLEMS

1. History of headaches. Patient has had significant, prolonged headaches. Some 10 or 15 years ago, I referred him to a clinic for evaluation of his headaches. At that time, migraine versus vascular headache was considered. Patient is asymptomatic presently.

2. History of azotemia. Patient has had mild azotemia, and he was evaluated for this in the Monroe University's Department of Nephrology. No significant abnormality was found, and he remains under observation.

3. History of hyperlipidemia. Mild hyperlipidemia is present, controlled with Zocor 10 mg daily. He has remained asymptomatic on the Zocor.

4. History of microcytosis. This condition has been found on a couple of occasions in the past, but patient has had no significant abnormality and remains under observation. CBC was drawn and results are pending.

PROFESSIONAL HISTORY

A retired coal miner, no other significant exposure.

ALLERGIES AND IDIOSYNCRASIES

None known.

REVIEW OF SYSTEMS

EYES, EARS, NOSE, THROAT: No complaints. Wears glasses.

GASTROINTESTINAL: No anorexia or early satiety. No abdominal pain, hematemesis, melena, or hematochezia.

MUSCULOSKELETAL: No arthralgia or bone pain.

CARDIOVASCULAR: No chest pain or palpitations.

The remainder of the ROS is negative and noncontributory.

PHYSICAL EXAMINATION

VITAL SIGNS: Blood pressure 130/60, pulse 60 and regular, afebrile, respiratory rate 20.

HEENT: Normocephalic, atraumatic. Nares patent. Tympanic membranes clear. Oropharynx without erythema, buccal mucosa clear. Pupils equal, round, react to light and accommodation. Extraocular movements intact. Sclerae anicteric.

NECK: No bruits, jugular venous distention, or adenopathy.

CHEST: Clear to auscultation, percussion, and palpation.

HEART: Point of maximum impulse in the midline. Regular S1 and S2. No S3 or S4 present.

ABDOMEN: Soft, nontender. No visceromegaly, masses, rebound, or guarding. Bowel sounds present in all four quadrants.

(continued)

HISTORY AND PHYSICAL EXAMINATION
Patient Name: Harold Rivers
PCP: A. Leigh Wells, MD
Date of Exam: 06/15/2014
Page 3

NEUROLOGIC EXAM: Alert and oriented x3. Deep tendon reflexes symmetrical. No patholog**ic** reflexes.

PSYCHIATRIC: Mood and affect upbeat.

DIAGNOSES
1. Spondylolisthesis.
2. History of headaches.
3. Mild azotemia.
4. Hyperlipidemia.

NOTE: I find no clinical evidence to preclude Mr. Rivers from undergoing the planned neurologic procedure for his spondylolisthesis.

_____

A. Leigh Wells, MD

Internal Medicine

ALW:xx

D:06/15/2014

T:06/16/2014

C: T. Washington King, MD

1. **-emia** _____

_____

Spelled Correctly? ☐ Yes ☐ No _____
2. **-logy** _____

_____

Spelled Correctly? ☐ Yes ☐ No _____
3. **-osis** _____

_____

Spelled Correctly? ☐ Yes ☐ No _____
4. **-algia** _____

_____

Spelled Correctly? ☐ Yes ☐ No _____
5. **-ile** _____

_____

Spelled Correctly? ☐ Yes ☐ No _____

(continued)

6. **-ory** _____

_____

Spelled Correctly? ☐ Yes ☐ No _____

7. **-pathy** _____

_____

Spelled Correctly? ☐ Yes ☐ No _____

8. **-ion** _____

_____

Spelled Correctly? ☐ Yes ☐ No _____

9. **-megaly** _____

_____

Spelled Correctly? ☐ Yes ☐ No _____

10. **-ic** _____

_____

Spelled Correctly? ☐ Yes ☐ No _____

Number correct _____ × *10 points/correct answer: Your score* _____ *%*

Whole Body Terminology

CHAPTER CONTENT

OBJECTIVES

Upon completing this chapter and the review exercises at the end of the chapter, the learner should be able to:

1. List the five body cavities identified in this chapter.

2. List the organs contained within the five body cavities as identified in the chapter reading.

3. Define at least 10 general terms relating to the body as a whole.

4. Correctly spell and pronounce terms listed on the Written and Audio Terminology Review, using the phonetic pronunciations provided.

59

5. Identify the nine body regions studied in this chapter.

6. Identify at least eight terms relating to the structural organization of the body.

7. Identify at least 10 directional terms relating to the body as a whole.

8. Create at least 10 medical terms relating to the body as a whole.

Overview

So far we have discussed prefixes that are placed at the beginning of a word, suffixes that are placed at the end of a word, and word roots that are the foundation of a word. We have also reviewed the word building rules used to construct medical terms, using any combination of prefixes, word roots, and suffixes.

In addition to the ability to build medical terms that relate to the various body systems and particular diseases, disorders, and treatments, it is important to know terms that relate to the body as a whole. Whole body terms are an important part of medical terminology because they help define the makeup of the various body systems.

Medical terms are used to describe the structural organization of the body, from the cellular level to the systemic level. They are used to describe body cavities; divisions of the spinal column; regions, quadrants, and planes of the body. In addition, whole body terms provide information about position, direction, and location of organs in relation to each other within the body. By reading a medical report, one can determine the exact location being referred to. Knowledge of whole body terminology provides the necessary foundation for a better understanding of the body systems that follow.

Structural Organization

Although the organization of the body begins at the chemical level, our discussion of terms begins at the cellular level and builds from that point. Cells grouped together to perform specialized functions are known as **tissue**. Tissues arranged together to perform a special function are known as an **organ**. Organs that work together to perform the many functions of the body as a whole are called **systems**.

Cells

The **cell** is the smallest and most numerous structural unit of living matter. Refer to *Figure 4-1*. All cells are surrounded by a **(1) cell membrane**, which is the cell's outer covering. The **cell membrane** is a semipermeable barrier that allows certain substances to pass through while blocking others. The **cell membrane** is also known as the plasma **membrane**. The central controlling body within a living cell is the **(2) nucleus**, which

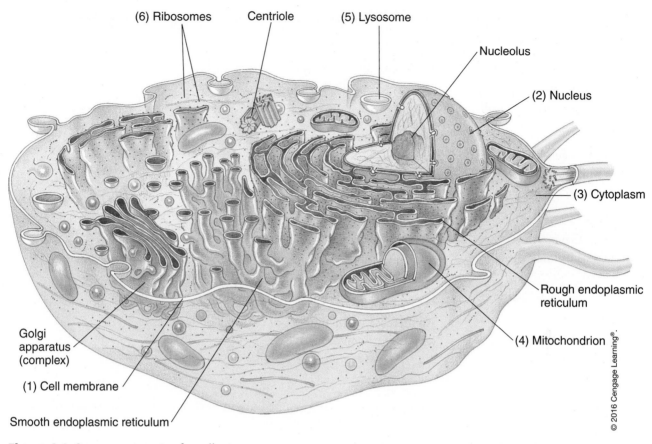

Figure 4-1 Component parts of a cell

is enclosed within the **cell membrane**. The **nucleus** is made up of threadlike structures called **chromosomes** (molecules of deoxyribonucleic acid, or DNA) that control the functions of growth, repair, and reproduction for the body. The **chromosomes** contain segments or regions called **genes** that transmit hereditary characteristics. Each body cell, with the exception of the female ovum and the male spermatozoa, contains 23 pairs of **chromosomes** that determine its genetic makeup. The female ovum (egg) and the male spermatozoa (sperm) each contain only 23 **chromosomes**. When the female ovum and the male sperm unite, resulting in fertilization of the ovum, the newly formed embryo contains 23 pairs of **chromosomes** (half coming from the ovum and half coming from the sperm).

Surrounding the **nucleus** of the cell is the **(3) cytoplasm**. The **cytoplasm** is a gel-like substance containing cell organs (called organelles) that carry out the essential functions of the cell. A few examples of organelles are **(4) mitochondria** (which provide the energy needed by the cell to carry on its essential functions) and **(5) lysosomes**, which contain various types of enzymes that function in intracellular digestion. When bacteria enter the cells, the lysosome enzymes destroy the bacteria by digesting them. The **(6) ribosomes**, which synthesize proteins, are often called the cell's "protein factories." The following terms relate to cellular growth.

Word	Meaning
anaplasia (an-ah-**PLAY**-zee-ah) ana- = not, without -plasia = formation, growth	A change in the structure and orientation of cells, characterized by a loss of differentiation and reversion to a more primitive form.
aplasia (ah-**PLAY**-zee-ah) a- = without, not -plasia = formation, growth	A developmental failure resulting in the absence of any **organ** or **tissue**.
dysplasia (dis-**PLAY**-zee-ah) dys- = bad, difficult, painful, disordered -plasia = formation, growth	Any abnormal development of cells, tissues or organs ("disordered formation").
hyperplasia (**high**-per-**PLAY**-zee-ah) hyper- = excessive -plasia = formation, growth	An increase in the number of cells of a body part ("excessive formation").
hypoplasia (**high**-poh-**PLAY**-zee-ah) hypo- = under, below, beneath, less than normal -plasia = formation, growth	Incomplete or underdeveloped **organ** or **tissue**, usually the result of a decrease in the number of cells.
neoplasia (**nee**-oh-**PLAY**-zee-ah) neo- = new -plasia = formation, growth	The new and abnormal development of cells that may be benign or malignant.

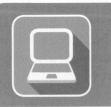

Media Link

Increase your understanding of the cell. Watch the **Typical Cell** animation on the Student Companion Site.

Tissues

Tissue is composed of groups of similar cells that perform specialized or common functions. The four main types of **tissue** are connective, epithelial, muscle, and nervous.

1. **Connective tissue** supports and binds other body **tissue** and parts. **Connective tissue** may be liquid (as in blood), fatty (as in protective padding), fibrous (as in tendons and ligaments), cartilage (as in the rings of the trachea), or solid (as in bone).

2. **Epithelial tissue** covers the internal and external organs of the body. It also lines the vessels, body cavities, glands, and body organs.

3. **Muscle tissue** is capable of producing movement of the parts and organs of the body through the contraction and relaxation of its fibers. The three types of muscle tissue in the body are (a) **skeletal muscle**, which is attached to bone and is responsible for the movement of the skeleton, (b) **smooth muscle** (also known as **visceral muscle**), which is found in the walls of the hollow internal organs of the body such as the stomach and intestines, and (c) **cardiac muscle**, which makes up the muscular wall of the heart.

4. **Nervous tissue** transmits impulses throughout the body, thereby activating, coordinating, and controlling the many functions of the body.

The term *membrane* describes a thin layer of **tissue** that covers a surface, lines a cavity, or divides a space, such as the **abdominal** membrane that lines the abdominal wall. A specific **membrane**, the **peritoneum**, is an extensive serous **membrane** that covers the entire abdominal wall of the body and is reflected over the contained viscera.

A medical specialist in the study of tissues is known as a **histologist**. The study of cells is known as **cytology**.

Organs

Organs are made up of tissues arranged together to perform a particular function. Examples of various organs are the liver, spleen, stomach, and ovaries. The term *visceral* refers to the internal organs. In the remaining chapters of this textbook, the various organs of the body are discussed in their specific **system** chapter.

Systems

The organization of various organs so they can perform the many functions of the body as a whole is known as **systems**. Most of the remaining chapters in this textbook focus on the primary body systems, including:

integumentary	cardiovascular
skeletal	respiratory
muscles and joints	digestive
nervous	urinary
special senses	male reproductive
endocrine	female reproductive
blood and lymphatic	

Body Planes

To identify the position of various parts of the body in the study of anatomy, the body can be visually divided into areas called planes. These imaginary slices, or cuts, are made as if a dividing sheet were passed through the body at a particular angle and in a particular direction. For example, if you were physically able to use a vertical plane to divide the body into unequal right and left portions, you would create the sagittal plane. Then if you were physically able to divide the body straight down the middle into equal right and left halves, you would create the **midsagittal plane**. If you separated those two halves of the body, laying them open like a book, you could view the inner structures of the body on the left side and on the right side. The **midsagittal plane** divides the body or structure into equal right and left portions. See *Figure 4-2*.

The imaginary line created when the body is divided into equal right and left halves is referred to as the **midline** of the body. The **long axis** of the body is defined as the imaginary line created by directing a vertical line through the middle of the body from the top of the head to a space equidistant between the feet, essentially the midline of the body. When we discuss directional terms, notice that many of the terms are described in relation to the **midline** of the body and the imaginary lines created by the various planes of the body. The following is a list of the planes of the body.

Vertical Planes

A vertical plane is an imaginary slice through the body (running from the head to the feet) that is perpendicular to the horizon.

frontal plane	Any of the vertical planes passing through the body from the head to the feet, perpendicular to the sagittal planes and dividing the body into front and back portions (also known as the coronal plane). See *Figure 4-3*.

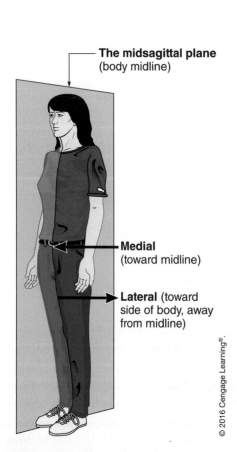

Figure 4-2 Midsagittal plane

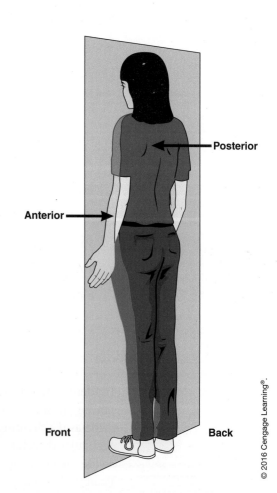

Figure 4-3 Frontal (coronal) plane

midsagittal plane

The **midsagittal plane** is a vertical plane through the middle of the body that divides the body into equal right and left halves; also known as the median plane. See *Figure 4-2*.

As stated previously, the imaginary line created by the **midsagittal plane** is known as the **midline** of the body. The **midline** of the body may also be referred to as the long axis of the body. The long axis runs the same direction as the **midsagittal plane** and distributes the weight of the body equally on each side of the line. It is interesting to note that swimming strokes are referred to as long axis strokes (backstroke and freestyle) or short axis strokes (breaststroke and butterfly) based on how the body moves against the axis of the body.

Horizontal Plane

A horizontal plane is an imaginary slice through the body (running from side to side across the body) that is parallel to the horizon.

transverse plane

Any of the planes cutting across the body, perpendicular to the sagittal and the frontal planes and dividing the body into **superior** (upper) and **inferior** (lower) portions. See *Figure 4-4*.

Although we can visualize the cuts through the body that create the various planes (based on our sense of direction and our knowledge of anatomy), medical technology has advanced to the point that computers can produce a cross-sectional image of the body. This image, produced by computerized axial tomography (or CAT scan), represents a detailed cross section of the **tissue** structure being examined. (CAT scans are discussed in later chapters.)

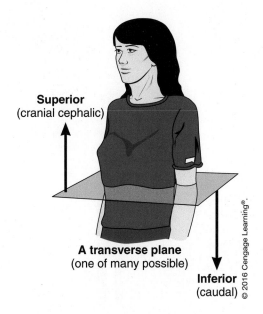

Superior
(cranial cephalic)

A transverse plane
(one of many possible)

Inferior
(caudal)

© 2016 Cengage Learning®.

Figure 4-4 Transverse plane

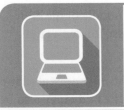

Media Link

See the planes in 3D in the **Body Planes** animation on the Student Companion Site.

Body Regions and Quadrants

In addition to planes, areas of the body can be further divided into regions and quadrants. Anatomists have divided the abdomen into nine imaginary sections (called regions) that are helpful in identifying the location of particular **abdominal** organs. Moreover, regions are useful for describing the location of pain.

Figure 4-5 shows the nine **abdominal** regions, which are identified from the left to the right, moving from top to bottom one row at a time. The most **superficial** organs in these regions are also identified.

region 1	**Right hypochondriac region** Located in the upper-right section of the abdomen, beneath the cartilage of the lower ribs, the **superficial** organs visible in the right hypochondriac region include the right lobe of the liver and the gallbladder.

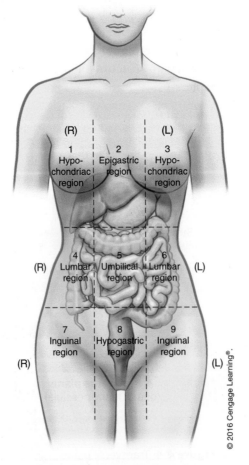

Figure 4-5 Abdominal regions

© 2016 Cengage Learning®.

region 2	**Epigastric region** Located between the right and left hypochondriac regions in the upper section of the abdomen, beneath the cartilage of the lower ribs; the **superficial** organs visible in the **epigastric region** include parts of the right and left lobes of the liver and a major portion of the stomach.
region 3	**Left hypochondriac region** Located in the upper-left section of the abdomen, beneath the cartilage of the lower ribs; the **superficial** organs visible in the left hypochondriac region include a small portion of the stomach and a portion of the large intestine.
region 4	**Right lumbar region** Located in the middle-right section of the abdomen, beneath the right hypochondriac region; the **superficial** organs visible in the right lumbar region include portions of the large and small intestines.
region 5	**Umbilical region** Located in the middle section of the abdomen, between the right and left lumbar regions and directly beneath the **epigastric region**; the **superficial** organs visible in the **umbilical region** include a portion of the transverse colon and portions of the small intestine.
region 6	**Left lumbar region** Located in the middle-left section of the abdomen, beneath the left hypochondriac region; the **superficial** organs visible in the left lumbar region include portions of the small intestine and part of the colon.
region 7	**Right inguinal (iliac) region** Located in the lower-right section of the abdomen, beneath the right lumbar region; the **superficial** organs visible in the right inguinal region include portions of the small intestine and the cecum.
region 8	**Hypogastric region** Located in the lower-middle section of the abdomen, beneath the **umbilical region**; the **superficial** organs visible in the hypogastric region include the urinary bladder, portions of the small intestine, and the appendix.
region 9	**Left inguinal (iliac) region** Located in the lower-left section of the abdomen, beneath the left lumbar region; the **superficial** organs visible in the left inguinal region include portions of the colon and the small intestine.

Anatomists have also divided the abdomen into quadrants. These four imaginary divisions provide reference points for physicians and health professionals when describing the location of abdominopelvic pain or when locating areas of involvement in certain diseases or conditions. The landmark on the

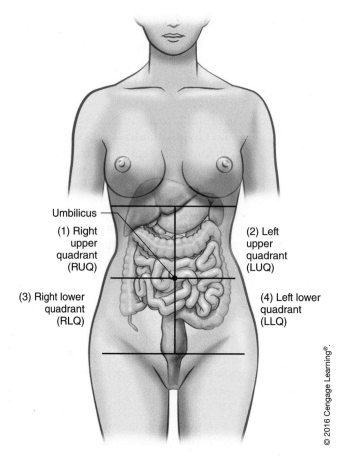

Umbilicus

(1) Right upper quadrant (RUQ)

(2) Left upper quadrant (LUQ)

(3) Right lower quadrant (RLQ)

(4) Left lower quadrant (LLQ)

© 2016 Cengage Learning®.

Figure 4-6 Abdominal quadrants

external abdominal wall for dividing the abdomen into quadrants is the **umbilicus**, or **navel** (sometimes referred to as the belly button). To divide the abdomen into quadrants, an imaginary line is drawn vertically and horizontally through the **umbilicus**, creating the four **abdominal** quadrants: **(1) right upper quadrant (RUQ)**, **(2) left upper quadrant (LUQ)**, **(3) right lower quadrant (RLQ)**, and **(4) left lower quadrant (LLQ)**. *Figure 4-6* shows the four **abdominal** quadrants.

An additional reference point on the abdomen that uses the **umbilicus** as a landmark is **McBurney's point**. **McBurney's point** is located on the right side of the abdomen, about two-thirds of the distance between the **umbilicus** and the **anterior** bony prominence of the hip. When tenderness exists upon **McBurney's point**, a physician might suspect appendicitis (inflammation of the appendix).

Body Cavities

The body has two major cavities, or hollow spaces, which contain orderly arrangements of internal body organs. These main body cavities are the **ventral** cavity and the **dorsal** cavity. Each of these is further divided into smaller cavities containing specific organs. *Figure 4-7* provides a visual reference for the major body cavities and their subdivisions.

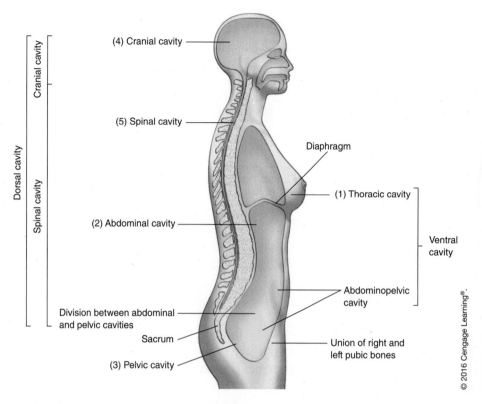

Figure 4-7 Major body cavities and subdivisions

Ventral Cavity Subdivisions

The **ventral** cavity (which contains the organs on the front, or "belly side," of the body) is subdivided into the **thoracic cavity** (chest cavity), the **abdominal cavity**, and the **pelvic cavity**. See *Figure 4-7* for a visual reference.

Feature Walk-Through

Some anatomy figures include numbers next to the structure names. These numbers correlate to the description of the structure within the text. As an example, note that the thoracic cavity label is preceded by a (1) in *Figure 4-7*. Likewise, there is a (1) before the *thoracic cavity* term in the following paragraph. This correlation helps you synthesize the written description with an image of the structure, encouraging a complete understanding of the anatomical structure.

---

(1) thoracic cavity
thorac/o = chest
-ic = pertaining to

The **thoracic cavity** contains the lungs, heart, aorta, esophagus, and trachea.

---

(2) abdominal cavity
-abdomin/o = abdomen
-al = pertaining to

The **abdominal cavity** is separated from the **thoracic cavity** by the diaphragm (the muscle that aids in the process of breathing). The **abdominal cavity** contains the liver, gallbladder, spleen, stomach, pancreas, intestines, and kidneys.

---

(3) pelvic cavity
pelv/i = pelvis
-ic = pertaining to

The **pelvic cavity** contains the urinary bladder and reproductive organs. The **pelvic cavity** and the **abdominal cavity** are often addressed collectively as the **abdominopelvic cavity**, which refers to the space between the diaphragm and the groin.

Dorsal Cavity Subdivisions

The **dorsal** cavity, which contains the organs of the back side of the body, is subdivided into the **cranial cavity** and the **spinal cavity**. See *Figure 4-7* for a visual reference.

(4) cranial cavity crani/o = skull -al = pertaining to	The **cranial cavity** contains the brain.
(5) spinal cavity spin/o = spine -al = pertaining to	The **spinal cavity** contains the nerves of the spinal cord.

Divisions of the Back

The back is subdivided into five sections that relate to the proximity (nearness) of each section to the vertebrae of the spinal column. The sections are named for the vertebrae located in that particular area of the back, as shown in *Figure 4-8*.

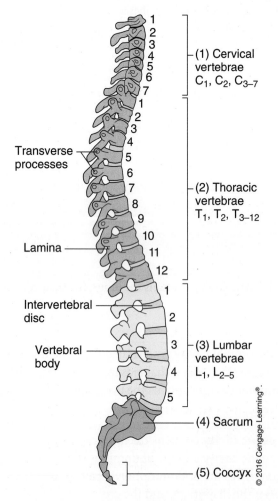

Figure 4-8 Divisions of the back

(1) cervical vertebrae cervic/o = neck -al = pertaining to	The **cervical vertebrae**, consisting of the first seven segments of the spinal column, make up the bones of the neck (cervic/o = neck). The abbreviations for the **cervical vertebrae** range from C1 to C7. These abbreviations are used to pinpoint the exact area of involvement with the **cervical vertebrae**.
(2) thoracic vertebrae thorac/o = chest -ic = pertaining to	The **thoracic vertebrae**, consisting of the next 12 segments (or vertebrae of the spinal column) make up the vertebral bones of the chest (thorac/o = chest or thorax). The abbreviations for the thoracic vertebrae range from T1 to T12. These abbreviations are also used to pinpoint the exact area of or involvement with the thoracic vertebrae.
(3) lumbar vertebrae lumb/o = loins, lower back -ar = pertaining to	The **lumbar vertebrae** consist of five large segments of the movable part of the spinal column. Identified as L1 through L5, the lumbar vertebrae are the largest and strongest of the vertebrae of the spinal column.
(4) sacrum sacr/o = sacrum -um = noun ending	The **sacrum**, located below the **lumbar vertebrae**, is the fourth segment of the spinal column. This single, triangular-shaped bone is a result of the fusion of the five individual sacral bones in the child.
(5) coccyx (COCK-siks)	The fifth segment of the **vertebral column** is the **coccyx**. It is located at the very end of the **vertebral column** and is also called the tailbone. The adult **coccyx** is a single bone that is the result of the fusion of the four individual **coccygeal** bones in the child.

Direction

Directional terms are used by health professionals to define the specific location of a structure, to increase understanding when stating the relationship between body areas, and to indicate the position of the body for particular procedures. The standard reference position for the body as a whole, which gives meaning to these directional terms, is known as **anatomical position**. Anatomical position means that the person is standing with the arms at the sides and the palms turned forward. The individual's head and feet are also pointing forward. Directional terms often use the anatomical position and the **midline** of the body as reference points. *Figure 4-9* is a visual reference for the anatomical position and the directional terms.

The following is a list of the most commonly used directional terms (and definitions) that use the anatomical position and/or the **midline** of the body as reference points.

Word	Meaning
superficial*	Pertaining to the surface of the body or near the surface.
deep	Away from the surface and toward the inside of the body.

*The terms marked with an asterisk (*) are immediately followed by a term with the opposite meaning.

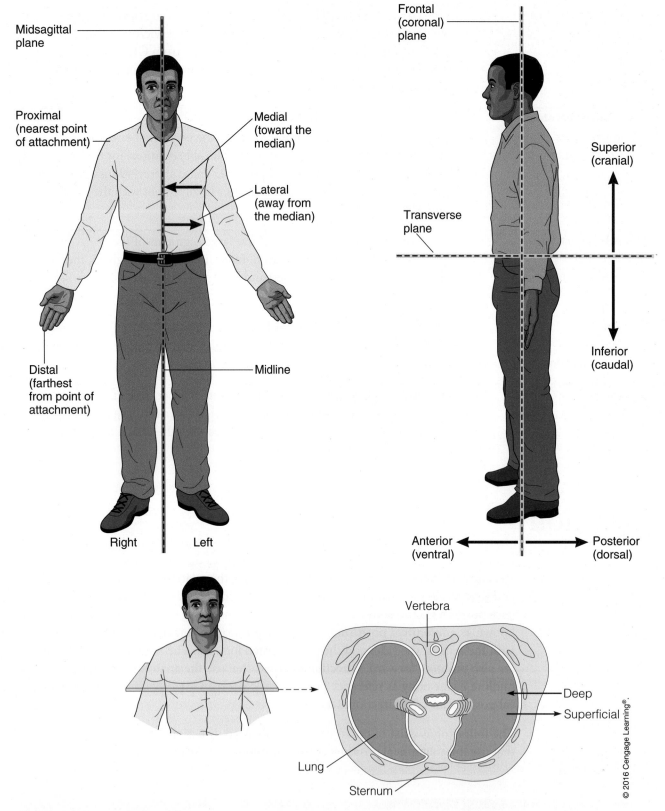

Figure 4-9 Anatomical position

Word	Meaning
anterior* (an-**TEE**-ree-or)	Pertaining to the front of the body or toward the belly of the body.
posterior (poss-**TEE**-ree-or)	Pertaining to the back of the body.
ventral* (**VEN**-tral) ventr/o = belly, front side -al = pertaining to	Of or pertaining to a position toward the belly of the body; frontward; **anterior**.
dorsal (**DOR**-sal) dors/o = back -al = pertaining to	Pertaining to the back or **posterior**.
medial* (**MEE**-dee-al) medi/o = middle -al = pertaining to	Toward the **midline** of the body.
lateral (**LAT**-er-al) later/o = side -al = pertaining to	Toward the side of the body, away from the **midline** of the body.
superior* (soo-**PEE**-ree-or)	Above or upward toward the head.
inferior (in-**FEE**-ree-or)	Below or downward toward the tail or feet.
cranial* (**KRAY**-nee-al) crani/o = skull -al = pertaining to	Pertaining to the head.
caudal (**KAWD**-al)	Pertaining to the tail.
distal* (**DISS**-tal)	Away from or farthest from the trunk of the body or farthest from the point of attachment of a body part.
proximal (**PROCK**- sih-mal) proxim/o = near -al = pertaining to	Toward or nearest to the trunk of the body or nearest to the point of attachment of a body part.

*The terms marked with an asterisk (*) are immediately followed by a term with the opposite meaning.

Word	Meaning
supine* (soo-**PINE**) © 2016 Cengage Learning®. **Figure 4-10A** Supine position	The following terms do not use the **midline** of the body as a reference point. Lying horizontally on the back, face up. (see *Figure 4-10A*).
prone (**PROHN**) © 2016 Cengage Learning®. **Figure 4-10B** Prone position	Lying facedown on the abdomen (see *Figure 4-10B*).
supination* (**soo**-pin-**AY**-shun)	A movement that allows the palms of the hands to turn upward or forward.
pronation (proh-**NAY**-shun)	A movement that allows the palms of the hands to turn downward and backward.
plantar* (**PLANT**-ar)	Pertaining to the sole or bottom of the foot.
dorsum (**DOR**-sum)	The back or posterior surface of a part; in the foot, the top of the foot.

*The terms marked with an asterisk (*) are immediately followed by a term with the opposite meaning.

Feature Walk-Through

The **Vocabulary** section presents terms from the chapter that are frequently used when discussing the human body. Study this section to learn what each term means, including the word parts that form each term. Word parts are shown in blue and are followed by their definition.

VOCABULARY

Word	Definition

abdominal cavity
    abdomin/o = abdomen
    -al = pertaining to
	The cavity beneath the **thoracic cavity** that is separated from the **thoracic cavity** by the diaphragm; contains the liver, gallbladder, spleen, stomach, pancreas, intestines, and kidneys.

abdominopelvic cavity
    abdomin/o = abdomen
    pelv/i = pelvis
    -ic = pertaining to
	A term that describes the abdominal and **pelvic cavity** collectively; refers to the space between the diaphragm and the groin.

Word	Definition
anaplasia (**an**-ah-**PLAY**-zee-ah) ana- = not, without -plasia = formation, growth	A change in the structure and orientation of cells, characterized by a loss of differentiation and reversion to a more primitive form.
anatomical position	The standard reference position for the body as a whole: the person is standing with arms at the sides and palms turned forward; the individual's head and feet are also pointing forward.
anterior (an-**TEE**-ree-or)	Pertaining to the front of the body or toward the belly of the body.
aplasia (ah-**PLAY**-zee-ah) a- = without, not -plasia = formation, growth	A developmental failure resulting in the absence of any **organ** or **tissue**.
cardiac muscle cardi/o = heart -ac = pertaining to	The muscle that makes up the muscular wall of the heart.
caudal (**KAWD**-al)	Pertaining to the tail.
cell	The smallest and most numerous structural unit of living matter.
cell membrane	The semipermeable barrier that is the outer covering of a cell.
cervical vertebrae (**SER**-vic-al **VER**-teh-bray) cervic/o = neck -al = pertaining to	The first seven segments of the spinal column; identified as C1 through C7.
chromosomes (**KROH**-moh- sohmz)	The threadlike structures within the **nucleus** that control the functions of growth, repair, and reproduction for the body.
coccyx (**COCK**-siks)	The tailbone. Located at the end of the **vertebral column**, the **coccyx** results from the fusion of four individual **coccygeal** bones in the child.
connective tissue	**Tissue** that supports and binds other body **tissue** and parts.
cranial (**KRAY**-nee-al) crani/o = skull -al = pertaining to	Pertaining to the skull or cranium.
cranial cavity crani/o = skull -al = pertaining to	The cavity that contains the brain.

Word	Definition
cytology (sigh-**TOL**-oh-jee) cyt/o = cell -logy = the study of	The study of cells.
cytoplasm (**SIGH**-toh-plazm) cyt/o = cell -plasm = living substance	A gel-like substance that surrounds the **nucleus** of a cell. The **cytoplasm** contains cell organs, called organelles, which carry out the essential functions of the cell.
deep	Away from the surface and toward the inside of the body.
distal (**DISS**-tal)	Away from or farthest from the trunk of the body or farthest from the point of attachment of a body part.
dorsal dors/o = back -al = pertaining to	Pertaining to the back.
dorsum dors/o = back -um = noun ending	The back or **posterior** surface of a part; in the foot, the top of the foot.
dysplasia (dis-**PLAY**-zee-ah) dys- = bad, difficult, painful, disordered -plasia = formation, growth	Any abnormal development of tissues or organs.
epigastric region (ep-ih-**GAS**-trik **REE**-jun) epi- = upon, over gastr/o = stomach -ic = pertaining to	The region of the abdomen located between the right and left hypochondriac regions in the upper section of the abdomen, beneath the cartilage of the ribs.
epithelial tissue (**ep**-ih-**THEE**-lee-al **TISH**-yoo)	The **tissue** that covers the internal and external organs of the body; it also lines the vessels, body cavities, glands, and body organs.
frontal plane	Any of the vertical planes passing through the body from the head to the feet, perpendicular to the sagittal planes and dividing the body into front and back portions.
genes	Segments of **chromosomes** that transmit hereditary characteristics.
histologist (hiss-**TOL**-oh-jist) hist/o = tissue -logist = one who specializes	A medical scientist who specializes in the study of tissues.

Word	Definition

hyperplasia (**high**-per-**PLAY**-zee-ah)
  hyper- = excessive
  -plasia = formation, growth
	An increase in the number of cells of a body part.

hypochondriac region (**high**-poh-**KON**-dree-ak **REE**-jun)
  hypo- = under, below, beneath,
          less than normal
  chondr/i = cartilage
  -ac = pertaining to
	The right and left regions of the upper abdomen, beneath the cartilage of the lower ribs; located on either side of the **epigastric region**.

hypogastric region (**high**-poh-**GAS**-trik **REE**-jun)
  hypo- = under, below, beneath,
          less than normal
  gastr/o = stomach
  -ic = pertaining to
	The middle section of the lower abdomen, beneath the **umbilical region**.

hypoplasia (**high**-poh-**PLAY**-zee-ah)
  hypo- = under, below, beneath,
          less than normal
  -plasia = formation, growth
	Incomplete or underdeveloped **organ** or **tissue**, usually the result of a decrease in the number of cells.

inferior	Below or downward toward the tail or feet.

inguinal region (**ING**-gwih-nal)
  inguin/o = groin
  -al = pertaining to
	The right and left regions of the lower section of the abdomen; also called the iliac region.

intervertebral disc (in-ter-**VER**-teh-bral disk)
  inter- = between
  vertebr/o = vertebra
  -al = pertaining to
	A flat, circular, plate-like structure of cartilage that serves as a cushion (or shock absorber) between the vertebrae.

lateral
  later/o = side
  -al = pertaining to
	Toward the side of the body, away from the **midline** of the body.

long axis	The long axis of the body; the imaginary line created by directing a vertical line through the middle of the body from the top of the head to a space equidistant between the feet; essentially the midline of the body.

lumbar region
  lumb/o = loins
  -ar = pertaining to
	The right and left regions of the middle section of the abdomen.

Word	Definition
lumbar vertebrae 　lumb/o = loins, lower back 　-ar = pertaining to	The largest and strongest of the vertebrae of the spinal column, located in the lower back. The **lumbar vertebrae** consist of five large segments of the movable part of the spinal column; identified as L1 through L5.
lysosomes (**LIGH**-soh-sohmz)	Cell organs (or organelles) that contain various types of enzymes that function in intracellular digestion. **Lysosomes** destroy bacteria by digesting them.
McBurney's point	A point on the right side of the abdomen, about two-thirds of the distance between the **umbilicus** and the **anterior** bony prominence of the hip.
medial (**MEE**-dee-al) 　medi/o = middle 　-al = pertaining to	Toward the **midline** of the body.
mediolateral (**MEE**-dee-oh-**LAT**-er-al) 　medi/o = middle 　later/o = side 　-al = pertaining to	Pertaining to the middle and side of a structure.
membrane	A thin layer of **tissue** that covers a surface, lines a cavity, or divides a space, such as the periotneum that lines the abdominal wall.
midline of the body	The imaginary "line" created when the body is divided into equal right and left halves.
midsagittal plane (mid-**SADJ**-ih-tal)	The **plane** that divides the body (or a structure) into right and left equal portions.
mitochondria (my-toh-**KON**-dree-ah)	Cell organs (or organelles), which provide the energy needed by the cell to carry on its essential functions.
muscle tissue	The **tissue** capable of producing movement of the parts and organs of the body by contracting and relaxing its fibers.
navel (**NAY**-vel)	The **umbilicus**; the belly button.
neoplasia (nee-oh-**PLAY**-zee-ah) 　neo- = new 　-plasia = formation, growth	The new and abnormal development of cells that may be benign or malignant.
nervous tissue	Tissue that transmits impulses throughout the body, thereby activating, coordinating, and controlling the many functions of the body.
nucleus (**NOO**-klee-us) 　nucle/o = nucleus 　-us = noun ending	The central controlling body within a living cell that is enclosed within the **cell membrane**.

Word	Definition
organ	Tissues arranged together to perform a special function.
pelvic cavity pelv/i = pelvis -ic = pertaining to	The lower front cavity of the body, located beneath the **abdominal at cavity**; contains the urinary bladder and reproductive organs.
peritoneum (**pair**-ih-toh-**NEE**-um) peritone/o = peritoneum -um = noun ending	A specific serous **membrane** that covers the entire abdominal wall of the body and is reflected over the contained viscera.
plane	Imaginary slices (or cuts) made through the body as if a dividing sheet were passed through the body at a particular angle and in a particular direction, permitting a view from a different angle.
plantar (**PLANT**-ar)	Pertaining to the sole or bottom of the foot.
posterior (poss-**TEE**-ree-or)	Pertaining to the back of the body.
pronation (proh-**NAY**-shun)	A movement that allows the palms of the hands to turn downward and backward.
prone (**PROHN**)	Lying facedown on the abdomen.
proximal (**PROCK** sih-mal) proxim/o = near -al = pertaining to	Toward or nearest to the trunk of the body or nearest to the point of attachment of a body part.
ribosomes (**RYE**-boh-sohmz)	Cell organs (or organelles) that synthesize proteins; often called the cell's "protein factories."
sacrum (**SAY**-krum) sacr/o = sacrum -um = noun ending	The singular triangular-shaped bone that results from the fusion of the five individual sacral bones of the child.
skeletal muscle (**SKELL**-eh-tal) skelet/o = skeleton -al = pertaining to	Muscle that is attached to bone and is responsible for the movement of the skeleton.
smooth muscle	Muscle found in the walls of the hollow internal organs of the body such as the stomach and intestines.
spinal cavity spin/o = spine -al = pertaining to	The cavity that contains the nerves of the spinal cord; also known as the spinal canal.

Word	Definition
superficial	Pertaining to the surface of the body or near the surface.
superior (soo-**PEE**-ree-or)	Above or upward toward the head.
supination (soo-pin-**AY**-shun)	A movement that allows the palms of the hands to turn upward or forward.
supine (soo-**PINE**)	Lying horizontally on the back, face up.
system	Organs that work together to perform the many functions of the body as a whole.
thoracic cavity (**thoh-RASS**-ik) thorac/o = chest -ic = pertaining to	The chest cavity, which contains the lungs, heart, aorta, esophagus, and trachea.
thoracic vertebrae (**thoh-RASS**-ik) thorac/o = chest -ic = pertaining to	The second segment of 12 vertebrae that make up the vertebral bones of the chest; identified as T1 through T12.
tissue	A group of cells that performs specialized functions.
transverse plane (trans-**VERS**)	Any of the planes cutting across the body perpendicular to the sagittal and the frontal planes, dividing the body into **superior** (upper) and **inferior** (lower) portions.
umbilical region umbilic/o = navel -al = pertaining to	The region of the abdomen located in the middle section of the abdomen, between the right and left lumbar regions and directly beneath the **epigastric region**.
umbilicus umbilic/o = navel -us = noun ending	The **navel**; also called the belly button.
ventral ventr/o = belly, front side -al = pertaining to	Pertaining to the front; belly side.
visceral viscer/o = internal organs -al = pertaining to	Pertaining to the internal organs.
visceral muscle viscer/o = internal organs -al = pertaining to	See *smooth muscle*.

Feature Walk-Through

Study and work through the **Word Elements** to learn more about prefixes, combining forms, and suffixes. It is important to notice how pronunciations differ when the same word part is used in a complete term.

The following word elements pertain to the body as a whole. As you review the list, pronounce each word element aloud twice and then check the "Say It" box. Pronouncing the word elements aloud will help you remember how they sound, which can also help you spell terms correctly when you hear them pronounced by your instructor, by a health care professional, or on a transcription tape. An example term is listed below each word element. Pronounce the example term and then write the definition. You may use your medical dictionary. Some of the example terms you will find in the chapter and some you will find only in your medical dictionary. This is intentional to make you aware of and allow you practice using this valuable resource, which will help you find the meaning of terms you do not already know.

WORD ELEMENTS

Word Element	Pronunciation	"Say It"	Meaning
abdomin/o **abdomin**al	ab-**DOM**-ih-no ab-**DOM**-ih-nal	☐	abdomen
ana- **ana**plasia	**AN**-ah an-ah-**PLAY**-zee-ah	☐	not, without
anter/o **anter**ior	an-**TEE**-roh an-**TEE**-ree-or	☐	front
cervic/o **cervic**al	**SER**-vih-ko **SER**-vih-kal	☐	neck; cervix
coccyg/o **coccyg**eal vertebrae	**COCK**-sih-goh cock-**SIJ**-ee-al **VER**-teh-bray	☐	**coccyx**
crani/o **crani**al	**KRAY**-nee-oh **KRAY**-nee-al	☐	skull, cranium
cyt/o **cyt**ology	**SIGH**-toh sigh-**TOL**-oh-jee	☐	cell
dors/o **dors**um	**DOR**-so **DOR**-sum	☐	back
dys- **dys**plasia	**DISS** dis-**PLAY**-zee-ah	☐	bad, difficult, painful, disordered
epi- **epi**gastric	**EP**-ih ep-ih-**GAS**-trick	☐	upon, over
hist/o **hist**ologist	**HISS**-toh his-**TOL**-oh-jist	☐	**tissue**
hypo- **hypo**chondriac region	**HIGH**-poh high-poh-**KON**-dree-ak	☐	under, below, beneath, less than normal
-iac card**iac** muscle	**EE**-ak **CAR**-dee-ak	☐	pertaining to

Word Element	Pronunciation	"Say It"	Meaning
ili/o **ili**ac	**ILL**-ee-oh **ILL**-ee-ak	☐	ilium
inguin/o **inguin**al region	**ING**-gwih-no **ING**-gwih-nal	☐	groin
inter- **inter**vertebral	**IN**-ter **in**-ter-**VER**-teh-bral	☐	between
-ion supina**tion**	**SHUN** soo-pin-**AY**-shun	☐	action, process
later/o **later**al	**LAT**-er-oh **LAT**-er-al	☐	side
lumb/o **lumb**ar	**LUM**-boh **LUM**-bar	☐	loins, lower back
medi/o **medi**olateral	**MEE**-dee-oh **MEE**-dee-oh-**LAT**-er-al	☐	middle
nucle/o **nucle**ic acid	**NOO**-klee-oh noo-**KLEE**-ic	☐	**nucleus**
pelv/i **pelv**ic cavity	**PELL**-vih **PELL**-vik	☐	pelvis
-plasm neo**plasm**	**PLAZM** **NEE**-oh-plazm	☐	living substance
poster/o **poster**ior	**POSS**-tee-roh poss-**TEE**-ree-or	☐	back
proxim/o **proxim**al	**PROK**-sim-oh **PROCK**-sih-mal	☐	near
sacr/o **sacr**um	**SAY**-kroh **SAY**-krum	☐	**sacrum**
-some chromo**some**	**SOHM** **KROH**-moh-sohm	☐	"a body" of a specified type
spin/o **spin**al canal	**SPY**-noh **SPY**-nal	☐	spine
thorac/o **thorac**ic vertebrae	**THOH**-rah-koh **thoh**-**RASS**-ik **VER**-teh-bray	☐	chest
umbilic/o **umbilic**al region	um-**BILL**-ih-koh um-**BILL**-ih-kal	☐	**navel**
ventr/o **ventr**al	**VEN**-troh **VEN**-tral	☐	belly, front side

Word Element	Pronunciation	"Say It"	Meaning
vertebr/o **vertebr**al column	**VER**-teh-broh **VER**-teh-bral	☐	vertebra
viscer/o **viscer**al cavity	**VISS**-er-oh **VISS**-er-al	☐	internal organs

COMMON ABBREVIATIONS

Abbreviation	Meaning	Abbreviation	Meaning
RUQ	right upper quadrant	**RLQ**	right lower quadrant
LUQ	left upper quadrant	**LLQ**	left lower quadrant

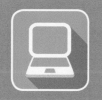

Online Resources

For comprehensive Quick Access Abbreviation Tables, go to the Student Companion Website. These tables are a valuable study tool and quick reference for learning abbreviations. Search by abbreviation or by the definition of the abbreviation.

WRITTEN AND AUDIO TERMINOLOGY REVIEW

Review each of the following terms from the chapter. Study the spelling of each term, and write the definition in the space provided. Check definitions by looking the term up in the glossary.

Term	Pronunciation	Definition
abdominal	☐ ab-**DOM**-ih-nal	_____
abdominal cavity	☐ ab-**DOM**-ih-nal **CAV**-ih-tee	_____
abdominopelvic cavity	☐ ab-**dom**-ih-noh-**PEL**-vik **CAV**-ih-tee	_____
anaplasia	☐ **an**-ah-**PLAY**-zee-ah	_____
anterior	☐ an-**TEE**-ree-or	_____
aplasia	☐ ah-**PLAY**-zee-ah	_____
cardiac muscle	☐ **CAR**-dee-ak **MUS**-sul	_____
caudal	☐ **KAWD**-al	_____

Term	Pronunciation	Definition
cell membrane	☐ SELL MEM-brayn	_____
cervical vertebrae	☐ SER-vih-kal VER-teh-bray	_____
chromosomes	☐ KROH-moh-sohmz	_____
coccygeal	☐ cock-SIJ-ee-al	_____
coccyx	☐ COCK-siks	_____
connective tissue	☐ kon-NEK-tiv TISH-yoo	_____
cranial	☐ KRAY-nee-al	_____
cranial cavity	☐ KRAY-nee-al CAV-ih-tee	_____
cytology	☐ sigh-TOL-oh-jee	_____
cytoplasm	☐ SIGH-toh-plazm	_____
distal	☐ DISS-tal	_____
dorsal	☐ DOR-sal	_____
dorsum	☐ DOR-sum	_____
dysplasia	☐ dis-PLAY-zee-ah	_____
epigastric region	☐ ep-ih-GAS-trik REE-jun	_____
epithelial tissue	☐ ep-ih-THEE-lee-al TISH-yoo	_____
frontal plane	☐ FRONT-al plane	_____
genes	☐ JEENS	_____
histologist	☐ hiss-TOL-oh-jist	_____
hyperplasia	☐ high-per-PLAY-zee-ah	_____
hypoplasia	☐ high-poh-PLAY-zee-ah	_____
inferior	☐ in-FEE-ree-or	_____
inguinal region	☐ ING-gwih-nal REE-jun	_____
intervertebral disc	☐ in-ter-VER-teh-bral DISK	_____
lateral	☐ LAT-er-al	_____
lumbar vertebrae	☐ LUM-bar VER-teh-bray	_____
lysosomes	☐ LIGH-soh-sohmz	_____
McBurney's point	☐ Mc-BURN-eez POINT	_____
medial	☐ MEE-dee-al	_____
mediolateral	☐ mee-dee-oh-LAT-er-al	_____
membrane	☐ MEM-brayn	_____
midline	☐ MID-line	_____
midsagittal plane	☐ mid-SADJ-ih-tal plane	_____

Term	Pronunciation	Definition
mitochondria	☐ **my**-toh-**KON**-dree-ah	_____
navel	☐ **NAY**-vel	_____
neoplasia	☐ **nee**-oh-**PLAY**-zee-ah	_____
nucleus	☐ **NOO**-klee-us	_____
organ	☐ **OR**-gan	_____
pelvic cavity	☐ **PELL**-vik **CAV**-ih-tee	_____
peritoneum	☐ **pair**-ih-toh-**NEE**-um	_____
plane	☐ **PLANE**	_____
plantar	☐ **PLANT**-ar	_____
posterior	☐ poss-**TEE**-ree-or	_____
pronation	☐ proh-**NAY**-shun	_____
prone	☐ **PROHN**	_____
proximal	☐ **PROCK**-sih-mal	_____
ribosomes	☐ **RYE**-boh-sohmz	_____
sacrum	☐ **SAY**-krum	_____
skeletal muscle	☐ **SKELL**-eh-tal **MUS**-sul	_____
smooth muscle	☐ **SMOOTH MUS**-sul	_____
spinal cavity	☐ **SPY**-nal **CAV**-ih-tee	_____
superficial	☐ **soo**-per-**FISH**-al	_____
superior	☐ soo-**PEE**-ree-or	_____
supination	☐ **soo**-pin-**AY**-shun	_____
supine	☐ soo-**PINE**	_____
system	☐ **SIS**-tem	_____
thoracic cavity	☐ **thoh**-**RASS**-ik **CAV**-ih-tee	_____
tissue	☐ **TISH**-yoo	_____
transverse plane	☐ trans-**VERS** plane	_____
umbilical region	☐ um-**BILL**-ih-kal **REE**-jun	_____
umbilicus	☐ um-**BILL**-ih-kus	_____
ventral	☐ **VEN**-tral	_____
vertebral column	☐ **VER**-teh-bral **KOL**-um	_____
visceral	☐ **VISS**-er-al	_____
visceral muscle	☐ **VISS**-er-al **MUS**-sul	_____

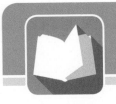

Review Checkpoint

Apply what you have learned in this chapter by completing the exercises in your workbook.

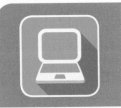

Online Resources

For additional study tools, including comprehensive Quick Access Abbreviation Tables, PowerPoint® slides, and animations, go to the Student Companion Website.

Chapter Review Exercises

The following exercises provide a more in-depth review of the chapter material. Your goal in these exercises is to complete each section at a minimum 80% level of accuracy. A space has been provided for your score at the end of each section.

A. Term to Definition

Define each term by writing the definition in the space provided. Check the box if you are able to complete this exercise correctly the first time (without referring to the answers). Each correct answer is worth 10 points. Record your score in the space provided at the end of the exercise.

☐ 1. prone_____

☐ 2. cervical vertebrae _____

☐ 3. cytology_____

☐ 4. dorsum _____

☐ 5. epigastric _____

☐ 6. supination _____

☐ 7. pronation _____

☐ 8. lateral _____

☐ 9. mediolateral _____

☐ 10. supine _____

Number correct _____ **× 10 points/correct answer: Your score** _____ **%**

B. Labeling

Label the nine regions of the body. Each correct response is worth 10 points. If you get all nine regions correct without referring to your textbook, give yourself a bonus of 10 points for a total of 100 points. Record your score in the space provided at the end of the exercise.

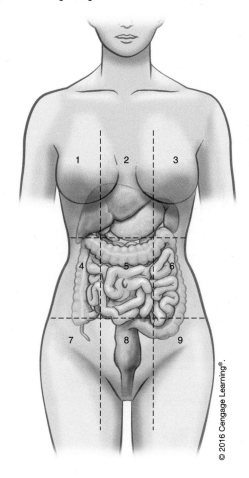

© 2016 Cengage Learning®.

1. _____

2. _____

3. _____

4. _____

5. _____

6. _____

7. _____

8. _____

9. _____

Number correct _____ × 10 points/correct answer: subtotal _____

10-point bonus for getting all answers correct + _____

Total number of points earned _____

C. Crossword Puzzle

Each crossword answer is worth 10 points. When you have completed the crossword puzzle, total your points and enter your score in the space provided.

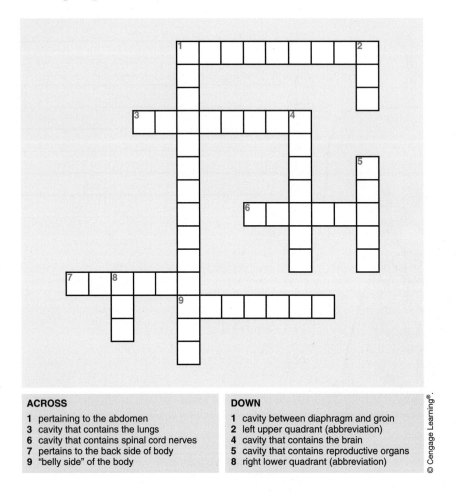

ACROSS

1 pertaining to the abdomen
3 cavity that contains the lungs
6 cavity that contains spinal cord nerves
7 pertains to the back side of body
9 "belly side" of the body

DOWN

1 cavity between diaphragm and groin
2 left upper quadrant (abbreviation)
4 cavity that contains the brain
5 cavity that contains reproductive organs
8 right lower quadrant (abbreviation)

© Cengage Learning®.

Number correct _____ × 10 points/correct answer: Your score _____%

D. Completion

Complete each sentence with the most appropriate answer. Each correct answer is worth 10 points. Record your score in the space provided at the end of the exercise.

1. The fourth segment of the spinal column is a fused, triangular-shaped bone that in the child consisted of five individual bones; it is called the _____.

2. The tailbone is known as the _____.

3. The smallest and most numerous unit of living matter is the _____.

4. The semipermeable barrier that surrounds the cell is known as the _____.

5. The central controlling body within a living cell is known as the _____.

6. The gel-like substance that surrounds the nucleus of the cell is the _____.

7. The term that describes any abnormal development of tissues or organs is _____.

8. The term that describes new and abnormal development of cells that may be benign or malignant is _____.

9. The term that refers to a developmental failure resulting in the absence of any organ or tissue is

_____

10. The term that refers to an increase in the number of cells of a body part is _____.

Number correct _____ **× 10 points/correct answer: Your score** _____**%**

E. Matching the Directional Terms

Match the descriptions on the right with the applicable directional term on the left. Each correct answer is worth 10 points. Record your answers in the space provided at the end of the exercise.

_____ 1. superficial   a. pertaining to the head

_____ 2. anterior   b. toward the side of the body, away from the midline of the body

_____ 3. dorsal   c. pertaining to the surface of the body or near the surface

_____ 4. medial   d. below or downward toward the tail or feet

_____ 5. lateral   e. pertaining to the back or posterior

_____ 6. superior   f. pertaining to the tail

_____ 7. inferior   g. above or upward toward the head

_____ 8. cranial   h. away from or farthest from the trunk of the body

_____ 9. caudal   i. pertaining to the front of the body or toward the belly of the body

_____ 10. distal   j. toward the midline of the body

Number correct _____ **× 10 points/correct answer: Your score** _____**%**

F. Spelling

Circle the correctly spelled term in each pairing of words. Each correct answer is worth 10 points. Record your score in the space provided at the end of the exercise.

1. coccyx   coccyxx
2. midsaggital   midsagittal
3. MacBurney's   McBurney's
4. mediolateral   medialateral
5. peritoneum   peritoneim
6. ribosomes   ribysomes
7. viseral   visceral
8. umbilicus   umbillicus
9. navul   navel
10. dysplasia   dysplacia

Number correct _____ **× 10 points/correct answer: Your score** _____**%**

G. Definition of Term

Identify and provide the medical term to match the definition provided. Each correct answer is worth 10 points. Record your score in the space provided at the end of the exercise.

1. Pertaining to the abdomen.

   _____

2. The study of cells.

   _____

3. Without development.

   _____

4. One who specializes in the study of tissues.

   _____

5. New and abnormal development of cells that may be benign or malignant.

   _____

6. Pertaining to the sole or bottom of the foot.

   _____

7. The threadlike structures within the nucleus of the cell that control the functions of growth, repair, and reproduction for the body.

   _____

8. Pertaining to the skull or cranium.

   _____

9. The umbilicus; the belly button.

   _____

10. Tissues arranged together to perform a special function.

   _____

Number correct _____ × *10 points/correct answer: Your score* _____%

H. Multiple Choice

Read each statement carefully and select the correct answer from the options listed. Each correct answer is worth 10 points. Record your score in the space provided at the end of the exercise.

1. A change in the structure and orientation of cells, characterized by a loss of differentiation to a more primitive form ("without formation"), is known as:
   a. neoplasia
   b. anaplasia
   c. dysplasia
   d. hypoplasia

2. The new and abnormal development of cells that may be benign or malignant ("new formation") is known as:
   a. neoplasia
   b. anaplasia
   c. dysplasia
   d. hypoplasia

3. A developmental failure resulting in the absence of any organ or tissue ("without formation") is known as:

    a. hyperplasia

    b. hypoplasia

    c. aplasia

    d. neoplasia

4. Any abnormal development of tissues ("disordered formation") is known as:

    a. neoplasia

    b. aplasia

    c. dysplasia

    d. anaplasia

5. An increase in the number of cells of a body part ("excessive formation") is known as:

    a. hyperplasia

    b. hypoplasia

    c. aplasia

    d. neoplasia

6. Incomplete or underdeveloped organ or tissue, usually the result of a decrease in the number of cells ("less than, under formation"), is known as:

    a. hyperplasia

    b. hypoplasia

    c. aplasia

    d. neoplasia

7. When a person is standing with the arms at the sides and the palms turned forward, with the head and feet pointing forward, the individual is said to be in what position?

    a. supine

    b. anatomical

    c. prone

    d. lateral

8. The medical term that means "pertaining to the tail" is:

    a. caudal

    b. cranial

    c. dorsal

    d. ventral

9. The imaginary "line" created when the body is divided into equal right and left halves is called the:

    a. transverse plane

    b. midline of the body

    c. frontal plane

    d. coronal plane

10. The navel, or belly button, is also known as the:

    a. umbilicus

    b. nucleus

    c. Munro's point

    d. McBurney's point

Number correct _____ *× 10 points/correct answer: Your score* _____%

I. Word Element Review

The following words relate to the chapter text. The prefixes, suffixes, and combining vowels have been provided. Read the definition carefully and complete the word by filling in the space, using the word elements provided in the chapter. Each correct answer is worth 10 points. Record your score in the space provided at the end of the exercise.

1. Pertaining to the abdomen

    _____/ al

2. Pertaining to the neck

    _____/ al

3. The study of cells

    _____/ o / logy

4. Pertaining to the side

    _____/ al

5. Pertaining to the belly or front side

    _____/ al

6. A new growth ("cell or tissue substance")

    neo /_____

7. Without formation or growth

    _____/ plasia

8. Pertaining to the skull

    _____/ al

9. Pertaining to between the vertebrae

    _____/ vertebral

10. Pertaining to internal organs

    _____/ al

Number correct _____ × 10 points/correct answer: Your score _____%

J. Labeling

The following figures illustrate directional terms and various planes of the body. Study the figures carefully and label the numbered items appropriately. Each correct response is worth 10 points. Record your score in the space provided at the end of the exercise.

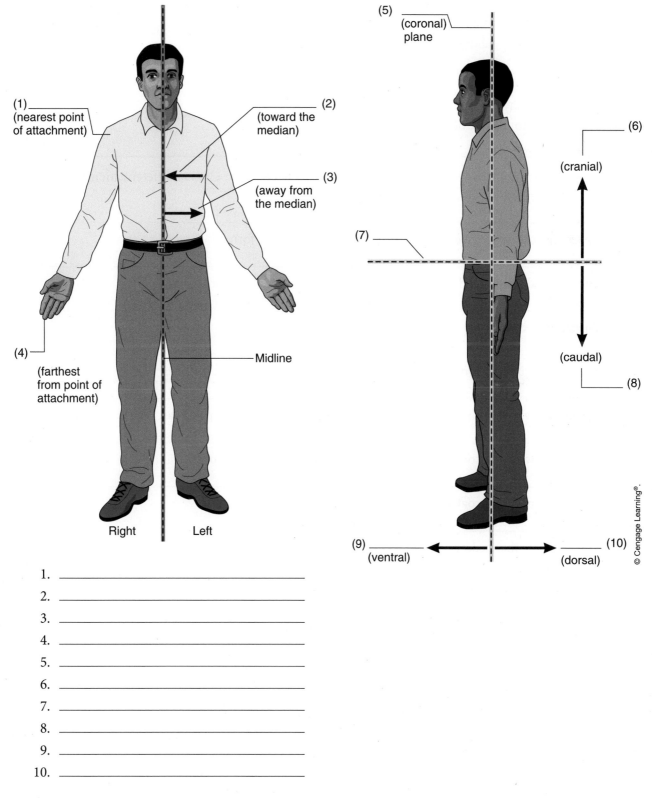

(1) (nearest point of attachment)

(2) (toward the median)

(3) (away from the median)

(4) (farthest from point of attachment)

Midline

Right   Left

(5) (coronal) plane

(6) (cranial)

(7)

(caudal)

(8)

(9) (ventral)   (10) (dorsal)

© Cengage Learning®.

1. _____
2. _____
3. _____
4. _____
5. _____
6. _____
7. _____
8. _____
9. _____
10. _____

Number correct _____ **× *10 points/correct answer: Your score*** _____%

K. Word Search

Read each definition carefully and identify the applicable word from the list that follows. Enter the word in the space provided and then find it in the puzzle and circle it. The words may be read up, down, diagonally, across, or backward. Each correct answer is worth 10 points. Record your score in the space provided at the end of the exercise.

plantar	pelvic	neoplasia
anaplasia	abdominal	histologist
cytology	cranial	dysplasia
thoracic	cervical	

Example: Pertaining to the sole or bottom of the foot.

plantar

1. A change in the structure and orientation of cells, characterized by a loss of differentiation and reversion to a more primitive form.

2. Any abnormal development of tissues or organs ("disordered formation").

3. The new and abnormal development of cells that may be benign or malignant.

4. The study of cells.

5. The body cavity that contains the lungs, heart, aorta, esophagus, and trachea.

6. The body cavity that contains the liver, gallbladder, spleen, stomach, pancreas, intestines, and kidneys.

7. The body cavity that contains the urinary bladder and reproductive organs.

8. The body cavity that contains the brain.

9. The vertebrae that make up the bones of the neck.

10. A medical scientist who specializes in the study of tissues.

E	P	E	L	V	I	C	I	S	L	S	L	I	M	L
A	L	A	G	A	O	I	L	D	U	S	I	U	S	T
M	A	N	A	P	L	A	S	I	A	L	P	V	L	V
C	N	F	Y	S	E	R	O	L	A	I	N	A	R	C
I	T	S	S	C	L	D	L	I	E	O	C	I	G	I
R	A	H	E	E	Y	T	Y	G	O	L	O	T	Y	C
C	R	O	A	S	N	E	E	S	M	A	T	C	L	L
U	R	R	T	S	L	N	E	I	P	R	E	A	O	E
M	A	R	R	A	T	I	G	I	R	L	P	L	T	S
C	E	R	V	I	C	A	L	N	S	E	A	U	A	C
E	N	T	C	S	A	S	C	I	N	E	D	S	M	L
N	U	E	H	A	R	C	H	I	T	R	Y	A	I	E
C	E	R	U	L	E	N	T	A	C	D	H	L	E	A
N	L	E	N	P	P	I	L	E	A	A	Y	C	D	O
C	A	B	D	O	M	I	N	A	L	U	R	L	E	C
E	I	N	E	E	H	C	N	U	T	U	R	O	S	I
F	I	S	S	N	R	E	A	S	M	E	M	N	H	S
P	G	S	I	H	I	S	T	O	L	O	G	I	S	T

© Cengage Learning®.

Number correct _____ × *10 points/correct answer: Your score* _____%

L. Opposites

Write the opposite meaning for the directional terms that follow. Place your answer in the space provided. Each correct answer is worth 10 points. Record your score in the space provided at the end of the exercise.

1. superficial   _____
2. anterior   _____
3. ventral   _____
4. medial   _____
5. superior   _____
6. cranial   _____
7. distal   _____
8. supine   _____
9. supination   _____
10. plantar   _____

Number correct _____ × *10 points/correct answer: Your score* _____%

CHAPTER CONTENT

OBJECTIVES

Upon completing this chapter and the review exercises at the end of the chapter, the learner should be able to:

1. Identify the major structures of the skin.

2. List five functions of the skin.

3. Identify and define 20 pathological conditions of the integumentary system.

4. Identify at least 10 diagnostic techniques, treatments, or procedures used in assessing disorders of the integumentary system.

5. Correctly spell and pronounce terms listed in the Written and Audio Terminology Review, using the phonetic pronunciations provided.

6. Identify at least 10 skin lesions, based on their descriptions.

7. Create at least 10 medical terms related to the integumentary system, and identify the applicable combining form(s) for each term.

8. Identify at least 20 abbreviations common to the integumentary system.

Overview

One of the body's most important organs is the skin. This protective covering is part of the **integumentary system**, which consists of the skin, hair, nails, sweat glands, and oil glands. Also known as the **integument** or the **cutaneous membrane**, the skin has five basic functions:

1. The skin protects the body against invasion by microorganisms and protects underlying body structures and delicate tissues from injury. The pigment **melanin**, which provides color to the skin, further protects the skin from the harmful effects of the ultraviolet rays of the sun.

2. The skin regulates body temperature by protecting the body from excessive loss of heat and fluids from underlying tissues. **Sweat glands**, which are located under the skin, secrete a watery fluid that cools the body as it evaporates from the surface of the skin.

3. The skin serves as a sensory receptor for sensations such as touch, pressure, pain, and temperature. These sensations are detected by the nerve endings within the skin and relayed to the brain. The appearance of the skin, in the form of facial expressions (e.g., grimaces, shivering, frowns, or smiles), is sometimes visible evidence of the sensations felt by the skin.

4. The skin provides for elimination of body wastes in the form of perspiration. Substances such as water, salts, and some fatty substances are excreted through the **pores** (openings) of the skin.

5. The skin is responsible for the first step in the synthesis of vitamin D, which is essential for bone growth and development. When exposed to the ultraviolet rays of the sun, molecules within the skin are converted to a chemical that is transported in the blood to the liver and kidneys, where it is converted into vitamin D.

The study of the skin is known as **dermatology**. The physician who specializes in the treatment of diseases and disorders of the skin is known as a **dermatologist**.

Anatomy and Physiology

The main structures of the skin include the **epidermis**, **dermis**, and subcutaneous layers. As we discuss these structures, refer to *Figure 5-1* for a visual reference.

Epidermis

The **(1) epidermis**, the outer layer of the skin, contains no blood or nerve supply. It consists of squamous epithelial cells, which are flat, scalelike, and arranged in layers (strata). The **epidermis** actually has about five different layers of **stratified** epithelium

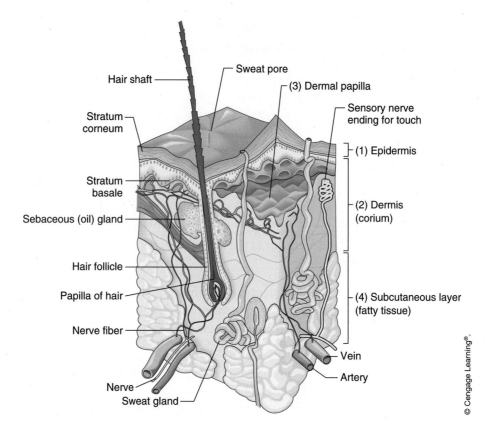

Figure 5-1 Layers and structures of the skin

cells, each carrying on specific functions. The two layers of the **epidermis** that will be mentioned here are the **stratum basale** and the **stratum corneum**. The **basal layer (stratum basale)** is where new cells are continually being reproduced, pushing older cells toward the outermost surface of the skin. It is the innermost, or deepest, layer of the **epidermis**. The **basal layer** also contains **melanocytes**, which provide color to the skin and some protection from the harmful effects of the ultraviolet rays of the sun. The outermost layer of the **epidermis** is the **stratum corneum**, where the dead skin cells are constantly being shed and replaced. When the cells reach the outermost layer of the **epidermis** and die, they become filled with a hard water-repellant protein called **keratin**. This characteristic of **keratin** (waterproofing the body) creates a barrier, or a first line of defense for the body, by not allowing water to penetrate the skin or to be lost from the body—and by not allowing microorganisms to penetrate the unbroken skin. If the skin is injured and the barrier layer is damaged, microorganisms and other contaminants can easily pass through the **epidermis** to the lower layers of the skin, and fluids can escape the body (as occurs with burns).

Dermis

The **(2) dermis** is the inner thicker layer of skin lying directly beneath the **epidermis**. It is also known as the **corium**. It protects the body against mechanical injury and compression and serves as a reservoir (storage area) for water and electrolytes. Composed of living tissue, the **dermis** contains capillaries, lymphatic channels, and nerve endings. The hair follicles, sweat glands, and **sebaceous** (oil) **glands** are also embedded in the **dermis**. The **dermis** contains both connective tissue and elastic fibers to give it strength and elasticity. If the elastic fibers of the **dermis** are overstretched as a result of rapid increase in size of the abdomen (for example, due to obesity or during pregnancy), the fibers will weaken and tear. These linear tears in the **dermis** are known as **stretch marks** or **striae**. They begin as pinkish-blue streaks with jagged edges and may be accompanied by itching. As they heal and lose their color, the striae remain as silvery-white scar lines.

The thickness of the **dermis** varies from the very thin delicate layers of the eyelids to the thicker layers of the palms of the hands and soles of the feet. Look at your hands and notice the distinct pattern of ridges on your fingertips. These ridges provide friction for grasping objects and are a result of the papillae (projections) of the superficial layer of the **dermis** that extend into the **epidermis**. The thin layer of the **epidermis** conforms to the ridges of the **(3)** dermal papillae, forming the characteristic ridges you are observing on your fingertips. In each of us, these ridges form a unique pattern that is genetically determined. These patterns are the basis of fingerprints and footprints.

Subcutaneous Layer

The **(4) subcutaneous tissue**, which lies just beneath the **dermis**, consists largely of loose connective tissue and adipose (fatty) tissue that connects the skin to the surface muscles. It is sometimes called the superficial fascia or subcutaneous fascia. The subcutaneous, or fatty, tissue serves as insulation for the body and protects the deeper tissues. It is rich in nerves and nerve endings, including those that supply the **dermis** and **epidermis**. The major blood vessels that supply the skin pass through the subcutaneous layer, and sweat glands and hair roots extend from the **dermis** down into the subcutaneous layer. The thickness of the subcutaneous layer varies, from the thinnest layer over the eyelids to the thickest layer over the abdomen.

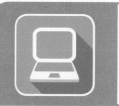

Media Link

To see the structures of the skin up close, view the **Skin** animation on the Student Companion Website.

Accessory Structures

The accessory structures of the skin consist of the hair, nails, and glands.

Hair

A strand of hair (*Figure 5-2*) is a long slender filament of **keratin** that consists of a **(1) hair root**, which is embedded in the **(2) hair follicle**, and a **(3) hair shaft** (which is the visible part of the hair). Each hair develops within the hair follicle, with any new hair forming from the **keratin** cells located at the bottom of the follicles.

Hair covers most of the human body, with the exception of the palms of the hands, the soles of the feet, the lips, the nipples, and some areas of the genitalia. Toward the end of the second trimester of pregnancy (about the fifth month), the developing fetus is almost completely covered with a soft downy (very fine) hair known as **lanugo**. This

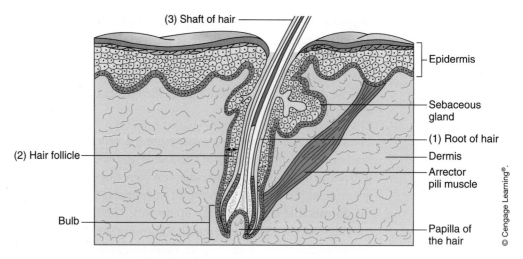

Figure 5-2 Structure of the hair

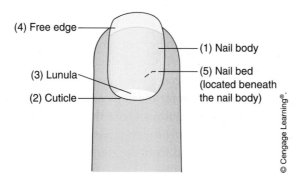

Figure 5-3 Structure of the nail

hairy coating is almost completely gone by birth, with any remaining **lanugo** disappearing shortly after birth. When present at birth, **lanugo** appears as a very fine velvety coating of hair over the baby's skin.

Hair gets its color from the **melanocytes** (darkly pigmented cells) that surround the core of the hair shaft. These cells produce **melanin**, which gives hair a black or brown color depending on the amount produced. A unique type of **melanin** containing iron is responsible for red hair. When hair turns gray or white, usually due to the aging process, the amount of **melanin** has decreased significantly in the hair.

Nails

The fingernails and toenails are protective coverings for the tips of the fingers and toes. These hard keratinized nail beds cover the dorsal surface of the last bone of each finger or toe. See *Figure 5-3*.

The visible part of the nail is called the **(1) nail body**. The fold of skin at the base of the nail body is known as the **(2) cuticle**. Beneath the cuticle is the extension of the nail body known as the root of the nail. It lies in a groove hidden by the cuticle. At the base of the nail body nearest the root is a crescent-shaped white area known as the **(3) lunula**. The **(4) free edge** of the nail extends beyond the tip of the fingertip or toe. Nails grow approximately 0.5 mm per week. The nail body is nourished by the **(5) nail bed**, which is an epithelial layer located directly beneath it. The rich supply of blood vessels contained in the nail bed generate the pink color you can see through the translucent nail bodies.

Glands

The glands of the skin complete the accessory structures of the skin. Refer to *Figure 5-4*.

The (1) **sweat**, or **sudoriferous**, **gland** is a small structure that originates deep within the **dermis** and ends at the surface of the skin with a tiny opening called a (2) **pore**. The sweat glands are found on almost all body surfaces, particularly the palms of the hands, soles of the feet, forehead, and armpits (axillae). Two main functions of the sweat glands are to cool the body by evaporation and to eliminate waste products through their pores.

The sweat glands produce a clear watery fluid known as **sweat** (or **perspiration**), which travels from the gland to the surface of the skin (where it is excreted through the pores). As the sweat evaporates from the surface of the skin into the air, it creates a cooling effect on the body.

In addition to being clear or colorless, sweat is odorless. It is made up of mostly water containing a small amount of dissolved substances such as salts, ammonia, uric acid, urea, and other waste products. These waste products are eliminated from the body through the pores of the sweat glands. As the sweat comes in contact with the bacteria present on the surface of the skin, it becomes contaminated and decomposes. This interaction of the sweat with the bacteria found on the surface of the skin creates the odor we often associate with sweating.

The (3) **sebaceous gland**, also known as the **oil gland**, secretes a substance necessary for lubricating the hair and keeping the skin soft and waterproof. This substance, known as **sebum**, is secreted along the shaft of the hair follicles and directly onto the skin through ducts that open directly onto the **epidermis**.

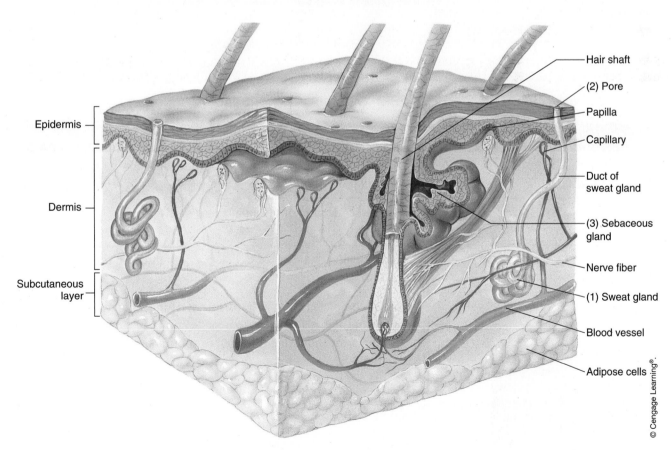

Figure 5-4 Glands of the skin

Secretion of **sebum** is influenced by the sex hormones and increases during adolescence. As a result of this increased secretion of **sebum**, the sebaceous gland ducts often become blocked and a **pimple** or **blackhead** may develop. The sebaceous glands (present throughout most of the body) are more numerous on the scalp, forehead, face, and chin. They are absent on the palms of the hands and the soles of the feet.

The **ceruminous gland** is actually classified as a modified sweat gland. Opening onto the free surface of the external ear canal, the ceruminous glands lubricate the skin of the ear canal with a yellowish-brown waxy substance called **cerumen** (also known as ear wax).

Feature Walk-Through

The **Review Checkpoint** system focuses on learning smaller amounts of material rather than waiting until the end of the chapter to review *all* of the content in the chapter. Here's how it works. Read and study the section content and when prompted by the Review Checkpoint, stop and complete the exercises for that section in the workbook. This review system allows you to feel confident about the material in each section before moving ahead and helps prepare you for the review exercises and medical scenario at the end of the chapter.

Review Checkpoint

Check your understanding of this section by completing the **Anatomy and Physiology** exercises in your workbook.

VOCABULARY

The following vocabulary terms are frequently used when discussing the integumentary system.

Word	Definition
abrasion (ah-**BRAY**-zhun)	A scraping or rubbing away of skin or mucous membrane as a result of friction to the area.
abscess (**AB**-sess)	A localized collection of pus in any part of the body.
albino (al-**BYE**-noh)	An individual with a marked deficiency of pigment in the eyes, hair, and skin.
alopecia (**al**-oh-**PEE**-she-ah) 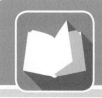	Partial or complete loss of hair; baldness. **Alopecia** may result from normal aging, a reaction to a medication such as anticancer medications, an endocrine disorder, or some skin disease. See *Figure 5-5.* **Figure 5-5** Alopecia *(Courtesy of Robert A. Silverman, M.D., Clinical Associate Professor, Department of Pediatrics, Georgetown University)*

Word	Definition
amputation (am-pew-**TAY**-shun)	The surgical removal of a part of the body or a limb or a part of a limb; performed to treat recurrent infections or **gangrene** of a limb.
basal layer (**BAY**-sal layer)	The deepest of the five layers of the **epidermis**.
blackhead	An open **comedo**, caused by accumulation of **keratin** and **sebum** within the opening of a hair follicle.
blister	A small thin-walled skin **lesion** containing clear fluid; a **vesicle**.
boil	A localized pus-producing infection originating deep in a hair follicle; a **furuncle**.
bruise	A bluish-black discoloration of an area of the skin or mucous membrane caused by an escape of blood into the tissues as a result of an injury to the area; see *ecchymosis*.
bulla (**BULL**-ah)	A large blister.
carbuncle (**CAR**-bung-kul)	A circumscribed inflammation of the skin and deeper tissues that contains pus, which eventually discharges to the skin surface.
cellulitis (sell-yoo-**LYE**-tis) 	A diffuse acute infection of the skin and **subcutaneous tissue**, characterized by localized heat, deep redness, pain, and swelling. See *Figure 5-6*. **Figure 5-6** Cellulitis (This child developed a secondary staphylococcal infection at the smallpox vaccination site. Note the signs of cellulitis, including spreading erythema that envelopes the smallpox vaccination site, swelling, and accompanying areas of cutaneous purulency.) *(Courtesy of the Centers for Disease Control and Prevention, Allen W. Mathies, MD/ California Emergency Preparedness Office (Calif/EPO), Immunization Branch)*
cerumen (seh-**ROO**-men)	Ear wax.
ceruminous gland (seh-**ROO**-mih-nus gland)	A modified sweat gland that lubricates the skin of the ear canal with a yellowish-brown waxy substance called **cerumen** (or ear wax).
cicatrix (**SIK**-ah-trix *or* sik-**AY**-trix)	A scar; the pale, firm tissue that forms in the healing of a wound.
circumscribed (**SIR**-kum-skrybd)	Confined to a limited space or well-defined area (as if a circle were drawn around it).
collagen (**KOL**-ah-jen)	The protein substance that forms the glistening inelastic fibers of connective tissue such as tendons, ligaments, and fascia.
comedo (**KOM**-ee-doh)	The typical **lesion** of **acne vulgaris**, caused by accumulation of **keratin** and **sebum** within the opening of a hair follicle (closed **comedo** = whitehead; open **comedo** = blackhead).

Word	Definition
contusion (kon-**TOO**-zhun)	An injury to a part of the body without a break in the skin.
corium (**KOH**-ree-um)	The **dermis**; the layer of the skin just under the **epidermis**.
cryosurgery (cry-oh-**SER**-jer-ee) cry/o = cold	A noninvasive treatment that uses subfreezing temperature to freeze and destroy the tissue. Coolants such as liquid nitrogen are used in the metal probe.
curettage (kyoo-reh-**TAHZH**)	The process of scraping material from the wall of a cavity or other surface for the purpose of removing abnormal tissue or unwanted material.
cutaneous membrane (kew-**TAY**-nee-us) cutane/o = skin -ous = pertaining to	The skin. See *integument*.
cuticle (**KEW**- tih-kul)	A fold of skin that covers the root of the fingernail or toenail.
cyanosis (sigh-ah-**NOH**-sis) cyan/o = blue -osis = condition	A condition of a bluish discoloration of the skin.
cyst (**SIST**)	A closed sac or pouch in or within the skin that contains fluid, semifluid, or solid material.
debridement (dah-**BREED**-ment)	Removal of debris, foreign objects, and damaged or necrotic tissue from a wound in order to prevent infection and to promote healing.
dermatitis (der-mah-**TYE**-tis) dermat/o = skin -itis = inflammation 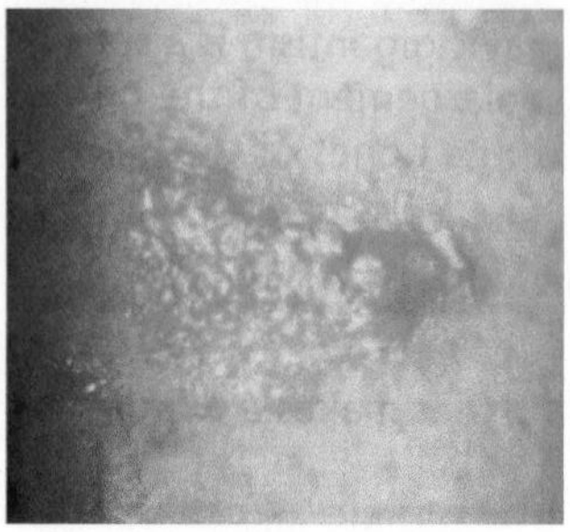 **Figure 5-7** Dermatitis *(Courtesy of Timothy G. Berger, M.D., Clinical Professor, Department of Dermatology, University of California, San Francisco)*	Inflammation of the skin. See *Figure 5-7*.
dermatologist (der-mah-**TOL**-oh-jist) dermat/o = skin -logist = specialist in the study of	A physician who specializes in the treatment of diseases and disorders of the skin.

Word	Definition
dermatology (der-mah-**TOL**-oh-jee) dermat/o = skin -logy = the study of	The study of the skin.
dermis (**DER**-mis) derm/o = skin -is = noun ending	The layer of skin immediately beneath the **epidermis**; the **corium**.
diaphoresis (**dye**-ah-foh-**REE**-sis)	The secretion of sweat.
ecchymosis (**ek**-ih-**MOH**-sis) 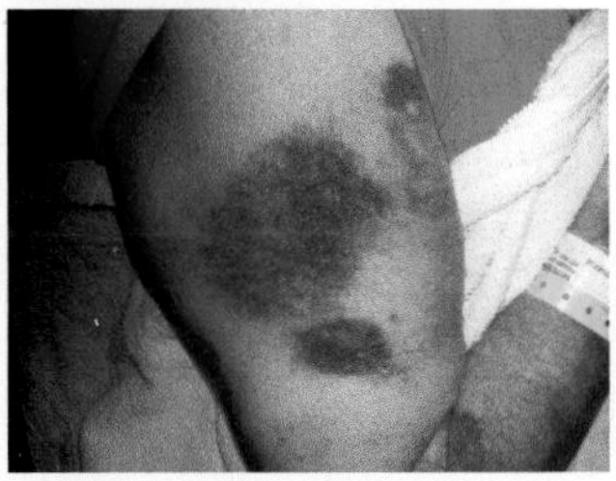 © Cengage Learning®. **Figure 5-8** Ecchymosis	A bluish-black discoloration of an area of the skin or mucous membrane caused by an escape of blood into the tissues as a result of injury to the area; also known as a bruise or a black-and-blue mark. See *Figure 5-8*.
electrodesiccation (ee-lek-troh-**des**-ih-**KAY**-shun)	A technique that uses an electrical spark to burn and destroy tissue; used primarily for the removal of surface lesions.
epidermis (ep-ih-**DER**-mis) epi- = upon, over derm/o = skin -is = noun ending	The outermost layer of the skin.
epidermoid cyst (ep-ih-**DER**-moid) epi- = upon, over derm/o = skin -oid = resembling	A **cyst** filled with a cheesy material composed of **sebum** and epithelial debris that has formed in the duct of a sebaceous gland; also known as a **sebaceous cyst**.
epithelium (ep-ih-**THEE**-lee-um)	The tissue that covers the internal and external surfaces of the body.
erythema (eh-rih-**THEE**-mah)	Redness of the skin due to capillary dilation. An example of **erythema** is nervous blushing or a mild sunburn.
erythremia (**er**-ih-**THREE**-mee-ah) erythr/o = red -emia = blood condition	An abnormal increase in the number of red blood cells; polycythemia vera.

Word	Definition
erythroderma (eh-**rith**-roh-**DER**-mah) erythr/o = red derm/o = skin -a = noun ending	See *erythema*.
excoriation (eks-koh-ree-**AY**-shun)	An injury to the surface of the skin caused by trauma, such as scratching or abrasions.
exfoliation (eks-foh-lee-**AY**-shun)	Peeling or sloughing off of tissue cells, as in peeling of the skin after a severe sunburn.
fissure (**FISH**-ur)	A cracklike sore or groove in the skin or mucous membrane.
fistula (**FISS**-tyoo-lah)	An abnormal passageway between two tubular organs (e.g., rectum and vagina) or from an organ to the body surface.
furuncle (**FYOO**-rung-kul) 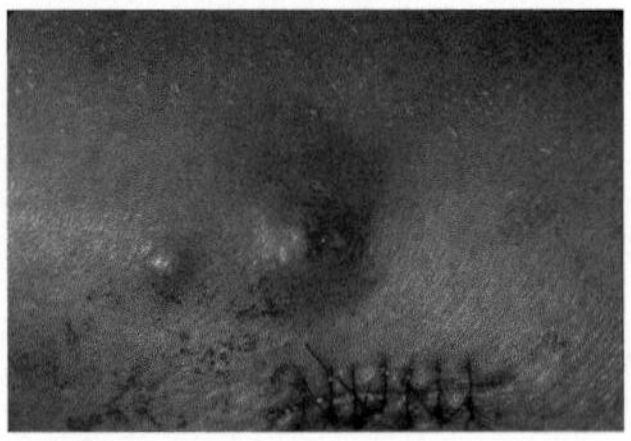 **Figure 5-9** Furuncle *(Courtesy of Robert A. Silverman, M.D., Clinical Associate Professor, Department of Pediatrics, Georgetown University)*	A localized pus-producing infection originating deep in a hair follicle; a boil. See *Figure 5-9*.
gangrene (**GANG**-green)	Death of tissue, most often involving the extremities. **Gangrene** is usually the result of ischemia (loss of blood supply to an area), bacterial invasion, and subsequent putrefaction (decaying) of the tissue.
hair follicle (**FOL**-ih-kul)	The tiny tube within the **dermis** that contains the root of a hair shaft.
hair root	The portion of a strand of hair that is embedded in the hair follicle.
hair shaft	The visible part of the hair.
hemangioma (hee-**man**-jee-**OH**-mah) hem/o = blood angi/o = vessel -oma = tumor 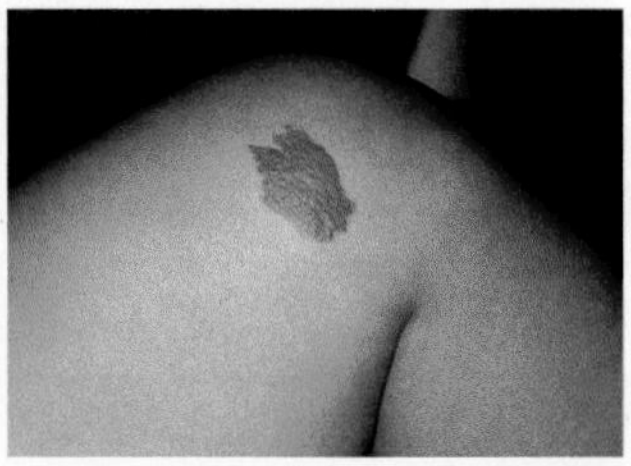 © Cengage Learning®. **Figure 5-10** Hemangioma	A benign (nonmalignant) tumor that consists of a mass of blood vessels and has a reddish-purple color. See *Figure 5-10*.

Word	Definition
heparin (**HEP**-er-in)	A natural anticoagulant substance produced by the body tissues; **heparin** is also produced in laboratories for therapeutic use as heparin sodium.
hirsutism (**HER**-soot-izm)	Excessive body hair in an adult male distribution pattern, occurring in women.
histamine (**HISS**-tah-min *or* **HISS**-tah-meen)	A substance (found in all cells) that is released in allergic inflammatory reactions.
histiocyte (**HISS**-tee-oh-sight) histi/o = tissue -cyte = cell	**Macrophage**; a large phagocytic cell (cell that ingests microorganisms, other cells, and foreign particles) occurring in the walls of blood vessels and loose connective tissue.
hives	Circumscribed, slightly elevated lesions of the skin that are paler in the center than its surrounding edges; see *wheal*.
hydrocele (**HIGH**-droh-seel) hydr/o = water -cele = swelling or herniation	A collection of fluid located in the area of the scrotal sac in the male.
ichthyosis (**ik**-thee-**OH**-sis) ichthy/o = fishlike, scaly -osis = condition	An inherited dermatological condition in which the skin is dry, hyperkeratotic (hardened), and fissured—resembling fish scales.
integument (in-**TEG**-you-ment)	The skin. See *cutaneous membrane*.
integumentary system (in-teg-you-**MEN**-tah-ree **SIS**-tem)	The body system consisting of the skin, hair, nails, sweat glands, and sebaceous glands.
keratin (**KAIR**-ah-tin)	A hard fibrous protein found in the **epidermis**, hair, nails, enamel of the teeth, and horns of animals.
keratolytic (**kair**-ah-toh-**LIT**-ic) kerat/o = hard, horny; also refers to cornea of the eye -lytic = destruction	An agent used to break down or loosen the horny (hardened) layer of the skin.
laceration (**lass**-er-**AY**-shun)	A tear in the skin.
lanugo (lan-**NOO**-go)	Soft, very fine hair that covers the body of the developing fetus; this hairy coating is almost completely gone by birth.
lesion (**LEE**-zhun)	Any visible damage to the tissues of the skin, such as a wound, sore, rash, or boil.

Word	Definition
lipedema (**lip**-eh-**DEE**-mah) lip/o = fat -edema = swelling	An abnormal condition in which there is swelling/enlargement of the lower extremities due to an irregular distribution of fat and fluid deposits in the subcutaneous tissue; accompanied by tenderness in the affected area. The lower extremities are disproportionately larger than the upper portion of the body. This condition usually affects women (up to 11%). The exact cause of this chronic condition is unknown.
lipocyte (**LIP**-oh-sight) lip/o = fat -cyte = cell	A fat cell.
lunula (**LOO**-noo-lah)	The crescent-shaped pale area at the base of the fingernail or toenail.
macrophage (**MACK**-roh-fayj) macr/o = large phag/o = to eat -e = noun ending	A large phagocytic cell (cell that ingests microorganisms, other cells, and foreign particles) occurring in the walls of blood vessels and loose connective tissue; see *histiocyte*.
macule (**MACK**-yool)	A small, flat discoloration of the skin that is neither raised nor depressed.
mast cell	A cell (found within the connective tissue) that contains **heparin** and **histamine**; these substances are released from the mast cell in response to injury and infection.
melanin (**MEL**-an-in) melan/o = black	A black or dark pigment (produced by **melanocytes** within the **epidermis**) that contributes color to the skin and helps filter ultraviolet light.
melanocytes (**MEL**-an-oh-sights *or* mel-**AN**-oh-sights) melan/o = black -cyte = cell	Cells responsible for producing **melanin**.
melanoma (**mel**-ah-**NOH**-mah) melan/o = black -oma = tumor	Darkly pigmented tumor
nail body	The visible part of the nail.
necrotizing fasciitis (**NECK**-roh-tiz-ing **fas**-ee-**EYE**-tis) necr/o = death fasci/o = band of fibrous tissue -itis = inflammation	A rare, but serious infection caused by bacteria (such as Group A streptococci) that can destroy skin, fat, and the tissue covering the muscles within a very short time. The bacteria enter the body through a skin wound. The symptoms start suddenly after an injury or wound and are more severe than they would normally be with the wound or injury. Immediate medical attention is essential as the infection can spread rapidly and can quickly become life-threatening. Necrotizing fasciitis is sometimes is called flesh-eating bacteria.

Word	Definition
nodule (**NOD**-yool)	A small, circumscribed swelling protruding above the skin.
oil gland	One of the many small glands located in the **dermis**; its secretions provide oil to the hair and surrounding skin; see *sebaceous gland*.
onycholysis (**on**-ih-**KOL**-ih-sis) onych/o = nail -lysis = destruction or detachment	Separation of a fingernail from its bed, beginning at the free margin. This condition is associated with **dermatitis** of the hand, **psoriasis**, and fungal infections.
onychomycosis (**on**-ih-koh-my-**KOH**-sis) onych/o = nail myc/o = fungus -osis = condition	Any fungal infection of the nails.
onychophagia (**on**-ih-koh-**FAY**-jee-ah) onych/o = nail -phagia = to eat	The habit of biting the nails.
pachyderma (pak-ee-**DER**-mah) pachy = thick derm/o = skin -a = noun ending	Abnormal thickening of the skin.
papule (**PAP**-yool)	A small, solid, circumscribed elevation on the skin.
paronychia (**par**-oh-**NIK**-ee-ah) par/o = beside, beyond, near onych/o = nail -ia = condition 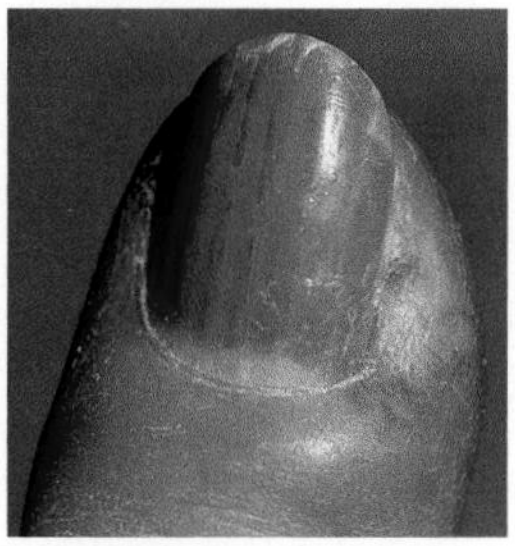 © Cengage Learning®. **Figure 5-11** Paronychia	Inflammation of the fold of skin surrounding the fingernail; also called runaround. See *Figure 5-11*.
pediculosis (pee-dik-you-**LOH**-sis)	Infestation with lice.
perspiration	The clear, watery fluid produced by the sweat glands; see *sweat*.
petechia (pee-**TEE**-kee-ah)	Small, pinpoint hemorrhages of the skin.

Word	Definition
pimple	A **papule** or **pustule** of the skin.
polyp (**POL**-ip)	A small, stalk-like growth that protrudes upward or outward from a mucous membrane surface, resembling a mushroom stalk.
pores	Openings of the skin through which substances such as water, salts, and some fatty substances are excreted.
pressure ulcer 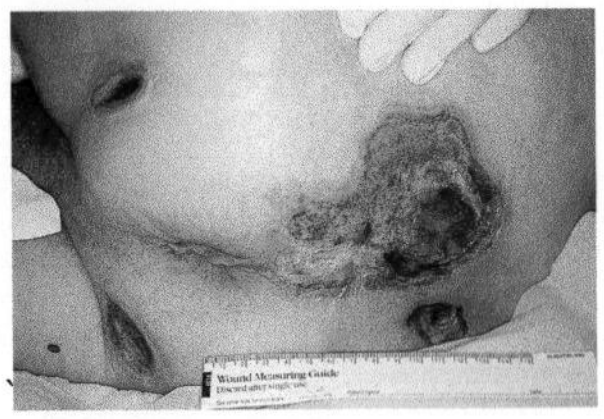 **Figure 5-12** Stage IV pressure sore *(Photo Courtesy of Hollister Wound LLC, Libertyville, Illinois)*	An inflammation, sore, or **ulcer** in the skin over a bony prominence of the body, resulting from loss of blood supply and oxygen to the area due to prolonged pressure on the body part; also known as a decubitus **ulcer** or pressure sore. See *Figure 5-12.*
pruritus (proo-**RYE**-tus)	Itching.
purpura (**PER**-pew-rah)	A group of bleeding disorders characterized by bleeding into the skin and mucous membranes; small, pinpoint hemorrhages are known as **petechia** and larger hemorrhagic areas are known as ecchymoses or bruises.
pustule (**PUS**-tyool)	A small elevation of the skin filled with pus; a small **abscess**.
scales	Thin flakes of hardened **epithelium** shed from the **epidermis**.
sebaceous cyst (see-**BAY**-shus **SIST**) 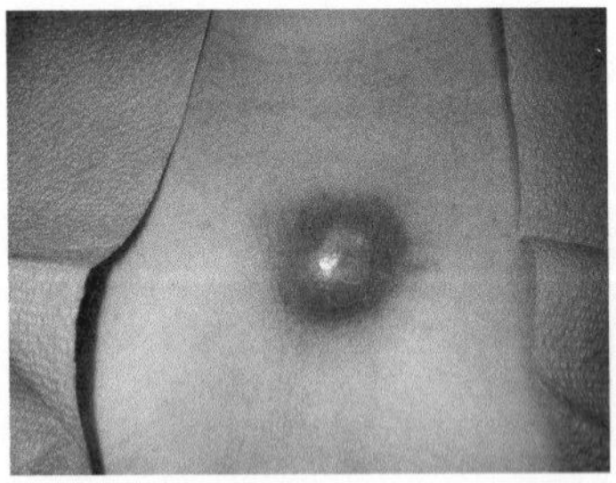 **Figure 5-13** Sebaceous cyst	A **cyst** filled with a cheesy material consisting of **sebum** and epithelial debris that has formed in the duct of a sebaceous gland; also known as an epidermoid cyst. *Figure 5-13* shows an infected **sebaceous cyst** in the mid-sternal area of the chest.
sebaceous gland (see-**BAY**-shus)	An **oil gland** located in the **dermis**; its secretions provide oil to the hair and surrounding skin.
seborrhea (**seb**-or-**EE**-ah) seb/o = sebum -rrhea = flow, drainage	Excessive secretion of **sebum**, resulting in excessive oiliness or dry scales.
sebum (**SEE**-bum) seb/o = sebum -um = noun ending	The oily secretions of the sebaceous glands.

Word	Definition
skin tags	A small brownish or flesh-colored outgrowth of skin occurring frequently on the neck; also known as a cutaneous papilloma.
squamous epithelial cells (**SKWAY**-mus **ep**-ih-**THEE**-lee-ul)	Flat scalelike cells arranged in layers (strata).
squamous epithelium (**SKWAY**-mus **ep**-ih-**THEE**-lee-um)	The single layer of flattened platelike cells that cover internal and external body surfaces.
stratified (**STRAT**-ih-fyd)	Layered; arranged in layers.
stratum (**STRAT**-um)	A uniformly thick sheet or layer of cells.
stratum basale (**STRAT**-um **BAY**-sil)	The layer of skin where new cells are continually being reproduced, pushing older cells toward the outermost surface of the skin.
stratum corneum (**STRAT**-um **COR**-nee-um)	The outermost layer of the **epidermis** (consisting of dead cells that have converted to **keratin**), which continually sloughs off or flakes away; known as the keratinized (or "horny") cell layer (kerat/o = horn).
stretch marks	Linear tears in the **dermis** that result from overstretching from rapid growth. They begin as pinkish-blue streaks with jagged edges and may be accompanied by itching. As they heal and lose their color, they remain as silvery-white scar lines, also known as striae.

subcutaneous tissue (**sub**-kew-**TAY**-nee-us)
  sub- = beneath, under, below
  cutane/o = skin
  -ous = pertaining to
	The fatty layer of tissue located beneath the **dermis**.

subungual hematoma (sub-**UNG**-gwall hee-mah-**TOH**-mah)
  sub = beneath, under, below
  ungu/o = nail
  hemat/o = blood
  -oma = tumor
	A collection of blood beneath a nail bed, usually the result of trauma (injury).

sudoriferous gland (**soo**-door-**IF**-er-us)	A sweat gland.
sweat	The clear, watery fluid produced by the sweat glands; also known as perspiration.
sweat gland	One of the tiny structures within the **dermis** that produces sweat, which carries waste products to the surface of the skin for excretion; also known as a **sudoriferous gland**.

Word	Definition
telangiectasia (tell-**an**-jee-ek-**TAY**-zee-ah)	The permanent dilation of groups of superficial capillaries and venules. These dilated vessels may be visible through the skin as tiny red lines. Common causes include but are not limited to **rosacea**, elevated estrogen levels, and actinic damage.
ulcer (**ULL**-ser)	A circumscribed, open sore or **lesion** of the skin that is accompanied by inflammation.
urticaria (**ur**-tih-**KARE**-ree-ah) 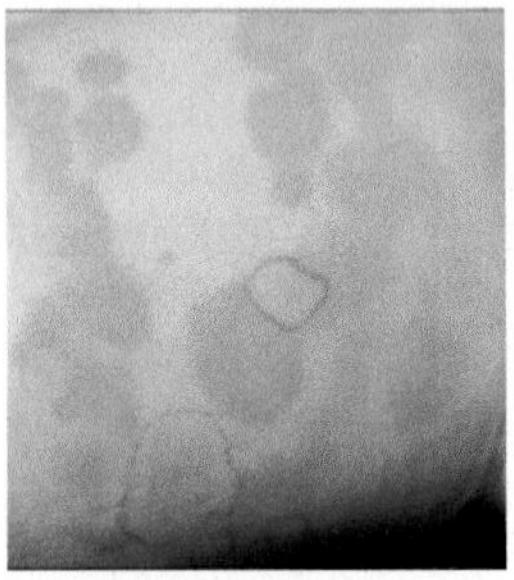 **Figure 5-14** Urticaria *(Courtesy of Robert A. Silverman, M.D., Clinical Associate Professor, Department of Pediatrics, Georgetown University)*	A reaction of the skin in which there is an appearance of smooth, slightly elevated patches (wheals) that are redder or paler than the surrounding skin and often accompanied by severe itching (**pruritus**). See *Figure 5-14.*
vesicle (**VESS**-ih-kul)	A small thin-walled skin **lesion** containing clear fluid; a blister.
vitiligo (**vit**-ih-**LYE**-goh)	A skin disorder characterized by nonpigmented white patches of skin of varying sizes that are surrounded by skin with normal pigmentation.
wheal (**WHEEL**)	A circumscribed, slightly elevated **lesion** of the skin that is paler in the center than its surrounding edges; hives.
whitehead	A closed **comedo** caused by accumulation of **keratin** and **sebum** within the opening of a hair follicle; the content within is not easily expressed.
xanthoderma (**zan**-thoh-**DER**-mah) xanth/o = yellow derm/o = skin -a = noun ending	Any yellow coloration of the skin.
xeroderma (**zee**-roh-**DER**-mah) xer/o = dry derm/o = skin -a = noun ending	A chronic skin condition characterized by roughness and dryness.

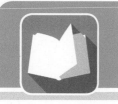

Review Checkpoint

Check your understanding of this section by completing the **Vocabulary** exercises in your workbook.

WORD ELEMENTS

The following word elements pertain to the integumentary system. As you review the list, pronounce each word element aloud twice and check the box after you "say it." Write the definition for the example term given for each word element. Use your medical dictionary to find the definitions of the example terms.

Word Element	Pronunciation	"Say It"	Meaning
adip/o **adip**ofibroma	**ADD**-ih-poh **add**-ih-poh-fih-**BROH**-mah	☐	fat
albin/o **albin**ism	al-**BYE**-noh **AL**-bin-izm	☐	white
caut/o **caut**ery	**KAW**-toh **KAW**-ter-ree	☐	burn
cutane/o sub**cutane**ous	kew-**TAY**-nee-oh sub-kew-**TAY**-nee-us	☐	skin
derm/o **derm**abrasion	**DERM**-oh **der**-mah-**BRAY**-zhun	☐	skin
dermat/o **dermat**itis	der-**MAT**-oh **der**-mah-**TYE**-tis	☐	skin
-edema lip**edema**	eh-**DEE**-mah **lip**-eh-**DEE**-mah	☐	Swelling
erythr/o **erythr**algia	eh-**RIH**-thro **eh**-rih-**THRAL**-jee-ah	☐	red
fasci/o **fasci**itis	**FASH**-ee-oh **fas**-ee-**EYE**-tis	☐	band of fibrous tissue
hidr/o **hidr**osis	**HIGH**-droh high-**DROH**-sis	☐	sweat

Word Element	Pronunciation	"Say It"	Meaning
hist/o, histi/o **hist**ology	**HISS**-toh hiss-**TOL**-oh-jee	☐	tissue
ichthy/o **ichthy**osis	**IK**-thee-oh **ik**-thee-**OH**-sis	☐	fish
kerat/o **kerat**osis	**KERR**-ah-toh **kerr**-ah-**TOH**-sis	☐	hard, horny; also refers to cornea of the eye
leuk/o **leuk**oderma	**LOO**-koh **loo**-koh-**DER**-mah	☐	white
lip/o **lip**ocyte	**LIP**-oh **LIP**-oh-sight	☐	fat
lip/o **lip**ohypertrophy	**LIP**-oh **lip**-oh-**high**-**PER**-troh-fee	☐	fat
melan/o **melan**oma	mell-**AH**-noh **mell**-ah-**NOH**-mah	☐	black
myc/o **myc**osis	**MY**-koh my-**KOH**-sis	☐	fungus
necr/o **necr**osis	**NECK**-roh neh-**KROH**-sis	☐	death
onych/o **onych**ogryposis	**ON**-ih-koh **on**-ih-koh-grih-**POH**-sis	☐	nails
pil/o **pil**onidal	**PYE**-loh **pye**-loh-**NYE**-dal	☐	hair
scler/o **scler**oderma	**SKLEHR**-oh **sklehr**-oh-**DER**-mah	☐	hard; also refers to sclera of the eye
squam/o **squam**ous epithelium	**SKWAY**-moh **SKWAY**-mus ep-ih-**THEE**-lee-um	☐	scales
trich/o **trich**iasis	**TRIK**-oh trik-**EYE**-ah-sis	☐	hair
xanth/o **xanth**osis	**ZAN**-thoh zan-**THOH**-sis	☐	yellow
xer/o **xer**oderma	**ZEE**-roh **zee**-roh-**DER**-mah	☐	dryness

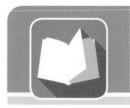

Review Checkpoint

Check your understanding of this section by completing the **Word Elements** exercises in your workbook.

Skin Lesions

A skin **lesion** is any circumscribed area of injury to the skin or a wound to the skin. The following are the most commonly known skin lesions.

abrasion (ah-**BRAY**-zhun)	A scraping or rubbing away of skin or mucous membrane as a result of friction to the area. An example of an **abrasion** is "carpet burn," which can occur in children who run and slide across a carpet on their knees.
abscess (**AB**-sess)	A localized collection of pus in any body part that results from invasion of pus-forming bacteria. The area is surrounded by inflamed tissue; a small **abscess** on the skin is also known as a **pustule**.
blister	A small thin-walled skin **lesion** containing clear fluid; a **vesicle**.
bulla (**BULL**-ah)	A large blister.
carbuncle (**CAR**-bung-kul)	A **circumscribed** inflammation of the skin and deeper tissues that contains pus, which eventually discharges to the skin surface. The **lesion** begins as a painful node covered by tight, reddened skin. The skin later thins out and perforates, discharging pus through several small openings. Treatment may include administration of antibiotics and use of warm compresses.
comedo (**KOM**-ee-doh)	The typical **lesion** of **acne vulgaris**, caused by the accumulation of **keratin** and **sebum** within the opening of a hair follicle. When a **comedo** is closed, it is called a **whitehead**, and the content within is not easily expressed. When a **comedo** is open, it is called a **blackhead**, and the oily content is easily expressed. Both forms of comedos are usually located on the face but may also appear on the back and chest.

cyst (**SIST**)	A closed sac or pouch in or within the skin that contains fluid, semifluid, or solid material.
	A common example of a fluid-filled **cyst** is a **hydrocele**, which is a collection of fluid located in the area of the scrotal sac in the male. A common example of a solid-filled **cyst** is a **sebaceous cyst**, which is a **cyst** filled with a cheesy material consisting of **sebum** and epithelial debris that has formed in the duct of a sebaceous gland; also known as an epidermoid cyst. Sebaceous cysts frequently form on the scalp and may grow quite large.
fissure (**FISH**-ur) 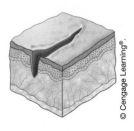 **Figure 5-15** Fissure	A cracklike sore or groove in the skin or mucous membrane.
	An example of a **fissure** is the cracklike sore in the skin that occurs with athlete's foot or the groovelike sore, known as an anal **fissure**, that occurs in the mucous membrane near the anus. For an example of a **fissure** in the mucous membrane, see *Figure 5-15*.
fistula (**FISS**-tyoo-lah)	An abnormal passageway between two tubular organs (such as the rectum and vagina) or from an organ to the body surface.
	Some fistulas are created surgically for therapeutic purposes, and others may be the result of congenital defects, infection, or injury to the body. An example of a surgically created **fistula** is an arteriovenous **fistula** created for the purpose of hemodialysis. (See the discussion of hemodialysis in Chapter 15.) A rectovaginal **fistula** results from an abnormal passageway between the rectum and vagina. This opening allows feces from the rectum or anal canal to escape into the vaginal canal. The rectovaginal **fistula** can result from trauma during childbirth.
furuncle (**FYOO**-rungkul)	A localized pus-producing (pyogenic) infection originating deep in a hair follicle, characterized by pain, redness, and swelling; also known as a boil. See *Figure 5-9*.
	Because a **furuncle** is caused by a staphylococcal infection, it is important to avoid squeezing or irritating the **lesion**, in order to prevent the possible spread of the infection to surrounding tissue.
hives	Circumscribed, slightly elevated lesions of the skin that are paler in the center than its surrounding edges; see *wheal*.
laceration (**lass**-er-**AY**-shun)	A tear in the skin; a torn, jagged wound.

© Cengage Learning®.

macule (**MACK**-yool)	A small, flat discoloration of the skin that is neither raised nor depressed.
	Some common examples of macules are **bruises**, freckles, and the rashes of measles and roseola. See *Figure 5-16*.

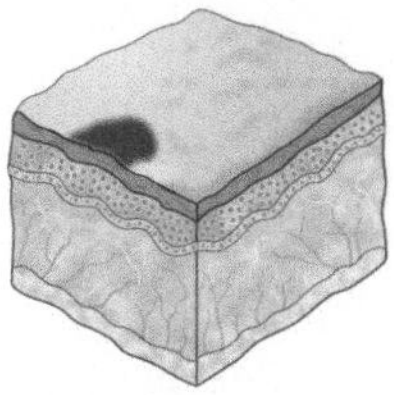

© Cengage Learning®.

Figure 5-16 Macule

nodule (**NOD**-yool)	A small, circumscribed swelling protruding above the skin; a small node.

papule (**PAP**-yool)	A small, solid, circumscribed elevation on the skin.
	Examples of a **papule** include a pimple, a wart, and an elevated **nevus** (mole). See *Figure 5-17*.

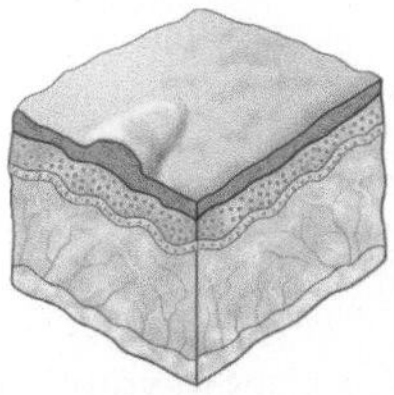

© Cengage Learning®.

Figure 5-17 Papule

polyp (**POL**-ip)	A small, stalk-like growth that protrudes upward or outward from a mucous membrane surface, resembling a mushroom stalk.
	An example of a **polyp** is a nasal polyp.

pressure ulcer (**PRESH**-ur **ULL**-ser)	An inflammation, sore, or **ulcer** in the skin over a bony prominence of the body, resulting from loss of blood supply and oxygen to the area due to prolonged pressure on the body part. Also known as a decubitus ulcer or pressure sore. See *Figure 5-12*.

pustule (**PUS**-tyool)	A small elevation of the skin filled with pus; a small **abscess** on the skin.

scales	Thin flakes of hardened **epithelium** that are shed from the **epidermis**.

ulcer (**ULL**-ser)	A circumscribed, open sore or **lesion** of the skin that is accompanied by inflammation.
	A decubitus ulcer, also known as a bedsore, is the breakdown of skin and underlying tissues resulting from constant pressure to bony prominences of the skin and inadequate blood supply and oxygenation to the area.

vesicle	A small thin-walled skin **lesion** containing clear fluid; a blister.
(**VESS**-ih-kul)	The small fluid-filled blisters that occur with poison ivy are vesicles. See *Figure 5-18*.

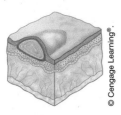

Figure 5-18 Vesicle

wheal	A circumscribed, slightly elevated **lesion** of the skin that is paler in the center than its surrounding edges; hives.
(**WHEEL**)	A **wheal** is usually accompanied by intense itching and is of short duration. A mosquito bite is an example of a **wheal**. An allergic reaction to something may result in numerous wheals of varying sizes and intense itching, which is known as **urticaria**.

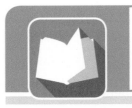

Review Checkpoint

Check your understanding of this section by completing the **Skin Lesions** exercises in your workbook.

Pathological Conditions

Feature Walk-Through

The arrangement of medical terms in each chapter permits you to learn a **basic definition** of a term followed by a more detailed description. The medical term and the basic definition are highlighted with a green background. The more detailed description follows in regular type. This **Simple to Complex Definition** presentation lets you tailor learning to your specific needs.

Note that the study of **word elements** is integrated throughout the book. Word elements are repeated in each chapter to reinforce their meaning again and again. The medical term appears in the left-hand column, usually with a phonetic pronunciation directly beneath the term, including a breakdown of the component parts of the term, shown in blue, when appropriate. This format allows you to learn the medical term in context while continuing to reinforce the word elements.

acne vulgaris	A common inflammatory disorder seen on the face, chest, back, and neck; appears as papules, pustules, and comedos; commonly known as acne. See *Figure 5-19*.
(**ACK**-nee vul-**GAY**-ris)	**Acne vulgaris** typically begins during adolescence due to the influence of sex hormones, largely androgens. Because it is a major cosmetic concern for the teenage population, acne should never be dismissed as trivial. This condition is characterized by:

1. the formation of comedos, papules, and pustules on the face, chest, back, and neck;

2. the increased secretion of **sebum** as evidenced by greasy skin; and

3. hyperkeratosis at the opening of the hair follicle, which blocks the discharge of **sebum** and promotes the colonization of anaerobic bacteria.

The formation of **blackheads** (open comedos) and **whiteheads** (closed comedos) occurs as a result of the growth of anaerobic bacteria, which can live without air. The degree of involvement varies from the small comedos to obstruction of the entire follicle when large pustules or abscesses form. Picking, scratching, or pressing of these lesions can lead to secondary infections and scarring. Although there is no cure for acne, treatment is directed at the following:

1. keeping the skin free of excess oil and bacteria through frequent cleansing,

2. avoiding heavy makeup and creams that can clog up the pores,

3. controlling infection with local antibiotics, and

4. decreasing the keratinization (hardening) of follicles by using **keratolytic** agents or *retinoic acid*.

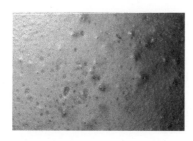

Figure 5-19 Acne scarring
(Courtesy of Robert A. Silverman, M.D., Clinical Associate Professor, Department of Pediatrics, Georgetown University)

| **albinism** | A condition characterized by absence of pigment in the skin, hair, and eyes. |

(**AL**-bin-izm)
    albin/o = white
    -ism = condition

Individuals with **albinism** lack the inherited ability to produce a brown skin coloring pigment, **melanin**. Persons with this inherited disorder:

1. are hypersensitive to light (photophobia),

2. are susceptible to skin cancer,

3. are prone to visual disturbances such as nearsightedness,

4. have pink or very pale blue eyes,

5. must avoid the sun to protect their eyes and skin from burning.

The widespread incidence of **albinism** is 1 in 20,000 births, equally male and female. The prevalence of **albinism** is higher in African Americans than in Caucasians.

| **burns** | Tissue injury produced by flame, heat, chemicals, radiation, electricity, or gases. The extent of the damage to the underlying tissue is determined by the mode and duration of exposure, the thermal intensity or temperature, and the anatomic site of the burn. Burn degree is classified according to the depth of injury. See *Figures 5-20A through* C. |

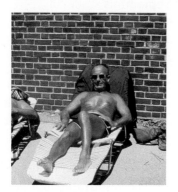

Figure 5-20A First-degree burn

First-degree (superficial) burns:

1. produce redness and swelling of the **epidermis**,

2. are painful, and

3. heal spontaneously with peeling in about three to six days and produce no scar.

An example of a first-degree or superficial burn is sunburn. See *Figure 5-20A*.

Second-degree (partial-thickness) burns:

1. exhibit a blistering pink to red color and some swelling,
2. involve the **epidermis** and upper layer of the **dermis**,
3. are very sensitive and painful, and
4. heal in approximately two weeks without a scar if no wound infection or trauma occurs during the healing process.

An example of a second-degree or partial-thickness burn is flash contact with hot objects, such as boiling water. See *Figure 5-20B*.

Third-degree (full-thickness) burns:

1. cause tissue damage according to the duration and temperature of the heat source,
2. involve massive necrosis of the **epidermis** and entire **dermis**, and may include part of the **subcutaneous tissue** or muscle,
3. appear brown, black, tan, white, or deep cherry red (will not blanch) and are wet or dry, sunken, with eschar (dry crust) and coagulated capillaries,
4. produce pain according to the amount of nerve tissue involved (where nerve endings are destroyed, pain will be absent), and
5. will take a long time to heal and will likely require **debridement**(s) and grafting. See *Figure 5-20C*.

The classification of burns as first, second, or third degree helps evaluate the severity of the burn. However, other factors influence the severity, such as:

1. the age of person burned,
2. the percentage of body surface burned,
3. the location of burn on the body, and
4. concurrent injuries.

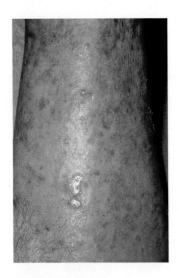

Figure 5-20B Second-degree burn

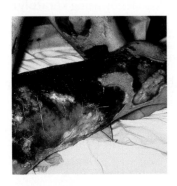

Figure 5-20C Third-degree burn

(A, B, and C Courtesy of the Phoenix Society for Burn Survivors, Inc.)

callus	A common (usually painless) thickening of the **epidermis** at sites of external pressure or friction, such as the weight-bearing areas of the feet and on the palmar surface of the hands. This localized hyperplastic area of up to 1 inch in size is also known as a callosity.
(**CAL**-us)	

A **callus** may be caused by pressure or friction from ill-fitting shoes, deformities of the foot, or improper weight bearing. It may also be the result of repeated trauma to the skin such as that which occurs with manual labor or strumming a string instrument (guitar, banjo, etc.).

Treatment for calluses involves relieving the pressure or friction points on the skin. Metatarsal pads may also provide relief. The best treatment is prevention (i.e., by wearing shoes that fit well and avoiding unnecessary trauma to the hands and feet).

carcinoma, basal cell

(**car**-sih-**NOH**-mah, **BAY**-sal sell)

carcin/o = cancer

-oma = tumor

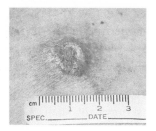

Figure 5-21 Basal cell carcinoma

(Courtesy of Robert A. Silverman, MD, Pediatric Dermatology, Georgetown University)

A malignant epithelial cell tumor that begins as a slightly elevated **nodule** with a depression or ulceration in the center that becomes more obvious as the tumor grows. As the depression enlarges, the tissue breaks down, crusts, and bleeds. See *Figure 5-21*.

Basal cell carcinoma is the most common malignant tumor of the epithelial tissue, occurring most often on areas of the skin exposed to the sun (usually between the hairline and the upper lip). If not treated, the basal cell carcinomas will invade surrounding tissue, which can lead to destruction of body parts (such as a nose). Treatment includes surgical excision, **curettage and electrodesiccation**, **cryosurgery**, or radiation therapy (see the section on diagnostic tests and procedures for descriptions of these). Basal cell carcinomas rarely metastasize, but they tend to recur—especially those that are larger than 2 cm in diameter.

carcinoma, squamous cell

(**kar**-sih-**NOH**-mah, **SKWAY**-mus sell)

carcin/o = cancer

-oma = tumor

squam/o = scales

-ous = pertaining to

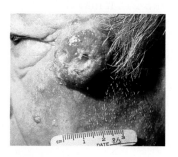

Figure 5-22 Squamous cell carcinoma

(Courtesy of Robert A. Silverman, MD, Pediatric Dermatology, Georgetown University)

A malignancy of the squamous (or scalelike) cells of the epithelial tissue, which is a much faster growing cancer than **basal cell carcinoma** and which has a greater potential for metastasis if not treated. See *Figure 5-22*.

These squamous cell lesions are seen most frequently on sun-exposed areas such as the:

1. top of the nose,

2. forehead,

3. margin of the external ear,

4. back of the hands, and

5. lower lip.

The squamous cell **lesion** begins as a firm, flesh-colored or red **papule**, sometimes with a crusted appearance. As the **lesion** grows, it may bleed or ulcerate and become painful. When **squamous cell carcinoma** recurs, it can be quite invasive and create an increased risk of metastasis.

Treatment is surgical excision with the goal of removing the tumor completely, along with a margin of healthy surrounding tissue. **Cryosurgery** for low-risk squamous cell carcinomas is also common.

dermatitis

(**der**-mah-**TYE**-tis)

dermat/o = skin

-itis = inflammation

Inflammation of the skin, seen in several forms. **Dermatitis** may be acute or chronic, contact or seborrheic.

Contact dermatitis occurs as the skin responds to an irritant or allergen with redness, **pruritus** (itching), and various skin lesions. Two forms of contact dermatitis are allergic contact dermatitis and irritant contact dermatitis.

Allergic contact dermatitis develops by sensitization. When coming in contact with a substance for the first time, no immediate inflammation occurs, but future exposure to this substance will result in severe acute inflammation with pruritic red vesicular oozing lesions at the area of contact. Common causes of allergic contact dermatitis include plants such as poison oak (refer

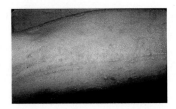

Figure 5-23 Allergic contact dermatitis

(Courtesy of the Centers for Disease Control and Prevention

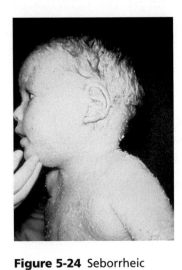

Figure 5-24 Seborrheic dermatitis

(Courtesy of Robert A. Silverman, MD, Pediatric Dermatology Clinical Associate Professor, Department of Pediatrics, Georgetown University)

back to *Figure 5-7*) and poison ivy; drugs; some metals such as copper, silver, mercury, and jewelry; and many industrial cleaners. See *Figure 5-23*.

Irritant contact dermatitis occurs following repeated exposure of a mild irritant or initial exposure of a strong irritant. This severe inflammatory reaction is characterized by a fine, itchy rash of clearly defined red papules and vesicles. The chronic features of irritant contact dermatitis are dryness and scaling with a dull reddened appearance. Some of the common causes of irritant contact dermatitis are soaps, detergents, oven cleaners, and bleaches.

Seborrheic (seb-oh-REE-ik) dermatitis is a very common inflammatory condition seen in areas where the oil glands are most prevalent, such as the:

1. scalp,
2. area behind the ears,
3. eyebrows,
4. sides of the nose,
5. eyelids, and
6. middle of the chest.

The skin affected by **seborrheic dermatitis** appears reddened with a greasy, yellowish crusting or scales. If itching occurs, it is usually mild. The most common form of **seborrheic dermatitis** is seen in infants from birth to 12 months of age and is called cradle cap (see *Figure 5-24*). It may also occur in adults, and statistics show it is higher in persons:

1. with disorders of the central nervous system, such as Parkinson's disease,
2. recovering from a stressful medical crisis, such as a heart attack,
3. confined for long periods of time in the hospital or a long-term care facility, and
4. with disorders of the immune system, such as AIDS.

eczema (**EK**-zeh-mah)	An acute or chronic inflammatory skin condition characterized by **erythema**, papules, vesicles, pustules, scales, crusts, or scabs and accompanied by intense itching.

These lesions may occur alone or in any combination. They may be dry or they may produce a watery discharge with resultant itching.

Long-term effects of **eczema** may result in thickening and hardening of the skin, known as lichenification, which is due to irritation caused from repeated scratching of the itchy area. Redness and scaling of the skin may also accompany this. Severe itching predisposes the areas to secondary infections and possible invasion by viruses.

An estimated 9% to 12% of the population is affected by **eczema**, occurring most commonly during infancy and childhood. The incidence decreases in adolescence and adulthood. No exact cause is known. However, statistics support a convincing genetic component in that children whose mother and father are affected have an 80% chance of developing **eczema**. This inflammatory response is believed to be initiated by **histamine** release, with lesions usually occurring on the flexor surfaces of the arms and legs, the hands, the feet, and the upper trunk of the body.

Although there is no specific treatment to cure **eczema**, local and systemic medications may be prescribed to prevent itching. It is important to stress daily skin care and avoidance of known irritants. Chronic **eczema** is often frustrating to control and may recur throughout most of the individual's life.

exanthematous viral diseases (eks-an-**THEM**-ah-tus **VYE**-ral dih-**ZEEZ**-ez)	A skin eruption or rash accompanied by inflammation, having specific diagnostic features of an infectious viral disease.

There are more than 50 known viral agents that cause exanthems (eruptions of the skin accompanied by inflammation). The most common viral agents cause childhood communicable infections such as:

1. rubella (German measles),

2. roseola infantum,

3. rubeola (measles), and

4. erythema infectiosum (fifth disease).

These childhood diseases are discussed further in Chapter 19.

gangrene (**GANG**-green)	Tissue death due to the loss of adequate blood supply, invasion of bacteria, and subsequent decay of enzymes (especially proteins), producing an offensive, foul odor.

Gangrene can occur in two forms:

1. **dry gangrene**, seen in an extremity that is dry, cold, and shriveled, and which has a blackening appearance (late complication of diabetes mellitus)

2. **moist gangrene** follows the cessation of blood flow to tissue after a crushing injury, embolism, tourniquet, or tight bandage. If untreated, it will progress quickly to death.

The necrotic tissue must be removed through **debridement** or **amputation** to restore healing. Treatment should be aimed at the prevention of **gangrene**.

herpes zoster (shingles) (**HER**-peez **ZOS**-ter)	An acute viral infection characterized by painful vesicular eruptions on the skin following along the nerve pathways of underlying spinal or cranial nerves.

Ten to twenty percent of the population are affected by **herpes zoster**, with the highest incidence in adults over 50. This acute eruption is caused by reactivation of latent varicella virus (the same virus that causes chickenpox). See *Figure 5-25*.

Symptoms of **herpes zoster** include:

1. severe pain before and during eruption,

2. fever,

3. itching,

4. gastrointestinal disturbances,

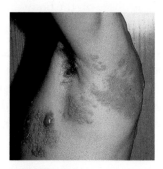

Figure 5-25 Herpes zoster
(Courtesy of Robert A. Silverman, MD, Clinical Associate Professor, Pediatric Dermatology, Georgetown University)

5. headache,

6. general tiredness, and

7. increased sensitivity of the skin around the area.

The lesions usually take three to five days to erupt and then progress to crusting and drying (with recovery in approximately three weeks). Treatment involves the use of antiviral medications, analgesics, and sometimes corticosteroids (which aid in decreasing the severity of symptoms).

hyperkeratosis (**high**-per-**kerr**-ah-**TOH**-sis) hyper- = excessive kerat/o = hard, horny; also refers to cornea of the eye -osis = condition	An overgrowth of the horny layer of the **epidermis**.

This overgrowth occurs when the keratinocyte moves from the basal cell to the **stratum corneum** in 7 days instead of the normal 14 days, resulting in the formation of thick, flaky scales, along with excess growth of the cornified layer of **epithelium**. This process occurs in **psoriasis** and in the formation of calluses and corns.

impetigo (**im**-peh-**TYE**-goh *or* im-peh-**TEE**-goh)	Contagious superficial skin infection characterized by serous vesicles and pustules filled with millions of staphylococcus or streptococcus bacteria, usually forming on the face. See *Figure 5-26*.

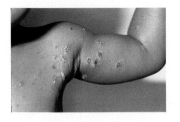

Figure 5-26 Impetigo
(Courtesy of Robert A. Silverman, MD, Clinical Associate Professor, Pediatric Dermatology, Georgetown University)

Impetigo progresses to pruritic erosions and crusts with a honey-colored appearance. The discharge from the lesions allows the infection to be highly contagious. Treatment includes:

1. cleaning lesions with antibacterial soap and water, using individual washcloths,

2. administration of oral and topical antibiotics,

3. Burrow's solution compresses, and

4. good handwashing.

It is important to instruct the individual to complete the entire regime of systemic antibiotics to prevent the possibility of complications due to secondary infections such as acute glomerulonephritis and/or rheumatic fever.

Kaposi's sarcoma (**CAP**-oh-seez sar-**KOH**-mah) sarc/o = flesh -oma = tumor	Vascular malignant lesions that begin as soft purple-brown nodules or plaques on the face and oral cavity but can occur anywhere on the body and gradually spread throughout the skin.

This systemic disease also involves the gastrointestinal tract and lungs. **Kaposi's sarcoma** occurs most often in men, and there is an increased incidence in men infected with AIDS. It is also associated with diabetes and malignant lymphoma. Radiotherapy and chemotherapy are usually recommended as methods of treatment. **Kaposi's sarcoma** may also be treated with **cryosurgery** or laser surgery. (A visual reference may be seen in Chapter 21.)

keloid (**KEE**-loyd) kel/o = fibrous growth -oid = resembling	An enlarged, irregularly shaped, and elevated scar that forms due to the presence of large amounts of **collagen** during the formation of the scar.

keratosis (**kerr**-ah-**TOH**-sis) kerat/o = hard, horny; also refers to cornea of the eye -osis = condition	Skin condition in which there is a thickening and overgrowth of the cornified **epithelium**.
seborrheic keratosis (**seb**-oh-**REE**-ik **kerr**-ah-**TOH**-sis)	Appears as brown or waxy yellow wartlike **lesion**(s), 5 to 20 mm in diameter, loosely attached to the skin surface. Seborrheic keratosis is also known as senile warts.
actinic keratosis (ak-**TIN**-ic **kerr**-ah-**TOH**-sis)	A premalignant, gray or red-to-brown, hardened **lesion** caused by excessive exposure to sunlight. Also called solar keratosis.
leukoplakia (**loo**-koh-**PLAY**-kee-ah) leuk/o = white	White, hard, thickened patches firmly attached to the mucous membrane in areas such as the mouth, vulva, or penis. Oral **leukoplakia** varies in size and occurs gradually over a period of several weeks. It begins without symptoms, but eventually develops sensitivity to hot or highly seasoned foods. Causes of oral **leukoplakia** vary from irritating tobacco smoke to friction caused by a rough tooth or dentures. A biopsy should be performed when oral **leukoplakia** persists for more than two to three weeks because approximately 3% develop into cancerous lesions.
malignant melanoma (mah-**LIG**-nant **mel**-ah-**NOH**-mah) melan/o = black, dark -oma = tumor	Malignant skin tumor originating from **melanocytes** in preexisting nevi, freckles, or skin with pigment; darkly pigmented cancerous tumor. These tumors have irregular surfaces and borders, have variable colors, and are generally located on the trunk in men and on the legs in women. The diameter of most malignant melanomas measures more than 6 mm. Around the primary **lesion**, small satellite lesions 1 to 2 cm in diameter are often noted. Persons at risk for malignant melanomas include those with a family history of melanoma and those with fair complexions. There is also an increased risk to develop particular forms of malignant melanomas with excessive sun exposure. Generally, most melanomas are extremely invasive and spread first to the lymphatic system and then metastasize throughout the body to any organ (with fatal results). All nevi and skin should be inspected and self-examined regularly, remembering the ABCDs of **malignant melanoma**: *Asymmetry*—any pigmented **lesion** that has flat and elevated parts should be considered potentially malignant. *Borders*—any leakage across the borders of brown pigment or margins irregularly shaped are suspicious. *Color*—variations whether red, black, dark brown, or pale are suspicious. *Diameter*—any lesions with the preceding characteristics measuring more than 6 mm in diameter should be removed.

Treatment is surgical removal and, for distant metastases, chemotherapy and radiation therapy. The depth of surgical dissection and the prognosis depends on the staging classification of the tumor. The five-year survival rate is approximately 60% for all forms of malignant melanomas.

nevus (mole) (**NEE**-vus)	A visual accumulation of **melanocytes**, creating a flat or raised rounded **macule** or **papule** with definite borders.

Nevi should be monitored for changes in size, color, thickness, itching, or bleeding. When any of these changes are noted, immediate professional assessment should be sought because of the potential for developing **malignant melanoma**.

onychocryptosis
(**on**-ih-koh-krip-**TOH**-sis)
  onych/o = nail
  crypt/o = hidden
  -osis = condition
	Ingrown nail. The nail pierces the lateral fold of skin and grows into the **dermis**, causing swelling and pain.

Ingrown nails most commonly involve the large toe.

onychomycosis
(**on**-ih-koh-my-**KOH**-sis)
  onych/o = nail
  myc/o = fungus
  -osis = condition
	A fungal infection of the nails.

The nail becomes opaque, white, thickened, and friable (easily broken).

pediculosis (pee-**dik**-you-**LOH**-sis)	A highly contagious parasitic infestation caused by blood-sucking lice.

Pediculosis may occur on any of the following parts of the body:

1. head (pediculosis capitis),
2. body (pediculosis corporis),
3. eyelashes and eyelids (pediculosis palpebrarum), and
4. pubic hair (pediculosis pubis).

With all types of **pediculosis**, a rash or wheals, intense **pruritus**, and the presence of louse eggs (nits) on the skin, hair shafts, or clothing are characteristic. When nits are present on the hair shaft, they appear as tiny silvery-gray beads that cling to the hair strand. When thumping the hair strand, the nit will not fall from the strand (as would dandruff). **Pediculosis** can be spread directly through close physical contact or indirectly through articles of clothing, brushes, bed linens, and towels.

Treatment includes use of a special shampoo followed by removal of the nits with a fine-tooth comb. The treatment must be repeated weekly until nits are no longer present. Lice on the eyelid and lashes require a special ophthalmic ointment. Due to the intense itching, secondary infections can be a concern requiring antibiotic treatment.

pemphigus (**PEM**-fih-gus)	A rare incurable disorder manifested by blisters in the mouth and on the skin, which spread to involve large areas of the body, including the chest, face, umbilicus, back, and groin.

These painful blisters ooze, form crusts, and put off a musty odor. The serious risk is the secondary infection with the large areas of skin involved. Treatment involves administration of drugs, prevention of excessive fluid loss, and prevention of infection.

pilonidal cyst (**pye**-loh-**NYE**-dal)	A closed sac located in the sacrococcygeal area of the back, sometimes noted at birth as a dimple.

The **cyst** causes no symptoms unless it becomes acutely infected. When the **pilonidal cyst** is infected, an incision and drainage are indicated, followed by removal of the **cyst** or sac.

psoriasis (soh-**RYE**-ah-sis)	A common, noninfectious, chronic disorder of the skin manifested by silvery-white scales covering round, raised, reddened plaques producing itching (**pruritus**).

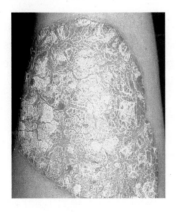

The process of hyperkeratosis produces various-sized lesions occurring mainly on the scalp, ears, extensor surfaces of the extremities, bony prominences, and perianal and genital areas. See *Figure 5-27* for a visual reference. There is no cure for **psoriasis**. Treatment for **psoriasis** includes topical application of various medications, phototherapy, and ultraviolet light therapy in an attempt to slow the hyperkeratosis.

Figure 5-27 Psoriasis
(Courtesy of Robert A. Silverman, MD, Pediatric Dermatology, Georgetown University)

rosacea (roh-**ZAY**-she-ah)	**Rosacea** is a chronic inflammatory skin disease that mainly affects the skin of the middle third of the face. The individual has persistent redness over the areas of the face, nose, and cheeks.

The small blood vessels of the cheeks enlarge and become visible through the skin, appearing as tiny red lines (known as **telangiectasia**). Pimples may also be present with **rosacea**, resembling teenage acne.

Rosacea occurs most often in adults between the ages of 30 to 50, especially those with fair skin. **Rosacea** may be mistaken for rosy cheeks, sunburn, or acne. However, it differs from acne in that no blackheads or whiteheads are present.

Treatment is directed at controlling the symptoms. Individuals may be advised to avoid situations (i.e., stress, sunlight, spicy foods, hot beverages, alcohol, and exposure to extreme heat or cold) that could trigger blushing or flushing of the skin, since this is thought to aggravate **rosacea**. Treatment may also involve both oral and topical antibiotics. Individuals with **rosacea** are also advised to use mild facial cleansers and moisturizers and sunscreens that do not contain alcohol. There is no cure for **rosacea**, but it can be controlled with proper regular treatment.

scabies (**SKAY**-beez)	A highly contagious parasitic infestation caused by the "human itch mite," resulting in a rash, **pruritus**, and slightly raised thread-like skin lines.

Scabies is seen most frequently on the genital area, armpits, waistline, hands, and breasts. **Scabies** can be spread directly through close physical contact or indirectly through articles of clothing, brushes, bed linens, and towels.

Treatment includes the use of special sulfur preparations, shampoos, and topical ointments. Due to the intense itching, secondary infections can be a concern requiring antibiotic treatment.

scleroderma (**sklair**-oh-**DER**-mah) scler/o = hard; also refers to sclera of the eye derm/o = skin -a = noun ending	A gradual thickening of the **dermis** and swelling of the hands and feet to a state in which the skin is anchored to the underlying tissue.

The severity of this disease varies from a mild localized form only affecting the skin (seen in persons in the 30- to 50-year age group) to a generalized form known as progressive systemic scleroderma (PSS) with progressive systemic involvement (persons die from pulmonary, cardiac, GI, renal, or pulmonary involvement).

No cure is available for **scleroderma**. Therefore, the treatment is aimed at decreasing symptoms and treating the involved system with medications appropriate to the dysfunction. Physiotherapy may be recommended for some patients to restore and maintain musculoskeletal function as much as possible.

systemic lupus erythematosus (sis-**TEM**-ic **LOO**-pus air-ih-them-ah-**TOH**-sus)	A chronic, multisystem, inflammatory disease characterized by lesions of the nervous system and skin, renal problems, and vasculitis. A red rash known as the "butterfly rash" is often seen on the nose and face.

Skin lesions may also spread to the mucous membranes or other tissues. Pain and swelling of the joints (along with weakness, weight loss, and fatigue) are symptoms of the disease process. Treatment consists of the use of the systemic steroids, topical steroids on skin lesions, salicylates or non-steroidal anti-inflammatory drugs (NSAIDs) to relieve joint pain and swelling, and protection from sunlight.

tinea (**TIN**-ee-ah)	More commonly known as ringworm, a chronic fungal infection of the skin that is characterized by scaling, itching, and sometimes painful lesions. The lesions are named according to the body part affected. See *Figures 5-28A through* C.

tinea capitis (**TIN**-ee-ah **CAP**-ih-tis) capit/o = head -is = noun ending	Ringworm of the scalp (more common in children).

The infection may lead to hair loss. Symptoms of **tinea capitis** include small, round, elevated patches, severe itching and scaling of the scalp. Treatment with topical antifungal agents is sufficient for clearing the condition. See *Figure 5-28A.*

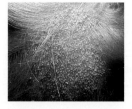

Figure 5-28A Tinea capitis
(Courtesy of Robert A. Silverman, M.D., Clinical Associate Professor, Department of Pediatrics, Georgetown University)

tinea corporis
 	
(**TIN**-ee-ah **COR**-poh-ris)
 	
  corpor/o = body
  -is = noun ending
 	
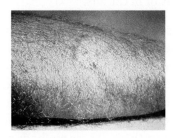
	Ringworm of the body is characterized by round patches with elevated red borders of pustules, papules, or vesicles that affect the nonhairy skin of the body. The **lesion** actually looks like a circle and is raised. See *Figure 5-28B*.
	
	Ringworm of the body is most common in hot, humid climates and in rural areas. **Tinea corporis** can be spread through skin contact with an infected person or skin contact with an infected domestic animal, especially cats.
	
	Figure 5-28B Tinea corporis
	(Courtesy of the Centers for Disease Control and Prevention [CDC]).

tinea cruris
 	
(**TIN**-ee-ah **KROO**-ris)
 	
  crur/o = leg or thigh
  -is = noun ending
	Ringworm of the groin; also known as jock itch.
	
	This type of ringworm occurs more commonly in adult males. It is characterized by red, raised, vesicular patches in the groin area that are accompanied by **pruritus**.
	
	Tinea cruris is more likely to occur during the hot, humid summer months and is aggravated by heat, physical activity, tight-fitting clothes, and perspiration. Topical antifungal agents are recommended for treatment.

tinea pedis
 	
(**TIN**-ee-ah **PED**-is)
 	
  ped/o = foot
  -is = noun ending
 	
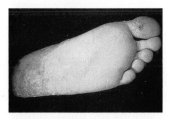
 	
Figure 5-28C Tinea pedis
(Courtesy of the Centers for Disease Control and Prevention [CDC])
	Ringworm of the foot; also known as athlete's foot.
	
	It affects the space between the toes and the soles of the feet, with lesions varying from dry and peeling to draining painful fissures with a foul odor and **pruritus**. Adults are most susceptible to **tinea pedis**. See *Figure 5-28C*.
	
	Drying the feet well after bathing and applying powder between the toes will keep the moisture from building up and help prevent the recurrence of the fungal infection. Treatment with topical antifungal agents is helpful in clearing the condition, although recurrence is common.
	
	Treatment for all types of **tinea** that are severe or resistant to the topical antifungal agents includes the administration of oral antifungal medications that act systemically. If this becomes necessary, the drug of choice is griseofulvin.

wart (verruca; verrucae [pl.]) (veh-**ROO**-kah; veh-**ROO**-kee)	A benign, circumscribed, elevated skin **lesion** that results from hypertrophy of the **epidermis**; caused by the human papilloma virus. See *Figure 5-29*. The virus can be spread by touch or contact with the skin shed from a wart. They may occur alone or in clusters. The **common wart** (verruca vulgaris) occurs on the face, elbow, fingers, or hands. These are seen largely in children and young adults. **Plantar warts** occur either singly or in clusters on the sole of the foot. These warts can be painful, causing individuals to feel as if they have a stone in their shoe. **Plantar warts** occur primarily at points of pressure, such as over the metatarsal heads and the heel of the foot.

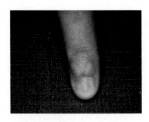

Figure 5-29 Verruca vulgaris (wart)
(Courtesy of Robert A. Silverman, MD, Clinical Associate Professor, Pediatric Dermatology, Georgetown University)

Condyloma acuminata (or **venereal warts**) are transmitted via sexual contact and are found on the female genitalia, the penis, or the rectum. These warts develop near the mucous membrane/skin junctures on the prepuce of the penis or on the female vulva. The growths appear as small, soft, moist, pinkish or purplish projections that appear singly or in clusters.

Seborrheic warts or **seborrheic keratoses** are seen in the elderly population. These are benign, circumscribed, slightly raised lesions that occur on the face, neck, chest, or upper back and are often accompanied by itching. The lesions range from yellowish-tan to dark brown and are covered with either a greasy scale or a rough, dry scale depending on the location. Treatment for **seborrheic warts** includes **curettage**, cryotherapy, or **electrodesiccation** in conjunction with a local anesthetic. These methods of treatment are discussed later in the chapter.

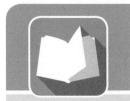

Review Checkpoint

Check your understanding of this section by completing the **Pathological Conditions** exercises in your workbook.

Diagnostic Techniques, Treatments, and Procedures

allergy testing	Various procedures used to identify specific allergens in an individual by exposing the person to a very small quantity of the allergen.
	The intradermal, patch, and scratch tests are among the most common allergy tests used.
	A more advanced, convenient way of testing for allergies is the ImmunoCAP® Allergy Blood Test. This blood test is the first allergy test cleared by the FDA as a truly quantitative test for pinpointing allergens. A small blood sample is drawn and sent to a laboratory to determine the exact amount of IgE antibodies present in the patient's blood for each specific allergen. (The IgE antibody circulates in the blood when the body is fighting an allergen.) This test is accurate and reliable and allows the doctor to assess an individual's reaction to particular food and environmental allergens and to determine whether the symptoms are due to an allergy or another medical condition. The physician can use the results to tailor treatment strategies appropriately for the patient or refer the patient to an allergy specialist.
cautery (**KAW**-ter-ree)	Heat or caustic substances that burn and scar the skin (coagulation of tissue).

cryosurgery

(**cry**-oh-**SER**-jer-ee)

cry/o = cold

A noninvasive treatment that uses subfreezing temperature to freeze and destroy the tissue.

A local anesthetic is applied to the surface of the **lesion**, followed by the application of liquid nitrogen, which freezes and destroys tumor tissue. **Cryosurgery** is used for low-risk squamous cell malignancies and primary basal cell carcinomas. This procedure causes very little pain and has good cosmetic results. It may also be used to remove warts. **Cryosurgery** requires a prolonged healing time, during which the wound tends to be painful and swollen (with some inflammation and blistering).

curettage and electrodesiccation

(kew-reh-**TAHZH** and ee-**lek**-troh-des-ih-**KAY**-shun)

A combination procedure of **curettage** that involves scraping away abnormal tissue and **electrodesiccation**, which involves destroying the tumor base with a low-voltage electrode.

This treatment is used for basal cell cancers that are superficial, recur due to poor margin control, or are less than 2 cm in diameter. It is also used to treat primary squamous cell carcinomas with distinct edges when the diameter is less than 1 cm.

Good cosmetic results and preservation of normal tissue have been noted as advantages of **curettage and electrodesiccation**. Disadvantages are that healing time is longer and it is very difficult to confirm that all tumor margins have been excised.

debridement

(dah-**BREED**-ment)

Removal of debris, foreign objects, and damaged or necrotic tissue from a wound to prevent infection and to promote healing.

This may be a surgical or medical procedure. When debriding a burn, it may be done along with hydrotherapy.

dermabrasion

(**der**-mah-**BRAY**-zhun)

Removal of the **epidermis** and a portion of the **dermis** with sandpaper or brushes to eliminate superficial scars or unwanted tattoos.

A chemical is used to cause light freezing of the skin prior to the use of the brushes and sandpaper.

dermatoplasty

(**DER**-mah-toh-**plas**-tee)

dermat/o = skin

-plasty = surgical repair

Skin transplantation to a body surface damaged by injury or disease.

electrodesiccation

(ee-lek-troh-**des**-ih-**KAY**-shun)

A technique using an electrical spark to burn and destroy tissue; used primarily for the removal of surface lesions.

Electrodesiccation involves the destruction of tissue by burning it with an electrical spark upon contact. The spark desiccates (dries) the tissue by dehydration. Although it is used primarily for removing small surface lesions, it may also be used to eliminate abnormal tissue deeper in the skin using a local anesthetic; also known as **fulguration**.

electrosurgery (ee-**lek**-troh-**SER**-jer-ee)	The removal or destruction of tissue with an electrical current. The variety of electrosurgeries include: 1. **electrodesiccation**, which is destruction of superficial tissue; 2. electrocoagulation, which is destruction of deeper tissue; and 3. electrosection, which is cutting through skin and tissue.
escharotomy (**es**-kar-**OT**-oh-mee)	An incision made into the necrotic tissue resulting from a severe burn. This scab (or dry crust) that forms after a severe full-thickness burn is known as an eschar. Removal of this necrotic tissue is necessary to prevent a wound infection of the burn site. The eschar is incised with a scalpel or by electrocautery for relief of tightness in the affected area. This sterile surgical incision allows for expansion of tissue created by the edema and aids in promoting blood flow to the area and preventing **gangrene**.
fulguration (**ful**-goo-**RAY**-shun)	See *electrodesiccation*.
liposuction (**LIP**-oh-suck-shun) lip/o = fat	Aspiration of fat through a suction cannula or curette to alter the body contours. **Liposuction** is usually done on younger persons because of the elasticity of their skin. A pressure dressing is applied after the procedure to aid the skin in adapting to the new tissue size.
skin biopsy (**BYE**-op-see)	The removal of a small piece of tissue from a skin **lesion** for the purpose of examining it under a microscope to confirm or establish a diagnosis. Types of skin biopsies are: 1. **excisional biopsy**, which is removal of the complete tumor or **lesion** for analysis; 2. **incisional biopsy**, in which a portion of the **lesion** is removed with a scalpel; 3. **punch biopsy**, which is removal of a small specimen of tissue in the "cookie cutter" fashion, and 4. **shave biopsy**, which uses the scalpel or a razor blade to shave lesions elevated above the skin.
skin graft	A process of placing tissue on a recipient site, taken from a donor site, to provide the protective mechanisms of skin to an area unable to regenerate skin (as in third-degree burns).

Skin grafting is successful when the base of the wound aids the donor tissue in developing a new blood supply and is found to be effective in wounds:

1. that are free of infection,

2. that have a good blood supply, and

3. in which bleeding can be controlled.

Full-thickness (both **epidermis** and **dermis**) or split-thickness (**epidermis** with a segment of **dermis**) grafts may be used. Types of grafting include:

1. **autografting**, in which the donor tissue comes from the person receiving the graft (transplanting tissue from one part of the body to another location in the same individual),

2. **homografting** or **allografting**, in which the donor tissue is harvested from a cadaver, and

3. **heterograft** or **xenograft**, in which the donor tissue is obtained from an animal.

Wood's lamp	An ultraviolet light used to examine the scalp and skin for the purpose of observing fungal spores.

The light causes hairs infected with a fungus, such as ringworm of the scalp (**tinea capitis**), to appear as a bright fluorescent blue-green color; also called Wood's light, black light, or Wood's rays.

The procedure is performed in a darkened room, and the light beam is focused on the affected area. If the fungal spores are present, they will appear brilliantly fluorescent (as described).

Review Checkpoint

Check your understanding of this section by completing the **Diagnostic Techniques, Treatments, and Procedures** exercises in your workbook.

COMMON ABBREVIATIONS

Abbreviation	Meaning	Abbreviation	Meaning
Bx, bx	biopsy	PPD	purified protein derivative
decub.	decubitus (ulcer); pressure sore	PSS	progressive systemic scleroderma
DLE	discoid lupus erythematosus		
EAHF	eczema, asthma, and hay fever	SLE	systemic lupus erythematosus
FANA	fluorescent antinuclear antibody	subq.	subcutaneous
		TENS	transcutaneous electrical nerve stimulation
FS	frozen section		
ID	intradermal	ung.	ointment
I&D	incision and drainage	UV	ultraviolet (light)
LE	(systemic) lupus erythematosus	XP, XDP	xeroderma pigmentosum

Review Checkpoint

Check your understanding of this section by completing the **Common Abbreviations** exercises in your workbook.

WRITTEN AND AUDIO TERMINOLOGY REVIEW

Review each of the following terms from this chapter. Study the spelling of each term, and write the definition in the space provided. Check definitions by looking the term up in the glossary.

Term	Pronunciation	Definition
abrasion	☐ ah-**BRAY**-zhun	_____
abscess	☐ **AB**-sess	_____
acne vulgaris	☐ **ACK**-nee vul-**GAY**-ris	_____
actinic keratosis	☐ ak-**TIN**-ic **kerr**-ah-**TOH**-sis	_____

Term	Pronunciation	Definition
adipofibroma	☐ **add**-ih-poh-fib-**BROH**-mah	_____
albinism	☐ **AL**-bin-izm	_____
alopecia	☐ **al**-oh-**PEE**-she-ah	_____
amputation	☐ **am**-pew-**TAY**-shun	_____
basal cell carcinoma	☐ **BAY**-sal sell **kar**-sih-**NOH**-mah	_____
basal layer	☐ **BAY**-sal layer	_____
bulla	☐ **BULL**-ah	_____
callus	☐ **CAL**-us	_____
carbuncle	☐ **CAR**-**bung**-kul	_____
cautery	☐ **KAW**-ter-ree	_____
cellulitis	☐ sell-yoo-**LYE**-tis	_____
cerumen	☐ seh-**ROO**-men	_____
ceruminous gland	☐ seh-**ROO**-mih-nus gland	_____
cicatrix	☐ sik-**AY**-trix or **SIK**-ah-trix	_____
collagen	☐ **KOL**-ah-jen	_____
comedo	☐ **KOM**-ee-doh	_____
condyloma acuminata	☐ **con**-dih-**LOH**-mah ah-**kew**-min-**AH**-tah	_____
contusion	☐ kon-**TOO**-zhun	_____
corium	☐ **KOH**-ree-um	_____
cryosurgery	☐ **cry**-oh-**SER**-jer-ee	_____
curettage	☐ **kyoo**-reh-**TAHZH**	_____
curettage and electrodesiccation	☐ **kew**-reh-**TAHZH** and ee-**lek**-troh-**des**-ih-**KAY**-shun	_____
cyanosis	☐ **sigh**-ah-**NOH**-sis	_____
cyst	☐ **SIST**	_____
debridement	☐ dah-**BREED**-ment	_____
dermabrasion	☐ **der**-mah-**BRAY**-zhun	_____
dermatitis	☐ **der**-mah-**TYE**-tis	_____
dermatology	☐ **der**-mah-**TOL**-oh-jee	_____
dermatoplasty	☐ **DER**-mah-toh-**plas**-tee	_____
dermis	☐ **DER**-mis	_____

Term	Pronunciation	Definition
diaphoresis	☐ **dye**-ah-foh-**REE**-sis	_____
ecchymosis	☐ **ek**-ih-**MOH**-sis	_____
eczema	☐ **EK**-zeh-mah	_____
electrodesiccation	☐ ee-**lek**-troh-**des**-ih-**KAY**-shun	_____
electrosurgery	☐ ee-**lek**-troh-**SIR**-jeh-ree	_____
epidermis	☐ **ep**-ih-**DER**-mis	_____
epithelium	☐ **ep**-ih-**THEE**-lee-um	_____
erythema	☐ **eh**-rih-**THEE**-mah	_____
erythralgia	☐ **eh**-rih-**THRAL**-jee-ah	_____
erythremia	☐ **er**-ih-**THREE**-mee-ah	_____
erythroderma	☐ eh-**rith**-roh-**DER**-mah	_____
escharotomy	☐ es-**kar**-**OT**-oh-mee	_____
exanthematous viral diseases	☐ **eks**-an-**THEM**-ah-tus **VYE**-ral dih-**ZEEZ**-ez	_____
excoriation	☐ eks-**koh**-ree-**AY**-shun	_____
exfoliation	☐ **eks**-foh-lee-**AY**-shun	_____
fissure	☐ **FISH**-ur	_____
fistula	☐ **FISS**-tyoo-lah	_____
fulguration	☐ ful-goo-**RAY**-shun	_____
furuncle	☐ **FYOO**-rung-kul	_____
gangrene	☐ **GANG**-green	_____
hemangioma	☐ hee-**man**-jee-**OH**-mah	_____
heparin	☐ **HEP**-er-in	_____
herpes zoster	☐ **HER**-peez **ZOS**-ter	_____
hidrosis	☐ high-**DROH**-sis	_____
hirsutism	☐ **HER**-soot-izm	_____
histamine	☐ **HISS**-tah-min _or_ **HISS**-tah-meen	_____
histiocyte	☐ **HISS**-tee-oh-sight	_____
histology	☐ hiss-**TOL**-oh-jee	_____
hydrocele	☐ **HIGH**-droh-seel	_____
ichthyosis	☐ **ik**-thee-**OH**-sis	_____
impetigo	☐ im-peh-**TYE**-goh _or_ im-peh-**TEE**-goh	_____

Term	Pronunciation	Definition
integument	☐ in-**TEG**-you-ment	_____
integumentary system	☐ in-**teg**-you-**MEN**-tah-ree **SIS**-tem	_____
Kaposi's sarcoma	☐ **CAP**-oh-seez sar-**KOH**-mah	_____
keloid	☐ **KEE**-loyd	_____
keratin	☐ **KAIR**-ah-tin	_____
keratolytic	☐ **kair**-ah-toh-**LIT**-ic	_____
keratosis	☐ **kerr**-ah-**TOH**-sis	_____
laceration	☐ **lass**-er-**AY**-shun	_____
lanugo	☐ lan-**NOO**-go	_____
lesion	☐ **LEE**-zhun	_____
leukoderma	☐ **loo**-koh-**DER**-mah	_____
leukoplakia	☐ **loo**-koh-**PLAY**-kee-ah	_____
lipedema	☐ **lip**-eh-**DEE**-mah	_____
lipocyte	☐ **LIP**-oh-sight	_____
lipohypertrophy	☐ **lip**-oh-high-**PER**-troh-fee	_____
liposuction	☐ **LIP**-oh-**suck**-shun	_____
lunula	☐ **LOO**-noo-lah	_____
macule	☐ **MACK**-yool	_____
malignant melanoma	☐ mah-**LIG**-nant **mel**-ah-**NOH**-mah	_____
melanin	☐ **MEL**-an-in	_____
melanocytes	☐ mel-**AN**-oh-sightz *or* **MEL**-an-oh-sightz	_____
mycosis	☐ my-**KOH**-sis	_____
necrotizing fasciitis	☐ **NECK**-roh-tiz-ing **fas**-ee-**EYE**-tis	_____
nevus	☐ **NEE**-vus	_____
nodule	☐ **NOD**-yool	_____
onychocryptosis	☐ **on**-ih-koh-krip-**TOH**-sis	_____
onychogryposis	☐ **on**-ih-koh-grih-**POH**-sis	_____
onycholysis	☐ **on**-ih-**KOL**-ih-sis	_____
onychomycosis	☐ **on**-ih-koh-my-**KOH**-sis	_____
onychophagia	☐ **on**-ih-koh-**FAY**-jee-ah	_____

Term	Pronunciation	Definition
pachyderma	☐ **pak**-ee-**DER**-mah	_____
papule	☐ **PAP**-yool	_____
pediculosis	☐ pee-**dik**-you-**LOH**-sis	_____
pemphigus	☐ **PEM**-fih-gus	_____
petechia	☐ pee-**TEE**-kee-ah	_____
pilonidal cyst	☐ **pye**-loh-**NYE**-dal cyst	_____
plantar warts	☐ **PLAN**-tar warts	_____
polyp	☐ **POL**-ip	_____
pruritus	☐ proo-**RYE**-tus	_____
psoriasis	☐ soh-**RYE**-ah-sis	_____
purpura	☐ **PER**-pew-rah	_____
pustule	☐ **PUS**-tyool	_____
rosacea	☐ roh-**ZAY**-she-ah	_____
scabies	☐ **SKAY**-beez	_____
scleroderma	☐ **sklair**-oh-**DER**-mah	_____
sebaceous cyst	☐ see-**BAY**-shus **SIST**	_____
seborrhea	☐ **seb**-or-**EE**-ah	_____
seborrheic dermatitis	☐ **seb**-oh-**REE**-ik der-mah-**TYE**-tis	_____
seborrheic keratoses	☐ **seb**-oh-**REE**-ik **kair**-ah-**TOH**-seez	_____
seborrheic warts	☐ **seb**-oh-**REE**-ik warts	_____
sebum	☐ **SEE**-bum	_____
skin biopsy	☐ skin **BYE**-op-see	_____
squamous cell carcinoma	☐ **SKWAY**-mus sell **kar**-sih-**NOH**-mah	_____
squamous epithelium	☐ **SKWAY**-mus ep-ih-**THEE**-lee-um	_____
stratified	☐ **STRAT**-ih-fyed	_____
stratum	☐ **STRAT**-um	_____
stratum basale	☐ **STRAT**-um **BAY**-sil	_____
stratum corneum	☐ **STRAT**-um **COR**-nee-um	_____
subcutaneous tissue	☐ **sub**-kew-**TAY**-nee-us tissue	_____
subungual hematoma	☐ sub-**UNG**-gwall hee-mah-**TOH**-mah	_____
sudoriferous gland	☐ soo-door-**IF**-er-us gland	_____

Term	Pronunciation	Definition
systemic lupus erythematosus	☐ sis-**TEM**-ic **LOO**-pus air-ih-them-ah-**TOH**-sus	_____
tinea	☐ **TIN**-ee-ah	_____
tinea capitis	☐ **TIN**-ee-ah **CAP**-ih-tis	_____
tinea corporis	☐ **TIN**-ee-ah **COR**-poh-ris	_____
tinea cruris	☐ **TIN**-ee-ah **KROO**-ris	_____
tinea pedis	☐ **TIN**-ee-ah **PED**-is	_____
trichiasis	☐ trik-**EYE**-ah-sis	_____
ulcer	☐ **ULL**-ser	_____
urticaria	☐ er-tih-**KAIR**-ree-ah	_____
verruca	☐ ver-**ROO**-kah	_____
vesicle	☐ **VESS**-ih-kul	_____
vitiligo	☐ **vit**-ih-**LYE**-goh	_____
wheal	☐ **WHEEL**	_____
xanthoderma	☐ **zan**-thoh-**DER**-mah	_____
xanthosis	☐ zan-**THOS**-sis	_____
xeroderma	☐ **zee**-roh-**DER**-mah	_____

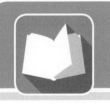

Review Checkpoint

Apply what you have learned in this chapter by completing the **Putting It All Together** exercise in your workbook.

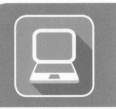

Online Resources

For additional study tools, including PowerPoint® slides and animations, go to the Student Companion Website.

Chapter Review Exercises

The following exercises provide a more in-depth review of the chapter material. Your goal in these exercises is to complete each section at a minimum 80% level of accuracy. A space has been provided for your score at the end of each section.

A. Spelling

Circle the correctly spelled term in each pairing of words. Each correct answer is worth 10 points. Record your score in the space provided at the end of the exercise.

1.	alopecia	alopeshea	6.	petechii	petechia
2.	eccymosis	ecchymosis	7.	pruritus	pruritis
3.	gangreen	gangrene	8.	sudoriferous	sudoiferous
4.	hirsutism	hirtsutism	9.	xanthoderma	zanthoderma
5.	icthyosis	ichthyosis	10.	histocyte	histiocyte

Number correct _____ × *10 points/correct answer: Your score* _____ *%*

B. Term to Definition

Define each term by writing the definition in the space provided. Check the box if you are able to complete this exercise correctly the first time (without referring to the answers). Each correct answer is worth 10 points. Record your score in the space provided at the end of the exercise.

☐ 1. pruritus _____

☐ 2. vitiligo _____

☐ 3. sudoriferous gland _____

☐ 4. onycholysis _____

☐ 5. keratin _____

☐ 6. hirsutism _____

☐ 7. erythema _____

☐ 8. exfoliation _____

☐ 9. ecchymosis _____

☐ 10. cellulitis _____

Number correct _____ × *10 points/correct answer: Your score* _____ *%*

C. Matching Abbreviations

Match the abbreviations on the left with the applicable definition on the right. Each correct response is worth 10 points. Record your score in the space provided at the end of the exercise.

_____	1. Bx	a.	ointment
_____	2. decub.	b.	dermatology
_____	3. TENS	c.	purified protein derivative
_____	4. PPD	d.	fluorescent antinuclear antibody

_____ 5. FANA   e. subcutaneous

_____ 6. FS   f. frozen section

_____ 7. ID   g. ultraviolet (light)

_____ 8. SLE   h. decubitus ulcer; bedsore

_____ 9. PSS   i. progressive systemic scleroderma

_____ 10. ung.   j. biopsy

                      k. transcutaneous electric nerve stimulation

                      l. systemic lupus erythematosus

                      m. intradermal

Number correct _____ *× 10 points/correct answer: Your score* _____ *%*

D. Crossword Puzzle

Each crossword answer is worth 10 points. When you have completed the crossword puzzle, total your points and enter your score in the space provided.

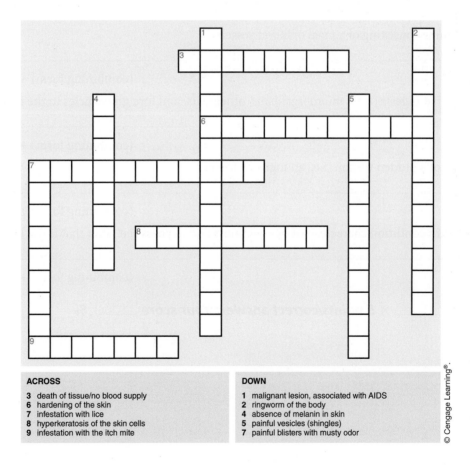

ACROSS

3 death of tissue/no blood supply
6 hardening of the skin
7 infestation with lice
8 hyperkeratosis of the skin cells
9 infestation with the itch mite

DOWN

1 malignant lesion, associated with AIDS
2 ringworm of the body
4 absence of melanin in skin
5 painful vesicles (shingles)
7 painful blisters with musty odor

© Cengage Learning®.

Number correct _____ *× 10 points/correct answer: Your score* _____ *%*

E. Definition to Term

Identify and provide the medical term to match the following definitions. Write the term in the first space and the applicable combining form for the word in the second space. Each correct answer is worth 5 points. Record your score in the space provided at the end of the exercise.

1. Inflammation of the skin

   _____   _____
   (word)   (combining form)

2. Condition of bluish discoloration

   _____   _____
   (word)   (combining form)

3. Layer of skin immediately beneath the epidermis

   _____   _____
   (word)   (combining form)

4. Abnormal increase in the number of red blood cells (hint: "blood condition")

   _____   _____
   (word)   (combining form)

5. Benign tumor consisting of a mass of blood vessels

   _____   _____
   (word)   (combining form) + (combining form)

6. Large cell that ingests (eats) microorganisms, other cells, and foreign particles in the blood vessels

   _____   _____
   (word)   (combining form) + (combining form)

7. Condition of a hidden toenail (i.e., an ingrown toenail)

   _____   _____
   (word)   (combining form) + (combining form)

8. Chronic skin condition characterized by roughness and dryness (i.e., skin that is dry)

   _____   _____
   (word)   (combining form) + (combining form)

Number correct _____ × *5 points/correct answer: Your score* _____ %

F. Labeling

Label the following structures of the skin and nails by writing your answers in the spaces provided. Each correct answer is worth 10 points. When you have completed this exercise, record your score in the space provided at the end of the exercise.

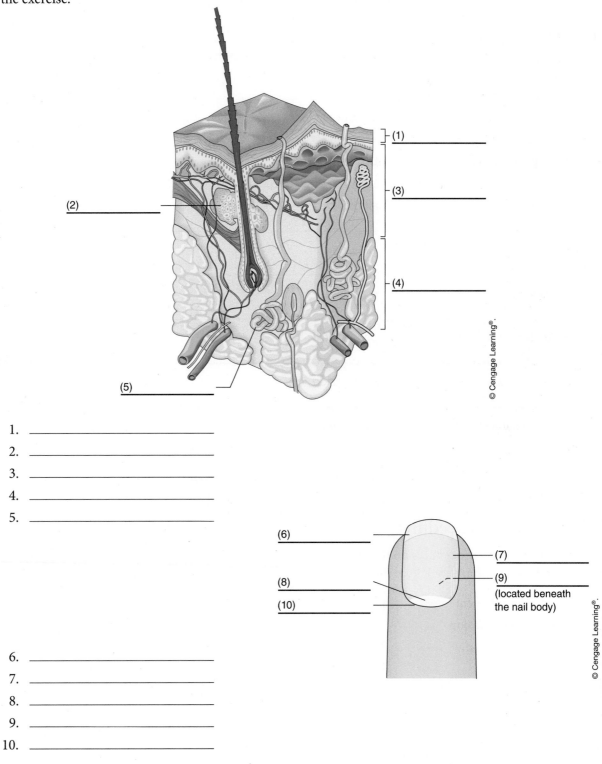

© Cengage Learning®.

1. _____
2. _____
3. _____
4. _____
5. _____

(6) _____
(7) _____
(8) _____
(9) _____
(located beneath the nail body)
(10) _____

© Cengage Learning®.

6. _____
7. _____
8. _____
9. _____
10. _____

Number correct _____ *× 10 points/correct answer: Your score* _____ *%*

G. Identify and Define

Circle the correct spelling of each word and then write the definition for the correctly spelled word in the space provided. Refer to your text for assistance with definitions. Each correct answer is worth 5 points. Record your answer in the space provided at the end of the exercise.

1. psoriasis   poriasis

   _____

2. infantigo   impetigo

   _____

3. cryiosurgery   cryosurgery

   _____

4. hyperkeratosis   hyperkarotosis

   _____

5. albinism   albinoism

   _____

6. gangreen   gangrene

   _____

7. exzema   eczema

   _____

8. pediculosis   peddiculosis

   _____

9. leukaplakia   leukoplakia

   _____

10. melonama (malignant)   melanoma (malignant)

    _____

Number correct _____ × *5 points/correct answer: Your score* _____ *%*

H. Matching Procedures

Match the following procedures on the left with their descriptions on the right. Each correct answer is worth 10 points. When you have completed the exercise, record your score in the space provided at the end of the exercise.

_____ 1. debridement

_____ 2. dermabrasion

_____ 3. escharotomy

_____ 4. cautery

_____ 5. allergy testing

_____ 6. curettage

_____ 7. cryosurgery

_____ 8. electrodesiccation

_____ 9. skin biopsy

a. an incision made into the eschar with a scalpel or by electrocautery for relief of tightness in a person with a burn

b. removal of small pieces of tissue from skin lesions for diagnosis

c. destruction of a tumor base with a low-voltage electrode

d. removal of foreign objects and damaged or necrotic tissue from a wound in order to prevent infection and promote healing

e. a process of placing tissue on a recipient site taken from a donor site

f. scraping away abnormal tissue

g. heat or caustic substances that burn and scar the skin

_____ 10. skin graft

  h. removal of the epidermis and a portion of the dermis with sandpaper or brushes

  i. procedures used to identify specific allergens in an individual by exposing the person to a very small quantity of the allergen

  j. a noninvasive treatment for nonmelanoma skin cancer by using liquid nitrogen

Number correct _____ × 10 points/correct answer: Your score _____ %

I. Completion

The following statements describe various pathological conditions of the integumentary system. Complete each sentence with the most appropriate pathological condition. Each correct answer is worth 10 points. Record your score in the space provided at the end of the exercise.

1. The most common malignant tumor of the epithelial tissue is:

_____

2. An inflammatory skin reaction characterized by intense itching, predisposing the person to secondary infections and long-term chronic lichenification, is known as:

_____

3. Rash or wheals, intense pruritus, and the presence of louse eggs (nits) on the skin, hair shafts, or clothing is known as:

_____

4. An inflammatory disorder (seen on the face, chest, back, and neck) that appears as papules, pustules, and comedos is known as:

_____

5. Skin tumors with irregular surfaces, uneven borders, and variable colors (originating from melanocytes) are known as:

_____

6. Blisters form (with some swelling, involving the epidermis and upper layer of the dermis) that are very sensitive and painful when this condition occurs:

_____

7. The noninfectious chronic disorder of the skin that is manifested by silvery-white scales over round, raised, reddened plaques producing pruritus is:

_____

8. A contagious skin infection characterized by serous vesicles and pustules filled with millions of staphylococci or streptococcal bacteria is known as:

_____

9. A skin cancer with scale-like cells that has a potential for metastasis if not treated is:

_____

10. A condition that involves massive necrosis of the epidermis and entire dermis, and may include part of the subcutaneous tissue, is known as:

_____

Number correct _____ × 10 points/correct answer: Your score _____ %

J. Matching Skin Lesions

Match the skin lesions on the left with the applicable description on the right. Each correct answer is worth 10 points. Record your score in the space provided at the end of the exercise.

_____ 1. abrasion

_____ 2. bulla

_____ 3. fissure

_____ 4. furuncle

_____ 5. macule

_____ 6. polyp

_____ 7. pustule

_____ 8. scales

_____ 9. vesicle

_____ 10. ulcer

a. a circumscribed, open sore or lesion of the skin that is accompanied by inflammation

b. a small elevation of the skin filled with pus

c. a small stalk-like growth that protrudes upward or outward from a mucous membrane surface

d. a blister

e. thin flakes of hardened epithelium that are shed from the epidermis

f. a crack-like sore or groove in the skin or mucous membrane

g. a large blister

h. a small flat discoloration of the skin that is neither raised nor depressed

i. a boil

j. a scraping or rubbing away of skin or mucous membrane as a result of friction to the area

Number correct _____ **× 10 points/correct answer: Your score** _____ **%**

K. Word Search

Read each definition carefully and identify the applicable word from the list that follows. Enter the word in the space provided and then find it in the puzzle and circle it. The words may be read up, down, diagonally, across, or backward. Each correct answer is worth 10 points. Record your score in the space provided at the end of the exercise.

bulla	epidermis	abscess	cuticle
cerumen	cellulitis	fissure	lunula
lipocyte	decubitus	dermatology	

Example: A large blister.

bulla _____

1. A localized collection of pus in any part of the body.

_____

2. An inflammation, sore, or ulcer in the skin over a bony prominence of the body is known as a _____ ulcer; also known as a pressure ulcer.

_____

3. A fold of skin that covers the root of the fingernail or toenail.

_____

4. Another name for earwax.

_____

5. A diffuse, acute infection of the skin and subcutaneous tissues characterized by localized heat, deep redness, pain, and swelling.

_____

6. The term that means "the study of the skin."

_____

7. The outermost layer of the skin.

_____

8. A crack-like sore or groove in the skin or mucous membrane.

_____

9. A fat cell.

_____

10. The crescent-shaped pale area at the base of the fingernail or toenail.

_____

Number correct _____ **× 10 points/correct answer: Your score** _____ **%**

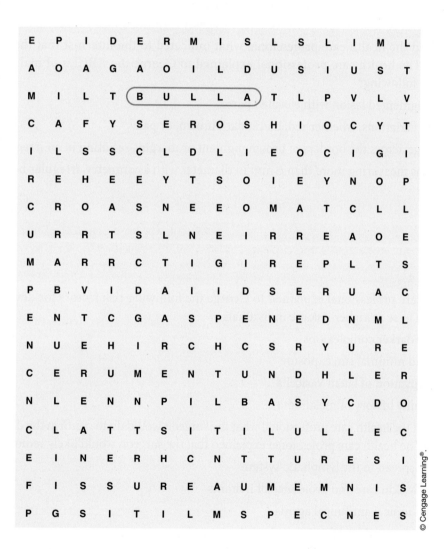

L. Medical Scenario

The following medical scenario presents information on one of the pathological conditions discussed in this chapter. Read the scenario carefully and select the most appropriate answer for each question that follows. Each correct answer is worth 20 points. Record your score in the space provided at the end of the exercise.

George Banister, a 55-year-old patient, visited his internist today for a physical exam. During the visit, George asked the physician about a mole on his back. George's internist is referring him to a surgeon to follow up on

(continued)

removing the lesion because he suspects it to be a malignant melanoma. As George is leaving the office, he asks several questions about malignant melanomas.

1. George asked the health care professional to explain what malignant melanoma means. The best explanation would be:

   a. malignancy of the squamous (or scale-like) cells of the epithelial tissue that is seen most frequently on the top of the nose, forehead, or lower lip

   b. the most common malignant tumor of the epithelial tissue, which rarely metastasizes but tends to recur—especially those that are larger than 2 cm in diameter

   c. a darkly pigmented malignant skin tumor originating from melanocytes in preexisting moles, freckles, or skin pigment with the potential to invade throughout the body to any organ

   d. contagious superficial skin infection characterized by serous vesicles and pustules filled with millions of staphylococcus or streptococcus bacteria, usually forming on the face

2. George asked the health care professional what indicated to the internist that this lesion was likely a melanoma. The health care professional explained to George the ABCDs of malignant melanoma as which of the following?

   1. any flat pigmented lesion with elevated parts

   2. any color variations, whether red, black, dark brown, or pale

   3. any leakage across the borders of brown pigment or margins resulting in an irregular shape

   4. any lesions measuring more than 6 mm in diameter with asymmetry, irregular borders, and color variations

      a. 1, 2

      b. 2, 3

      c. 2, 3, 4

      d. 1, 2, 3, 4

3. The health care professional explained to George the following risk factors for developing a malignant melanoma. Those at higher risk are individuals:

   a. who have darker complexions

   b. having had minimal sun exposure

   c. with reactivation of latent varicella

   d. with a family history of melanoma

4. George asked the health care professional what the surgeon would do to confirm the diagnosis of malignant melanoma. The health care professional explained that the surgeon would likely remove the lesion and:

   a. check for spread to the lymphatic system

   b. stress daily skin care and avoidance of irritants

   c. treat with topical antifungal agents

   d. treat with antivirals, analgesics, and corticosteroids

5. The health care professional explained that if there is evidence of distant metastases, the treatment will most likely include:

   a. aggressive use of corticosteroids

   b. oral antifungal agents that act systemically

   c. chemotherapy and radiation therapy

   d. physiotherapy to maintain and restore musculoskeletal function

Number correct _____ *× 20 points/correct answer: Your score* _____ *%*

M. Proofreading Skills

Example:

dysphagia   *difficulty swallowing*

Spelled correctly?   ☑ Yes   ☐ No _____

Feature Walk-Through

The **Proofreading Skills** exercise gives you practice reading actual medical reports and learning to be aware of potentially misspelled terms. Read the following History and Physical Examination Report. For each **boldface** term, provide a brief definition and then verify the spelling by placing a check mark in the Yes or No box. If the term is misspelled, write the correct spelling. Each correct answer is worth 10 points. Ask your instructor for the answers and then record your score in the space provided at the end of the exercise.

HISTORY AND PHYSICAL EXAMINATION

Hillcrest
medical center

PATIENT NAME: Gloria Ramos

PATIENT ID: 132462

ROOM NO.: 541

DATE OF ADMISSION
06/22/2014

ADMITTING PHYSICIAN
Leon Medina, MD

ADMITTING DIAGNOSIS
Stomatitis, possibly methotrexate related.

CHIEF COMPLAINT
Swelling of lips causing difficulty swallowing.

HISTORY OF PRESENT ILLNESS
This patient is a 57-year-old white Cuban woman with a long history of rheumatoid arthritis. She has received methotrexate on a weekly basis as an outpatient for many years. Approximately 2 weeks ago, she developed a respiratory infection for which she received antibiotics. She developed 1 large **ulcer** and several small ulcerations in her mouth and was instructed to discontinue the methotrexate approximately 10 days ago.

She showed some initial improvement but over the past 3 to 5 days has had malaise, a low-grade fever, and severe oral ulcerations with difficulty in swallowing, although she can drink liquids with less difficulty.

The patient denies any other problems at this point except for a flare-up of arthritis since discontinuing the methotrexate. She has rather diffuse pain involving both large and small joints.

MEDICATIONS
Prednisone 10 mg p.o. daily, Premarin 0.625 mg p.o. daily, and diflunisol 1000 mg p.o. daily, recently discontinued because of questionable allergic reaction. Hydrochlorothiazide 25 mg p.o. every other day. Oral calcium supplements. In the past, she has been on penicillamine, azathioprine, and hydroxychloroquine, but she has not had Azulfidine, cyclophosphamide, or chlorambucil.

(continued)

HISTORY AND PHYSICAL EXAMINATION
Patient Name: Gloria Ramos
Patient ID: 132462
Admission Date: 06/22/2014
Page 2

ALLERGIES
None by history.

FAMILY AND SOCIAL HISTORY
Noncontributory.

PHYSICAL EXAMINATION
GENERAL: This is a chronically ill-appearing female, alert, oriented, and cooperative. She moves with great difficulty because of fatigue and malaise.

VITAL SIGNS: Blood pressure 107/80, heart rate 100 and regular, respirations 22.

HEENT: Normocephalic. No scalp **leisions**. Dry eyes with conjunctival injection. Mild exophthalmos. Dry nasal mucosa. Marked cracking and bleeding of her lips with erosions of the mucosa. She has a large ulceration of the mucosa at the bite margin on the left. She has some scattered ulceration on her hard and soft palate. She has difficulty opening her mouth because of pain.

SKIN: She has an area of mild **ecchymosis** on her skin and some **erythema**; she has some **scales** and **papuels** located on the flexor surfaces of the arms, but no obvious skin breakdown. No vesicles noted on the skin. One small skin **laceration** noted on the left forearm. She has a small **fissher** in the buttocks crease.

PULMONARY: Clear to percussion and auscultation.

CARDIOVASCULAR: No murmurs or gallops noted.

ABDOMEN: Protuberant, no organomegaly, and positive bowel sounds.

NEUROLOGIC EXAM: Cranial nerves II through XII are grossly intact. Diffuse hyporeflexia.

MUSCULOSKELETAL: Erosive, destructive changes in the elbows, wrists, and hands consistent with rheumatoid arthritis. She also has bilateral total knee replacements with stovepipe legs and perimalleolar pitting edema 2+. I feel no pulses distally in either leg.

PROBLEMS
1. Swelling of lips and **dysphagia** with questionable early Stevens-Johnson syndrome.
2. Rheumatoid arthritis, class III, stage IV.
3. Flare-up of arthritis after discontinuing methotrexate.
4. Osteoporosis with compression fracture.
5. Mild dehydration.
6. Nephrolithiasis.

PLAN
Patient is admitted for IV hydration and treatment of oral ulcerations. We will obtain a **dermatology** consult. IV leucovorin will be started, and the patient will be put on high-dose corticosteroids.

Leon Medina, MD

LM:xx

D:06/22/2014

T:06/23/2014

1. **ulcer** _____

_____

Spelled Correctly?   ☐ Yes   ☐ No _____

2. **leisions** _____

_____

Spelled Correctly?   ☐ Yes   ☐ No _____

3. **ecchymosis** _____

_____

Spelled Correctly?   ☐ Yes   ☐ No _____

4. **erythema** _____

_____

Spelled Correctly?   ☐ Yes   ☐ No _____

5. **scales** _____

_____

Spelled Correctly?   ☐ Yes   ☐ No _____

6. **papuels** _____

_____

Spelled Correctly?   ☐ Yes   ☐ No _____

7. **vesicles** _____

_____

Spelled Correctly?   ☐ Yes   ☐ No _____

8. **laceration** _____

_____

Spelled Correctly?   ☐ Yes   ☐ No _____

9. **fissher** _____

_____

Spelled Correctly?   ☐ Yes   ☐ No _____

10. **dermatology** _____

_____

Spelled Correctly?   ☐ Yes   ☐ No _____

Number correct _____ *× 10 points/correct answer: Your score* _____ *%*

CHAPTER CONTENT

OBJECTIVES

Upon completing this chapter and the review exercises at the end of the chapter, the learner should be able to:

1. Identify five functions of the skeletal system.

2. Identify four classifications of bones.

3. Correctly identify 10 different bone markings.

4. Correctly identify at least 10 major bones of the body by labeling the skeletal diagram provided in the chapter review exercises.

5. Define at least 10 pathological conditions of the skeletal system.

6. Identify and define at least 10 different types of bone fractures.

7. Correctly spell and pronounce terms listed on the Written and Audio Terminology Review, using the phonetic pronunciations provided.

8. Correctly construct words relating to the skeletal system.

9. Identify at least 10 abbreviations common to the skeletal system.

Overview

The thigh bone's connected to the knee bone, the knee bone's connected to the leg bone, the leg bone's connected to the ankle bone, and on, and on, and on. . . . If you've ever heard the words of the song about "them bones," you will often be reminded of it as you discuss the skeletal system. You will also discover that in the human skeleton the thigh bone (**femur**) *is* connected to the knee bone (**patella**), and the knee bone *is* connected to the leg bone (**fibula** and the **tibia**), and on, and on, and on . . . !

The human skeleton, which consists of 206 bones, performs several important functions. First, the bones of the skeleton serve as the supporting framework of the body. They provide shape and alignment to the body and support to the soft tissues. Second, the hard bones of the skeleton protect the vital internal organs from injury. The brain, for example, is protected by the bones of the skull—and the spinal cord is protected by the bones of the **vertebrae**. Third, the skeleton plays an important role in movement by providing points of attachment for muscles, ligaments, and tendons. This connection of muscles to bones allows for movement of the jointed bones as the muscles contract or relax. Fourth, the bones of the skeleton serve as a reservoir for storing minerals. The principal minerals stored in the bone are calcium and phosphorus. Fifth, the red marrow of the bones is responsible for blood cell formation. This process of blood cell formation is known as **hematopoiesis**.

The bones of the skeleton are classified according to their shape as long, short, flat, irregular, or sesamoid. **Long bones** are longer than they are wide, with distinctively shaped ends. Examples of long bones are the bones of the upper arm (**humerus**), lower arm (**radius** and **ulna**), thigh (**femur**), lower leg (**tibia** and **fibula**), and the fingers and toes (**phalanges**). **Short bones** are about as long as they are wide, with a somewhat box-shaped structure. Examples of short bones are the bones of the wrist (**carpals**) and the ankle (**tarsals**). **Flat bones** are broad and thin, having a flat (sometimes curved) surface. Examples of flat bones are the breastbone (sternum), ribs, shoulder blade (scapula), and pelvis. **Irregular bones** come in various sizes and shapes, and they are often clustered in groups. Examples of irregular bones are the bones of the spinal column (**vertebrae**) and the face. **Sesamoid bones** are unique, irregular bones embedded in the substance of tendons and usually located around a joint. Only the few tendons subjected to compression or unusual exertion-type stress have these bones. The kneecap is a good example of a sesamoid bone. In addition to the kneecap, the most common locations for **sesamoid bones** are around the hand-to-finger joints (metacarpophalangeal joints) and the foot-to-toe joints (metatarsophalangeal joints).

The medical specialty that deals with the prevention and correction of disorders of the musculoskeletal system is **orthopedics**. The physician who specializes in orthopedics is an **orthopedist**. A health care profession that deals with the diagnosis, treatment, and prevention of mechanical disorders of the musculoskeletal system, with special emphasis on the spinal column, is **chiropractic**. Chiropractic treatment uses manipulation of body structures, such as the spinal column, so that pressure on nerves coming from the spinal cord due to displacement of a vertebral body may be relieved. A practitioner certified and licensed to provide chiropractic care is a **chiropractor**.

Anatomy and Physiology

Bone Structure

As we discuss the structure of a long bone, look at *Figure 6-1* to identify each part.

The **(1) diaphysis** is the main shaft-like portion of a long bone. It has a hollow, cylindrical shape and consists of thick compact bone. The **(2) epiphysis** is located at each end of a long bone. The epiphyses have a bulblike shape that provides ample space for muscle attachments. The epiphyseal plate **(3) epiphyseal line** is a layer of cartilage that separates the **diaphysis** from the **epiphysis** of the bone. In children and young adults, the epiphyseal cartilage provides the means for the bone to increase in length. During periods of growth, the epiphyseal cartilage multiplies and thickens, generating new cartilage. When this occurs, the edges of the epiphyseal cartilage nearest the **diaphysis** are replaced by new bony tissue. Because the older cartilage is replaced with new bony tissue, the bone as a whole grows in length. When skeletal growth is complete, the epiphyseal cartilage will have been completely replaced by bone, causing the **epiphyseal line** to disappear on X-rays.

The **(4) periosteum** is the thick white fibrous membrane that covers the surface of the long bone except at joint surfaces (i.e., at the ends of the epiphyses). These joint surfaces are covered with **(5) articular cartilage**. The **articular cartilage** is a thin layer of cartilage that covers the ends of the long bones and the surfaces of the joints.

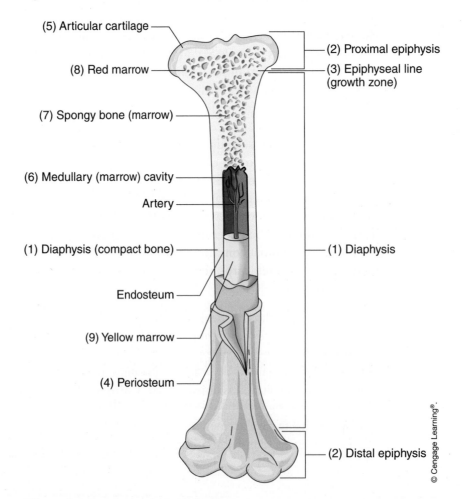

Figure 6-1 Structure of a long bone

Bones differ not only in size and shape but in the types of bone tissue found in them. Look again at *Figure 6-1* as we take a closer look at the structural components of bone.

Compact bone is the hard outer shell of the bone. It lies just under the **periosteum**. The **diaphysis**, or shaft, of a long bone consists of a hollow cylinder of compact bone. Within the center of this hollow area is the **(6) medullary (marrow) cavity**, which contains yellow marrow. Compact bone has a system of small canals (called the **haversian canals**) that extends lengthwise through the bone. The **haversian canals** contain blood vessels, lymphatic vessels, and nerves. The blood vessels transport nutrients and oxygen to the bone cells. **Cancellous bone**, also called **(7) spongy bone** or **trabecular bone**, is not as dense as compact bone. The **trabeculae** are needlelike bony spicules that give the **cancellous bone** its spongy appearance. They are arranged along lines of stress, giving added strength to the bone.

The spaces between the **trabeculae** are filled with **(8) red bone marrow**. It is in the red marrow that blood cell production occurs throughout one's life. In an infant or child, almost all of the bones contain red marrow. In the adult, the bones that still contain red marrow include the ribs, the **vertebrae**, the epiphyses of the **humerus** (upper arm bone) and the **femur** (thigh bone), the sternum (breastbone), and the pelvis. The red marrow that was present in childhood is gradually replaced with yellow marrow as the individual grows into adulthood. The **(9) yellow marrow** stores fat and is not an active site for blood cell production in the adult.

Bone Formation

Now that we know how many bones we have and the structure of bones from the outside to the inner core, let's take it a step further. How are the bones formed?

The bones of the human skeleton begin their formation before birth. They begin as soft, flexible bones consisting of mostly cartilage and fibrous connective tissue. The cartilage and fibrous connective tissue are gradually replaced by stronger calcified bone tissue as the skeleton continues to develop. Calcium salts are deposited into the gel-like matrix of the developing bones through the action of various enzymes, and **osteoblasts** (immature bone cells) actively produce the bony tissue that replaces the cartilage. The conversion of the fibrous connective tissue and cartilage into bone or a bony substance is known as **ossification**.

Bone is living tissue that is constantly being replaced and remodeled throughout life. This constant altering of bones occurs through growth in length and diameter. Earlier we discussed the bone's growth in length, occurring at the **epiphyseal line**. Bones also grow in diameter by the combined action of the **osteoblasts** and the **osteoclasts**. The **osteoclasts** are large cells that digest, or absorb, bony tissue. They help hollow out the central portion of the bone by eating away at—or destroying the old bone tissue from— the inner walls of the **medullary cavity**, thus enlarging the diameter of the **medullary cavity**. This process of removing the old bone tissue, or destroying it so that its components can be absorbed into the circulation, is known as **resorption**. At the same time **resorption** is occurring through the action of the **osteoclasts**, the **osteoblasts** from the inner layer of the **periosteum** are depositing new bone around the outside of the bone. This concurrent process forms a larger bone structure from the smaller one. **Osteoblasts** become mature bone cells when the surrounding intercellular material hardens around them. They are then called **osteocytes** (mature bone cells). These **osteocytes** are living cells that continue to maintain the bone without producing new bone tissue.

Bone Markings

Now that we have discussed the structure and formation of bone, let's examine some of the specific features of individual bones (known as **bone markings**). These markings, which create characteristic features, include enlargements that extend out from the bone and openings or hollow regions within the bone. These areas may serve as points of attachment for muscles and tendons, join one bone to another, or provide cavities and passage for nerves and blood vessels.

Bone processes are projections or outgrowths of bone. They help form joints or serve as points of attachment for muscles and tendons. Here are some of the more commonly known bone processes (see *Figure 6-2*).

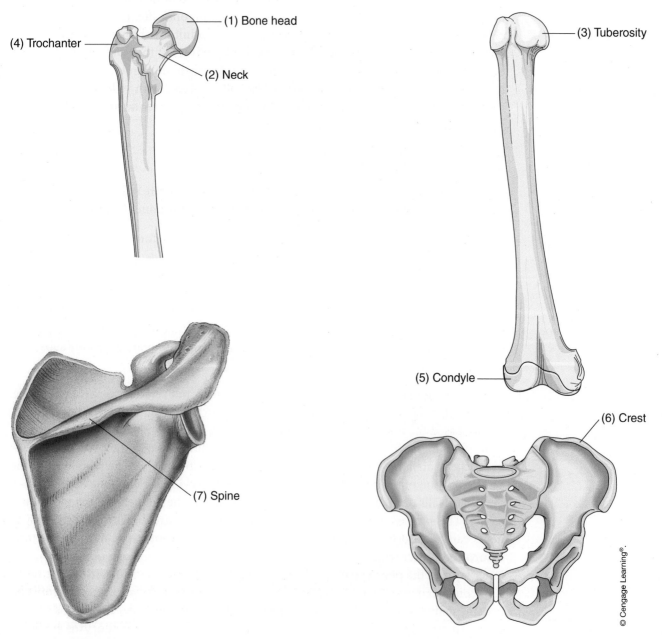

Figure 6-2 Bone processes

(1) bone head	A rounded, knoblike end of a long bone, separated from the shaft of the bone by a narrow portion (the neck of the bone).
(2) neck	A constricted or narrow section that connects with the head, as in the neck connecting to the head or the neck of the **femur**.
(3) **tuberosity** (too-ber-**OSS**-ih-tee)	An elevated, broad, rounded process of a bone—usually for attachment of muscles or tendons.
(4) **trochanter** (tro-**KAN**-ter)	Large bony process located below the neck of the **femur**, for attachment of muscles.
(5) **condyle** (**CON**-dial)	A knucklelike projection at the end of a bone; usually fits into a **fossa** of another bone to form a joint.
(6) **crest**	A distinct border or ridge; an upper elevated edge, as in the upper part of the hip bone (the **iliac** crest); generally a site for muscle attachment.
(7) **spine**	A sharp projection from the surface of a bone, similar to a crest; for example, the spine of the scapula (shoulder blade) used for muscle attachment. **Bone depressions** are concave (indented) areas, or openings, in a bone. They help form joints or serve as points of attachment for muscle.
sulcus (**SULL**-kus)	A groove or depression in a bone; a **fissure**.
sinus (**SIGH**-nus)	An opening or hollow space in a bone, as in the paranasal sinuses or the frontal sinus.
fissure (**FISH**-er)	Same as *sulcus*.
fossa (**FOSS**-ah)	A hollow or shallow concave depression in a bone.
foramen (for-**AY**-men)	A hole within a bone that allows blood vessels or nerves to pass through, as in the **foramen** magnum of the skull that allows the spinal cord to pass through it.

Specific Skeletal Bones

Thus far, we have discussed the structure and formation of bones and their distinguishing markings. Let's now study specific bones of the skeletal system. These bones are discussed in order from the head to the toe, and include the majority of the bones of the skeleton. Throughout this section, refer to the figures for visual reinforcement about the bones being discussed.

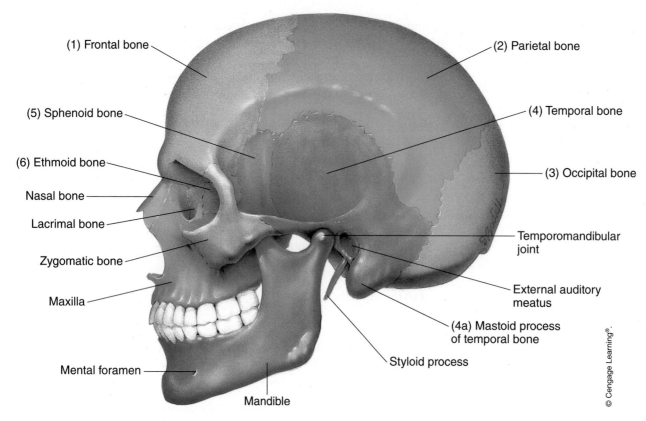

(1) Frontal bone

(2) Parietal bone

(5) Sphenoid bone

(4) Temporal bone

(6) Ethmoid bone

(3) Occipital bone

Nasal bone

Lacrimal bone

Temporomandibular joint

Zygomatic bone

External auditory meatus

Maxilla

(4a) Mastoid process of temporal bone

Mental foramen

Styloid process

Mandible

© Cengage Learning®.

Figure 6-3 Cranial bones

Cranial Bones

The cranium is the bony skull that envelops the brain. It consists of eight bones, which are immovable. The borders of the cranial bones meet to form **sutures**, or immovable joints. Refer to *Figure 6-3* as you study the bones of the cranium.

(1) frontal bone	The frontal bone forms the forehead (front of the skull) and the upper part of the bony cavities that contain the eyeballs. The frontal sinuses are located in this bone, just above the area where the frontal bone joins the nasal bones.
(2) **parietal bones** (pah-**REYE**-eh-tal)	Moving toward the back of the head, just behind the frontal bones ("posterior to the frontal bones") are the two **parietal bones**. They form most of the top and the upper sides of the cranium.
(3) **occipital bone** (ock-**SIP**-ih-tal)	The single **occipital bone** forms the back of the head and the base of the skull (the back portion of the floor of the cranial cavity). The **occipital bone** contains the **foramen** magnum (a large opening in its base), through which the spinal cord passes.
(4) **temporal** bones (**TEM**-por-al)	The two **temporal** bones form the lower sides and part of the base of the skull (cranium). These bones contain the middle and inner ear structures. They also contain the mastoid sinuses. Immediately behind the external part of the ear is the **temporal** bone, which projects downward to form the **(4a) mastoid process**, which serves as a point of attachment for muscles.

(5) sphenoid bone
(**SFEE**-noyd)
sphen/o = wedge
-oid = resembling

The **sphenoid bone** is a bat-shaped bone (resembling a bat with out-stretched wings) located at the base of the skull in front of the **temporal** bones. It extends completely across the middle of the cranial floor, joining with and anchoring the frontal, parietal, occipital, **temporal**, and ethmoid bones. The sphenoid bones form part of the base of the eye orbits.

(6) ethmoid bone
(**ETH**-moyd)

The **ethmoid bone** lies just behind the nasal bone, in front of the **sphenoid bone**. It also forms the front of the base of the skull, part of the eye orbits, and the nasal cavity. The **ethmoid bone** also contains the ethmoid sinuses.

As mentioned, the adult cranial bones are fused by immovable joints known as **sutures**, permitting no movement of the cranial bones. This is different in the newborn. See *Figure 6-4*.

Within the cranial bones of a newborn are two points of union where a space is present between the bones. These spaces are called fontanelles ("soft spots"), also spelled **fontanel**. A **fontanelle** is a space between bones of an infant's cranium that is covered by a tough membrane. The **(1) anterior fontanelle**, also called the **frontal fontanelle**, is the diamond-shaped space between the frontal and the **parietal bones**. It normally closes between 18 and 24 months of age. The **(2) posterior fontanelle**, also called the **occipital fontanelle**, is the space between the **occipital** and **parietal bones** and is much smaller than the anterior **fontanelle**. It normally closes within 2 months after birth.

The fontanelles in the newborn permit the bones of the roof of the skull to override one another during the birth process, narrowing the skull slightly as the head is exposed to the pressures within the birth canal. This may mold the newborn's head into an asymmetrical shape during the birthing process. The head generally assumes its normal shape in a week. The complete **ossification** of the cranial **sutures** (making them immovable joints) does not occur for some years after birth. The cranial bones are held together by fibrous connective tissue until **ossification** occurs, allowing some movement of the infant's skull bones. This feature permits additional growth of the skull to accommodate the normal development of the brain.

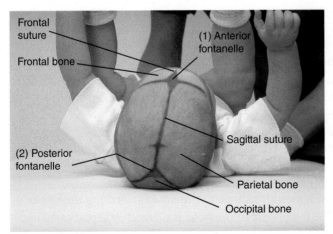
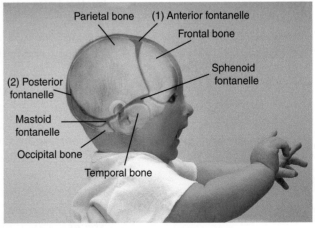

Figure 6-4 Fontanels in the newborn cranium

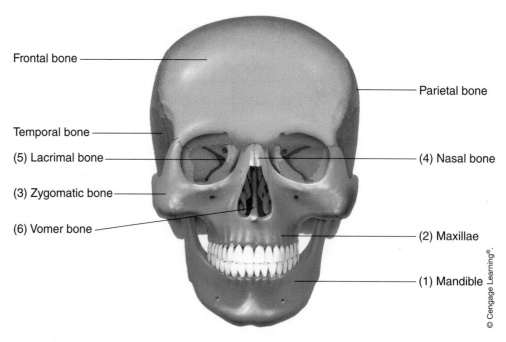

Figure 6-5 Facial bones

Facial Bones

The facial part of the skull is given its distinctive shape by two bones: the maxillae (upper jaw bones) and the mandible (lower jaw bone). These bones and 12 others make up the facial bones. All of the facial bones are connected by immovable joints (**sutures**) with the exception of the mandible (the only movable joint of the skull). Refer to *Figure 6-5* as you study the facial bones.

(1) mandibular bone (man-**DIB**-yoo-lar)	The **mandibular** bone, or mandible, is the lower jaw bone. It is the largest, strongest bone of the face and is the only movable bone of the skull. The **mandibular** bone meets the **temporal** bone in a movable joint called the **temporomandibular joint**, or **TMJ**. The mandible contains sockets for the teeth along its upper margin.
(2) maxillary bones (**MACK**-sih-**ler**-ee)	The two **maxillary** bones (maxillae) are the bones of the upper jaw. They are fused in the midline by a suture. These two bones form not only the upper jaw but the hard palate (front part of the roof of the mouth). The **maxillary** bones contain the **maxillary** sinuses and the sockets for the teeth along the lower margin.
(3) zygomatic bones (zeye-go-**MAT**-ik)	The two **zygomatic** bones—one on each side of the face—form the high part of the cheek and the outer border of the eye orbits.
(4) nasal bones (**NAYZ**-al)	The two slender nasal bones give shape to the nose by forming the upper part of the bridge. The lower part of the nose is formed by septal cartilage. The nasal bones meet at the midline of the face. They also join the frontal bone, the **ethmoid bone**, and the maxillae.

(5) lacrimal bones (**LACK**-rim-al)	The two small **lacrimal bones** are paper thin and shaped somewhat like a fingernail. They are located at the inner corner of each eye, forming the sidewall of the nasal cavity and the middle wall of the eye orbit. The **lacrimal bones** join the cheek bones on each side to form the **fossa**, which houses the tear (or lacrimal) duct.
(6) vomer (**VOH**-mer)	The **vomer** is a thin, flat bone that forms the lower portion of the nasal septum. It joins with the sphenoid, palatine, ethmoid, and **maxillary** bones. Other facial bones that are not shown in the illustration include the following:
palatine bones (**PAL**-ah-tine)	The two **palatine bones** are shaped like the letter L: they have a vertical and a horizontal portion. The vertical portion of the **palatine bones** forms the sidewall of the back of the nasal cavity. The horizontal portion of the **palatine bones** joins in the midline to form the back (posterior) part of the roof of the mouth, or hard palate. The **palatine bones** also join with the maxillae and **sphenoid bone**.
nasal conchae (**NAYZ**-al **KONG**-kee)	The two inferior **nasal conchae** bones help complete the nasal cavity by forming the side and lower wall. These bones connect with the maxilla, lacrimal, ethmoid, and **palatine bones**.

Hyoid Bone

The **hyoid** (**HIGH**-oyd) **bone** is located just above the larynx and below the mandible (see *Figure 6-6*). It does not connect with any other bone to form a joint but is suspended from the **temporal** bone by ligaments. The **hyoid bone** serves as points of attachment for muscles of the tongue and throat.

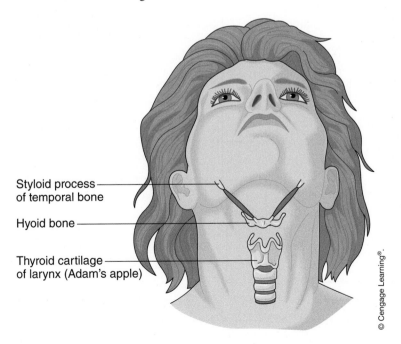

Styloid process
of temporal bone

Hyoid bone

Thyroid cartilage
of larynx (Adam's apple)

© Cengage Learning®.

Figure 6-6 The hyoid bone

Vertebral Bones

The bones of the vertebral column form the long axis of the body. Also referred to as the spinal column or the "backbones," the vertebral column consists of 24 **vertebrae**, the **sacrum**, and the **coccyx**. It offers protection to the spinal cord as it passes through the central opening of each vertebra for the length of the column. The vertebral column (which connects with the skull, the ribs, and the pelvis) is divided into five segments, or divisions. The first three of these segments—the cervical, thoracic, and **lumbar vertebrae**—provide some flexibility in movement to the spinal column because each vertebra is separated by a cartilaginous disk. As you study the divisions of the vertebral column, refer to *Figure 6-7*.

(1) cervical vertebrae

(**SIR**-vih-kal **VER**-teh-bray)

The first segment of the vertebral column is the **cervical vertebrae**, which consists of the first seven bones of the vertebral column. These are neck bones that do not communicate with the ribs. The **cervical vertebrae** are identified specifically as C1 through C7. The first cervical vertebra (which connects the spine with the **occipital bone** of the head) is also known as "atlas," after the Greek god Atlas, who supported the world on his shoulders. The second cervical vertebra is known as "axis" because atlas rotates about this bone, providing the rotating movements of the head.

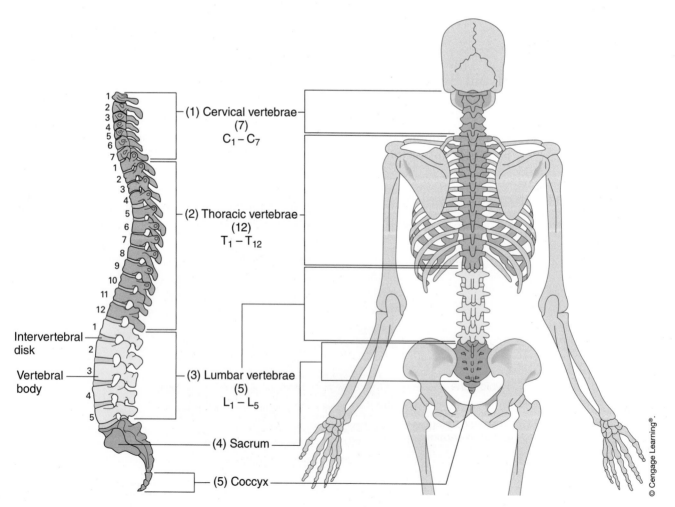

Figure 6-7 Divisions of a vertebral column

(2) thoracic vertebrae (tho-**RASS**-ik **VER**-teh-bray)	Progressing down the vertebral column, the second segment is the **thoracic vertebrae**, consisting of the next 12 **vertebrae**. These **vertebrae** connect with the 12 pairs of ribs and are identified specifically as T1 through T12.
(3) lumbar vertebrae (**LUM**-bar **VER**-teh-bray)	The third segment is the **lumbar vertebrae**, consisting of the next five **vertebrae**. The **lumbar vertebrae** are larger and heavier than the other **vertebrae** and support the back and lower trunk of the body. These **vertebrae** do not communicate with the ribs. They are identified specifically as L1 through L5.
(4) sacrum (**SAY**-crum)	The fourth segment of the vertebral column—the **sacrum**—is located below the **lumbar vertebrae**. The adult **sacrum** is a single triangular-shaped bone that resulted from the fusion of the five individual sacral bones of the child. The **sacrum** is wedged between the two hip bones and is attached to the pelvic girdle.
(5) coccyx (**COCK**-siks)	The fifth segment of the vertebral column is the **coccyx** (also called the "tailbone"), located at the very end of the vertebral column. The adult **coccyx** is a single bone that resulted from the fusion of four individual **coccygeal** bones in the child.

We shall now examine the vertebral column more closely by taking a look at the structure of a vertebra. Refer to *Figure 6-8* as you read.

Although the **vertebrae** within the spinal column vary considerably from segment to segment, they do have basic similarities. For example, each vertebra has a body called the **(1) vertebral body**. This thick anterior portion of the vertebra is drum-shaped and serves as the weight-bearing part of the spinal column. Each of the vertebral bodies of the spinal column is separated by a disk of cartilage called the **intervertebral disk**. These cartilaginous disks are flat, circular, platelike structures that serve as shock absorbers (or cushions) between the vertebral bodies. The disks also provide some flexibility to the spinal column. With the exception of the **sacrum** and the **coccyx**, the center of each vertebra contains a large opening called the **(2) vertebral foramen**, which serves as a passageway for the spinal cord. The vertebral column, as a unit, forms a bony spinal canal that protects the spinal cord. The posterior part of the vertebra is called the **(3) vertebral arch**, which consists of a **(4) spinous process** projecting from the midline of the back of the vertebral arch; a **(5) transverse process**, which extends laterally from the vertebral arch; and a space between the transverse process and the spinous process

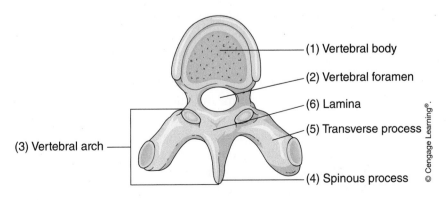

(3) Vertebral arch

(1) Vertebral body

(2) Vertebral foramen

(6) Lamina

(5) Transverse process

(4) Spinous process

© Cengage Learning®.

Figure 6-8 Structure of a thoracic vertebra

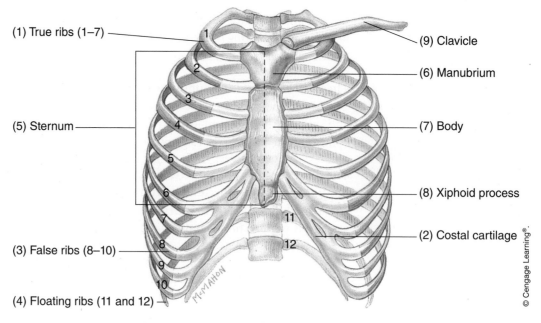

(1) True ribs (1–7)

(5) Sternum

(3) False ribs (8–10)

(4) Floating ribs (11 and 12)

(9) Clavicle

(6) Manubrium

(7) Body

(8) Xiphoid process

(2) Costal cartilage

© Cengage Learning®.

Figure 6-9 Bones of the thorax

known as the **(6) lamina**. The spinous and transverse processes of the **vertebrae** serve as points of attachment for muscles and ligaments.

Bones of the Thorax

The bones that create the shape of the thoracic cavity (chest cavity) are the ribs and the sternum, with the **thoracic vertebrae** forming the center back support. As you study these bones, refer to *Figure 6-9.*

The 12 pairs of ribs that shape the thorax are divided into three categories: true ribs, false ribs, and floating ribs. The **(1) true ribs** are the first seven pairs of ribs (ribs 1 through 7). They are called true ribs because they attach to the sternum in the front and to the **vertebrae** in the back. The ribs attach to the sternum by means of **(2) costal cartilage**, which extends from each individual rib. The **(3) false ribs** consist of the next three pairs of ribs (ribs 8 through 10). They have the name false ribs because they connect in the back to the **vertebrae** but not with the sternum in the front. Instead, they attach to the cartilage of the rib above (the seventh rib). The last two pairs of ribs (11 and 12) are called **(4) floating ribs**. Although these ribs attach to the **vertebrae** in the back, they are completely free of attachment in the front. The spaces between the ribs (called the intercostal spaces) contain the blood vessels, nerves, and muscles.

The **(5) sternum** is also called the breastbone. It is a flat, elongated bone (somewhat sword-shaped) that forms the midline portion of the front of the thorax. The broad upper end of the sternum is called the **(6) manubrium**. It connects with each clavicle (collarbone), whereas the sides of the manubrium connect with the first pair of ribs. The elongated **(7) body** of the sternum connects on its sides with the second through seventh pair of ribs. The lower portion of the sternum is called the **(8) xiphoid process**. The **(9) clavicle**, also called the collarbone, is a slender bone with two shallow curves that helps support the shoulder by connecting laterally to the scapula and anteriorly to the sternum.

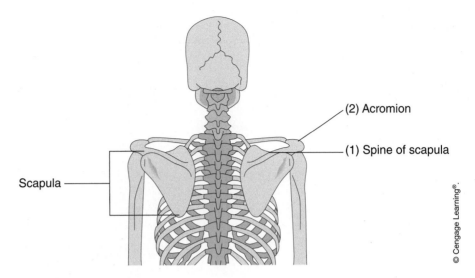

(2) Acromion

(1) Spine of scapula

Scapula

© Cengage Learning®.

Figure 6-10 The scapula

The **scapula**, a large, triangular-shaped bone, is also called the shoulder blade (see *Figure 6-10*). The portion of the scapula that can be felt in the back, behind the shoulder, is the raised ridge called the **(1) spine**. This area serves as points of attachment for muscles. The **(2) acromion** is the somewhat spoon-shaped projection of the scapula that connects with the clavicle to form the highest point of the shoulder.

Bones of the Upper Extremities

The bones of the upper extremities, shown in *Figure 6-11*, include the following.

(1) humerus (**HYOO**-mer-us)	The **humerus** is the upper arm bone. It joins the scapula above and the **radius** and **ulna** below.
(2) radius (**RAY**-dee-us)	The **radius** is one of the two lower arm bones that joins the **humerus** above and the wrist bones below. It is on the lateral, or thumb, side of the arm.
(3) ulna (**UHL**-nah)	The **ulna** is the second of the two lower arm bones that joins the **humerus** above and the wrist bones below. It is on the medial, or little finger, side of the arm. The **ulna** has a large projection at its end called the **olecranon** process. It is the **olecranon** that forms the point of the elbow.
(4) carpals (**CAR**-pals)	The bones of the wrist are known as the **carpals**. Each wrist has eight carpal bones (two rows of four bones each).
(5) metacarpals (met-ah-**CAR**-pals)	The bones of the hand are known as the **metacarpals**. They form the bones of the hand. The word *metacarpal* literally means "beyond the carpals." The **metacarpals** join with the **carpals** at their upper (proximal) end, and with the **phalanges** (fingers) at their lower (distal) end.
(6) phalanges (fah-**LAN**-jeez)	The bones of the fingers are known as the **phalanges** (as are the bones of the toes). Each finger has three phalangeal bones. The thumb has only two.

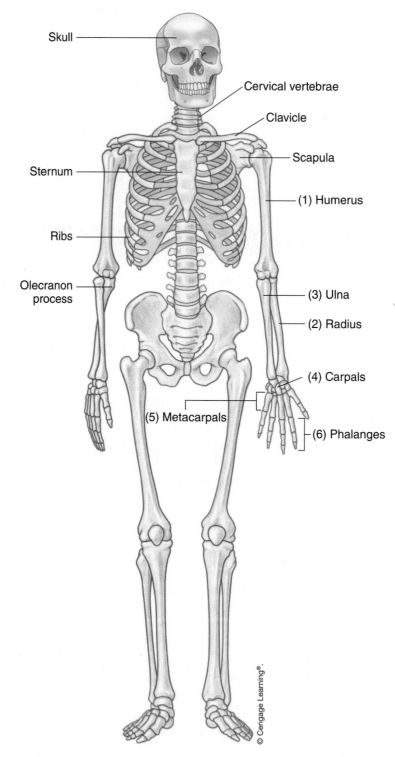

Skull

Cervical vertebrae

Clavicle

Scapula

Sternum

(1) Humerus

Ribs

Olecranon
process

(3) Ulna

(2) Radius

(4) Carpals

(5) Metacarpals

(6) Phalanges

© Cengage Learning®.

Figure 6-11 Bones of the upper extremities

Pelvic Bones

The **pelvis**, shown in *Figure 6-12*, is the bony structure formed by the hip bones (the ilium, ischium, and pubis), the **sacrum**, and the **coccyx**. The pelvis is the lower part of the trunk of the body and serves as a support for the vertebral column and as a connection with the lower extremities. The term *pelvic girdle* refers to the bony ring formed by the hip bones, the **sacrum**, and the **coccyx**—the bony ring that forms the walls of the pelvis.

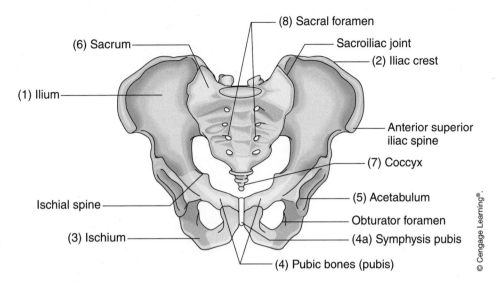

Figure 6-12 Bones of the pelvis

If you place your hand just below your waist, on your hip, the bone your hand is resting on is the ilium. The **(1) ilium** is the largest of the three hip bones. It is the upper flared portion of the hip bones. The **(2) iliac crest** is the upper curved edge of the ilium. The **iliac crest** has an anterior projection (toward the front of the body) called the **anterior iliac crest**, or the **anterior iliac spine**. It also has a posterior projection that is not as prominent. As you look at the illustration, notice the broad shape of the ilium. This flat bone is a good source for red bone marrow, as we studied earlier.

The **(3) ischium** is the lowest part of the hip bones and is the strongest of the pelvic bones. If you are sitting in a chair as you read this material, the bony part of your body that rests on the seat of the chair is your ischium (unless, of course, you are sitting on your feet!). The ischium has a projection on either side, at the back of the pelvic outlet, known as the **ischial** spine. The **ischial** spine takes on a great degree of importance in determining the adequacy of the diameter of the pelvic outlet for childbirth. It also serves as a point of reference in relation to how far a baby's head has progressed down the birth canal during labor.

The pubis is the anterior (front) part of the hip bones. The two bones of the pubis meet at the anterior midline of the pelvis and are connected by a cartilaginous joint. This point of connection of the two **(4) pubic** bones is called the **(4a) symphysis pubis**.

Segments of the ilium, ischium, and pubis form the **(5) acetabulum**, which is the socket that serves as the connecting point for the **femur** (thigh bone) and the hip. This is also known as the hip joint. The **(6) sacrum** and the **(7) coccyx** are actually part of the vertebral column and have been discussed earlier. They are, however, noted in *Figure 6-12* to show their correlation with the pelvis. The small openings in the fused segments of the **sacrum** through which the sacral nerves pass are known as the **(8) sacral foramen**.

Bones of the Lower Extremities

As you study the bones of the lower extremities, refer to *Figure 6-13* for a visual reference. The bones of the lower extremities include the following.

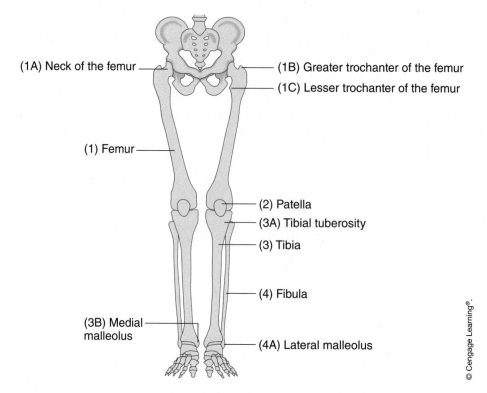

(1A) Neck of the femur
(1B) Greater trochanter of the femur
(1C) Lesser trochanter of the femur
(1) Femur
(2) Patella
(3A) Tibial tuberosity
(3) Tibia
(4) Fibula
(3B) Medial malleolus
(4A) Lateral malleolus

© Cengage Learning®.

Figure 6-13 Bones of the lower extremities

(1) femur (**FEE**-mer)	The **femur** is the thigh bone. It is the longest, heaviest, and strongest bone in the body. The proximal end of the **femur** (the end nearest the pelvis) has a large rounded head (somewhat ball-shaped) that fits into the acetabulum of the hip bones, forming the hip joint. The (1A) neck of the **femur** connects the head with the shaft of the bone. The (1B) greater **trochanter** is the large lateral projection at the point where the neck and the shaft meet. This projection, and the (1C) lesser **trochanter**, serves as a site for muscle attachment. The greater **trochanter** takes on significant importance as a landmark when selecting the site for the ventrogluteal intramuscular injection.
(2) patella (pah-**TELL**-ah)	The **patella** is the knee bone, or kneecap. It is the largest sesamoid bone in the body. Located in the tendon of the large anterior thigh muscle (quadriceps femoris), the **patella** covers and protects the knee joint, which is the point of connection between the thigh bone (**femur**) and one of the lower leg bones (**tibia**).
(3) tibia (**TIB**-ee-ah)	The **tibia** is the larger and stronger of the two lower leg bones. Also called the shin bone, the **tibia** is located on the great toe side of the lower leg. If you move your hand down the center front of your lower leg, you will feel the sharp anterior crest of the **tibia**. The proximal end of the **tibia** connects with the **femur** to form the knee joint. The (3A) tibial **tuberosity** serves as an anchoring point for the tendons of the muscles from the thigh (those that enclose the **patella**). The distal end of the **tibia** connects with the tarsal bones. It has a downward projection

called the (3B) medial malleolus, which is the bony prominence on the inner aspect of the ankle. (Place your hand on the inside of your ankle to feel this bony prominence.)

(4) fibula

(**FIB**-yoo-lah)

The **fibula** is the more slender of the two lower leg bones and is lateral to the **tibia**. The proximal end of the **fibula** connects with the lateral **condyle** of the **tibia**. The distal end of the **fibula** projects downward to form the (4A) lateral malleolus, which is the bony prominence on the outer aspect of the ankle. (Place your hand on the outside of your ankle to feel this bony prominence.) The **fibula** connects again with the **tibia** just above the lateral malleolus and is therefore not a weight-bearing bone.

The bones of the ankle (shown in *Figure 6-14A*) are known as the **(1) tarsals.** There are seven tarsal bones. The largest is the **(2) calcaneus.** The calcaneus, also known as the heel bone, serves as a point of attachment for several of the muscles of the calf. Just above the calcaneus is the **(3) talus** bone, which joins with the **tibia** and **fibula** to form the ankle joint. The impact of a person's entire body weight is received by the talus bone at this point of connection and is then distributed to the other tarsal bones. The posterior part of the foot, consisting of the talus and calcaneus, is also known as the hind foot.

The bones of the foot (also shown in *Figure 6-14A*) are known as the **(4) metatarsals.** The heads of the metatarsal bones form the ball of the foot. The metatarsal bones, plus the tarsal bones, form the arch of the foot. The structural design of the arches of the foot, along with support from strong ligaments and tendons, makes the tarsal and metatarsal bones architecturally sound for weight bearing. The bones of the toes (shown in *Figure 6-14B*) are known as the **(5) phalanges** (as are the bones of the fingers). Each toe has three phalangeal bones, except for the great toe (which has only two).

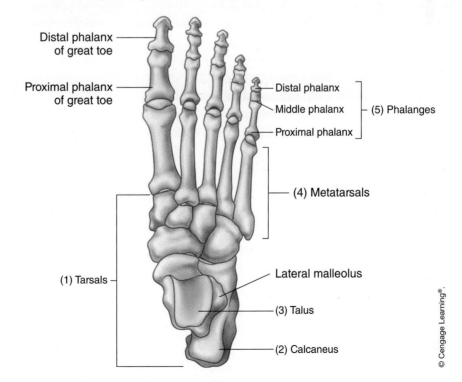

Distal phalanx of great toe
Proximal phalanx of great toe
Distal phalanx
Middle phalanx
Proximal phalanx
(5) Phalanges
(4) Metatarsals
(1) Tarsals
Lateral malleolus
(3) Talus
(2) Calcaneus

© Cengage Learning®.

Figure 6-14A Bones of the ankle and foot

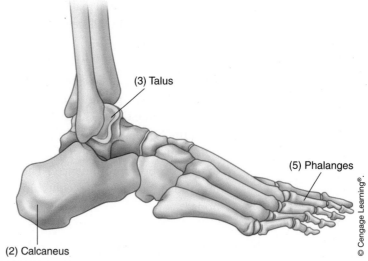

(3) Talus

(5) Phalanges

© Cengage Learning®.

(2) Calcaneus

Figure 6-14B Bones of the ankle and foot

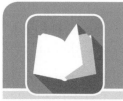

Review Checkpoint

Check your understanding of this section by completing the **Anatomy and Physiology** exercises in your workbook.

VOCABULARY

The following vocabulary words are frequently used when discussing the skeletal system.

Word	Definition
allogenic (**al**-oh-**JEN**-ick) all/o- = difference from -genic = pertaining to formation, producing	Pertaining to originating from a different origin, as in a transplant of tissue from a matching donor but not of the individual (recipient).
ankylosing spondylitis (**ang**-kih-**LOH**-sing **spon**-dih-**LYE**-tis) ankyl/o = stiff spondyl/o = spine, vertebra -itis = inflammation	A type of arthritis that affects the vertebral column and causes deformities of the spine. *For additional information refer to Chapter 7.*
arthrodesis (**ar**-throh-**DEE**-sis) arthr/o = joint -desis = binding or surgical fusion	The surgical fusion of a joint

Word	Definition
articular cartilage (ar-**TIK**-yoo-lar **CAR**-tih-lij)	Thin layer of cartilage that covers the ends of the long bones and the surfaces of the joints.
bone depressions	Concave, indented areas or openings in bones.
bone markings	Specific features of individual bones.
bone processes	Projections or outgrowths of bones.
cancellous bone (**CAN**-sell-us)	Spongy bone, not as dense as compact bone.
cervical vertebrae (**SIR**-vih-kal **VER**-teh-bray) cervic/o = neck -al = pertaining to	**Vertebrae** or bones of the neck, C1 through C7.
compact bone	Hard outer shell of the bone.
condyle (**CON**-dial)	Knucklelike projection at the end of a bone.
costochondritis (**koss**-toh-kon-**DRIGH**-tis) cost/o = ribs chondr/o – cartilage -itis = inflammation	Inflammation of the rib cartilage of the anterior chest wall; characterized by pain and tenderness in the area.
crest	Distinct border or ridge, as in **iliac** crest.
diaphysis (**dye-AFF**-ih-sis)	Main shaftlike portion of a bone.
epiphyseal line (**ep**-ih-**FIZZ**-ee-al)	A layer of cartilage that separates the **diaphysis** from the **epiphysis** of a bone; also known as the epiphyseal plate.
epiphysis (eh-**PIFF**-ih-sis)	The end of a bone.
false ribs	Rib pairs 8 through 10, which connect to the **vertebrae** in the back but not to the sternum in the front, because they join the seventh rib in the front.
fissure (**FISH**-er)	A groove or depression in a bone; a **sulcus**.
flat bones	Bones that are broad and thin with flat or curved surfaces, such as the sternum.
floating ribs	Rib pairs 11 and 12, which connect to the **vertebrae** in the back but are free of any attachment in the front.
fontanelle *or* **fontanel** (**fon**-tah-**NELL**)	Space between the bones of an infant's cranium; "soft spot."
foramen (for-**AY**-men)	Hole in a bone through which blood vessels or nerves pass.
fossa (**FOSS**-ah)	Hollow or concave depression in a bone.

Word	Definition
haversian canals (ha-**VER**-shan)	System of small canals within compact bone that contain blood vessels, lymphatic vessels, and nerves.
hematopoiesis (**hem**-ah-toh-poy-**EE**-sis) hemat/o = blood -poiesis = formation of	The normal formation and development of blood cells in the bone marrow.
hemopoietic, hematopoietic (**hee**-moh-poy-**ET**-ick) hem/o = blood -poietic = pertaining to formation of	Pertaining to the formation of blood cells. Hemopoietic/ hematopoietic is the adjective form of the word hemopoiesis/ hematopoiesis, which means the production of the formed elements in the blood (this occurs in the red bone marrow throughout one's life).
intercostal spaces (in-ter-**COS**-tal) inter- = between cost/o = ribs -al = pertaining to	Spaces between the ribs.
intervertebral disk (in-ter-**VER**-teh-bral disk) inter- = between vertebr/o = vertebra -al = pertaining to	A flat, circular, platelike structure of cartilage that serves as a cushion (or shock absorber) between the **vertebrae**.
long bones	Bones that are longer than they are wide and with distinctive shaped ends, such as the **femur**.
lumbar vertebrae (**LUM**-bar **VER**-teh-bray) lumb/o = loins, lower back -ar = pertaining to vertebr/o = vertebra	The **vertebrae** of the lower back, L1 through L5.
medullary cavity (**MED**-u-lair-ee)	The center portion of the shaft of a long bone containing the yellow marrow.
ossification (**oss**-sih-fih-**KAY**-shun)	The conversion of cartilage and fibrous connective tissue to bone; the formation of bone.
osteoblasts (**OSS**-tee-oh-blasts) oste/o = bone -blast = immature, embryonic	Immature bone cells that actively produce bony tissue.
osteoclasts (**OSS**-tee-oh-clasts) oste/o = bone -clast = something that breaks	Large cells that absorb or digest old bone tissue.
osteocytes (**OSS**-tee-oh-sites) oste/o = bone -cyte = cell	Mature bone cells.

Word	Definition

osteonecrosis
 (**oss**-tee-oh-neh-**KROH**-sis)
   oste/o = bone
   necr/o = death
   -osis = condition
	The death of bone tissue; possibly from trauma or some disease process.

periosteum
 (pair-ee-**AH**-stee-um)
   peri- = around
   oste/o = bone
   -um = noun ending
	The thick, white, fibrous membrane that covers the surface of a long bone.

red bone marrow	The soft, semifluid substance located in the small spaces of **cancellous bone** that is the source of blood cell production.
resorption (ree-**SORP**-shun)	The process of removing or digesting old bone tissue.
sesamoid bones (**SES**-a-moyd bones)	Irregular bones imbedded in tendons near a joint, as in the kneecap.
short bones	Bones that are about as long as they are wide and somewhat box-shaped, such as the wrist bone.
sinus (**SIGH**-nuss)	An opening or hollow space in a bone; a cavity within a bone.
spine	A sharp projection from the surface of a bone, similar to a crest.

stenosis
 (stin-**OH**-sis)
   sten/o = short, contracted, or narrow
   -osis = condition
	An abnormal condition characterized by a narrowing or restriction of an opening or passageway in a body structure.

subluxation (**sub**-luck-**SAY**-shun)	An incomplete dislocation (of a bone from the joint).
sulcus (**SULL**-kus)	A groove or depression in a bone; a fissure.
sutures (**SOO**-cherz)	Immovable joints, such as those of the cranium.

synovectomy
 (**sin**-oh-**VECK**-toh-mee)
   synov/o = synovial membrane, synovial
           fluid
   -ectomy = surgical removal
	Surgical removal of the synovial membrane from a joint

thoracic vertebrae
 (tho-**RASS**-ik **VER**-teh-bray)
   thorac/o = chest
   -ic = pertaining to
   vertebr/o = vertebra
	The 12 **vertebrae** of the chest, T1 through T12.

Word	Definition
trabeculae (trah-**BEK**-yoo-lay)	Needlelike bony spicules within **cancellous bone** that contribute to the spongy appearance. Their distribution along lines of stress adds to the strength of the bone.
trochanter (tro-**CAN**-ter)	Large bony process located below the neck of the **femur**.
true ribs	The first seven pairs of ribs, which connect to the **vertebrae** in the back and to the sternum in the front.
tubercle (**TYOO**-ber-kal)	A small rounded process of a bone.
tuberosity (too-ber-**OSS**-ih-tee)	An elevated, broad, rounded process of a bone.
vertebral foramen (**VER**-teh-bral for-**AY**-men)	A large opening in the center of each vertebra that serves as a passageway for the spinal cord.
yellow marrow	Located in the **diaphysis** of long bones, yellow marrow consists of fatty tissue and is inactive in the formation of blood cells.

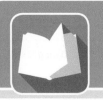

Review Checkpoint

Check your understanding of this section by completing the **Vocabulary** exercises in your workbook.

WORD ELEMENTS

The following word elements pertain to the skeletal system. As you review the list, pronounce each word element aloud twice and check the box after you "say it." Write the definition for the example term given for each word element. Use your medical dictionary to find the definitions of the example terms.

Word Element	Pronunciation	"Say It"	Meaning
acetabul/o **acetabul**ar	**ass**-eh-**TAB**-yoo-loh **ass**-eh-**TAB**-yoo-lar	☐	acetabulum
ankyl/o **ankyl**osis	**ANG**-kih-loh ang-kih-**LOH**-sis	☐	stiff
arthr/o **arthr**itis	**AR**-throh ar-**THRYE**-tis	☐	joint

Word Element	Pronunciation	"Say It"	Meaning
-blast, blast/o **osteo**blast	**BLAST**-oh **OSS**-stee-oh-blast	☐	embryonic stage of development
calc/o, calc/i hypo**calc**emia	**KALK**-oh, **KALK**-sigh **high**-poh-kal-**SEE**-mee-ah	☐	calcium
calcane/o **calcane**odynia	kal-**KAY**-nee-oh kal-**kay**-nee-oh-**DIN**-ee-ah	☐	heel bone
carp/o **carp**al	**CAR**-poh **CAR**-pal	☐	wrist
chondr/i, chondr/o **chondr**itis	kon-**DRIGH**, kon-**DROH** kon-**DRIGH**-tis	☐	cartilage
-clast, -clastic osteo**clast**	**CLAST,CLAST**-ic **OSS**-stee-oh-clast	☐	to break
clavicul/o supra**clavicul**ar	klah-**VIK**-yoo-loh **soo**-prah-klah-**VIK**-yoo-lar	☐	collarbone
coccyg/o **coccyg**eal	**COCK**-si-goh cock-**SIJ**-ee-al	☐	**coccyx**
cost/o **cost**ochondral	**KOSS**-toh **koss**-toh-**CON**-dral	☐	ribs
crani/o **crani**otomy	**KRAY**-nee-oh kray-nee-**OTT**-oh-mee	☐	skull, cranium
-desis arthro**desis**	**DEE**-sis **ar**-throh-**DEE**-sis	☐	to bind, tie together
femor/o **femor**al	**FEM**-or-oh **FEM**-or-al	☐	**femur**
fibul/o **fibul**ar	**FIB**-yoo-loh **FIB**-yoo-lar	☐	**fibula**
gen/o osteo**gen**esis	**JEN**-oh oss-tee-oh-**JEN**-eh-sis	☐	to produce
humer/o **humer**al	**HYOO**-mor-oh **HYOO**-mor-al	☐	**humerus**
ili/o **ili**ac	**ILL**-ee-oh **ILL**-ee-ac	☐	ilium
ischi/o **ischi**al	**ISS**-kee-oh **ISS**-kee-al	☐	ischium
kyph/o **kyph**osis	**KI**-foh kye-**FOH**-sis	☐	humpback; pertaining to a hump

Word Element	Pronunciation	"Say It"	Meaning
lamin/o **lamin**ectomy	**LAM**-ih-no **lam**-ih-**NEK**-toh-mee	☐	lamina
lord/o **lord**osis	**LOR**-doh lor-**DOH**-sis	☐	swayback; bent
lumb/o **lumb**ar	**LUM**-boh **LUM**-bar	☐	loins, lower back
malac/o **malac**otomy	mah-**LAY**-coh mal-ah-**COT**-oh-me	☐	softening
-malacia osteo**malacia**	mah-**LAY**-she-ah **oss**-tee-oh-mah-**LAY**-she-ah	☐	softening
mandibul/o **mandibul**ar	man-**DIB**-yoo-loh man-**DIB**-yoo-lar	☐	mandible (lower jaw bone)
mastoid/o **mastoid**itis	mass-**TOYD**-oh mass-toyd-**EYE**-tis	☐	mastoid process
maxill/o **maxill**ary	**MACK**-sih-loh **MACK**-sih-**ler**-ee	☐	upper jaw
metacarp/o **metacarp**als	met-ah-**CAR**-poh met-ah-**CAR**-pals	☐	hand bones
metatars/o **metatars**algia	met-ah-**TAR**-soh met-ah-tar-**SAL**-jee-ah	☐	foot bones
myel/o osteo**myel**itis	**MY**-ell-oh **oss**-tee-oh-**my**-ell-**EYE**-tis	☐	spinal cord or bone marrow
olecran/o **olecran**on	oh-**LEK**-ran-oh oh-**LEK**-ran-on	☐	elbow
orth/o **orth**opedics	**OR**-thoh or-thoh-**PEE**-diks	☐	straight
oste/o **oste**oma	**OSS**-tee-oh oss-tee-**OH**-mah	☐	bone
patell/o, patell/a **patell**ar	pah-**TELL**-oh, pah-**TELL**-ah pah-**TELL**-ar	☐	kneecap
pelv/i **pelv**imetry	**PELL**-vigh pell-**VIM**-eh-tree	☐	pelvis
phalang/o **phalang**itis	fal-**AN**-goh **fal**-an-**JYE**-tis	☐	fingers, toes
-physis dia**physis**	**FIH**-sis dye-**AFF**-ih-sis	☐	growth, growing

Word Element	Pronunciation	"Say It"	Meaning
por/o osteo**por**otic	**POR**-row oss-tee-oh-poh-**ROT**-ic	☐	cavity, opening, passage, or pore
-porosis osteo**porosis**	por-**ROW**-sis **oss**-tee-oh-por-**ROW**-sis	☐	porous; lessening in density
pub/o **pub**ic	**PYOO**-boh **PYOO**-bik	☐	pubis
rach/i **rach**itis	**RAH**-kigh rah-**KIGH**-tis	☐	spinal column
radi/o **radi**al	**RAY**-dee-oh **RAY**-dee-al	☐	radiation; also refers to the **radius**
scapul/o **scapul**ar	**SKAP**-yoo-loh **SKAP**-yoo-lar	☐	shoulder blade
scoli/o **scoli**osis	**SKOH**-lee-oh skoh-lee-**OH**-sis	☐	crooked, bent
spondyl/o **spondyl**osis	**SPON**-dih-loh spon-dih-**LOH**-sis	☐	vertebra
sten/o **sten**osis	**STIN**-oh	☐	short, contracted, or narrow
stern/o sub**stern**al	**STER**-noh sub-**STER**-nal	☐	sternum
synovi/o, synov/o **synovi**al	sin-**OH**-vee-oh, sin-**OH**-voh sin-**OH**-vee-al	☐	synovial membrane, synovial fluid
tars/o **tars**als	**TAR**-soh **TAR**-sulz	☐	ankle bones
tempor/o **tempor**al	**TEM**-por-oh **TEM**-por-al	☐	temples of the head
vertebr/o inter**vertebr**al	ver-**TEE**-broh in-ter-ver-**TEE**-bral	☐	vertebra

Review Checkpoint

Check your understanding of this section by completing the **Word Elements** exercises in your workbook.

Pathological Conditions

As you study the pathological conditions of the skeletal system, note that the **basic definition** is in a green shaded box, followed by a detailed description in regular print. The phonetic pronunciation is directly beneath each term, and a breakdown of the component parts of the term appear where appropriate.

osteoporosis

(**oss**-tee-oh-poh-**ROW**-sis)

   poste/o = bone

   -porosis = porous, lessening in
                  density

Osteoporosis literally means porous bones; that is, bones that were once strong become fragile due to loss of bone density.

The patient is more susceptible to fractures, especially in the wrist, hip, and vertebral column. **Osteoporosis** occurs most frequently in postmenopausal women, in sedentary or immobilized individuals, and in patients on long-term steroid treatment.

A major factor in **osteoporosis** is hormonal: postmenopausal women are at a high risk for **osteoporosis** because estrogen production and bone calcium storage decrease with menopause. Significant risk has been reported in persons of all ethnic backgrounds. White and Asian women have the lowest general bone density and are at greater risk.

Classic characteristics of **osteoporosis** are fractures that occur in response to normal activity or minimal trauma, a loss of standing height of greater than 2 inches, and the development of the typical cervical **kyphosis** (dowager's hump). See *Figure 6-15*.

Treatment includes (but is not limited to) prescribing drug therapy such as estrogen replacement therapy and calcium supplements, promoting calcium intake, and promoting active weight-bearing exercises.

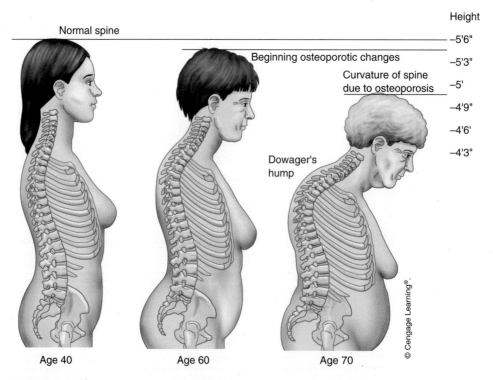

Figure 6-15 Structural changes due to osteoporosis

osteomalacia

(**oss**-tee-oh-mah-**LAY**-she-ah)

oste/o = bone

-malacia = softening

Osteomalacia is a disease in which the bones become abnormally soft due to a deficiency of calcium and phosphorus in the blood (which is necessary for bone mineralization). This disease results in fractures and noticeable deformities of the weight-bearing bones. When the disease occurs in children, it is called rickets.

The deficiency of these minerals is due to a lack of vitamin D, which is necessary for the absorption of calcium and phosphorus by the body. The vitamin D deficiency may be caused by a diet lacking in vitamin D, by a lack of exposure to sunlight or by a metabolic disorder causing **malabsorption**.

Treatment includes daily administration of vitamin D and a diet sufficient in calcium and phosphorus, as well as protein. Supplemental calcium may also be prescribed.

osteomyelitis

(**oss**-tee-oh-my-ell-**EYE**-tis)

oste/o = bone

myel/o = bone marrow

-itis = inflammation

Osteomyelitis is a local or generalized infection of the bone and bone marrow, resulting from a bacterial infection that has spread to the bone tissue through the blood.

Osteomyelitis is most frequently caused by a staphylococcal infection, but it may also be caused by a viral or fungal infection. The infection usually spreads from adjacent infected tissue to the bone marrow. It may also be introduced directly into the bone tissue as a result of injury or surgery.

Although symptoms vary with individuals, generalized symptoms of **osteomyelitis** include a sudden onset of fever (above 101° F), pain or tenderness, **erythema** (redness) and swelling over the affected bone, **anorexia** (loss of appetite), headaches, and general **malaise** (vague feeling of discomfort). There may be an open wound in the skin over the affected bone, with **purulent** (pus-containing) drainage.

Treatment for **osteomyelitis** includes bed rest and administration of intravenous or intramuscular antibiotics for four to six weeks. If the antibiotic therapy is not effective, surgical treatment may be necessary to drain the bone of pus and to remove any dead bone tissue.

Ewing's sarcoma

(**YOO**-wings sar-**KOH**-mah)

sarc/o = related to the flesh

-oma = tumor

Ewing's sarcoma is a malignant tumor of the bones common to young adults, particularly adolescent boys.

It usually develops in the long bones or the pelvis and is characterized by pain, swelling, fever, and **leukocytosis**. Treatment includes **chemotherapy**, **radiation**, and surgery to remove the tumor. Patients who respond well to this therapy may not lose the extremity to amputation. The **prognosis** with the combination therapies is about a 65% cure rate.

osteogenic sarcoma

(**oss**-tee-oh-**JEN**-ic sar-**KOH**-mah)

oste/o = bone

genic = pertaining to formation, producing

sarc/o = related to the flesh

-oma = tumor

Osteogenic sarcoma is a malignant tumor arising from bone. Also known as osteosarcoma, it is the most common malignant bone tumor, with common sites being the distal **femur** (just above the knee), the proximal **tibia** (just below the knee), and the proximal **humerus** (just below the shoulder joint).

Early complaint of pain is often described as an intermittent and dull aching. Night pain is common. As the disease rapidly progresses, the pain increases in intensity and duration. Other symptoms include weight loss, general malaise, and loss of appetite (anorexia).

Bone biopsy, X-ray films, **bone scan**, and **MRI** are the most common methods used to confirm the diagnosis and determine the location and size of the tumor.

Treatment includes radiation, chemotherapy, and surgery to remove the tumor. Patients who respond well to this combination therapy may not lose the extremity to amputation (which has historically been the treatment of choice). The prognosis for **osteogenic sarcoma** has improved with the combination therapies.

osteochondroma (**oss**-tee-oh-kon-**DROH**-mah) oste/o = bone chondr/o = cartilage -oma = tumor	An **osteochondroma** is the most common benign bone tumor. The **femur** and the **tibia** are most frequently involved.

Usually located within the bone marrow cavity, osteochondromas are covered by a cartilaginous cap. The onset of an osteochondroma is usually in childhood, but it may not be diagnosed until adulthood. Approximately 10% of all osteochondromas develop into malignant tumors (sarcomas).

Paget's disease (**PAJ**-ets dih-**ZEEZ**) **osteitis deformans** (oss-tee-**EYE**-tis de-**FOR**-manz) oste/o = bone -itis = inflammation	A nonmetabolic disease of the bone, characterized by excessive bone destruction (breakdown of bone tissue by the **osteoclasts**) and unorganized bone formation by the **osteoblasts**. The bone is weak and prone to fractures. After symptoms are present, the diseased bone takes on a characteristic mosaic pattern that can be detected with X-ray or bone scan; also known as osteitis deformans.

Paget's disease may occur in one bone or in several sites. The most common areas of occurrence are the **vertebrae, femur, tibia**, pelvis, and skull. Individuals with symptoms may develop pathological fractures, may complain of bone pain, and may experience skeletal deformity such as bowing of the leg bones (**tibia** or **femur**) or **kyphosis**.

The exact cause of this disease is unknown. Paget's disease more commonly affects persons of middle age and the elderly, with a higher incidence in men than women.

spinal stenosis (**SPIGH**-nal stin-**OH**-sis) spin/o = spine -al = pertaining to -sten/o = short, contracted, or narrow -osis = condition	Spinal stenosis is a narrowing of the vertebral canal, nerve root canals, or intervertebral foramini (openings) of the **lumbar** spinal canal. The narrowing causes pressure on the nerve roots prior to their exit from the foramini.

Symptoms include (but may not be limited to) numbness and tingling pain in the buttocks, thighs, or calves when walking, running, or climbing stairs. Standing still does not relieve the pain, but sitting or flexing the back may provide relief.

This condition may be congenital or due to spinal degeneration. If conservative measures (improved posture, abdominal muscle strengthening, and weight loss) fail to correct the problem, surgery may be indicated to relieve the pressure on the area nerves.

talipes equinovarus	**Clubfoot.** See *Figure 6-16*.

(**TAL**-ih-peez eh-kwine-oh-**VAIR**-us)

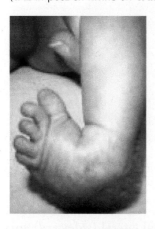

The infant's foot is fixed in plantar flexion (turned downward) and deviates medially (turned inward), and the heel is in an elevated position. Therefore, the infant's foot cannot remain in normal position with the sole of the foot firmly on the floor.

Figure 6-16 Talipes equinovarus (clubfoot)
(*Courtesy of the Centers for Disease Control and Prevention, James W. Hanson, MD*)

abnormal curvature of the spine	In this section, we define three abnormal curvatures of the spine.

For a visual reference, refer to *Figure 6-17*.

(A) Kyphosis (kye-**FOH**-sis) **is an abnormal outward curvature of a portion of the spine, commonly known as humpback or hunchback.**

(B) Lordosis (lor-**DOH**-sis) **is an abnormal inward curvature of a portion of the spine, commonly known as swayback.**

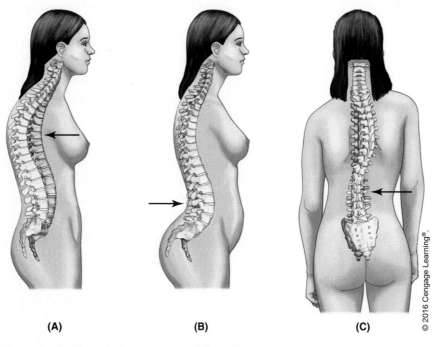

(A)   (B)   (C)

© 2016 Cengage Learning®.

Figure 6-17 Abnormal curvatures of the spine

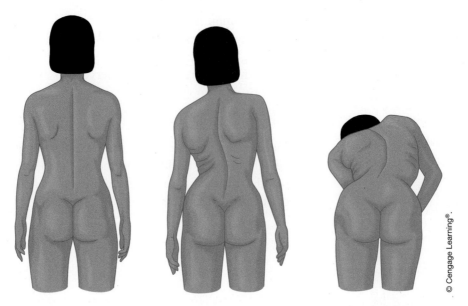

© Cengage Learning®.

Figure 6-18 Scoliosis screening: (A) Normal spine; (B) Patient with scoliosis standing erect (iliac crests are not symmetrical); (C) Patient with scoliosis bending forward (shoulders are symmetrical)

(C) Scoliosis (skoh-lee-OH-sis) **is an abnormal lateral (sideward) curvature of a portion of the spine. The curvature may be to the left or to the right.**

These abnormal curvatures of the spine may affect children or adults. The cause may be unknown (**idiopathic**), or it may be due to defects of the spine at birth (**congenital**) or some disease process (**pathological**).

Symptoms of any one of these abnormal curvatures of the spine may range from complaining of chronic fatigue and backache, to noticing that a skirt/dress hemline is longer on one side than the other, to noticing that shoulders are uneven. **Scoliosis** is sometimes picked up in a general health screening by performing a **scoliosis** screening. The individual should not be wearing shoes and should be disrobed, at least from the waist up. While the patient is standing erect (and then while the patient is bending forward), the health professional looks for symmetry of the shoulders, **iliac** crests, and normal alignment of the spinal column (see *Figure 6-18*).

If **scoliosis** is suspected, an X-ray will confirm or deny the suspicion. Treatment for abnormal curvature of the spine depends on the type and severity of the curvature. It may vary from physical therapy, exercises, or back braces to surgical intervention for correcting the deformity.

fracture	A fracture is a broken bone; a sudden breaking of a bone.

As you read about the different types of fractures, refer to the various illustrations provided. Fractures are classified according to the severity of the break. A **closed fracture** (*Figure 6-19A*) is also known as a simple fracture. There is a break in a bone but no open wound in the skin. An **open fracture** (*Figure 6-19B*) is also known as a compound fracture. There is a break in a bone, as well as an open wound in the skin. A **complete fracture** is a break that extends through the entire thickness of the bone.

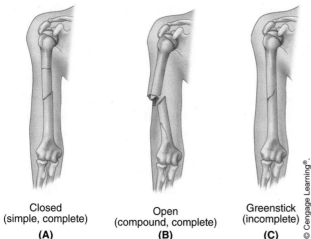

Closed
(simple, complete)
(A)

Open
(compound, complete)
(B)

Greenstick
(incomplete)
(C)

© Cengage Learning®.

Figure 6-19 (A) Closed fracture (simple, complete);
(B) Open (compound, complete); (C) Greenstick fracture
(incomplete)

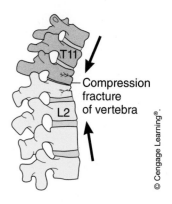

Compression
fracture
of vertebra

© Cengage Learning®.

Figure 6-20 Compression
fracture

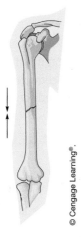

© Cengage Learning®.

Figure 6-21 Impacted
fracture

An incomplete fracture is also known as a **greenstick fracture** (*Figure 6-19C*). It is a break that does not extend through the entire thickness of the bone; that is, one side of the bone is broken and one side of the bone is bent. An incomplete fracture has the name greenstick fracture because its break is similar to trying to snap a "green stick or branch" from a tree. The break is incomplete, with one side breaking and the other side bending considerably but not breaking.

A **compression fracture** is caused by bone surfaces being forced against each other, as in the compression of one vertebra against another. Compression fractures are often associated with **osteoporosis**. See *Figure 6-20*.

An **impacted fracture** occurs when a direct force causes the bone to break, forcing the broken end of the smaller bone into the broken end of the larger bone. See *Figure 6-21*.

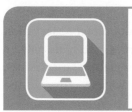

Media Link

View the **Direct Force** animation on the Student Companion Website.

A **comminuted fracture** occurs when the force is so great that it splinters or crushes a segment of the bone. See *Figure 6-22*.

A **Colles' fracture** occurs at the lower end of the **radius**, within 1 inch of connecting with the wrist bones. See *Figure 6-23*.

A **hairline fracture** is also known as a **stress fracture**. It is a minor fracture in which the bone continues to be in perfect alignment. The fracture appears on an X-ray as a very thin "hair line" between the two segments. It does not extend through the entire surface of the bone. This type of

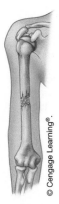

Figure 6-22 Comminuted fracture

fracture may occur in runners who run too much or too fast on hard surfaces or who wear improper shoe support. The hairline fracture usually is not visible until three to four weeks after the onset of symptoms. A **pathological fracture** occurs when a bone, which is weakened by a preexisting disease, breaks in response to a force that would not cause a normal bone to break. Examples of some underlying causes of pathological fractures include but are not limited to rickets, **osteomalacia**, and **osteoporosis**. An **occult fracture** is a fracture that cannot be detected by X-ray until several weeks after the injury (a "hidden" fracture). The individual may experience pain and swelling as a result of the injury. The occult fracture is most likely to occur in the ribs, **tibia, metatarsals**, or navicular bones (small bones in the hand or foot).

Treatment of Fractures

The specific method of treatment for fractures depends on the type of fracture sustained, its location, and any related injuries. An X-ray may be used to confirm and determine the severity of the fracture.

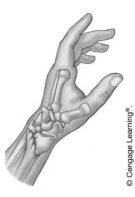

Figure 6-23 Colles' fracture

When a bone breaks, the normal anatomic alignment of the bone is displaced. To restore the bone to normal alignment, the fracture must be "reduced"; that is, the fragmented bone ends must be brought back together into a straight line, eliminating or "reducing" the fracture. The reduction of a fracture may be accomplished through closed reduction or open reduction.

Closed reduction of a fracture consists of aligning the bone fragments through manual manipulation or traction without making an incision into the skin. See *Figure 6-24*.

Once the fracture is reduced, the bone is immobilized to maintain the position of the bone until healing occurs. Examples of devices used to stabilize the realigned bone are a cast, splint, or immobilizer. These devices protect the realignment of the fractured bone and maintain support. The immobilization also aids in reducing the pain. It is important with casting and splinting to check for swelling and/or loss of sensation in the extremity. See *Figure 6-25* for immobilization devices.

Open reduction of a fracture consists of realigning the bone under direct observation during surgery. See *Figure 6-26*. Devices such as screws, pins, wires, and nails may be used internally to maintain the bone alignment while healing takes place. These devices, known as **internal fixation devices**, are more commonly used with fractures of the **femur** and fractures of joints See *Figure 6-27*.

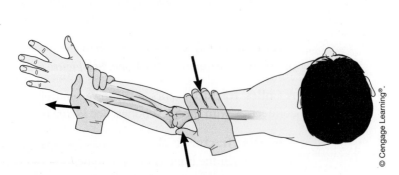

Figure 6-24 Closed reduction of a fracture

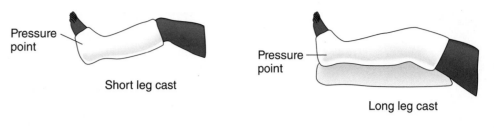

Pressure point — Short leg cast

Pressure point — Long leg cast

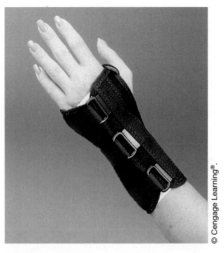

Figure 6-25 Devices used to stabilize fractures

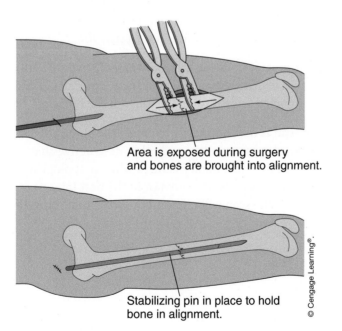

Area is exposed during surgery and bones are brought into alignment.

Stabilizing pin in place to hold bone in alignment.

Figure 6-26 Open reduction of a fracture

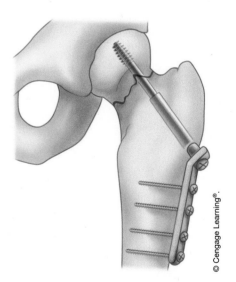

Figure 6-27 Internal fixation devices

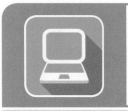

Media Link

View the **Internal Fixation of Fractures** animation on the Student Companion Website.

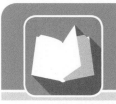

Review Checkpoint

Check your understanding of this section by completing the **Pathological Conditions** exercises in your workbook.

Diagnostic Techniques, Treatments, and Procedures

bone scan

A bone scan involves the intravenous injection of a radioisotope, which is absorbed by bone tissue. After approximately 3 hours, the skeleton is scanned with a gamma camera (scanner) moving from one end of the body to the other. The scanner detects the areas of radioactive concentration (areas where the bone absorbs the isotope) and converts the radioactive image to a screen on which the concentrations show up as pinpoint dots cast in the image of a skeleton.

Areas of greater concentration of the radioisotope appear darker than other areas of distribution and are called "hot spots." Follow-up X-rays are then conducted to determine the cause of the hot spots. See *Figure 6-28*.

A bone scan is used primarily to detect the spread of cancer to the bones (metastasis), **osteomyelitis**, and other destructive changes in the bone. It can be used to detect bone fractures when pathological fractures are suspected and multiple X-rays are not in the best interest of the patient. The hot spots on the scan will pinpoint the areas needing X-ray.

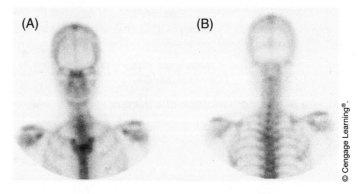

Figure 6-28 A bone scan of the head, shoulders, and upper spine (A) anterior view (B) posterior view

© Cengage Learning®.

bone marrow aspiration	A bone marrow aspiration is the process of removing a small sample of bone marrow from a selected site with a needle for the purpose of examining the specimen under a microscope.

This common method of obtaining a bone marrow sample is used to diagnose specific blood disorders such as severe anemia, acute leukemia, neutropenia (decreased number of white blood cells; i.e., neutrophils), and thrombocytopenia (decreased number of platelets). The preferred sites for bone marrow aspiration are (1) the sternum, (2) the **iliac** crest, and (3) the broad end of the **tibia**. See *Figure 6-29*.

A bone marrow aspiration is performed using sterile technique to prevent **osteomyelitis**. After the skin has been **anesthetized** (numbed), the aspiration needle is inserted through the skin down to the **periosteum**.

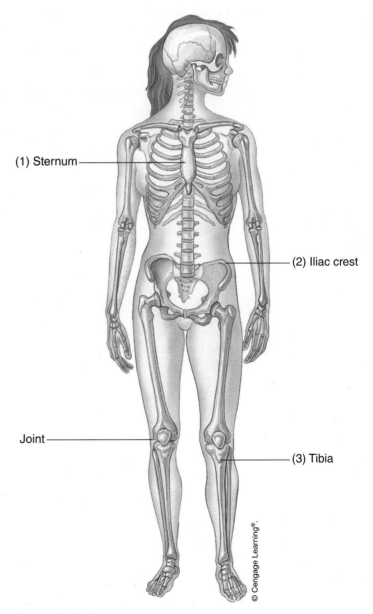

Figure 6-29 Sites for bone marrow aspiration

The **periosteum** is then anesthetized to lessen the pain of the procedure. When the marrow cavity is entered, the marrow stylet (a long, closed cylinder that keeps the lumen of the aspiration needle closed during entry) is removed, and a sterile syringe is attached to the needle for aspiration of the marrow specimen.

When a larger specimen of bone marrow is required, a bone marrow biopsy is performed using a larger lumen biopsy needle designed to obtain a core of bone marrow. The procedure is basically the same as for a bone marrow aspiration.

Bone Density Evaluation

The measurement of bone mineral density is important in providing helpful information regarding treatment and prevention of **osteoporosis**. The most commonly used procedure to evaluate bone density is **dual energy X-ray absorptiometry** (DEXA). Other procedures, such as quantitative computed tomography (QCT) and peripheral bone density testing, may be used but have limitations.

dual energy X-ray absorptiometry (DEXA) (ab-sorp-she-**AHM**-eh-tree)	**Dual energy X-ray absorptiometry** (DEXA) is a noninvasive procedure that measures bone density. In the DEXA procedure, an X-ray machine generates the energy photons that pass through the bones. A computer then evaluates the amount of radiation absorbed by the bones, and the findings are interpreted by a physician.

This procedure measures the bone density more accurately than the dual photon absorptiometry, takes less time, and emits less radiation to the patient. It is the "gold standard" for bone density measurement.

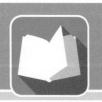

Review Checkpoint

Check your understanding of this section by completing the **Diagnostic Techniques, Treatments, and Procedures** exercises in your workbook.

COMMON ABBREVIATIONS

Abbreviation	Meaning	Abbreviation	Meaning
C1, C2, C3, …	cervical vertebra 1, 2, 3, etc.	RLE	right lower extremity
		RUE	right upper extremity
DEXA	**dual energy X-ray absorptiometry**	S1	**sacrum** (When transcribing, you may hear a medical report refer to the disk space between the last lumbar vertebra and the **sacrum** as L5–S1.)
DIP	distal interphalangeal (joint)		
Fx	fracture		
L1, L2, L3, …	lumbar vertebra 1, 2, 3, etc.	T1, T2, T3, …	thoracic vertebra 1, 2, 3, etc.
		THA	total hip arthroplasty
LLE	left lower extremity	THR	total hip replacement
LUE	left upper extremity	TKA	total knee arthroplasty
MCP	metacarpophalangeal (joint)	TKR	total knee replacement
		TMJ	temporomandibular joint
MTP	metatarsophalangeal (joint)		
PIP	proximal interphalangeal (joint)		

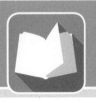

Review Checkpoint

Check your understanding of this section by completing the **Common Abbreviations** exercises in your workbook.

WRITTEN AND AUDIO TERMINOLOGY REVIEW

Review each of the following terms from this chapter. Study the spelling of each term and write the definition in the space provided. Check definitions by looking the term up in the glossary.

Term	Pronunciation	Definition
acetabular	☐ **ass**-eh-**TAB**-yoo-lar	_____
allogenic	☐ **al**-oh-**JEN**-ick	_____
ankylosing spondylitis	☐ **ang**-kih-**LOH**-sing **spon**-dih-**LYE**-tis	_____
arthrodesis	☐ **ar**-throh-**DEE**-sis	_____
articular cartilage	☐ ar-**TIK**-yoo-lar **CAR**-tih-laj	_____
calcaneodynia	☐ kal-**kay**-nee-oh-**DIN**-ee-ah	_____
cancellous bone	☐ **CAN**-sell-us bone	_____
carpals	☐ **CAR**-pals	_____
cervical vertebrae	☐ **SIR**-vih-kal **VER**-teh-bray	_____
coccygeal	☐ cock-**SIJ**-ee-al	_____
coccyx	☐ **COCK**-six	_____
condyle	☐ **CON**-dial	_____
costochondral	☐ koss-toh-**CON**-dral	_____
costochondritis	☐ **koss**-toh-kon-**DRIGH**-tis	_____
craniotomy	☐ kray-nee-**OTT**-oh-mee	_____
diaphysis	☐ dye-**AFF**-ih-sis	_____
dual energy X-ray absorptiometry	☐ dual energy X-**RAY** ab-sorp-she-**AHM**-eh-tree	_____
epiphyseal line	☐ ep-ih-**FIZZ**-e-al line	_____
epiphysis	☐ eh-**PIFF**-ih-sis	_____
ethmoid bone	☐ **ETH**-moyd bone	_____
Ewing's sarcoma	☐ **YOO**-wings sar-**KOH**-mah	_____
femoral	☐ **FEM**-or-al	_____
femur	☐ **FEE**-mer	_____
fibula	☐ **FIB**-yoo-lah	_____

Term	Pronunciation	Definition
fibular	☐ **FIB**-yoo-lar	_____
fissure	☐ **FISH**-er	_____
fontanelle or fontanel	☐ fon-tah-**NELL**	_____
foramen	☐ foh-**RAY**-men	_____
fossa	☐ **FOSS**-ah	_____
haversian canals	☐ ha-**VER**-shan canals	_____
hematopoiesis	☐ **hem**-ah-toh-poy-**EE**-sis	_____
hemopoietic, hematopoietic	☐ **hee**-moh-poy-**ET**-ick, **hee**-mah-toh-poy-**ET**-ick	_____
humeral	☐ **HYOO**-mer-al	_____
humerus	☐ **HYOO**-mer-us	_____
hyoid bone	☐ **HIGH**-oyd bone	_____
iliac	☐ **ILL**-ee-ak	_____
intervertebral disk	☐ in-ter-**VER**-teh-bral disk	_____
ischial	☐ **ISS**-kee-al	_____
kyphosis	☐ kye-**FOH**-sis	_____
lacrimal bones	☐ **LACK**-rim-al bones	_____
laminectomy	☐ lam-ih-**NEK**-toh-mee	_____
lordosis	☐ lor-**DOH**-sis	_____
lumbar	☐ **LUM**-bar	_____
lumbar vertebrae	☐ **LUM**-bar **VER**-teh-bray	_____
mandibular	☐ man-**DIB**-yoo-lar	_____
mastoiditis	☐ mass-toyd-**EYE**-tis	_____
maxillary	☐ **MACK**-sih-**ler**-ee	_____
medullary cavity	☐ **MED**-u-lair-ee cavity	_____
metacarpals	☐ met-ah-**CAR**-pals	_____
metatarsalgia	☐ **met**-ah-tar-**SAL**-jee-ah	_____
metatarsals	☐ met-ah-**TAR**-sulz	_____
nasal conchae	☐ **NAYZ**-l **KONG**-kee	_____
occipital bone	☐ ock-**SIP**- ih-tal bone	_____
olecranon	☐ oh-**LEK**-ran-on	_____
orthopedics	☐ or-thoh-**PEE**-diks	_____
ossification	☐ **oss**-sih-fih-**KAY**-shun	_____
osteoblasts	☐ **OSS**-tee-oh-blasts	_____

Term	Pronunciation	Definition
osteoclasts	☐ **OSS**-tee-oh-clasts	_____
osteocytes	☐ **OSS**-tee-oh-sites	_____
osteogenic sarcoma	☐ oss-tee-oh-**JEN**-ic sar-**KOH**-mah	_____
osteoma	☐ oss-tee-**OH**-mah	_____
osteomalacia	☐ **oss**-tee-oh-mah-**LAY**-she-ah	_____
osteonecrosis	☐ **oss**-tee-oh-neh-**KROH**-sis	_____
osteoporosis	☐ oss-tee-oh-poh-**ROW**-sis	_____
palatine bones	☐ **PAL**-ah-tine bones	_____
parietal bones	☐ pah-**REYE**-eh-tal bones	_____
patella	☐ pah-**TELL**-ah	_____
patellar	☐ pah-**TELL**-ar	_____
pelvimetry	☐ pell-**VIM**-eh-tree	_____
periosteum	☐ pair-ee-**AH**-stee-um	_____
phalanges	☐ fah-**LAN**-jeez	_____
phalangitis	☐ fal-an-**JYE**-tis	_____
pubic	☐ **PYOO**-bik	_____
rachitis	☐ rah-**KIGH**-tis	_____
radial	☐ **RAY**-dee-al	_____
radius	☐ **RAY**-dee-us	_____
resorption	☐ re-**SORP**-shun	_____
sacrum	☐ **SAY**-crum	_____
scapular	☐ **SKAP**-yoo-lar	_____
scoliosis	☐ skoh-lee-**OH**-sis	_____
sesamoid bones	☐ **SES**-a-moyd bones	_____
sinus	☐ **SIGH**-nuss	_____
sphenoid bone	☐ **SFEE**-noyd bone	_____
spondylosis	☐ spon-dih-**LOH**-sis	_____
subluxation	☐ **sub**-luck-**SAY**-shun	_____
substernal	☐ sub-**STER**-nal	_____
sulcus	☐ **SULL**-kuss	_____
supraclavicular	☐ **soo**-prah-klah-**VIK**-yoo-lar	_____
sutures	☐ **SOO**-cherz	_____
synovectomy	☐ **sin**-oh-**VECK**-toh-mee	_____
talipes equinovarus	☐ **TAL**-ih-peez **eh**-kwine-oh-**VAIR**-us	_____
tarsals	☐ **TAR**-sulz	_____
temporal	☐ **TEM**-por-al	_____

Term	Pronunciation	Definition
thoracic vertebrae	☐ tho-**RASS**-ik **VER**-teh-bray	_____
tibia	☐ **TIB**-ee-ah	_____
trabeculae	☐ trah-**BEK**-yoo -lay	_____
trochanter	☐ tro-**KAN**-ter	_____
tubercle	☐ **TYOO**-ber-kal	_____
tuberosity	☐ too-ber-**OSS**-ih-tee	_____
ulna	☐ **UHL**-nah	_____
vertebrae	☐ **VER**-teh-bray	_____
vertebral foramen	☐ **VER**-teh-bral for-**AY**-men	_____
vomer	☐ **VOH**-mer	_____
zygomatic bones	☐ zeye-go-**MAT**-ik bones	_____

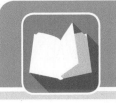

Review Checkpoint

Apply what you have learned in this chapter by completing the **Putting It All Together** exercise in your workbook.

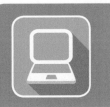

Online Resources

For additional study tools, including PowerPoint® slides and animations, go to the Student Companion Website.

Chapter Review Exercises

The following exercises provide a more in-depth review of the chapter material. Your goal in these exercises is to complete each section at a minimum 80% level of accuracy. A space has been provided for your score at the end of each section.

A. Labeling

Write the names of the bones in the applicable spaces. Each correct bone name is worth 10 points. When you have completed the exercise, total your points and record your score in the space provided at the end of the exercise.

(continued)

Name of Bone

1. _____

2. _____

3. _____

4. _____

5. _____

6. _____

7. _____

8. _____

9. _____

10. _____

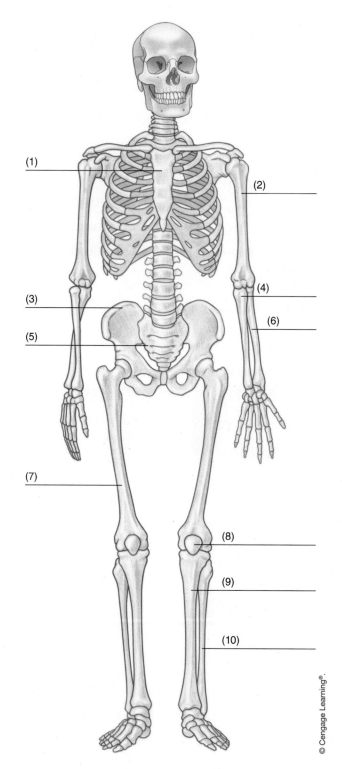

(1)

(2)

(3)

(4)

(5)

(6)

(7)

(8)

(9)

(10)

© Cengage Learning®.

Number correct _____ × ***10 points/correct answer: Your score*** _____ ***%***

B. Completion

The following is a discussion of the structure and formation of bone. Complete the sentences with the most appropriate word. Each correct answer is worth 10 points. Record your score in the space provided at the end of the exercise.

1. The main shaft-like portion of a bone is the _____.
2. When skeletal growth is complete, the _____ will not show up on X-ray.
3. The _____ is the thick white fibrous membrane that covers the surface of the long bones.
4. Dense bone tissue that is the hard outer shell of the bone is known as _____.
5. Compact bone has a system of small canals that contain blood vessels, lymphatic vessels, and nerves. These canals are called the _____ canals.
6. _____ are the immature bone cells that are actively producing bony tissue that replaces cartilage.
7. The conversion of fibrous connective tissue and cartilage into bone or a bony substance is known as _____.
8. _____ are large cells that digest (or absorb) bony tissue, helping to hollow out the central portion of the bone.
9. A mature bone cell is called an _____.
10. Blood cell formation occurs in the _____.

Number correct _____ × 10 points/correct answer: Your score _____ %

C. Matching

Match the following bone markings in the left column with the applicable description on the right. Each correct answer is worth 10 points. Record your score in the space provided at the end of the exercise.

_____ 1. trochanter

_____ 2. crest

_____ 3. fissure

_____ 4. fossa

_____ 5. foramen

_____ 6. sinus

_____ 7. condyle

_____ 8. neck

_____ 9. tuberosity

_____ 10. spine

a. an elevated, broad, rounded process of a bone, usually for muscle or tendon attachment

b. a sharp projection from the surface of a bone

c. a constricted or narrow section that connects with the head

d. the large bony process located below the neck of the femur; for muscle

e. an opening or hollow space in a bone

f. a distinct border or ridge; an upper, elevated edge

g. a groove or depression in a bone

h. a hole within a bone through which blood vessels or nerves pass

i. a sharp projection from the surface of a bone, similar to a crest; used for muscle attachment

j. a knuckle-like projection at the end of a bone

k. a hollow or shallow concave depression in a bone

Number correct _____ × 10 points/correct answer: Your score _____ %

D. Spelling

Circle the correctly spelled term in each pairing of words. Each correct answer is worth 10 points. Record your score in the space provided at the end of the exercise.

1. sinus   sinous
2. temperal   temporal
3. mandibuler   mandibular
4. thoracic   thoraxic
5. xiphoid   zyphoid
6. acromian   acromion
7. meticarpals   metacarpals
8. acetabelum   acetabulum
9. maleolus   malleolus
10. condyle   condile

Number correct _____ × *10 points/correct answer: Your score* _____ %

E. Multiple Choice

Read each statement carefully and select the correct answer from the options listed. Each correct answer is worth 10 points. Record your score in the space provided at the end of the exercise.

1. A disease in which the bones become abnormally soft due to a deficiency of calcium and phosphorus in the blood is known as:
   a. osteoporosis
   b. osteomalacia
   c. osteomyelitis
   d. Ewing's sarcoma

2. Bones that are longer than they are wide and with distinctive-shaped ends, such as the femur, are known as:
   a. compact bones
   b. sesamoid bones
   c. short bones
   d. long bones

3. A flat, circular, platelike structure of cartilage that serves as a cushion (or shock absorber) between the vertebrae is known as:
   a. intercostal space
   b. intervertebral disk
   c. epiphyseal line
   d. bone process

4. A hollow or concave depression in a bone is called a:
   a. fossa
   b. foramen
   c. crest
   d. spine

5. The large bony process located below the neck of the femur is the:

   a. tuberosity

   b. trabeculae

   c. trochanter

   d. condyle

6. A disease characterized by bones that were once strong becoming fragile due to loss of bone density is called:

   a. osteomalacia

   b. osteoporosis

   c. osteomyelitis

   d. osteochondroma

7. The medical term for an abnormal outward curvature of a portion of the spine, commonly known as humpback or hunchback, is:

   a. scoliosis

   b. lordosis

   c. kyphosis

   d. osteochondroma

8. The medical term for an abnormal inward curvature of a portion of the spine, commonly known as swayback, is:

   a. osteochondroma

   b. kyphosis

   c. lordosis

   d. scoliosis

9. The medical term for an abnormal lateral (sideward) curvature of a portion of the spine to the left or to the right is:

   a. lordosis

   b. scoliosis

   c. kyphosis

   d. osteochondroma

10. A layer of cartilage that separates the diaphysis from the epiphysis of a bone is the:

   a. epiphyseal line

   b. intervertebral disk

   c. crest

   d. cancellous bone

Number correct _____ × *10 points/correct answer: Your score* _____ %

F. Proofreading Skills

Read the following History and Physical Exam Report. For each bold term, provide a brief definition and indicate if the term is spelled correctly. If it is misspelled, provide the correct spelling. Each correct answer is worth 10 points. Record your score in the space provided at the end of the exercise.

Example:

midclavicular: _pertaining to the midpoint of the clavicle bone._

Spelled Correctly?   ✔ Yes   ☐ No _____

HISTORY AND PHYSICAL EXAMINATION

Hillcrest
medical center

PATIENT NAME: Emma Parker

PATIENT ID: 112591

ROOM NO.: 444

DATE OF ADMISSION:
09/25/2014

ADMITTING PHYSICIAN:
Sherman Loyd, MD

ADMITTING DIAGNOSIS
Acute intertrochanteric **fracture** of right **femur**.

The history below was obtained from the patient, and physical examination was performed with her stated verbal understanding and consent. She was alert, oriented x3 with reasonable thought content. She understood questions well and was in no acute distress.

CHIEF COMPLAINT
Right hip injury.

HISTORY OF PRESENT ILLNESS
I was called to see this 69-year-old black female patient, well known to me, who was brought to the ER after she sustained an injury of her right hip. She states she was walking when her right leg just "gave out," and she fell onto the right hip. She complained of mild pain in the right hip, and mild edema was noted in the ER. In addition, she had external **rotation** of the right leg.

Initial x-ray demonstrated findings of intertrochanteric fracture, nondisplaced, of the right hip; and a **hairline fracture** of the right **ileac crest**. Consultation was obtained from Dr. Dodd, chief **orthapedist** for the hospital, who concurred with the diagnosis, and treatment recommendations were made. She was subsequently admitted to the hospital for further evaluation and treatment, including surgical repair of the hip.

PAST MEDICAL HISTORY
Usual childhood diseases. She denies previous rheumatic fever or polio. The only surgical history was an appendectomy in the past and repair of a fractured left **tibia** in approximately 1993.

SOCIAL HISTORY
She lives at home with her husband, who is rather feeble. Denies the use of tobacco or alcohol.

(continued)

HISTORY AND PHYSICAL EXAMINATION
Patient Name: Emma Parker
Patient ID: 112591
Admission Date: 09/25/2014
Page 2

FAMILY HISTORY
Noncontributory.

REVIEW OF SYSTEMS
Otherwise unremarkable.

PHYSICAL EXAMINATION
GENERAL: This is an alert black female patient appropriate for stated chronologic age who is in no acute distress.

SKIN: Multiple senile keratotic lesions noted.

HEENT: Normocephalic. Normal hair distribution. Pupils equal, round, reactive to light and accommodation (PERRLA). Extraocular movements intact (EOMI). Sclerae anicteric. Funduscopic exam essentially benign other than some mild cataract formation. Ear canals are clear. Tympanic membranes normal. Buccal mucosa is moist. Oropharynx noninflamed. Teeth are present but in disrepair.
History and Physical Examination

NECK: Soft and supple with no palpable nodes or masses noted.

LUNGS: Clear in all fields without wheezes, rales, or rhonchi.

CHEST: Symmetrically moving chest cage upon respiratory excursions.

HEART: Rate regular with no murmur, click, gallop, or rub. Point of maximal impulse (PMI) in left fifth **intercostal space**, **midclaviculer** line.

ABDOMEN: Soft without tenderness, masses, or organomegaly.

GENITORECTAL/BREASTS: Deferred at this time. Not felt to be indicated.

EXTREMITIES: External rotation of right leg is noted; peripheral pulses found to be symmetrically intact. Mild tenderness is noted over the outer aspect of the right **acetabulum**. No frank deformity is noted.

NEUROLOGIC: Grossly intact with no focal deficits appreciated.

IMPRESSION:

Right intertrochanteric **femarul** fracture.

PLAN
Admit the patient in Buck's traction. IV fluids. Type and cross x2 for anticipated surgery in the a.m. Call Dr. Carol Dodd for **orthopedic** consultation.

Sherman Loyd, MD

SL:xx

D:09/25/2014

T:09/27/2014

(continued)

1. **fracture** _____

   _____

   Spelled Correctly? ☐ Yes   ☐ No _____

2. **femur** _____

   Spelled Correctly? ☐ Yes   ☐ No _____

3. **hairline fracture** _____

   Spelled Correctly? ☐ Yes   ☐ No _____

4. **ileac crest** _____

   Spelled Correctly? ☐ Yes   ☐ No _____

5. **orthapedist** _____

   Spelled Correctly? ☐ Yes   ☐ No _____

6. **intercostal** _____

   Spelled Correctly? ☐ Yes   ☐ No _____

7. **acetabulum** _____

   Spelled Correctly? ☐ Yes   ☐ No _____

8. **femarul** _____

   Spelled Correctly? ☐ Yes   ☐ No _____

9. **tibia** _____

   Spelled Correctly? ☐ Yes   ☐ No _____

10. **orthopedic** _____

    Spelled Correctly? ☐ Yes   ☐ No _____

Number correct _____ × *10 points/correct answer: Your score* _____ %

G. Crossword Puzzle

Each crossword answer is worth 10 points. When you have completed the crossword puzzle, total your points and enter your score in the space provided.

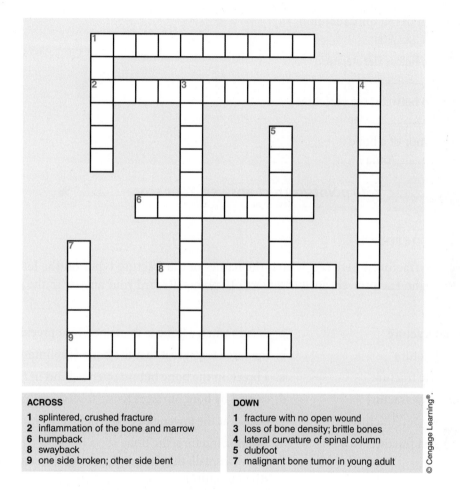

ACROSS
1 splintered, crushed fracture
2 inflammation of the bone and marrow
6 humpback
8 swayback
9 one side broken; other side bent

DOWN
1 fracture with no open wound
3 loss of bone density; brittle bones
4 lateral curvature of spinal column
5 clubfoot
7 malignant bone tumor in young adult

© Cengage Learning®.

Number correct _____ × *10 points/correct answer: Your score* _____ %

H. Word Element Review

The following words relate to the skeletal system. The prefixes and suffixes have been provided. Read the definition carefully and complete the word by filling in the space with the word elements provided in this chapter. If you have forgotten your word building rules, see Chapter 1. Each correct word is worth 10 points. Record your score in the space provided at the end of the exercise.

1. Pertaining to the acetabulum
   _____/ar

2. Low blood calcium level
   hypo /_____/emia

3. Pertaining to the cartilage and the ribs
   _____/chondr/al

4. Incision into the skull
   _____/otomy

(continued)

5. Softening of bone tissue

   _____/_____

6. Pertaining to the jaw bone

   _____/ar

7. Inflammation of the spinal column

   _____/itis

8. Pertaining to below the sternum

   sub/_____/al

9. Pertaining to between the vertebrae

   inter/_____/al

10. A benign tumor of a bone

   _____/oma

Number correct _____ × 10 points/correct answer: Your score _____ %

I. Matching Fractures

Can you name these fractures? Let's see! Match the names of the fracture types on the left with the applicable description on the right. Each correct answer is worth 10 points. Record your answer in the space provided at the end of the exercise.

_____ 1. closed fracture

_____ 2. open fracture

_____ 3. complete fracture

_____ 4. greenstick fracture

_____ 5. compression fracture

_____ 6. impacted fracture

_____ 7. comminuted fracture

_____ 8. Colles' fracture

_____ 9. hairline fracture

_____ 10. pathological fracture

a. occurs when a bone is weakened by a preexisting disease

b. the force is so great that the bone is splintered or crushed

c. a break in the bone but no open wound in the skin

d. caused by bone surfaces being forced against each other

e. occurs at the lower end of the radius, within 1 inch of the wrist

f. a minor fracture; the bone stays in perfect alignment; X-ray shows a small, thin line at the site of the fracture (also called a stress fracture)

g. the force of the break causes the broken end of the smaller bone to be jammed into the broken end of the larger bone

h. one side of the bone is broken and the other side is bent; an incomplete fracture

i. a break that extends through the entire thickness of the bone

j. a break in the bone and an open wound in the skin

Number correct _____ × 10 points/correct answer: Your score _____ %

J. Matching Abbreviations

Match the abbreviations on the left with the correct definition on the right. Each correct answer is worth 20 points. Record your score in the space provided at the end of the exercise.

_____ 1. Fx

_____ 2. DEXA

a. temporomandibular joint

b. dual energy X-ray absorptiometry

_____ 3. C1, C2, C3, . . .   c. total knee replacement

_____ 4. TMJ   d. cervical vertebra 1, 2, 3, etc.

_____ 5. THR   e. lumbar vertebra 1, 2, 3, etc.

f. fracture

g. total hip replacement

Number correct _____ *× 20 points/correct answer: Your score* _____ *%*

K. Word Search

Read each definition carefully and identify the applicable word from the list that follows. Enter the word in the space provided, and then find it in the puzzle and circle it. The words may be read up, down, diagonally, across, or backward. Each correct answer is worth 10 points. Record your score in the space provided at the end of the exercise.

fossa	floating	condyle	true
foramen	sutures	epiphysis	spine
sesamoid	osteocytes	trochanter	

Example: A hollow or concave depression in a bone.

fossa _____

1. The type of rib pairs 11 and 12 that connect to the vertebrae in the back but are free of any attachment in the front.

_____

2. A knucklelike projection at the end of a bone.

_____

3. The first seven pairs of ribs that connect to the vertebrae in the back and to the sternum in the front.

_____

4. Immovable joints, such as those of the cranium.

_____

5. Mature bone cells.

_____

6. A hole in a bone through which blood vessels or nerves pass.

_____

7. The end of a bone.

_____

8. The large bony process located below the neck of the femur.

_____

9. A sharp projection from the surface of a bone, similar to a crest.

_____

10. The type of irregular bones imbedded in tendons near a joint, as in the kneecap.

_____

(continued)

```
F  L  O  A  T  I  N  G  I  O  L  E  M  I  C
A  C  Y  N  G  E  S  M  S  I  D  A  S  T  T
M  I  O  T  T  M  N  M  E  T  T  R  N  V  R
C  A  O  N  E  E  O  O  S  D  I  C  C  B  O
I  L  C  S  D  T  N  L  I  E  O  O  I  T  S
N  U  H  E  I  Y  T  T  O  T  E  L  N  L  T
C  R  O  P  H  L  L  B  I  U  A  E  C  O  E
O  U  S  T  N  P  N  E  M  A  R  O  F  E  O
N  U  R  R  P  O  I  P  I  A  T  E  O  E  C
T  U  V  O  D  A  I  I  N  D  E  Y  S  M  Y
E  A  L  C  G  R  S  P  I  N  E  C  S  E  T
N  I  E  H  A  R  C  H  I  S  I  S  A  I  E
E  S  P  A  D  R  U  Y  A  R  D  I  S  G  S
N  U  L  N  I  R  E  S  I  D  U  A  L  D  T
C  R  A  T  B  L  O  I  I  U  A  T  C  O  A
E  E  N  E  R  H  C  S  U  T  U  R  E  S  A
F  R  E  R  U  U  R  I  S  M  E  M  N  I  C
P  E  R  I  T  O  N  D  I  O  M  A  S  E  S
```

Number correct _____ *× 10 points/correct answer: Your score* _____ %

L. Medical Scenario

The following medical scenario presents information on one of the pathological conditions discussed in this chapter. Read the scenario carefully and select the most appropriate answer for each question that follows. Each correct answer is worth 20 points. Record your score in the space provided at the end of the exercise.

Ginger Black, a 15-year-old patient, is visiting her pediatrician today for a physical. The health care professional explains to Ginger and her mother that Ginger will be screened for scoliosis today during her physical exam.

1. Ginger's mother asks the health care professional to explain what scoliosis screening means. The best explanation would be that she will need to be undressed from the waist up and remove her shoes and:

   a. the physician will look at her back while she is standing erect and when she bends over (He will be observing for symmetry of shoulders, iliac crests, and normal alignment of the spinal column.)

   b. the physician will beam a minimal amount of radiation from radioactive isotopes through the bones of her back, shoulders, and spinal column to check bone density

   c. her height and weight will be measured and compared to previous heights and weights

   d. her feet will be assessed to observe for plantar flexion and medial deviation

2. The health care professional further explains to Ginger and her mother that scoliosis is:

   a. the most common benign bone tumor frequently involving the femur and tibia

   b. a malignant tumor of the spine common to young adults, particularly adolescent girls

   c. an abnormal outward curvature of a portion of the spine, commonly known as humpback or hunchback

   d. an abnormal lateral curvature of a portion of the spine that may cause a skirt/dress hemline to be longer on one side

3. Ginger asks the health care professional if there are any symptoms of scoliosis. The health care professional would respond by explaining to Ginger and her mother that symptoms of scoliosis are:

   a. weight loss, general malaise, and anorexia

   b. chronic fatigue, backache, and uneven shoulders

   c. sudden onset of fever, pain, erythema, and swelling over the affected bone

   d. loss of standing height greater than 2 inches and presence of a dowager's hump

4. The health care professional explains to Ginger and her mother that when scoliosis is suspected, the diagnosis is confirmed or denied through a:

   a. spinal X-ray

   b. spinal bone marrow aspiration

   c. dual energy absorptiometry

   d. dual photon absorptiometry

5. The health care professional explains that if there is evidence of scoliosis, the treatment depends on the type and severity, which may entail:

   a. realigning the fracture through closed or open reduction

   b. radiation, chemotherapy, or surgery to remove the tumor

   c. physical therapy, exercises, back braces, or surgical intervention

   d. physiotherapy, bed rest, or administration of intravenous or intramuscular antibiotics for four to six weeks

Number correct _____ × 20 points/correct answer: Your score _____ %

CHAPTER
7

Muscles and Joints

CHAPTER CONTENT

OBJECTIVES

Upon completing this chapter and the review exercises at the end of the chapter, the learner should be able to:

1. Identify three different types of muscles and indicate the control under which each type functions.

2. Correctly identify at least five major muscles of the body by labeling the muscle diagram provided in the chapter review exercises.

3. Define at least 10 pathological conditions of the muscles and joints.

4. Identify a minimum of 10 abbreviations common to the muscles and joints.

5. Demonstrate the ability to create at least 10 medical words pertaining to the muscles and joints.

6. Define 10 different range-of-motion movements of the skeletal muscles.

7. Identify at least five diagnostic techniques used in evaluating patients with disorders of the muscles or joints.

8. Proof and correct one transcription exercise relative to the muscles and joints.

9. Correctly spell and pronounce terms listed on the Written and Audio Terminology Review, using the phonetic pronunciations provided.

Overview of Muscular System

When you picked up this book, opened it, and turned the pages to this chapter on the muscles and joints, you used *many* of the more than 600 skeletal muscles of your body without much thought about muscle movement! If you were to close this book, put it down, and decide *not* to read this chapter on muscles and joints, you would still use many of the muscles you used when you picked it up. So let's keep it open and continue reading!

The skeleton, as we have studied, provides points of attachment and support for the muscles. However, it cannot move itself; it must have help. The ability of the muscles to **contract** and extend produces body movement, allowing us to move about freely. In addition to movement of the body, the muscles have two other important functions.

Muscles support and maintain body posture through a low level of continual contraction, that is, a continual pull against gravity keeps the body in good alignment. Good body posture places the least amount of strain on the body's muscles, **ligaments**, and bones. Skeletal muscles also have a great effect on body temperature because they produce a substantial amount of heat when they contract. Think about the last time you were cold and you shivered. You used the energy generated by the contraction of your muscles to raise your body temperature. This response is controlled by your "built-in thermostat," the hypothalamus, which is an endocrine gland discussed in Chapter 13.

In this chapter, we concentrate on the major muscles of the body, leaving the detailed study of the muscular system to anatomy and physiology textbooks. We also study the articulations (joints) of the body and how they create the possibility for movement by the muscles.

Anatomy and Physiology (Muscles)

Types of Muscles

The body contains three types of muscles: **skeletal muscle**, smooth muscle, and **cardiac muscle**. Skeletal muscles attach to the bones of the skeleton. They are also known as **voluntary muscles** because they operate under conscious control. Not all voluntary muscles, however, are skeletal muscles. Some voluntary muscles are not attached to the skeleton. They are responsible for movement of the face, eyes, tongue, and pharynx. Skeletal muscles are also called **striated muscles** because they have a striped appearance when viewed under a microscope. However, not all striated muscle is skeletal. As will be discussed later, cardiac muscle is also striated in appearance.

Many of the skeletal muscles work in pairs, creating coordinated movement through the opposing actions of **contraction** and relaxation. For example, when muscle A contracts (or shortens) to flex the arm, muscle B must relax. This action brings the arm closer to the body. Conversely, to extend the arm muscle, muscle A must relax (returning to its normal resting length) while muscle B contracts. This action moves the arm away from the body.

Smooth muscles (also called **visceral muscles**) are found in the walls of hollow organs and tubes such as the stomach, intestines, respiratory passageways, and blood vessels. When viewed under a microscope, smooth muscles lack the striations (stripes) visible in striated muscles. Smooth muscles are *not* under the conscious control of the individual. Accordingly, they are also known as **involuntary muscles**. The contraction of smooth, or involuntary, muscles is regulated by hormones and the autonomic nervous system. The autonomic nervous system regulates involuntary vital function, including the activity of the **cardiac muscle**, smooth muscles, and glands.

Cardiac muscle is a specialized type of muscle that forms the wall of the heart. As previously mentioned, it is controlled by the autonomic nervous system and is an involuntary muscle. When viewed through a microscope, **cardiac muscle** is striated in appearance.

Attachment of Muscles

Each **skeletal muscle** consists of individual muscle cells called **muscle fibers**. These fibers are held together by thin sheets of fibrous connective tissue called **fascia**, which penetrate and cover the entire muscle. The **fascia** and the partitions within the muscle extend to form a strong fibrous band of tissue called a **tendon**. The **tendon** attaches the muscle to the bone as it becomes continuous with the periosteum of the bone.

The attachments of muscles to bones are strategically placed so that muscles can cause movement of the bones when they contract or relax. Most of our muscles cross at least one joint, attaching to both of the bones forming the **articulation**. When movement occurs, one of the bones moves more freely than the other. The point of attachment of the muscle to the bone that is *less movable* is called the **origin**. (The name of that particular bone will name the "point of origin" for the muscle.) The point of attachment of the muscle to the bone it *moves* is called the **insertion**. (The name of that particular bone will name the point of **insertion** for the muscle.) See *Figure 7-1*.

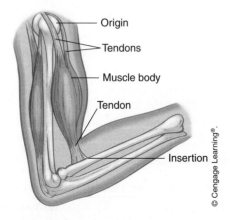

Origin

Tendons

Muscle body

Tendon

Insertion

© Cengage Learning®.

Figure 7-1 Origin and insertion points of a muscle

Groups of Muscles

This chapter concentrates on several of the major muscles near the body surface.

Note: This discussion does not cover all of the muscles of the body.

Many of the muscles discussed here will take on greater importance when you study administration of medications by injection, range-of-motion exercises, and other medical procedures. Although these muscles are generally described in the singular form, most of them are present on both sides of the body. Each description, when possible, includes a "Do this" section designed to have you locate the muscle being discussed by participating in the exercise.

Muscles That Move the Head and Neck

For a visual reference, as you study these muscles, refer to *Figure 7-2*.

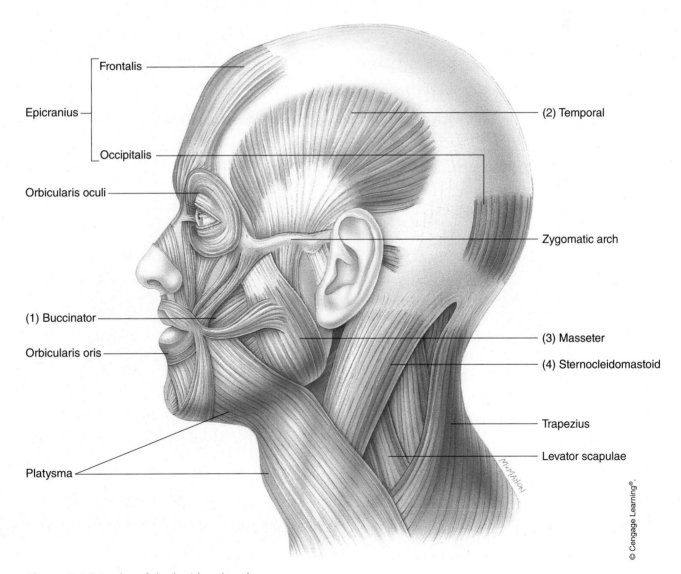

Figure 7-2 Muscles of the head and neck

(1) **buccinator** (**BUCK**-sin-ay-tor) bucc/o = cheek	The **buccinator** muscle is located in the fleshy part of the cheek. (*Do this: Suck in your cheeks. Now release them. Blow as if you were blowing out a candle. Now whistle. Smile! You have used your **buccinator** muscle to respond to each of these commands.*)
(2) **temporal** (**TEM**-po-ral) tempor/o = temporal	The **temporal** muscle is located above and near the ear. (*Do this: Open and close your jaws as if you were biting and chewing a piece of meat. To do this, you have used your **temporal** muscle.*)
(3) **masseter** (mass-**SEE**-ter)	The **masseter** muscle, located at the angle of the jaw, also raises the mandible and closes the jaw. It is used when biting and chewing.
(4) sternocleidomastoid (**stir**-noh-**klye**-doh-**MASS**-toyd) stern/o = sternum mastoid/o = mastoid process	The **sternomastoid** muscle is sometimes called the **sternocleidomastoid** muscle. It extends from the sternum upward along the side of the neck to the mastoid process. (*Do this: Bend your neck, bringing your chin toward your chest. Now raise your head back to normal position and turn your head from side to side. You are using your **sternomastoid** muscle.*)

Muscles That Move the Upper Extremities

For a visual reference, as you study these muscles, refer to *Figure 7-3*.

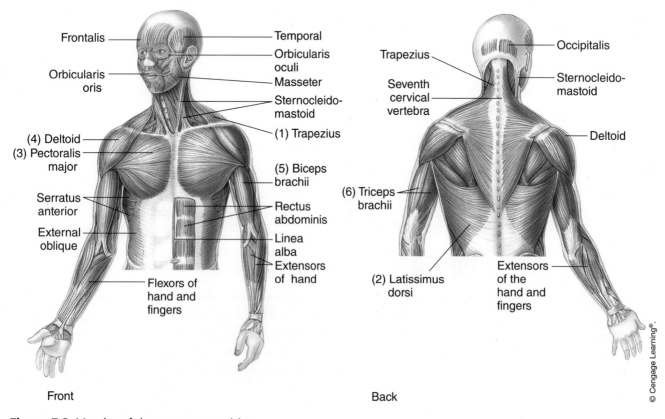

Front

Back

© Cengage Learning®.

Figure 7-3 Muscles of the upper extremities

(1) trapezius (trah-**PEE**-zee-us)	The **trapezius** muscle is a triangular-shaped muscle that extends across the back of the shoulder, covers the back of the neck, and inserts on the clavicle and scapula. *(Do this: Raise your shoulders as if you were shrugging them. Now pull them back. You have just used your **trapezius** muscles to accomplish this movement.)*
(2) latissimus dorsi (lah-**TIS**-ih-mus **DOR**-sigh) dors/o = back	The **latissimus dorsi** muscle originates from the vertebrae of the lower back, crosses the lower half of the thoracic region, and passes between the humerus and scapula to insert on the anterior surface of the humerus. It forms the posterior border of the axilla (armpit). *(Do this: Lean slightly forward. Straighten or extend your arms over your head, and begin moving your arms in a swimming motion. This **extension** of the arms and bringing them down forcibly is accomplished by using the **latissimus dorsi** muscle.)*
(3) pectoralis major (**peck**-toh-**RAY**-lis) pector/o = chest	The **pectoralis major** muscle is a large, fan-shaped muscle that crosses the upper part of the front of the chest. It originates from the sternum and crosses over to the humerus. It forms the anterior border of the axilla (armpit). *(Do this: Cross your right arm over your chest, and touch the back part of your left shoulder. To do this, your pectoralis major muscle flexed, causing the arm to adduct [come toward the body], pulling the arm across the shoulder.)*
(4) deltoid (**DELL**-toyd)	The **deltoid** muscle covers the shoulder joint. It originates from the clavicle and the scapula and inserts on the lateral side of the humerus. The **deltoid** muscle is one of the muscles used for intramuscular injections. *(Do this: Hold your left arm straight down beside your body. Now raise your left arm out, away from your body, until it is in a horizontal position. The contraction of the **deltoid** muscle is responsible for abducting the arm [moving it away from the body].)*
(5) biceps brachii (**BYE**-seps **BRAY**-kee-eye) bi- = two	The **biceps brachii** muscle has two heads, both of which originate from the scapula and insert on the radius. *(Do this: Bend your right elbow to bring your lower arm up toward the right upper arm, holding the position tightly enough to flex your muscle. Now relax your right arm and then extend it out in front of you and turn your palm up. Your **biceps brachii** muscle was responsible for flexing your lower arm and for supinating your palm, that is, turning the palm up.)*
(6) triceps brachii (**TRY**-seps **BRAY**-kee-eye) tri- = three	The **triceps brachii** muscle has three heads, which originate from the scapula and the humerus and insert onto the olecranon process of the ulna (at the elbow). *(Do this: Extend your right arm, straightening your elbow as if to throw a boxing blow. Be sure no one is near enough to receive that blow! Your **triceps brachii** muscle is responsible for straightening the elbow.)*

Muscles of the Trunk of the Body

The **trunk** is the main part of the body, to which the head and the extremities are attached. It is also called the **torso**. The muscles of the trunk include the **diaphragm** and the muscles of the abdomen and perineum. A discussion of these muscles can be found in most anatomy textbooks.

Muscles That Move the Lower Extremities

The muscles of the lower extremities (which are longer and stronger than those of the upper extremities) provide strength, stability, and movement to the lower extremities. The **perineum** is the lower end of the trunk, between the thighs. In the male, the perineum is identified as the space between the scrotum and the anus, and in the female, as the space between the vaginal opening and the anus. The perineal muscles control actions such as assisting in the erection of the penis (male) or the clitoris (female), emptying the urethral canal, constricting the urethra, and tightening the anal sphincter. As you study the muscles that move the lower extremities, refer to *Figure 7-4* for a visual reference.

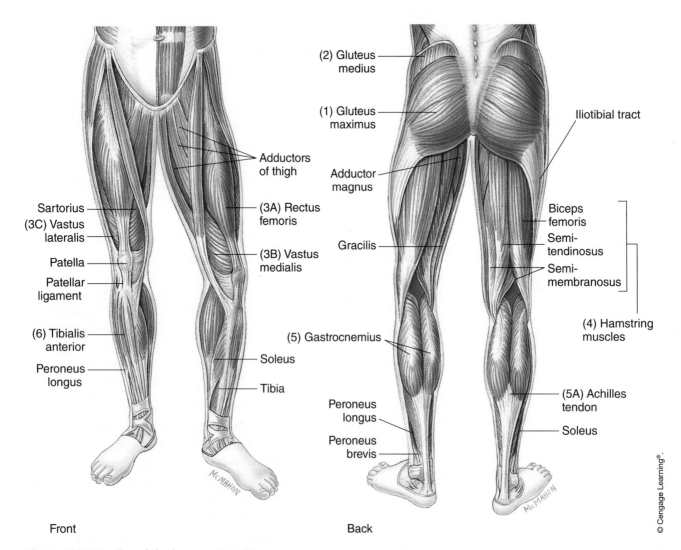

Front

Back

© Cengage Learning®.

Figure 7-4 Muscles of the lower extremities

(1) gluteus maximus (**GLOO**-tee-us **MACKS**-ih-mus)	The gluteus maximus muscle forms most of the fleshy part of the buttock. It is a large muscle that offers support when an individual is standing. This muscle originates from the ilium and inserts in the femur. It is responsible for causing the thigh to rotate, or turn, outward; that is, it extends the thigh. If you are sitting properly in a chair as you read this material, you are sitting on your gluteus maximus muscle.
(2) gluteus medius (**GLOO**-tee-us **MEE**-dee-us)	The gluteus medius muscle is a smaller muscle located above the upper outer quadrant of the gluteus maximus muscle. It originates from the posterior part of the ilium and inserts in the greater trochanter of the femur. The gluteus medius muscle also helps abduct the thigh, rotating it outward. The gluteus medius muscle is one of the muscles used for an intramuscular injection.
(3) **quadriceps femoris** (**KWAHD**-rih-seps **FEM**-or-iss)	The anterior part of the thigh has five muscles that work together to extend the thigh, as in extending the leg to kick a ball. Four of these muscles are actually part of one large muscle (the **quadriceps femoris**), even though they are named individually. For study purposes, we will discuss them individually. The (**3A**) **rectus femoris** muscle covers the center of the anterior part of the thigh. Originating from the ilium, it inserts on the patellar tendon. The rectus femoris muscle is used as an intramuscular injection site. The (**3B**) **vastus medialis** is located on the inner side of the femur. The (**3C**) **vastus lateralis** is located on the outer side of the femur. It is often used as a site for intramuscular injections. The fourth head of the **quadriceps femoris** muscle is the **vastus intermedius**, which is deeper in the center of the thigh. Each of these muscle heads, except the rectus femoris, originates from the femur and inserts on the patellar tendon.
(4) **hamstring muscles** (**HAM**-string muscles)	Located in the posterior part of the thigh are the **hamstring muscles** (biceps femoris, semimembranosus, and the semitendinosus), which are responsible for flexing the leg on the thigh (as in kneeling). They also extend the thigh. These muscles originate from the ischium and insert on the fibula and the tibia. If you feel the area behind your knee, you can feel the hamstring muscle tendons.
(5) **gastrocnemius** (**gas**-trok-**NEE**-mee-us)	The **gastrocnemius** muscle is the main muscle of the calf. It attaches to the calcaneus (heel bone) by way of the (**5A**) **Achilles tendon**. The **gastrocnemius** muscle is used in standing on tiptoe (plantar flexing the foot) and in flexing the toes. If you are a ballerina you will certainly exercise your **gastrocnemius** muscle!
(6) **tibialis anterior** (tib-ee-**AY**-lis an-**TEER**-ee-or)	The **tibialis anterior** muscle is positioned on the front of the leg. It is responsible for turning the foot inward (inversion) and for dorsiflexing the foot (i.e., pulling the foot back up toward the leg). If you choose to walk on your heels, raising the ball of your foot and your toes up off the ground, you will be using your **tibialis anterior** muscle.

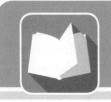

Review Checkpoint

Check your understanding of this section by completing the **Anatomy and Physiology** exercises in your workbook.

VOCABULARY (MUSCLES)

The following vocabulary terms are frequently used when discussing the muscular system.

Word	Definition
arthralgia (ar-**THRAL**-jee-ah) arthr/o = joint -algia = pain	Pain in the joints; symptom present in many joint diseases.
ataxia (ah-**TAK**-see-ah) a- = without, not tax/o = order -ia = condition	Without muscular coordination
atrophy (**AT**-roh-fee) a = without troph/o = development -y = noun ending	Wasting away; literally "without development."
bradykinesia (**brad**-ee-kih-**NEE**-zee-ah) brady- = slow -kinesia = movement	Abnormally slow movement
cardiac muscle (**CAR**-dee-ack muscle) cardi/o = heart -ac = pertaining to	Specialized type of muscle that forms the wall of the heart. **Cardiac muscle** is a type of involuntary muscle.
contract/contraction (con-**TRAK**-shun)	A reduction in size, especially of muscle fibers.
contracture (con-**TRAK**-cher)	An abnormal (usually permanent) bending of a joint into a fixed position; usually caused by **atrophy** and shortening of muscle fibers.

Word	Definition
dyskinesia (**dis**-kih-**NEE**-zee-ah) dys- = bad, difficult, painful, disordered kines/o = movement -ia = condition	A condition in which there is impairment of voluntary movement; "bad or difficult movement"
epicondylitis (**ep**-ih-**kon**-dih-**LYE**-tis) epi- = upon, over condyl/o = condyle -itis = inflammation	Painful inflammation of the tissues surrounding the elbow; also known as tennis elbow.
fascia (**FASH**-ee-ah)	Thin sheets of fibrous connective tissue that penetrate and cover the entire muscle, holding the fibers together.
fibromyalgia (**figh**-broh-my-**AL**-jee-ah) fibr/o = fiber my/o = muscle -algia = pain	A chronic condition that is characterized by widespread muscle and pain throughout much of the body, muscle spasms, fatigue, and muscle stiffness. The pain may begin gradually or have a sudden onset. The condition affects women more than men.
hemiparesis (**hem**-ee-pah-**REE**-sis) hemi- = half -paresis = paralysis	Slight or partial paralysis of one half of the body (i.e. left or right side)
hemiplegia (**hem**-ee-**PLEE**-jee-ah) hemi- = half -plegia = paralysis	Paralysis of one half of the body (i.e. left or right side)
insertion (in-**SIR**-shun)	The point of attachment of a muscle to a bone it moves.
involuntary muscles	Muscles that act without conscious control. They are controlled by the autonomic nervous system and hormones.
muscle fiber	The name given to the individual muscle cell.
myocele (**MY**-oh-seel) my/o = muscle -cele = swelling or herniation	Herniation of muscle through the muscular sheath (fascia) surrounding it
myoparesis (**my**-oh-pah-**REE**-sis) my/o = muscle -paresis = paralysis	Slight or partial paralysis of a muscle
origin	The point of attachment of a muscle to a bone that is less movable (i.e., the more fixed end of attachment).

Word	Definition
paraplegia (**par**-ah-**PLEE**-jee-ah) para- = near, beside, beyond, two like parts -plegia = paralysis	Paralysis of the lower extremities of the body, usually due to spinal cord injuries.
pelvic girdle weakness (**PELL**-vik **GER**-dul **WEAK**-ness)	Weakness of the muscles of the **pelvic girdle** (the muscles that extend the hip and the knee). In **muscular dystrophy**, the **pelvic girdle weakness** causes the child to use one or both hands to assist in rising from a sitting position by "walking" the hands up the lower extremities until he or she is in an upright position.
pseudohypertrophic muscular dystrophy (**soo**-doh-**high**-per-**TROH**-fic **MUSS**-kew-lar **DIS**-troh-fee) pseud/o = false hyper- = excessive troph/o = development -ic = pertaining to	A form of **muscular dystrophy** that is characterized by progressive weakness and muscle fiber degeneration without evidence of nerve involvement or degeneration of nerve tissue; also known as Duchenne's muscular dystrophy.
quadriplegia (**kwad**-rih-**PLEE**-jee-ah) quadr/i = four -plegia = paralysis	Paralysis of all four extremities and the trunk of the body; caused by injury to the spinal cord at the level of the cervical vertebrae
sarcopenia (**sar**-koh-**PEE**-nee-ah) sarc/o = flesh -penia = decrease in; deficiency	A loss of skeletal muscle mass that occurs with aging; it is seen more in people who are inactive. Prevention and treatment measures that have been shown to be useful are resistance training or strength training exercises.
skeletal muscle (**SKELL**-eh-tal muscle)	Muscles that attach to the bones of the skeleton. **Skeletal muscles** act voluntarily.
smooth muscle	Muscles found in the walls of hollow organs and tubes such as the stomach, intestines, respiratory passageways, and blood vessels; also known as visceral muscles. Smooth muscles act involuntarily.
striated muscle (**STRY**-ay-ted muscle)	Muscles that have a striped appearance when viewed under a microscope. Skeletal and cardiac muscles are examples.
tendon (**TEN**-dun)	A strong fibrous band of tissue that extends from a muscle, attaching it to the bone by becoming continuous with the periosteum of the bone.
torso (**TOR**-soh)	See *trunk.*
trunk	The main part of the body, to which the head and the extremities are attached; also called the **torso.**

Word	Definition

visceral muscle
(**VISS**-er-al muscle)
   viscer/o = pertaining to the internal
          organs of the body
   -al = **pertaining to**
	Muscles of the internal organs. See also *smooth muscle*.

voluntary muscle (**VOL**-un-**ter**-ee muscle)	Muscles (such as skeletal muscles) that operate under conscious control. Those that are responsible for movement of the face, eyes, tongue, and pharynx are under voluntary control.

Review Checkpoint

Check your understanding of this section by completing the **Vocabulary** exercises in your workbook.

WORD ELEMENTS (MUSCLES)

The following word elements pertain to the muscular system. As you review the list, pronounce each word element aloud twice and check the box after you "say it." Write the definition for the example term given for each word element. Use your medical dictionary to find the definitions of the example terms.

Word Element	Pronunciation	"Say It"	Meaning
bi- **bi**cep	**BYE** **BYE**-sep	☐	twice, double, two
bi- **bi**ceps	**BYE** **BYE**-seps	☐	two, double
bucc/o **bucc**al	**BUCK**-oh **BUCK**-al	☐	cheek
-cele myo**cele**	**SEEL** **MY**-oh-seel	☐	swelling or herniation
dors/o **dors**al	**DOR**-soh **DOR**-sal	☐	back
dys- **dys**kinesia	**DISS** **dis**-kih-**NEE**-zee-ah	☐	bad. Difficult, painful, disordered

Word Element	Pronunciation	"Say It"	Meaning
dys- **dyst**onia	**DIS** dis-**TOH**-nee-ah	☐	bad, difficult, painful, disordered
electr/o **electr**omyogram	ee-**LEK**-troh ee-**lek**-troh-**MY**-oh-gram	☐	electrical, electricity
fasci/o **fasci**otomy	**FASH**-ee-oh fash-ee-**OTT**-oh-mee	☐	band of fibrous tissue
fibr/o **fibr**oma	**FIH**-broh fih-**BROH**-mah	☐	fiber
-graphy electroneuromyo**graphy**	**GRAH**-fee ee-**lek**-troh-**noo**-roh-my-**OG**-rah-fee	☐	process of recording
-itis fasci**itis**	**EYE**-tis fas-ee-**EYE**-tis	☐	inflammation
kinesi/o, kines/o **kinesi**ology	kigh-**NEE**-zee-oh, kigh-**NEE**-zoh **kigh**-nee-zee-**OL**-oh-jee	☐	movement
leiomy/o **leiomy**ofibroma	lye-oh-**MY**-oh **lye**-oh-**my**-oh-fye-**BROH**-mah	☐	smooth muscle
my/o **my**algia	**MY**-oh my-**AL**-jee-ah	☐	muscle
myos/o **myos**itis	my-**OH**-so my-oh-**SIGH**-tis	☐	muscle
pector/o **pector**al	peck-**TOR**-oh **PECK**-toh-ral	☐	pertaining to the chest
-plegia hemi**plegia**	**PLEE**-jee-ah hem-ee-**PLEE**-jee-ah	☐	paralysis
rhabdomy/o **rhabdomy**osarcoma	rab-**DOH**-my-oh **rab**-doh-**my**-oh-sar-**KOH**-mah	☐	**striated muscle; skeletal muscle**
tax/o a**tax**ia	**TACK**-soh ah-**TACK**-see-ah	☐	coordination, order
tri- **tri**ceps	**TRY** **TRY**-seps	☐	three
troph/o dys**trophy**	**TROH**-foh **DIS**-troh-fee	☐	development

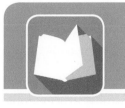

Review Checkpoint

Check your understanding of this section by completing the **Word Elements** exercises in your workbook.

Pathological Conditions (Muscles)

Diseases and disorders of the muscles may occur at any age. Some conditions are chronic and may require medications, treatments, and possibly surgery to correct the injury. Others may be disease conditions with which the individual will live throughout his or her life. As you study the pathological conditions of the muscular system, note that the **basic definition** is in a green shaded box followed by a detailed description in regular print. The phonetic pronunciation is directly beneath each term, as well as a breakdown of the component parts of the term where applicable.

muscular dystrophy

(**MUSS**-kew-lar **DIS**-troh-fee)

  dys- = bad, difficult, painful, disordered

  troph/o = development

  -y = noun ending

Muscular dystrophy is a group of genetically transmitted disorders characterized by progressive symmetrical wasting of skeletal muscles; there is no evidence of nerve involvement or degeneration of nerve tissue. The onset of **muscular dystrophy** is early in life.

Muscle weakness is characteristic of all types of **muscular dystrophy**. Diagnostic tests are performed to confirm the diagnosis of **muscular dystrophy**. These findings include elevated enzyme tests (CPK), abnormal **muscle biopsy** results, and an abnormal **electromyogram**.

There are numerous types of **muscular dystrophy**. One of the most common types is **Duchenne's muscular dystrophy**, with symptoms generally appearing by the age of three. As the disease progresses, the muscles **atrophy** (waste away) and contractures form. Muscle tissue is replaced with fat as the muscle fibers degenerate. The muscle weakness may first appear as pelvic girdle weakness and then progress to include weakness of the shoulder muscles. It will finally involve extreme weakness of all muscles, including those controlling respiration. Scoliosis is common in the late stages of **muscular dystrophy**.

Treatment is aimed at controlling the symptoms and includes exercise programs, possible corrective surgery for the scoliosis, braces to support the weakened muscles, and breathing exercises. Additionally, corticosteroid therapy may be used to decrease muscular destruction and improve muscle strength. There is no known cure for muscular dystrophy, and death usually results from respiratory complications occurring in late adolescence. Research has revealed that stem cell injections are proving to considerably slow the disease progression in muscular dystrophy.

polymyositis

(**pol**-ee-my-oh-**SIGH**-tis)

  poly- = many, much, excessive

  myos/o = muscle

  -itis = inflammation

Polymyositis is a chronic, progressive disease affecting the skeletal (striated) muscles. It is characterized by muscle weakness of hips and arms and degeneration (**atrophy**).

The disease is termed *dermatomyositis* when the patient also has a rash on the face, neck, shoulders, chest, and upper extremities. This chronic disease is also characterized by periods of remission ("symptom free") and relapse (symptoms return).

The onset of **polymyositis** is gradual, with patients first experiencing weakness of the hips and shoulders. They may have difficulty getting out of a chair or the bathtub, difficulty climbing stairs, or difficulty reaching for things on the upper shelf of a cabinet or closet. They may experience **arthralgia** (painful joints) accompanied by edema. As the disease progresses, the neck muscles may become so weak that the patient may not be able to raise his or her head from the pillow.

The cause of **polymyositis** is unknown. It is thought to be caused by an autoimmune reaction. It occurs twice as often in women as in men and appears most commonly between the ages of 40 and 60.

Treatment includes high doses of corticosteroids and immunosuppressive drugs, along with reduction of the patient's activities until the inflammation subsides. Response to treatment has resulted in long satisfactory periods of remission in some patients and recovery in others.

rotator cuff tear

(**ROH**-tay-tor kuff **TAIR**)

A tear in the muscles that form a "cuff" over the upper end of the arm (head of the humerus). See *Figure 7-5*. The rotator cuff helps lift and rotate the arm, and hold the head of the humerus in place during **abduction** of the arm.

The individual may experience sudden acute pain, a snapping sensation, and weakness in the arm if a rotator cuff tear develops acutely due to an injury. If the tear has a gradual onset due to repetitive overhead activity or wear and degeneration of the **tendon**, the pain may be mild at first

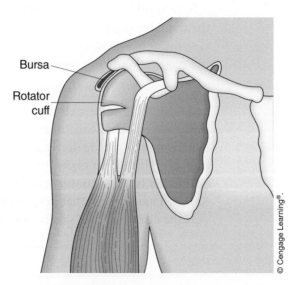

Bursa

Rotator cuff

© Cengage Learning®

Figure 7-5 Rotator cuff tear

and noticeable only with the overhead activities. The pain may become more evident over time, and raising the arm to reach to overhead level may become difficult.

Work activities that cause the individual to raise the arms overhead (such as construction work, painting, or stocking shelves, and physical activities such as swimming, pitching, and playing tennis) may cause rotator cuff tears. It is more common in people over the age of 40, but may also occur in younger individuals following acute trauma or the repetitive work or physical activities described previously.

Treatment may consist of conservative measures such as rest and limited overhead activity, placing the arm in a sling, use of nonsteroidal anti-inflammatory medications, and ice/heat applications while the tear heals. Recovery may take several weeks or months. Cortisone injections (to reduce inflammation) serve as a line of defense between conservative treatment and surgery. If conservative measures are not successful or there is a complete tear, surgery is indicated to repair the tear. After surgery, the individual's arm is usually immobilized with a sling for several weeks. Progressive physical therapy is started toward the end of the first week to restore full use of the arm.

strains	A strain is an injury to the body of the muscle or attachment of the **tendon**, resulting from overstretching, overextension, or misuse (i.e., a "muscle pull").

Vigorous exercise may cause intense muscle strain when the individual is unaccustomed to this type of activity. Chronic muscle strain may result from repetitious muscle overuse.

Strains may vary from mild to severe. Patient symptoms may vary from the gradual onset of muscle spasms, some discomfort, and decreased motion of the affected area (with no bruising) to severe muscle spasms, intense pain and tenderness, a sensation of a "sudden tearing" in the area, and swelling. An X-ray of the affected area may be ordered to rule out the possibility of a fracture.

Treatment includes rest, ice packs to the affected area for the first 24 to 48 hours to decrease the swelling, compression of the area with an elastic bandage to prevent swelling, and elevation of the affected part. Muscle relaxants may be prescribed if the muscle spasms continue after the injury.

The healing process for a muscle strain may take four to six weeks. Activity should be limited during this time to avoid a recurrence of injury. For a comparison of sprains and strains, see *Table 7-1*, page 236.

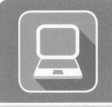

Media Link

Learn more about strains by watching the **Hamstring Strain** animation on the Student Companion Website.

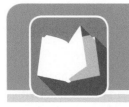

Review Checkpoint

Check your understanding of this section by completing the **Pathological Conditions** exercises in your workbook.

Diagnostic Techniques, Treatments, and Procedures (Muscles)

muscle biopsy

(muscle **BYE**-op-see)

Muscle biopsy is the extraction of a specimen of muscle tissue, through either a biopsy needle or an incisional biopsy, for the purpose of examining it under a microscope.

Muscle biopsy may be performed for the purpose of diagnosing muscle **atrophy** (as in **muscular dystrophy**) or for diagnosing inflammation (as in **polymyositis**).

If an **incisional biopsy** of muscle tissue is needed, the procedure is carried out under local anesthesia. A surgical incision is made and the desired specimen is obtained. A pressure dressing is applied after the procedure. The affected extremity is immobilized for a period of 12 to 24 hours after the procedure. The biopsy is usually taken from the **deltoid** or quadriceps muscles.

If a **needle biopsy** of muscle tissue is needed, the procedure is carried out under local anesthesia. The biopsy needle is inserted, the inner trocar is removed, and the specimen is aspirated. Usually a bandage over the biopsy site is the only dressing needed.

electromyography

(ee-**LEK**-troh-my-**OG**-rah-fee)

electr/o = electrical, electricity

my/o = muscle

-graphy = the process of recording

Electromyography is the process of recording the strength of the contraction of a muscle when it is stimulated by an electric current.

The procedure is performed using either a surface electrode applied to the skin or a needle electrode inserted into the muscle. The muscle is electrically stimulated, and the response is recorded with an oscilloscope (an instrument that displays a visual representation of electrical variations on a fluorescent screen).

Review Checkpoint

Check your understanding of this section by completing the **Diagnostic Techniques, Treatments, and Procedures** exercises in your workbook.

COMMON ABBREVIATIONS (MUSCLES)

Abbreviation	Meaning	Abbreviation	Meaning
IM	intramuscular	DTR	deep **tendon** reflexes
MD	muscular dystrophy	EMG	electromyography

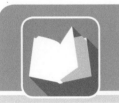

Review Checkpoint

Check your understanding of this section by completing the **Common Abbreviations** exercises in your workbook.

Overview of Joints

We have discussed the skeletal system (our means of support and structure) and the muscular system, our means of movement. Now let's take a look at the system that determines our degree of movement: the joints of the body. A joint is a point at which two individual bones connect. It is also called an **articulation**. The type of joint present between the bones determines the range of motion for that body part. When we think of the joints of the body, we usually think of those that permit considerable movement, making it possible for us to perform the many activities of our day-to-day life. Some of the joints, however, allow no movement. Sutures are immovable joints. Their purpose is to bind bones together. Other joints permit only limited motion. For example, the joints between the vertebrae of the spinal column provide strong support to the spinal column while allowing a narrow range of movement. Let's continue our study by discussing some of the different classifications of joints.

Classifications of Joints

Joints may be classified according to their structure or according to their function. The structural classification is based on the type of connective tissue that joins the bones or by the presence of a fluid-filled joint capsule. The functional classification is based on the degree of movement allowed. Examples of the joint classifications follow.

Structural Classification

The following is a listing of joints according to the type of connective tissue that joins the bones together.

fibrous joint

(**FYE**-bruss)

In a **fibrous joint**, the surfaces of the bones fit closely together and are held together by fibrous connective tissue (as in a **suture** between the skull bones). This is an immovable joint. See *Figure 7-6*.

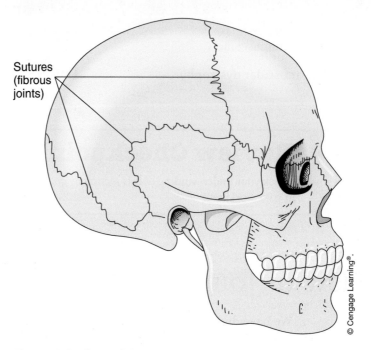

Figure 7-6 Fibrous joint

cartilaginous joint

(car-tih-**LAJ**-ih-nus)

In a **cartilaginous joint**, the bones are connected by cartilage, as in the symphysis (joint between the pubic bones of the pelvis). This type of joint allows limited movement. See *Figure 7-7*.

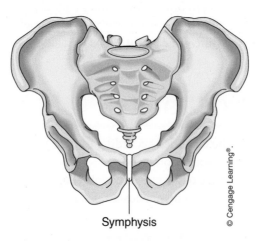

Figure 7-7 Cartilaginous joint

synovial joint

(sin-**OH**-vee-al)

In a **synovial joint** (*Figure 7-8*), the bones have a space between them called the **(1)** joint cavity. The joint cavity is lined with a **(2)** **synovial membrane**, which secretes a thick lubricating fluid called the **synovial fluid**. The bones of the synovial joint are held together by **ligaments**. The surfaces of the connecting bones are protected by a thin layer of cartilage called the **(3)** **articular cartilage**. A synovial joint allows free movement.

Located near some synovial joints are small sacs containing **synovial fluid**. Each sac, called a **(4)** **bursa**, lubricates the area around the joint where friction is most likely to occur. A **bursa** tends to be associated with bony prominences, such as the elbow, knee, or shoulder.

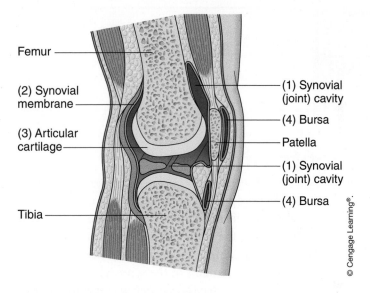

Figure 7-8 Synovial joint and bursa

Functional Classification

The synovial joints are the freely movable joints. The action of these joints allows us to bend, stand, turn, run, jump, and walk—all movements necessary in carrying out our day-to-day routines of life. Two types of synovial joints (based on the amount of movement they permit) are the **hinge joint** and the ball-and-socket joint.

hinge joint

(**HINJ** joint)

A **hinge joint** allows movement in one direction—a back-and-forth type of motion. An example of a **hinge joint** is the elbow. See *Figure 7-9*.

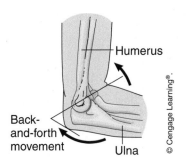

Figure 7-9 Hinge joint

ball-and-socket joint

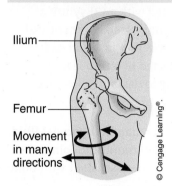

Ilium

Femur

Movement in many directions

© Cengage Learning®.

A **ball-and-socket joint** allows movements in many directions around a central point. A ball-shaped head that fits into the concave depression of another bone allows the bone with the ball-shaped head to move in many directions. Examples of ball-and-socket joints are the shoulder joint and the hip joint. See *Figure 7-10*.

Figure 7-10 Ball-and-socket joint

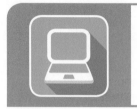

Media Link

View the animation on **Synovial Joints** on the Student Companion Website.

Movements of Joints

The coordination of the muscular contractions and the range of motion of the joints allow for the many movements of the body. The joints allow the bending or extending of the elbow, the stooping to pick up an object from the floor, the fine finger grasp to pick up a small object, the turning of one's head, and so on. Let's take a look at some of the various movements of the synovial joints. Each description includes a "Do this" section designed to have the learner perform the range-of-motion exercise being discussed by participating in the exercise. For a visual reference, as you study these movements, refer to *Figures 7-11A through F*.

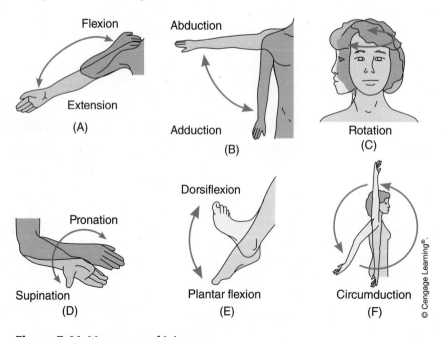

Flexion
Extension
(A)

Abduction
Adduction
(B)

Rotation
(C)

Pronation
Supination
(D)

Dorsiflexion
Plantar flexion
(E)

Circumduction
(F)

© Cengage Learning®.

Figure 7-11 Movement of joints

flexion (**FLEK**-shun)	**Flexion** is a bending motion. It decreases the angle between two bones. *(Do this: Bend your right elbow and touch the side of your neck with your fingertips. By bending the elbow, you decreased the angle between the lower arm bones and the upper arm bone by bringing them closer together. Keep your arm in this position as you read the next movement description.)*
extension (eks-**TEN**-shun)	**Extension** is a straightening motion. It increases the angle between two bones. *(Do this: Remove your fingertips from the side of your neck and straighten your right arm, extending it as if you were going to shake someone's hand. You may now relax your arm. By completing this movement, you increased the angle between the lower arm bones and the upper arm bone by moving them farther apart.)*
abduction (ab-**DUCK**-shun)	**Abduction** is the movement of a bone away from the midline of the body. *(Do this: Raise your left arm out from your side until it is almost parallel with your left shoulder. You may now relax your arm. This action moved your arm away from the midline of your body, thus accomplishing the movement of **abduction**.)*
adduction (ad-**DUCK**-shun)	**Adduction** is the movement of a bone toward the midline of the body. *(Do this: First, place both of your hands on top of your head. Now remove your hands from the top of your head and return them to your side. This action moved your arms toward the midline of your body, thus accomplishing the movement of **adduction**.)*
rotation (roh-**TAY**-shun)	**Rotation** is the movement that involves the turning of a bone on its own axis. *(Do this: Turn your head from side to side as if to say "no." This twisting or turning of the head accomplishes the movement of **rotation**, that is, **rotation** of the neck.)*
supination (soo-pin-**NAY**-shun)	**Supination** is the act of turning the palm up or forward. *(Do this: Place your right hand out, as if to receive change from a cashier. This upward turning of your palm is called **supination**. Next, place your hands by your side, arms relaxed; turn your palms so they face forward. This forward turning of your palms is also called **supination**.)*
pronation (proh-**NAY**-shun)	**Pronation** is the act of turning the palm down or backward. *(Do this: Place your left hand out, as if to show a ring you are wearing. This downward turning of your palm is called **pronation**. Next, place your hands by your side, arms relaxed. Turn your palms so that they face backward. This backward turning of your palms is also called **pronation**.)*

dorsiflexion (dor-sih-**FLECK**-shun)	**Dorsiflexion** of the foot narrows the angle between the leg and the top of the foot (i.e., the foot is bent backward, or upward, at the ankle).
plantar flexion (**PLAN**-tar **FLEK**-shun)	**Plantar flexion** of the foot increases the angle between the leg and the top of the foot (i.e., the foot is bent downward at the ankle, with the toes pointing downward, as in ballet dancing).
circumduction (sir-kum-**DUCK**-shun)	**Circumduction** is the movement of an extremity around in a circular motion. This motion can be performed with ball-and-socket joints, as in the shoulder and hip. *(Do this: Extend your right arm out beside your body and move your arm around in a circular motion. When you do this, you are performing a **circumduction** motion using your shoulder joint.)*

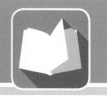

Review Checkpoint

Check your understanding of this section by completing the **Anatomy and Physiology** exercises in your workbook.

VOCABULARY (JOINTS)

The following vocabulary terms are frequently used when discussing the Joints.

Word	Definition
abduction (ab-**DUCK**-shun) ab- = from, away from	Movement of a bone away from the midline of the body.
adduction (ad-**DUCK**-shun) ad- = toward, increase	Movement of a bone toward the midline of the body.

arthralgia
(ar-**THRAL**-jee-ah)
  arthr/o = joint
  -algia = pain
	Joint pain.

articular cartilage (ar-**TIK**-yoo-lar **CAR**-tih-laj)	Thin layer of cartilage protecting and covering the connecting surfaces of the bones.

Word	Definition
articulation (ar-tik-yoo-**LAY**-shun)	The point at which two bones come together; a joint.
ball-and-socket joint	A joint that allows movements in many directions around a central point.
bunion	Abnormal enlargement of the joint at the base of the great toe.
bunionectomy (bun-yun-**ECK**-toh-mee) -ectomy = surgical removal	Surgical removal of a **bunion**; removing the bony overgrowth and the **bursa**.
bursa (**BER**-sah) burs/o = bursa -a = noun ending	A small sac that contains **synovial fluid** for lubricating the area around the joint where friction is most likely to occur.
closed manipulation	The manual forcing of a joint back into its original position without making an incision; also called closed reduction.
closed reduction	See *closed manipulation*.
crepitation (crep-ih-**TAY**-shun)	Clicking or crackling sounds heard upon joint movement.
dorsiflexion (dor-sih-**FLECK**-shun) dors/i = back	Dorsiflexion of the foot is bending the foot backward, or upward, at the ankle.
extension (eks-**TEN**-shun)	A straightening motion that increases the angle between two bones.
flexion (**FLEK**-shun)	A bending motion that decreases the angle between two bones.
ganglionectomy (gang-lee-on-**ECK**-toh-mee) ganglion/o = ganglion -ectomy = surgical removal	Surgical removal of a **ganglion**.
hinge joint (**HINJ** joint)	A joint that allows movement in one direction; a back-and-forth motion.
joint cavity	The space between two connecting bones.
kyphosis (kye-**FOH**-sis) kyph/o = humpback; pertaining to a hump -osis = condition	Humpback.

Word	Definition
ligaments (**LIG**-ah-ments)	Connective tissue bands that join bone to bone, offering support to the joint.
malaise (mah-**LAYZ**)	A vague feeling of weakness.
needle aspiration (needle ass-per-**AY**-shun)	The **insertion** of a needle into a cavity for the purpose of withdrawing fluid.
photosensitivity (**foh**-toh-**sen**-sih-**TIH**-vih-tee)	Increased reaction of the skin to exposure to sunlight.
plantar flexion (**PLAN**-tar **FLEK**-shun)	**Plantar flexion** of the foot is bending the foot downward, at the ankle, as in ballet dancing.
pronation (proh-**NAY**-shun)	The act of turning the palm down or backward.
rotation (roh-**TAY**-shun)	The turning of a bone on its own axis.
sciatica (sigh-**AT**-ih-kah)	Inflammation of the sciatic nerve, marked by pain and tenderness along the path of the nerve through the thigh and leg.
subluxation (**sub**-luks-**AY**-shun)	An incomplete **dislocation**.
supination (soo-pin-**AY**-shun)	The act of turning the palm up or forward.
suture (**soo**-cher)	An immovable joint.
synovial fluid (sin-**OH**-vee-al)	A thick lubricating fluid located in synovial joints.
synovial membrane (sin-**OH**-vee-al **MEM**-brayn)	The lining of a synovial joint cavity.
viscous (**VISS**-kus)	Sticky; gelatinous.

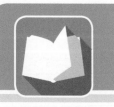

Review Checkpoint

Check your understanding of this section by completing the **Vocabulary** exercises in your workbook.

WORD ELEMENTS (JOINTS)

The following word elements pertain to the joints. As you review the list, pronounce each word element aloud twice and check the box after you "say it." Write the definition for the example term given for each word element. Use your medical dictionary to find the definitions of the example terms.

Word Element	Pronunciation	"Say It"	Meaning
ankyl/o **ankyl**osis	**ANG**-kih-loh ang-kih-**LOH**-sis	☐	stiff
arthr/o **arthr**itis	**AR**-throh ar-**THRYE**-tis	☐	joint
articul/o **articul**ar	ar-**TIK**-yoo-loh ar-**TIK**-yoo-lar	☐	joint
burs/o **burs**itis	**BER**-soh ber-**SIGH**-tis	☐	**bursa**
-centesis arthro**centesis**	sen-**TEE**-sis ar-throh-sen-**TEE**-sis	☐	surgical puncture
-desis arthro**desis**	**DEE**-sis ar-throh-**DEE**-sis	☐	binding or surgical fusion
-gram arthro**gram**	**GRAM** **AR**-thro-gram	☐	record or picture
-graphy arthro**graphy**	**GRAH**-fee ar-**THROG**-rah-fee	☐	process of recording
-itis tendin**itis**	**EYE**-tis ten-din-**EYE**-tis	☐	inflammation
ligament/o **ligament**al	lig-ah-**MEN**-toh lig-ah-**MEN**-tal	☐	ligament
oste/o **oste**oarthritis	**OSS**-tee-oh oss-tee-oh-ar-**THRYE**-tis	☐	bone
-plasty arthro**plasty**	**PLAS**-tee **AR**-throh-**plas**-tee	☐	surgical repair
-scopy arthro**scopy**	**SKOH**-pee ar-**THROS**-koh-pee	☐	process of viewing with an endoscope
ten/o, tendin/o, tend/o **ten**osynovitis	**TEN**-oh, ten-**DIN**-oh, **TEN**-doh, **ten**-oh-**sin**-oh-**VYE**-tis	☐	**tendon**

Review Checkpoint

Check your understanding of this section by completing the **Word Elements** exercises in your workbook.

Pathological Conditions (Joints)

As you study the pathological conditions of the joints, note that the **basic definition** is in a green shaded box (followed by a detailed description in regular print). The phonetic pronunciation is directly beneath each term as well as a breakdown of the component parts of the term where applicable.

adhesive capsulitis

(add-**HE**- sive cap-sool-**EYE**-tis)

Adhesive capsulitis is a shoulder condition characterized by stiffness of the shoulder, limited shoulder movement, and pain; also known as "frozen shoulder." The condition may be idiopathic (cause unknown) or due to an underlying cause such as trauma, **osteoarthritis**, or systemic diseases. Adhesive capsulitis is divided into three stages: the painful stage, the adhesive stage, and the recovery stage.

- During the painful stage, the individual will experience pain with movement and increasing stiffness of the shoulder. He/she may actually notice a decreased ability to reach behind the back, as in fastening a garment or removing something from a back pocket. Muscle spasms may occur, and the individual may have increasing pain at night as well as at rest.

- During the adhesive stage of the condition, the individual usually experiences less pain but has increased stiffness and limitation of movement. The pain is less intense and may decrease at night and while at rest. However, discomfort may be noted with extreme ranges of shoulder movement.

- During the recovery stage, there is decreased pain (with noticeable restriction of shoulder movement). This phase is self-limiting (usually one to three months), and there is a gradual and spontaneous increase in range of motion in the shoulder.

The goal of treatment for adhesive capsulitis is to reduce the pain and restore the shoulder mobility. Treatment includes ice to decrease pain, nonsteroidal anti-inflammatory drugs (NSAIDs) to reduce inflammation, and physical therapy and exercise to enhance joint movement.

arthritis

(ar-**THRY**-tis)
arthr/o = joint
-itis = inflammation

Arthritis is inflammation of joints.

The discussion of **arthritis** will be limited to four types: **ankylosing spondylitis, gout, osteoarthritis, and rheumatoid arthritis** (entries are listed alphabetically).

ankylosing spondylitis	**Ankylosing spondylitis** is a type of **arthritis** that affects the vertebral column and causes deformities of the spine.

(**ang**-kih-**LOH**-sing **spon**-dih-**LYE**-tis)
  ankyl/o = stiff
  spondyl/o = spine; vertebra
  -itis = inflammation

It is also known as Marie-Strumpell disease and as rheumatoid spondylitis. Patient symptoms include other joint involvement, **arthralgia** (pain in the joints), weight loss, and generalized **malaise** (weakness). As the disease progresses, the spine becomes increasingly stiff with fusion of the spine into a position of **kyphosis** (humpback). Treatment includes anti-inflammatory medications to decrease the inflammation and relieve the pain, and physical therapy to keep the spine as straight as possible and promote mobility.

bunion (hallux valgus)	A **bunion**, or **hallux valgus**, is an abnormal enlargement of the joint at the base of the great toe. See *Figure 7-12*.

(**BUN**-yun) (**HAL**-uks **VAL**-gus)

The great toe deviates laterally, causing it either to override or undercut the second toe. As the condition worsens, the bony prominence enlarges at the base of the great toe, causing pain and swelling of the joint.

A **bunion** often occurs as a result of **arthritis** or of chronic irritation and pressure from wearing poorly fitting shoes, although it can be congenital. Treatment for a **bunion** may include application of padding between the toes or around the **bunion** to relieve pressure when wearing shoes, medications to relieve the pain and inflammation, or a **bunionectomy** (which involves removal of the bony overgrowth and the **bursa**).

dislocation	A **dislocation** is the displacement of a bone from its normal location within a joint, causing loss of function of the joint.

(diss-loh-**KAY**-shun)

If the **dislocation** is not complete (i.e., the bone is not completely out of its joint), it is termed a *partial dislocation* or *subluxation*. A **dislocation** can occur in any synovial joint but is more common in the shoulder, fingers, hip, and knee.

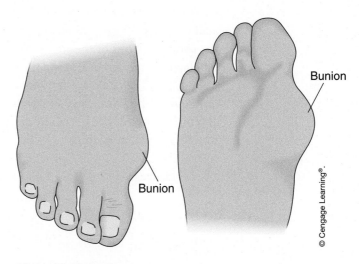

© Cengage Learning®.

Figure 7-12 Bunion

Dislocations are most often the result of an injury that exerts a force great enough to tear the joint **ligaments** (remember that the **ligaments** hold the bones in place at the joint). If this happens, the joint will be extremely painful, there will be rapid swelling at the site, the shape of the joint will be altered, and the patient will be unable to move the joint without severe pain.

Treatment involves the **closed manipulation**, or **reduction**, of the joint (forcing it back into its original position). This should be performed by a physician as soon after the **dislocation** as possible (within 30 minutes) because of the extensive swelling that occurs with a **dislocation**. Prior to the procedure, a sedative is administered intravenously to the patient. The procedure may be performed under local or general anesthesia. After the joint is returned to its normal position, it is immobilized with a cast, splint, or bandage until healing takes place.

ganglion (**GANG**-lee-on)	A **ganglion** is a cystic tumor developing on a **tendon**; sometimes occurring on the back of the wrist. See *Figure 7-13*.

The **ganglion**, which is filled with a jellylike substance, surfaces as a smooth lump just under the skin. It can be painless or somewhat bothersome to the wrist movements.

Treatment for a **ganglion** is unwarranted if the patient is not experiencing pain, disfigurement, or interference with wrist function. If, however, these symptoms are present and the patient is experiencing discomfort from the **ganglion**, a **ganglionectomy** (surgical removal of a **ganglion**) can be performed. The physician may favor a **needle aspiration** procedure to remove the fluid from within the cyst, followed by injection of cortisone.

gout (**GOWT**)	**Gout** is a form of acute **arthritis** that is most often characterized by inflammation of the first metatarsal joint of the great toe. It may also be found in the hands and in the spine. When gout is specifically isolated to the first metatarsal joint of the great toe, it is called podagra (poh-**DAG**-rah).

Gout is a hereditary disease in which the patient does not metabolize uric acid properly. Large amounts of uric acid accumulate in the blood and in the **synovial fluid** of the joints. (The body produces uric acid from metabolism of ingested purines in the diet, especially from eating red meats.) The uric acid crystals are responsible for the inflammatory reaction that develops in the joint, causing intense pain. The pain reaches a peak after several hours and then gradually declines. The attack may be accompanied by a slight fever and chills.

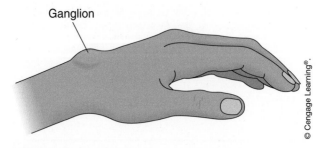

Figure 7-13 Ganglion

Treatment for **gout** may include bed rest, immobilization of the affected part, and application of a cold pack (if the area is not too painful to touch). Anti-inflammatory medications may be given to lessen the inflammation of the area; analgesics may be given to relieve the pain; and medications, such as allopurinol, may be prescribed to lower the uric acid level in the blood. The patient will be instructed to avoid eating foods high in purine (i.e., decrease the intake of red meat) and to increase fluid intake.

herniated disk (**HER**-nee-ay-ted **DISK**)	A **herniated disk** (herniated nucleus pulposus) is the rupture of the central portion, or nucleus, of the disk through the disk wall and into the spinal canal. A **herniated disk** is also called a ruptured disk. See *Figure 7-14*.

Herniation may occur as a result of injury, an abrupt movement, or a degeneration of the vertebrae, or it may be the result of accumulated trauma to the vertebrae. It occurs most often between the fourth and fifth lumbar vertebrae.

When a herniation occurs, the patient may experience a severe, burning, or knifelike pain that worsens on movement. This would indicate pressure on the spinal nerves. If the herniation occurs in the lumbar vertebrae, the pain will radiate down the buttocks and back of the leg following the path of the sciatic nerve. This is known as **sciatica**. If the herniation occurs in the cervical vertebrae, neck flexion or tilting may elicit pain that radiates down the arm, creating a stinging, burning sensation.

Treatment consists of conservative measures such as bed rest, analgesics to relieve the pain, muscle relaxants, physical therapy, and chiropractic manipulation. If this approach is not successful, surgical intervention may become necessary to remove the **herniated disk**.

Lyme disease (**LYME** dih-**ZEEZ**)	**Lyme disease** is an acute, recurrent, inflammatory infection transmitted through the bite of an infected deer tick.

It is characterized by a circular rash (a red, itchy rash with a circular center) and influenza-like symptoms: weakness, chills, fever, headaches,

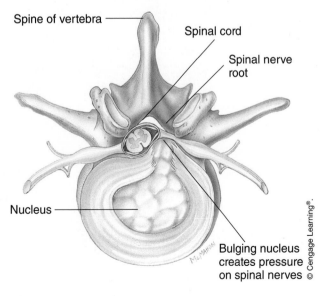

Figure 7-14 Herniated disk

and muscle or joint pain. If these symptoms occur following a camping or hiking trip, the possibility of **Lyme disease** should be considered. The individual should inspect his or her skin for the presence of a tick and remove it if one is found.

Treatment with antibiotics, such as tetracycline, is usually effective. Medications will also be given to relieve the fever, headaches, and muscle or joint pain.

osteoarthritis

(**oss**-tee-oh-ar-**THRYE**-tis)

  oste/o = bone

  arthr/o = joint

  -itis = inflammation

Osteoarthritis is also known as degenerative joint disease. It is the most common form of **arthritis** and results from wear and tear on the joints, especially weight-bearing joints such as the hips and knees.

As this chronic disease progresses, the repeated stress to the joints results in degeneration of the joint cartilage. The joint space becomes narrower, taking on a flattened appearance. See *Figure 7-15*.

Symptoms include joint soreness and pain; stiffness, especially in the mornings; and aching, particularly with changes in the weather. Joint movement may elicit clicking or crackling sounds, known as **crepitation**. The patient may also experience a decrease in the range of motion of a joint and increased pain with use of the joint.

The objectives of treatment for **osteoarthritis** are to reduce inflammation, lessen the pain, and maintain the function of the affected joints. **Osteoarthritis** cannot be cured. Medications may be prescribed to reduce the inflammation and to relieve the pain. Physical therapy may be prescribed to promote the function of the joint. If the condition becomes severe, joint replacement surgery may become necessary.

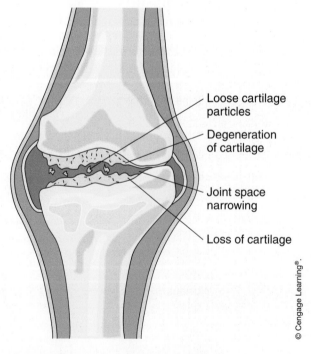

Loose cartilage particles

Degeneration of cartilage

Joint space narrowing

Loss of cartilage

© Cengage Learning®.

Figure 7-15 Osteoarthritis (knee joint)

rheumatoid arthritis

(**ROO**-mah-toyd ar-**THRYE**-tis)

arthr/o = joint

-itis = inflammation

Rheumatoid arthritis is a chronic, systemic, inflammatory disease that affects multiple joints of the body, mainly the small peripheral joints such as in those of the hands and feet.

Larger peripheral joints such as the wrists, elbows, shoulders, ankles, knees, and hips may also be affected. This disease usually occurs in people between the ages of 20 and 40 and is characterized by periods of remission and relapse. Women are affected two to three times more often than men.

Rheumatoid arthritis is characterized by joint pain, stiffness, limitation of movement, and fatigue. The patient usually experiences pain upon arising in the morning and after periods of idleness. The joints of the hands and feet are usually swollen and painful. Characteristic changes in the hands and fingers include ulnar deviation at the metacarpophalangeal (MCP) joints. A condition known as swan neck deformity is also associated with **rheumatoid arthritis**. It is characterized by hyperextension of the proximal interphalangeal (PIP) joint with compensatory **flexion** of the distal interphalangeal (DIP) joint. See *Figure 7-16*.

The main objectives of treatment for **rheumatoid arthritis** are to reduce the inflammation and pain in the joints, to maintain the function of the joints, and to prevent joint deformity. Treatment includes salicylates—such as aspirin to relieve the pain and inflammation (given in high doses)—rest, and physical therapy. If aspirin is not tolerated well, nonsteroidal anti-inflammatory medications may be given to relieve the inflammation. Joint replacement surgery may become necessary for advanced cases of **rheumatoid arthritis**.

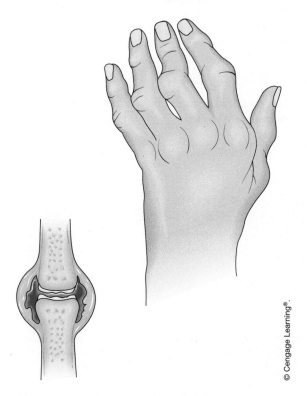

© Cengage Learning®.

Figure 7-16 Rheumatoid hand deformity

sprain	A sprain is an injury involving the **ligaments** that surround and support a joint, caused by a wrenching or twisting motion.

Movements, such as those associated with sports activities that overstress a joint or trying to break a fall, can be the cause of sprains to the upper extremities. Movements that twist the ankle, causing it to invert (turn inward), can be the cause of a sprained ankle. Movements such as whiplash (a sudden jerking or violent back-and-forth movement of the head and neck) can cause a cervical sprain.

A sprain can vary from mild (the ligament is not weakened because only a few fibers are torn) to severe (the ligament is completely torn, either away from its attachment or within itself, with resultant tissue bleeding). If the sprain is severe, the patient may indicate a feeling that something has snapped or torn, and that the joint feels loose. The affected area will be tender to the touch. Other symptoms include swelling, decreased motion, severe pain, and discoloration. Increased tissue swelling following the injury will result in disability of the affected area.

Immediate treatment includes elevating the injured joint and applying ice to the area to prevent swelling. An X-ray of the affected area may be ordered to rule out the possibility of a fracture. The joint may be immobilized with either a splint or a cast. For a less severe sprain, taping the joint may be sufficient.

The healing process for a severe sprain may take four to six weeks. The joint may be immobilized for three to four weeks. Activity should be limited during this time to avoid recurrence of injury. *Table 7-1* compares sprains and strains.

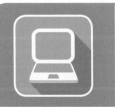

Media Link

Learn more about sprains by viewing the **Shoulder Injury** animation on the Student Companion Website.

Table 7-1 Sprains versus Strains

	Defined	Common Sites	Causes	Symptoms
Sprain	Injury involving the ligaments that surround and support a joint	Knee, ankle	Wrenching or twisting motion	Pain, swelling, decreased motion, and some disability of affected area
Strain	Injury to the body of the muscle or attachment of a tendon	Lower back, cervical regions of the spine	Overstretching, overextension, or misuse	Pain, localized tenderness, possible muscle spasms, and decreased motion of affected area

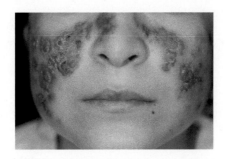

Figure 7-17 Butterfly rash often seen in SLE
(Courtesy of Robert A. Silverman, M.D., Clinical Associate Professor, Department of Pediatrics, Georgetown University)

systemic lupus erythematosus

(sis-**TEM**-ik **LOO**-pus
eh-**rih**-them-ah-**TOH**-sus)

Systemic lupus erythematosus (SLE) is a chronic inflammatory connective-tissue disease affecting the skin, joints, nervous system, kidneys, lungs, and other organs. The most striking symptom of the disease is the "butterfly rash" that appears on both cheeks, joined by a narrow band of rash across the nose. See *Figure 7-17.*

The disease may begin acutely with fever, arthritic joint pain, and weakness, or it may develop over the course of years with periodic fever and weakness. The butterfly rash covers both cheeks and connects by crossing the nose. The rash is aggravated by exposure to the sun (**photosensitivity**).

Mild cases of lupus may be treated with anti-inflammatory medicines, including aspirin, to control the joint pain and fever. More severe cases may be treated with corticosteroid medications.

Diagnostic Techniques, Treatments, and Procedures (Joints)

arthrocentesis

(ar-throh-sen-**TEE**-sis)

   arthr/o = joint
   -centesis = surgical puncture

An **arthrocentesis** is the surgical puncture of a joint with a needle for the purpose of withdrawing fluid for analysis.

A local anesthetic is used and the puncture needle is inserted using sterile technique. Normal **synovial fluid** is clear, straw colored, and slightly sticky. When mixed with glacial acetic acid, it will form a white **viscous** (sticky) clot. When inflammation is present, as in **rheumatoid arthritis**, the **synovial fluid** will be watery and cloudy. The mixture of **synovial fluid** with the glacial acetic acid will result in a clumplike clot that is easily broken.

arthrogram

(**AR**-throh-gram)

   arthr/o = joint
   -gram = record

An arthrogram is an X-ray of a joint after injection of a contrast medium.

arthrography

(ar-**THROG**-rah-fee)

  arthr/o = joint

  -graphy = process of recording

Arthrography is the process of X-raying the inside of a joint after a contrast medium (a substance that makes the inside of the joint visible) has been injected into the joint.

arthroplasty

(**AR**-throh-**plas**-tee)

  arthr/o = joint

  -plasty = surgical repair

Arthroplasty is the surgical reconstruction (repair) of a joint.

It involves the surgical reconstruction or replacement of a painful, degenerated repair joint to restore mobility. It is used as a treatment method for **osteoarthritis** and **rheumatoid arthritis** as well as to correct congenital deformities of the joint.

arthroscopy

(ar-**THROSS**-koh-pee)

  arthr/o = joint

  -scopy = process of viewing

Arthroscopy is the visualization of the interior of a joint by using an endoscope.

A specially designed endoscope is inserted through a small incision into the joint. This procedure is used primarily with knee problems and is useful for obtaining a biopsy of cartilage or **synovial membrane** for analysis. See *Figure 7-18.*

rheumatoid factor

(**ROO**-mah-toyd factor)

The **rheumatoid factor** test is a blood test that measures the presence of unusual antibodies that develop in a number of connective tissue diseases, such as **rheumatoid arthritis**.

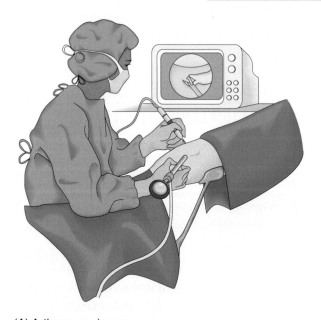

(A) Arthroscope in use

(B) Internal view of the knee during arthroscopy

© Cengage Learning®.

Figure 7-18 Arthroscopy of the knee

erythrocyte sed rate

(eh-**RITH**-roh-sight sed rate)

  erythr/o = red

  -cyte = cell

The **erythrocyte** sedimentation **(sed) rate** (ESR) is a blood test that measures the rate at which erythrocytes (red blood cells) settle to the bottom of a test tube filled with unclotted blood.

Elevated sed rates are associated with inflammatory conditions. The more elevated the sed rate, the more severe the inflammation. This test may be helpful in determining the degree of inflammation in **rheumatoid arthritis**.

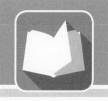

Review Checkpoint

Check your understanding of this section by completing the **Diagnostic Techniques, Treatments, and Procedures** exercises in your workbook.

COMMON ABBREVIATIONS (JOINTS)

Abbreviation	Meaning	Abbreviation	Meaning
DIP	distal interphalangeal (joint)	OA	osteoarthritis
ESR (sed rate)	erythrocyte sedimentation rate	PIP	proximal interphalangeal (joint)
HNP	herniated nucleus pulposus	RA	rheumatoid arthritis
MCP	metacarpophalangeal (joint)	RF	rheumatoid factor
MTP	metatarsophalangeal (joint)	SLE	systemic lupus erythematosus

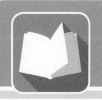

Review Checkpoint

Check your understanding of this section by completing the **Common Abbreviations** exercises in your workbook.

WRITTEN AND AUDIO TERMINOLOGY REVIEW

Review each of the following terms from this chapter. Study the spelling of each term and write the definition in the space provided. Check definitions by looking the term up in the glossary.

Term	Pronunciation	Definition
abduction	☐ ab-**DUCK**-shun	_____
adduction	☐ ad-**DUCK**-shun	_____
ankylosing spondylitis	☐ **ang**-kih-**LOH**-sing **spon**-dih-**LYE**-tis	_____
ankylosis	☐ **ang**-kih-**LOH**-sis	_____

Term	Pronunciation	Definition
arthralgia	☐ ar-**THRAL**-jee-ah	_____
arthritis	☐ ar-**THRYE**-tis	_____
arthrocentesis	☐ ar-throh-sen-**TEE**-sis	_____
arthrodesis	☐ ar-throh-**DEE**-sis	_____
arthrography	☐ ar-**THROG**-rah-fee	_____
arthroplasty	☐ **AR**-throh-**plas**-tee	_____
arthroscopy	☐ ar-**THROSS**-koh-pee	_____
articular	☐ ar-**TIK**-yoo-lar	_____
articular cartilage	☐ ar-**TIK**-yoo-lar **CAR**-tih-laj	_____
articulation	☐ ar-tik-yoo-**LAY**-shun	_____
ataxia	☐ ah-**TACK**-see-ah	_____
atrophy	☐ **AT**-troh-fee	_____
biceps	☐ **BYE**-seps	_____
biceps brachii	☐ **BYE**-seps **BRAY**-kee-eye	_____
bradykinesia	☐ **brad**-ee-kih-**NEE**-zee-ah	_____
buccal	☐ **BUCK**-al	_____
buccinator	☐ **BUCK**-sin-ay-tor	_____
bunion	☐ **BUN**-yun	_____
bunionectomy	☐ bun-yun-**ECK**-toh-mee	_____
bursa	☐ **BER**-suh	_____
bursitis	☐ ber-**SIGH**-tis	_____
cardiac muscle	☐ **CAR**-dee-ak muscle	_____
cartilaginous joint	☐ **car**-tih-**LAJ**-ih-nus joint	_____
circumduction	☐ **sir**-kum-**DUCK**-shun	_____
contracture	☐ con-**TRACK**-cher	_____
crepitation	☐ crep-ih-**TAY**-shun	_____
deltoid	☐ **DELL**-toyd	_____
diaphragm	☐ **DYE**-ah-fram	_____
dislocation	☐ **diss**-loh-**KAY**-shun	_____
dorsal	☐ **DOR**-sal	_____
dorsiflexion	☐ dor-sih-**FLEK**-shun	_____

Term	Pronunciation	Definition
dyskinesia	☐ **dis**-kih-**NEE**-zee-ah	_____
dystonia	☐ dis-**TOH**-nee-ah	_____
dystrophy	☐ **DIS**-troh-fee	_____
electromyogram	☐ ee-**lek**-troh-**MY**-oh-gram	_____
electromyography	☐ ee-**lek**-troh-my-**OG**-rah-fee	_____
electroneuromyography	☐ ee-**lek**-troh-**noo**-roh-my-**OG**-rah-fee	_____
epicondylitis	☐ **ep**-ih-**kon**-dih-**LYE**-tis	_____
erythrocyte sed rate	☐ eh-**RITH**-roh-sight SED RATE	_____
extension	☐ eks-**TEN**-shun	_____
fascia	☐ **FASH**-ee-ah	_____
fasciotomy	☐ fash-ee-**OTT**-oh-mee	_____
fibroma	☐ fye-**BROH**-mah	_____
fibromyalgia	☐ **figh**-broh-my-**AL**-jee-ah	_____
fibrous joint	☐ **FYE**-bruss joint	_____
flexion	☐ **FLEK**-shun	_____
ganglion	☐ **GANG**-lee-on	_____
gastrocnemius	☐ **gas**-trok-**NEE**-mee-us	_____
gout	☐ **GOWT**	_____
hallux valgus	☐ **HAL**-uks **VAL**-gus	_____
hamstring muscles	☐ **HAM**-string muscles	_____
hemiparesis	☐ **hem**-ee-pah-**REE**-sis	_____
hemiplegia	☐ **hem**-ee-**PLEE**-jee-ah	_____
herniated disk	☐ **HER**-nee-ay-ted disk	_____
hinge joint	☐ **HINJ** joint	_____
insertion	☐ in-**SIR**-shun	_____
latissimus dorsi	☐ lah-**TIS**-ih-mus **DOR**-sigh	_____
leiomyofibroma	☐ **lye**-oh-**my**-oh-fye-**BROH**-mah	_____
ligamental	☐ lig-ah-**MEN**-tal	_____
ligaments	☐ **LIG**-ah-ments	_____
Lyme disease	☐ **LYME** dih-**ZEEZ**	_____

Term	Pronunciation	Definition
masseter	☐ mass-**SEE**-ter	
muscle biopsy	☐ muscle **BYE**-op-see	
muscular dystrophy	☐ **MUSS**-kew-lar **DIS**-troh-fee	
myalgia	☐ my-**AL**-jee-ah	
myocele	☐ **MY**-oh-seel	
myoparesis	☐ **my**-oh-pah-**REE**-sis	
myositis	☐ my-oh-**SIGH**-tis	
needle aspiration	☐ needle ass-per-**AY**-shun	
osteoarthritis	☐ **oss**-tee-oh-ar-**THRYE**-tis	
paraplegia	☐ **par**-ah-**PLEE**-jee-ah	
pectoral	☐ **PECK**-toh-ral	
pelvic girdle	☐ **PELL**-vik **GER**-dul	
photosensitivity	☐ **foh**-toh-**sen**-sih-**TIH**-vih-tee	
plantar flexion	☐ **PLAN**-tar **FLEK**-shun	
polymyositis	☐ **pol**-ee-my-oh-**SIGH**-tis	
pronation	☐ proh-**NAY**-shun	
pseudohypertrophic muscular dystrophy	☐ **soo**-doh-**high**-per-**TROH**-fic **MUSS**-kew-ler **DIS**-troh-fee	
quadriceps femoris	☐ **KWAHD**-rih-seps **FEM**-or-iss	
quadriplegia	☐ **kwad**-rih-**PLEE**-jee-ah	
rhabdomyosarcoma	☐ **rab**-doh-**my**-oh-sar-**KOH**-mah	
rheumatoid arthritis	☐ **ROO**-mah-toyd ar-**THRYE**-tis	
rheumatoid factor	☐ **ROO**-mah-toyd factor	
rotation	☐ roh-**TAY**-shun	
sarcopenia	☐ **sar**-koh-**PEE**-nee-ah	
sciatica	☐ sigh-**AT**-ih-kah	
skeletal muscle	☐ **SKELL**-eh-tal muscle	
sternomastoid	☐ stir-no-**MASS**-toyd	
striated muscle	☐ **STRY**-ay-ted muscle	
subluxation	☐ sub-luks-**AY**-shun	

Term	Pronunciation	Definition
supination	☐ soo-pin-**NAY**-shun	_____
suture	☐ **SOO**-cher	_____
synovial fluid	☐ sin-**OH**-vee-al fluid	_____
synovial membrane	☐ sin-**OH**-vee-al **MEM**-brayn	_____
systemic lupus erythematosus	☐ sis-**TEM**-ik **LOO**-pus eh-**rih**-them-ah-**TOH**-sus	_____
temporal	☐ **TEM**-po-ral	_____
tendinitis	☐ **ten**-din-**EYE**-tis	_____
tendon	☐ **TEN**-dun	_____
tenosynovitis	☐ **ten**-oh-**sin**-oh-**VYE**-tis	_____
tibialis anterior	☐ tib-ee-**AY**-lis an-**TEER**-ee-or	_____
torso	☐ **TOR**-soh	_____
trapezius	☐ trah-**PEE**-zee-us	_____
triceps	☐ **TRY**-seps	_____
triceps brachii	☐ **TRY**-seps **BRAY**-kee-eye	_____
visceral muscle	☐ **VISS**-er-al muscle	_____
viscous	☐ **VISS**-kus	_____
voluntary muscle	☐ **VOL**-un-tair-ee muscle	_____

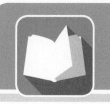

Review Checkpoint

Apply what you have learned in this chapter by completing the **Putting It All Together** exercise in your workbook.

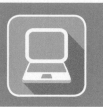

Online Resources

For additional study tools, including PowerPoint® slides and animations, go to the Student Companion Website.

Chapter Review Exercises

The following exercises provide a more in-depth review of the chapter material. Your goal in these exercises is to complete each section at a minimum 80% level of accuracy. A space has been provided for your score at the end of each section.

A. Matching Abbreviations

Match the abbreviations on the left with the correct definition on the right. Each correct answer is worth 20 points. Record your score in the space provided at the end of this exercise.

_____ 1. IM   a. rheumatoid arthritis

_____ 2. MD   b. intramuscular

_____ 3. EMG   c. systemic lupus erythematosus

_____ 4. RA   d. muscular dystrophy

_____ 5. SLE   e. electromyography

                          f. rheumatoid factor

                          g. sedimentation rate

                          h. deep tendon reflex

Number correct _____ **× 20 points/correct answer: Your score** _____**%**

B. Matching Terms

Match the terms on the left with the most appropriate description on the right. Each correct answer is worth 10 points. Record your score in the space provided at the end of the exercise.

_____ 1. skeletal muscle

_____ 2. insertion

_____ 3. origin

_____ 4. striated muscle

_____ 5. visceral muscle

_____ 6. involuntary muscle

_____ 7. voluntary muscle

_____ 8. muscle fiber

_____ 9. fascia

_____ 10. tendon

a. thin sheets of fibrous connective tissue covering a muscle

b. found in the walls of hollow organs and tubes such as the stomach, intestines, blood vessels, and respiratory passageways

c. attached to the bones of the skeleton; responsible for moving the bones of the skeleton

d. strong fibrous band of tissue that attaches muscle to bone

e. point of attachment of the muscle to the bone that it moves

f. acts under the control of the autonomic nervous system

g. has a striped appearance when viewed under the microscope

h. point of attachment of the muscle to the bone that is less movable

i. individual muscle cells

j. so named because it acts under conscious control

Number correct _____ **× 10 points/correct answer: Your score** _____ **%**

C. Labeling

Label the following diagrams for the muscles by writing your answers in the spaces provided. Each correct response is worth 10 points. Record your score in the space provided at the end of the exercise.

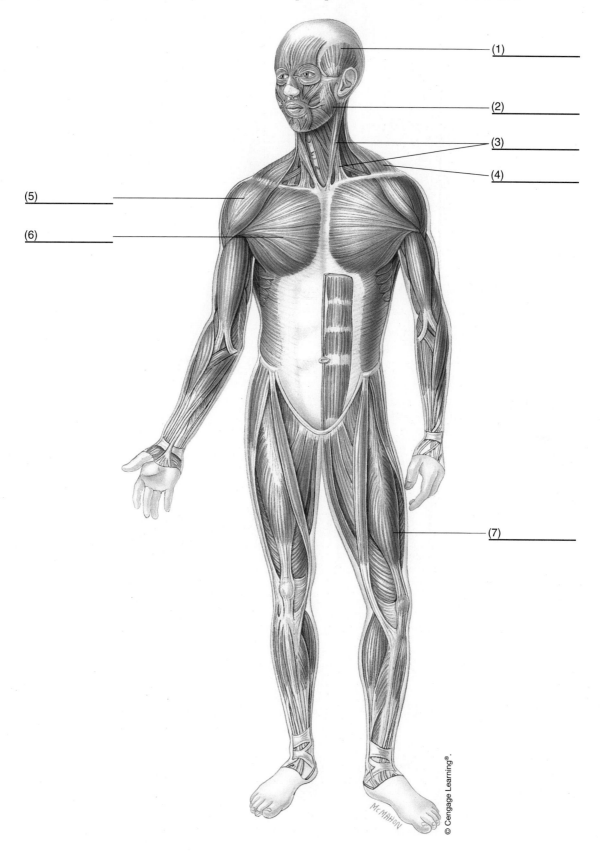

(1) _____

(2) _____

(3) _____

(4) _____

(5) _____

(6) _____

(7) _____

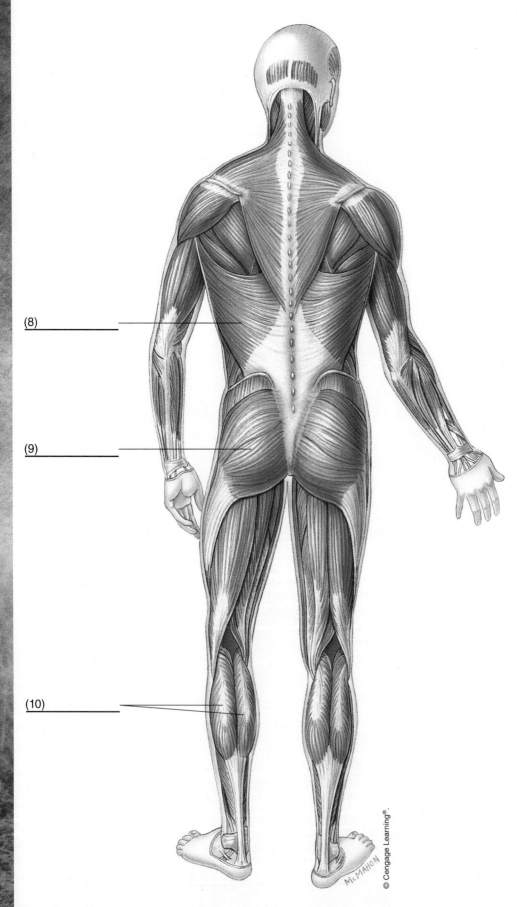

(8) _____

(9) _____

(10) _____

© Cengage Learning®.

1. _____ _____
2. _____ _____
3. _____ _____
4. _____ _____
5. _____ _____
6. _____ _____
7. _____ _____
8. _____ _____
9. _____ _____
10. _____ _____

Number correct _____ **× 10 points/correct answer: Your score** _____ **%**

D. Spelling

Circle the correctly spelled term in each pairing of words. Each correct answer is worth 10 points. Record your score in the space provided at the end of the exercise.

1. brachi   brachii
2. dystrophy   dystrophe
3. polymyocytis   polymyositis
4. arthritis   artheritis
5. viscos   viscous
6. visceral   viceral
7. adduction   aduction
8. soupination   supination
9. rheumatoid   rumatoid
10. siatica   sciatica

***Number correct* _____ × *10 points/correct answer: Your score* _____ %**

E. Crossword Puzzle

The topic of this crossword puzzle is pathological conditions of the muscles and joints. Each crossword answer is worth 10 points. When you have completed the crossword puzzle, total your points and enter your score in the space provided.

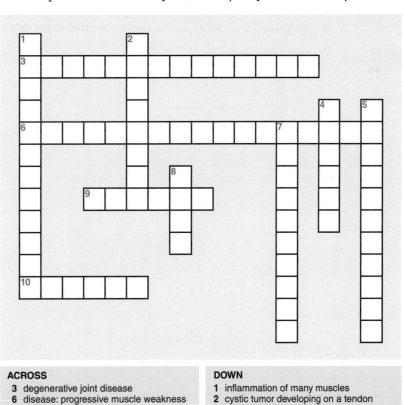

ACROSS
  3 degenerative joint disease
  6 disease: progressive muscle weakness
  9 enlargement of joint of great toe
10 injury to the body of a muscle

DOWN
  1 inflammation of many muscles
  2 cystic tumor developing on a tendon
  4 injury involving twisted ligaments
  5 transmitted by infected deer tick
  7 arthritis affecting small joints
  8 due to accumulations of uric acid

© Cengage Learning®.

***Number correct* _____ × *10 points/correct answer: Your score* _____ %**

F. Completion

Complete each sentence with the most appropriate word. Each correct answer is worth 10 points. Record your score in the space provided at the end of the exercise.

1. Pain in the joints is termed _____.
2. The point of attachment of a muscle to the bone it moves is called _____.
3. Another name for an individual muscle cell is a(n) _____.
4. The muscles that attach to the bones of the skeleton are known as the _____ muscles.
5. The main part of the body to which the head and the extremities are attached is the _____.
6. Another name for a joint is a(n) _____.
7. A clicking or crackling sound heard upon joint movement is known as _____.
8. A small sac (located near a joint) that contains synovial fluid for lubricating areas of increased friction is known as a(n) _____.
9. The proper term for an incomplete dislocation of a joint is _____.
10. An immovable joint is called a(n) _____.

Number correct _____ **× 10 points/correct answer: Your score** _____ **%**

G. Word Element Review

The following words relate to the muscles and joints. The prefixes and suffixes have been provided. Read the definition carefully and complete the word by filling in the space, using the word elements provided in the chapter. Each correct answer is worth 10 points. Record your score in the space provided at the end of this exercise.

1. Pertaining to the cheek
   _____ /al
2. A fibrous tumor
   _____ /oma
3. A painful muscle
   _____ /algia
4. Pertaining to the chest
   _____ /al
5. Bad, or poor, development
   dys/_____ /y
6. Condition of stiffness, as in a stiff joint
   _____ /osis
7. Surgical puncture of a joint
   arthro/_____
8. Inflammation of a tendon
   _____ /itis
9. Surgical repair of a joint
   arthro/_____
10. The process of viewing the interior of a joint with a scope
    arthro/_____

Number correct _____ **× 10 points/correct answer: Your score** _____ **%**

H. Word Search

Read each definition carefully and identify the applicable word from the list that follows. Enter the word in the space provided and then find it in the puzzle and circle it. The words may be read up, down, diagonally, across, or backward. Each correct answer is worth 10 points. Record your score in the space provided at the end of the exercise.

flexion	ambulation	rotation
pronation	dorsiflexion	plantarflexion
adduction	extension	abduction
supination	circumduction	

Example: Another word for walking: _ambulation_ _____

1. A bending motion that decreases the angle between two bones: _____
2. The act of turning the palm up or forward: _____
3. A straightening motion that increases the angle between two bones: _____
4. The movement of a bone toward the midline of the body: _____
5. A movement that involves turning a bone on its own axis: _____
6. The act of turning the palm down or backward: _____
7. The movement of a bone away from the midline of the body: _____
8. A foot movement that bends the foot downward, as in ballet dancing: _____
9. A foot movement that bends the foot upward toward the leg: _____
10. Movement of an extremity around in a circular motion: _____

C	A	D	O	R	S	I	F	L	E	X	I	O	N	A
B	I	S	N	O	I	T	A	N	O	R	P	C	D	M
A	O	R	U	E	T	L	I	M	B	R	I	C	E	B
D	N	E	C	P	F	L	E	X	I	O	N	A	R	U
D	A	X	N	U	I	N	O	I	T	A	T	O	R	L
U	T	T	O	I	M	N	E	X	T	E	N	S	I	A
C	I	E	I	R	C	D	A	R	O	T	A	T	I	T
T	O	N	T	A	L	Y	U	T	A	D	D	U	C	I
I	N	S	C	D	O	R	S	C	I	P	R	O	N	O
O	S	I	U	I	R	C	U	M	T	O	S	U	P	N
N	O	O	D	F	L	E	X	I	O	I	N	R	A	T
D	U	N	B	S	U	P	I	N	A	T	O	N	I	L
E	R	O	A	D	O	R	S	I	F	L	E	N	X	N
P	L	A	N	T	A	R	F	L	E	X	I	O	N	O

© Cengage Learning®.

Number correct _____ **× *10 points/correct answer: Your score*** _____ **%**

I. Proofreading Skills

Read the following Operative Report. For each bold term, provide a brief definition and indicate if the term is spelled correctly. If it is misspelled, provide the correct spelling. Each correct answer is worth 10 points. Record your score in the space provided at the end of the exercise.

Example:

hemiplegia: *paralysis of one side of the bone*

Spelled Correctly?   ☑ Yes   ☐ No _____

OPERATIVE REPORT

Hillcrest
medical center

PATIENT NAME: Smith, John

PATIENT ID: 436725

SURGEON: Martin Agnew, MD

DATE OF OPERATION: 10/21/2014

PREOPERATIVE DIAGNOSES
1. Cerebral palsy, with spastic **hemiplegia**, right.
2. Internal rotation and flexion deformity, right lower leg and knee.

POSTOPERATIVE DIAGNOSES
1. Cerebral palsy, with spastic hemiplegia, right.
2. Internal **rotation** and **flexion** deformity, right lower leg and knee.
3. Bunion, first metatarsophalangeal joint of great toe, left foot.

PROCEDURE
1. Transfer of gracilis and semitendinosus tendons to the lateral aspect of the femur.
2. Lengthening of the posterior tibial **tendon** on the right lower leg.
3. **Bunionectomy**, left great toe.

SURGEON
Martin Agnew, MD

ANESTHESIOLOGISTS
Mark Norman, CRNA
Joseph Rimmer, MD

ANESTHESIA
General.

(continued)

OPERATIVE REPORT
Patient Name: Smith, John
Patient ID: 436725
Surgeon: Martin Agnew, MD
Date of Operation: 10/21/2014
Page 2

PROCEDURE IN DETAIL
Under general anesthesia, the semitendinosus and gracilis tendons were identified on the medial aspect of the thigh by entering through a longitudinal incision over the distal end of these muscles. The muscles were resected from their distal **insertion** point and the **fascia** around the muscles was stripped to allow transfer to the right outer portion of the femur. An incision was made over the lateral aspect of the thigh, and by entering the thigh in the interval between the **vastus lateralis** and the **hamstring muscles** the femur was identified. Drill holes were made in the femur, and the tendons were transferred and sutured in place with #2-0 chromic suture. The fascia was then closed with interrupted # 2-0 chromic suture and the subcutaneous tissue, and both incisions were closed with #3-0 plain suture. The skin was closed with #4-0 nylon.

A bunionectomy was then performed on the left foot. The bony overgrowth and **bursa** were removed without difficulty. The subcutaneous tissue was closed with interrupted #3-0 plain suture, and the skin was closed with interrupted #4-0 nylon. A pressure dressing was applied to the area.

The posterior tibial tendon was exposed by making a longitudinal incision over the distal portion of the medial aspect of the right leg. By sharp dissection, this tendon was identified and lengthened and was then resutured with #2-0 chromic suture. The subcutaneous tissue was closed with interrupted #3-0 plain suture, and the skin was closed with interrupted #4-0 nylon. A short-leg plaster cast was then applied, holding the foot in neutral position.

The patient tolerated the procedure well and was taken to the recovery room in good condition.

_____

Martin Agnew, MD

MA:TR

D:10/28/2014

T:10/29/2014

1. **rotation** _____

_____

Spelled Correctly? ☐ Yes ☐ No _____
2. **flexion** _____

_____

Spelled Correctly? ☐ Yes ☐ No _____
3. **bunion** _____

_____

Spelled Correctly? ☐ Yes ☐ No _____
4. **tendon** _____

_____

Spelled Correctly? ☐ Yes ☐ No _____

(continued)

5. **bunionectomy** _____

_____

Spelled Correctly? ☐ Yes ☐ No _____

6. **insertion** _____

_____

Spelled Correctly? ☐ Yes ☐ No _____

7. **fascia** _____

_____

Spelled Correctly? ☐ Yes ☐ No _____

8. **vastus lateralis** _____

_____

Spelled Correctly? ☐ Yes ☐ No _____

9. **hamstring muscles** _____

_____

Spelled Correctly? ☐ Yes ☐ No _____

10. **bursa** _____

_____

Spelled Correctly? ☐ Yes ☐ No _____

Number correct _____ × *10 points/correct answer: Your score* _____ *%*

J. Matching Diagnostics

Match the diagnostic techniques or tests on the left with the most applicable definition on the right. Each correct response is worth 20 points. Record your score in the space provided at the end of this exercise.

_____ 1. muscle biopsy

_____ 2. electromyography

_____ 3. arthrocentesis

_____ 4. arthroscopy

_____ 5. ESR

a. measures the rate at which red blood cells settle to the bottom of a test tube filled with unclotted blood

b. surgical puncture of a joint for the purpose of withdrawing fluid

c. extraction of a specimen of muscle tissue for the purpose of diagnosis

d. the process of recording the strength of the contraction of a muscle when it is stimulated by an electric current

e. the process of viewing the interior of a joint by using an endoscope

Number correct _____ × *20 points/correct answer: Your score* _____ *%*

K. Medical Scenario

The following medical scenario presents information on one of the pathological conditions discussed in this chapter. Read the scenario carefully and select the most appropriate answer for each question that follows. Each correct answer is worth 20 points. Record your score in the space provided at the end of the exercise.

Sarah Sisk, a 49-year-old patient, has a scheduled visit with her internist today. She attended a health fair yesterday, where a physician suggested she follow up with her primary physician due to a possible diagnosis of polymyositis. The health care professional was not familiar with polymyositis, so when preparing for Sarah's visit, she looked it up to become more familiar with the signs and symptoms, cause, and treatment.

1. The health care professional found that *polymyositis* means:

   a. an acute injury to the body of the muscle or attachment of the tendon, resulting from overstretching, overextension, or misuse

   b. a chronic, progressive, disease affecting the skeletal muscles characterized by muscle weakness and degeneration

   c. a genetically transmitted disorder characterized by progressive weakness and muscle fiber degeneration without evidence of nerve involvement or degeneration of nerve tissue

   d. a chronic disease in which the muscles and bones become abnormally soft due to deficiency of calcium and phosphorus in the blood, resulting in fractures and noticeable deformities of the weight-bearing bones

2. The health care professional identifies that polymyositis is characterized by the patient initially complaining of weakness in the hips and shoulders and difficulty:

   1. breathing

   2. climbing stairs

   3. reaching for things on the upper shelf

   4. in getting out of a chair or the bathtub

      a. 1, 2

      b. 2, 3

      c. 2, 3, 4

      d. 1, 2, 3, 4

3. The health care professional learns that polymyositis is a disease that is:

   a. chronic, characterized by periods of remission and relapse

   b. incurable with death resulting from respiratory complications

   c. acute, requiring about four to six weeks to be resolved

   d. terminal with treatment of radiation and chemotherapy

4. The health care professional gained knowledge that polymyositis occurs twice as often in:

   a. men between the ages of 20 and 40

   b. men between the ages of 40 and 60

   c. women between the ages of 20 and 40

   d. women between the ages of 40 and 60

5. The health care professional discovers that treatment for polymyositis includes:

   a. bed rest for one week and administration of chemotherapy agents and antibiotics

   b. reduction of activities during inflammation, and high doses of corticosteroids and immunosuppressive drugs

   c. physiotherapy to maintain musculoskeletal function, and radiation therapy

   d. chemotherapy and radiation with possible amputation of affected extremity

Number correct _____ × *20 points/correct answer: Your score* _____ %

The Nervous System

CHAPTER CONTENT

OBJECTIVES

Upon completing this chapter and the review exercises at the end of the chapter, the learner should be able to:

1. Correctly identify at least 10 anatomical terms relating to the nervous system.

2. Identify the structures common to the central nervous system.

3. Correctly spell and pronounce terms listed on the Written and Audio Terminology Review, using the phonetic pronunciations provided.

4. Demonstrate the ability to create at least 10 medical words pertaining to the nervous system.

5. Identify the structures of the brain by labeling them on the diagrams provided in the chapter review exercises.

6. Identify at least 10 abbreviations common to the nervous system.

7. Identify at least 10 diagnostic procedures common to the nervous system.

8. Identify at least 30 pathological conditions common to the nervous system.

9. State the difference between afferent and efferent nerves.

10. List the structures of the central nervous system and the peripheral nervous system.

11. Correctly form the plurals of words ending in *-ion*, *-ite*, and *-us* by completing the appropriate chapter review exercise.

Overview

Think of the computer with all of its many wires throughout the system that enable it to perform its many functions. This massive system of wires and networks sends and receives messages. There are numerous wires that are twisted together into a braid, called the power cable, which connects the computer to the electricity that gives it the necessary power to operate.

Now think of the nervous system with all of its many nerves throughout the body that enable the body to carry on its many functions. This system of nerves sends and receives messages. There are many nerve fibers that are twisted together into bundles called nerves that connect the brain and the spinal cord with various parts of the body, relaying messages back and forth. Complicated? Yes!

The nervous system is perhaps the most intricate of all body systems. Consisting of the brain, spinal cord, and nerves, the nervous system functions to regulate and coordinate all body activities and to detect changes in the internal and external environment, evaluate the information, and respond to the stimuli by bringing about bodily responses. It is the center of all mental activity, including thought, learning, and memory.

The study of the nervous system and its disorders is known as **neurology**. The physician who specializes in treating the diseases and disorders of the nervous system is known as a **neurologist**. Any surgery involving the brain, spinal cord, or peripheral nerves is known as **neurosurgery**, and the physician who specializes in surgery of the brain, spinal cord, or peripheral nerves is known as a **neurosurgeon**.

Anatomy and Physiology

The nervous system is divided into two subdivisions: the **central nervous system (CNS)**, consisting of the brain and spinal cord, and the **peripheral nervous system (PNS)**, consisting of 12 pairs of cranial nerves and 31 pairs of spinal nerves. The central nervous system is responsible for processing and storing **sensory** and motor information and for controlling consciousness. The **peripheral nervous system** is responsible for transmitting **sensory** and motor impulses back and forth between the CNS and the rest of the body.

The Peripheral Nervous System

The PNS is made up of nerves and ganglia. A **nerve** is a cordlike bundle of nerve fibers that transmits impulses to and from the brain and spinal cord to other parts of the body. A nerve is macroscopic (i.e., able to be seen without the aid of a microscope). A **ganglion** is a knotlike mass of nerve cell bodies located outside the CNS.

The PNS contains **afferent** (sensory) **nerves** (which carry impulses from the body to the CNS) and **efferent** (motor) **nerves**, which carry impulses from the CNS to the muscles and glands, causing the target organs to do something in response to the commands received.

The PNS is further broken down into the **somatic nervous system** and the **autonomic nervous system**. The **somatic nervous system (SNS)** provides voluntary control over skeletal muscle contractions, and the **autonomic nervous system (ANS)** provides involuntary control over smooth muscle, cardiac muscle, and glandular activity and secretions in response to the commands of the CNS. The ANS contains two types of nerves: sympathetic and parasympathetic. **Sympathetic nerves** regulate essential involuntary body functions such as increasing the heart rate, constricting blood vessels, and raising the blood pressure. Responding to the "fight-or-flight response," the body prepares to deal with immediate threats to the internal environment. The **parasympathetic nerves** regulate essential involuntary body functions such as slowing the heart rate, increasing peristalsis of the intestines, increasing glandular secretions, and relaxing sphincters—thus serving as a complement to the SNS and returning the body to a more restful state. *Figure 8-1* illustrates the divisions of the nervous system.

Cells of the Nervous System

There are two main types of cells found in the nervous system tissue: neurons and **neuroglia**. The **neuron**, known as the functional unit, is the actual nerve cell. It transmits the impulses of the nervous system. A **neuron** consists of three basic parts: a cell

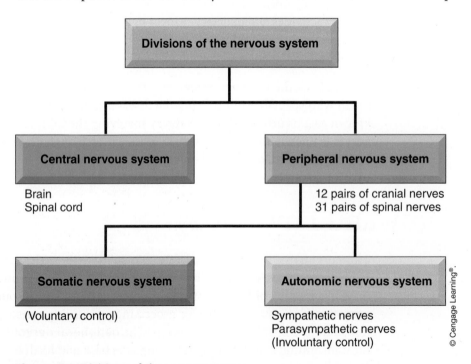

Figure 8-1 Divisions of the nervous system

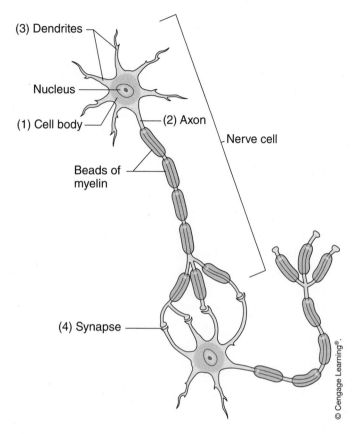

Figure 8-2 The neuron

body, one **axon**, and one or more dendrites. As you read about the structure of the **neuron**, refer to *Figure 8-2*.

The **(1)** cell body is the structure that contains the nucleus and cytoplasm, as do other cells. The **(2)** axon is a single slender projection that extends from the cell body. Axons conduct impulses away from the cell body. Some axons are covered with a **myelin sheath**, which protects the **axon** and speeds the transmission of the impulses. Axons covered with this **myelin sheath** appear white, making up the **white matter** of the nervous system. Axons not covered with the myelin sheath appear gray, making up the **gray matter** of the nervous system. The **(3)** dendrites branch extensively from the cell body, somewhat like tiny trees. The dendrites conduct impulses toward the cell body. Neurons are not continuous with one another throughout the body. Instead, a small space exists between the **axon** of one **neuron** and the **dendrite** of another **neuron**. This space between the two nerves over which the impulse must cross is known as a **(4)** synapse. Chemical substances are released into the **synapse** to activate or inhibit the transmission of nerve impulses across the synapses. These substances are known as neurotransmitters.

Nerves are classified according to the direction in which they transmit impulses. **Afferent nerves** transmit impulses toward the brain and spinal cord. They are also known as **sensory nerves**. **Efferent nerves** transmit impulses away from the brain and spinal cord. They are also known as **motor nerves**. The CNS also contains connecting neurons that conduct impulses from afferent nerves to (or toward) **motor nerves**. These are known as **interneurons**.

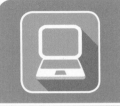

Media Link

See neurotransmitters in action. Watch the **Neurotransmitters** animation on the Student Companion Website.

The **neuroglia**, a special type of connective tissue for the nervous system, provide a support system for the neurons. **Neuroglia** do not conduct impulses; they protect the nervous system through **phagocytosis** by engulfing and digesting any unwanted substances. There are three types of **neuroglia** cells: astrocytes, **microglia**, and **oligodendrocytes** (see *Figure 8-3*). **(1) Astrocytes** are star-shaped cells with numerous radiating processes for attachment. They are the largest and most numerous of the neuroglial cells and are found only in the CNS. The astrocytes wrap themselves around the brain's blood capillaries, forming a tight sheath. This sheath, plus the wall of the capillary, forms the **blood–brain barrier** that prevents the passage of harmful substances from the bloodstream into the brain tissue or **cerebrospinal fluid. (2) Microglia** are small interstitial cells that have slender branched processes stemming from their bodies.

Microglial cells are phagocytic in nature and engulf cellular debris, waste products, and pathogens within the nerve tissue. During times of injury or infection of the nerve tissue, the number of microglial cells dramatically increase, and these cells migrate to the damaged or infected area.

(3) Oligodendrocytes are found in the interstitial nervous tissue. They are smaller than astrocytes and have fewer processes. The processes of the **oligodendrocytes** fan out from the cell body and coil around the axons of many neurons to form the protective

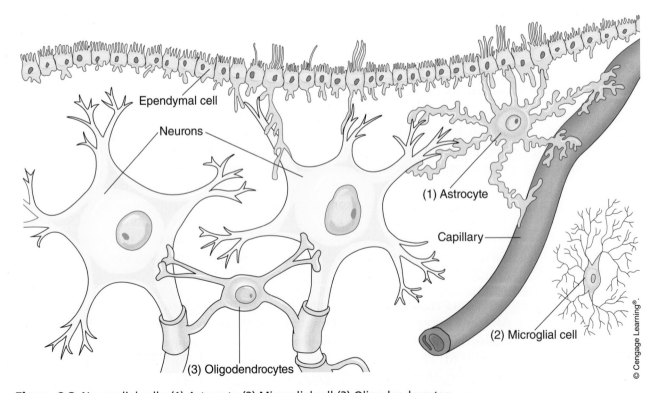

© Cengage Learning®.

Figure 8-3 Neuroglial cells: (1) Astrocyte (2) Microglial cell (3) Oligodendrocytes

myelin sheath that covers the axons of many nerves in the body. The **myelin sheath** acts as an electrical insulator and helps to speed the conduction of nerve impulses.

The Central Nervous System

The CNS, consisting of the brain and the spinal cord, is highly complex in structure and function. We will first discuss the protective coverings of the brain and spinal cord and then will concentrate on the structures of the brain.

The spinal cord and the brain are surrounded by bone for protection. The brain is enclosed in the cranium (skull), and the spinal cord is protected by the vertebrae of the spinal column. In addition to the protection offered by the cranium and the vertebrae, the brain and spinal cord are surrounded by connective tissue membranes (called **meninges**) and by **cerebrospinal fluid**.

The **meninges** are three layers of protective membranes that surround the brain and spinal cord. See *Figure 8-4*. The outermost layer of the **meninges** is called the **(1) dura mater**, which is a tough white connective tissue. Located beneath the **dura**

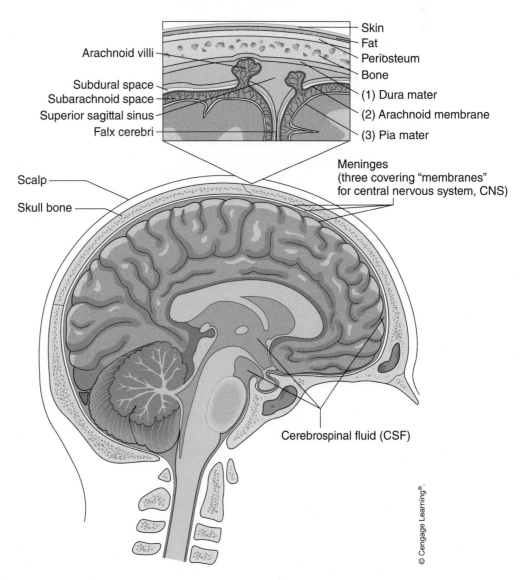

Figure 8-4 The meninges

mater is a cavity called the **subdural space**, which is filled with serous fluid. There is also a space immediately outside the **dura mater** called the **epidural space**. This space contains a supporting cushion of fat and other connective tissues. The middle layer of the **meninges** is called the **(2) arachnoid membrane**, which resembles a spider web in appearance. This thin layer has numerous threadlike strands that attach to the innermost layer of the **meninges**. The space immediately beneath the **arachnoid membrane** is the **subarachnoid space**, which contains **cerebrospinal fluid (CSF)**. This fluid provides additional protection for the brain and spinal cord by serving as a shock absorber. The innermost layer of the **meninges** is the **(3) pia mater**, which is tightly bound to the surface of the brain and spinal cord.

The cushion of **cerebrospinal fluid** flows in and around the organs of the CNS: from the blood, through the ventricles of the brain, the central canal of the spinal cord, the subarachnoid spaces around the brain and the spinal cord, and back into the blood. The **cerebrospinal fluid** contains proteins, glucose, urea, salts, and some white blood cells. It provides some nutritive substances to the CNS. A constant volume of CSF is maintained within the CNS because the fluid is absorbed as rapidly as it is formed. Any interference with the absorption of the CSF will result in an abnormal collection of fluid within the brain, which is termed *hydrocephaly* (or **hydrocephalus**). This condition is discussed in the pathological conditions section.

Structures of the Brain

The brain is one of the largest organs in adults. It weighs approximately 3 pounds in most adults. The brain grows rapidly during the first 9 years or so of life, reaching full size by approximately 18 years of life. This very complex structure, which coordinates almost every physical and mental activity of the body, is divided into four major divisions for discussion: (1) the **cerebrum**, (2) the **cerebellum**, (3) the **diencephalon**, and (4) the brain stem. *Figures 8-5A* and *B* serve as a visual reference to our discussion of the brain.

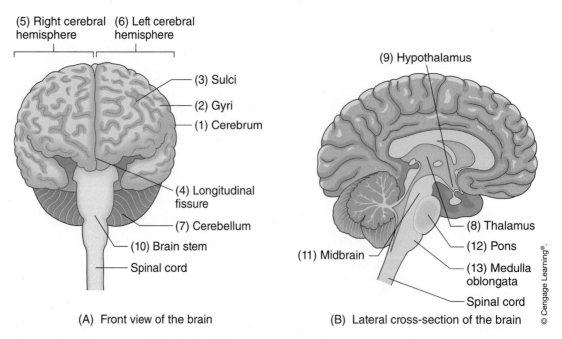

(A) Front view of the brain

(5) Right cerebral hemisphere
(6) Left cerebral hemisphere
(3) Sulci
(2) Gyri
(1) Cerebrum
(4) Longitudinal fissure
(7) Cerebellum
(10) Brain stem
Spinal cord

(B) Lateral cross-section of the brain

(9) Hypothalamus
(8) Thalamus
(11) Midbrain
(12) Pons
(13) Medulla oblongata
Spinal cord

© Cengage Learning®.

Figure 8-5 Structures of the brain: (A) Front view of the brain (B) Lateral cross-section of the brain

The **(1) cerebrum** is the largest part (and the uppermost portion) of the brain. It controls consciousness, memory, sensations, emotions, and voluntary movements. The surface of the **cerebrum** is known as the **cerebral cortex**. The striking feature of the **cerebral cortex** is the presence of convolutions, or elevations, known as **(2) gyri** (singular: *gyrus*), which are separated by grooves known as **(3) sulci** (singular: *sulcus*). The gyri give the appearance of encased sausage folded upon itself many times. The **cerebrum** is divided by a deep **(4) longitudinal fissure** into the two hemispheres: the **(5) right cerebral hemisphere** and the **(6) left cerebral hemisphere**.

The **(7) cerebellum** is attached to the brain stem. It has an essential role in maintaining muscle tone and coordinating normal movement and balance.

The **diencephalon** is located between the **cerebrum** and the **midbrain**. It consists of several structures, with the main ones being the **thalamus**, **hypothalamus**, and the pineal gland. The **(8) thalamus** receives all **sensory** stimuli (except those of smell) and relays them to the **cerebral cortex**. The **(9) hypothalamus** (a small region located just below the **thalamus**) is responsible for activating, controlling, and integrating the peripheral autonomic nervous system, endocrine system processes, and many **sensory** functions such as body temperature, sleep, and appetite. The **pineal body** is a small cone-shaped structure that extends from the posterior portion of the **diencephalon**. The **pineal body**, also known as the pineal gland, is thought to be involved in regulating the body's biological clock. It also produces **melatonin**, which is an important hormone believed to regulate day/night cycles and the onset of puberty and the menstrual cycle.

The **(10) brain stem** is the region between the **diencephalon** and the spinal cord. It consists of the **midbrain**, pons, and **medulla oblongata**. The **(11) midbrain** is the upper part of the brain stem. The **(12) pons** is located between the **midbrain** and the medulla. The **(13) medulla oblongata** is the lowest part of the brain stem and is continuous with the spinal cord. The brain stem serves as a pathway for conduction of impulses between the brain and spinal cord. It controls such vital functions as respiration, blood pressure, and heart rate.

The Spinal Cord

The spinal cord is the pathway for impulses traveling to and from the brain. It carries 31 pairs of spinal nerves that affect the limbs and lower part of the body. The spinal cord is protected by CSF, the three layers of the **meninges**, and the bony encasement of the cervical, thoracic, and lumbar vertebrae.

Review Checkpoint

Check your understanding of this section by completing the **Anatomy and Physiology** exercises in your workbook.

VOCABULARY

The following vocabulary words are frequently used when discussing the nervous system.

Word	Definition
absence seizure (**AB**-senz **SEE**-zyoor)	A small seizure in which there is a sudden temporary loss of consciousness lasting only a few seconds.
acetylcholine (ah-seh-till-**KOH**-leen)	A chemical substance in the body tissues that facilitates the transmission of nerve impulses from one nerve to another. It has a stimulant (or excitatory) effect on some parts of the body (such as the skeletal muscles) and a depressant (or inhibitory) effect on other parts of the body (such as the heart muscle); also known as a **neurotransmitter**.
afferent nerves (**AFF**-er-ent nerves)	Transmitters of nerve impulses toward the CNS; also known as **sensory nerves**.
agnosia (ag-**NOH**-zee-ah) a- = without, not gnos/o = to know -ia = condition	Loss of mental ability to understand **sensory** stimuli (such as sight, sound, or touch) even though the **sensory** organs themselves are functioning properly (e.g., the inability to recognize or interpret the images the eye is seeing is known as optic agnosia).
agraphia (ah-**GRAFF**-ee-ah) a- = without, not graph/o = record -ia = condition	The inability to convert one's thoughts into writing.
alexia (ah-**LEK**-see-ah) a- = without, not -lexia = reading	The inability to understand written words.
analgesia (an-al-**JEE**-zee-ah) an- = without, not -algesia = sensitivity to pain	Without sensitivity to pain.
anesthesia (an-ess-**THEE**-zee-ah) an- = without, not -esthesia = feeling, sensation	Without feeling or sensation.

Word	Definition
Anesthetic (**an**-es-**THET**-ick) an- = without esthet/o = feeling, nervous sensation or sense of perception -ic = pertaining to	Pertaining to partially or completely numbing or eliminating sensitivity with or without loss of consciousness
aneurysm (**AN**-yoo-rizm)	A localized dilatation in the wall of an artery that expands with each pulsation of the artery; usually caused by hypertension or atherosclerosis.
aphasia (ah-**FAY**-zee-ah) a- = without, not -phasia = speech	Inability to communicate through speech, writing, or signs because of an injury to or disease in certain areas of the brain.
apraxia (ah-**PRAK**-see-ah) a- = without, not -praxia = perform	Inability to perform coordinated movements or use objects properly; not associated with **sensory** or motor impairment or paralysis.
arachnoid membrane (ah-**RAK**-noyd **MEM**-brayn)	The weblike middle layer of the three membranous layers surrounding the brain and spinal cord.
astrocyte (**ASS**-troh-sight) astr/o = star-shaped -cyte = cell	A star-shaped neuroglial cell found in the CNS.
astrocytoma (ass-troh-sigh-**TOH**-mah) astr/o = star-shaped cyt/o = cell -oma = tumor	A tumor of the brain or spinal cord composed of astrocytes.
ataxia (ah-**TAK**-see-ah) a- = without, not tax/o = order -ia = condition	Without muscular coordination.
aura (**AW**-rah)	The sensation an individual experiences prior to the onset of a **migraine headache** or an epileptic seizure. It may be a sensation of light or warmth and may precede the attack by hours or only a few seconds.
autonomic nervous system (aw-toh-**NOM**-ik **NER**-vus **SIS**-tem)	The part of the nervous system that regulates the involuntary vital functions of the body, such as the activities involving the heart muscle, smooth muscles, and the glands. The **autonomic nervous system** has two divisions: the SNS and the PNS (defined separately).

Word	Definition
axon (**AK**-son)	The part of the nerve cell that transports nerve impulses away from the nerve cell body.
blood–brain barrier (**BLUD-BRAIN BAIR**-ree-er)	A protective characteristic of the capillary walls of the brain that prevents the passage of harmful substances from the bloodstream into the brain tissue or CSF.
bradykinesia (**brad**-ee-kih-**NEE**-zee-ah) brady- = slow -kinesia = movement	Abnormally slow movement.
brain stem	The stemlike portion of the brain that connects the cerebral hemisphere with the spinal cord. The brain stem contains the **midbrain**, the **pons**, and the **medulla oblongata**.
Brudzinski's sign (broo-**JIN**-skeez **SIGN**)	A positive sign of **meningitis**, in which there is an involuntary flexion of the arm, hip, and knee when the patient's neck is passively flexed.
burr hole	A hole drilled into the skull using a form of drill.
cauda equina (**KAW**-dah ee-**KWY**-nah)	The lower end of the spinal cord and the roots of the spinal nerves that occupy the spinal canal below the level of the first lumbar vertebra; so named because it resembles a horse's tail.
causalgia (kaw-**ZAL**-jee-ah) caus/o = burn -algia = pain	A sensation of an acute burning pain along the path of a peripheral nerve, sometimes accompanied by erythema of the skin; due to injury to peripheral nerve fibers.
cell body	The part of the cell that contains the nucleus and the cytoplasm.
central nervous system	One of the two main divisions of the nervous system, consisting of the brain and the spinal cord.
cephalalgia (**seff**-ah-**LAL**-jee-ah) cephal/o = head -algia = pain	Pain in the head; headache.
cerebellum (ser-eh-**BELL**-um)	The part of the brain responsible for coordinating voluntary muscular movement; located behind the brain stem.
cerebral concussion (ser-**REE**-bral con-**KUSH**-shun) cerebr/o = brain; cerebrum -al = pertaining to	A brief interruption of brain function, usually with a loss of consciousness lasting for a few seconds. This transient loss of consciousness is usually caused by blunt trauma (a blow) to the head.

Word	Definition
cerebral contusion (seh-**REE**-bral con-**TOO**-zhun) cerebr/o = brain; cerebrum -al = pertaining to	Small scattered venous hemorrhages in the brain; better described as a "bruise" of the brain tissue occurring when the brain strikes the inner skull.
cerebral cortex (seh-**REE**-bral **COR**-teks) cerebr/o = brain; cerebrum -al = pertaining to	The thin outer layer of nerve tissue, known as gray matter, that covers the surface of the **cerebrum**.
cerebrospinal fluid (ser-eh-broh-**SPY**-nal **FLOO**-id) cerebr/o = brain; cerebrum spin/o = spine -al = pertaining to	The fluid flowing through the brain and around the spinal cord that protects them from physical blow or impact.
cerebrum (seh-**REE**-brum) cerebr/o = brain; cerebrum -um = noun ending	The largest and uppermost part of the brain. It controls consciousness, memory, sensations, emotions, and voluntary movements.
cervical radiculopathy (**SIR**-vick-al rah-**dick**-you-**LOP**-ah-thee) cervic/o = neck -al = pertaining to radicul/o = root -pathy = disease	Any disease of the spinal nerve roots in the neck; caused by pressure on the nerve roots.
Cheyne-Stokes respirations (**CHAIN-STOHKS** res-pir-**AY**-shunz)	An abnormal pattern of breathing characterized by periods of apnea followed by deep rapid breathing.
coma (**COH**-mah)	A deep sleep in which the individual cannot be aroused and does not respond to external stimuli.
comatose (**COH**-mah-tohs)	Pertains to being in a **coma**.
contracture (kon-**TRAK**-chur)	A permanent shortening of a muscle causing a joint to remain in an abnormally flexed position, with resultant physical deformity.
convolution (kon-voh-**LOO**-shun)	One of the many elevated folds of the surface of the **cerebrum**; also called a **gyrus**.

Word	Definition
craniotomy (kray-nee-**OTT**-oh-mee) crani/o = skull -tomy = incision into	A surgical incision into the cranium or skull.
deficit (**DEFF**-ih-sit)	Any deficiency or variation of the normal, as in a weakness deficit resulting from a **cerebrovascular accident** (CVA).
dementia (dee-**MEN**-shee-ah)	A progressive irreversible mental disorder in which the person has deteriorating memory, judgment, and ability to think.
demyelination (dee-**MY**-eh-lye-**NAY**-shun)	Destruction or removal of the **myelin sheath** that covers a nerve or nerve fiber.
dendrite (**DEN**-dright)	A projection that extends from the nerve cell body. It receives impulses and conducts them on to the cell body.
diencephalon (**dye**-en-**SEFF**-ah-lon)	The part of the brain located between the **cerebrum** and the **midbrain**. Its main structures consist of the **thalamus**, **hypothalamus**, and pineal gland.
diplopia (dip-**LOH**-pee-ah) dipl/o = double -opia = vision	Double vision; also called ambiopia.
dura mater (**DOO**-rah **MAH**-ter)	The outermost of the three membranes (**meninges**) surrounding the brain and spinal cord.
dyslexia (dis-**LEK**-see-ah) dys- = bad, difficult, painful, disordered -lexia = reading	A condition characterized by an impairment of the ability to read. Letters and words are often reversed when reading.
dysphasia (dis-**FAY**-zee-ah) dys- = bad, difficult, painful, disordered -phasia = speech	Difficult speech.
efferent nerves (**EE**-fair-ent nerves)	Transmitters of nerve impulses away from the CNS; also known as **motor nerves**.
embolism (**EM**-boh-lizm)	An abnormal condition in which a blood clot (embolus) becomes lodged in a blood vessel, obstructing the flow of blood within the vessel.
epidural space (**ep**-ih-**DOO**-ral space) epi- = upon	The space immediately outside the **dura mater** that contains a supporting cushion of fat and other connective tissues.

Word	Definition
epilepsy (**EP**-ih-lep-see)	A neurological condition characterized by recurrent episodes of sudden brief attacks of seizures. The seizure may vary from mild and unnoticeable to full-scale convulsive seizures.
fissure (**FISH**-er)	A deep groove on the surface of an organ.
fontanelle or **fontanel** (fon-tah-**NELL**)	A space covered by tough membrane between the bones of an infant's cranium, called a "soft spot."
gait (**GAYT**)	The style of walking.
ganglion (**GANG**-lee-on)	A knotlike mass of nerve tissue found outside the brain or spinal cord (plural: ganglia).
gray matter	The part of the nervous system consisting of axons that are not covered with **myelin sheath**, giving a gray appearance.
gyrus (**JYE**-rus)	One of the many elevated folds of the surface of the **cerebrum** (plural: *gyri*).
hemiparesis (hem-ee-pah-**REE**-sis) hemi- = half -paresis = paralysis	Slight or partial paralysis of one half of the body (i.e., left or right side).
hemiplegia (hem-ee-**PLEE**-jee-ah) hemi- = half -plegia = paralysis	Paralysis of one half of the body (i.e., left or right side).
herpes zoster (**HER**-peez **ZOSS**-ter)	An acute infection caused by the same virus that causes chickenpox, characterized by painful vesicular lesions along the path of a spinal nerve; also called **shingles**.
hyperesthesia (**high**-per-ess-**THEE**-zee-ah) hyper- = excessive -esthesia = feeling, sensation	Excessive sensitivity to **sensory** stimuli, such as pain or touch.
hyperkinesis (**high**-per-kigh-**NEE**-sis) hyper- = excessive -kinesis = movement	Excessive muscular movement and physical activity; hyperactivity.
hypochondriasis (**high**-poh-kon-**DRY**-ah-sis) hypo- = under, below, beneath, less than normal chondr/o = cartilage -iasis = presence of an abnormal condition	A chronic abnormal concern about the health of the body, characterized by extreme anxiety, depression, and an unrealistic interpretation of real or imagined physical symptoms as indications of a serious illness or disease despite rational medical evidence that no disorder is present.

Word	Definition
hypothalamus (**high**-poh-**THAL**-ah-mus)	A part of the brain located below the **thalamus** that controls many functions, such as body temperature, sleep, and appetite.
interneurons (**in**-ter-**NOO**-rons)	Connecting nuerons that conduct impulses from **afferent nerves** to or toward **motor nerves**.
Kernig's sign (**KER**-nigz sign)	A diagnostic sign for meningitis marked by the person's inability to extend the leg completely when the thigh is flexed upon the abdomen and the person is sitting or lying down.
kinesiology (kih-**nee**-see-**OL**-oh-jee) kinesi/o = movement -logy = the study of	The study of muscle movement.
lethargy (**LETH**-ar-jee)	A state of being sluggish. See *stupor*.
longitudinal fissure (**lon**-jih-**TOO**-dih-nal **FISH**-er)	A deep groove in the middle of the **cerebrum** that divides the **cerebrum** into the right and left hemispheres.
medulla oblongata (meh-**DULL**-ah **ob**-long-**GAH**-tah)	One of the three parts of the brain stem. The **medulla oblongata** is the most essential part of the brain in that it contains the cardiac, vasomotor, and respiratory centers of the brain.
meninges (men-**IN**-jeez) mening/o = meninges -es = noun ending	The three layers of protective membranes that surround the brain and spinal cord.
microglia (my-**KROG**-lee-ah)	Small neuroglial cells found in the interstitial tissue of the nervous system that engulf cellular debris, waste products, and pathogens within the nerve tissue.
midbrain	The uppermost part of the brain stem.
motor nerves (**MOH**-tor nerves)	See *efferent nerves*.
myelin sheath (**MY**-eh-lin **SHEETH**)	A protective sheath that covers the axons of many nerves in the body. It acts as an electrical insulator and helps speed the conduction of nerve impulses.
narcolepsy (**NAR**-koh-**lep**-see) narc/o = sleep -lepsy = seizure, attack	Uncontrolled, sudden attacks of sleep.

Word	Definition
nerve	A cordlike bundle of nerve fibers that transmit impulses to and from the brain and spinal cord to other parts of the body. A nerve is macroscopic (i.e., able to be seen without the aid of a microscope).
nerve block	The injection of a local anesthetic along the course of a nerve or nerves to eliminate sensation to the area supplied by the nerve(s); also called conduction anesthesia.
neuralgia (noo-**RAL**-jee-ah) neur/o = nerve -algia = pain	Severe, sharp, spasmlike pain that extends along the course of one or more nerves.
neuritis (noo-**RYE**-tis) neur/o = nerve -itis = inflammation	Inflammation of a nerve.
neuroglia (noo-**ROG**-lee-ah) neur/o = nerve gli/o = gluey substance -a = noun ending	The supporting tissue of the nervous system.
neurologist (noo-**ROL**-oh-jist) neur/o = nerves -logist = one who specializes in the study of	A physician who specializes in treating the diseases and disorders of the nervous system.
neurology (noo-**ROL**-oh-jee) neur/o = nerves -logy = the study of	The study of the nervous system and its disorders.
neuron (**NOO**-ron) neur/o = nerve -on = noun ending	A nerve cell.
neurosurgeon (noo-roh-**SIR**-jun)	A physician who specializes in surgery of the nervous system.
neurosurgery (noo-roh-**SIR**-jer-ee)	Any surgery involving the nervous system (i.e., of the brain, spinal cord, or peripheral nerves).
neurotransmitter (noo-roh-**TRANS**-mit-er)	A chemical substance within the body that activates or inhibits the transmission of nerve impulses at synapses.

Word	Definition
nuchal rigidity (**NOO**-kal rih-**JID**-ih-tee)	Rigidity of the neck. The neck is resistant to flexion. This condition is seen in patients with **meningitis**.
occlusion (oh-**KLOO**-zhun)	Blockage.

oligodendrocyte
(all-ih-goh-**DEN**-droh-sight)
  olig/o = few, little, scanty
  dendr/o = tree, branches
  -cyte = cell
	A type of neuroglial cell found in the interstitial tissue of the nervous system. Its **dendrite** projections coil around the axons of many neurons to form the **myelin sheath**.

palliative (**PAL**-ee-ah-tiv)	Soothing.

paraplegia
(par-ah-**PLEE**-jee-ah)
  para- = near, beside, beyond, two
        like parts
  -plegia = paralysis
	Paralysis of the lower extremities and trunk, usually due to spinal cord injuries.

parasympathetic nerves (pair-ah-sim-pah-**THET**-ik)	Nerves of the ANS that regulate essential involuntary body functions such as slowing the heart rate, increasing peristalsis of the intestines, increasing glandular secretions, and relaxing sphincters.
parasympathomimetic (**pair**-ah-**sim**-pah-thoh-mim-**ET**-ik)	Copying or producing the same effects as those of the **parasympathetic nerves**; "to mimic" the **parasympathetic nerves**.
paresthesia **pair**-es-**THEE**-zee-ah	A sensation of numbness or tingling.
peripheral nervous system (per-**IF**-er-al nervous system)	The part of the nervous system outside the CNS, consisting of 12 pairs of cranial nerves and 31 pairs of spinal nerves.

phagocytosis
(fag-oh-sigh-**TOH**-sis)
  phag/o = to eat
  cyt/o = cell
  -osis = process; condition
	The process by which certain cells engulf and destroy microorganisms and cellular debris.

pia mater (**PEE**-ah **MAH**-ter)	The innermost of the three membranes (**meninges**) surrounding the brain and spinal cord.
pineal body (**PIN**-ee-al body)	A small cone-shaped structure (located in the **diencephalon** of the brain) thought to be involved in regulating the body's biological clock and that produces melatonin; also called the pineal gland.
pineal gland (**PIN**-ee-al gland)	See *pineal body*.

Word	Definition
plexus (**PLEKS**-us)	A network of interwoven nerves.
pons (**PONZ**)	The part of the brain located between the **medulla oblongata** and the **midbrain**. It acts as a bridge to connect the **medulla oblongata** and the **cerebellum** to the upper portions of the brain.
quadriplegia (kwad-rih-**PLEE**-jee-ah) quadri- = four -plegia = paralysis	Paralysis of all four extremities and the trunk of the body; caused by injury to the spinal cord at the level of the cervical vertebrae.
radiculotomy (rah-dick-yoo-**LOT**-oh-mee) radicul/o = root -tomy = process of cutting	The surgical resection of a spinal nerve root (a procedure performed to relieve pain); also called a **rhizotomy**.
receptor (ree-**SEP**-tor)	A sensory nerve ending (i.e., a nerve ending that receives impulses and responds to various types of stimulation).
rhizotomy (rye-**ZOT**-oh-mee) rhiz/o = root -tomy = process of cutting	The surgical resection of a spinal nerve root (a procedure performed to relieve pain); also called a radiculotomy.
sciatica (sigh-**AT**-ih-kah)	Inflammation of the sciatic nerve; characterized by pain along the course of the nerve, radiating through the thigh and down the back of the leg.
sensory (**SEN**-soh-ree)	Pertaining to sensation.
sensory nerves (**SEN**-soh-ree nerves)	Transmitters of nerve impulses toward the CNS; also known as **afferent nerves**.
shingles	See *herpes zoster*.
shunt	A tube or passage that diverts or redirects body fluid from one cavity or vessel to another; may be a congenital defect or artificially constructed for the purpose of redirecting fluid, as a shunt used in **hydrocephalus**.
somatic nervous system (soh-**MAT**-ik nervous system)	The part of the PNS that provides voluntary control over skeletal muscle contractions.
stimulus (**STIM**-yoo-lus)	Any agent or factor capable of initiating a nerve impulse.

Word	Definition
stupor (**STOO**-per)	A state of **lethargy**. The person is unresponsive and seems unaware of his or her surroundings.
subarachnoid space (sub-ah-**RAK**-noyd space)	The space located just under the **arachnoid membrane** that contains **cerebrospinal fluid**.
subdural space (sub-**DOO**-ral space)	The space located just beneath the **dura mater** that contains serous fluid.
sulcus (**SULL**-kuss)	A depression or shallow groove on the surface of an organ; as a **sulcus** that separates any of the convolutions of the cerebral hemispheres (plural: *sulci*).
sympathetic nerves (sim-pah-**THET**-ik)	Nerves of the ANS that regulate essential involuntary body functions such as increasing the heart rate, constricting blood vessels, and raising the blood pressure.
sympathomimetic (sim-pah-thoh-mim-**ET**-ik)	Copying or producing the same effects as those of the **sympathetic nerves**; "to mimic" the **sympathetic nerves**.
synapse (**SIN**-aps)	The space between the end of one nerve and the beginning of another, through which nerve impulses are transmitted.
syncope (**SIN**-koh-pee)	Fainting.
thalamus (**THAL**-ah-mus)	The part of the brain located between the cerebral hemispheres and the **midbrain**. The **thalamus** receives all **sensory** stimuli, except those of smell, and relays them to the **cerebral cortex**.
thrombosis (throm-**BOH**-sis) thromb/o = clot -osis = condition	An abnormal condition in which a clot develops in a blood vessel.
tonic-clonic seizure (**TON**-ik-**CLON**-ik SEE-zhur)	A seizure characterized by the presence of muscle contraction or tension followed by relaxation, creating a "jerking" movement of the body.
ventricle (brain) (**VEN**-trih-kul)	A small hollow within the brain that is filled with **cerebrospinal fluid**.
whiplash	An injury to the cervical vertebrae and their supporting structures due to a sudden back-and-forth jerking movement of the head and neck. Whiplash may occur as a result of an automobile being struck suddenly from the rear.
white matter	The part of the nervous system consisting of axons covered with **myelin sheath**, giving a white appearance.

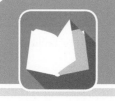

Review Checkpoint

Check your understanding of this section by completing the **Vocabulary** exercises in your workbook.

WORD ELEMENTS

The following word elements pertain to the nervous system. As you review the list, pronounce each word element aloud twice and check the box after you "say it." Write the definition for the example term given for each word element. Use your medical dictionary to find the definitions of the example terms.

Word Element	Pronunciation	"Say It"	Meaning
a- **a**phasia	**AH** ah-**FAY**-zee-ah	☐	without, not
an- **an**encephaly	**AN** an-en-**SEFF**-ah-lee	☐	without, not
-algesia an**algesia**	al-**JEE**-zee-ah an-al-**JEE**-zee-ah	☐	sensitivity to pain
alges/o an**alges**ic	**AL**-jee-soh an-al-**JEE**-sik	☐	sensitivity to pain
-algia cephal**algia**	**AL**-jee-ah seff-ah-**LAL**-jee-ah	☐	pain
-asthenia my**asthenia** gravis	ass-**THEE**-nee-ah my-ass-**THEE**-nee-ah **GRAV**-iss	☐	strength
brady- **brady**esthesia	**BRAD**-ee brad-ee-ess-**THEE**-zee-ah	☐	slow
cerebell/o **cerebell**ospinal	ser-eh-**BELL**-oh ser-eh-bell-oh-**SPY**-nal	☐	**cerebellum**
cerebr/o **cerebr**itis	ser-**EE**-broh ser-eh-**BRYE**-tis	☐	**cerebrum**
crani/o **crani**otomy	**KRAY**-nee-oh kray-nee-**OTT**-oh-mee	☐	skull, cranium
encephal/o **encephal**ography	en-**SEFF**-ah-loh en-**SEFF**-ah-**LOG**-rah-fee	☐	brain

Word Element	Pronunciation	"Say It"	Meaning
-esthesia an**esthesia**	ess-**THEE**-zee-ah an-ess-**THEE**-zee-ah	☐	sensation or feeling
esthesi/o an**esthesi**ologist	ess-**THEE**-zee-oh an-ess-thee-zee-**OL**-oh-jist	☐	feeling, sensation
esthet/o an**esthet**ic	es-**THET**-oh **an**-es-**THET**-ick	☐	feeling, nervous sensation or sense of perception
gli/o **gli**oma	**GLEE**-oh glee-**OH**-mah	☐	**neuroglia** or gluey substance
hypo- = **hypo**esthesia	**HIGH**-poh **high**-poh-es-**THEE**-zee-ah	☐	under, below, beneath, less than normal
-kinesia brady**kinesia**	kih-**NEE**-see-ah brad-ee-kih-**NEE**-see-ah	☐	movement
kinesi/o **kinesi**ology	kih-**NEE**-see-oh kih-**NEE**-see-**OL**-oh-jee	☐	movement
-lepsy narco**lepsy**	**LEP**-see **NAR**-koh-**lep**-see	☐	seizure, attack
-lexia dys**lexia**	**LEK**-see-ah dis-**LEK**-see-ah	☐	reading
mening/o **mening**itis	men-**IN**-go men-in-**JYE**-tis	☐	**meninges**
myel/o **myel**ocele	**MY**-eh-loh **MY**-eh-loh-seel	☐	spinal cord or bone marrow
narc/o **narc**osis	**NAR**-koh nar-**KOH**-sis	☐	sleep
neur/o **neur**opathy	**NOO**-roh noo-**ROP**-ah-thee	☐	nerve
-paresis hemi**paresis**	par-**EE**-sis hem-ee-pah-**REE**-sis	☐	partial paralysis
-phasia dys**phasia**	**FAY**-zee-ah dis-**FAY**-zee-ah	☐	speech
-plegia para**plegia**	**PLEE**-jee-ah par-ah-**PLEE**-jee-ah	☐	paralysis
-praxia a**praxia**	**PRAK**-see-ah ah-**PRAK**-see-ah	☐	perform

Word Element	Pronunciation	"Say It"	Meaning
radicul/o **radicul**opathy	rah-**DICK**-you-loh rah-**dick**-you-**LOP**-ah-thee	☐	root
thec/o intra**thec**al	**THEE**-koh in-trah-**THEE**-kal	☐	sheath
ton/o dys**ton**ia	**TON**-oh dis-**TON**-ee-ah	☐	tension, tone
ventricul/o **ventricul**ostomy	ven-**TRIK**-yoo-loh ven-trik-yoo-**LOSS**-toh-mee	☐	**ventricle** of the heart or brain

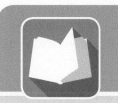

Review Checkpoint

Check your understanding of this section by completing the **Word Elements** exercises in your workbook.

Pathological Conditions

As you study the pathological conditions of the nervous system, note that the **basic definition** is in a green shaded box followed by a detailed description in regular print. The phonetic pronunciation is directly beneath each term, along with a breakdown of the component parts of the term where applicable.

The pathological conditions for the nervous system are listed in alphabetical order for easy reference. The pathological conditions fall into the following categories: **congenital** disorders (those occurring at birth); degenerative, functional, and seizure disorders; infectious disorders; **intracranial tumors** and traumatic disorders; vascular disorders; peripheral nerve disorders; and disk disorders. As each disorder is discussed, its category is identified.

Alzheimer's disease

(**ALTS**-high-merz dih-**ZEEZ**)

Deterioration of a person's intellectual functioning. **Alzheimer's disease** (AD) is progressive and extremely debilitating. It begins with minor memory loss and progresses to complete loss of mental, emotional, and physical functioning, frequently occurring in persons over 65 years of age.

This process occurs through three identified stages over a number of years. **Stage 1** lasts for approximately 1 to 3 years and includes loss of short-term memory; decreased ability to pay attention or learn new information; gradual personality changes such as increased irritability, denial, and depression; and difficulties in depth perception. People with AD in stage 1 often recognize and attempt to adjust or cover up mental errors.

Stage 2 lasts approximately 2 to 10 years, during which time the person loses the ability to write, to identify objects by touch, to accomplish purposeful movements, and to perform simple tasks such as getting dressed. During this progressive deterioration, safety is a major concern. Also during the second stage, the person with AD loses the ability to communicate socially with others. He or she uses the wrong words in conversation, tends to repeat phrases, and may eventually develop total loss of language function (called **aphasia**).

Stage 3 lasts for 8 to 10 years, during which time the person with AD has very little (if any) communication skills due to disorientation to time, place, and person. Bowel and bladder incontinence, posture flexion, and limb rigidity also are noted during this stage. This increasing deterioration tends to render the person with AD dependent on others to provide for basic needs. The individual may be cared for by family members or need placement in a long-term care facility. The person with AD is prone to additional complications such as malnutrition, dehydration, and pneumonia.

It has been identified that both chemical and structural changes in the brain cause the symptoms of AD. However, there is no single clinical test for identifying AD. Before a diagnosis is made, other conditions that mimic the symptoms must be excluded. A clinical diagnosis of Alzheimer's is then based on tests such as physical, psychological, neurological, and psychiatric examinations plus various laboratory tests. With today's new diagnostic tools and criteria, it is possible for physicians to make a positive clinical diagnosis of Alzheimer's with approximately 90% accuracy. A confirmation of the diagnosis of AD is not possible until death because biopsy or autopsy examination of the brain tissue is required for a diagnosis.

Treatment for AD includes the use of tacrine hydrochloride (Cognex), which is approved for use in mild to moderate cases due to its ability to improve memory in approximately 40% of persons with AD. Antidepressants and tranquilizers are also frequently used to treat symptoms. The persons/families experiencing AD need a great deal of education and support to endure this difficult disease.

amyotrophic lateral sclerosis (ALS) (ah-**my**-oh-**TROH**-fick **LAT**-er-al skleh-**ROH**-sis) a- = without, not my/o = muscle troph/o = development -ic = pertaining to scler/o = hard; also refers to clera of the eye -osis = condition	**Amyotrophic lateral sclerosis (ALS)** is a severe weakening and wasting of the involved muscle groups, usually beginning with the hands and progressing to the shoulders, upper arms, and legs. It is caused by decreased nerve innervation to the muscle groups.

This lack of muscle innervation is due to the loss of motor neurons in the brain stem and spinal cord. This is specifically a motor deficit and does not involve cognitive (mental thinking) or **sensory** (hearing, vision, and sensation) changes. As the muscle masses weaken and lose innervation, the person with ALS begins to complain of worsening fatigue with resulting uncoordinated movements, spasticity, and eventually paralysis.

As the brain stem involvement increases, the person with ALS experiences severe wasting of the muscles in the tongue and face, causing speech, chewing, and swallowing difficulties. In addition, other manifestations of ALS include difficulty clearing airway and breathing and loss of temperament control (with fluctuating emotions). Complications of ALS include loss of verbal communication, loss of ability to provide self-care, total immobility, depression, malnutrition, pneumonia, and inevitable respiratory failure.

There is no cure for ALS, and the primary care focuses on support of the person and family to meet their physical and emotional needs, especially as this physically debilitating disease progresses. The course of ALS varies according to the individual, but approximately 50% die within 3 to 5 years of diagnosis. ALS is also called Lou Gehrig's disease.

anencephaly
(**an**-en-**SEFF**-ah-lee)
 	
  an- = without, not
  encephal/o = brain
  -y = noun ending
	Anencephaly is an absence of the brain and spinal cord at birth, a congenital disorder.

The condition is incompatible with life. It can be detected through an amniocentesis or ultrasonography early in pregnancy.

Bell's palsy (**BELLZ PAWL**-zee)	**Bell's palsy** is a temporary or permanent unilateral weakness or paralysis of the muscles in the face following trauma to the face, an unknown infection, or a tumor pressing on the facial nerve rendering it paralyzed.

Symptoms include drooling, inability to close the eye or regulate salivation on the affected side (with a distorted facial appearance), and loss of appetite and taste perception. Treatment includes gentle massage; applying warm, moist heat; facial exercises to activate muscle tone; prednisone to reduce swelling; and analgesics to relieve pain. Early treatment is important for a complete recovery.

brain abscess (**BRAIN AB**-sess)	A **brain abscess** is a localized accumulation of pus located anywhere in the brain tissue due to an infectious process—either a primary local infection or an infection secondary to another infectious process in the body (such as bacterial endocarditis, sinusitis, otitis, or dental abscess).

The initial symptom is a complaint of a headache that results from the increase in intracranial pressure (ICP). Other symptoms follow according to the location of the abscess. They include vomiting, visual disturbances, seizures, neck stiffness, and unequal pupil size. A computerized tomography (CT) scan and/or an electroencephalogram (EEG) will verify the diagnosis and location.

A **brain abscess** is treated aggressively with intravenous antibiotics. With signs and symptoms of ICP, mannitol (an osmotic diuretic) may be given in addition to steroids to reduce cerebral edema and thus decrease the intracranial pressure. If treatment response is not good in a short period of time and there is an increased intracranial pressure, surgical drainage may be required to preserve cerebral functioning.

carpal tunnel syndrome (**CAR**-pal **TUN**-el **SIN**-drom)	**Carpal tunnel syndrome** is a pinching or compression of the median nerve within the carpal tunnel due to inflammation and swelling of the tendons, causing intermittent or continuous pain that is greatest at night.

The carpal tunnel is a narrow passage from the wrist to the hand housing blood vessels, tendons, and the median nerve. This tendon inflammation occurs largely as a result of repetitious overuse of the fingers, hands, or wrists.

Treatment involves anti-inflammatory medications, splints, physical therapy, and stopping the repetitive overuse. When medical treatment fails to relieve the pain, surgical intervention may be necessary to relieve pressure on the median nerve.

cerebral concussion (seh-**REE**-bral con-**KUSH**-un)	**Cerebral concussion** is a brief interruption of brain function, usually with a loss of consciousness lasting for a few seconds.

This transient loss of consciousness is usually caused by blunt trauma (a blow) to the head. With a severe concussion, the individual may experience unconsciousness for a longer period of time, a seizure, respiratory arrest, or hypotension.

The individual experiencing a **cerebral concussion** will likely have a headache after regaining consciousness and will not be able to remember the events surrounding the injury. Other symptoms often associated with a **cerebral concussion** include blurred vision, drowsiness, confusion, visual disturbances, and dizziness.

The individual will need to be observed for signs of increased intracranial pressure or signs of intracranial bleeding during the period of unconsciousness and for several hours after consciousness is resumed. These signs indicate an injury requiring further treatment.

cerebral contusion (seh-**REE**-bral con-**TOO**-zhun)	**Cerebral contusion** is a small, scattered venous hemorrhage in the brain (or better described as a "bruise" of the brain tissue) occurring when the brain strikes the inner skull.

The contusion will likely cause swelling of the brain tissue (called cerebral edema). Cerebral edema will be at its height 12 to 24 hours after the injury.

Symptoms vary according to the size and location of the contusion. Some symptoms include increased ICP, combativeness, and altered level of consciousness.

Treatment includes close observation for secondary effects, including signs of increasing intracranial pressure and altered levels of consciousness. Hospitalization is usually required to monitor ICP, maintain cerebral perfusion, and administer corticosteroids and osmotic diuretics.

cerebral palsy (seh-**REE**-bral **PAWL**-zee) cerebr/o = brain; **cerebrum** -al = pertaining to	**Cerebral palsy** (CP) is a collective term used to describe congenital (at birth) brain damage that is permanent but not progressive. It is characterized by the child's lack of control of voluntary muscles.

The lack of voluntary muscle control in CP is due to injuries to the **cerebrum** which occur before birth, during birth, or during the first 3 to 5 years of a child's life. The specific symptoms and types of CP will vary according to the area of the **cerebrum** involved. The four major types of CP are as follows:

1. **Spastic** results from damage to the cortex of the brain, causing tense muscles and very irritable muscle tone. A very tense heel cord that forces a child to walk on his or her toes is an example of the spastic type of CP. This is the most common type.

2. **Ataxic** results from damage to the **cerebellum** and involves tremors, a disturbed equilibrium, loss of coordination, and abnormal movements. This type of CP will force the child to stagger when walking.

3. **Athetoid** (or dyskinetic) is due to damage to the basal ganglia, which causes abnormal movements such as twisting or sudden jerking. This jerking may result from any **stimulus**, including the increased intensity brought on by stress.

4. **Mixed** CP is a combination of **symptoms** of the three types of CP previously cited.

Intellectual function may range from extremely bright normal to severe mental retardation. Other common handicaps associated with CP include oculomotor impairment, convulsive disorder(s), and hearing and speech impairments.

cerebrovascular accident (CVA) (seh-**REE**-broh-**VASS**-kyoo-lar **AK**-sih-dent) cerebr/o = brain; **cerebrum**	A **cerebrovascular accident (CVA)** involves death of a specific portion of brain tissue, resulting from a decrease in blood flow (ischemia) to that area of the brain; also called stroke.

Causes of a **cerebrovascular accident** include cerebral hemorrhage, **thrombosis** (clot formation), and **embolism** (dislodging of a clot). **Transient ischemic attacks (TIAs)** are brief periods of ischemia in the brain, lasting from minutes to hours, which can cause a variety of symptoms. TIAs (or "mini-strokes") often precede a full-blown thrombotic CVA. The neurological symptoms range according to the amount of ischemia and the location of the vessels involved. The person experiencing a TIA may complain of numbness or weakness in the extremities or corner of the mouth as well as difficulty communicating. The person may also experience a visual disturbance. Sometimes the symptoms are vague and difficult to describe. The person may simply complain of a "funny feeling."

Cerebral **thrombosis** (clot), also called thrombotic CVA, makes up 50% of all CVAs and occurs largely in individuals older than 50 years of age and often during rest or sleep. The cerebral clot is typically caused by atherosclerosis, which is a thickened fibrotic vessel wall that causes the diameter of the vessel to be decreased or completely closed off from the buildup of plaque. The thrombotic CVA is often preceded by one or many TIAs. The occurrence of the CVA caused by a cerebral **thrombosis** is rapid, but the progression is slow. It is often called a "stroke-in-evolution," sometimes taking three days to become a "completed stroke" (wherein the maximum neurological dysfunction becomes evident and the affected area of the brain is swollen and necrotic).

Cerebral **embolism** occurs when an embolus or fragments of a blood clot, fat, bacteria, or tumor lodge in a cerebral vessel and cause an **occlusion**. This **occlusion** renders the area supplied by this vessel ischemic. A heart problem may lead to the occurrence of a cerebral embolus such as endocarditis, atrial fibrillation, and valvular conditions. A piece of a clot may break off in the carotid artery and move into the circulation, causing a cerebral **embolism**. A fat embolus can occur from the fracture of a long bone. The cerebral emboli will cause immediate neurological dysfunction. If the embolus breaks up and is consumed by the body, the dysfunction will disappear. If the embolus does not break up, the dysfunction will remain. Even when the embolus breaks up, the vessel wall is often left weakened, increasing the possibility of a cerebral hemorrhage at this site.

Cerebral hemorrhage occurs when a cerebral vessel ruptures, allowing bleeding into the CSF, brain tissue, or the **subarachnoid space**. High blood pressure is the most common cause of a cerebral hemorrhage. The symptoms occur rapidly and generally include a severe headache along with other neurological dysfunctions (related to the area involved).

Symptoms of a CVA may vary from going unnoticed; to numbness, confusion, and dizziness; to more severe disabilities such as impaired consciousness (ranging from **stupor** to **coma**, paralysis, and **aphasia**). The symptoms of a CVA will differ widely according to the degree of involvement, the amount of time the blood flow is decreased or stopped, and the region of the brain involved.

Treatment of CVA depends on the cause and effect of the stroke. The prognosis, or predicted outcome, for a stroke victim depends on the degree of damage to the affected area of the brain and how quickly treatment is initiated.

degenerative disk (deh-**JEN**-er-ah-tiv **DISK**)	**Degenerative disk** is the deterioration of the intervertebral disk, usually due to constant motion and wear on the disk.

A vertebral misalignment will result in constant rubbing on the disk, with gradual wasting and inflammation that results in **degenerative disk** disease. Pain is the primary symptom and occurs in the regions served by the spinal nerves of the disk space involved. The pain is described as burning and continuous, sometimes radiating down the leg(s). There may be some motor function loss as well. The person with **degenerative disk** disease is often unable to carry on normal daily activities due to the pain and/or motor loss. Treatment includes bed rest, bracing the back, nonsteroidal anti-inflammatory drugs (NSAIDs), analgesics, **transcutaneous electrical nerve stimulation (TENS)**, and finally surgical interventions (spinal fusion or freeing compressed spinal nerve roots).

encephalitis (en-**seff**-ah-**LYE**-tis) encephal/o = brain -itis = inflammation	**Encephalitis** is the inflammation of the brain largely caused by a virus that enters the CNS when the person experiences a viral disease such as measles or mumps or through the bite of a mosquito or tick.

Encephalitis may also (but less often) be caused by parasites, rickettsia, fungi, or bacteria. Whatever the causative organism, it becomes invasive and destructive to the brain or spinal cord tissue involved.

Encephalitis is characterized by symptoms similar to **meningitis**. However, there is no buildup of exudate (as there is with **meningitis**). Small hemorrhages occur in the CNS tissue, causing the tissue to become necrotic.

Symptoms include restlessness, seizure, headache, fever, stiff neck, altered mental function, and decreased level of consciousness. The person with **encephalitis** may also experience facial weakness, difficulty communicating and understanding verbal communication, a change in personality, or weakness on one side of the body. The deterioration of nerve cells and the increase of cerebral edema may eventually result in permanent neurological problems and/or a **comatose** state. The outcome varies related to the degree of inflammation, the age and condition of the individual experiencing **encephalitis**, and the cause.

Treatment for **encephalitis** includes administering medications, treating symptoms, and preventing complications. Administration of mild analgesics for pain, antipyretics for fever, anticonvulsants for seizure activity, antibiotics for intercurrent infections, and corticosteroids or osmotic diuretics to control cerebral edema are all part of the treatment regimen as indicated according to the symptoms.

epilepsy (**EP**-ih-**lep**-see)	**Epilepsy** is a syndrome of recurring episodes of excessive irregular electrical activity of the brain resulting in involuntary muscle movements called seizures.

These seizures may occur with a diseased or structurally normal CNS, and this abnormal electrical activity may involve a part or all of the person's brain. Epileptic seizures may affect consciousness level, skeletal motor function, sensation, and autonomic function of the internal organs. Severe seizures may produce a decrease of oxygen in the blood circulating through the body as well as acidosis and respiratory arrest. Seizures are classified according to the area of the brain or the focus, the cause, and the clinical signs and symptoms experienced. The categories include:

1. **Partial seizures**, arising from a focal area that may be **sensory**, motor, or even a diverse complex focus.

2. **Generalized seizures**, commonly resulting in loss of consciousness and involving both cerebral hemispheres. Grand mal and petit mal seizures are the most common types of generalized seizures.

Anticonvulsant medications can reduce or control most seizure activity. Diagnostic testing performed to confirm a diagnosis of seizures includes (but may not be limited to) the following: complete neurological exam, ambulatory electroencephalogram, MRI, and CT scan. A discussion of the ambulatory encephalogram appears in the section on diagnostic techniques and procedures.

grand mal seizure (grand **MALL SEE**-zyoor)	A **grand mal seizure** is an epileptic seizure characterized by a sudden loss of consciousness and by generalized involuntary muscular contraction, vacillating between rigid body extension and an alternating contracting and relaxing of muscles.

The **grand mal seizure**, also called **tonic-clonic seizure**, is the most common seizure in adults and children. Persons experiencing tonic-clonic seizures may describe an **aura** (indication of some type) preceding the onset of the tonic phase of the seizure.

The tonic phase begins with a sudden loss of consciousness, followed by the person's falling to the floor (with muscle contractions causing rigid extension of the head, legs, and arms, and clenching of the teeth). The eyes roll back and the pupils are dilated and fixed. As the diaphragm contracts, and air is forced through closed vocal chords, a cry is often heard and breathing is stopped. Both urinary and bowel incontinence may happen. This phase may last up to 1 minute, but the average duration is 15 seconds before the clonic phase begins.

The clonic phase is characterized by contraction and relaxation of muscle groups in arms and legs, with rapid shallow breathing called hyperventilation. Excessive salivation occurs during the clonic phase, but subsides gradually within an average of 45 to 90 seconds.

The person experiencing a **grand mal seizure** can remain unconscious for up to 30 minutes after the clonic phase has stopped. There is confusion and disorientation as consciousness is regained. The person will not remember the seizure itself but will feel very tired and complain of muscle soreness and fatigue. If an **aura** occurs with a seizure, that is usually the last memory recalled. Protection of the person during the tonic-clonic phase is the priority of care.

petit mal seizure (pet-**EE MALL SEE**-zyoor)	A **petit mal seizure** is a small seizure in which there is a sudden temporary loss of consciousness lasting only a few seconds; also known as an **absence seizure**.

The individual may have a blank facial expression and may experience repeated blinking of the eyes during this brief period of time. There is no loss of consciousness and the episode often goes unnoticed by the individual. The duration of the seizure is 5 to 10 seconds. Petit mal seizures occur more frequently in children prior to puberty, beginning most often about the age of 5.

Guillain-Barré syndrome (**GHEE**-yon bah-**RAY SIN**-drom)	**Guillain-Barré syndrome** is acute polyneuritis ("inflammation of many nerves") of the PNS in which the myelin sheaths on the axons are destroyed, resulting in decreased nerve impulses, loss of reflex response, and sudden muscle weakness, which usually follows a viral gastrointestinal or respiratory infection.

This polyneuritis usually begins with symmetric motor and **sensory** loss in the lower extremities, which ascends to the upper torso, upper extremities, and cranial nerves. The person with **Guillain-Barré syndrome** retains complete mental ability and consciousness while experiencing pain, weakness, and numbness. Approximately 25% of persons with **Guillain-Barré syndrome** will experience respiratory dysfunction requiring ventilatory assistance. In most persons, this disease begins to resolve itself in several weeks, but the patient may take several months to 2 years to regain complete muscle strength. Treatment is symptomatic, supportive, and aimed at preventing complications related to extended immobility, pain, anxiety, powerlessness, and respiratory dysfunction.

headache (cephalalgia)
(**seff**-ah-**LAL**-jee-ah)
  cephal/o = head
  -algia = pain
	Cephalalgia involves pain (varying in intensity from mild to severe) anywhere within the cranial cavity. It may be chronic or acute and may occur as a result of a disease process or be totally benign. The majority of headaches are transient and produce mild pain relieved by a mild **analgesic**.

Disturbances in cranial circulation produce two of the three most common types of headaches: migraines and clusters. Tension headaches caused by muscle contraction comprise the other common type.

migraine headache (**MY**-grain headache)	A **migraine headache** is a recurring, pulsating, vascular headache usually developing on one side of the head. It is characterized by a slow onset that may be preceded by an **aura**, during which a **sensory** disturbance occurs such as confusion or some visual interference (e.g., flashing lights).

The pain intensity gradually becomes more severe and may be accompanied by nausea, vomiting, irritability, fatigue, sweating, or chills. Migraines occur at any age, with more frequency in females and those with a positive family history for migraine headaches. There is an increase in migraine headaches during periods of stress and crisis as well as a correlation with the menstrual cycle.

Migraines are often called vascular headaches. Dilation of the vessels in the head along with a drop in the serotonin level (which acts as a vasoconstrictor and a **neurotransmitter**, aiding in nerve transmission) occur at the onset of the migraine, which may last for hours or for days. Treatment for migraine headaches includes medications to prevent the onset of the headaches and medications to relieve the headache and diminish or reduce the severity of the symptoms.

cluster headache (**KLUSS**-ter headache)	A **cluster headache** occurs typically two to three hours after falling asleep; described as extreme pain around one eye that wakens the person from sleep.

There are usually no prodromal (or early) signs. However, the associated symptoms include a discharge of nasal fluid, tearing, sweating, flushing, and facial edema. The duration of a **cluster headache** is 30 minutes to several hours, and the episodes are clustered (occurring every day for several days or weeks). Then there may be a period of time with no headaches (lasting for months), until there is a return of the daily cluster headaches.

tension headache (**TEN**-shun headache)	A **tension headache** occurs from long, endured contraction of the skeletal muscles around the face, scalp, upper back, and neck.

Tension headaches make up the majority of headaches and occur in relation to excessive emotional tension such as anxiety and stress. The continued contraction of these skeletal muscles results in pain varying in intensity and duration. The onset of tension headaches is often during adolescence, but they occur most often in middle age. The headache is described as viselike, pressing, or tight.

Mild analgesics such as acetaminophen or aspirin are used to relieve the tension headache. Tranquilizers may be used to reduce muscle tension.

hematoma, epidural (hee-mah-**TOH**-mah, **eh**-pih-**DOO**-ral) epi- = upon, over dur/o = **dura mater** -al = pertaining to hemat/o = blood -oma = tumor	Epidural hematoma is a collection of blood (**hematoma**) located above the **dura mater** and just below the skull. The **hematoma** is blood collected from a torn artery, usually the middle meningeal artery, or from an injury such as a skull fracture or contusion. The initial symptom is a brief loss of consciousness. This brief period is followed by a period in which the individual is extremely rational (lucid). This lucid period may last for one to two hours or up to one to two days. When the lucid period is over, a rapid decline in consciousness occurs, accompanied by one or all of the following: progressively severe headache, drowsiness, confusion, seizures, paralysis, one fixed pupil, an increase in blood pressure, a decrease in pulse rate, and even **coma**. The epidural hematoma develops rapidly. Therefore, timely treatment is necessary to save the individual's life. A craniology is performed to repair the damaged blood vessels and remove pooled blood. **Burr holes** drilled into the skull can often be used to accomplish the clot evacuation and ligation of the artery.
hematoma, subdural (hee-mah-**TOH**-mah, **sub**-doo-ral) sub- = below, under dur/o = **dura mater** -al = pertaining to hemat/o = blood -oma = tumor	Subdural hematoma is a collection of blood below the **dura mater** and above the arachnoid layer of the **meninges**. This collection of blood usually occurs as a result of a closed head injury, an acceleration–deceleration injury, a cerebral atrophy noted in older adults, use of anticoagulants, a contusion, and/or chronic alcoholism. Subdural hematomas largely occur as a result of venous bleeding. They vary in the rate of development from the acute subdural hematoma (which occurs in minutes to hours of an injury) to a chronic subdural hematoma, which can evolve over weeks to months. Symptoms include agitation, drowsiness, confusion, headache, dilation and sluggishness of one pupil, possible seizures, signs of increased intracranial pressure (IICP), and paralysis. Treatment for large subdural hematomas includes diuretic medications to control brain swelling and surgical evacuation. The acute subdural hematoma may be removed through burr holes, but the chronic subdural hematoma is usually removed by a **craniotomy** because the blood collects so slowly it tends to solidify (preventing aspiration through burr holes).
herniated disk (**HER**-nee-**ay**-ted disk)	**Herniated disk** is rupture or herniation of the disk center (nucleus pulposus) through the disk wall and into the spinal canal, causing pressure on the spinal cord or nerve roots.

The herniation may be caused by trauma or by sudden straining or lifting in an unusual position. An intervertebral disk is a flexible pad of cartilage located between every vertebra to provide shock absorption and flexibility for movement.

Herniated intervertebral disks occur most frequently in the lumbosacral area, causing symptoms of **sciatica**: pain radiating from the back to the hip and down the leg. Herniation of the cervical disks occurs occasionally, causing shoulder pain radiating down the arm to the hand, stiffness of the neck, and **sensory** loss in the fingers. The diagnosis is usually confirmed with a CT scan, MRI, or a myelogram.

Conservative medical treatment such as bed rest, local application of heat, muscle relaxants, anti-inflammatory agents, and analgesics is usually the initial therapy. If back pain and **sciatica** are persistent and not relieved by the conservative medical treatment or if neurological dysfunctions are increasing, surgical intervention is indicated.

Huntington's chorea
(**HUNT**-ing-tonz koh-**REE**-ah)

Huntington's chorea is an inherited neurological disease characterized by rapid, jerky, involuntary movements and increasing **dementia** due to the effects of the basal ganglia on the neurons.

There is no cure for this progressive degenerative disease. Beginning about the age of 30 to 40, the early effects include irritability, periods of alternating emotions, posture and positioning problems, protruding tongue, speech problems, restlessness, and complaints of a "fidgety" feeling. These abnormal movements (which gradually increase to involve all muscles and the inability to be still for more than several minutes) are aggravated by attempts to perform voluntary movements, by stress, and by emotional situations. As the disease progresses, movement of the diaphragm becomes impaired, making the person with **Huntington's chorea** susceptible to choking, aspiration, poor oxygenation, and malnutrition. Other late effects include loss of mental skills and total dependence on others for care. Death typically occurs approximately 15 to 20 years after the onset of symptoms due to an infectious process or aspiration pneumonia.

Because there is no cure for **Huntington's chorea**, the supportive care includes education of the disease process for the person and family (along with genetic counseling). The emotional and psychological needs of the person and family are great and require much support.

hydrocephalus
(high-droh-**SEFF**-ah-lus)
  hydro- = water
  cephal/o = head
  -us = noun ending

Hydrocephalus is an abnormal increase of **cerebrospinal fluid** in the brain that causes the ventricles of the brain to dilate, resulting in an increased head circumference in the infant with open **fontanel**(s); a congenital disorder.

The increase in **cerebrospinal fluid** (CSF) may be due to an increased production of CSF, a decreased absorption of CSF, or a blockage in the normal flow of CSF. The infant may also show frontal bossing (forehead protrudes out), which may cause the "setting sun" sign in which the sclerae (whites of the eyes) above the irises are visible when the eyes are directed downward. The infant will demonstrate other signs of increased pressure, such as a high-pitched cry, a bulging **fontanel**, extreme irritability, and an inability to sleep for long periods of time.

Hydrocephalus in the young infant may be indicated by increased head circumference, resulting in an abnormal graphing curve. This may be detected when checking the head circumference of the infant on well-baby checkups in the physician's office. (This procedure is discussed in Chapter 19.) Along with checking head circumference, the infant should be assessed for any signs and symptoms of increased intracranial pressure (IICP).

When the diagnosis of **hydrocephalus** is made, treatment to relieve or remove the obstruction is initiated. When there is no obstruction, a **shunt** is generally required to relieve the intracranial pressure. The excess CSF is shunted into another body space, thus preventing permanent damage to the brain tissue. As the child grows, the shunt must be replaced with a longer one.

Hydrocephalus is often a complication of another disease or disorder. The infant with **spina bifida cystica** may develop **hydrocephalus**. It can also occur as a result of an intrauterine infection due to diseases such as rubella or syphilis.

intracranial tumors
(in-trah-**KRAY**-nee-al **TOO**-morz)
  intra- = within
  crani/o = skull; cranium
  -al = pertaining to
	Intracranial tumors occur in any structural region of the brain. They may be malignant or benign, classified as primary or secondary, and are named according to the tissue from which they originate.

An intracranial tumor causes the normal brain tissue to be displaced and compressed, leading to progressive neurological deficiencies. The clinical symptoms of **intracranial tumors** include headaches, dizziness, vomiting, problems with coordination and muscle strength, changes in personality, altered mental function, seizures, paralysis, and **sensory** disturbances.

Surgical removal is the desired treatment when possible. Radiation and/or chemotherapy are used according to location, classification, and type.

primary intracranial tumors (**PRIGH**-mah-ree in-trah-**KRAY**-nee-al **TOO**-morz)	**Primary intracranial tumors** arise from gliomas, malignant glial cells that are a support for nerve tissue, and from tumors that arise from the **meninges**.

Gliomas constitute about one-half of all brain tumors and are classified according to the principal cell type, shape, and size, as follows:

1. *Glioblastoma multiformes* are the most frequent and aggressive intracranial tumors. This type of tumor arises in the cerebral hemisphere and is the most rapidly growing of the gliomas.

2. *Astrocytomas* are the most common type of primary brain tumor. They are slow-growing usually noncancerous primary tumors made up of astrocytes (star-shaped cells). Astrocytomas tend to invade surrounding structures and over time become more anaplastic (i.e., they revert to a more primitive form). A highly malignant glioblastoma may develop within the tumor mass.

3. *Ependymomas* comprise approximately 6% of all **intracranial tumors**. They commonly arise from the ependymomal cells that line the fourth

ventricle wall and often extend into the spinal cord. An ependymoma occurs more commonly in children and adolescents and is usually encapsulated and benign.

4. *Oligodendrogliomas* comprise approximately 5% of all **intracranial tumors** and are usually slow growing. At times the oligodendrogliomas imitate the glioblastomas with rapid growth. Oligodendrogliomas occur most often in the frontal lobe.

5. *Medulloblastomas* are the most common type of childhood brain cancer and occur most frequently in children between 5 and 9 years of age. They affect more boys than girls and typically arise in the **cerebellum**, growing rapidly. The prognosis is poor.

Meningiomas are benign and comprise approximately 15% of all **intracranial tumors**. They originate from the **meninges**, grow slowly, and are vascular. Meningiomas largely occur most often in adults.

metastatic intracranial tumors (secondary) (met-ah-**STAT**-ikin-trah-**KRAY**-nee-al **TOO**-morz) intra- = within crani/o = skull; cranium -al = pertaining to	**Metastatic intracranial tumors** occur as a result of metastasis from a primary site such as the lung or breast. They occur more frequently than primary neoplasms.

Brain metastasis, most frequently arising from lung and breast cancers, is a common occurrence, comprising approximately 15% of **intracranial tumors**. The tissue in the brain reacts intensely to the presence of a metastatic tumor, which usually progresses rapidly. Surgical removal of a single metastasis to the brain can be achieved if the tumor is located in an operable region. The removal may provide the individual with several months or years of life.

meningitis (acute bacterial) (men-in-**JYE**-tis ah-**KYOOT** back-**TEE**-ree-al) mening/o = meninges -itis = inflammation	**Meningitis (acute bacterial)** is a serious bacterial infection of the **meninges**—the covering of the brain and spinal cord—that can have residual debilitating effects or even a fatal outcome if not diagnosed and treated promptly with appropriate antibiotic therapy.

The bacteria enters the **meninges** by way of the bloodstream from an infection in another part of the body (e.g., an upper respiratory infection) or through a penetrating wound such as an operative procedure, a skull fracture, or a break in the skin covering a structural defect such as a **meningomyelocele**. Once the bacteria invades the **meninges** (causing inflammation), there is a rapid multiplication of the bacteria leading to swelling in the brain tissue, congestion in the blood circulation of the CNS, and formation of clumps of exudate that may collect around the base of the brain and have the potential to occlude CSF circulation.

These alterations lead to an increase in intracranial pressure as well as the following symptoms: irritability; extremely stiff neck (**nuchal rigidity**); headache in the older infant, child, or adult; fever; pain with eye movement; light sensitivity (photophobia); nausea and vomiting; diarrhea; drowsiness; confusion; and possibly seizures. Other specific characteristics in the infant include resistance to being diapered or cuddled, crying with position changes, high-pitched cry, decreased activity, bulging tense **fontanel**, and poor feeding and sleeping.

Prior to beginning the antibiotic therapy, cultures of CSF, urine, blood, and the nasopharynx are obtained in an attempt to identify the causative bacterial organism. A **lumbar puncture** (LP) is done to obtain the CSF on infants with open **fontanel** or others who show no signs of long-standing increased intracranial pressure (papilledema noted when optic fundi observed). In the individual with bacterial meningitis, the CSF obtained from the **lumbar puncture** will generally appear cloudy, showing the presence of white blood cells (WBCs) as well as a decrease in glucose and an increase in protein.

The treatment for bacterial meningitis includes intravenous antibiotics for at least 10 days, according to organism(s) identified in cultures. The individual will likely be hospitalized initially and placed on isolation for 24 to 48 hours. The environment should be kept dark and quiet with very little stimuli.

The outcome of bacterial meningitis varies from complete recovery to miscellaneous physical and mental disabilities. These outcomes are related to the age of the individual and to the interval between onset of symptoms and the beginning of treatment. The diagnosis of bacterial meningitis in the infant is often difficult to identify because of the lack of verbal communication and the vagueness of physiological symptoms (e.g., in the infant less than one month of age, the temperature may go up or down). The long-term complications include mild learning disabilities to severe mental and physical handicaps, cranial nerve malfunctions, peripheral circulatory collapse, arthritis, and subdural effusion.

Acute meningitis may also be caused by viruses. Viral meningitis, also known as aseptic meningitis, is usually clinically mild, and spontaneous recovery without complications is normal.

multiple sclerosis (MS)	**Multiple sclerosis (MS)** is a degenerative inflammatory disease of the CNS attacking the **myelin sheath** in the spinal cord and brain, leaving it sclerosed (hardened) or scarred and interrupting the flow of nerve impulses.
(**MULL**-tih-pal **SKLEH**-roh-sis)	
scler/o = hard (also refers to sclera of the eye)	
-osis = condition	

MS largely affects young adults between the ages of 20 and 40, with females being affected more often than males. The course for this disease varies greatly in that the initial onset can be gradual over weeks, months, or years or within minutes or hours. The common duration of MS is approximately 30 years, although there are documented cases of persons dying within several months after the beginning of the disease. This disease can follow two types: the exacerbation–remitting type (in which the exacerbation or onset of symptoms is followed by a complete remission) or the chronic progressive type, in which there is a steady loss of neurological function. The scarring of the **myelin sheath** either slows the transmission of nerve impulses or completely inhibits the transmission of stimuli to the spinal cord and brain. The areas involved affect different systems and cause many symptoms, such as:

1. Unsteady balance, poor coordination with shaky irregular movements, and vertigo

2. Numbness and/or weakness of one or more extremities

3. Speech, visual, and auditory disturbance

4. Urinary incontinence or urgency

5. Facial pain or numbness and difficulty chewing and swallowing

6. Fatigue, spasticity, and muscular wasting or atrophy

7. Impaired sensation to temperature

8. Impotence in males

9. Emotional disturbances

The person experiencing MS is at risk for the following complications: seizures and **dementia**, blindness, recurring urinary tract infections (UTIs), bowel and bladder incontinence, respiratory infections, and injuries from falls.

There is no cure for MS. However, specific medications have helped to prolong remissions and decrease the exacerbations of ambulatory persons. The goals of drug therapy are to decrease inflammation, slow the immune response, and promote muscle relaxation. The goal of care for the person with MS is to relieve and decrease the severity of symptoms and promote independence as much as possible for as long as possible.

myasthenia gravis (my-ass-**THEE**-nee-ah **GRAV**-iss) **my/o** = muscle **-asthenia** = loss of strength	**Myasthenia gravis** is a chronic progressive neuromuscular disorder causing severe skeletal muscle weakness (without atrophy) and fatigue, which occurs at different levels of severity.

The muscles are weak because the nerve impulse is not transmitted successfully to the muscle cell from the nerve cell, and these episodes occur periodically (with remissions between). **Myasthenia gravis** is considered to be an autoimmune disease in which antibodies block or destroy some **acetylcholine** receptor sites. It occurs more often in women than in men, with the onset usually between the ages of 20 and 40. In men, the onset is between the ages of 50 and 60.

Symptoms of **myasthenia gravis** may occur gradually or suddenly. Facial muscle weakness may be the most noticeable symptom, owing to drooping eyelids, difficulty with swallowing, and difficulty speaking. The periods of muscle weakness generally occur late in the day or after strenuous exercise. Rest does refresh the tired weak muscles. The weakness eventually becomes so severe that paralysis occurs.

In addition to medications, treatment for **myasthenia gravis** may require restricted activity and a soft or liquid diet. The care provided for the person and family is supportive and symptomatic.

narcolepsy (**NAR**-koh-**lep**-see) **narc/o** = sleep **-lepsy** = seizure, attack	**Narcolepsy** is a rare syndrome of uncontrolled sudden attacks of sleep. The main features of **narcolepsy** are daytime sleepiness and cataplexy.

Medications may be used to treat **narcolepsy**, with the goal of achieving normal alertness with minimal side effects. A polysomnogram (polly-**SOHM**-no-gram) may be performed to evaluate sleep disorders such as **narcolepsy**. This test is discussed in the section on diagnostic techniques and procedures.

Excessive daytime sleepiness is usually the first symptom to appear in individuals who have **narcolepsy**. Attacks are likely to occur in monotonous conditions conducive to normal sleep but may also occur in situations that could prove to be dangerous, such as working with machinery and/or while driving. The individual may feel refreshed upon awakening from the sleep episode but may fall asleep again within a few minutes.

The attacks can occur at any time and may be frequent and happen almost instantaneously. The attacks might last from minutes to hours. The individual could have a few episodes to many in a single day.

Cataplexy is a sudden loss of muscle tone (momentary paralysis without loss of consciousness) initiated by emotional stimuli such as surprise, anger, or laughter. This weakness can be confined to the extremities or involve all muscles, causing the individual to collapse.

neuroblastoma
(**noo**-roh-blass-**TOH**-mah)
  neur/o = nerve
  blast/o = embryonic stage of
           development
  -oma = tumor
	Neuroblastoma is a highly malignant tumor of the sympathetic nervous system.
	
	It most commonly occurs in the adrenal medulla, with early metastasis spreading widely to liver, lungs, lymph nodes, and bone.

Parkinson's disease (**PARK**-in-sons dih-**ZEEZ**)	**Parkinson's disease** is a degenerative, slowly progressive deterioration of nerves in the brain stem's motor system characterized by a gradual onset of symptoms such as a stooped posture with the body flexed forward; a bowed head; a shuffling **gait**; pill-rolling gestures; an expres sionless, masklike facial appearance; muffled speech; and swallowing difficulty.

The cause of **Parkinson's disease** is not known. However, a **neurotransmitter** deficiency (dopamine) has been clinically noted in persons with **Parkinson's disease**. **Parkinson's disease** is seen more often in males, with the onset of symptoms beginning between the ages of 50 and 60. The clinical symptoms can be divided into three groups:

1. **Motor dysfunction** demonstrated by the nonintentional tremors (pill rolling), slowed movements, inability to start voluntary movements, speech problems, muscle rigidity, and **gait** and posture disturbances.

2. **Autonomic system dysfunction** demonstrated by mottled skin, problems from seborrhea and excess sweating on the upper neck and face and absence of sweating on the lower body, abnormally low blood pressure when standing, heat intolerance, and constipation.

3. **Mental and emotional dysfunction** demonstrated by loss of memory, declining mental processes, lack of problem-solving skills, uneasiness, and depression.

Treatment for **Parkinson's disease**, in addition to drug therapy, consists of control of symptoms and supportive measures with physical therapy playing an important role in keeping the person's mobility maximized.

A recent surgical technique used for the person with **Parkinson's disease** is a pallidotomy. This procedure involves the destruction of the involved tissue in the brain to reduce tremors and severe dyskinesia. The goal of this procedure, to restore a more normal ambulatory function to the individual, is not always successful.

peripheral neuritis

(per-**IF**-er-al noo-**RYE**-tis)

neur/o = nerve

-itis = inflammation

Peripheral neuritis is a general term indicating inflammation of one or more peripheral nerves, the effects being dependent on the particular nerve involved.

The peripheral nerve disorders discussed in this chapter are **trigeminal neuralgia** (*tic douloureux*), **Bell's palsy**, and **carpal tunnel syndrome**. Each has been listed alphabetically.

poliomyelitis

(poh-lee-oh-**my**-eh-**LYE**-tis)

poli/o = gray matter, in
       nervous system

myel/o = spinal cord;
       bone marrow

-itis = inflammation

Poliomyelitis is an infectious viral disease entering through the upper respiratory tract and affecting the ability of spinal cord and brain motor neurons to receive stimulation. Muscles affected become paralyzed without the motor nerve stimulation (i.e., respiratory paralysis requires ventilatory support).

This once dreaded crippling disease has been nearly eliminated due to the vaccine and immunization programs of Salk and Sabin. The clinical symptoms include excessive nasal secretions, low-grade fever, progressive muscle weakness, nausea and vomiting, stiff neck, and flaccid paralysis of the muscles involved. Muscle atrophy then occurs with decreased reflexes, followed by joint and muscle deterioration.

Treatment for **poliomyelitis** is supportive, including medications for fever and pain relief, bed rest, physical therapy, and respiratory support as indicated. Prevention of this infectious disease is the strategy for today, with the use of Sabin trivalent oral vaccine (which provides immunity for all three forms of **poliomyelitis**).

postpolio syndrome

(**POST-POH**-lee-oh **SIN**-drom)

post- = after, behind

poli/o = gray matter (in the
       nervous system)

syn- = together, joined

-drome = that which runs together

Postpolio syndrome is progressive weakness occurring at least 30 years after the initial **poliomyelitis** attack.

It involves already affected muscles in which there is uncontrolled, uncoordinated twitching. These muscle groups begin to waste and the person experiences extreme weakness. The treatment for **postpolio syndrome** is supportive.

Reye's syndrome

(**RISE SIN**-drom)

syn- = together, joined

-drome = that which runs together

Reye's syndrome is an acute brain encephalopathy along with fatty infiltration of the internal organs that may follow acute viral infections; occurs in children under the age of 18, often with a fatal result. There are confirmed studies linking the onset of **Reye's syndrome** to aspirin administration during a viral illness.

The symptoms of **Reye's syndrome** typically follow a pattern through stages:

1. Sudden, continuous vomiting, confusion, and **lethargy** (sluggishness and apathy)
2. Irritability, hyperactive reflexes, delirium, and hyperventilation

3. Changes in level of consciousness progressing to **coma**, and sluggish pupillary response

4. Fixed, dilated pupils; continued loss of cerebral function; and periods of absent breathing

5. Seizures, loss of deep tendon reflexes, and respiratory arrest

The prognosis is directly related to the stage of **Reye's syndrome** at the time of diagnosis and treatment. Treatment includes decreasing intracranial pressure to prevent seizures, controlling cerebral edema, and closely monitoring the child for changes in level of consciousness. In some cases, respiratory support and/or dialysis is necessary.

shingles (herpes zoster) (**SHING**-ulz **HER**-peez **ZOSS**-ter)	**Shingles (herpes zoster)** is an acute viral infection seen mainly in adults who have had chicken pox, characterized by inflammation of the underlying spinal or cranial nerve pathway (producing painful vesicular eruptions on the skin along these nerve pathways). See *Figure 8-6.*

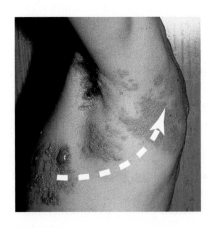

Of the population, 10% to 20% are affected by **herpes zoster**, with the highest incidence in adults over 50. Symptoms include severe pain before and during eruption, fever, itching, GI disturbances, headache, general tiredness, and increased sensitivity of the skin around the area. The lesions usually take three to five days to erupt and then progress to crusting and drying (with recovery in approximately three weeks). Treatment with antiviral medications, analgesics, and sometimes corticosteroids aids in decreasing the severity of symptoms.

Figure 8-6 Shingles-vesicles follow a nerve pathway
(Photo courtesy of Robert A. Silverman, MD, Clinical Associate Professor, Pediatric Dermatology, Georgetown University)

skull fracture (depressed) (**SKULL FRAK**-chur, deh-**PREST**)	A broken segment of the skull bone thrust into the brain as a result of a direct force, usually a blunt object, is a skull fracture.

Automobile and industrial accidents are two potential causes of this type of injury. The manifestations of a depressed skull fracture depend on the section of the brain injured and the extent of damage to the underlying vessels. The greater the involvement of vessels, the higher the risk for hemorrhage. Damage to the motor area will likely result in some form of paralysis.

Treatment includes a **craniotomy** to remove the depressed segment(s) of bone and raise it (them) back into position. Preoperative and postoperative treatment is directed at relieving intracranial pressure (ICP). Postoperative care may include wearing head protection until there is partial healing of the fracture.

spina bifida cystica (**SPY**-nah **BIFF**-ih-dah **SISS**-tih-kah)	**Spina bifida cystica** is a congenital defect of the CNS in which the back portion of one or more vertebrae is not closed normally and a cyst protrudes through the opening in the back, usually at the level of the fifth lumbar or first sacral vertebrae.

Two types of **spina bifida cystica**—**meningocele** and **meningomyelocele**—are discussed in the following entries.

meningocele

(meh-**NING**-goh-**seel**)

mening/o = meninges

-cele = swelling or herniation

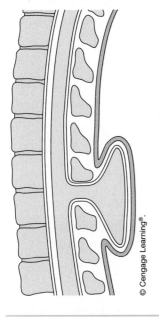
© Cengage Learning®.

Meningocele is a cystlike sac covered with skin or a thin membrane protruding through the bony defect in the vertebrae containing **meninges** and CSF. See *Figure 8-7*.

Some spinal nerve roots may be displaced, but their function is still sound. Neurological complications occur rarely and are not as severe as those noted with the **meningomyelocele**.

Hydrocephalus is a possible complication occurring after surgical closure of the **meningocele**. Extreme care must be taken to protect the cystlike sac from injury prior to the surgical closure owing to the increased risk of an infection.

Figure 8-7 Meningocele

meningomyelocele

(men-**in**-goh-my-**ELL**-oh-seel)

mening/o = meninges

myel/o = spinal cord or bone marrow

-cele = swelling or herniation

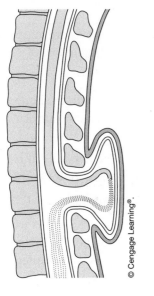
© Cengage Learning®.

Meningomyelocele is a cystlike sac covered with skin or a thin membrane protruding through the bony defect in the vertebrae that contains **meninges**, CSF, and spinal cord segments. See *Figure 8-8*.

Due to the involvement of the spinal cord segments, there are neurological symptoms such as weakness or paralysis of the legs as well as altered bowel and bladder control. **Hydrocephalus** is generally present. Extreme care must be taken to protect the sac from injury or rupture prior to surgical closure owing to the increased risk of an infection.

Figure 8-8 Meningomyelocele

spina bifida occulta (**SPY**-nah **BIFF**-ih-dah oh-**KULL**-tah) 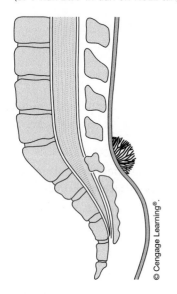	**Spina bifida occulta** is a congenital defect of the CNS in which the back portion of one or more vertebrae is not closed. A dimpling over the area may occur. See *Figure 8-9*. Other symptoms include hair growing out of this area, a port wine nevus (pigmented blemish) over the area, and/or a subcutaneous lipoma (fatty tumor) in the area. This defect can occur anywhere along the vertebral column but usually occurs at the level of the fifth lumbar or first sacral vertebrae. There are usually very few neurological symptoms present. Without symptoms there is no treatment recommended.

Figure 8-9 Spina bifida occulta

spinal cord injuries (**paraplegia** and **quadriplegia**)	Severe injuries to the spinal cord, such as vertebral dislocation or vertebral fractures, resulting in impairment of spinal cord function below the level of the injury. Spinal cord injuries are generally the result of trauma caused by motor vehicle accidents, falls, diving in shallow water, or accidents associated with contact sports. Spinal cord injuries are seen most often in the male adolescent and young adult population. Trauma to the spinal cord occurring above the level of the third to fourth cervical vertebrae (C3 and C4) often results in a fatality due to the loss of innervation to the diaphragm and intercostal muscles, which maintain respirations.

paraplegia
 	
(par-ah-**PLEE**-jee-ah)
 	
  para- = near, beside, beyond, two
        like parts
  -plegia = paralysis
	Paraplegia (paralysis of the lower extremities) is caused by severe injury to the spinal cord in the thoracic or lumbar region, resulting in loss of **sensory** and motor control below the level of injury.
	
	Other common problems occurring with spinal cord injury to the lumbar and thoracic regions include loss of bladder, bowel, and sexual control.

quadriplegia
 	
(**kwad**-rih-**PLEE**-jee-ah)
  quadri- = four
  -plegia = paralysis
	Quadriplegia follows severe trauma to the spinal cord between the fifth and seventh cervical vertebrae, generally resulting in loss of motor and **sensory** function below the level of injury.
	
	Paralysis in **quadriplegia** includes the trunk, legs, and pelvic organs with partial or total paralysis in the upper extremities. The higher the trauma the more debilitating the motor and **sensory** impairments. **Quadriplegia** may also be characterized by cardiovascular complications, low body temperature, impaired peristalsis, inability to perspire, and loss of control of bladder, bowel, and sexual functions.

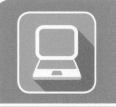

Media Link

View the **Spinal Cord Injuries** animation on the Student Companion Website.

Diagnosis and extent of injury with spinal cord injuries is confirmed with physical assessment, spinal X-rays, CT scans, and MRI scans. Emergency treatment should be started at the scene of the injury to provide stabilization of the normal alignment to prevent additional injury. Further stabilization of the vertebrae will be accomplished at an acute-care setting.

Tay-Sachs disease

(**TAY-SACKS** dih-**ZEEZ**)

Tay-Sachs disease is a congenital disorder caused by altered lipid metabolism, resulting from an enzyme deficiency.

An accumulation of a specific type of lipid occurs in the brain and leads to progressive neurological deterioration with both physical and mental retardation. The symptoms of neurological deterioration begin around the age of six months. Deafness, blindness with a cherry red spot on each retina, convulsions, and paralysis all occur in the child with **Tay-Sachs disease** until death occurs around the age of 2 to 4 years. There is no specific therapy for this condition. Therefore, supportive and symptomatic care are indicated.

Tay-Sachs disease occurs most frequently in families of Eastern European Jewish origin, specifically the Ashkenazic Jews. This disease can be diagnosed in utero through amniocentesis.

trigeminal neuralgia

(*tic douloureux*)

(try-**JEM**-ih-nal noo-**RAL**-jee-ah, *tik* **DOO**-*loh-roo*)

Short periods of severe unilateral pain, which radiates along the fifth cranial nerve, is **trigeminal neuralgia** (*tic douloureux*).

There are three branches of the fifth cranial nerve (trigeminal nerve), each of which can be affected. Pain in the eye and forehead is experienced when the ophthalmic branch is affected. The mandibular branch causes pain in the lower lip, the section of the cheek closest to the ear, and the outer segment of the tongue. The upper lip, nose, and cheek are painful when the maxillary branch is affected.

Heat, chewing, or touching of the affected area activates the pain. Analgesics are used to control the pain. Persons who smoke are encouraged to quit. The nerve roots can be dissected through a surgical procedure when no other options have relieved the pain.

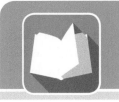

Review Checkpoint

Check your understanding of this section by completing the **Pathological Conditions** exercises in your workbook.

Diagnostic Techniques, Treatments, and Procedures

Babinski's reflex

(bah-**BIN**-skeez **REE**-fleks)

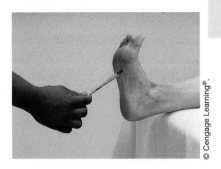
© Cengage Learning®.

Babinski's reflex can be tested by stroking the sole of the foot, beginning at midheel and moving upward and lateral to the toes. A positive Babinski's occurs when there is dorsiflexion of the great toe and fanning of the other toes. See *Figure 8-10*.

Although a normal reflex in newborns, the **Babinski's reflex** is abnormal when found in children and adults. A positive **Babinski's reflex** in an adult represents upper motor neuron disease of the pyramidal tract.

Figure 8-10 Assessment of Babinski reflex

brain scan

A brain scan is a nuclear counter scanning of cranial content two hours after an intravenous injection of radioisotopes.

Normally, blood does not cross the **blood–brain barrier** and come in contact with brain tissue. However, in localized pathological situations, this barrier is disrupted, allowing isotopes to gather. These isotopes concentrate in abnormal tissue of the brain, indicating a pathological process. The scanner can localize any abnormal tissue where the isotopes have accumulated.

The brain scan assists in diagnosing abnormal findings such as an acute cerebral infarction, cerebral neoplasm, cerebral hemorrhage, **brain abscess**, aneurysms, cerebral **thrombosis**, hematomas, **hydrocephalus**, cancer metastasis to the brain, and bleeds.

cerebral angiography

(seh-**REE**-bral **an**-jee-**OG**-rah-fee)

cerebr/o = brain; **cerebrum**

-al = pertaining to

angi/o = vessel

-graphy = process of recording

Cerebral angiography is visualization of the cerebral vascular system via X-ray after the injection of a radiopaque contrast medium into an arterial blood vessel (carotid, femoral, or brachial).

The arterial, capillary, and venous recording structures are outlined as the contrast medium flows through the brain. Through the **cerebral angiography**, cerebral circulation abnormalities such as occlusions or aneurysms are visualized. Vascular and nonvascular tumors can be noted as well as hematomas and abscesses.

cerebrospinal fluid analysis

(ser-eh-broh-**SPY**-nal **FLOO**-id an-**AL**-ah-sis)

cerebr/o = brain; **cerebrum**

spin/o = spine

-al = pertaining to

CSF obtained from a **lumbar puncture** is analyzed for the presence of bacteria, blood, or malignant cells as well as for the amount of protein and glucose present.

Normal CSF is clear and colorless without blood cells, bacteria, or malignant cells. The normal protein level is 15 to 45 mg/dL but may be as high as 70 mg/dL in children and elderly adults. The normal glucose level is 50 to 70 mg/dL.

CT scan of the brain	Computed tomography (CT) is the analysis of a three-dimensional view of brain tissue obtained as X-ray beams pass through successive horizontal layers of the brain; also called computerized axial tomography (CAT scan).

The images provided are as though you were looking down through the top of the head. The computer detects the radiation absorption and the variation in tissue density in each layer. From this detection of radiation absorption and tissue density, a series of anatomic pictures are produced in varying shades of gray.

When contrast is indicated, intravenous (IV) iodinated dye is injected via a peripheral IV site. If receiving the contrast, the person should have nothing by mouth (n.p.o.) for four hours prior to the study because the contrast dye can cause nausea and vomiting.

CT scans are helpful in identifying **intracranial tumors**, cerebral infarctions, ventricular displacement or enlargement, cerebral aneurysm, intracranial bleeds, **multiple sclerosis, hydrocephalus,** and **brain abscess.** CT scans are not limited to scans of the brain but may also be used to detect abnormalities such as blood clots, cysts, fractures, infections, and tumors in internal structures. In addition, they may be used to examine structures within the abdomen, pelvis, chest, head, spine, nerves, and blood vessels.

chordotomy
 	
 (kor-**DOT**-oh-mee)
 	
   chord/o = string, cord
   -tomy = incision into
	Chordotomy is a neurosurgical procedure for pain control accomplished through a **laminectomy,** in which there is surgical interference of pathways within the spinal cord that control pain.

The intent of this surgical procedure is to interrupt tracts of the nervous system that relay pain sensations from their point of origin to the brain to relieve pain.

cisternal puncture (sis-**TER**-nal **PUNK**-chur)	**Cisternal puncture** involves insertion of a short, beveled spinal needle into the cisterna magna (a shallow reservoir of CSF between the medulla and the **cerebellum**) to drain CSF or to obtain a CSF specimen.

The needle is inserted between the first cervical vertebrae and the foramen magnum. Immediately after the procedure, the person should be observed for cyanosis, difficulty breathing, or absence of breathing. Complications are rare.

craniotomy
 	
 (kray-nee-**OTT**-oh-mee)
 	
   crani/o = skull; cranium
   -tomy = incision into
	Craniotomy is a surgical procedure that makes an opening into the skull.

A **craniotomy** may be accomplished by creating a bone flap in which one side remains hinged with muscles and other structures to the skull. Another technique to allow entry into the skull is through a free-form flap whereby a portion of the bone is completely removed from its attachments. A third type of **craniotomy** is an enlarging **burr hole** that allows the brain to be exposed for the procedure.

echoencephalography

(**eck**-oh-en-**sef**-ah-**LOG**-rah-fee)

  echo- = sound

  encephal/o = brain

  -graphy = process of recording

Ultrasound used to analyze the intracranial structures of the brain is termed **echoencephalography**.

Ventricular dilation or a vital shift of midline structures are usually picked up on the **echoencephalography**. These findings may indicate an enlarging lesion. There is a great chance of error in administering and interpreting the test. Therefore, limitations must be considered.

electroencephalography (EEG)

(ee-**leck**-troh-en-**sef**-ah-**LOG**-rah-fee)

  electr/o = electricity

  encephal/o = brain

  -graphy = process of recording

Measurement of electrical activity produced by the brain and recorded through electrodes placed on the scalp is termed **electroencephalography**.

The electrodes are connected to a machine that amplifies the electrical activity and records it on moving paper. During the recording of the EEG, the person must remain very still and relaxed. This is usually achieved in a quiet room with subdued lighting. If a sleep EEG recording is ordered, the person is given a sedative and the EEG is recorded as the person falls asleep.

A **sleep-deprived EEG** is performed after the individual has been deprived of sleep for 24 hours before the test. The individual should not smoke cigarettes or consume any beverages containing caffeine for 24 hours before the test. During sleep deprivation, EEG abnormalities may show up. These abnormalities can occur under stress such as fatigue and drowsiness. The EEG recording is conducted while the patient is awake and while asleep.

An **ambulatory EEG** may be performed to confirm a diagnosis of **epilepsy**. If **epilepsy** waves occur in the brain only once every three or four hours or if they happen only after an hour or so of sleep, the routine EEG may appear normal. The ambulatory EEG will provide prolonged readings of the electrical activity of the brain over a 24-hour period while the individual is awake and asleep. The scalp electrodes are attached using a special glue that holds them in place for an extended period. The small portable recorder can be worn around the waist. Most recorders have an "event" button that can be pressed if the individual experiences any symptoms indicative of a seizure. The patient usually keeps a diary of his/her activities during the day to assist the doctor in identifying the cause of any abnormal activity that may appear on the recording.

An EEG provides information helpful in evaluating individuals with cranial neurological problems, epileptic seizures, focal damage in the cortex, psychogenic unresponsiveness, and cerebral death.

electromyography

(ee-**lek**-troh-my-**OG**-rah-fee)

  electr/o = electricity

  my/o = muscle

  -graphy = process of recording

Electromyography (EMG) is the process of recording the electrical activity of muscle by inserting a small needle into the muscle and delivering a small current that stimulates the muscle.

The activity is recorded on a computer and is interpreted by a doctor trained in electrodiagnostic medicine. The EMG records the electrical activity in muscle tissue and is used to distinguish **neuropathy** (nerve disease) from myopathy (muscle disease).

EMG and nerve conduction studies (NCS) are often used in combination and are referred to as EMG/NCS. They are used to test for any dysfunction of nerve and muscle such as pinching or compression of a specific nerve or any inherited or acquired nerve or muscle dysfunction. The NCS records the speed at which impulses travel along the nerve and measures the electrical responses.

laminectomy
 (**lam**-ih-**NEK**-toh-mee)
   lamin/o = lamina
   -ectomy = surgical removal
	Laminectomy is the surgical removal of the bony arches from one or more of the vertebrae to relieve pressure on the spinal cord.

This surgical procedure is done under general **anesthesia**. The pressure on the spinal cord may be caused by a degenerated or a displaced disk or may be from a displaced bone from an injury. If more than one vertebrae is involved, a fusion may be required to maintain stability of the spine.

lumbar puncture (**LUM**-bar **PUNK**-chur)	**Lumbar puncture** involves the insertion of a hollow needle and stylet into the **subarachnoid space**, generally between the third and fourth lumbar vertebrae below the level of the spinal cord under strict aseptic technique.

A **lumbar puncture** permits CSF to be withdrawn for further examination or to decrease ICP, **intrathecal** injections (material injected into the lumbar **subarachnoid space** for circulation through the CSF) to be made, and access for further assessment.

A written consent for a **lumbar puncture** is required in most agencies due to the possible hazards of the procedure. Hazards include discomfort during the procedure, postpuncture headache, possible morbidity or mortality, infection, intervertebral disk damage, and respiratory failure.

A **lumbar puncture** takes only a few minutes and is performed with the person lying on his or her side with chin tucked down to chest and legs pulled into the abdomen. The person must be completely still to avoid damage by the needle. To decrease discomfort, a local anesthetic is normally injected prior to introduction of the needle and stylet.

A **lumbar puncture** is valuable in the diagnosis of **meningitis**, brain tumors, spinal cord tumors, **encephalitis**, and cerebral bleeding. The **lumbar puncture** is contraindicated in the presence of greatly increased intracranial pressure due to the potential abrupt release of pressure, which could cause compression of the brain stem and sudden death.

magnetic resonance **imaging (MRI)**	MRI is a noninvasive scanning procedure that provides visualization of fluid, soft tissue, and bony structures without the use of radiation.

The person is placed inside an electromagnetic, tubelike machine where specific radio frequency signals change the alignment of hydrogen atoms in the body. The absorbed radio frequency energy is analyzed by a computer, and an image is projected on the screen. See *Figure 8-11*.

The MRI provides far more precision and accuracy than most diagnostic tools. Those persons with implanted metal devices cannot undergo an MRI due to the strong magnetic field and the possibility of dislodging a chip or rod. MRI scans are not limited to scans of the brain. They may be performed on any part of the body and produce detailed images of soft tissues and. organs. MRI scans can be used to examine the abdomen, chest, joints, nervous system, pelvis, and spinal column.

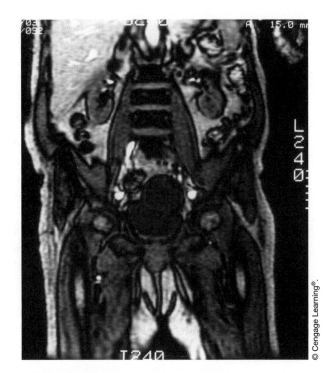

© Cengage Learning®.

Figure 8-11 Coronal image of abdomen acquired during a breath hold in this magnetic resonance image

An **open MRI** scanner does not place the patient in a tubelike machine. Instead, the patient is placed in a much less confining space. Open MRI scanners are particularly helpful with patients who suffer from claustrophobia ("fear of enclosed spaces"), pediatric patients, and larger patients who might not fit in the conventional MRI scanner.

myelography
 	
(my-eh-**LOG**-rah-fee)
 	
  myel/o = spinal cord, bone marrow
  -graphy = process of recording
	Myelography is the introduction of contrast medium into the lumbar **subarachnoid space** through a **lumbar puncture** to visualize the spinal cord and vertebral canal through X-ray examination.
	
	Roughly 10 mL of CSF is removed, and a radiopaque substance is injected slowly into the lumbar **subarachnoid space**. **Myelography** is accomplished on a tilt table in the radiology department to visualize the spinal canal in various positions. After a series of films are taken of the vertebral canal viewing various parts, the contrast medium is removed. **Myelography** aids in the diagnosis of adhesions and tumors producing pressure on the spinal canal or of intervertebral disc abnormalities.

neurectomy
 	
(noo-**REK**-toh-mee)
 	
  neur/o = nerve
  -ectomy = surgical removal
	A **neurectomy** is a neurosurgical procedure to relieve pain in a localized or small area by incision of cranial or peripheral nerves.
	
	In relieving pain, the intent of this surgical procedure is to interrupt tracts of the nervous system that relay pain sensations from their point of origin to the brain.

polysomnogram

(polly-**SOHM**-no-gram)

poly- = many

somn/o = sleep

-gram = record or recording

A polysomnogram (PSG) is a sleep study or sleep test that evaluates physical factors affecting sleep. Physical activity and level of sleep are monitored by a technician while the patient sleeps. See *Figure 8-12*.

Small electrodes are attached to parts of the patient's head and body. Flexible wiring attached to the electrodes is then connected to a central monitoring unit. While the patient sleeps, the electrodes monitor and record various physical activities that occur such as heart rate and activity, breathing, eye movements, muscle activity, and leg movements.

The patient is observed and monitored through the night by a technician. Activities such as snoring, kicking during sleep, periodic movements, and sleep stages are monitored. A polysomnogram is useful in evaluating sleep disorders such as sleep apnea, sleepwalking, night terrors, restless leg syndrome, insomnia, and **narcolepsy**.

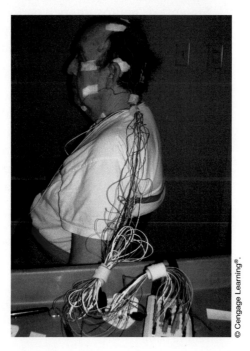

Figure 8-12 Patient being prepared for polysomnogram

positron emission tomography (PET)

(**POZ**-ih-tron ee-**MISH**-un toh-**MOG**-rah-fee)

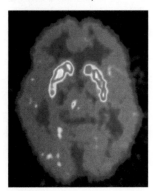

A **positron emission tomography (PET)** scan produces computerized radiographic images of various body structures when radioactive substances are inhaled or injected. See *Figure 8-13*.

The metabolic activity of the brain and numerous other body structures are shown through computerized color-coded images that indicate the degree and intensity of the metabolic process. The PET scan exposes persons to very little radiation because the radioactive substances used are very short-lived.

Figure 8-13 PET scan shows that cocaine binds to specific brain locations primarily at dopamine-uptake

(From "Addiction Brain Mechanisms and Their Related Implications," by D.J. Nutt, 1996, The Lancet, 347, pp. 33–35)

PET scans are used in assessing **dementia**, brain tumors, cerebral vascular disease, and brain tumors. In addition, there is a growing employment of the procedure in the study of biochemical activity of the brain and the study and diagnosis of cancer.

Romberg test (**ROM**-berg test)	The **Romberg test** is used to evaluate cerebellar function and balance. The person is asked to stand quietly with feet together and hands at the side and to attain equilibrium. The following step is to evaluate if the person can close his or her eyes and maintain equilibrium without swaying or falling. The next part of the evaluation is to assess if the person can lift the hands to shoulder height and then close eyes without hands drifting downward. If these two evaluations are completed successfully, the balance and cerebellar function are intact.
stereotaxic neurosurgery (**ster**-eh-oh-**TAK**-sik **noo**-roh-**SER**-jer-ee)	**Stereotaxic neurosurgery** is performed on a precise location of an area within the brain that controls specific function(s) and may involve destruction of brain tissue with various agents such as heat, cold, and sclerosing or corrosive fluids. This destruction may interrupt pathways of electrical activity or destroy specific nuclei. The precise location is calculated preoperatively. A small hole is drilled in the skull, and the tip of a needle or probe is guided accurately to the exact location. The complications of **stereotaxic neurosurgery** relate to the site of the surgical approach and potential bleeding. It is possible for these tiny lesions to create lasting pain relief.
sympathectomy (**sim**-pah-**THEK**-toh-mee)	**Sympathectomy** is a surgical procedure used to interrupt a portion of the sympathetic nerve pathway for the purpose of relieving chronic pain.
tractotomy (trak-**TOT**-oh-mee)	A **tractotomy** involves a **craniotomy**, through which the anterolateral pathway in the brain stem is surgically divided in an attempt to relieve pain. Morbidity and mortality rates connected with this procedure are high.

transcutaneous electrical nerve stimulation (TENS)
 	
(**tranz**-kyoo-**TAY**-nee-us
ee-**LEK**-trih-kul nerve
stim-yoo-**LAY**-shun)
  trans- = across, through
  cutane/o = skin
  -ous = pertaining to
	Transcutaneous electrical nerve stimulation (TENS) is a form of cutaneous stimulation for pain relief that supplies electrical impulses to the nerve endings of a nerve close to the pain site.
	
	This is accomplished by placing electrodes on the skin and connecting them to a stimulator by flexible wires. Electrical impulses produced are much like the body's impulses but are distinct enough to hinder transmission of pain signals to the brain.
	
	The person wearing a TENS unit is responsible for controlling the pulsation and voltage of the electrical impulses. The person wearing the TENS must clean the electrodes and skin every eight hours along with reapplying the electrode jelly. One use of the TENS is with persons experiencing back pain and/or **sciatica**.

Review Checkpoint

Check your understanding of this section by completing the **Diagnostic Techniques, Treatments, and Procedures** exercises in your workbook.

COMMON ABBREVIATIONS

Abbreviation	Meaning	Abbreviation	Meaning
ACTH	adrenocorticotrophic hormone	**MSLT**	multiple sleep latency test
ALS	amyotrophic lateral sclerosis	**NCS**	nerve conduction study
ANS	autonomic nervous system	**NPH**	normal-pressure hydrocephalus
CAT	computerized axial tomography		
CNS	central nervous system	**NREM**	non-rapid eye movement (stage of sleep)
CSF	cerebrospinal fluid		
CT	computed tomography	**PET**	positron emission tomography
CVA	cerebrovascular accident; stroke	**PNS**	peripheral nervous system
ECT	electroconvulsive therapy		
EEG	electroencephalogram	**PSG**	polysomnogram
EMG	electromyography	**REM**	rapid eye movement (stage of sleep)
ICP	intracranial pressure		
LOC	level of consciousness	**RT**	reading test
LP	lumbar puncture	**SNS**	somatic nervous system
MRI	magnetic resonance imaging	**TENS**	transcutaneous electrical nerve stimulation
MS	multiple sclerosis	**TIA**	transient ischemic attack

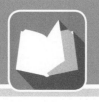

Review Checkpoint

Check your understanding of this section by completing the **Common Abbreviations** exercises in your workbook.

WRITTEN AND AUDIO TERMINOLOGY REVIEW

Review each of the following terms from this chapter. Study the spelling of each term and write the definition in the space provided. Check definitions by looking up the term in the glossary.

Term	Pronunciation	Definition
absence seizure	AB-senz SEE-zyoor	
acetylcholine	ah-seh-till-KOH-leen	
afferent nerves	AFF-er-ent nerves	
agnosia	ag-NOH-zee-ah	
agraphia	ah-GRAFF-ee-ah	
alexia	ah-LEK-see-ah	
Alzheimer's disease	ALTS-high-merz dih-ZEEZ	
amyotrophic lateral sclerosis (ALS)	ah-my-oh-TROFF-ik LAT-er-al skleh-ROH-sis	
analgesia	an-al-JEE-zee-ah	
analgesic	an-al-JEE-zik	
anencephaly	an-en-SEFF-ah-lee	
anesthesia	an-ess-THEE-zee-ah	
anesthesiologist	an-ess-thee-zee-OL-oh-jist	
anesthetic	an-es-THET-ick	
aneurysm	AN-yoo-rizm	
aphasia	ah-FAY-zee-ah	
apraxia	ah-PRAK-see-ah	
arachnoid membrane	ah-RAK-noyd MEM-brayn	
astrocyte	ASS-troh-sight	
astrocytoma	ass-troh-sigh-TOH-mah	
ataxia	ah-TAK-see-ah	
aura	AW-rah	
autonomic nervous system	aw-toh-NOM-ik NER-vus SIS-tem	
axon	AK-son	

Term	Pronunciation	Definition
Babinski's reflex	☐ bah-**BIN**-skeez **REE**-fleks	_____
Bell's palsy	☐ **BELLZ PAWL**-zee	_____
blood–brain barrier	☐ **BLUD-BRAIN BAIR**-ree-er	_____
bradyesthesia	☐ **brad**-ee-ess-**THEE**-zee-ah	_____
bradykinesia	☐ **brad**-ee-kih-**NEE**-zee-ah	_____
brain abscess	☐ **BRAIN AB**-sess	_____
Brudzinski's sign	☐ broo-**JIN**-skeez SIGN	_____
burr hole	☐ **BURR HOLE**	_____
carpal tunnel syndrome	☐ **CAR**-pal **TUN**-el **SIN**-drom	_____
cauda equina	☐ **KAW**-dah ee-**KWY**-nah	_____
causalgia	☐ kaw-**ZAL**-jee-ah	_____
cephalalgia	☐ **seff**-ah-**LAL**-jee-ah	_____
cerebellospinal	☐ **ser**-eh-**bell**-oh-**SPY**-nal	_____
cerebellum	☐ **ser**-eh-**BELL**-um	_____
cerebral angiography	☐ **SER**-eh-bral (seh-**REE**-bral) **an**-jee-**OG**-rah-fee	_____
cerebral concussion	☐ seh-**REE**-bral con-**KUSH**-shun	_____
cerebral contusion	☐ seh-**REE**-bral con-**TOO**-zhun	_____
cerebral cortex	☐ seh-**REE**-bral **KOR**-teks	_____
cerebral palsy	☐ seh-**REE**-bral **PAWL**-zee	_____
cerebritis	☐ **ser**-eh-**BRYE**-tis	_____
cerebrospinal fluid	☐ seh-**ree**-broh-**SPY**-nal **FLOO**-id	_____
cerebrovascular accident (CVA)	☐ seh-**ree**-broh-**VASS**-kyoo-lar **AK**-sih-dent	_____
cerebrum	☐ seh-**REE**-brum	_____
cervical radiculopathy	☐ **SIR**-vick-al rah-**dick**-you-**LOP**-ah-thee	_____
Cheyne-Stokes respirations	☐ **CHAIN-STOHKS** res-pir-**AY**-shunz	_____
chordotomy	☐ kor-**DOT**-oh-mee	_____
cisternal puncture	☐ sis-**TER**-nal **PUNK**-chur	_____
cluster headache	☐ **KLUSS**-ter headache	_____
coma	☐ **COH**-mah	_____
comatose	☐ **COH**-mah-tohs	_____

Term	Pronunciation	Definition
contracture	☐ kon-**TRAK**-chur	_____
convolution	☐ **kon**-voh-**LOO**-shun	_____
craniotomy	☐ **kray**-nee-**OTT**-oh-mee	_____
degenerative disk	☐ dee-**JEN**-er-ah-tiv **DISK**	_____
dementia	☐ dee-**MEN**-shee-ah	_____
demyelination	☐ dee-**my**-eh-lye-**NAY**-shun	_____
dendrite	☐ **DEN**-dright	_____
diencephalon	☐ **dye**-en-**SEFF**-ah-lon	_____
diplopia	☐ dip-**LOH**-pee-ah	_____
dura mater	☐ **DOO**-rah **MAH**-ter	_____
dyslexia	☐ dis-**LEK**-see-ah	_____
dysphasia	☐ dis-**FAY**-zee-ah	_____
dystonia	☐ dis-**TON**-ee-ah	_____
echoencephalography	☐ **eck**-oh-en-**sef**-ah-**LOG**-rah-fee	_____
efferent nerves	☐ **EE**-fair-ent nerves	_____
electroencephalography	☐ ee-**leck**-troh-en-**sef**-ah-**LOG**-rah-fee	_____
embolism	☐ **EM**-boh-lizm	_____
encephalitis	☐ en-**seff**-ah-**LYE**-tis	_____
epidural space	☐ **ep**-ih-**DOO**-rall space	_____
epilepsy	☐ **EP**-ih-**lep**-see	_____
fissure	☐ **FISH**-er	_____
fontanelle or fontanel	☐ **fon**-tah-**NELL**	_____
gait	☐ **GAYT**	_____
ganglion	☐ **GANG**-lee-on	_____
glioma	☐ glee-**OH**-mah	_____
grand mal seizure	☐ grand **MALL SEE**-zyoor	_____
Guillain-Barré syndrome	☐ **GHEE**-yon bah-**RAY SIN**-drom	_____
gyrus	☐ **JYE**-rus	_____
hematoma	☐ hee-mah-**TOH**-mah	_____
hemiparesis	☐ **hem**-ee-pah-**REE**-sis	_____
hemiplegia	☐ **hem**-ee-**PLEE**-jee-ah	_____
herniated disk	☐ **HER**-nee-**ay**-ted disk	_____
herpes zoster	☐ **HER**-peez **ZOSS**-ter	_____

Term	Pronunciation	Definition
Huntington's chorea	☐ **HUNT**-ing-tonz koh-**REE**-ah	_____
hydrocephalus	☐ **high**-droh-**SEFF**-ah-lus	_____
hypochondriasis	☐ **high**-poh-kon-**DRY**-ah-sis	_____
hyposthenia	☐ **high**-poss-**THEE**-nee-ah	_____
hypothalamus	☐ **high**-poh-**THAL**-ah-mus	_____
interneurons	☐ **in**-ter-**NOO**-rons	_____
intracranial tumors	☐ **in**-trah-**KRAY**-nee-al **TOO**-morz	_____
intrathecal	☐ **in**-trah-**THEE**-cal	_____
kinesiology	☐ kih-**nee**-see-**OL**-oh-jee	_____
laminectomy	☐ **lam**-ih-**NEK**-toh-mee	_____
lethargy	☐ **LETH**-ar-jee	_____
longitudinal fissure	☐ **lon**-jih-**TOO**-dih-nal **FISH**-er	_____
lumbar puncture	☐ **LUM**-bar **PUNK**-chur	_____
medulla oblongata	☐ meh-**DULL**-ah **ob**-long-**GAH**-tah	_____
meninges	☐ men-**IN**-jeez	_____
meningitis (acute bacterial)	☐ **men**-in-**JYE**-tis (ah-**KYOOT** back-**TEE**-ree-al)	_____
meningocele	☐ meh-**NING**-goh-**seel**	_____
meningomyelocele	☐ men-**in**-goh-my-**ELL**-oh-seel	_____
metastatic intracranial tumors	☐ **met**-ah-**STAT**-ik **in**-trah-**KRAY**-nee-al **TOO**-morz	_____
microglia	☐ my-**KROG**-lee-ah	_____
midbrain	☐ **MID**-brain	_____
migraine headache	☐ **MY**-grain headache	_____
motor nerves	☐ **MOH**-tor nerves	_____
multiple sclerosis (MS)	☐ **MULL**-tih-pal skleh-**ROH**-sis (MS)	_____
myasthenia gravis	☐ **my**-as-**THEE**-nee-ah **GRAV**-iss	_____
myelin sheath	☐ **MY**-eh-lin **SHEETH**	_____
myelocele	☐ **MY**-eh-loh-seel	_____
myelography	☐ **my**-eh-**LOG**-rah-fee	_____
narcolepsy	☐ **NAR**-koh-**lep**-see	_____
narcosis	☐ nar-**KOH**-sis	_____
neuralgia	☐ noo-**RAL**-jee-ah	_____

Term	Pronunciation	Definition
neurectomy	☐ noo-**REK**-toh-mee	_____
neuritis	☐ noo-**RYE**-tis	_____
neuroblastoma	☐ **noo**-roh-blass-**TOH**-mah	_____
neuroglia	☐ noo-**ROG**-lee-ah	_____
neurologist	☐ noo-**ROL**-oh-jist	_____
neurology	☐ noo-**ROL**-oh-jee	_____
neuron	☐ **NOO**-ron	_____
neuropathy	☐ noo-**ROP**-ah-thee	_____
neurosurgeon	☐ **noo**-roh-**SIR**-jun	_____
neurosurgery	☐ **noo**-roh-**SIR**-jer-ee	_____
neurotransmitter	☐ **noo**-roh-**TRANS**-mit-er	_____
nuchal rigidity	☐ **NOO**-kal rih-**JID**-ih-tee	_____
occlusion	☐ oh-**KLOO**-zhun	_____
oligodendrocytes	☐ **ol**-ih-goh-**DEN**-droh-sights	_____
palliative	☐ **PAL**-ee-ah-tiv	_____
paraplegia	☐ **par**-ah-**PLEE**-jee-ah	_____
parasympathetic nerves	☐ **pair**-ah-**sim**-pah-**THET**-ik nerves	_____
parasympathomimetic	☐ **pair**-ah-**sim**-pah-thoh-mim-**ET**-ik	_____
paresthesia	☐ **pair**-es-**THEE**-zee-ah	_____
Parkinson's disease	☐ **PARK**-in-sons dih-**ZEEZ**	_____
peripheral nervous system	☐ per-**IF**-er-al nervous system	_____
peripheral neuritis	☐ per-**IF**-er-al noo-**RYE**-tis	_____
petit mal seizure	☐ pet-**EE MALL SEE**-zyoor	_____
phagocytosis	☐ **fag**-oh-sigh-**TOH**-sis	_____
pia mater	☐ **PEE**-ah **MAH**-ter	_____
pineal body	☐ **PIN**-ee-al body	_____
plexus	☐ **PLEKS**-us	_____
poliomyelitis	☐ **poh**-lee-oh-**my**-eh-**LYE**-tis	_____
pons	☐ **PONZ**	_____
positron emission tomography (PET)	☐ **POZ**-ih-tron ee-**MISH**-un toh-**MOG**-rah-fee	_____
postpolio syndrome	☐ **POST-POH**-lee-oh **SIN**-drom	_____

Term	Pronunciation	Definition
primary intracranial tumors	☐ **PRIGH**-mair-ree in-trah-**KRAY**-nee-al **TOO**-morz	_____
quadriplegia	☐ **kwad**-rih-**PLEE**-jee-ah	_____
receptor	☐ ree-**SEP**-tor	_____
Reye's syndrome	☐ **RISE SIN**-drom	_____
rhizotomy	☐ rye-**ZOT**-oh-mee	_____
Romberg test	☐ **ROM**-berg test	_____
sciatica	☐ sigh-**AT**-ih-kah	_____
sensory	☐ **SEN**-soh-ree	_____
sensory nerves	☐ **SEN**-soh-ree nerves	_____
shingles	☐ **SHING**-ulz	_____
somatic nervous system	☐ soh-**MAT**-ik nervous system	_____
spina bifida cystica	☐ **SPY**-nah **BIFF**-ih-dah **SISS**-tih-kah	_____
spina bifida occulta	☐ **SPY**-nah **BIFF**-ih-dah oh-**KULL**-tah	_____
stereotaxic neurosurgery	☐ **stair**-eh-oh-**TAK**-sik **noo**-roh-**SER**-jer-ee	_____
stimulus	☐ **STIM**-yoo-lus	_____
stupor	☐ **STOO**-per	_____
subarachnoid space	☐ **sub**-ah-**RAK**-noyd space	_____
subdural space	☐ sub-**DOO**-ral space	_____
sulcus	☐ **SULL**-kuss	_____
sympathectomy	☐ **sim**-pah-**THEK**-toh-mee	_____
sympathetic nerves	☐ **sim**-pah-**THET**-ik nerves	_____
sympathomimetic	☐ **sim**-pah-thoh-mim-**ET**-ik	_____
synapse	☐ **SIN**-aps	_____
syncope	☐ **SIN**-koh-pee	_____
Tay-Sachs disease	☐ **TAY-SACKS** dih-**ZEEZ**	_____
thalamus	☐ **THAL**-ah-mus	_____
thrombosis	☐ throm-**BOH**-sis	_____
tonic-clonic seizure	☐ **TON**-ik-**KLON**-ik **SEE**-zhur	_____
tractotomy	☐ trak-**TOT**-oh-mee	_____
transcutaneous electrical nerve stimulation (TENS)	☐ **tranz**-kyoo-**TAY**-nee-us ee-**LEK**-trih-kul nerve **stim**-yoo-**LAY**-shun (TENS)	_____

Term	Pronunciation	Definition
trigeminal neuralgia (*tic douloureux*)	☐ try-**JEM**-ih-nal noo-**RAL**-jee-ah (*tik* **DOO**-*loh-roo*)	_____
ventricle	☐ **VEN**-trih-kul	_____
ventriculostomy	☐ ven-**trik**-yoo-**LOSS**-toh-mee	_____

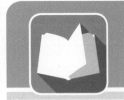

Review Checkpoint

Apply what you have learned in this chapter by completing the **Putting It All Together** exercise in your workbook.

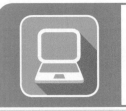

Online Resources

For additional study tools, including PowerPoint® slides and animations, go to the Student Companion Website.

Chapter Review Exercises

The following exercises provide a more in-depth review of the chapter material. Your goal in these exercises is to complete each section at a minimum 80% level of accuracy. A space has been provided for your score at the end of each section.

A. Form the Plurals

Write the plural form and definition of each word listed. If you have forgotten how to form plurals, you may wish to refer to the section on forming plurals in Chapter 3. Each correct answer is worth 10 points. Record your score in the space provided at the end of the exercise.

a. ganglion

    1. Plural: _____

    2. Definition: _____

    _____

b. gyrus

    3. Plural: _____

    4. Definition: _____

    _____

c. dendrite

   5. Plural: _____

   6. Definition: _____

          _____

d. stimulus

   7. Plural: _____

   8. Definition: _____

e. sulcus

   9. Plural: _____

  10. Definition: _____

Number correct _____ **× 10 points/correct answer: Your score** _____ **%**

B. Spelling

Circle the correctly spelled term in each pairing of words. Each correct answer is worth 10 points. Record your score in the space provided at the end of the exercise.

1. aneurysm   anurysm
2. automonic   autonomic
3. cephoalgia   cephalalgia
4. efferent   eferent
5. girus   gyrus
6. narcolepsy   narcrolepsy
7. thalamus   thalmus
8. myalin   myelin
9. nuckle   nuchal
10. sciatica   siatica

Number correct _____ **× 10 points/correct answer: Your score** _____ **%**

C. Crossword Puzzle

The terms in the following crossword puzzle pertain to the anatomy and physiology of the nervous system. Each correct answer is worth 10 points. When you have completed the puzzle, total your points and enter your score in the space provided.

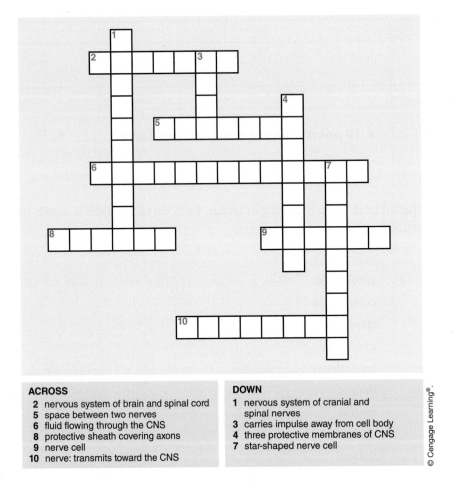

ACROSS

2 nervous system of brain and spinal cord
5 space between two nerves
6 fluid flowing through the CNS
8 protective sheath covering axons
9 nerve cell
10 nerve: transmits toward the CNS

DOWN

1 nervous system of cranial and spinal nerves
3 carries impulse away from cell body
4 three protective membranes of CNS
7 star-shaped nerve cell

© Cengage Learning®.

Number correct _____ *× 10 points/correct answer: Your score* _____ *%*

D. Term to Definition

Define each term by writing the definition in the space provided. Check the box if you are able to complete this exercise correctly the first time (without referring to the answers). Each correct answer is worth 10 points. Record your score in the space provided at the end of the exercise.

☐ 1. syncope: _____

☐ 2. sciatica: _____

☐ 3. paresthesia: _____

☐ 4. palliative: _____

☐ 5. occlusion: _____

☐ 6. neuritis: _____

☐ 7. lethargy: _____

☐ 8. hemiparesis: _____

☐ 9. fissure: _____

☐ 10. coma: _____

Number correct _____ × *10 points/correct answer: Your score* _____ *%*

E. Matching Structures

Match the structures of the CNS listed on the left with the most appropriate definition on the right. Each correct answer is worth 10 points. Record your score in the space provided at the end of the exercise.

_____ 1. arachnoid

_____ 2. brain stem

_____ 3. cerebellum

_____ 4. cerebrum

_____ 5. diencephalon

_____ 6. dura mater

_____ 7. medulla oblongata

_____ 8. hypothalamus

_____ 9. pons

_____ 10. ventricle

a. a small hollow within the brain that is filled with cerebrospinal fluid

b. controls body temperature, sleep, and appetite

c. stemlike portion of the brain that connects the cerebral hemispheres with the spinal cord

d. contains the cardiac, vasomotor, and respiratory centers of the brain

e. the weblike, middle layer of the meninges

f. outermost layer of the meninges

g. located between the cerebrum and the midbrain (consists of the thalamus, hypothalamus, and pineal gland)

h. responsible for coordinating voluntary muscular movement

i. controls consciousness, memory, sensations, etc.

j. acts as a bridge to connect the medulla oblongata and the cerebellum to the upper portions of the brain

Number correct _____ × *10 points/correct answer: Your score* _____ *%*

F. Definition to Term

Use the definitions to identify and provide the appropriate medical word. Write the word in the first space and its combining form in the second space. Each correct answer is worth 5 points. Record your score in the space provided at the end of the exercise.

1. Pain in the head ("headache"):

   _____   _____
   (word)   (combining form)

2. A condition in which there is abnormally slow movement:

   _____   _____
   (word)   (combining form)

3. Difficult speech:

   _____   _____
   (word)   (combining form)

(*continued*)

4. The study of the nervous system and its disorders:

_____   _____

(word)   (combining form)

5. Paralysis of all four extremities of the body:

_____   _____

(word)   (combining form)

6. An abnormal condition in which a clot develops in a blood vessel:

_____   _____

(word)   (combining form)

7. Inflammation of the meninges:

_____   _____

(word)   (combining form)

8. "Without speech":

_____   _____

(word)   (combining form)

9. Incision into the skull:

_____   _____

(word)   (combining form)

10. Uncontrolled, sudden attacks of sleep:

_____   _____

(word)   (combining form)

Number correct _____ × **5 points/correct answer: Your score** _____ **%**

G. Labeling

Label the following diagrams by identifying the appropriate structures. Place your answers in the spaces provided. Each correct answer is worth 10 points. Record your score in the space provided at the end of the exercise.

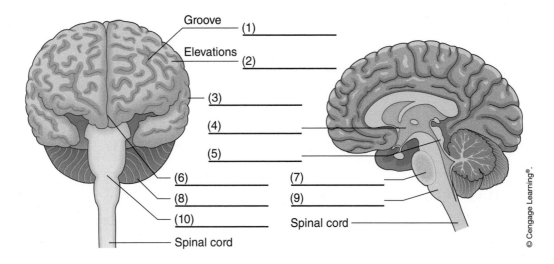

1. _____

2. _____

3. _____

4. _____

5. _____

6. _____

7. _____

8. _____

9. _____

10. _____

Number correct _____ **× 10 points/correct answer: Your score** _____ **%**

H. Matching Abbreviations

Match the abbreviations on the left with the applicable definition on the right. Each correct response is worth 10 points. Record your score in the space provided at the end of the exercise.

_____ 1. ANS   a. electrocardiogram

_____ 2. CSF   b. level of consciousness

_____ 3. CVA   c. computed tomography

_____ 4. EEG   d. transient ischemic attacks

_____ 5. ICP   e. autonomic nervous system

(*continued*)

_____ 6. MRI   f. lumbar puncture

_____ 7. REM   g. cerebrospinal fluid

_____ 8. TIA   h. cardiovascular accident

_____ 9. LOC   i. rapid eye movement

_____ 10. LP   j. magnetic resonance imaging

                                 k. intracranial pressure

                                 l. adrenocorticotropic hormone serum

                                 m. electroencephalogram

                                 n. cerebrovascular accident

Number correct _____ **× 10 points/correct answer: Your score** _____ **%**

I. Definition to Term

Use the following definition to identify and provide the correct procedure. Each correct answer is worth 10 points. Record your score in the space provided at the end of the exercise.

1. Visualization of the cerebrovascular system via X-ray after the injection of a radiopaque contrast medium into an artery.

   _____

2. A noninvasive scanning procedure that provides a computer projected image of fluid, soft tissue, or bony structures without the use of radiation.

   _____

3. Measurement of electrical activity produced by the brain and recorded through electrodes placed on the scalp.

   _____

4. Insertion of a hollow needle and stylet into the subarachnoid space generally between the third and fourth lumbar vertebrae.

   _____

5. A three-dimensional view of brain tissue obtained as X-ray beams pass through successive horizontal layers of the brain.

   _____

6. A surgical procedure that makes an opening into the skull.

   _____

7. A positive finding in an adult represents upper motor neuron disease of the pyramidal tract.

   _____

8. An evaluation of cerebellar function and balance.

   _____

9. Surgical removal of bony arches from one or more vertebrae to relieve pressure from the spinal cord.

   _____

10. Introduction of contrast medium into the lumbar subarachnoid space through a lumbar puncture to visualize the spinal cord and vertebral canal through X-ray examination.

   _____

Number correct _____ **× 10 points/correct answer: Your score** _____ **%**

J. Word Search

Read each definition carefully and identify the applicable word from the list that follows. Enter the word in the space provided and then find it in the puzzle and circle it. The words may be read up, down, diagonally, across, or backward. Each correct answer is worth 10 points. Record your score in the space provided at the end of the exercise.

aphasia	paraplegia	encephalitis
syncope	migraine	hydrocephalus
neurology	epilepsy	cephalalgia
cerebral palsy		Alzheimer's

Example: The inability to speak.

*aphasia*_____

1. Congenital brain damage that is permanent but not progressive; characterized by the child's lack of control of voluntary muscles.

   _____

2. Many times, this condition requires the use of a shunt to remove CSF and decrease intracranial pressure.

   _____

3. Paralysis of the lower extremities and trunk, usually due to spinal cord injury.

   _____

4. A degenerative disease that progresses through three stages, ending with the deterioration of mental, emotional, and physical functioning.

   _____

5. A syndrome of recurring episodes of excessive irregular electrical activity of the CNS; also called seizures.

   _____

6. A type of headache often preceded by an aura.

   _____

7. The study of the nervous system.

   _____

8. Inflammation of the brain or spinal cord tissue.

   _____

9. Another name for fainting.

   _____

10. The medical term for pain in the head; headache.

    _____

Number correct _____ × *10 points/correct answer: Your score* _____ *%*

M	E	(A	P	H	A	S	I	A)	I	O	N	S	T	I
U	A	I	G	E	L	P	A	R	A	P	I	A	P	S
L	D	B	Y	A	C	U	T	E	I	T	G	E	N	E
C	E	P	H	A	L	A	L	G	I	A	E	A	S	P
I	A	D	H	R	S	I	F	L	E	X	I	L	N	O
P	C	S	Y	N	I	T	A	N	O	R	P	Z	D	C
L	O	E	D	E	T	H	I	M	B	R	I	H	E	N
E	N	E	R	P	P	L	E	X	I	O	N	E	R	Y
S	A	X	O	E	I	N	O	I	T	A	P	I	R	S
C	T	T	C	I	B	N	E	X	T	I	N	M	I	A
L	I	N	E	R	C	R	A	R	L	T	A	E	I	T
E	E	N	P	A	L	Y	A	E	A	D	D	R	C	I
R	N	S	H	D	R	R	P	L	I	P	R	S	N	O
O	S	I	A	I	E	S	U	M	P	O	S	U	P	N
S	O	O	L	S	Y	D	S	H	C	A	S	Y	A	T
I	U	N	U	S	E	N	E	U	R	O	L	O	G	Y
S	R	O	S	D	S	R	S	I	F	L	E	S	X	N
P	L	A	N	M	I	G	R	A	I	N	E	O	Y	O

© Cengage Learning®.

K. Matching Pathological Conditions

Match the pathological conditions on the left with the most applicable definition on the right. Each correct answer is worth 10 points. Record your score in the space provided at the end of the exercise.

_____ 1. cerebral embolism

_____ 2. glioblastoma multiforme

_____ 3. cerebral concussion

_____ 4. epidural hematoma

_____ 5. cerebrovascular accident

_____ 6. cerebral contusion

_____ 7. subdural hematoma

_____ 8. depressed skull fracture

_____ 9. hydrocephalus

_____ 10. spina bifida occulta

a the most rapidly growing glioma, comprising 20% of all intracranial tumors

b. a collection of arterial blood located above the dura mater and just below the skull

c. a broken segment of the skull thrust into the brain as a result of direct force

d. a brief interruption of brain function, usually with a loss of consciousness lasting a few seconds

e. a collection of venous blood below the dura mater and above the arachnoid layer of the meninges

f. neurological deficits resulting from cerebral ischemia to a specific localized area in the brain; stroke

g. an increased amount of CSF in the brain

h. a congenital defect of the CNS in which the back portion of one or more vertebrae is not closed

i. small, scattered, venous hemorrhages in the brain tissue

j. fragment of blood clot, fat, bacteria, or tumor that lodges in a cerebral vessel

Number correct _____ **× 10 points/correct answer: Your score** _____ **%**

L. Completion

Complete the following statements with the most appropriate answer. Each correct answer is worth 10 points. Record your score in the space provided at the end of the exercise.

1. A congenital defect of the CNS in which the back portion of one or more vertebrae is not closed normally and a cyst protrudes through the opening in the back, usually at the level of L5 or S1.

   _____

   (three words)

2. Also called tonic-clonic, these begin with sudden loss of consciousness, followed by muscle contractions and rigid extension of the head and arms, followed by a brief absence of respirations.

   _____

   (three words)

3. Occurring in any structural region of the brain, these may be malignant or benign, causing normal brain tissue to be displaced and compressed.

   _____

   (two words)

4. This follows severe trauma to the spinal cord between the fifth and eighth cervical vertebrae, generally resulting in loss of motor and sensory function below the level of the injury.

   _____

   (one word)

5. A very brief period of ischemia in the brain, lasting from minutes to hours, which can cause a variety of symptoms.

   _____

   (three words)

6. A rupture of the nucleus pulposus through the disk wall and into the spinal canal, causing pressure on the spinal cord or nerve roots.

   _____

   (three words)

7. This condition is characterized by intermittent or continuous pain in the hand, wrist, and arm due to the pinching of the median nerve and inflammation and swelling of tendons.

   _____

   (three words)

8. This condition occurs when a cerebral vessel ruptures, allowing blood into the CSF, brain tissue, or subarachnoid space.

   _____

   (two words)

(continued)

9. This condition is characterized by temporary or permanent unilateral weakness or paralysis to the muscles in the face following trauma to the face, an unknown infection, or a tumor pressing on the facial nerve.

_____

(two words)

10. These occur as a result of metastasis from a primary site such as the lung or breast.

_____

(three words)

Number correct _____ **× 10 points/correct answer: Your score** _____ **%**

M. Medical Scenario

The following medical scenario presents information on one of the pathological conditions discussed in this chapter. Read the scenario carefully and select the most appropriate answer for each question that follows. Each correct answer is worth 20 points. Record your score in the space provided at the end of the exercise.

Laverne Hopps is a 65-year-old patient visiting her internist. Laverne was discharged from the hospital two days ago following a stroke, which began while she was resting and progressed over two days. She had experienced TIAs prior to the occurrence of this stroke. She will be attending outpatient rehabilitation for physical therapy, occupational therapy, and speech therapy. Laverne's husband asks the health care professional some questions about his wife's stroke and her prognosis.

1. The health care professional bases her response to his questions about strokes on the basis that a stroke is also called:

   a. a cerebral concussion and is a brief interruption of brain function, usually with a loss of consciousness lasting for a few seconds

   b. a cerebrovascular accident and involves death of a specific portion of brain tissue, resulting from ischemia to that area of the brain

   c. Huntington's chorea and is an inherited neurological disease characterized by rapid, jerky, involuntary movements and increasing dementia due to the effects of the basal ganglia on the neurons

   d. multiple sclerosis and is a degenerative inflammatory disease of the central nervous system attacking the myelin sheath in the spinal cord and brain, leaving it sclerosed or scarred

2. From the information given about Mrs. Hopps's stroke, the health care professional realizes that it was most likely caused by a:

   a. cerebral hemorrhage

   b. fat emboli

   c. subarachnoid hemorrhage

   d. cerebral thrombosis

3. The health care professional discussed the occurrence of strokes with Mr. Hopps. She explained to him that the type of stroke Mrs. Hopps experienced is typically:

   a. a result of a virus that enters the CNS

   b. a result of atherosclerosis

   c. due to high blood pressure

   d. from a fracture of a long bone

4. Mr. Hopps asked the health care professional about his wife's symptoms and prognosis. She discussed with him that the deficits and prognosis depend on the degree of:

   a. hydrocephalus

   b. peripheral neuritis

   c. damage and the specific area of the brain affected

   d. inflammation of the spinal cord tissue

5. Mr. Hopps asked the health care professional what the speech therapist will help his wife accomplish. The health care professional explains that the speech therapist will assist Mrs. Hopps with her aphasia by working to improve her:

   a. ability to perform coordinated movements

   b. communication through speech and writing

   c aura

   d. gait

Number correct _____ *× 20 points/correct answer: Your score* _____ *%*

N. Proofreading Skills

Read the following Radiology Report. For each bold term, provide a brief definition and indicate if the term is spelled correctly. If it is misspelled, provide the correct spelling. Each correct answer is worth 20 points. Record your score in the space provided at the end of the exercise.

Example:

> **CT** *computed tomography* _____
> Spelled Correctly? ☑ Yes ☐ No _____

RADIOLOGY REPORT

Hillcrest
medical center

PATIENT NAME: Lydia Cruz

PATIENT ID: 11723

X-RAY NO.: 03-7946

ADMITTING PHYSICIAN
Tomas Burgos, MD

PROCEDURE:
Lumbar **myalography** and post myelogram CT.

DATE
05/26/2014

CLINICAL INFORMATION
Previous **CT** evidence of disk bulging. Patient experiencing **sciatica**, right side.

(continued)

RADIOLOGY REPORT
Patient Name: Lydia Cruz
Patient ID: 11723
X-Ray NO.: 03-7946
Date: 05/26/2014
Page 2

Lumbar puncture was done by Dr. Mann. Water-soluble contrast media was instilled into the **subrachnoid space** . After obtaining lumbar myelogram films, the patient was moved to the CT scanner where angled cuts were done at all levels. The images were recorded with the bone and soft tissue technique.

The L1-2 and L2-3 levels are unremarkable. The L3-4 level does show some facet arthropathy on the right with some spurring on the anterior aspect of the right facets. There is some relative narrowing of the entire canal at the L3-4 level due to this spurring, some prominence of the ligamentum flavum, and slight disk bulging.

The L4-5 level reveals changes of moderate facet arthropathy with, again, relative stenosis of the canal on the same basis as above. The lumbosacral level reveals facet arthropathy changes of a mild degree with no definite **herniated disk** or remarkable degree of disk bulging.

IMPRESSION
CT scan showing facet arthropathy changes at lower 3 interspaces, most marked at the L4-5 level.

Relative stenosis of the canal at the L3-4 and L4-5 levels due to facet arthropathy, some ligamentum flavum prominence, and low-grade disk bulging.

_____

Howard Mann, MD

HM:xx

D:05/26/2014

T:05/26/2014

1. **myalography** _____

   _____

   Spelled Correctly? ☐ Yes ☐ No _____
2. **sciatica** _____

   _____

   Spelled Correctly? ☐ Yes ☐ No _____
3. **lumbar puncture** _____

   _____

   Spelled Correctly? ☐ Yes ☐ No _____
4. **subrachnoid space** _____

   _____

   Spelled Correctly? ☐ Yes ☐ No _____
5. **herniated disk** _____

   _____

   Spelled Correctly? ☐ Yes ☐ No _____

Number correct _____ **× 20 points/correct answer: Your score** _____ **%**

The Blood and Lymphatic Systems

CHAPTER CONTENT

OBJECTIVES

Upon completing this chapter and the review exercises at the end of the chapter, the learner should be able to:

1. List the major functions of the blood and of the lymphatic system as identified in the chapter overview of each system.

2. Identify and define 30 pathological conditions of the blood and lymphatic systems.

3. Identify at least 10 diagnostic techniques used in the diagnosis and treatment of disorders of the blood and lymphatic systems.

4. Correctly spell and pronounce terms listed on the Written and Audio Terminology Review, using the phonetic pronunciations provided.

5. Identify and define at least 10 medical terms related to the blood and lymphatic systems.

6. Identify at least 10 abbreviations common to the blood and lymphatic systems.

7. Identify at least 10 combining forms related to the blood and lymphatic systems.

Overview of the Blood System

The cells of the body depend on a steady supply of oxygen and nutrients to carry out their normal metabolic functions. They also depend on a means of disposing metabolic waste products to maintain a balanced internal environment. What system does the body use to achieve the transportation of oxygen and nutrients to the body cells and the transportation of waste products away from the body cells? The blood system.

Blood is the liquid pumped by the heart through the arteries, veins, and capillaries. It is much more than the simple liquid it seems to be; it is composed of a straw-colored fluid called **plasma**, the formed elements (cells and cell fragments), and a series of cell types with different functions. Two major functions of the blood are to transport oxygen and nutrients to the cells and to remove carbon dioxide and other waste products from the cells for elimination. You may have heard of the saying "blood is thicker than water" when referring to family relationships. The words are true: Blood *is* thicker than water. The term *viscosity* refers to the thickness of a fluid as compared with water; and compared with water, blood is about five times thicker. The viscosity of blood remains relatively constant, but it changes if the number of blood cells changes or if the concentration of plasma proteins changes. An example of an increase in the viscosity of blood (i.e., the stickiness of the blood) would be an increase in the number of erythrocytes (red blood cells), which would result in an increase in blood volume and thickness.

The total blood volume in an average adult male is 5 to 6 liters; in an average adult female, 4 to 5 liters. Blood accounts for approximately 8% of one's total body weight. It is slightly alkaline, having a pH of 7.35 to 7.45 (using water as the standard for a neutral liquid, with a pH of 7.0).

The scientific study of blood and blood-forming tissues is known as **hematology**. A medical specialist in the study of **hematology** is a **hematologist**.

Anatomy and Physiology (Blood)

The anatomy and physiology section in this chapter concentrates on the composition of blood (liquid and solid components), the blood types, and the mechanisms of blood clotting.

Composition of Blood

The liquid portion of blood is known as **plasma**; that is, whole blood minus the formed elements. **Plasma** is essential for transporting the cellular elements (solid components) of blood throughout the circulatory system. **Plasma** is a yellow or straw-colored fluid that is about 90% water. The remaining portion consists of the following **solutes** (substances dissolved in a solution): electrolytes, proteins, fats, glucose, **bilirubin**, and gases. The most abundant of the solutes are the **plasma proteins**. These plasma proteins, which are manufactured mainly by the liver, are grouped into three major classes: albumins, globulins, and **fibrinogen**.

1. **Albumin** constitutes approximately 60% of the plasma proteins. Albumins help maintain the normal blood volume and blood pressure. Because of their abundance, albumins attract water into the vessels through the capillaries by **osmosis** (fluid flows from a lesser concentration of solute to a greater concentration of solute). When this happens, the balance between the fluid in the blood and the fluid in the interstitial tissues is maintained; that is, the fluid will remain in the blood vessels as it should and will not leak out into the surrounding tissues. If this balance (osmotic pressure) is upset, the fluid will leave the blood vessels, seep into the surrounding tissue spaces, and result in swelling of the tissues (**edema**).

2. **Globulin** constitutes approximately 36% of the plasma proteins. There are three types of globulins: alpha, beta, and gamma. The alpha and beta globulins serve primarily to transport lipids (fats) and fat-soluble vitamins in the blood. Gamma globulins are the **antibodies** that function in **immunity**.

3. **Fibrinogen** constitutes approximately 4% of the plasma proteins. It is the largest of the plasma proteins. **Fibrinogen** is essential in the process of blood clotting. The process of blood clotting, or **coagulation**, is discussed in detail in another section of this chapter.

The solid components of the blood are the formed elements, or the cells and cell fragments, suspended in the **plasma**. The production of the formed elements in the blood is termed *hemopoiesis*. After birth, most of the production of blood cells occurs in the red bone marrow in specific regions of the body (skull, sternum, ribs, vertebrae, pelvis), with all types of blood cells developing from undifferentiated (unspecialized) stem cells called **hemocytoblasts**. As the blood cells develop from the hemocytoblast stage and undergo **differentiation** or become specialized in function, they mature into one of seven cell lines—with each cell line having a different purpose. These seven lines of specialized cells are grouped into three classifications: erythrocytes, leukocytes, and thrombocytes. Refer to *Figure 9-1* for a visual reference of the formed elements of the blood as the discussion continues.

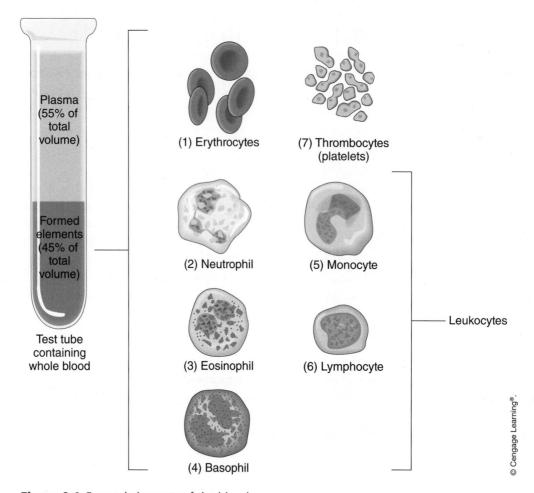

Figure 9-1 Formed elements of the blood

Erythrocytes

An (**1**) **erythrocyte** is a tiny biconcave-shaped disk that is thinner in the center than around the edges. They are also known as red blood cells (RBCs). Mature red blood cells do not have a **nucleus**. They have an average life span of approximately 120 days. The main component of the red blood cell is **hemoglobin**, which consists of **heme** (iron) and **globin** (protein). The biconcave shape of the red blood cell provides a maximum surface area for the bonding of oxygen to the **hemoglobin** to form **oxyhemoglobin**. Oxyhemoglobin is responsible for the bright red color of blood and is formed when the blood circulates through the lungs. Most of the oxygen used by the body cells is transported to the cellular level as oxyhemoglobin.

The primary function of the red blood cell is to transport oxygen to the cells of the body. Once the oxygen has been released to the cells, the biconcave shape of the red blood cell enables it to absorb carbon dioxide (a waste product of cellular metabolism). When this deoxygenated blood is returned to the lungs, the carbon dioxide is released through the process of exhalation and more oxygen is combined with the **hemoglobin** and distributed to the body cells.

The normal range of erythrocytes for a healthy adult male is 4.5 to 6 million per cubic millimeter of blood and slightly fewer for a healthy adult female (about 4.8 million per cubic millimeter of blood). The erythrocytes are the most numerous of the formed elements in the blood.

Leukocytes

Leukocytes are larger than erythrocytes but are fewer in number. They are also called white blood cells (WBCs). A mature **leukocyte** does not lose its **nucleus**, and it does not possess **hemoglobin**. Leukocytes (five types) are grouped into two categories: **granulocytes** and agranulocytes.

Granulocytes

Granulocytes consist of neutrophils, eosinophils, and basophils. They have granules in their cytoplasm that absorb various dyes (as when prepared for a slide for viewing under a microscope). The various colors, as well as the shapes of the nuclei, help identify the different white blood cells under the microscope. The (2) neutrophils constitute approximately 60% to 70% of all white blood cells. They have multilobed nuclei. Neutrophils are **phagocytic** in nature; that is, they respond to infections and tissue damage by engulfing and destroying bacteria. Neutrophils do not absorb acid or base dye very well; they remain a fairly neutral color. The (3) eosinophils constitute approximately 2% to 4% of all white blood cells. They have a **nucleus** with two lobes. Eosinophils increase in number in response to allergic reactions. Eosinophils will stain a rosy color with an acid dye. The (4) basophils constitute less than 1% of all white blood cells. They have a **nucleus** with two lobes. Basophils secrete histamine (released during allergic reactions) and **heparin**, which is a natural anticoagulant (prevents clotting). Basophils will stain a dark blue with a base dye.

Agranulocytes

Agranulocytes consist of monocytes and lymphocytes. They do not have granules in their cytoplasm and do not stain a dark color when prepared for a slide for viewing under a microscope. Agranulocytes have a large **nucleus** that is not multilobed. The (5) monocytes constitute approximately 3% to 8% of all white blood cells. They are the largest of the white blood cells and have a kidney bean–shaped **nucleus**. Monocytes are phagocytic in nature. The (6) lymphocytes constitute approximately 20% to 25% of all white blood cells. They have a large, spherical-shaped **nucleus**. Lymphocytes play an important role in the **immune** process: some lymphocytes are phagocytic in that they attack the bacteria directly, whereas other lymphocytes produce **antibodies** that destroy bacteria.

Thrombocytes

A (7) **thrombocyte** (also known as a **platelet**) is a small, disk-shaped fragment of a very large cell called **megakaryocyte**. Platelets contain no **hemoglobin**. They are essential for the normal clotting (**coagulation**) of blood. The average **platelet** count ranges from 250,000 to 500,000 platelets per cubic milliliter of blood.

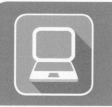

Media Link

See the components of blood in 3-D. View **The Blood** animation on the Student Companion Website.

Blood Types

When discussing blood types, it is important to understand the relationship between **antigens** and **antibodies**. An antigen, also called an **agglutinogen**, is a substance present on the red blood cell that can stimulate the body to make **antibodies**. An **antibody** is a substance present in the **plasma** that reacts in some way with the antigen that stimulated its formation. Once the **antibodies** become established, they will be programmed to recognize the antigen as "foreign to the body" in the future and will "attack it" if they come in contact with it again. In some cases, the antigen–antibody combination will result in **agglutination**, or clumping of the red blood cells. Because of this, it is critically important to match the **antigens** and **antibodies** of the blood donor and the blood recipient to prevent the possibility of **agglutination**. This is accomplished through clinical laboratory tests called blood typing and cross-matching.

The **antigens** on the red blood cells are organized into blood groups. Each person's blood belongs to one of the following four blood types: A, B, AB, or O. The letter designating the blood type indicates the type of antigen present on the red blood cell. For example, type A blood has the A antigen present on its red blood cells. This means that the particular individual was born with the A antigen present on his or her red blood cells and that this individual will not have any anti-A antibodies present in his or her **plasma** that would destroy the A antigen. The **plasma** would, however, have anti-B antibodies present that would cause **agglutination** if the individual received type B blood instead of its expected type A. A breakdown of the antigen–antibody combinations for the four ABO blood types is outlined in *Table 9-1*.

The presence or absence of a specific antigen on the red blood cell will make a difference in the type of blood that a person can receive in a transfusion. The person who gives blood is called the **donor**. The person who receives the blood is called the **recipient**. For example, type O-negative blood is considered the "universal donor blood" because it does not have A antigens or B antigens present on its red blood cells. Consequently, any anti-A or anti-B antibodies present in the recipient's **plasma** will not cause **agglutination** of the red blood cells of the donor blood. Type AB blood is considered the "universal recipient blood" because it contains no anti-A or anti-B antibodies in its **plasma** and will not clump any donor blood that contains either A or B antigens on its red blood cells. When blood is transfused from one individual to another, however, it should not be done without first **cross-matching**; that is, mixing the donor blood with the recipient blood and observing the mixture for **agglutination** of the donor's red blood cells.

Another important antigen located on the surface of the red blood cells is the **Rh factor**. This antigen is named "Rh" because it was first studied in the rhesus monkey.

Table 9-1 ABO Blood Types

Blood Type	Antigen Present on RBC	Antibody Present in Plasma
A	A	Anti-B antibody
B	B	Anti-A antibody
AB	AB	No antibodies present
O	No antigens present	Both anti-A and anti-B antibodies

Individuals who have the Rh factor present on their red blood cells are said to be **Rh positive (Rh+)**. People who do not have the Rh factor present on their red blood cells are said to be **Rh negative (Rh−)**. There are two major concerns with Rh− individuals: (1) if an Rh− individual is exposed to Rh+ blood through a transfusion, the Rh− individual will develop anti-Rh antibodies that will cause a transfusion reaction (**agglutination**) should the Rh− individual receive Rh+ blood a second time, and (2) if an Rh− mother gives birth to an Rh+ baby, and the Rh− and Rh+ bloods mix during the birth process (from ruptured vessels in the placenta), the Rh− mother's body will develop anti-Rh antibodies that will cause problems with future pregnancies. Specifically, if the Rh− mother has a subsequent pregnancy with an Rh+ baby, the anti-Rh antibodies that have been formed in her blood will recognize the Rh+ blood as foreign to her body and will pass through the placenta and react with the Rh antigens on the red blood cells of the fetus. The result will be **agglutination** and destruction of the fetal red blood cells.

To prevent the possibility of future complications from the Rh negative–Rh positive interaction, the Rh− mother is given an injection of Rh immune globulin (RhoGAM) during week 28 of pregnancy. This special preparation of anti-Rh globulin prevents the development of anti-Rh antibodies in the Rh− mother's blood.

Mechanisms of Blood Clotting

The clotting of blood is known as **coagulation**. Its purpose is to plug ruptured blood vessels to stop bleeding. There are many steps involved in the mechanism of blood clotting. These chemical reactions take place in a definite and rapid sequence, resulting in the formation of a clot that stops the bleeding. The steps involved in the process of blood clotting are as follows:

1. There must be some type of injury to a blood vessel that creates a roughened area in the vessel.

2. Some of the blood platelets disintegrate as they flow over the rough spot in the blood vessel, releasing a substance called **thromboplastin**.

3. The **thromboplastin** converts **prothrombin** (a blood protein) into the active enzyme **thrombin**. This occurs in the presence of calcium ions and other clotting factors.

4. The **thrombin** converts **fibrinogen** (another blood protein) into **fibrin**. This also occurs in the presence of calcium ions. The resulting **fibrin** threads form a mesh that adheres to the tissue of the damaged vessel to form a clot.

As mentioned, the normal mechanisms of clotting of blood are designed to stop bleeding. This occurs in response to injury to a blood vessel (as described previously). Unfortunately, clots sometimes form in uninjured blood vessels. This type of clot formation is abnormal and has the potential for stopping the flow of blood to a vital organ. The abnormal formation of clots can be life threatening. A clot that forms and stays in place in a blood vessel is known as a **thrombus**. The abnormal vascular condition in which a **thrombus** develops is called **thrombosis**. An abnormal circulatory condition in which a clot dislodges from its place and travels through the bloodstream is called an **embolism**. The dislodged, circulating clot is known as an **embolus**. In addition to a blood clot, an embolus may be a small bit of fatty tissue or air that travels through the bloodstream until it becomes lodged in a vessel.

Review Checkpoint

Check your understanding of this section by completing the **Anatomy and Physiology** exercises in your workbook.

VOCABULARY (BLOOD)

The following vocabulary words are frequently used when discussing the blood.

Word	Definition
agglutination (ah-**gloo**-tih-**NAY**-shun)	The clumping of cells as a result of interaction with specific **antibodies** called agglutinins. Agglutinins are used in blood typing and in identifying or estimating the strength of immunoglobulins or **immune** serums.
albumin (al-**BYOO**-min)	A plasma protein. Various albumins are found in practically all animal tissues and in many plant tissues. In blood, **albumin** helps maintain blood volume and blood pressure.
allergen (**AL**-er-jin)	A substance that can produce a hypersensitive reaction in the body.
allergy (**AL**-er-jee)	A hypersensitive reaction to normally harmless **antigens**, most of which are environmental.
anaphylaxis (**an**-ah-fih-**LAK**-sis)	An exaggerated, life-threatening **hypersensitivity** reaction to a previously encountered antigen.
anisocytosis (an-**ih**-soh-sigh-**TOH**-sis) aniso = unequal cyt/o = cell -osis = condition	An abnormal condition of the blood characterized by red blood cells of variable and abnormal size.
antibodies (**AN**-tih-bod-eez)	Substances produced by the body in response to bacteria, viruses, or other foreign substances. Each class of antibody is named for its action.
antigens (**AN**-tih-jenz)	A substance, usually a protein, that causes the formation of an antibody and reacts specifically with that antibody.
ascites (ah-**SIGH**-teez)	An abnormal intraperitoneal (within the peritoneal cavity) accumulation of a fluid containing large amounts of protein and electrolytes.
basophil (**BAY**-soh-fill)	A granulocytic white blood cell characterized by cytoplasmic granules that stain blue when exposed to a basic dye. Basophils represent 1% or less of the total white blood cell count.

Word	Definition
bilirubin (bill-ih-**ROO**-bin)	The orange-yellow pigment of bile formed principally by the breakdown of **hemoglobin** in red blood cells after termination of their normal life span.
candidiasis (**kan**-dih-**DYE**-ah-sis) -iasis = abnormal condition	A type of yeast infection (most often from the fungi *Candida albicans*). Affected sites may be skin, oral mucosa, respiratory tract or vagina. The characteristic symptom with candidiasis is severe itching (pruritus) and a milky-white discharge. This condition is usually treated with topical or oral antifungal agents.

carcinoma
(**kar**-sih-**NOH**-mah)
  carcin/o = cancer
  -oma = tumor
	A malignant neoplasm.

coagulation (koh-**ag**-yoo-**LAY**-shun)	The process of transforming a liquid into a solid, especially of the blood.
corpuscle (**KOR**-pus-ul)	Any cell of the body; a red or white blood cell.
cytokines (**SIGH**-toh-kyens) cyt/o = cell	A group of proteins that are produced primarily by white blood cells; they are involved in cell-to-cell communication to coordinate antibody and immune responses.

cytotoxic
(**sigh**-toh-**TOK**-sick)
  cyt/o = cell
  tox/o = poison
  -ic = pertaining to
	Pertaining to being destructive to cells.

differentiation (**diff**-er-en-she-**AY**-shun)	A process in development in which unspecialized cells or tissues are systemically modified and altered to achieve specific and characteristic physical forms, physiologic functions, and chemical properties.
dyscrasia (dis-**KRAY**-zee-ah)	An abnormal condition of the blood or bone marrow, such as **leukemia**, **aplastic anemia**, or prenatal Rh incompatibility.
edema (eh-**DEE**-ma)	The abnormal accumulation of fluid in interstitial spaces of tissues.

electrophoresis
(ee-**lek**-troh-for-**EE**-sis)
  electr/o- = electrical; electricity
  -phoresis = transmission
	The movement of charged suspended particles through a liquid medium in response to changes in an electric field. Charged particles of a given substance migrate in a predictable direction and at a characteristic speed.

embolus
(**EM**-boh-lus)
  embol/i = to throw
  -us = noun ending
	A dislodged, circulating blood clot.

Word	Definition
embolism (**EM**-boh-lizm) embol/i = to throw -ism = condition	An abnormal condition in which a blood clot (embolus) becomes lodged in a blood vessel, obstructing the flow of blood within the vessel.
enzyme (**EN**-zime)	An organic substance that initiates and accelerates a chemical reaction.
eosinophil (**ee**-oh-**SIN**-oh-fill) eosin/o = red, rosy	A granulocytic, bilobed **leukocyte** somewhat larger than a **neutrophil** characterized by large numbers of coarse, refractile, cytoplasmic granules that stain with the acid dye eosin.
erythremia (ehr-rih-**THREE**-mee-ah) erythr/o = red -emia = blood condition	An abnormal increase in the number of red blood cells.
erythroblast (eh-**RITH**-roh-blast) erythr/o = red -blast = immature cell	An immature red blood cell.
erythrocyte (eh-**RITH**-roh-sight) erythr/o = red -cyte = cell	A mature red blood cell.
erythropoiesis (eh-**rith**-roh-**poy**-**EE**-sis) erythr/o = red -poiesis = formation	The process of red blood cell production.
erythropoietin (eh-**rith**-roh-**POY**-eh-tin)	A hormone synthesized mainly in the kidneys and released into the bloodstream in response to anoxia (lack of oxygen). The hormone acts to stimulate and regulate the production of erythrocytes and is thus able to increase the oxygen-carrying capacity of the blood.
fibrin (**FYE**-brin)	A stringy, insoluble protein that is the substance of a blood clot.
fibrinogen (fye-**BRIN**-oh-jen)	A plasma protein converted into fibrin by **thrombin** in the presence of calcium ions.
globin (**GLOH**-bin)	A group of four **globulin** protein molecules that become bound by the iron in **heme** molecules to form **hemoglobin**.
globulin (**GLOB**-yoo-lin)	A plasma protein made in the liver. **Globulin** helps in the synthesis of **antibodies**.
granulocyte (**GRAN**-yoo-loh-sight) granul/o = granules -cyte = cell	A type of **leukocyte** characterized by the presence of cytoplasmic granules.

Word	Definition

hematologist
(hee-mah-**TOL**-oh-jist)
  hemat/o = blood
  -logist = one who specializes in
       the study of
	A medical specialist in the field of **hematology**.

hematology
(**hee**-mah-**TOL**-oh-jee)
  hemat/o = blood
  -logy = the study of
	The scientific study of blood and blood-forming tissues.

heme (**HEEM**)	The pigmented, iron-containing, nonprotein portion of the **hemoglobin** molecule. **Heme** binds with and carries oxygen in the red blood cells, releasing it to tissues that give off excess amounts of carbon dioxide.
hemoglobin (**hee**-moh-**GLOH**-bin)	A complex protein–iron compound in the blood that carries oxygen to the cells from the lungs and carbon dioxide away from the cells to the lungs.

hemolysis
(**hee**-**MALL**-ih-sis)
  hem/o = blood
  -lysis = destruction or
       detachment
	The breakdown of red blood cells and the release of **hemoglobin** that occurs normally at the end of the life span of a red cell.

hemorrhage
(**HEM**-eh-rij)
  hem/o = blood
  -rrhage = excessive flow or
       discharge
	A loss of a large amount of blood in a short period of time, either externally or internally. **Hemorrhage** may be arterial, venous, or capillary.

hemostasis
(**hee**-moh-**STAY**-sis)
  hem/o = blood
  -stasis = stopping or controlling
	The termination of bleeding by mechanical or chemical means or by the complex **coagulation** process of the body, consisting of vasoconstriction, **platelet** aggregation, and **thrombin** and fibrin synthesis.

heparin (**HEP**-er-in)	A naturally occurring anticlotting factor present in the body.

hyperalbuminemia
(high-per-al-**byoo**-mih-**NEE**-mee-ah)
  hyper- = excessive
  albumin/o = protein (**albumin**)
  -emia = blood condition
	An increased level of **albumin** in the blood.

hyperbilirubinemia (high-per-**bill**-ih-roo-bin-**EE**-mee-ah)	Greater than normal amounts of the bile pigment, **bilirubin**, in the blood.

Word	Definition
hyperlipemia (**high**-per-lip-**EE**-mee-ah) hyper- = excessive lip/o = fat -emia = blood condition	An excessive level of blood fats, usually caused by a lipoprotein lipase deficiency or a defect in the conversion of low-density lipoproteins to high-density lipoproteins; also called **hyperlipidemia.**
hyperlipidemia (**high**-per-lip-**id**-**EE**-mee-ah)	See *hyperlipemia.*
ion (**EYE**-on)	An electrically charged particle.
leukocyte (**LOO**-koh-sight) leuk/o = white -cyte = cell	A white blood cell, one of the formed elements of the circulating blood system.
leukocytopenia (**loo**-koh-**sigh**-toh-**PEE**-nee-ah) leuk/o = white cyt/o = cell -penia = decrease in; deficiency	An abnormal decrease in number of white blood cells to fewer than 5,000 cells per cubic millimeter.
lymphedema (**lim**-feh-**DEE**-mah) lymph/o = lymph -edema = swelling	Swelling of a part of the body due to an abnormal accumulation of tissue fluid within the interstitial spaces.
lymphoscintigraphy (**lim**-foh-sin-**TIH**-grah-fee) lymph/o = lymph scint/i = -graphy = process of recording	A special type of nuclear medicine imaging that provides pictures of the lymphatic system; used to detect metastatic tumors in lymph nodes.
megakaryocyte (**meg**-ah-**KAIR**-ee-oh-sight) mega- = large kary/o = nucleus -cyte = cell	An extremely large bone marrow cell.
metastasize (meh-**TAS**-tah-sighz) meta- = beyond, after	To spread to distant parts of the body, as in the spread of tumor cells from one site to another.
monocyte (**MON**-oh-sight) mono- = one -cyte = cell	A large mononuclear **leukocyte.**

Word	Definition
myeloid (**MY**-eh-loyd) myel/o = bone marrow, spinal cord -oid = resembling	Of or pertaining to the bone marrow or the spinal cord.
neutrophil (**NOO**-troh-fill)	A polymorphonuclear (multilobed nucleus) granular **leukocyte** that stains easily with neutral dyes.
pancytopenia (**pan**-sigh-toh-**PEE**-nee-ah) pan- = all cyt/o = cell -penia = deficiency	A marked reduction in the number of the red blood cells, white blood cells, and platelets.
pica (**PIE**-kah)	A craving to eat unusual substances (non-food substances), including but not limited to things such as clay, dirt, starch, chalk, glue, ice, and hair. This appetite disorder occurs with some nutritional deficiency states such as iron deficiency anemia. It may also occur in pregnancy.
plasma (**PLAZ**-mah)	The watery, straw-colored, fluid portion of the **lymph** and the blood in which the leukocytes, erythrocytes, and platelets are suspended.
platelet (**PLAYT**-let)	A clotting cell; a **thrombocyte**.
prothrombin (proh-**THROM**-bin)	A plasma protein precursor of **thrombin**. It is synthesized in the liver if adequate vitamin K is present.
reticulocyte (reh-**TIK**-yoo-loh-sight)	An immature **erythrocyte** characterized by a meshlike pattern of threads and particles at the former site of the **nucleus**.
sarcoma (sar-**KOH**-mah) sarc/o = flesh -oma = tumor	A malignant neoplasm of the connective and supportive tissues of the body, usually first presenting as a painless swelling.
septicemia (sep-tih-**SEE**-mee-ah)	Systemic infection in which **pathogens** are present in the circulating bloodstream, having spread from an infection in any part of the body.
seroconversion (**see**-roh-con-**VER**-zhun)	A change in serologic tests from negative to positive as **antibodies** develop in reaction to an infection or vaccine.
serology (see-**RALL**-oh-jee)	The branch of laboratory medicine that studies blood **serum** for evidence of infection by evaluating antigen–antibody reactions.
serum (**SEE**-rum)	Also called blood **serum**. The clear, thin, and sticky fluid portion of the blood that remains after **coagulation**. **Serum** contains no blood cells, platelets, or fibrinogen.

Word	Definition

splenomegaly
(**splee**-noh-**MEG**-ah-lee)
  splen/o = spleen
  -megaly = enlargement
	An abnormal enlargement of the spleen.

staphylococci
(**staf**-ih-loh-**KOCK**-sigh)
  staphyl/o = grapelike clusters
  -cocci = a group of bacteria
	A group of bacteria that grow in grapelike cluster formation; responsible for pyogenic (pus-producing) infections such as boils, carbuncles, and abscesses.

stem cell	A formative cell; a cell whose daughter cells may give rise to other cell types.

streptococci
(**strep**-toh-**KOCK**-sigh)
  strept/o = twisted chain
  -cocci = a group of bacteria
	A group of bacteria that grow in a twisted, chainlike formation. Streptococci can cause human infections such as strep throat, meningitis, endocarditis, neonatal sepsis, and necrotizing fasciitis.

teletherapy
(**tel**-eh-**THER**-ah-pee)
  tel/e- = distance
  -therapy = treatment
	Radiation therapy administered by a machine positioned at some distance from the patient.

thrombin (**THROM**-bin)	An enzyme formed from **prothrombin**, calcium, and **thromboplastin** in **plasma** during the clotting process. It causes fibrinogen to change to fibrin, which is essential in the formation of a clot.

thrombocyte
(**THROM**-boh-sight)
  thromb/o = clot
  -cyte = cell
	A clotting cell; a **platelet**.

thrombocytopenia
(**throm**-boh-**sigh**-toh-**PEE**-nee-ah)
  thromb/o = clot
  cyt/o = cell
  -penia = decrease in; deficiency
	An abnormal hematologic condition in which the number of platelets is reduced.

thromboplastin (**throm**-boh-**PLAST**-in)	A complex substance that initiates the clotting process by converting **prothrombin** into **thrombin** in the presence of calcium ion.

thrombosis
(throm-**BOH**-sis)
  thromb/o = clot
  -osis = condition
	The formation or existence of a blood clot.

thrombus
(**THROM**-bus)
  thromb/o = clot
  -us = noun ending
	A clot.

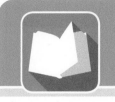

Review Checkpoint

Check your understanding of this section by completing the **Vocabulary** exercises in your workbook.

WORD ELEMENTS (BLOOD)

The following word elements pertain to the blood system. As you review the list, pronounce each word element aloud twice and check the box after you "say it." Write the definition for the example term given for each word element. Use your medical dictionary to find the definitions of the example terms.

Word Element	Pronunciation	"Say It"	Meaning
agglutin/o **agglutin**ation	ah-**GLOO**-tin-oh ah-**gloo**-tin-**NAY**-shun	☐	to clump
aniso- **aniso**cytosis	**AN**-ih-soh an-**ih**-soh-sigh-**TOH**-sis	☐	unequal
bas/o **bas**ophil	**BAY**-soh **BAY**-soh-fill	☐	base
blast/o, -blast **blast**ocyte	**BLAST**-oh, **BLAST** **BLAST**-oh-sight	☐	embryonic stage of development
carcin/o **carcin**ogen	kar-**SIH**-noh **kar**-sih-**NOH**-jen	☐	cancer
chrom/o **chrom**ophilic	**KROH**-moh kroh-moh-**FILL**-ik	☐	color
coagul/o **coagul**ation	koh-**AG**-yoo-loh koh-**ag**-yoo-**LAY**-shun	☐	clotting
-cocci staphylo**cocci**	**KOCK**-sigh **staf**-ih-loh-**KOCK**-sigh	☐	a group of bacteria
cyt/o **cyt**ogenesis	**SIGH**-toh **sigh**-toh-**JEN**-ess-is	☐	cell
-emia polycyth**emia**	**EE**-mee-ah **pol**-ee-sigh-**THEE**-mee-ah	☐	blood condition
eosin/o **eosin**ophilia	ee-oh-**SIN**-oh **ee**-oh-sin-oh-**FILL**-ee-ah	☐	red, rosy
erythr/o **erythr**ocytopenia	eh-**RITH**-roh eh-**rith**-roh-**sigh**-toh-**PEE**-nee-ah	☐	red

Word Element	Pronunciation	"Say It"	Meaning
-globin hemo**globin**	**GLOH**-bin **hee**-moh-**GLOH**-bin	☐	containing protein
hem/o **hem**ogram	**HEE**-moh **HEE**-moh-gram	☐	blood
hemat/o **hemat**ologist	hee-**MAH**-toh hee-mah-**TOL**-oh-jist	☐	blood
is/o **is**otonic	**EYE**-soh **eye**-soh-**TON**-ik	☐	equal
kary/o **kary**ocyte	**KAIR**-ee-oh **KAIR**-ee-oh-sight	☐	**nucleus**
leuk/o **leuk**ocyte	**LOO**-koh **LOO**-koh-sight	☐	white
-lytic hemo**lytic**	**LIT**-ik **hee**-moh-**LIT**-ik	☐	destruction
mono- **mono**cytopenia	**MON**-oh **mon**-oh-**sigh**-toh-**PEE**-nee-ah	☐	one
morph/o **morph**ology	**MOR**-foh mor-**FOL**-oh-jee	☐	form, shape
myel/o **myel**oblast	**MY**-ell-oh **MY**-ell-oh-blast	☐	bone marrow or spinal cord
nucle/o **nucle**us	**NOO**-klee-oh **NOO**-klee-us	☐	**nucleus**
-oid spher**oid**	**OYD** **SFEE**-royd	☐	resembling
-oma lymph**oma**	**OH**-mah lim-**FOH**-mah	☐	tumor
-osis erythrocy**tosis**	**OH**-sis eh-**rith**-roh-sigh-**TOH**-sis	☐	condition
-penia pancyto**penia**	**PEE**-nee-ah **pan**-sigh-toh-**PEE**-nee-ah	☐	decrease in; deficiency
-phage macro**phage**	**FAYJ** **MAK**-roh-fayj	☐	to eat
phag/o **phag**ocyte	**FAG**-oh **FAG**-oh-sight	☐	to eat
-philia hemo**philia**	**FILL**-ee-ah **hee**-moh-**FILL**-ee-ah	☐	attraction to

Word Element	Pronunciation	"Say It"	Meaning
-phoresis electro**phoresis**	for-**EE**-sis ee-**lek**-troh-for-**EE**-sis	☐	transmission
-poiesis erythro**poiesis**	poy-**EE**-sis eh-**rith**-roh-poy-**EE**-sis	☐	formation
poikil/o **poikil**ocytosis	**POY**-kill-oh **poy**-kill-oh-sigh-**TOH**-sis	☐	varied; irregular
sider/o **sider**oblast	**SID**-er-oh **SID**-er-oh-**blast**	☐	iron
spher/o **spher**ocytosis	**SFEE**-roh **sfee**-roh-sigh-**TOH**-sis	☐	round; sphere
staphyl/o **staphyl**ococcal	**STAF**-ee-loh staf-ee-loh-**KOCK**-al	☐	grapelike clusters
-stasis hemo**stasis**	**STAY**-sis **hee**-moh-**STAY**-sis	☐	stopping or controlling
strept/o **strept**ococcal	**STREP**-toh strep-toh-**KOCK**-al	☐	twisted chains
tel/e **tel**etherapy	**TEL**-ee **tel**-eh-**THER**-ah-pee	☐	distance
-therapy immuno**therapy**	**THER**-ah-pee im-yoo-noh-**THER**-ah-pee	☐	treatment
thromb/o **thromb**osis	**THROM**-boh throm-**BOH**-sis	☐	clot
tox/o cyto**tox**ic	**TOK**-soh **sigh**-toh-**TOK**-sick	☐	poison

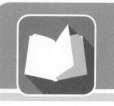

Review Checkpoint

Check your understanding of this section by completing the **Word Elements** exercises in your workbook.

Pathological Conditions (Blood)

As you study the pathological conditions of the blood, note that the **basic definition** is in a green shaded box, followed by a detailed description in regular print. The phonetic pronunciation is directly beneath each term, as well as a breakdown of the component parts of the term where applicable.

anemia
 	
(an-**NEE**-mee-ah)
 	
   an- = without
   -emia = blood condition
	Anemia describes a condition in which there is a decrease in **hemoglobin** in the blood to levels below the normal range, resulting in a deficiency of oxygen being delivered to the cells.

	There are various classifications of anemias. Each is named according to the cause. The following are some clinical manifestations common to all types of **anemia**: fatigue, paleness of the skin, headache, fainting, tingling sensations and numbness, loss of appetite, swelling in the lower extremities, and difficulty breathing.

anemia, aplastic
 	
(ah-**NEE**-mee-ah, ay-**PLAS**-tik)
 	
   an- = without
   -emia = blood condition
   a- = without
   plast/o = formation, development
   -ic = pertaining to
	Also called bone marrow depression anemia, **aplastic anemia** is characterized by **pancytopenia**—an inadequacy of the formed blood elements (RBCs, WBCs, and platelets).

	The lack of formation of the blood elements is believed to be due to an insult to the bone marrow's **stem cells**. The cause of **aplastic anemia** is not known in at least two-thirds of cases. It may develop simultaneously with infections or following an injury to the bone marrow. **Aplastic anemia** may occur because of a neoplastic disorder of the bone marrow, chemotherapy drugs, certain antibiotics (chloramphenicol) and other medications, or exposure to radiation or certain toxic chemicals.
	The person with **aplastic anemia** will be treated with blood transfusions until his or her bone marrow is capable of forming new cells. In some persons, the preferred treatment is a **bone marrow transplant** from a close tissue match (usually an identical twin or sibling).

anemia, hemolytic
 	
(an-**NEE**-mee-ah, **hee**-moh-**LIT**-ik)
 	
   an- = without
   -emia = blood condition
   hem/o = blood
   -lytic = destruction
	Hemolytic anemia is characterized by the extreme reduction in circulating RBCs due to their destruction.

	The destruction of the RBCs may occur because of intrinsic or extrinsic causes. Cell membrane weaknesses and structural defects in the **hemoglobin** are examples of intrinsic causes. Extrinsic examples include infections, drugs, toxins, chemicals, trauma, and artificial heart valves.

anemia, iron deficiency
 	
(an-**NEE**-mee-ah, **EYE**-urn
dee-FIH-shen-see)
 	
   an- = without
   -emia = blood condition
	Iron deficiency anemia is characterized by deficiency of **hemoglobin** level due to a lack of iron in the body. There is a greater demand on the stored iron than can be supplied by the body.

	In addition to the general symptoms associated with **anemia**, individuals with chronic iron deficiency anemia may suffer from brittle spoon-shaped nails, cracks at the corners of the mouth (cheilosis), a sore tongue, and a craving for unusual substances (such as clay or starch). This craving for unusual substances is known as **pica**.
	Iron deficiency anemia is the most common type of **anemia**. It may be due to loss of iron or to inadequate intake or absorption of iron in the digestive system. Chronic blood loss can lead to this type of **anemia** and may occur as the result of loss of blood due to chronic bleeding (e.g., gastrointestinal bleeding, heavy menstrual periods). It is particularly common in older adults. Treatment is aimed at the underlying cause and may include increasing foods high in iron content and oral iron supplements.

anemia, pernicious

(an-**NEE**-mee-ah, per-**NISH**-us)

an- = without

-emia = blood condition

Pernicious anemia results from a deficiency of mature RBCs and the formation and circulation of megaloblasts (large, nucleated, immature, poorly functioning RBCs) with marked **poikilocytosis** (RBC shape variation) and **anisocytosis** (RBC size variation)

The formation of these distorted RBCs is due to a lack of vitamin B_{12} absorption necessary for proper maturation of the RBCs. Vitamin B_{12} chemically binds with the intrinsic factor (a protein secreted by the stomach), which protects the vitamin B_{12} until it is absorbed in the ileum. A shortage or absence of the intrinsic factor (normally found in gastric acids) results in an inadequate amount of vitamin B_{12}, **erythroblast** destruction, and ineffective **erythropoiesis**. There may also be a mild reduction in the production of mature WBCs and platelets.

Pernicious anemia typically occurs in persons over 60 years of age and is believed to be related to an autoimmune response. Along with loss of appetite, fatigue, irritability, and shortness of breath, the person experiencing **pernicious anemia** may also complain of a sore tongue. The destruction of the erythroblasts may result in elevated **bilirubin** levels in the blood and a jaundiced (yellowish) appearance to the skin. Treatment is lifelong vitamin B_{12} administration.

anemia, sickle cell

(an-**NEE**-mee-ah, **SIK**-ul **SELL**)

an- = without, not

-emia = blood condition

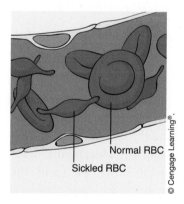

© Cengage Learning®.

Normal RBC

Sickled RBC

Figure 9-2 Regular and Sickled RBCs

Sickle cell anemia is a chronic hereditary form of **hemolytic** anemia in which the RBCs become shaped like a crescent in the presence of low oxygen concentration. See *Figure 9-2*.

These elongated, crescent-shaped RBCs clump, forming thromboses (clots), which occlude small blood vessels and cause areas of infarction (loss of oxygen), creating a great deal of pain for the individual. The pain is usually located in the hands, feet, and abdominal cavity. As oxygen concentration is reestablished, the crescent-shaped cells begin to resume their unsickled shape. It is the frequency of the changes in shape that renders the RBCs weakened, which then leads to **hemolysis**.

This disorder is inherited by the presence of one gene (sickle cell trait) or two genes (sickle cell disease), most typically among persons of African descent. Complications of **sickle cell anemia** include heart murmurs, congestive heart failure, enlarged liver, jaundice, gallstones, reduced urine concentration, hematuria, osteomyelitis, lower extremity ulcers, and problems with the eyes.

granulocytosis

(**gran**-yoo-loh-sigh-**TOH**-sis)

granul/o = granules

cyt/o = cell

-osis = condition

Granulocytosis is an abnormally elevated number of **granulocytes** in the circulating blood as a reaction to any variety of inflammation or infection.

In particular allergic conditions such as parasitic infections or asthma, there is a spiraling of eosinophilic granulocytes called **eosinophilia**. In particular types of **leukemia**, the number of basophilic granulocytes are increased, a condition called basophilia.

hemochromatosis	Hemochromatosis is a rare iron metabolism disease characterized by iron deposits throughout the body, usually as a complication of one of the **hemolytic** anemias.
(**hee**-moh-**kroh**-mah-**TOH**-sis)	
hem/o = blood	Typically seen in men over 40, the person with **hemochromatosis** has an enlarged liver and a bronze skin pigmentation. Congestive heart failure or diabetes mellitus are frequent secondary complications of **hemochromatosis**. Treatment is multiple blood transfusions.
chromat/o = color	
-osis = condition	

hemophilia	Hemophilia involves different hereditary inadequacies of **coagulation** factors resulting in prolonged bleeding times.
(**hee**-moh-**FILL**-ee-ah)	
hem/o = blood	**Hemophilia A**, also called classic hemophilia, is the most common type (accounts for approximately 83%) and is the result of a deficiency or absence of antihemophilic factor VIII. This factor VIII deficiency results in traumatic or spontaneous bleeding. Nearly all cases are reported in males and are characterized by bleeding in the joints, gums, or mouth. Hematuria is a common characteristic. Repeated joint bleeding produces extreme pain and deformity. The bleeding tendency can be relieved by transfusing factor VIII or fresh **plasma**.
phil/o = attraction to	
-ia = condition	
	Hemophilia B, also called Christmas disease, is the deficiency of a **coagulation** factor called factor IX and accounts for approximately 10% to 15% of the cases of hemophilia. Hemophilia B is only distinguishable from hemophilia A through laboratory **differentiation** of factor deficiencies. Other less common forms of **hemophilia** are Von Willebrand's disease and Rosenthal's disease.

leukemia (ALL, AML, CML)	Leukemia is an excessive uncontrolled increase of immature WBCs in the blood eventually leading to infection, anemia, and **thrombocytopenia** (decreased number of platelets).
(loo-**KEE**-mee-ah)	
leuk/o = white	The course of **leukemia** is subclassified as acute or chronic. Acute leukemia has a rapid onset and swiftly progresses to severe **thrombocytopenia**, progressive anemia, infective lesions in the throat and mouth, high fever, and severe infection. Affecting adults and the elderly, the onset of chronic leukemia is gradual and its progression slower than with the acute form. **Leukemia** is classified further according to tissue type and cell involvement.
-emia = blood condition	

- **Acute myelogenous leukemia (AML)** is predominated by immature **granulocytes**.
- **Acute lymphocytic leukemia (ALL)** is predominated by immature lymphocytes and develops most frequently in children and adolescents.
- **Chronic myelogenous leukemia (CML)** has immature and mature **granulocytes** existing in the bloodstream and bone marrow.
- **Chronic lymphocytic leukemia (CLL)** is predominated by exceptional amounts of lymphocytes found in the spleen, bone marrow, and lymph nodes that are abnormal, small, and mature.

The symptoms of all types of **leukemia** are similar and occur because the bone marrow produces large numbers of nonfunctioning leukocytes and decreased production of platelets and RBCs. Symptoms characteristic of nonfunctioning leukocytes include nail and skin infections, fever, throat and mouth ulcers, pneumonia, cystitis, and **septicemia**.

Symptoms characteristic of decreased RBCs (**anemia**) include fatigue, lethargy, pallor, rapid pulse, and difficulty breathing. Symptoms characteristic of decreased platelets include petechiae (pinpoint hemorrhages), epistaxis, hematuria, bruising, hematomas, and scleral or retinal hemorrhage.

Along with the CBC results and a thorough history, a bone marrow aspiration is completed to confirm the diagnosis of **leukemia**. Treatment for all forms of **leukemia** focuses on the relief of symptoms and the achievement of remission through the use of radiation therapy, chemotherapy, and bone marrow transplantation.

multiple myeloma **(plasma cell myeloma)** (**MULL**-tih-pul my-eh-**LOH**-mah) myel/o = bone marrow, spinal cord -oma = tumor	A malignant plasma cell neoplasm, **multiple myeloma** causes an increase in the number of both mature and immature plasma cells, which often entirely replace the bone marrow and destroy the skeletal structure.

The bones grow so fragile that the slightest movement can result in a fracture. An abnormal protein, called the Bence Jones protein, is found almost exclusively in the urine of individuals with **multiple myeloma**. Other characteristics include increased susceptibility to infections, **anemia**, hypercalcemia, and renal damage. The survival statistics for **multiple myeloma** are poor and depend strongly on the individual's response to chemotherapy.

polycythemia vera (**pol**-ee-sigh-**THEE**-mee-ah **VAIR**-ah) poly- = many, much, excessive -cythemia = condition involving cells of the blood	**Polycythemia vera** is an abnormal increase in the number of RBCs, **granulocytes**, and thrombocytes, leading to an increase in blood volume and viscosity (thickness).

The exact cause of **polycythemia vera** is unknown. The increased viscosity of the blood results in congestion of the spleen and liver with RBCs as well as stasis and **thrombosis** in other areas.

The clinical manifestations of **polycythemia vera** include light-headedness, headaches, visual disturbances, vertigo, ruddy cyanosis of the face, and eventual congestive failure due to the increased work load on the heart. Treatment includes removal of blood through a phlebotomy (to decrease the blood volume) and administration of myelotoxic drugs to suppress the bone marrow's production of cells.

purpura (**PURR**-pew-rah) purpur/o = purple -a = noun ending	**Purpura** is a collection of blood beneath the skin in the form of pinpoint hemorrhages appearing as red-purple skin discolorations.

These small hemorrhages are caused from a decreased number of circulating platelets (**thrombocytopenia**). The body may produce an antiplatelet factor that will damage its own platelets.

Idiopathic thrombocytopenic purpura is a disorder in which **antibodies** are made by the individual that destroys his or her own platelets. The cause of the prolonged **bleeding time** is unknown. Corticosteroids are administered, and many times the individuals require the removal of the spleen to stop **platelet** destruction. **Purpura** is also seen in persons with low **platelet** counts for other associated reasons such as drug reactions and **leukemia**.

thalassemia	**Thalassemia** is a hereditary form of **hemolytic** anemia in which the alpha or beta hemoglobin chains are defective and the production of **hemoglobin** is deficient, creating hypochromic microcytic RBCs.
(thal-ah-**SEE**-mee-ah)	

This form of **anemia** is most frequently seen in persons of Mediterranean descent. In the severe form of **thalassemia**, blood transfusions are necessary to sustain life. As a result of these frequent transfusions, there is an accumulation of iron in the liver, heart, and pancreas, which eventually leads to failure of these organs.

Review Checkpoint

Check your understanding of this section by completing the **Pathological Conditions** exercises in your workbook.

Diagnostic Techniques, Treatments, and Procedures (Blood)

direct antiglobulin test	The **direct antiglobulin** (blood) **test** is used to discover the presence of antierythrocyte antibodies present in the blood of an Rh-negative woman. The production of these **antibodies** is associated with an Rh incompatibility between a pregnant Rh-negative woman and her Rh-positive fetus.
(Coomb's test)	
(dih-**RECT** an-tih-**GLOB**-yew-lin **TEST**)	

If these **antibodies** are present in the Rh-negative woman's blood, it indicates that her red blood cells (which lack the Rh antigen) will be stimulated to produce the antierythrocyte antibodies if they come in contact with Rh-positive blood (which could happen if any of the blood from the fetus should pass through the umbilical cord into maternal circulation during the pregnancy). If this interaction occurs between the Rh-positive and Rh-negative blood, the maternal **antibodies** can cause severe **hemolysis** of the fetal blood (resulting in high levels of **bilirubin** by the time of birth). A Coomb's test can also be performed on an individual who has suffered from a **blood transfusion** reaction to determine the causative factor.

bleeding time	Measurement of the time required for bleeding to stop.

The normal bleeding time, according to one of the more common methods to evaluate bleeding time (the Ivy method), is 1 to 9 minutes. Prolonged times may be seen in the following situations: decreased number of platelets, overactivity of the spleen, **leukemia**, bone marrow failure, and bone marrow infiltration with primary or metastatic tumor.

blood transfusion (blood trans-**FEW**-zhun)	An administration of blood or a blood component to an individual to replace blood lost through surgery, trauma, or disease.

It is critical that **antibodies** to the donor's RBCs are not present in the recipient and **antibodies** to the recipient's RBCs are not present in the donor. A **hypersensitivity** reaction (mild fever to severe **hemolysis**) will occur if either of these situations is present. These types of reactions are kept to a minimum by typing for major Rh and ABO antigens.

In addition to typing, the blood is cross-matched to distinguish mismatches caused by minor **antigens**. The process of cross-matching includes the mixing of the donor's RBCs and the recipient's **serum** in saline solution and performing the indirect Coomb's test by adding Coomb's **serum**. When a person receives blood or a blood component that has been previously collected from that person through a reinfusion, it is called an **autologous transfusion**.

bone marrow biopsy (bone marrow **BY**-op-see)	The microscopic exam of bone marrow tissue, which fully evaluates hematopoiesis by revealing the number, shape, and size of the RBCs and WBCs and platelet precursors.

The bone marrow samples are obtained through aspiration or surgical removal. The **bone marrow biopsy** procedure is a valuable tool in assessing and diagnosing abnormal blood conditions such as leukemias, anemias, and conditions involving elevated and/or decreased platelet counts.

bone marrow transplant	After receiving an intravenous infusion of aggressive chemotherapy or total-body irradiation to destroy all malignant cells and to inactivate the **immune** system, a donor's bone marrow cells are infused intravenously into the recipient.

There must be a close match of the donor's tissue and blood cells to that of the recipient. The desired effect is for the infused marrow to repopulate the marrow space of the recipient with normal cells. This procedure is performed on persons with **leukemia**, myeloma, lymphomas, and **aplastic anemia**.

Complications of a bone marrow transplant include serious infections, potential for rejection of the donor's cells by the recipient's cells (graft versus host), and relapse of the original disease. Transplant recipients are placed on immunosuppressant medications to lessen the possibility of bone marrow transplant rejection.

complete blood cell count (CBC)	A series of tests performed on peripheral blood, which inexpensively screens for problems in the hematologic system as well as in several other organ systems.

Included in the CBC are:

1. **RBC count** (measures the number of RBCs per cubic millimeter of blood)
2. **Hemoglobin** (measures the number of grams of **hemoglobin** per 100 mL of blood)
3. **Hematocrit** (measures the percent volume of the RBCs in whole blood)
4. **RBC indices** (measures **erythrocyte** size and **hemoglobin** content)
5. **WBC count** (measures the number of white blood cells in a cubic millimeter of blood)
6. **WBC differential** (determines the proportion of each of the five types of white blood cells in a sample of 100 WBCs)
7. **Blood smear** (an examination of the peripheral blood to determine variations and abnormalities in RBCs, WBCs, and platelets)
8. **Platelet count** (measures the number of platelets in a cubic millimeter of blood)

erythrocyte sedimentation rate (ESR)
 	
(eh-**RITH**-roh-sight sed-ih-men-**TAY**-shun **RATE**)
  erythr/o = red
  -cyte = cell
	Erythrocyte sedimentation rate (ESR) is a test performed on the blood, which measures the rate at which red blood cells settle out in a tube of unclotted blood. The ESR is determined by measuring the settling distance of RBCs in normal saline over one hour.

The protein content of **plasma** is increased in the presence of inflammation. Therefore, the RBCs tend to clump on top of one another, raising their weight and thus increasing the ESR. The ESR will be increased in the following conditions: pneumonia, acute myocardial infarction (heart attack), severe anemia, and cancer. The ESR will be decreased in congestive heart failure, **sickle cell anemia**, **polycythemia vera**, and angina pectoris.

hematocrit (hee-**MAT**-oh-krit) hemat/o = blood	An assessment of RBC percentage in the total blood volume.

Typically, the **hematocrit** point percentage is roughly three times the **hemoglobin** when the RBCs contain average quantities of **hemoglobin** and are standard size. Certain factors may interfere with the **hematocrit** values, such as hemodilution or dehydration, abnormal RBC size, excessive WBC count, pregnancy, high altitudes, and certain drugs.

Increased levels are seen in congenital heart disease, dehydration, **polycythemia vera**, burns, shock, surgery, trauma, and severe diarrhea. Decreased levels are seen with **anemia**, **leukemia**, **hemorrhage**, hemolytic anemia, dietary deficiency, bone marrow failure, malnutrition, **multiple myeloma**, and organ failure.

hemoglobin test (hee-moh-**GLOH**-bin **TEST**) hem/o = blood -globin = containing protein	Concentration measurement of the **hemoglobin** in the peripheral blood. As a vehicle for transport of oxygen and carbon dioxide, **hemoglobin** levels provide information about the body's ability to supply tissues with oxygen.
	There are increased levels of **hemoglobin** in congenital heart disease, **polycythemia vera**, chronic obstructive pulmonary disease (COPD), congestive heart failure, dehydration, and severe burns. Decreased levels of **hemoglobin** are noted in **anemia**, **hemolysis**, **sickle cell anemia**, enlargement of the spleen (**splenomegaly**), cancer, severe **hemorrhage**, and nutritional deficiency.
lipid profile (**LIP**-id) lip/o = fat	A **lipid profile** measures the lipids in the blood.
	The standard concentration of total lipids in the blood is 400 to 800 mg/dL; triglycerides, 40 to 150 mg/dL; cholesterol, less than 200 mg/dL is desirable; phospholipids, 150 to 380 mg/dL; fatty acids, 9 to 15 mmol/L. Lipids that are insoluble in water are found in foods and stored in the body, where their reserve serves as a concentrated source of energy. High levels of cholesterol and triglycerides are identified with an increased risk for atherosclerosis.
partial thromboplastin time (PTT) (throm-boh-**PLAST**-tin)	A blood test used to evaluate the common pathway and system of clot formation within the body.
	The **PTT** assesses various blood clotting factors such as **fibrinogen** (factor I), **prothrombin** (factor II), and factors V, VIII, IX, X, XI, and XII. The PTT is prolonged if there is an insufficient quantity of any of these factors. **Heparin** will prolong the PTT by inactivating factor II and interfering with the formation of **thromboplastin**. The PTT is used to monitor the effectiveness of **heparin** therapy. Normal PTT is 60 to 70 seconds. The critical value is greater than 100 seconds.
	Increased PTT levels may be the result of vitamin K deficiency, **leukemia**, **heparin** administration, cirrhosis, disseminated intravascular coagulation, or clotting factor deficiencies. Decreased PTT levels are usually the result of disseminated intravascular coagulation in the early stages of extensive cancer.
platelet count (**PLAYT**-let **COUNT**)	The count of platelets per cubic millimeter of blood.
	Counts of 150,000 to 400,000/mm^3 are deemed normal. **Thrombocytopenia** is indicated at counts less than 100,000/mm^3. Counts greater than 400,000/mm^3 indicate thrombocytosis. This increase in the number of platelets (thrombocytosis) may cause organ tissue death due to loss of blood supply, and spontaneous **hemorrhage** can occur with **thrombocytopenia** (decreased number of platelets).
	Thrombocytopenia may occur due to **leukemia**, liver disease, kidney disease, **pernicious anemia**, hemolytic anemia, cancer chemotherapy, and **hemorrhage**. Thrombocytosis typically occurs with malignant disorders, **polycythemia vera**, **leukemia**, cirrhosis, and trauma.

prothrombin time (PT) (proh-**THROM**-bin)	Prothrombin time (PT) is a blood test used to evaluate the common pathway and extrinsic system of clot formation.
	The PT assesses the clotting proficiency of factors I and II (**fibrinogen** and **prothrombin**), and factors V, VII, and X. If there is an insufficient quantity of any of these factors, the PT is prolonged. Anticoagulants (e.g., coumadin) will prolong the PT. The PT is used to monitor the effectiveness of coumadin therapy. Normal PT is 10 to 13.4 seconds. A client with a PT greater than 30 is at high risk for **hemorrhage**.
red blood cell count (RBC)	The measurement of the circulating number of RBCs in 1 mm³ of peripheral blood.
	The standard time a functioning RBC remains in the peripheral blood is an average of 120 days, during which time the RBCs enable oxygen and carbon dioxide to be transported and exchanged. The spleen extracts the hemolyzed RBCs as well as abnormal RBCs from the circulation. Intravascular trauma to the RBCs caused from atherosclerotic plaques and artificial heart valves will shorten the life span of the RBC. **Anemia** is present with a 10% decrease in value of the RBCs. The standard concentration of RBCs in whole blood of females is 4.2 to 5.5 million/cubic millimeter and in males is 4.6 to 6.2 million/cubic millimeter.
	Increased levels of RBCs are seen in persons experiencing dehydration/hemoconcentration, **polycythemia vera**, high altitudes, pulmonary fibrosis, and congenital heart disease. Decreased levels are found in persons with overhydration/hemodilution, **anemia**, advanced cancer, antineoplastic chemotherapy, organ failure, dietary deficiency, **hemorrhage**, and bone marrow fibrosis.
red blood cell morphology (mor-**FOL**-oh-jee)	**Red blood cell morphology** is an examination of the RBC on a stained blood smear that enables the examiner to identify the form and shape of the RBCs.
	RBCs that are hypochromic (have a reduced **hemoglobin** content) can be seen as well as the identification of RBCs that are sickled, abnormally shaped, and have an abnormal size. **Poikilocytosis** (irregular-shaped red blood cells) and **anisocytosis** (inequality of red blood cell size) can also be distinguished.
reticulocyte count (reh-**TIK**-yoo-loh-sight)	**Reticulocyte count** is a measurement of the number of circulating reticulocytes, immature erythrocytes, in a blood specimen.
	Reticulocyte count is a direct indication of the bone marrow's production of RBCs. Increased levels may be caused by hemolytic anemia, leukemias, **sickle cell anemia**, pregnancy, or three to four days post-hemorrhage. A decreased level of reticulocytes is seen in persons with **pernicious anemia**, **aplastic anemia**, cirrhosis of the liver, folic acid deficiency, bone marrow failure, and chronic infection as well as in those who have received radiation therapy.
rouleaux (roo-**LOH**)	**Rouleaux** is an aggregation of RBCs viewed through the microscope that may be an artifact or may occur with persons with **multiple myeloma** as a result of abnormal proteins.

Schilling test	A diagnostic analysis for **pernicious anemia.**
	Orally administered radioactive cobalt is tagged with vitamin B_{12} and the gastrointestinal absorption is evaluated by the radioactivity of the urine samples collected over a 24-hour period. The standard level of radioactive B_{12} within 24 hours is 8% to 40%. In the person with **pernicious anemia,** the percentage of radioactive B_{12} will be decreased as a result of the inability to absorb vitamin B_{12}.

white blood cell (WBC) count	The measurement of the circulating number of WBCs in 1 cubic millimeter of peripheral blood.
	An elevated WBC count (leukocytosis) typically indicates inflammation, infection, leukemic neoplasia, or tissue necrosis. Physical or emotional stress or trauma may increase the total WBC count. A reduction in the WBC count (leukopenia) results from bone marrow failure, which may occur following chemotherapy or radiation therapy, with an overwhelming infection, autoimmune diseases, drug toxicity, or dietary deficiencies.

white blood cell differential (**diff**-er-**EN**-shal)	The **white blood cell differential** is a measurement of the percentage of each specific type of circulating WBCs present in 1 cubic millimeter of peripheral blood drawn for the WBC count.
	The specific types measured are neutrophils, lymphocytes, monocytes, eosinophils, and basophils. Lymphocytes and neutrophils comprise 75% to 90% of the total WBCs.
	The standard time a functioning **neutrophil** remains in the peripheral blood is an average of six hours, during which time it is responsible for digesting and killing bacterial microorganisms. The standard percentage of segmented neutrophils is 50% to 70%. Trauma and acute bacterial infections prompt **neutrophil** production, which results in an elevated WBC count and sometimes a life span of two hours or less. Immature forms of neutrophils enter the circulation early as a result of the increased production and are called "stab" cells or "band" cells (the standard percentage is only 0% to 5%). This process indicates an ongoing acute bacterial infection, also called a "shift to the left."
	The life span of the lymphocytes varies immensely from a few days, months, or years. The lymphocytes are responsible for fighting acute viral infections and chronic bacterial infections. The differential count combines the number of the **T cells** and the B cells and the normal count is 20% to 40%. The **T cells** are dedicated to cellular-type **immune** responses and the B cells are committed to antibody production or taking part in cellular **immunity.**
	Monocytes have a standard life span in the circulation of about 36 hours. These phagocytic cells are capable of fighting bacteria similarly to neutrophils but are manufactured more rapidly and occupy more time in the circulation. The normal percentage of monocytes is 1% to 6%. The standard percentage of eosinophils is 1% to 4%, and of basophils is 0% to 1%. Both of these types of WBCs are involved in the allergic response or parasitic infestations

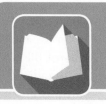

Review Checkpoint

Check your understanding of this section by completing the **Diagnostic Techniques, Treatments, and Procedures** exercises in your workbook.

COMMON ABBREVIATIONS (BLOOD)

Abbreviation	Meaning	Abbreviation	Meaning
Ab	antibody	HDL	high-density lipoprotein
Ag	antigen	Hgb	hemoglobin (also Hbg)
ABO	blood groups: A, AB, B, and O	IgA, IgD, IgE, IgG, IgM	immunoglobulin A, D, E, G, and M, respectively
AHF	antihemophilic factor (blood coagulation factor VIII)	LDL	low-density lipoprotein
AHG	antihemolytic globulin	lymph	lymphocyte
ALL	acute lymphatic leukemia	MCH	mean cell hemoglobin
AML	acute myelogenous leukemia	MCHC	mean cell hemoglobin concentration
BMT	bone marrow transplantation	MCV	mean cell volume
CBC	complete blood (cell) count	mono.	monocyte
CLL	cholesterol-lowering lipid chronic lymphocytic leukemia	poly.	polymorphonuclear leukocyte
diff. diag.	differential diagnosis	PMN	polymorphonuclear neutrophil (leukocytes)
eos.	eosinophil	PA	pernicious anemia
ESR	erythrocyte sedimentation rate	PT	prothrombin time
G-CSF	granulocyte colony-stimulating factor	PTT	partial thromboplastin time
GM-CSF	granulocyte-macrophage colony-stimulating factor	RBC	red blood cell (erythrocyte)
		segs	segmented neutrophils
Hb	hemoglobin	VLDL	very-low-density lipoprotein
Hbg	hemoglobin (also Hgb)	WBC	white blood cell (leukocyte)
Hct	hematocrit		

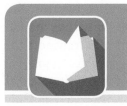

Review Checkpoint

Check your understanding of this section by completing the **Common Abbreviations** exercises in your workbook.

Overview of the Lymphatic System

The lymphatic system is often considered a part of the circulatory system because it consists of a moving fluid—**lymph**—which comes from the blood and returns to the blood by way of vessels (the lymphatic vessels). The lymphatic system consists of **lymph fluid** (which stems from the blood and tissue fluid), **lymph vessels** (which are similar to blood vessels and are designed to return the tissue fluid to the bloodstream), **lymph nodes** (which are located along the path of the collecting vessels), and specialized lymphatic organs such as the **thymus**, **spleen**, and the **tonsils**. The lymph vessels differ from the vessels of the cardiovascular system in that they do not form a closed circuit as do the vessels of the cardiovascular system. Instead, they originate in the intercellular spaces of the soft tissues of the body.

The two most important functions of the lymphatic system are (1) to produce **antibodies** and lymphocytes that are important to **immunity** and (2) to maintain a balance of fluid in the internal environment. The lymphatic system is an important part of the **immune system**, which protects the body against disease-producing organisms and other foreign bodies. The **immune** system includes the bone marrow, thymus, lymphoid tissues, lymph nodes, spleen, and lymphatic vessels.

The state of being resistant to or protected from a disease is known as **immunity**. The individual is said to be **immune**. The process of creating **immunity** to a specific disease in an individual is known as **immunization**. The study of the reaction of tissues of the **immune** system of the body to antigenic stimulation is **immunology**. The health specialist whose training and experience is concentrated in **immunology** is an **immunologist**.

Anatomy and Physiology (Lymphatic)

The anatomy and physiology section on the lymphatic system includes a discussion of the lymph vessels, lymph nodes, thymus, spleen, and **tonsils**.

Lymph Vessels

The smallest lymphatic vessels are the **lymphatic capillaries**. The capillaries originate in the tissue spaces as blind-ended sacs. Water and solutes continually filter out of capillary blood into the interstitial spaces. As interstitial fluid begins to accumulate, it is picked up by the lymphatic capillaries and is eventually returned to the blood. Once the interstitial fluid enters the lymphatic vessels, it is known as **lymph**.

It is critical that the interstitial fluid be returned to the general circulation and not remain in the tissue spaces, because the accumulation of fluid within the tissue spaces would cause swelling (**edema**). The lymphatic capillaries transport the **lymph** into larger vessels known as **lymphatic vessels**, which have valves to prevent the backward flow of fluid. The lymphatic vessels, like the veins of the cardiovascular system, have valves. However, unlike the cardiovascular system veins, the lymphatic vessels transport fluid in only one direction, which is away from the tissues, toward the thoracic cavity.

The lymphatic vessels continue to merge to form larger vessels, eventually entering the two **lymphatic ducts**: the right lymphatic duct and the thoracic duct. See *Figure 9-3*.

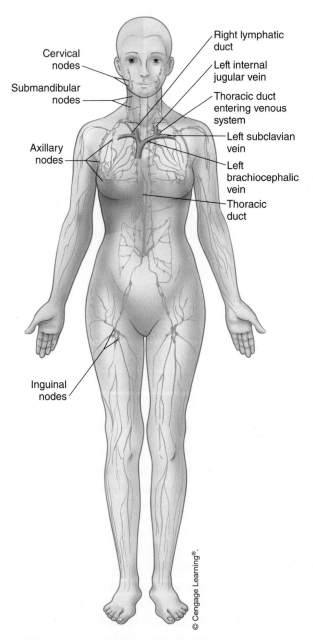

Cervical nodes

Submandibular nodes

Axillary nodes

Inguinal nodes

Right lymphatic duct

Left internal jugular vein

Thoracic duct entering venous system

Left subclavian vein

Left brachiocephalic vein

Thoracic duct

© Cengage Learning®.

Figure 9-3 Lymphatic ducts and nodes

These two ducts are the only points of entry of the **lymph** into the blood vessels of the body. **Lymph** drainage from the right side of the head and neck, the right upper extremity, and the right side of the chest flows into the **right lymphatic duct**. The right lymphatic duct empties into the right subclavian vein. **Lymph** drainage from the remaining regions of the body flows into the **thoracic duct**, which empties into the left subclavian vein.

Lymph Nodes

Located at various intervals along the course of the lymphatic system vessels are lymph nodes, which are collections of lymphatic tissue. The lymph nodes are also called the lymph glands. The major concentrations of lymph nodes throughout the body are the (1) cervical lymph nodes, (2) submandibular lymph nodes, (3) axillary lymph nodes, and (4) inguinal lymph nodes. See *Figure 9-3*. As the **lymph** passes through the stationary lymph nodes, two processes occur: old, dead cells and bacteria present in the **lymph** are filtered out so that they will not be emptied into the blood vessels, and phagocytes called macrophages engulf and destroy the bacteria (which are filtered out). This process of engulfing and destroying the bacteria is known as **phagocytosis**. Macrophages are special phagocytic cells involved in the defense against infection and in the disposal of the products of the breakdown of cells. They are found in the lymph nodes and in the liver, spleen, lungs, brain, and spinal cord. The lymph nodes also produce **antibodies** and lymphocytes, which are important to **immunity**.

Thymus

The **thymus** (also an endocrine gland) is a single gland located in the mediastinum, near the middle of the chest, just beneath the sternum. It secretes a hormone called thymosin, which stimulates the red bone marrow to produce **T lymphocytes (T cells)**, which are important in the **immune** response. The T lymphocytes mature in the thymus. Upon maturation, they enter the blood and circulate throughout the body (providing defense against disease by attacking foreign and/or abnormal cells). The thymus gland completes most of its essential work during childhood, decreasing significantly in size as one ages. It is quite small in older adults.

Spleen

The **spleen**, located in the left upper quadrant of the abdomen just below the diaphragm and behind the stomach, is the largest lymphatic organ in the body. The spleen plays an important role in the **immune** response by filtering blood in much the same way the lymph nodes filter the **lymph**. The macrophages of the spleen remove **pathogens** of all types from circulating blood. They also remove old red blood cells from circulation, breaking them down and forming bile that is returned to the liver to be excreted in bile. The spleen contains venous sinuses that serve as a storage reservoir for blood. In emergencies, such as **hemorrhage**, the spleen can release blood back into the general circulation. If the spleen should ever have to be removed, its functions can be performed by other lymphatic tissue and the liver. The removal of the spleen is called a **splenectomy**.

Tonsils

The **tonsils** are masses of lymphatic tissue located in a protective ring, just under the mucous membrane, surrounding the mouth and back of the throat. They are divided into three groups:

1. The **pharyngeal tonsils** (**adenoids**) are near the opening of the nasal cavity into the pharynx (throat).

2. When we speak of "the **tonsils**," we are usually referring to the **palatine tonsils** located on each side of the throat, near the opening of the oral cavity into the pharynx.

3. The **lingual tonsils** are located near the base of the tongue.

The **tonsils** help protect against bacteria and other harmful substances that may enter the body through the nose or mouth. Serving as the first line of defense from the external environment, the **tonsils** are subject to chronic infection or inflammation known as **tonsillitis**. Removal of the **tonsils** is known as a **tonsillectomy**.

Review Checkpoint

Check your understanding of this section by completing the **Anatomy and Physiology** exercises in your workbook.

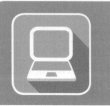

Media Link

View **The Lymphatic System** animation on the Student Companion Website for an overview of this system.

VOCABULARY (LYMPHATIC)

The following vocabulary words are frequently used when discussing the lymphatic system.

Word	Definition
acquired immunity (im-**YOO**-nih-tee)	**Immunity** that is a result of the body developing the ability to defend itself against a specific agent, as a result of having had the disease or from having received an **immunization** against a disease.
adenoids (**ADD**-eh-noydz)	Masses of lymphatic tissue located near the opening of the nasal cavity into the pharynx; also called the pharyngeal tonsils.

Word	Definition
edema (eh-**DEE**-mah)	The accumulation of fluid within the tissue spaces.
hypersensitivity (**high**-per-**sens**-ih-**TIV**-ih-tee)	An abnormal condition characterized by an excessive reaction to a particular stimulus.
immune reaction (**immune response**) (im-**YOON**)	A defense function of the body that produces **antibodies** to destroy invading **antigens** and malignancies.
immunity (im-**YOO**-nih-tee)	The state of being resistant to or protected from a disease. The individual is said to be "**immune**."
immunization (**im**-yoo-nigh-**ZAY**-shun)	The process of creating **immunity** to a specific disease.
immunologist (**im**-yoo-**NOL**-oh-jist)	The health specialist whose training and experience is concentrated in **immunology**.
immunology (**im**-yoo-**NOL**-oh-jee)	The study of the reaction of tissues of the **immune** system of the body to antigenic stimulation.
immunotherapy (**im**-yoo-no-**THAIR**-ah-pee)	A special treatment of allergic responses that administers increasingly large doses of the offending allergens to gradually develop **immunity**.
local reaction	A reaction to treatment that occurs at the site it was administered.
lymph (LIMF)	Interstitial fluid picked up by the lymphatic capillaries and eventually returned to the blood. Once the interstitial fluid enters the lymphatic vessels, it is known as **lymph**.
lymphadenopathy (lim-**fad**-eh-**NOP**-ah-thee) lymph/o = lymph aden/o = gland -pathy = disease	Any disorder of the lymph nodes or lymph vessels, characterized by localized or generalized enlargement.
lymphocyte (**LIM**-foh-sight) lymph/o = lymph -cyte = cell	Small, agranulocytic leukocytes originating from fetal stem cells and developing in the bone marrow.
macrophage (**MACK**-roh-fayj) macr/o = large phag/o = to eat -e = noun ending	Any phagocytic cell involved in the defense against infection and in the disposal of the products of the breakdown of cells. Macrophages are found in the lymph nodes, liver, spleen, lungs, brain, and spinal cord.
natural immunity (im-**YOO**-nih-tee)	**Immunity** with which we are born; also called genetic immunity.

Word	Definition
pathogens (**PATH**-oh-jenz) path/o = disease -gen = that which generates	Disease-producing microorganisms.
phagocytosis (**fag**-oh-sigh-**TOH**-sis) phag/o = to eat cyt/o = cell -osis = condition	The process of a cell engulfing and destroying bacteria.
resistance	The body's ability to counteract the effects of **pathogens** and other harmful agents.
susceptible (suh-**SEP**-tih-bul)	A state of having a lack of resistance to **pathogens** and other harmful agents. For example, the individual is said to be "**susceptible**."
T cells (**T SELLS**)	Cells important to the **immune** response. They mature in the thymus. Upon maturation, the **T cells** enter the blood and circulate throughout the body, providing defense against disease by attacking foreign and/or abnormal cells.
tonsils (**TON**-sills)	Masses of lymphatic tissue located in a protective ring, just under the mucous membrane, surrounding the mouth and back of the throat.

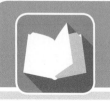

Review Checkpoint

Check your understanding of this section by completing the **Vocabulary exercises** in your workbook.

WORD ELEMENTS (LYMPHATIC)

The following word elements pertain to the lymphatic system. As you review the list, pronounce each word element aloud twice and check the box after you "say it." Write the definition for the example term given for each word element. Use your medical dictionary to find the definitions of the example terms.

Word Element	Pronunciation	"Say It"	Meaning
cyt/o, -cyte **cyt**omegalovirus	**SIGH**-toh, **SIGHT** **sigh**-toh-**meg**-ah-loh-**VYE**-rus	☐	cell
hyper- **hyper**splenism	**HIGH**-per high-per-**SPLEN**-izm	☐	excessive

Word Element	Pronunciation	"Say It"	Meaning
immun/o **immun**odeficiency	im-**YOO**-noh **im**-yoo-noh-deh-**FISH**-en-see	☐	**immune**, protection
lymph/o **lymph**ocyte	**LIM**-foh **LIM**-foh-sight	☐	**lymph**
lymphaden/o **lymphaden**itis	lim-**FAD**-en-oh lim-**fad**-en-**EYE**-tis	☐	lymph gland
lymphangi/o **lymphangi**ogram	lim-**FAN**-jee-oh lim-**FAN**-jee-oh-gram	☐	lymph vessel
mon/o **mon**onucleosis	**MON**-oh mon-oh-noo-klee-**OH**-sis	☐	one
sarc/o Kaposi's **sarc**oma	**SAR**-koh **KAP**-oh-seez sar-**KOH**-mah	☐	flesh

Review Checkpoint

Check your understanding of this section by completing the **Word Elements** exercises in your workbook.

Immunity

As we have already learned, the lymphatic system is an important part of the **immune** system, which protects the body against disease-producing organisms (**pathogens**) and other foreign microorganisms to which it is continually exposed. **Immunity** is the state of being resistant to or being protected from a disease. This section discusses both natural and **acquired immunity**, with a greater concentration on **acquired immunity**. The purpose of **immunity** is to develop resistance to a disease or to harmful agents. The body's ability to counteract the effects of **pathogens** and other harmful agents is called **resistance**. If the body lacks resistance to **pathogens** and other harmful agents, it is said to be **susceptible**.

Natural immunity is that with which we are born. It is also called genetic immunity. Some **pathogens** cannot affect certain species. For example, humans do not suffer from canine distemper, nor do canines suffer from human measles. **Natural immunity** is considered a permanent form of **immunity** to a specific disease.

Acquired immunity is **immunity** indicating that the body has developed the ability to defend itself against a specific agent. This protection can occur as a result of having had the particular disease or from having received immunizations against a disease. **Acquired immunity** can be divided further into two categories: (1) passive acquired immunity and (2) active acquired immunity.

1. **Passive acquired immunity** is acquired artificially by injecting **antibodies** from the blood of other individuals or animals into a person's body to protect him or her from a specific disease. This type of **immunity** is immediate but short lived, lasting only a few weeks. An example of passive immunity is the administration of **gamma globulin** (a blood protein containing **antibodies**) to individuals who have been exposed to viruses such as measles and infectious hepatitis. Another example of passive immunity is the passage of the mother's **antibodies** through the placenta into the baby's blood. This provides the newborn infant with passive immunity for approximately the first year of life, during which time the infant begins to develop his or her own **antibodies**.

2. **Active acquired immunity** is either acquired naturally as a result of having had a disease or artificially by being inoculated with a vaccine, antigen, or toxoid. With **natural acquired immunity**, an individual who has a full-blown case of a disease such as measles will usually develop enough **antibodies** to prevent a recurrence of the disease. Another form of active acquired immunity may be developed over a period of time after repeated exposures to an illness or disease (with only mild symptoms). With **artificial acquired immunity**, an individual receives a vaccine, antigen, or toxoid to stimulate the formation of **antibodies** within his or her body. For example, when a child receives the measles–mumps–rubella vaccine, he or she receives a mild strength of the disease in the form of the vaccine administered. This vaccine then stimulates the production of **antibodies** within the child's body against measles, mumps, and rubella.

The process of creating **immunity** to a specific disease is known as **immunization**. This is accomplished through the administration of vaccines, **antigens**, or toxoids to stimulate the formation of **antibodies** within an individual's body. Children receive routine immunizations throughout their early years to provide adequate protection against childhood diseases. These are discussed in Chapter 19. An individual may receive various immunizations throughout his or her lifetime to provide continued **immunity** against a disease (as in a tetanus toxoid booster) or to provide **immunity** against diseases prevalent in other countries (as in overseas travel).

Immune Reaction

The **immune reaction (immune response)** is a defense function of the body that produces **antibodies** to destroy invading **antigens** and malignancies. **Antigens** trigger the **immune** response during interaction with innumerable cells within the body. The types of **immune** responses are humoral immune response (involving the B lymphocytes of the body) and cell-mediated immune response, involving the T lymphocytes of the body. Both of these specialized cells have been genetically programmed to recognize specific invading **antigens** and to destroy them.

B lymphocytes originate from bone marrow stem cells and migrate to the lymph nodes and other lymphoid tissue. In the **humoral immune response**, when the B lymphocytes come in contact with specific invading **antigens**, they produce **antibodies** known as **immunoglobulins. Antibodies** belong to a group of blood proteins called gamma globulins. The gamma globulins are divided into five categories of immunoglobulins: immunoglobulin M (IgM), immunoglobulin G (IgG), immunoglobulin E (IgE), immunoglobulin A (IgA), and immunoglobulin D (IgD). Most **antibodies** are immunoglobulin type G (IgG). These immunoglobulins migrate to the site of the infection and react with the antigen and destroy it.

T lymphocytes originate from bone marrow stem cells and mature in the thymus gland. Upon maturation, the T lymphocytes enter the blood and circulate throughout the body, providing defense against disease by attacking foreign and/or abnormal cells. They migrate to the lymph nodes and lymphoid organs. In the **cell-mediated immune response**, when the T lymphocytes come in contact with specific invading **antigens**, they multiply rapidly and engulf and digest the antigen. This multiplication of cells produces cells that help destroy the antigen and cells called **memory cells**. The memory cells, which remain in circulation for many years, provide the body with resistance to any disease to which it has previously been exposed. When these memory cells face subsequent exposure to the same antigen, they are stimulated to produce cells rapidly that destroy the invading antigen. **Immunity** depends on the action of the memory cells.

Immunology is the study of the reaction of tissues of the immune system of the body to antigenic stimulation. An **immunologist** is a health specialist whose training and experience are concentrated in **immunology**. **Immunotherapy** is a special treatment of allergic responses that administers increasingly large doses of the offending allergens to gradually develop **immunity**.

When something happens to an individual's **immune** system causing it to function abnormally, the body forms **antibodies** that react against its own tissues. This is known as an **autoimmune disorder**. Unable to distinguish between internal antigens that are normally present in the cells and external invading **antigens**, the body reacts against the internal cells to cause localized and systemic reactions. These reactions affect the epithelial and connective tissues of the body, causing a variety of symptoms. Autoimmune disorders are divided into two categories: the collagen diseases (connective tissue diseases) and the autoimmune **hemolytic** disorders. The collagen diseases include disorders such as systemic lupus erythematosus, scleroderma, and rheumatoid arthritis. The autoimmune **hemolytic** diseases include disorders such as idiopathic thrombocytopenic purpura and acquired **hemolytic** anemia.

Hypersensitivity

Hypersensitivity is an abnormal condition characterized by an excessive reaction to a particular stimulus. It occurs when the body's **immune** system fails to protect itself against foreign material. The **antibodies** formed irritate certain body cells, causing a hypersensitive or allergic reaction. The allergic response is triggered by an **allergen**. Examples of allergens include ingested foods, penicillin and other antibiotics, grass, ragweed pollen, and bee or wasp stings. These allergens stimulate the formation of **antibodies** that produce the characteristic allergic reactions.

Hypersensitive reactions vary from mild to severe and from local to systemic. A **local reaction** is one that occurs at the site where treatment or medication was administered. A **systemic reaction** is one that is evidenced by generalized body symptoms such as runny nose, itchy eyes, hives, and rashes.

A severe and sometimes fatal hypersensitive (allergic) reaction to a previously encountered antigen is called **anaphylaxis** or **anaphylactic shock**. It is the result of an

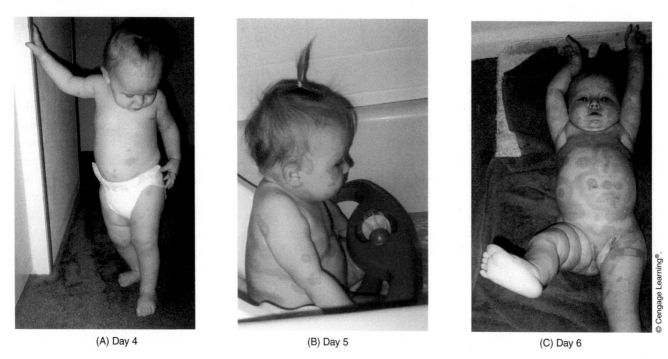

(A) Day 4   (B) Day 5   (C) Day 6

© Cengage Learning®.

Figure 9-4 Severe hypersensitive reaction to amoxicillin in a 13-month-old child (A) 4th day, (B) 5th day, (C) 6th day

antigen–antibody reaction that stimulates a massive secretion of histamine. **Anaphylaxis** can be caused by insect stings, contrast media containing iodide, aspirin, antitoxins prepared with animal **serum**, allergens used in testing and desensitizing patients who are hypersensitive, and other injected drugs. Penicillin injection is the most common cause of anaphylactic shock. *Figure 9-4* illustrates a severe reaction to penicillin. The series of pictures depict the child's reaction on days 4, 5, and 6 following oral administration of amoxicillin. This child received medication to counteract the reaction and did not require hospitalization.

Health care professionals should always ask patients if they are sensitive to any allergens or drugs to prevent adverse and sometimes fatal allergic responses to treatments or medications. Individuals with known hypersensitivities, or those receiving a first dose of injectable medication or penicillin, should remain in the physician's office for 15 to 20 minutes following the administration of medication or treatment. During this time, the individual should be observed for signs of possible **hypersensitivity**. Anaphylactic shock may occur within seconds or minutes after exposure to the sensitizing factor (**allergen**) and is commonly characterized by respiratory distress and vascular collapse. The first symptoms of anaphylactic shock are usually intense anxiety, weakness, sweating, and shortness of breath. This may be followed by hypotension, shock, arrhythmia, and respiratory congestion. Emergency treatment involves the immediate injection of epinephrine, which will raise the blood pressure through its vasoconstrictive action.

Individuals known to be hypersensitive to allergens and medications should wear a Medi-Alert tag around the neck or wrist. The presence of this tag will alert health care professionals or first-aid providers to the need for immediate action, informing them of either an **allergy** or a particular disease (such as diabetes).

Pathological Conditions (Lymphatic)

As you study the pathological conditions of the lymphatic system, note that the **basic definition** is in a green shaded box followed by a detailed description in regular print. The phonetic pronunciation is directly beneath each term, as well as a breakdown of the component parts of the term where applicable.

acquired immunodeficiency syndrome (AIDS) (**im-yoo**-noh-**dee-FIH**-shen-see **SIN**-drom)	**Acquired immunodeficiency syndrome (AIDS)** involves clinical conditions that destroy the body's **immune** system in the last or final phase of a human immunodeficiency virus (HIV) infection, which primarily damages helper T cell lymphocytes with CD_4 receptors.

HIV, a slow-growing virus, typically begins with an acute viral infection called the primary infection. This primary infection is systemic (in the bloodstream) and widespread (with seeding in the lymphatic system). In approximately eight weeks after onset, the CD_4 counts (normally 1,000) will have dropped by one-half (500), indicating a deficiency in the body's **immune** response. The signs and symptoms during this primary stage include headache, stiff neck, malaise, fatigue, fever, night sweats, rash, abdominal cramps, and diarrhea. By the twelfth week, the CD_4 counts will have rebounded to about 700. The measurable aspect of this primary infection is the presence of HIV antibodies. The ELISA and **western blot** tests are positive for **antibodies**.

During a latent period of approximately eight years, the CD_4 count usually declines steadily as the following signs and symptoms become more apparent: measurable presence of generalized **lymphadenopathy**, chronic diarrhea, weight loss, persistent fever, fatigue, night sweats, and oral thrush. **Kaposi's sarcoma** or hairy cell leukemia may appear during this latent stage.

When the CD_4 count reaches 200, "acquired immune deficiency" AIDS is clinically apparent. The person may or may not display signs and symptoms or develop an opportunistic neoplasm or infection. The CD_4 count will eventually reach 0, at which time the body has no **immune** defense and thus opportunistic infections and cancers will occur and affect all body systems.

About the 10th or 11th year after onset, the person will likely die from an overwhelming cancer or infection. HIV can be acquired via a blood transfusion, use of contaminated needles, or during unprotected sexual intercourse (especially anal sex). An unborn fetus can acquire HIV from the mother during pregnancy. Medical treatment includes various antiviral drugs and symptomatic management.

cytomegalovirus
 	
(**sigh**-toh-**meg**-ah-loh-**VYE**-rus)
  cyt/o = cell
  megal/o = enlarged
	Cytomegalovirus is a large species-specific herpes-type virus with a wide variety of disease effects. It causes serious illness in persons with AIDS, in newborns, and in individuals who are being treated with immunosuppressive drugs (as in individuals who have received an organ transplant). The virus usually results in retinal or gastrointestinal infection.

hypersensitivity	Tissue damage resulting from exaggerated **immune** responses.
(**high**-per-**sens**-sih-**TIV**-ih-tee)	The exaggerated responses are caused by one of the following four mechanisms.

1. **IgE-mediated type I hypersensitivity response** as occurs in allergic rhinitis, hives, allergic asthma, allergic conjunctivitis, and anaphylactic shock (acute systemic). The acute systemic response occurs as a result of the histamine and mediator release, causing increased capillary permeability, bronchial constriction, vasodilation, and smooth muscle contraction, which can lead to hypotension and impaired tissue perfusion, a state known as anaphylactic shock.

2. **Cytoxic type II hypersensitivity reaction** develops when **antibodies** bind to **antigens** on body cells. Causes of type II include transfusion reactions, autoimmune hemolytic anemia, and erythroblastosis fetalis.

3. **Immune complex-mediated type III sensitivity response** occurs when huge antibody, antigen, and complement proteins interact to form massive complexes (which accumulate in the tissues). Examples of type III hypersensitivity response include serum sickness, rheumatoid arthritis, systemic lupus erythematosus, and acute poststreptococcal glomerulonephritis.

4. **Delayed type IV hypersensitivity responses** are cell mediated rather than antibody mediated and involve **T cells**. Examples of type IV hypersensitivity response include contact dermatitis, graft-versus-host disease, and tuberculin reaction. A collection of skin tests may be used to assess and determine the causes of **hypersensitivity**.

hypersplenism	**Hypersplenism** is a syndrome involving a deficiency of one or more types of blood cells and an enlarged spleen.
(**high**-per-**SPLEN**-izm)	
hyper- = excessive	The causes of this syndrome are abundant. A few of the more common causes are hemolytic anemias, portal hypertension, lymphomas, tuberculosis, malaria, and several inflammatory and connective tissue diseases.
splen/o = spleen	
-ism = condition	

Symptoms of **hypersplenism** include left-sided abdominal pain and the feeling of fullness after a small intake. The enlarged spleen is easily palpated on physical examination. Treatment should begin with concentration on the underlying disorder, which may lead to the cure of the syndrome. A splenectomy is typically performed only for the individual with hemolytic anemia or the person with severe spleen enlargement (at high risk for a vascular accident).

Kaposi's sarcoma	**Kaposi's sarcoma** is a locally destructive malignant neoplasm of the blood vessels associated with AIDS, typically forming lesions on the skin, visceral organs, or mucous membranes. These lesions appear initially as tiny red to purple macules and evolve into sizable nodules or plaques.
(**CAP**-oh-seez sar-**KOH**-mah)	
sarc/o = flesh	
-oma = tumor	

The lesions occur due to an overgrowth of spindle-shaped cells and epithelial cells that result in the narrowing of the diameter of the vessels. The body responds by increasing the number of vessels in that area, thus causing more congestion.

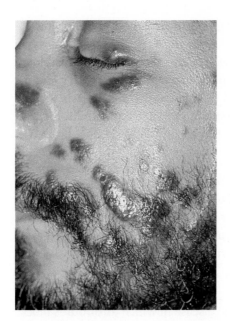

The signs and symptoms of **Kaposi's sarcoma** will vary but be specific according to the lesion site. Skin lesions were described previously. Gastrointestinal lesions may lead to mucosal bleeding, **anemia**, or obstruction. Pulmonary lesions may result in pulmonary effusion and shortness of breath. If the lesions are located in the lymphatics, there will be swollen lymph nodes and **edema**.

Kaposi's sarcoma is diagnosed with a biopsy of the lesion. With the pulmonary lesion, a chest X-ray is completed to confirm a pulmonary effusion. The treatment includes radiation therapy, chemotherapy, and laser cryotherapy. See *Figure 9-5*.

Figure 9-5 Kaposi's Sarcoma.
Courtesy of Robert A. Silverman, MD, Pediatric Dermatology, Georgetown University

---

lymphoma

(**LIM**-foh-mah)

  lymph/o = lymph

  -oma = tumor

Lymphoma is a lymphoid tissue neoplasm that is typically malignant, beginning with a painless enlarged lymph node(s) and progressing to **anemia**, weakness, fever, and weight loss.

The spleen and liver usually enlarge with widespread lymphoid tissue involvement. The development of lymphomas has a higher occurrence in the male population. Intensive chemotherapy and radiotherapy are the treatments with a **lymphoma**.

Burkitt's lymphoma is a malignant neoplasm in the jaw or abdomen and is seen chiefly in Central Africa. Rapid diagnosis and treatment typically results in quick shrinking of the lesion and complete cure of the disease.

Hodgkin's disease is characterized by progressive painless enlargement of a malignant tumor of the lymph tissue in the lymph nodes and spleen typically noted first in the cervical region. Males are affected twice as often as females. Clinical manifestations include enlarged lymph nodes, **splenomegaly**, low-grade fever, night sweats, anorexia, **anemia**, and leukocytosis. Diagnosis is made through the identification of a Reed-Sternberg cell (malignant cell in the lymph nodes). With localized disease, radiotherapy is the choice. However, with more extensive disease, chemotherapy or a combination of chemotherapy and radiation is used.

Non-Hodgkin's lymphoma is the classification of any type of malignant **lymphoma** other than Hodgkin's disease, including histiocytic lymphoma and lymphocytic lymphomas. Radiation and chemotherapy are administered to stop the growth and cure this disease.

---

mononucleosis

(**mon**-oh-**noo**-klee-**OH**-sis)

  mono- = one

  nucle/o = nucleus

  -osis = condition

Usually caused by the Epstein–Barr virus (EBV), **mononucleosis** typically is a benign, self-limiting acute infection of the B lymphocytes.

Young adults (15 to 20 years old) are primarily affected with this "kissing disease," as it is described due to the main mode of transmission (through saliva). The body's response to this B lymphocyte infection is the production of **antibodies** by the unaffected B lymphocytes and the T lymphocytes. As a result of this proliferation of B and T lymphocytes, the lymphoid tissue in the body becomes swollen. This swollen lymphoid tissue is most noted in enlarged, tender cervical lymph nodes and sometimes axillary and inguinal lymph nodes, the spleen, and the liver and typically lasts for one to three weeks. Other clinical manifestations include fever, chills, malaise, diaphoresis (profuse sweating), sore throat, profound fatigue, headache, red papular rash, and anorexia.

The diagnosis of **mononucleosis** is confirmed with a physical examination, elevated **lymphocyte** count and the presence of atypical lymphocytes, and a positive monospot test. Bed rest is the initial treatment, with administration of analgesics and corticosteroids as needed. A two- to three-week recovery period is needed, and many times the fatigue and debility last two to three months.

myasthenia gravis (my-as-**THEE**-nee-ah **GRAV**-is) my/o = muscle -asthenia = loss of strength	**Myasthenia gravis** is an autoimmune disease in which **antibodies** block or destroy some acetylcholine receptor sites.

Other structural problems cause the acetylcholine uptake to be decreased and therefore reduce neuromuscular transmissions. In approximately one-fifth of the cases, thymus gland involvement is noted.

Myasthenia gravis occurs more often in women than in men. In women, it usually occurs at the age of 20 to 40 years. In men, the onset of **myasthenia gravis** is between the ages of 50 and 60.

The symptoms may occur gradually or suddenly. Facial muscle weakness may be the most noticeable due to drooping eyelids, difficulty with swallowing, and difficulty speaking. The periods of muscle weakness generally occur late in the day or after strenuous exercise. Rest refreshes the tired, weak muscles. The weakness eventually becomes so severe that paralysis occurs.

Treatment for **myasthenia gravis** may require restricted activity, a soft or liquid diet, and administration of anticholinesterase drugs (Mestinon). Some individuals benefit from corticosteriods.

pneumocystis carinii pneumonia (PCP) (**noo**-moh-**SIS**-tis kah-**rye**-nee-eye noo-**MOH**-nee-ah) pneum/o = lungs; air cyst/o = sac -is = noun ending pneumon/o = lungs; air -ia = condition	**Pneumocystis carinii pneumonia** is caused by a common worldwide parasite, *Pneumocystis carinii,* for which most people have **immunity** if they are not severely immunocompromised.

The most frequent opportunistic infection occurring in persons with AIDS, **pneumocystis carinii pneumonia** (PCP) affects an estimated 75% to 80% of those individuals with AIDS. Individuals with PCP have severely impaired gas exchange as the disease progresses. The swollen, thickened air sacs of the lungs are filled with a protein-rich foamy fluid resulting in tachypnea; shortness of breath; fever; and a dry, nonproductive cough.

sarcoidosis
 	
(**sar**-koyd-**OH**-sis)
  sarc/o = flesh
  -oid = resembling
  -osis = condition
	Sarcoidosis is a systemic inflammatory disease resulting in the formation of multiple small, rounded lesions (granulomas) in the lungs (comprising 90%), lymph nodes, eyes, liver, and other organs.

	These granulomas can resolve spontaneously or may lead to fibrosis. The occurrence is highest in African American females between 20 and 40.
	Although the mortality rate is less than 3%, the disability caused by **sarcoidosis** of the respiratory, ocular, or other organs can be devastating to the individual. A biopsy of the granuloma may be needed to confirm the diagnosis. Corticosteroids are reserved for those persons experiencing severe manifestations or disabilities caused by the disease.
systemic lupus erythematosus (SLE)	An inflammatory connective tissue disease, chronic in nature, in which **immune** complexes are formed from the reaction of SLE autoantibodies and their corresponding **antigens**. These **immune** complexes are deposited in the connective tissues of lymphatic vessels, blood vessels, and other tissues.
	Local tissue damage occurs due to the inflammatory response when the **immune** complexes are deposited. These complexes are frequently deposited in the kidneys, causing damage to the tissue. Other tissues sometimes affected are the brain, lungs, skin, musculoskeletal system, heart, spleen, GI tract, and peritoneum.

Review Checkpoint

Check your understanding of this section by completing the **Pathological Conditions** exercises in your workbook.

Diagnostic Techniques, Treatments, and Procedures (Lymphatic)

enzyme-linked immunosorbent assay (ELISA) (**EN**-zym **LINK'T** im-yoo-noh-**SOR**-bent **ASS**-say)	**Enzyme-linked immunosorbent assay** (ELISA) is a blood test used for screening for an antibody to the AIDS virus. It may also be used to test for other diseases, such as Lyme disease.
	Positive outcome on this test indicates probable virus exposure but should be confirmed with the **western blot** test.
western blot	The **western blot** test detects the presence of the **antibodies** to HIV, the virus that causes AIDS, used to confirm validity of ELISA tests.
CT (CAT) scan	A collection of X-ray images taken from various angles following injection of a contrast medium.

Diagnosis of abnormalities in lymphoid organs are made in areas such as the spleen, thymus gland, and lymph nodes.

lymphangiogram	**Lymphangiogram** is an X-ray assessment of the lymphatic system following injection of a contrast medium into the lymph vessels in the hand or foot.
(lim-**FAN**-jee-oh-gram) lymph/o = lymph angi/o = vessel -gram = record, picture	

The path of **lymph** flow is noted moving into the chest region. This procedure is helpful in diagnosing and staging lymphomas.

Review Checkpoint

Check your understanding of this section by completing the **Diagnostic Techniques, Treatments, and Procedures** exercises in your workbook.

COMMON ABBREVIATIONS (LYMPHATIC)

Abbreviation	Meaning	Abbreviation	Meaning
ARC	AIDS-related complex	Histo	histology
AIDS	acquired immunodeficiency syndrome	HIV	human immunodeficiency virus
CDC	Centers for Disease Control and Prevention	HSV	herpes simplex virus
		ITP	idiopathic thrombocytopenic purpura
CMV	cytomegalovirus		
EBV	Epstein–Barr virus	KS	Kaposi's sarcoma
ELISA	enzyme-linked immunosorbent assay	SLE	systemic lupus erythematosus

Review Checkpoint

Check your understanding of this section by completing the **Common Abbreviations** exercises in your workbook.

WRITTEN AND AUDIO TERMINOLOGY REVIEW

Review each of the following terms from this chapter. Study the spelling of each term and write the definition in the space provided. Check definitions by looking the term up in the glossary.

Term	Pronunciation	Definition
acquired immunity	☐ acquired im-**YOO**-nih-tee	_____
acquired immunodeficiency syndrome (AIDS)	☐ acquired im-**yoo**-noh-**dee**-**FIH**-shen-see **SIN**-drom (**AIDS**)	_____
adenoids	☐ **ADD**-eh-noydz	_____
agglutination	☐ ah-**gloo**-tih-**NAY**-shun	_____
albumin	☐ al-**BYOO**-min	_____
allergen	☐ **AL**-er-jin	_____
allergy	☐ **AL**-er-jee	_____
anaphylaxis	☐ **an**-ah-fih-**LAK**-sis	_____
anemia	☐ an-**NEE**-mee-ah	_____
anisocytosis	☐ an-**ih**-soh-sigh-**TOH**-sis	_____
antibodies	☐ **AN**-tih-bod-eez	_____
antigens	☐ **AN**-tih-jenz	_____
aplastic anemia	☐ ah-**PLAST**-ik an-**NEE**-mee-ah	_____
ascites	☐ ah-**SIGH**-teez	_____
basophil	☐ **BAY**-soh-fill	_____
bilirubin	☐ bill-ih-**ROO**-bin	_____
blastocyte	☐ **BLAST**-oh-sight	_____
chromophilic	☐ kroh-moh-**FILL**-ik	_____
candidiasis	☐ **kan**-dih-**DYE**-ah-sis	_____
carcinoma	☐ **kar**-sih-**NOH**-mah	_____
coagulation	☐ koh-**ag**-yoo-**LAY**-shun	_____
corpuscle	☐ **KOR**-pus-ul	_____
cytogenesis	☐ **sigh**-toh-**JEN**-eh-sis	_____
cytokines	☐ **SIGH**-toh-kyens	_____

Term	Pronunciation	Definition
cytotoxic	☐ **sigh**-toh-**TOK**-sick	_____
cytomegalovirus	☐ **sigh**-toh-**meg**-ah-loh-**VYE**-rus	_____
differentiation	☐ **diff**-er-en-**she**-**AY**-shun	_____
direct antiglobulin test	☐ dih-**RECT an**-tih-**GLOB**-yoo-lin test	_____
dyscrasia	☐ dis-**KRAY**-zee-ah	_____
edema	☐ eh-**DEE**-ma	_____
electrophoresis	☐ ee-**lek**-troh-for-**EE**-sis	_____
enzyme-linked immunosorbent assay	☐ **EN**-zym **LINK'T im**-yoo-noh-**SOR**-bent **ASS**-say	_____
eosinophil	☐ **ee**-oh-**SIN**-oh-fill	_____
eosinophilia	☐ **ee**-oh-**sin**-oh-**FILL**-ee-ah	_____
erythremia	☐ **eh**-rih-**THREE**-mee-ah	_____
erythroblast	☐ eh-**RITH**-roh-blast	_____
erythrocyte	☐ eh-**RITH**-roh-sight	_____
erythrocyte sedimentation rate	☐ eh-**RITH**-roh-sight **sed**-ih-men-**TAY**-shun rate	_____
erythrocytopenia	☐ eh-**rith**-roh-**sigh**-toh-**PEE**-nee-ah	_____
erythrocytosis	☐ eh-**rith**-roh-sigh-**TOH**-sis	_____
erythropoiesis	☐ eh-**rith**-roh-poy-**EE**-sis	_____
erythropoietin	☐ eh-**rith**-roh-**poy**-**EE**-tin	_____
fibrin	☐ **FYE**-brin	_____
fibrinogen	☐ fye-**BRIN**-oh-jen	_____
globin	☐ **GLOH**-bin	_____
globulin	☐ **GLOB**-yoo-lin	_____
granulocytes	☐ **GRAN**-yoo-loh-sights	_____
granulocytosis	☐ **gran**-yoo-loh-sigh-**TOH**-sis	_____
hematocrit	☐ hee-**MAT**-oh-krit	_____
hematologist	☐ **hee**-mah-**TOL**-oh-jist	_____
hematology	☐ **hee**-mah-**TOL**-oh-jee	_____
heme	☐ **HEEM**	_____
hemochromatosis	☐ **hee**-moh-**kroh**-mah-**TOH**-sis	_____

3. Also called "bone marrow depression anemia," it is a form of anemia characterized by pancytopenia—an inadequacy of all the formed blood elements (RBCs, WBCs, and platelets).

   _____

   (two words)

4. A chronic hereditary form of hemolytic anemia in which the RBCs become shaped like crescents in the presence of low oxygen tension.

   _____

   (three words)

5. An abnormal proliferation of RBCs, granulocytes, and thrombocytes leading to an increase in blood volume and viscosity (thickness).

   _____

   (two words)

6. A term used to define different hereditary inadequacies of coagulation factors, which result in prolonged bleeding times.

   _____

   (one word)

7. Excessive uncontrolled increase of immature WBCs in the blood eventually leading to infection, anemia, and thrombocytopenia.

   _____

   (one word)

8. Collection of blood beneath the skin in the form of pinpoint hemorrhages appearing as red-purple skin discolorations.

   _____

   (one word)

9. An inflammatory connective tissue disease, chronic in nature, in which immune complexes are formed from the reaction of SLE autoantibodies and their corresponding antigens.

   _____

   (three words)

10. A syndrome presenting with immunodeficiency in the last or final phase of a human immunodeficiency virus (HIV) infection that primarily damages helper T cell lymphocytes with CD_4 receptors.

   _____

   (three words)

Number correct _____ × _10 points/correct answer: Your score_ _____ %

E. Word Search

Read each definition carefully and identify the applicable word from the list that follows. Enter the word in the space provided and then find it in the puzzle and circle it. The words may be read up, down, diagonally, across, or backward. Each correct answer is worth 10 points. Record your score in the space provided at the end of the exercise.

erythrocyte	Kaposi's sarcoma	ESR
lipid	acquired	CBC
hematocrit	sarcoidosis	PT
Schilling test	myasthenia gravis	

Example: The name for a red blood cell

erythrocyte

1. A systemic inflammatory disease resulting in the formation of multiple granulomas in the lungs (comprising 90%), lymph nodes, eyes, liver, and other organs.

2. A locally destructive malignant neoplasm of the blood vessels associated with AIDS typically forming lesions on the skin, visceral organs, or mucous membranes.

3. A diagnostic test performed to assess the percentage of red blood cells in the total volume of blood.

```
M  K  E  R  Y  T  H  R  O  C  Y  T  E  S  L
Y  A  S  R  E  T  S  O  P  O  R  E  T  N  A
A  P  R  Y  A  H  D  I  P  I  L  G  R  Y  S
S  O  I  S  P  E  C  S  T  S  S  U  T  N  I
T  S  O  I  T  D  I  B  L  E  I  I  T  A  S
H  I  H  Y  O  E  T  H  C  U  S  T  P  D  Y
E  S  R  D  E  R  E  I  M  B  I  I  A  I  L
N  S  M  E  U  I  O  N  X  R  T  N  R  O  A
I  A  O  A  V  U  N  G  C  T  N  P  G  P  N
A  R  M  C  T  Q  N  O  I  A  E  N  O  A  A
G  C  E  E  R  C  T  A  R  S  G  A  I  Q  C
R  O  U  L  E  A  U  X  J  I  O  R  D  U  I
A  M  I  T  M  T  A  E  R  C  N  A  A  E  R
V  A  I  E  I  A  S  R  M  L  I  S  R  V  T
I  J  H  L  S  Y  H  S  H  C  M  S  Y  A  I
S  I  S  O  D  I  O  C  R  A  S  M  Y  R  A
A  C  S  C  H  I  L  L  I  N  G  T  E  S  T
```

4. Immunity that occurs as a result of having had a disease or from having received an immunization against the disease.

_____

5. This is a diagnostic analysis for pernicious anemia.

_____

6. An abbreviation for a series of tests performed on peripheral blood that determines the number of red and white blood cells per cubic millimeter of blood.

_____

7. The name of a blood profile that measures triglycerides, cholesterol, phospholipids, fatty acids, and neutral fat.

_____

8. An autoimmune disease in which antibodies block or destroy some acetylcholine receptor sites, decreasing neuromuscular transmissions with resulting increased muscular weakness, extreme fatigue, and dysphagia.

_____

9. The abbreviation for the test that measures the rate at which red blood cells settle out in a tube of unclotted blood. The figure is expressed in millimeters per hour.

_____

10. The abbreviation for a one-stage blood test that detects certain plasma coagulation defects caused by a deficiency of various clotting factors, that is, factors V, VII, and X.

_____

Number correct _____ **× 10 points/correct answer: Your score** _____%

F. Matching Abbreviations

Match the abbreviations on the left with the most appropriate definition on the right. Each correct response is worth 10 points. When you have completed the exercise, record your score in the space provided at the end of the exercise.

_____	1. CMV	a. systemic lupus erythematosus
_____	2. ARC	b. Kaposi's sarcoma
_____	3. EBV	c. human immunodeficiency virus
_____	4. ITP	d. AIDS-related complex
_____	5. AIDS	e. autoimmune deficiency syndrome
_____	6. HSV	f. Epstein–Barr virus
_____	7. HIV	g. idiopathic thrombocytopenic purpura
_____	8. SLE	h. acquired immune deficiency syndrome
_____	9. KS	i. herpes simplex virus
_____	10. PTT	j. H-influenza virus
		k. cytomegalovirus
		l. The abbreviation for the blood test used to assess the clotting proficiency of factors I and II (fibrinogen and prothrombin), and factors V, VIII, IX, X, XI, and XII.

Number correct _____ **× 10 points/correct answer: Your score** _____ %

G. Spelling

Circle the correctly spelled term in each pairing of words. Each correct answer is worth 10 points. Record your score in the space provided at the end of the exercise.

1.	anaphylaxis	anaphlaxis	6.	hemorrage	hemorrhage
2.	acites	ascites	7.	hyperlipemia	hyperlypemia
3.	basophile	basophil	8.	myeloid	myloid
4.	dyscrasia	discrasia	9.	nutrophil	neutrophil
5.	fibrinogen	fibrinergen	10.	tonsills	tonsils

Number correct _____ *× 10 points/correct answer: Your score* _____ *%*

H. Completion

Complete each sentence with the most appropriate answer. Each correct answer is worth 10 points. Record your score in the space provided at the end of the exercise.

1. When someone has a lack of resistance to pathogens and other harmful agents, this individual is said to be:

   _____

2. Immunity with which we are born, also called genetic immunity, is known as:

   _____

3. An abnormal condition characterized by an excessive reaction to a particular stimulus is known as:

   _____

4. Immunity that is a result of the body's developing the ability to defend itself against a specific agent as a result of having had the disease or from having received an immunization against a disease is known as:

   _____

5. Another word for a platelet is:

   _____

6. The clear, thin, and sticky fluid portion of the blood that remains after coagulation is known as:

   _____

7. A systemic infection in which pathogens are present in the circulating bloodstream, having spread from an infection in any part of the body, is known as:

   _____

8. A naturally occurring anticlotting factor present in the body is:

   _____

9. The breakdown of red blood cells and the release of hemoglobin that occurs normally at the end of the life span of a red blood cell is known as:

   _____

10. A hormone that acts to stimulate and regulate the production of erythrocytes is:

    _____

Number correct _____ *× 10 points/correct answer: Your score* _____ *%*

I. Identify the Combining Form

For each word on the left, provide the applicable combining form and its definition in the blank space provided. Each correct answer is worth 10 points. Record your score in the space provided at the end of the exercise.

Medical Term	Combining Form	Definition
1. erythrocytosis	_____	_____
2. hematology	_____	_____
3. hyperlipemia	_____	_____
4. myeloid	_____	_____
5. pancytopenia	_____	_____
6. splenomegaly	_____	_____
7. thrombus	_____	_____
8. pathogens	_____	_____
9. electrophoresis	_____	_____
10. hemolysis	_____	_____

Number correct _____ *× 10 points/correct answer: Your score* _____*%*

J. Multiple Choice

Read each statement carefully and select the correct answer from the options listed. Each correct answer is worth 10 points. Record your score in the space provided at the end of the exercise.

1. The watery, straw-colored fluid portion of the lymph and blood in which leukocytes, erythrocytes, and platelets are suspended is the:
   a. plasma
   b. fibrin
   c. hemoglobin
   d. thrombin

2. A stringy, insoluble protein that is the substance of a blood clot is:
   a. plasma
   b. fibrin
   c. hemoglobin
   d. thrombin

3. The abnormal accumulation of fluid in interstitial spaces of tissues is known as:
   a. heme
   b. globin
   c. edema
   d. hemostasis

4. An abnormal condition of the blood or bone marrow (such as leukemia, aplastic anemia, or prenatal Rh incompatibility) is termed:
   a. dyscrasia

  b. ascites

  c. erythremia

  d. erythropoiesis

5. A naturally occurring anticlotting factor present in the body is:

  a. hemoglobin

  b. plasma

  c. heparin

  d. serum

6. The abbreviation for *hematocrit* is:

  a. Hb

  b. Ht

  c. Hct

  d. Hmt

7. A diagnostic analysis for pernicious anemia is the:

  a. white blood cell count

  b. Schilling test

  c. hematocrit

  d. lipid profile

8. An assessment of RBC percentage in the total blood volume is:

  a. white blood cell count

  b. Schilling test

  c. hematocrit

  d. lipid profile

9. An X-ray assessment of the lymphatic system following injection of a contrast medium into the lymph vessels in the hand or foot is known as a(n):

  a. lymphangiogram

  b. western blot

  c. ELISA

  d. Coomb's test

10. When a person receives blood or a blood component that has been previously collected from that person through a reinfusion it is called a(n):

  a. bone marrow transplant

  b. direct antiglobulin test

  c. autologous transfusion

  d. rouleaux

Number correct _____ × *10 points/correct answer: Your score* _____ %

K. Medical Scenario

The following medical scenario presents information on one of the pathological conditions discussed in this chapter. Read the scenario carefully and select the most appropriate answer for each question that follows. Each correct answer is worth 20 points. Record your score in the space provided at the end of the exercise.

Katrina Goodman, a 45-year-old patient, visited her internist last week, stating, "I'm so tired, and I have these bruises all over me." Katrina also complained of heavier than usual menstrual periods and mouth ulcers. Katrina's physician mentioned that she needed to complete a few tests to rule out leukemia. She started with a CBC blood test. The results were abnormal. Katrina is scheduled for a follow-up visit today and has many questions for the health care professional about this possible leukemia.

1. The health care professional bases her responses to Katrina's questions about leukemia on the fact that leukemia is a(n):

   a. hereditary form of hemolytic anemia in which the alpha or beta hemoglobin chains are defective and the production of hemoglobin is deficient, creating hypochromic microcytic RBCs

   b. malignant plasma cell neoplasm causing an increase in the number of both mature and immature plasma cells, which often entirely replace the bone marrow and destroy the skeletal structure

   c. excessive uncontrolled increase of immature WBCs in the blood, eventually leading to infection, anemia, and decreasing numbers of platelets

   d. abnormal increase in the number of RBCs, granulocytes, and thrombocytes, leading to an increase in the volume and viscosity of the blood

2. Katrina asks the health care professional how leukemia could cause the mouth ulcers. The health care professional would explain to Katrina that the increase:

   a. of immature WBCs would increase her susceptibility to infections

   b. of RBCs would predispose her to clot formation

   c. of platelets would reduce her defenses against infections

   d. in the hemoglobin would oversaturate the cells in her mouth

3. Katrina asks the health care professional how leukemia could cause all the bruises on her body. The health care professional would explain to Katrina that these are called purpura and are due to:

   a. an abnormal increase in the number of RBCs

   b. a decrease in the hemoglobin and hematocrit

   c. an increase in larger than usual WBCs

   d. a decrease in circulating platelets

4. Katrina also wanted the health care professional to explain why she had no energy and looked so pale. The health care professional explained to Katrina that these are the results of:

   a. anemia

   b. thrombocytopenia

   c. leukocytopenia

   d. hyperalbuminemia

5. Katrina inquired about how the physician would know for sure about the diagnosis of leukemia. The health care professional explained to Katrina that in most cases leukemia was diagnosed with the CBC results, a thorough history, and a:

   a. Schilling test

   b. white blood cell differential

   c. bone marrow aspiration

   d. erythrocyte sedimentation rate

Number correct _____ × *10 points/correct answer: Your score* _____%

L. Proofreading Skills

Read the following Consultation Report. For each bold term, provide a brief definition and indicate if the term is spelled correctly. If it is misspelled, provide the correct spelling. Each correct answer is worth 10 points. Record your score in the space provided at the end of the exercise.

Example:

    WBCs *white blood cells* _____

    Spelled correctly? ☑ Yes   ☐ No _____

HEMATOLOGY CONSULT

QUALI-CARE CLINIC

PATIENT NAME: Sabar Samaan

PCP: Patrick Keathley, MD

DATE OF BIRTH: August 10, 1971

AGE: 43

SEX: Male

DATE OF EXAM
June 20, 2014

HISTORY OF PRESENT ILLNESS
This 43-year-old Egyptian man was hospitalized in April at Hillcrest Medical Center under the care of Dr. Whitney of psychiatry because of a panic attack and clinical depression. At that time he was found to be anemic. He was unaware of having **aneemia**, and he apparently has no family history of anemia. He was being treated by Dr. Keathley, who is in the division of diabetes at the Florida Diabetes Institute. In May, his **WBCs** were 3400, **hgb** 11.7 grams, MCV 66.4, **platlets** 226,000. He developed a transient decrease in his testosterone and started losing weight. He was found to have adult-onset diabetes mellitus in September of last year. The patient had lost about 15 pounds before this diagnosis was made and some 20 pounds after the diagnosis of diabetes was made; however, his weight has been stable for the past month. His wife is concerned about his weight loss. The patient is referred to me for further evaluation and treatment of his anemia.

PAST HISTORY
As above. No history of heart disease. Has had no surgery.

MEDICATIONS
Glucophage 500 mg b.i.d. Blood sugars range from the low 100s to the 130s. Prozac and Wellbutrin per Dr. Whitney.

ALLERGIES
No known drug allergies.

(continued)

HEMATOLOGY CONSULT
Patient Name: Sabar Samaan
PCP: Patrick Keathley, MD
Date of Exam: June 20, 2014
Page 2

SOCIAL HISTORY

Married for 18 years, has 2 sons. A native of Egypt, he has lived in South Beach for 10 years. He had been a director of manufacturing in a fruit packing plant, but he now runs some convenience stores. Neither smokes cigarettes nor drinks alcohol.

FAMILY HISTORY

No family history of cancer, stroke, or anemia. Mother had heart disease and diabetes. Maternal aunts and uncles have had diabetes. Father is living and well in Egypt.

REVIEW OF SYSTEMS

CONSTITUTIONAL: No weakness, fever, sweats, rigors; weight loss as above.

EYES: Wears glasses. No blurred or double vision.

EARS, NOSE, MOUTH, THROAT: Decreased hearing, right ear. No tinnitus, epistaxis, vertigo, or oral ulcers.

NECK: No neck pain or masses.

CARDIOVASCULAR: No chest pain, palpitations, orthopnea, or paroxysmal nocturnal dyspnea.

RESPIRATORY: No dyspnea, chest pain, cough, or hemoptysis.

GI: No anorexia, bowel changes, melena, hematochezia, dyspepsia, or pain.

GU: No burning, frequency, or hematuria.

MUSCULOSKELETAL: No arthralgias or bone pain.

SKIN: No rash, itching, or lesions.

BREASTS: No breast, skin, or nipple changes.

NEUROLOGIC: No headaches, mental status changes, motor or sensory changes. No gait disturbances.

PSYCHIATRIC: See above.

ENDOCRINE: See above. No polyuria, polydipsia, cold or heat intolerance.

HEMATOLOGIC AND LYMPHATIC: No lymph node enlargement or skin bruising.

EXTREMITIES: No swelling, cyanosis, or weakness.

PHYSICAL EXAMINATION

VITAL SIGNS: T 97.1, P 67, BP 104/72.

GENERAL APPEARANCE: Well-developed, well-nourished Egyptian male in no obvious acute distress.

HEAD AND NECK: Normocephalic, atraumatic. Oropharynx without lesions. Nares patent. TMs not examined. Hearing aid in place on the right. Neck symmetrical without masses. Thyroid, no enlargement, masses, or tenderness. Eyes: Pupils round, reactive to light. Sclerae anicteric. Conjunctivae and lids normal. Funduscopic exam normal.

(continued)

HEMATOLOGY CONSULT
Patient Name: Sabar Samaan
PCP: Patrick Keathley, MD
Date of Exam: June 20, 2014
Page 3

CHEST: Respiratory effort normal. Clear to auscultation, percussion, and palpation.

CARDIOVASCULAR: Point of maximal impulse (PMI) normal location. Regular rhythm without murmur, gallop, or rub. Carotid, femoral, and pedal pulses not examined.

BREASTS: No masses, skin, or nipple changes.

ABDOMEN: No masses, hernias, visceromegaly, tenderness, or aortic enlargement. Bowel sounds normal.

GENITOURINARY: External genitalia showed normal testicles without masses.

RECTAL: I tried to do a rectal exam, but the patient was very uncomfortable. Exam was difficult, and I could not check his prostate adequately. No stool was obtained for Hemoccult.

LYMPHATIC: No abnormal lymph nodes in cervical, axillary, or groin areas.

MUSCULOSKELETAL: Exam of bones, joints, muscles of extremities; no tenderness of bones, full ROM at all joints without deformities, no muscle tenderness or wasting. No tenderness on percussion of spine.

EXTREMITIES: No cyanosis, clubbing, or edema.

SKIN: No rashes, lesions, or ulcerations.

NEUROLOGIC: Grossly intact. Gait and speech normal, fully oriented. Deep tendon reflexes (DTRs) and cranial nerves not tested. No pathologic reflexes. Sensation, strength, mental status normal.

PSYCHIATRIC: Mood and affect seem normal today.

Diagnostic studies from Dr. Keathley's office done in April of this year showed normal chemistries and a ferritin of 218, TIBC 228, % saturation 30%, reticulocyte count 1.3, and serum iron 68. TSH was low. He has had hepatitis studies and a Monospot test in the past that were negative.

IMPRESSION
1. Adult-onset diabetes mellitus.
2. Hypochromic, microcytic anemia. Target cells on his smear. Rule out blood loss, rule out hemoglobinopathy.
3. Weight loss of unclear etiology.
4. History of panic attacks and depression.

PLAN
1. Hemoglobin **electorphoresis** with A2 and F levels. **Reticulocyte** count, serum iron, total iron binding capacity, ferritin.
2. Three stool samples for occult blood.
3. PSA and CEA today.
4. Defer to Dr. Whitney for further psychiatric evaluation and treatment.

(*continued*)

HEMATOLOGY CONSULT
Patient Name: Sabar Samaan
PCP: Patrick Keathley, MD
Date of Exam: June 20, 2014
Page 4

COMMENT
This patient's anemia may be due to iron deficiency, thalassemia, or some combination of both. Certainly if he is iron deficient I would check his GI tract endoscopically; if we found something, it certainly could be a cause for his weight loss. This weight loss is probably related in part to his diabetes. The fact that it has leveled off may reflect the fact that his diabetes is under better control. Patient has had some depression. I will await the results of his studies at this point.

_____

David G. Cohmer, MD

Hematology/Oncology

DGC:xx

D:6/20/2014

T:6/22/2014

C: Austin Whitney, MD

   Patrick Keathley, MD

1. **aneemia** _____

_____

  Spelled Correctly? ☐ Yes ☐ No _____

2. **hgb** _____

_____

  Spelled Correctly? ☐ Yes ☐ No _____

3. **platlets** _____

_____

  Spelled Correctly? ☐ Yes ☐ No _____

4. **electorphoresis** _____

_____

  Spelled Correctly? ☐ Yes ☐ No _____

5. **reticulocyte** _____

_____

  Spelled Correctly? ☐ Yes ☐ No _____

Number correct _____ × *10 points/correct answer: Your score* _____ %

The Cardiovascular System

CHAPTER CONTENT

OBJECTIVES

Upon completing this chapter and the review exercises at the end of the chapter, the learner should be able to:

1. Identify and label the pathway of blood as it travels through the heart, to the lungs, and back through the heart.

2. List two major functions of the cardiovascular system.

3. Identify and label the structures of the heart by completing the exercise at the end of the chapter.

4. Define at least 10 common cardiovascular signs and symptoms.

5. Correctly spell and pronounce terms listed on the Written and Audio Terminology Review, using the phonetic pronunciations provided.

6. Define at least 20 common cardiovascular conditions.

7. Identify at least 20 abbreviations common to the cardiovascular system.

8. Identify four congenital heart diseases.

9. Identify at least three heart arrhythmias.

Overview

"And the beat goes on." Isn't it great that the beat of the heart *goes on* without conscious control? As we go about our busy schedules from day to day, the heart and the supporting structures of the cardiovascular system are responsible for pumping blood to the body tissues and cells, supplying these tissues and cells with oxygen and other nutrients, and removing carbon dioxide and other waste products of metabolism from the tissues and cells. The heart and blood vessels conjoin to pump and circulate the equivalent of 7,200 quarts of blood through the heart over a 24-hour period—approximately 5 quarts per minute or 2.5 ounces per beat, at the rate of 80 beats per minute!

The study of the heart is known as **cardiology**. The physician who specializes in the study of the diseases and disorders of the heart is known as a **cardiologist**.

Anatomy and Physiology

Heart

The heart is the center of the circulatory system. It lies within the **mediastinum** (in the thoracic cavity cradled between the lungs, just behind the sternum). Place your hand to the left of the midline of your chest cavity, just above the diaphragm, to locate the position of the heart. The area of the chest covering the heart is the **precordium**. Because the heart has a conelike shape, the broader upper portion is called the base, and the narrower lower tip of the heart is called the apex. The apex of the heart is located between the fifth and sixth ribs on a line perpendicular to the midpoint of the left clavicle. This position is usually just below the nipple. See *Figure 10-1*.

Apical pulses are taken on all children under two years of age and on patients with possible heart problems (the stethoscope is placed on the chest wall adjacent to the apex of the heart). The heart is described as being roughly the size of a clenched fist, weighing less than a pound (approximately 10.6 ounces). There are, however, other factors that influence heart weight and size (such as age, body weight, gender, frequency of physical activity, and heart disease). Using *Figure 10-2* as a guide, identify the linings and layers of the heart as described next.

The heart is enclosed by a thin, double-walled membranous sac called the **(1) pericardium**. The outer covering of this sac (which provides strength to the **pericardium**) is known as the **(2) parietal pericardium**. The inner layer of this membranous sac forms a thin, tight covering over the heart surface and is known as the **(3) visceral pericardium**, also known as the **epicardium**. Between these two layers

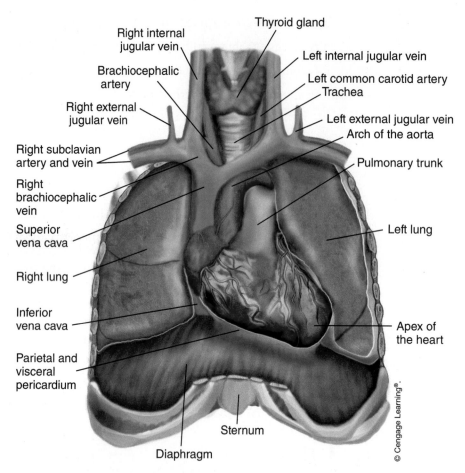

Figure 10-1 Apex/base of the heart

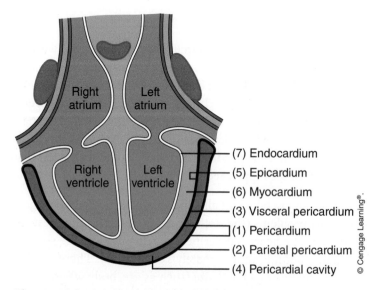

Figure 10-2 Linings and layers of the heart

is a small space called the **(4) pericardial cavity**. This cavity contains a very small amount of fluid that lubricates the surface of the heart and reduces friction during cardiac muscle contraction. The heart itself consists of three layers: the outer layer [known as the **(5) epicardium**]; the middle, muscular layer [known as the **(6) myocardium**]; and the inner layer, known as the **(7) endocardium**.

The heart functions as two pumps working simultaneously to move blood to all sites in the body. Divided into four chambers, the upper chambers—known as the **right** and **left atria** (singular: *atrium*)—are the receiving chambers. The lower chambers, known as the **right** and **left ventricles** (singular: *ventricle*), are the pumping chambers. The common wall between the right and left side of the heart is known as the **septum** (with the **interatrial septum** dividing the atria, and the **interventricular septum** dividing the ventricles). The varying thicknesses of the atrial and ventricular walls relate to the workload required by each chamber. The atrial walls are thinner than the ventricular walls because the atria receive blood, routing it on to the ventricles. The ventricular walls are thicker than those of the atria because the ventricles are responsible for pumping the blood through to the lungs (from the right ventricle) and throughout the entire body (from the left ventricle). Because the left ventricle has the greater workload of the two lower chambers, its muscle is approximately 2.5 to 3 times thicker than that of the right ventricle.

Circulation Through the Heart

Figure 10-3 identifies the parts of the heart and the vessels that transport blood. Refer to this figure as we discuss the flow pattern of the blood through the heart.

Deoxygenated blood enters the (**2**) **right atrium** from the (**1**) **superior vena cava**—which brings blood from the head, thorax, and upper limbs—and from the (**1**) **inferior vena cava**, which returns blood from the trunk, lower limbs, and abdominal viscera. From the right atrium, the deoxygenated blood passes through the (**3**) **tricuspid valve** into the (**4**) **right ventricle**. The right ventricle then contracts to pump the deoxygenated blood through the (**5**) **pulmonary valve** into the right and left (**6 and 7**) **pulmonary arteries**, which carry the oxygen-poor blood to the capillary network of the (**8**) **lungs**. The pulmonary arteries are the only arteries in the body that carry deoxygenated blood.

It is in the lungs where the exchange of gases takes place. Carbon dioxide leaves the bloodstream by way of the capillaries and passes into the alveoli of the lungs to be

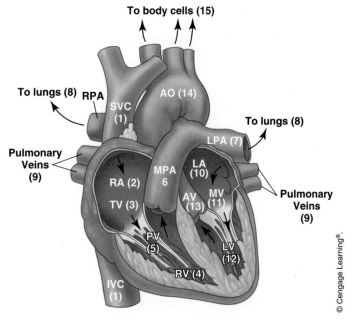

© Cengage Learning®.

Figure 10-3 Blood flow pattern through the heart

eliminated during respiration. Oxygen passes from the alveoli of the lungs through the capillaries into the bloodstream, oxygenating the blood. This circulation of the blood from the heart to the lungs for oxygenation and back to the heart is known as **pulmonary circulation**. The oxygenated blood is returned to the **(10) left atrium** of the heart by way of four **(9) pulmonary veins** (two from each lung). The pulmonary veins are the only veins in the body that carry oxygenated blood.

From the left atrium, the blood passes through the **(11) mitral (bicuspid) valve** into the **(12) left ventricle**. The left ventricle then pumps the blood through the **(13) aortic valve** into the **(14) aorta**. The aorta branches into arteries that distribute the freshly oxygenated blood to **(15) each body part** and region. This circulation of the blood from the heart to all parts of the body and back to the heart is known as **systemic circulation**. *Figure 10-4* illustrates both pulmonary and **systemic circulation**.

An important principle that determines the direction of the flow of blood in the heart is that fluid flows from a region of higher pressure to a region of lower pressure. When the left ventricle contracts, it creates increased pressure within the aorta, causing the blood to be forced progressively through the arteries and capillaries and into the veins. Skeletal muscle contractions promote the venous return of blood to the heart through their

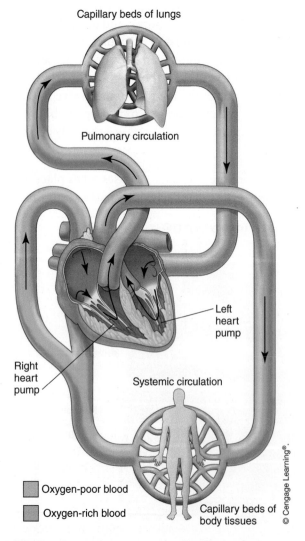

Figure 10-4 Pulmonary and systemic circulation

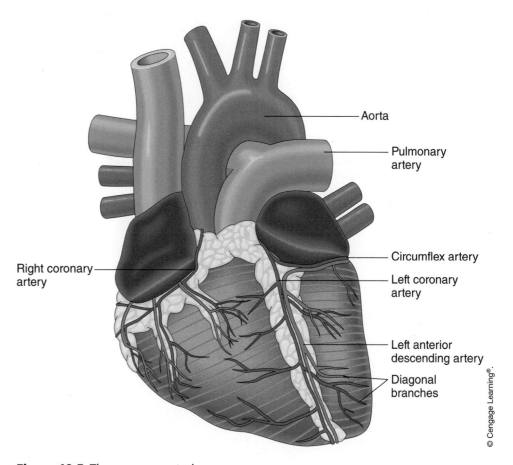

© Cengage Learning®.

Figure 10-5 The coronary arteries

contraction and relaxation actions, as discussed in the section on the supporting blood vessels. The blood eventually returns to the right atrium, where the pressure within the right atrium is less than the pressure within the vena cavae.

In addition to circulating blood throughout the body, arteries provide the blood supply to the heart muscle. The **coronary arteries** arise from the aorta near its origin at the left ventricle. These vessels supply blood to the heart muscle, which has a great need for oxygen and nutrients. The heart uses approximately three times more oxygen than other organs of the body. In this day and time, when there is great discussion of **coronary artery disease**, it is helpful to visualize the coronary arteries and realize their importance to effective myocardial function. See *Figure 10-5*.

Conduction System of the Heart

As stated previously, "the beat goes on"; but what is it that causes the heart to contract rhythmically to keep the blood flowing throughout the body? Orderly contraction of the heart occurs because the specialized cells of the conduction system methodically generate and conduct electrical impulses throughout the **myocardium**. The **sinoatrial node (SA node)**, a cluster of hundreds of cells, is located at the junction of the superior vena cava and the right atrium. The rate of impulses initiated by the sinoatrial node sets the rhythm for the entire heart. Therefore, the sinoatrial node is called the **pacemaker** of the heart. Once the impulse is initiated from the SA node, it travels across the atria, causing them to contract and forcing the blood into the ventricles of the heart.

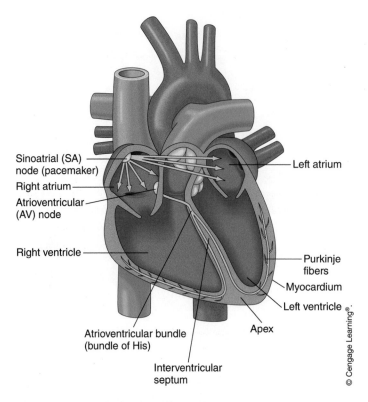

Sinoatrial (SA)
node (pacemaker)

Right atrium

Atrioventricular
(AV) node

Right ventricle

Left atrium

Purkinje
fibers

Myocardium

Left ventricle

Apex

Atrioventricular bundle
(bundle of His)

Interventricular
septum

© Cengage Learning®.

Figure 10-6 Conduction system of the heart

The wave of electricity continues traveling through the **myocardium** to the **atrioventricular node (AV node)**, which is located within the interatrial septum just above the junction of the atria and the ventricles. The AV node coordinates the incoming electrical impulses from the atria and relays the impulse to the ventricles through a bundle of specialized muscle fibers called the bundle of His.

The **bundle of His** enters the **septum** that separates the right and left ventricles (interventricular septum). It divides into **right** and **left bundle branches** that terminate in fibers called **Purkinje fibers**. The Purkinje fibers fan out into the muscles of the ventricles, forming the electrical impulse-conducting system of the heart. Receiving the electrical impulse from the bundle of His, the fibers cause the ventricles to contract.

To recap, the normal sequence of electrical impulses through the conduction system of the heart is as follows: SA node, through the atria to the AV node, from the AV node to the bundle of His, from the bundle of His to the bundle branches, and then to the Purkinje fibers. *Figure 10-6* illustrates the conduction system of the heart.

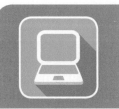

Media Link

Go to the Student Companion Website and watch the **Conduction System** animation.

Supporting Blood Vessels

Upon leaving the heart, the blood enters the vascular system (which is composed of many blood vessels). These blood vessels responsible for transporting blood to and from the heart and throughout the body are the arteries, arterioles, veins, venules, and capillaries.

Arteries are large, thick-walled vessels that carry the blood away from the heart. The walls of the aorta and large arteries are thicker than those of the veins, allowing them to withstand the force of the blood as the heartbeat propels it forward throughout the circulatory system. As the arteries continue on their path away from the heart, they branch into smaller vessels called arterioles. The **arterioles** have thinner walls than the arteries and are composed almost entirely of smooth muscle with very little elastic tissue. The arterioles carry the blood on to the minute blood vessels known as capillaries.

Capillaries have extremely thin walls, consisting of a single layer of endothelial cells. The thin walls of the capillaries allow for the exchange of materials between the blood and the tissue fluid surrounding the body cells. The exchange that takes place at the cellular level is one of the cells receiving the oxygen and nutrients for energy and nourishment and the blood vessels receiving the waste products of metabolism (carbon dioxide and urea) for removal from the body cells. These waste products are then transported by way of the cardiovascular system to their respective sites for elimination from the body: to the lungs for elimination of carbon dioxide and to the kidneys for elimination of urea. The capillaries connect the ends of the arterioles with the beginnings of the venules.

Venules are the smallest veins, which collect the deoxygenated blood from the cells for transport back to the heart. The venules branch into larger vessels known as veins. The **veins** have thinner walls than the arteries but thicker walls than the capillaries. The veins transport the blood from the venules to the heart. This is achieved by the contraction of the skeletal muscles, which creates a squeezing or "milking" action on the veins (keeping the blood moving in one direction: toward the heart). The valves within the veins support the flow of blood in one direction by closing when the skeletal muscles relax, thereby preventing the backflow of blood.

Cardiac Cycle

One cardiac cycle is equivalent to one complete heartbeat. As the heart carries out the function of propelling the blood through the blood vessels, it repeats two alternating phases: contraction—forcing blood out of the heart (**systole**)—and relaxation, allowing the heart to refill with blood (**diastole**).

During the **diastolic phase**, the ventricles relax and fill with blood. Deoxygenated blood enters the right atrium from the vena cavae and passes through the tricuspid valve to the right ventricle. The pulmonary valve is closed during this time, keeping the blood in the right ventricle. Simultaneously, oxygenated blood enters the left atrium from the **pulmonary vein** and passes through the mitral (bicuspid) valve into the left ventricle. The aortic valve is closed during this time, keeping the blood in the left ventricle.

Following this relaxation and filling period is the **systolic phase**, in which the ventricles contract. The right ventricle contracts to force the blood through the pulmonary valve into the **pulmonary artery**, which carries the blood to the lungs for oxygenation. The tricuspid valve is closed at this time to prevent the backflow of blood into the right atrium.

Simultaneously, the left ventricle contracts to force the blood through the aortic valve into the aorta, which then circulates the oxygenated blood to all parts of the body. The mitral (bicuspid) valve is closed at this time to prevent the backflow of blood into the left atrium.

With computerlike efficiency, the beat goes on, and the heart contracts every second of every day throughout one's life. The normal healthy heart beats continuously, resting only 0.4 second between beats.

Blood Pressure

Blood pressure is defined as the pressure exerted by the blood on the walls of the arteries. This pressure reaches its highest values in the left ventricle during **systole**. The maximum pressure reached within the ventricles is called **systolic pressure**, with the minimum pressure within the ventricles being called the **diastolic pressure**. Recording of these pressure changes within the heart is known as measuring the blood pressure. Blood pressure is measured with a **sphygmomanometer** and a **stethoscope**. The reading is recorded as a fraction, with the systolic reading on the top and the diastolic reading on the bottom: for example, "The patient had a blood pressure reading of 120/80." See *Figure 10-7*.

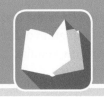

Review Checkpoint

Check your understanding of this section by completing the **Anatomy and Physiology** exercises in your workbook.

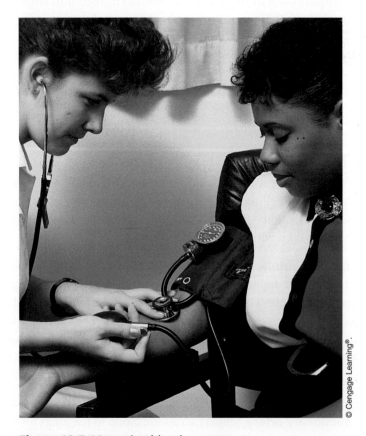

Figure 10-7 Measuring blood pressure

VOCABULARY

The following vocabulary words are frequently used when discussing the cardiovascular system.

Word	Definition
analgesic (**an**-al-**JEE**-sik) an- = without -algesic = sensitivity to pain	Pertaining to relieving pain; a medication that relieves pain.
anastomosis (ah-**nas**-toh-**MOH**-sis)	A surgical joining of two ducts, blood vessels, or bowel segments to allow flow from one to the other. **Anastomosis** of blood vessels may be performed to bypass an occluded area and restore normal blood flow to the area.
aneurysm (**AN**-yoo-rihzm) aneurysm/o = aneurysm	Localized dilation of a weakened area of the wall of an artery. The weakened area balloons out with every pulsation of the artery.
aneurysmectomy (**AN**-yoo-riz-**MEK**-toh-mee) aneurysm/o = aneurysm -ectomy = surgical removal	Surgical removal of the sac of an **aneurysm**.
anomaly (ah-**NOM**-ah-lee)	Deviation from normal; birth defect; for example, congenital **anomaly**.
anorexia (an-oh-**REK**-see-ah) an- = without -orexia = appetite	Lack or loss of appetite, resulting in the inability to eat. **Anorexia** is seen in individuals who are depressed, with the onset of **fever** and illness, with stomach disorders, or as a result of excessive intake of alcohol or drugs.
aplastic (ay-**PLAS**-tick) a- = without plast/o = formation, development -ic = pertaining to	without development
arthralgia (ar-**THRAL**-jee-ah) arthr/o = joint -algia = pain	Joint pain.
ascites (ah-**SIGH**-teez)	An abnormal collection of fluid within the peritoneal cavity (the peritoneum is the serous membrane that lines the entire abdominal cavity). This fluid contains large amounts of protein and electrolytes. General abdominal swelling occurs with **ascites**.

Word	Definition
asystole (a-**SIS**-toh-lee) 　a- = without 　-systole = contraction of the heart	Absence of contractions of the heart.
atherosclerosis (**ath**-er-**oh**-skleh-**ROH**-sis) 　ather/o = fatty 　scler/o = hardening 　-osis = condition	A form of **arteriosclerosis** (hardening of the arteries) characterized by fatty deposits building up within the inner layers of the walls of larger arteries.
benign (bee-**NINE**)	Noncancerous; not progressive.
bruit (brew-**EE**)	An abnormal sound or murmur heard with a stethoscope when listening to a carotid artery, organ, or gland; for example, during auscultation. (Plural pronunciation: brew-**EEZ**, **bruits**)
cardiologist (car-dee-**OL**-oh-jist) 　cardi/o = heart 　-logist = one who specializes in the 　　　　study of	One who specializes in the study of diseases and disorders of the heart.
cardiology (car-dee-**OL**-oh-jee) 　cardi/o = heart 　-logy = the study of	The study of the heart.
carditis (car-**DYE**-tis) 　card/o = heart 　-itis = inflammation	Inflammation of the heart muscles.
carotid endarterectomy (kah-**ROT**-id **end**-ar-ter-**ECK**-toh-mee) 　endo- = within 　arter/o = artery 　-ectomy = surgical removal	A surgical procedure performed to remove plaque buildup in the carotid arteries and facilitate blood flow; performed to reduce the risk of stroke caused by disruption of the blood flow.
claudication (**klaw**-dih-**KAY**-shun)	Cramplike pains in the calves of the legs caused by poor circulation to the muscles of the legs; commonly associated with **atherosclerosis**.
coronary artery (**KOR**-oh-nair-ree **AR**-ter-ee) 　coron/o = heart 　-ary = pertaining to 　arter/o = artery 　-y = noun ending	One of a pair of arteries that branch from the aorta. The coronary arteries and their branches supply blood and oxygen to the heart muscle (**myocardium**).

Word	Definition
cusp	Any one of the small flaps on the valves of the heart.
dependent edema (dependent eh-**DEE**-mah)	A fluid accumulation in the tissues influenced by gravity; usually greater in the lower extremities than in tissue levels above the level of the heart.
diastole (dye-**ASS**-toh-lee)	The period of relaxation of the heart, alternating with the contraction phase known as **systole**.
dysrhythmia (dis-**RITH**-mee-ah) dys- = bad, difficult, painful, disordered -rhythmia = rhythm	Abnormal rhythm.
echocardiogram (ek-oh-**CAR**-dee-oh-**gram**) echo- = sound cardi/o = heart -gram = record or picture	The graphic outline or record of movements of structures of the heart produced by ultrasonography (ultrasound).
edema (ee-**DEE**-mah)	The localized or generalized collection of fluid within the body tissues, causing the area to swell.
embolus (**EM**-boh-lus) embol/i = to throw -us = noun ending	A clot or part of a clot that has dislodged from another vessel and moved into a smaller vessel, possibly causing an obstruction to the flow of blood; an embolus may be solid, liquid, or gaseous.
endocarditis (**en**-doh-car-**DYE**-tis) endo- = within cardi/o = heart -itis = inflammation	Inflammation of the inner lining of the heart.
epicardium (**ep**-ih-**KARD**-ee-um) epi- = upon, over cardi/o = heart -um = noun ending	The inner layer of the **pericardium**, which is the double-folded membrane that encloses the heart.
hemostasis (**hee**-moh-**STAY**-sis) hem/o = blood -stasis – stopping; controlling	Stopping or controlling the flow of blood
hepatomegaly (**hep**-ah-toh-**MEG**-ah-lee) hepat/o = liver -megaly = enlarged	Enlargement of the liver.

Word	Definition
Homan's sign	Pain felt in the calf of the leg, or behind the knee, when the examiner is purposely dorsiflexing the foot of the patient (bending the toes upward toward the foot). If the patient feels pain, it is called a positive Homan's sign (indicating **thrombophlebitis**).
hyperlipidemia (**high**-per-lip-ih-**DEE**-mee-ah) hyper- = excessive -lipid/o = fat -emia = blood condition	An excessive level of fats in the blood.
hypertension (**high**-per-**TEN**-shun) hyper- = excessive	Elevated blood pressure persistently higher than 135/85 mmHg; high blood pressure; also known as arterial hypertension.
hypotension (**high**-poh-**TEN**-shun) hypo- = under, below, beneath, less than normal	Low blood pressure; less than normal blood pressure reading.
hypoxemia (**high**-pox-**EE**-mee-ah) hyp- = under, below, beneath, less than normal ox/o = oxygen -emia = blood condition	Insufficient oxygenation of arterial blood.
infarction (in-**FARC**-shun)	A localized area of necrosis (death) in tissue, a vessel, an organ, or a part resulting from lack of oxygen (anoxia) due to interrupted blood flow to the area.
ischemia (iss-**KEY**-mee-ah) -emia = blood condition	Decreased supply of oxygenated blood to a body part or organ.
lesion (**LEE**-zhun)	A wound, injury, or any pathological change in body tissue.
leukopenia (loo-koh-**PEE**-nee-ah) leuk/o = white -penia = decrease in; deficiency	An abnormal decrease in number of white blood cells to fewer than 5,000 cells per cubic millimeter; also called leukocytopenia.
lipid (**LIP**-id) lip/o = fat	Any of a group of fats or fatlike substances found in the blood. Examples of lipids are cholesterol, fatty acids, and triglycerides.
lumen (**LOO**-men)	A cavity or the channel within any organ or structure of the body; the space within an artery, vein, intestine, or tube.

Word	Definition
malaise (mah-**LAYZ**) mal- = bad, poor	A vague feeling of body **weakness** or discomfort, often indicating the onset of an illness or disease.
mediastinum (**mee**-dee-as-**TYE**-num)	The area between the lungs in the chest cavity that contains the heart, aorta, trachea, esophagus, and bronchi.
murmur	A low-pitched humming or fluttering sound, as in a "heart murmur," heard on auscultation.

megaloblastic anemia
(**MEG**-ah-loh-**blas**-tick
ah-**NEE**-mee-ah)
  megal/o = large
  blast/o = embryonic stage of
       development
  -ic = pertaining to
  an- = without, not, no
  -emia = blood condition
	A form of anemia characterized by excessive production of immature large erythrocytes (red blood cells), unable to carry on their normal function.

myelodysplastic syndrome
(**my**-eh-loh-dis-**PLAS**-tick
SIN-drohm)
  myel/o = spinal cord or bone marrow
  dys- = bad, difficult, painful, disordered
  plast/o = formation, development
  -ic = pertaining to
	A rare group of blood disorders that occur as a result of poorly formed or dysfunctional blood cells within the bone marrow; the bone marrow does not make enough healthy blood cells and there are abnormal (blast) cells in the blood and/or bone marrow.

myocardium
(**my**-oh-**CAR**-dee-um)
  my/o = muscle
  cardi/o = heart
  -um = noun ending
	The middle muscular layer of the heart.

nocturia
(nok-**TOO**-ree-ah)
  noct/o = night
  -uria = urine condition
	Urination at night.

occlusion (ah-**KLOO**-shun)	Closure, or state of being closed.

orthopnea
(**or**-**THOP**-nee-ah)
  orth/o = straight
  -pnea = breathing
	An abnormal condition in which a person sits up straight or stands up to breathe comfortably.

Word	Definition
pacemaker	The SA node (sinoatrial) of the heart located in the right atrium. It is responsible for initiating the heartbeat, influencing the rate and rhythm of the heartbeat. The cardiac pacemaker (artificial pacemaker) is an electric apparatus used for maintaining a normal heart rhythm by electrically stimulating the heart muscle to contract.
palpable (**PAL**-pah-bul)	Detectable by touch.
palpitation (**pal**-pih-**TAY**-shun)	A pounding or racing of the heart, associated with normal emotional responses or with heart disorders.
pericardial	Pertaining to the **pericardium**.
pericardium (**pehr**-ih-**KAR**-dee-um) peri- = around cardi/o = heart -um = noun ending	The double membranous sac that encloses the heart and the origins of the great blood vessels.
petechiae (peh-**TEE**-kee-ee)	Small, purplish, hemorrhagic spots on the skin; may be due to abnormality in the blood-clotting mechanism of the body.
phlebitis (fleh-**BYE**-tis) phleb/o = vein -itis = inflammation	Inflammation of a vein.
pitting edema (pitting ee-**DEE**-mah)	**Pitting edema** is swelling, usually of the skin of the extremities, that when pressed firmly with a finger will maintain the dent produced by the finger.
prophylactic (**proh**-fih-**LAK**-tik)	An agent that protects against disease.
pulmonary artery (**PULL**-moh-neh-ree **AR**-ter-ee) pulmon/o = lungs -ary = pertaining to arter/o = artery -y = noun ending	One of a pair of arteries that transports deoxygenated blood from the right ventricle of the heart to the lungs for oxygenation. The pulmonary arteries are the only arteries in the body to carry deoxygenated blood.
pulmonary circulation (**PULL**-moh-neh-ree) pulmon/o = lungs -ary = pertaining to	The circulation of deoxygenated blood from the right ventricle of the heart to the lungs for oxygenation and back to the left atrium of the heart; that is, from the heart, to the lungs, back to the heart.
pulmonary vein (**PULL**-moh-neh-ree vein) pulmon/o = lungs -ary = pertaining to	One of four large veins (two from each lung) that returns oxygenated blood from the lungs back to the left atrium of the heart. The pulmonary veins are the only veins in the body to carry oxygenated blood.

Word	Definition
SA node	Sinoatrial node; pacemaker of the heart; see *pacemaker*.
septicemia (**sep**-tih-**SEE**-mee-ah) -emia = blood condition	Systemic infection in which pathogens are present in the circulating bloodstream, having spread from an infection in any part of the body.
septum (**SEP**-tum)	A wall, or partition, that divides or separates two cavities. The interatrial septum separates the right and left atria, the atrioventricular septum separates the atria and the ventricles, and the interventricular septum separates the right and left ventricles.
serum sickness (**SEE**-rum)	A hypersensitivity reaction that may occur two to three weeks after administration of an antiserum. Symptoms include fever, enlargement of the spleen (splenomegaly), swollen lymph nodes, joint pain, and skin rash.
Sydenham's chorea (**SID**-en-hamz koh-**REE**-ah)	A form of chorea (involuntary muscle twitching) associated with **rheumatic fever**, usually occurring in childhood.
systemic circulation (sis-**TEM**-ik ser-kew-**LAY**-shun)	The circulation of blood from the left ventricle of the heart, throughout the body, and back to the right atrium of the heart. Oxygenated blood leaves the left ventricle of the heart and is distributed to the capillaries. Deoxygenated blood is picked up from the capillaries and is transported back to the right atrium of the heart.
systole (**SIS**-toh-lee)	The contraction phase of the heartbeat forcing blood into the aorta and the pulmonary arteries. **Systole** is marked by the first sound heard on auscultation, or the first pulse palpated, after the release of the blood pressure cuff (sphygmomanometer).
thrombosis (throm-**BOH**-sis) thromb/o = clot -osis = condition	The formation or existence of a blood clot.
vasoconstriction (**vaz**-oh-con-**STRIK**-shun)	Narrowing of the **lumen** of a blood vessel.
vegetation (vej-eh-**TAY**-shun)	An abnormal growth of tissue around a valve.

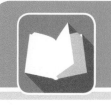

Review Checkpoint

Check your understanding of this section by completing the **Vocabulary** exercises in your workbook.

WORD ELEMENTS

The following word elements pertain to the cardiovascular system. As you review the list, pronounce each word element aloud twice and check the box after you "say it." Write the definition for the example term given for each word element. Use your medical dictionary to find the definitions of the example terms.

Word Element	Pronunciation	"Say It"	Meaning
aneurysm/o **aneurysm**ectomy	an-yoo-**RIZ**-moh **an**-yoo-riz-**MEK**-toh-mee	☐	aneurysm
angi/o **angi**ography	**AN**-jee-oh an-jee-**OG**-rah-fee	☐	vessel
arter/o, arteri/o **arteri**osclerosis	ar-**TEE**-roh, ar-**TEE**-ree-oh ar-**tee**-ree-oh-skleh-**ROH**-sis	☐	artery
arteriol/o **arteriol**e	ar-**tee**-ree-**OH**-loh ar-**TEE**-ree-ohl	☐	arteriole
ather/o **ather**oma	ah-**THAIR**-oh ah-thair-**OH**-ma	☐	fatty
blast/o erythro**blast**ocyte	**BLASS**-toh eh-**RITH**-roh-**blass**-toh-sight	☐	embryonic stage of development
cardi/o **cardi**ologist	**CAR**-dee-oh car-dee-**OL**-oh-jist	☐	heart
coron/o **coron**ary arteries	cor-**OH**-no **KOR**-oh-nair-ree **AR**-ter-eez	☐	heart
echo- **echo**cardiogram	**EH**-koh ek-oh-**CAR**-dee-oh-**gram**	☐	sound
electr/o **electr**ocardiogram	ee-**LEK**-troh ee-**lek**-troh-**CAR**-dee-oh-**gram**	☐	electrical, electricity
-emia an**emia**	**EE**-mee-ah ah-**NEE**-mee-ah	☐	blood condition
endo- **endo**carditis	**EN**-doh en-doh-car-**DYE**-tis	☐	within
-gram arterio**gram**	**GRAM** ar-**TEE**-ree-oh-**gram**	☐	record or picture

Word Element	Pronunciation	"Say It"	Meaning
-graphy electrocardio**graphy**	**GRAH**-fee ee-**lek**-troh-**CAR**-dee-**OG**-rah-fee	☐	process of recording
hem/o **hem**ostasis	**HEE**-moh **hee**-moh-**STAY**-sis	☐	blood
leuk/o **leuk**ocyte	**LOO**-koh **LOO**-koh-cyte	☐	white
megal/o **megalo**cardia	**MEG**-ah-loh **meg**-ah-loh-**CAR**-dee-ah	☐	enlarged
my/o **my**ocardium	**MY**-oh my-oh-**CAR**-dee-um	☐	muscle
-penia leukocyto**penia**	**PEE**-nee-ah **loo**-koh-**sigh**-toh-**PEE**-nee-ah	☐	decrease in; deficiency
-stasis veno**stasis**	**STAY**-sis **vee**-noh-**STAY**-sis	☐	stopping or controlling
ventricul/o **ventricul**ar	ven-**TRIK**-yoo-loh ven-**TRIK**-yoo-lar	☐	ventricle of the heart or brain

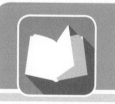

Review Checkpoint

Check your understanding of this section by completing the **Word Elements** exercises in your workbook.

Common Signs and Symptoms

A list of common complaints (signs and symptoms) that individuals with cardiovascular problems may describe when talking with the health professional follows. The observant health professional will listen carefully to all of the descriptions used by the patient. As you study the following terms, write each definition and word a minimum of three times (use a separate sheet of paper), pronouncing the word aloud each time. Note that the word and the **basic definition** are in a green shaded box, if you choose to learn only the abbreviated form of the definition. A more detailed description follows most words. Once you have mastered each word to your satisfaction, check the box provided beside the word.

☐ **anorexia**
(an-oh-**REK**-see-ah)
  an- = without
  -orexia = appetite
	Lack or loss of appetite.

☐ **anxiety** (ang-**ZIGH**-eh-tee)	A feeling of apprehension, worry, uneasiness, or dread, especially of the future. **Anxiety** is defined as a vague, uneasy feeling, the source of which is often nonspecific or unknown to the individual.

☐ **bradycardia**
(**brad**-ee-**KAR**-dee-ah)
  brady- = slow
  cardi/o = heart
  -ia = condition
	A slow heart rate characterized by a pulse rate under 60 beats per minute.
	
	The heart rate normally slows during sleep, and in some physically fit people the heart rate may be slow.

☐ **chest pain**	A feeling of discomfort in the chest area. This may be described as tightness, aching, squeezing, pressing, heaviness, crushing, strangling, indigestion, or burning or as a choking feeling in the throat.

☐ **cyanosis**
(sigh-ah-**NO**-sis)
  cyan/o = blueness
  -osis = condition
	Slightly bluish, grayish, slatelike, or dark discoloration of the skin due to the presence of abnormal amounts of reduced hemoglobin in the blood.
	
	Bluish discoloration of the skin and mucous membranes, especially of the lips, tongue, and fingernail beds.

☐ **dyspnea**
(**DISP**-nee-ah)
  dys- = bad, difficult, painful,
     disordered
  -pnea = breathing
	Difficult breathing; air hunger resulting in labored or difficult breathing, sometimes accompanied by pain (normal when caused by vigorous work or athletic activity).
	
	Audible labored breathing, distressed anxious expression, dilated nostrils, protrusion of abdomen and expanded chest, gasping, and marked **cyanosis** are among the symptoms of someone with **dyspnea**. The term refers to shortness of breath.

☐ **edema** (eh-**DEE**-mah)	A local or generalized condition in which the body tissues contain an excessive amount of tissue fluid; swelling. Generalized **edema** is sometimes called dropsy. **Pitting edema** is swelling, usually of the skin of the extremities, that when pressed firmly with a finger will maintain the dent produced by the finger. **Dependent edema** is a fluid accumulation in the tissues influenced by gravity; usually greater in the lower extremities than in tissue levels above the level of the heart.
☐ **fatigue** (**FAH**-teeg)	A feeling of tiredness or weariness resulting from continued activity or as a side effect from some psychotropic drug; A state of exhaustion or a loss of strength or endurance.

| □ **fever** | Elevation of temperature above the normal. |
| (**FEE**-ver) | The normal temperature taken orally is 98.6° F. However, it may be within the range of normal if it is one degree above or one degree below this value. |

| □ **headache** | A diffuse pain in different portions of the head and not confined to any nerve distribution area. |
| (**HED**-ache) | May be acute or chronic; may be frontal, temporal, or occipital; may be confined to one side of the head or to the region immediately over one eye. The pain may be dull and aching or acute and almost unbearable. It may be intermittently intense or throbbing or a pressure where the head feels as if it will burst. The medical term for a headache is *cephalalgia*. |

| □ **nausea** | Unpleasant sensation, usually preceding **vomiting**. |
| (**NAW**-see-ah) | Intense pain can cause **nausea**. |

| □ **pallor** | Lack of color, paleness; an unnatural paleness or absence of color in the skin. |
| (**PAL**-or) | |

| □ **palpitation** | Rapid, violent, or throbbing pulsation, as an abnormally rapid throbbing or fluttering of the heart. The **palpitation** is felt by the patient. |
| (pal-pih-**TAY**-shun) | |

| □ **sweat** | Perspiration; the liquid secreted by the sweat glands, having a salty taste. |
| (**SWET**) | The medical term for profuse sweating is *diaphoresis*. |

□ **tachycardia**	Abnormal rapidity of heart action, usually defined as a heart rate over 100 beats per minute.
(**tak**-ee-**CAR**-dee-ah)	
tachy- = rapid	
cardi/o = heart	
-ia = condition	

| □ **vomiting** | Ejection through the mouth of the gastric content. |
| (**VOM**-it-ing) | The forcible expulsion of the content of the stomach through the mouth; also called emesis. |

| □ **weakness** | Lacking physical strength or vigor (energy). |
| (**WEEK**-ness) | |

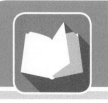

Review Checkpoint

Check your understanding of this section by completing the **Common Signs and Symptoms** exercises in your workbook.

Pathological Conditions

As you study the pathological conditions of the cardiovascular system, note that the **basic definition** is in a green shaded box followed by a detailed description in regular print. The phonetic pronunciation is directly beneath each term, as well as a breakdown of the component parts of the term where applicable.

The pathological conditions are grouped into four categories: pathological conditions of the heart, pathological conditions of the blood vessels, congenital heart diseases, and arrhythmias.

Pathological Conditions of the Heart

angina pectoris

(an-**JI**-nah *or* **AN**-jin-nah **PECK**-tor-is)

Angina pectoris is severe pain and constriction about the heart, usually radiating to the left shoulder and down the left arm, creating a feeling of pressure in the anterior chest.

Angina is caused by an insufficient supply of blood to the **myocardium**. This **ischemia** produces pain that can vary from substernal pressure to severe, agonizing pain. The person with an angina attack experiences classic signs such as burning, squeezing, and tightness in the chest that may radiate to the neck and left arm and shoulder blade. **Nausea** and vomiting sometimes accompany the pain. The individual may have a sense of impending death, an apprehension very characteristic of angina.

In susceptible individuals, angina attacks are frequently triggered by conditions that increase the oxygen demand of the **myocardium** (such as exertion or stress). An important characteristic of anginal pain is that it subsides when the precipitating cause is removed. An attack usually lasts less than 15 minutes and not more than 30 minutes. If the pain persists for more than 30 minutes, the individual should see a physician immediately because these symptoms could also be those of an impending **myocardial infarction** (heart attack).

Treatment of angina consists of improving the oxygen supply to the **myocardium** by administering vasodilators such as nitroglycerine preparations to relieve the pain. If the individual does not respond to these measures, further testing will be necessary to determine the appropriate method of treatment.

cardiac tamponade

(**CAR**-dee-ak **TAM**-poh-nod)

cardi/o = heart
-ac = pertaining to

Compression of the heart caused by the accumulation of blood or other fluid within the pericardial sac. (There is normally just enough fluid within this cavity to lubricate the area.) The accumulation of fluid in the pericardial cavity prevents the ventricles from adequately filling or pumping blood. **Cardiac tamponade** is a life-threatening emergency if untreated.

Cardiac tamponade is often associated with **pericarditis** (inflammation of the pericardial sac) caused by bacterial or viral infections. Other conditions that can lead to cardiac tamponade include (but may not be limited to) wounds to the heart, heart surgery, end-stage lung cancer, and acute myocardial infarction (heart attack).

The patient experiences symptoms such as **anxiety**, restlessness, chest pain that is worse with a deep breath, **dyspnea**, tachypnea, fainting, and light-headedness. Sometimes the chest pain may improve when the patient leans forward or sits up straight. Upon examination with a stethoscope, the patient's heart sounds may be weak, the blood pressure may be low, the peripheral pulses may be weak or absent, and the neck veins may be distended.

An echocardiogram, CT of the chest, or MRI of the chest may be ordered to confirm the fluid in the pericardial sac. Cardiac tamponade requires immediate intervention. Treatment is aimed at relieving the symptoms, improving heart function, and treating the tamponade to save the patient's life. The intervention of choice is a pericardiocentesis (surgical puncture of the sac around the heart) to remove the fluid from the pericardial sac and relieve the pressure.

cardiomyopathy (**CAR**-dee-oh-my-**OP**-ah-thee) cardi/o = heart my/o = muscle -pathy = disease	**Cardiomyopathy** is disease of the heart muscle itself, primarily affecting the pumping ability of the heart. This noninflammatory disease of the heart results in enlargement of the heart (cardiomegaly) and dysfunction of the ventricles of the heart.

The patient typically experiences symptoms similar to those of **congestive heart failure: fatigue**, **dyspnea**, rapid heartbeat (**tachycardia**), palpitations, and occasionally chest pain. Cardiomyopathy is divided into three groups: dilated, hypertrophic, and restrictive. This is based on the defects in structure and function of the diseased heart. Treatment is determined by the type of cardiomyopathy and is aimed at relieving the symptoms of congestion and reducing the workload of the heart.

congestive heart failure (kon-**JESS**-tiv heart failure)	Condition characterized by weakness, breathlessness, and abdominal discomfort. Edema in the lower portions of the body resulting from the flow of the blood through the vessels being slowed (venous stasis) and the outflow of blood from the left side of the heart is reduced. The pumping ability of the heart is progressively impaired to the point that it no longer meets bodily needs; also known as cardiac failure.

The principal feature in **congestive heart failure** is increased intravascular volume. Congestion of the tissues results from increased arterial and venous pressure due to decreased cardiac output in the failing heart.

Left-sided cardiac failure occurs when the left ventricle is unable to sufficiently pump the blood that enters it from the lungs. This causes increased pressure in the pulmonary circulation, which results in the forcing of fluid into the pulmonary tissues, creating pulmonary edema (congestion). The patient experiences dyspnea, cough (mostly moist sounding), **fatigue**, **tachycardia**, restlessness, and **anxiety**.

Right-sided cardiac failure occurs when the right side of the heart is unable to empty its blood volume sufficiently and cannot accommodate all of the blood it receives from the venous circulation. This results in congestion of the viscera and the peripheral tissues. The patient experiences **edema** of the lower extremities (**pitting edema**), weight gain, enlargement of the liver (**hepatomegaly**), distended neck veins, **ascites**, **anorexia**, **nocturia**, and weakness.

Treatment involves promoting rest to reduce the workload on the heart, medications to increase the strength and efficiency of the heartbeat, and medications to eliminate the accumulation of fluids within the body. Dietary sodium may also be restricted.

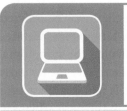

Media Link

Learn more about **congestive heart failure** by viewing the **CHF** animation on the Student Companion Website.

---

coronary artery disease

(**KOR**-oh-nair-ree **AR**-ter-ee dih-**ZEEZ**)

coron/o = heart
-ary = pertaining to
arter/o = artery
-y = noun ending

Coronary artery disease is the narrowing of the coronary arteries to the extent that adequate blood supply to the **myocardium** is prevented.

The narrowing is usually caused by **atherosclerosis**. It may progress to the point that the heart muscle is damaged due to lack of blood supply (**ischemia**) as the **lumen** of the **coronary artery** narrows. When the **lumen** of the artery is narrowed and the wall is rough, there is a great tendency for clots to form, creating the possibility for thrombotic occlusion of the vessel.

As a result of the **ischemia** of the myocardial muscle, the individual experiences a burning, squeezing tightness in the chest that may radiate to the neck, shoulder blade, and left arm. **Nausea**, vomiting, sweating, and **anxiety** may also accompany the pain.

Accepted treatments for occluded coronary arteries (that reduce or prevent sufficient flow of blood to the **myocardium**) include medications, percutaneous transluminal coronary angioplasty, directional coronary atherectomy, and coronary bypass surgery.

1. Medications may be used alone or in conjunction with other types of therapy.

2. **Percutaneous transluminal coronary angioplasty** is a nonsurgical procedure in which a catheter, equipped with a small inflatable balloon on the end, is inserted into the femoral artery and is threaded up the aorta (under X-ray visualization) into the narrowed **coronary artery**. When properly positioned, the balloon is carefully inflated, compressing the fatty deposits against the side of the walls of the artery and thus enlarging the opening of the artery to increase blood flow through the artery. Once the plaque is compressed against the

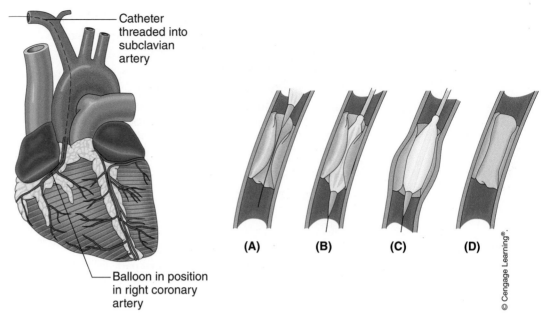

Catheter threaded into subclavian artery

(A)   (B)   (C)   (D)

© Cengage Learning®.

Balloon in position in right coronary artery

Figure 10-8 Balloon angioplasty (PTCA)

walls of the artery, the balloon-tipped catheter is then removed or replaced with a stent (a mesh tube used to hold the artery). Typically, a stent remains in place permanently unless re-occlusion occurs. This procedure is also called a balloon catheter dilation or a balloon angioplasty. See *Figure 10-8.*

3. **Directional coronary atherectomy** uses a catheter (AtheroCath), which has a small mechanically driven cutter that shaves the plaque and stores it in a collection chamber. See *Figure 10-9.*

The plaque is then removed from the artery when the device is withdrawn. This procedure usually lasts from one to three hours and requires overnight hospitalization.

During the atherectomy procedure, the patient remains awake but sedated. The catheter is inserted into the femoral artery and is advanced into position using X-ray visualization as a guide. Once in place, the catheter balloon is inflated, pressing the cutting device against the plaque on the opposite wall of the artery. This causes the plaque to protrude into the window of the cutting device. As this happens, the rotating blade of the cutting device then shaves off the plaque, storing it in the tip of the catheter until removal from the body. The process is repeated several times, using the cutting device, to widen the opening of the artery at the blockage site. If the medications, angioplasty, and atherectomy are not successful methods of treatment or the **coronary artery disease** is severe, coronary by pass surgery will then be the treatment of choice.

4. **Coronary bypass surgery** is designed to increase the blood flow to the myocardial muscle and involves bypass grafts to the coronary arteries that reroute the blood flow around the occluded area of the **coronary artery**. See *Figure 10-10.*

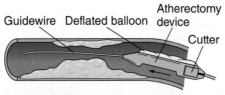

Guidewire   Deflated balloon   Atherectomy device   Cutter

1. In coronary atherectomy procedures, a special cutting device with a deflated balloon on one side and an opening on the other is pushed over a wire down the coronary artery.

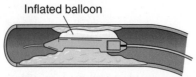

Inflated balloon

2. When the device is within a coronary artery narrowing, the balloon is inflated, so that part of the atherosclerotic plaque is "squeezed" into the opening of the device.

3. When the physician starts rotating the cutting blade, pieces of plaque are shaved off into the device.

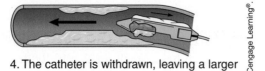

4. The catheter is withdrawn, leaving a larger opening for blood flow.

© Cengage Learning®.

Figure 10-9 Directional coronary atherectomy

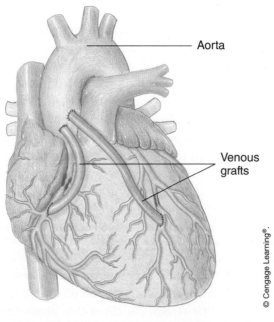

Aorta

Venous grafts

© Cengage Learning®.

Figure 10-10 Coronary artery bypass surgery

Grafts are made from veins taken from other parts of the body (usually the saphenous vein from the leg) and connected to the **coronary artery** above and below the **occlusion**. This **anastomosis** (plural: *anastomoses*) joins the two vessels, restoring the normal flow of oxygenated blood to the **myocardium**.

endocarditis
 	
(**en**-doh-car-**DYE**-tis)
  endo- = within
  cardi/o = heart
  -itis = inflammation
	Inflammation of the membrane lining of the valves and chambers of the heart caused by direct invasion of bacteria or other organisms and leading to deformity **of** the valve **cusps**. Abnormal growths called **vegetations** are formed on or within the membrane.

Endocarditis, also called bacterial endocarditis, is most frequently caused by infection from streptococcal bacteria. Other causative microorganisms include other bacteria, such as staphylococci, pneumococci, and enterococci; fungi; and rickettsiae. Patients who have rheumatic heart disease, who have had prosthetic valve surgery, or who have **mitral valve prolapse** are at greater risk for bacterial endocarditis.

The onset of bacterial endocarditis is misleading and may imitate many systemic diseases, with no early signs of cardiac involvement. There may be weakness and **fatigue**, an intermittent fever that persists for weeks, and night sweats. Chills, **malaise**, and **arthralgia** are also frequent complaints. A heart **murmur** may be heard that was not present initially.

The damage to the heart valves may cause lesions called vegetations that may break off into the bloodstream, forming **emboli** that lodge in other organs. If the emboli lodge in the small vessels of the skin, small pinpoint hemorrhages called **petechiae** may appear. The possibility of emboli lodging in other organs is also present with **endocarditis**.

Treatment involves the use of antibiotics to destroy the invading microorganism. Therapy will likely continue over the course of several weeks.

hypertensive heart disease (**high**-per-**TEN**-siv heart dih-**ZEEZ**)	**Hypertensive heart disease** is a result of long-term **hypertension**. The heart is affected because it must work against increased resistance due to increased pressure in the arteries.

The heart enlarges in an attempt to compensate for the increased cardiac workload. Cardiac failure can occur if the underlying **hypertension** is not treated. (**Hypertension** is discussed later in this chapter.)

mitral valve prolapse (**MY**-tral valve proh-**LAPS**)	**Mitral valve prolapse** is drooping of one or both cusps of the mitral valve back into the left atrium during ventricular systole (when the heart is pumping blood), resulting in incomplete closure of the valve mitral insufficiency.

Normally the mitral valve would completely close to prevent the backflow of blood into the left atrium during **systole**. Mitral valve prolapse is also known as click-murmur syndrome, Barlow's syndrome, and floppy mitral valve.

Many individuals are symptom free. The improper closing of the mitral valve produces an extra heart sound referred to as a mitral click, which can be heard on auscultation. Approximately 10% of the population has **mitral valve prolapse**.

The condition is relatively **benign**, with symptoms including atypical chest pain and palpitations. Treatment is directed at controlling the symptoms the patient is experiencing. Most patients with mitral valve prolapse no longer require routine pre-dentist antibiotics. The routine use of pre-dental antibiotics may be individualized based upon the particular heart condition and the recommendation of the patient's cardiologist.

myocardial infarction (**my**-oh-**CAR**-dee-al in-**FARC**-shun) my/o = muscle cardi/o = heart -al = pertaining to	Heart attack: a condition caused by **occlusion** of one or more of the coronary arteries. This life-threatening condition results when myocardial tissue is destroyed in areas of the heart that are deprived of an adequate blood supply due to the occluded vessels.

This condition, which is caused by **occlusion** of one or more of the coronary arteries, is a medical emergency that requires immediate attention. To wait may result in loss of life.

Symptoms of a **myocardial infarction** include prolonged heavy pressure or squeezing pain in the center of the chest behind the sternum. The pain may radiate to the shoulder, neck, arm, and fourth and fifth fingers of the left hand. The patient may describe the pain as "crushing" or "viselike," and may clench a fist and hold it over the heart to demonstrate the character of the pain.

Pain associated with a **myocardial infarction** may be similar to anginal pain but usually is severe and is *not* relieved by the same measures that relieve anginal pain. This pain is often accompanied by shortness of breath, **pallor**, cold, clammy skin, profuse sweating, dizziness, nausea, and vomiting.

Treatment involves measures directed at minimizing myocardial damage. This is accomplished by relieving the pain, providing rest, stabilizing the heart rhythm, and reducing the workload of the heart. The most critical period for a person who has suffered a **myocardial infarction** is the first 24 to 48 hours after the attack (the area of infarction can increase in size for several hours or days after the onset of the attack). The mortality rate for myocardial infarctions is approximately 35%, with most deaths occurring within the first 12 hours after the onset of the attack. A **myocardial infarction** may be called an MI, heart attack, or coronary occlusion.

myocarditis (**my**-oh-car-**DYE**-tis) my/o = muscle cardi/o = heart -itis = inflammation	**Inflammation of the myocardium** may be caused by viral or bacterial infections or may be a result of systemic diseases such as **rheumatic fever**. This may also be caused by fungal infections, **serum sickness**, or a chemical agent.

The signs and symptoms of uncomplicated **myocarditis** may be mild or absent and are often nonspecific. They may include symptoms such as **fatigue**, **dyspnea**, **fever**, and heart palpitations. A more complicated case of **myocarditis** can lead to **congestive heart failure**.

Treatment is specific to the underlying cause of **myocarditis** if it is known. Analgesics, oxygen, anti-inflammatory agents, and bed rest help until symptoms have disappeared.

pericarditis (**pair**-ih-kar-**DYE**-tis) peri = around cardi/o = heart -itis = inflammation	Inflammation of the **pericardium** (the saclike membrane that covers the heart muscle). It may be acute **or chronic**.

Pericarditis is usually caused by bacterial infection of the **pericardium**. Other causes include neoplasms, viruses, **rheumatic fever, myocardial infarction**, trauma, and tuberculosis.

The characteristic symptom of **pericarditis** is pain, usually over the precordium (area of the body overlying the heart and part of the lower thorax). The pericardial pain is aggravated by breathing, turning, or twisting of the body. It is relieved by sitting up (**orthopnea**). The characteristic sign of **pericarditis** is a pericardial friction rub that may be heard on auscultation (a grating sound heard as the heart beats).

Other symptoms include **dyspnea, tachycardia, malaise, fever**, and accumulation of fluid within the pericardial cavity. If the fluid accumulates rapidly, the pressure against the heart may result in shocklike symptoms: **pallor**; damp, moist skin; and a drop in blood pressure. The patient may appear extremely ill.

Treatment for **pericarditis** includes determining the underlying cause of **pericarditis** and treating it. If it is a result of bacterial invasion, treatment with antibiotics is in order. The patient is placed on bed rest until the **fever**, chest pain, and friction rub have disappeared. An **analgesic** may be prescribed for the pain.

rheumatic fever (roo-**MAT**-ic fever)	An inflammatory disease that may develop as a delayed reaction to insufficiently treated group A beta-hemolytic streptococcal infection of the upper respiratory tract.

This disorder usually occurs in school-age children (primarily ages 5 to 15) and may affect the joints, heart, central nervous system, skin, and other body tissues.

Early symptoms of **rheumatic fever** include **fever**, joint pains, nosebleeds, abdominal pain, and vomiting. Other symptoms include **polyarthritis, carditis**, and sometimes a late symptom of **Sydenham's chorea**. Mild cases of **rheumatic fever** may last for three to four weeks; severe cases, which include arthritis and **carditis**, may last two to three months. Except for the **carditis**, all of the symptoms of **rheumatic fever** usually subside without any permanent consequences.

Treatment includes bed rest and restriction of activities. Antibiotics are usually administered to ensure that no traces of group A streptococci remain in the body. Salicylates are given to reduce fever, joint pain, and swelling.

The prognosis for **rheumatic fever** depends on the degree of scarring and deformity that may have occurred to the heart valves if the patient developed **carditis**. Involvement of the heart may be evident during acute rheumatic fever, or it may be discovered long after the acute disease has subsided. The damage to the heart muscle and heart valves caused by episodes of **rheumatic fever** is known as **rheumatic heart disease**.

Pathological Conditions of the Blood Vessels

aneurysm (**AN**-yoo-rizm) aneurysm/o = aneurysm	A localized dilation of an artery formed at a weak point in the vessel wall. This weakened area balloons out with each pulsation of the artery. Once an **aneurysm** develops, the tendency is toward an increase in size. The danger of rupture is always a possibility and can lead to hemorrhage and ultimately to death. Aneurysms are most commonly caused by **atherosclerosis** and **hypertension**. Other (less frequent) causes include trauma to the wall of the artery, infection, and congenital defects. The most common site for an **aneurysm** is the aorta, and most of these occur below the renal arteries. Treatment of choice for a large abdominal, aortic aneurysm is surgery. The **aneurysmectomy** involves resection of the **aneurysm** and insertion of a bypass graft. During surgery, the **aneurysm** is removed and circulation is restored by suturing the synthetic graft to the aorta at one end and to the iliac arteries at the other end. *Figure 10-11* illustrates surgical treatment of a large abdominal aneurysm involving the iliac arteries.
arteriosclerosis (ar-**tee**-ree-oh-skleh-**ROH**-sis) arteri/o = artery scler/o = hard, also refers to 　　　　　sclera of the eye -osis = condition	An arterial condition in which there is thickening, hardening, and loss of elasticity of the walls of arteries, resulting in decreased blood supply, especially to the lower extremities and cerebrum. This is also called hardening of the arteries. Symptoms include intermittent **claudication**, changes in skin temperature and color, altered peripheral pulses, **bruits** over the involved artery, headache, dizziness, and memory defects (depending on the organ system involved). Some risk factors for **arteriosclerosis** include **hypertension**,

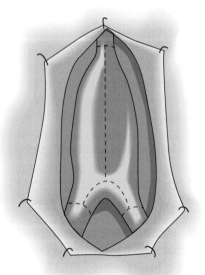 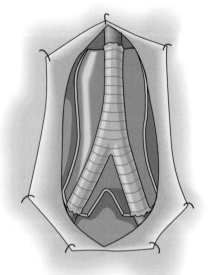

© Cengage Learning®.

Figure 10-11 Surgical repair of an abdominal aneurysm

increased blood lipids (particularly cholesterol and triglycerides), obesity, diabetes, cigarette smoking, inability to cope with stress, and family history of early-onset **atherosclerosis**. Treatment options may include a diet low in saturated fatty acids, medications to lower the blood lipid levels (in conjunction with the low-fat diet), proper rest and regular exercise, avoidance of stress, discontinuing cigarette smoking, and additional treatment specific to the condition for factors such as **hypertension**, diabetes, and obesity.

hypertension (**high**-per-**TEN**-shun) hyper- = excessive	A condition in which the patient has a higher blood pressure than that judged to be normal;

Characterized by elevated blood pressure persistently exceeding 140/90 mmHg; often asymptomatic.

Essential hypertension, (also called primary **hypertension**) accounting for approximately 90% of all **hypertension**, has no single known cause. Leading risk factors include hypercholesterolemia (high cholesterol level in the blood), obesity, high serum sodium level (high level of sodium in the blood), and a family history of high blood pressure.

There are also physical conditions that can cause **hypertension**, including complications of pregnancy and kidney disease. This type of **hypertension** is known as **secondary hypertension**, accounting for approximately 10% or less of all **hypertension**. Treatment of the primary condition can reduce the elevated blood pressure in secondary hypertension.

Malignant hypertension is a term given to **hypertension** that is severe and rapidly progressive. It is most common in African American men under the age of 40. Malignant hypertension is characterized by a diastolic pressure higher than 120 mmHg, severe headaches, confusion, and blurred vision. Unless medical treatment is successful, malignant hypertension may result in a cerebrovascular accident (stroke), fatal uremia (kidney failure), **myocardial infarction** (heart attack), or **congestive heart failure**.

Generally, treatment for **hypertension** includes medications designed to control the blood pressure, and a diet low in sodium, saturated fats, and calories for obesity. Patients are advised to exercise, to avoid stress, and to get proper rest.

peripheral arterial occlusive disease (per-**IF**-er-al ar-**TEE**-ree-al oh-**KLOO**-siv dih-**ZEEZ**)	Obstruction of the arteries in the extremities (predominantly the legs). The leading cause of this disease is **atherosclerosis**, which leads to narrowing of the **lumen** of the artery. The classic symptom of **peripheral arterial occlusive disease** is intermittent **claudication**, which is a cramplike pain in the muscles brought on by exercise and relieved by rest.

The patient may experience a feeling of coldness or numbness in the affected extremity. The extremity may appear pale when elevated or a ruddy, cyanotic color when allowed to dangle over the side of the bed. Observations of the color of the extremity, the feel (e.g., coolness) of the extremity, and the strength of the pulses is important for proper assessment of this condition. Unequal strength of pulses between extremities and absence of a pulse, which is normally **palpable**, are reliable signs of arterial occlusion.

Peripheral arterial disease is usually found in individuals over age 50 and most often in men. The obstructive lesions are essentially confined to segments of the arterial system in the lower extremities, extending from the abdominal aorta, below the renal arteries, to the popliteal artery (behind the knee). See *Figure 10-12*.

Treatment involves exercises designed to promote arterial blood flow in the extremities, avoidance of nicotine (which causes **vasoconstriction**), and measures necessary to control the contributing risk factors such as diabetes, **hyperlipidemia**, and **hypertension**.

If the condition is severe enough, surgical intervention may become necessary. The most common surgical procedure to improve the blood flow beyond the **occlusion** is a vascular bypass graft. This is the same type of bypass graft surgery discussed in the section on coronary artery disease, where the occluded area is "bypassed" with a graft attached above and below the blocked area (thus restoring a normal blood flow pattern to the vessel).

Raynaud's phenomenon (ray-**NOZ** feh-**NOM**-eh-non)	Intermittent attacks of **vasoconstriction** of the arterioles (causing **pallor** of the fingers or toes), followed by **cyanosis** and then redness before returning to normal color; initiated by exposure to cold or emotional disturbance.

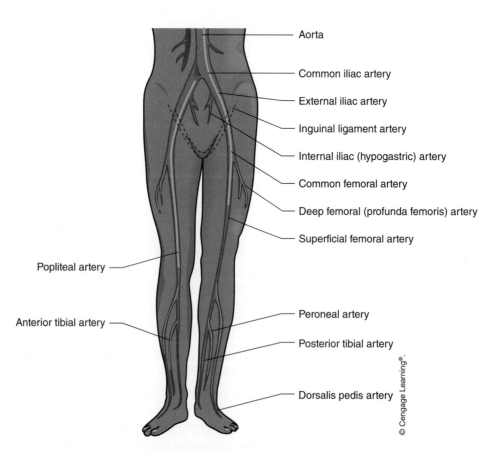

© Cengage Learning®.

Figure 10-12 Common sites for peripheral arterial occlusive disease

The characteristic color change of **Raynaud's phenomenon** is described as white (**pallor**), blue (cyanosis), and red (return of color). Numbness, tingling, and burning pain occur as the color changes. Normal color and sensation are restored by heat.

Raynaud's phenomenon can be secondary to physical conditions or idiopathic (cause unknown). It occurs most frequently in young women ages 18 to 30 and is usually treated by protecting the body and extremities from exposure to cold and sometimes use of medications to calm the individual and to dilate the blood vessels.

thrombophlebitis (**throm**-boh-fleh-**BY**-tis) thromb/o = clot phleb/o = vein -itis = inflammation	Inflammation of a vein associated with the formation of a thrombus (clot); usually occurs in an extremity, most frequently a leg.

Thrombophlebitis is classified as either superficial or deep. **Superficial thrombophlebitis** is usually obvious and is accompanied by a cordlike or thready appearance to the vessel, which is **palpable**. The vessel is extremely sensitive to pressure. The extremity may be pale, cold, and swollen. **Deep vein thrombosis (DVT)** occurs primarily in the lower legs, thighs, and pelvic area. It is not as evident as superficial thrombophlebitis and may be characterized by symptoms such as aching or cramping pain in the legs. *Figure 10-13* provides a visual reference for superficial versus deep veins in the development of phlebitis. **Homan's sign** (the pain experienced in the calf of the leg with forced dorsiflexion of the foot) is often evident in the physical examination of a person with suspected DVT. A diagnosis of DVT based only on the presenting clinical signs is often unreliable. A more accurate diagnosis can be achieved with the use of specific diagnostic procedures such as ultrasonography and venography in conjunction with the clinical signs.

Thrombophlebitis may be caused by poor venous circulation, which may be due to obesity, **congestive heart failure**, sitting in one position for long periods of time without exercising (as in riding in an automobile), immobility of an extremity for long periods of time, damage to the inner lining of the vein caused by trauma to the vessel (e.g., venipuncture); and a tendency of the blood to coagulate more rapidly than normal (hypercoagulability).

Treatment for **thrombophlebitis** of the leg involves complete bed rest and elevation of the affected extremity until the tenderness has subsided, which is usually five to seven days. Warm moist compresses may

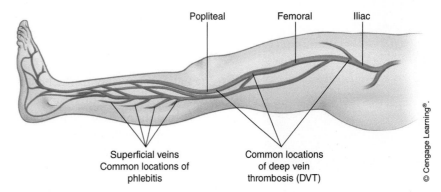

Popliteal   Femoral   Iliac

Superficial veins
Common locations of
phlebitis

Common locations
of deep vein
thrombosis (DVT)

© Cengage Learning®.

Figure 10-13 Superficial vs. deep veins in the development of phlebitis and thrombus

be applied to the affected area to help relieve some of the pain and to treat inflammation. Analgesics may be given for the pain. Vital signs are taken frequently and circulation of the affected extremity is checked. Anticoagulants are not routinely used for superficial thrombophlebitis but are used to treat deep vein thrombophlebitis. Elastic stockings, which support venous circulation (antiembolic stockings), are recommended when the patient becomes ambulatory.

| **varicose veins**
(**VAIR**-ih-kohs veins) | Enlarged, superficial veins; a twisted, dilated vein with incompetent valves. |

Veins have valves that keep the blood flowing in one direction only. In normal veins, the wall of the vein is strong enough to withstand the lateral pressure of the blood, and the blood flows through the valves in one direction. In **varicose veins**, however, the dilation of the vein from long periods of pressure prevents the complete closure of the valves, resulting in backflow of blood in the veins, creating the varicosities. See *Figure 10-14*.

Patients with **varicose veins** often complain of pain and muscle cramps, with a feeling of heaviness in the legs, moderate swelling, easy fatigability, minimal skin discoloration, and **palpable** distended veins (that may have a cordlike feel to them). Treatment includes conservative measures such as rest and elevation of the affected extremity along with the use of elastic stockings. Another nonsurgical treatment of **varicose veins** and spider veins is sclerotherapy.

Sclerotherapy is a form of treatment that involves the injection of a chemical irritant (sclerosing agent) into the varicosed vein. The sclerosing agent irritates the inner lining of the vein (causing localized inflammation of the vein), followed by formation of fibrous tissue (which closes the vein). Following the injections, compression bandages are applied to the leg (elastic leg wraps) and are worn for approximately five days. This is followed with the use of full therapeutic support hose for several weeks.

If the varicosities are severe enough, surgical intervention may become necessary. **Vein stripping** is a surgical procedure that consists of ligation (tying off) of the saphenous vein. A nylon wire is then inserted into the saphenous vein from an incision in the ankle and is threaded up the vein to the groin area. The wire is brought out of the vein in the groin area and is capped. It is then pulled downward to the ankle incision, "stripping" the vein.

The patient may stay in the hospital overnight following vein stripping surgery or may have this done on an outpatient basis. In either case, bed rest is maintained for 24 hours following surgery. Elastic compression bandages are applied to the leg, from the toe area to the groin, and remain on for approximately one week following surgery. It is important to promote exercise and movement of the legs and to elevate the head of the patient's bed to promote venous circulation. The patient will begin walking for short periods of time 24 to 48 hours after surgery.

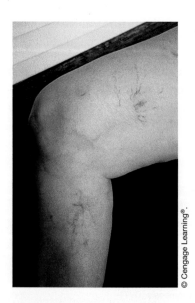

© Cengage Learning®.

Figure 10-14 Varicose veins (venous star)

venous insufficiency

(**VEE**-nuss in-soo-**FISH**-in-see)

ven/o = vein

-ous = pertaining to

An abnormal circulatory condition characterized by decreased return of venous blood from the legs to the trunk of the body.

Venous insufficiency occurs as a result of prolonged venous hypertension, which stretches the veins and damages the valves. Standing or sitting in one position for long periods of time, pregnancy, and obesity may cause chronically distended veins, which leads to damaged valves.

When damaged valves cause ongoing swelling in the legs, blood begins to pool in the veins. This can lead to chronic venous insufficiency (CVI), which can eventually cause ulcerations in the skin if not properly treated.

Swollen ankles are possibly the most common symptom. Individuals who stand or sit with their feet down for long periods of time may experience aching or a feeling of heaviness in the legs.

Treatment includes elevating the legs often; wiggling the toes, shifting the body position, and lifting oneself up on the balls of the feet if the individual must sit for long periods of time; daily exercise to promote circulation in the legs; and possible use of elastic stockings. Individuals are encouraged to avoid standing or sitting with the legs down for more than one hour at a time.

Congenital Heart Diseases

coarctation of the aorta

(**koh**-ark-**TAY**-shun)

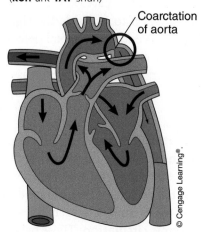

Coarctation of aorta

© Cengage Learning®.

Figure 10-15 Coarctation of the aorta

A congenital heart defect characterized by a localized narrowing of the aorta, which results in increased blood pressure in the upper extremities (area proximal to the defect) and decreased blood pressure in the lower extremities (area distal to the defect). See *Figure 10-15*.

The classic sign of **coarctation of the aorta** is a contrast in pulsations and blood pressures in the arms and legs. The femoral, popliteal, and pedal pulses are weak or delayed in comparison with the strong bounding pulses found in the arms and carotid arteries. See *Figure 10-18* for pulse points of the body. Surgical correction of the defect is curative if the disease is diagnosed early.

patent ductus arteriosus

(**PAY**-tent **DUCK**-tus ar-**TEE**-ree-**OH**-sis)

Patent ductus arteriosus is an abnormal opening between the **pulmonary artery** and the aorta caused by failure of the fetal ductus arteriosus to close after birth. This defect is seen primarily in premature infants. See *Figure 10-16*.

During the prenatal period, the ductus arteriosus serves as a normal pathway in the fetal circulatory system. It is a large channel between the **pulmonary artery** and the aorta, which is open, allowing fetal blood to bypass the lungs (passing from the **pulmonary artery** to the descending

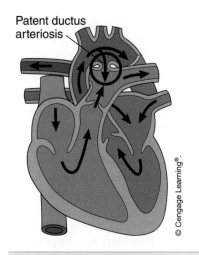

Patent ductus arteriosis

© Cengage Learning®.

aorta, and ultimately to the placenta). This passageway is no longer needed after birth and usually closes during the first 24 to 72 hours of life, once the normal circulatory pattern of the cardiovascular system is established.

If the ductus arteriosus remains open after birth, blood under pressure from the aorta is shunted into the **pulmonary artery**, resulting in oxygenated blood *recirculating* through the pulmonary circulation. A strain is placed on the heart due to the pumping of blood a second time through the pulmonary circulation. Treatment for **patent ductus arteriosus** is surgery to close the open channel.

Figure 10-16 Patent ductus arteriosus

tetralogy of Fallot (teh-**TROL**-oh-jee of fal-**LOH**)	A congenital heart **anomaly** that consists of four defects: pulmonary stenosis, interventricular septal defect, dextroposition (shifting to the right) of the aorta so that it receives blood from both ventricles, and hypertrophy of the right ventricle; named for the French physician, Etienne Fallot, who first described the condition.

(1) Pulmonary stenosis

(3) Overriding aorta

(2) Ventricular septal defect

(4) Right ventricular hypertrophy

© Cengage Learning®.

Figure 10-17 Tetralogy of Fallot

Further description of **tetralogy of Fallot** identifies the four defects in more detail: the (1) pulmonary stenosis (narrowing of the opening into the **pulmonary artery** from the right ventricle) restricts the flow of blood from the heart to the lungs; the (2) interventricular septal defect creates a right-to-left shunt between the ventricles, allowing deoxygenated blood from the right ventricle to communicate with the oxygenated blood in the left ventricle (which then exits the heart via the aorta); the (3) shifting of the aorta to the right causes it to override the right ventricle and thus communicate with the interventricular septal defect, allowing the oxygen-poor blood to pass more easily into the aorta; and the (4) hypertrophy of the right ventricle occurs because of the increased work required to pump blood through the obstructed **pulmonary artery**. See *Figure 10-17*.

Most infants born with **tetralogy of Fallot** display varying degrees of **cyanosis**, which may typically occur during activities that increase the need for oxygen such as crying, feeding, or straining with a bowel movement. The **cyanosis** develops as a result of the decreased flow of blood to the lungs for oxygenation and as a result of the mixing of oxygenated and deoxygenated blood released into the **systemic circulation**. These babies are termed "blue babies." Treatment for **tetralogy of Fallot** involves surgery to correct the multiple defects.

transposition of the great vessels (tranz-poh-**ZIH**-shun)	A condition in which the two major arteries of the heart are reversed in position, which results in two noncommunicating circulatory systems.

The aorta arises from the right ventricle (instead of the left) and delivers unoxygenated blood to the **systemic circulation**. This blood is returned from the body tissues back to the right atrium and right ventricle without being oxygenated because it does not pass through the lungs.

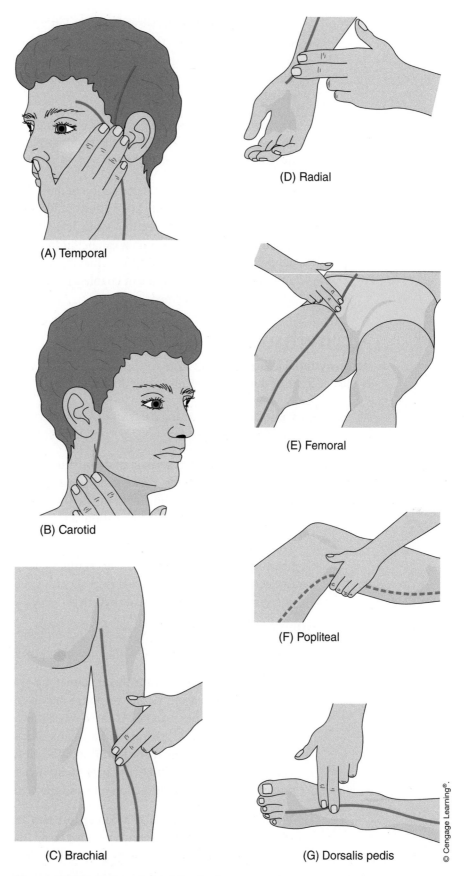

Figure 10-18 Pulse points of the body

(A) Temporal

(B) Carotid

(C) Brachial

(D) Radial

(E) Femoral

(F) Popliteal

(G) Dorsalis pedis

© Cengage Learning®.

The **pulmonary artery** arises from the left ventricle (instead of the right) and delivers blood to the lungs for oxygenation. The oxygenated blood returns from the lungs to the left atrium and the left ventricle and back to the lungs without sending the oxygenated blood throughout the **systemic circulation**.

This congenital **anomaly** creates an oxygen deficiency to the body tissues and an excessive workload on the right and left ventricles. The infant is usually severely cyanotic at birth.

Treatment involves surgical correction of the defect and repositioning of the vessels to reestablish a normal pattern of blood flow through the circulatory system. Surgical correction of the defect is delayed, if possible, until six months of age (when the infant can better tolerate the procedure). Immediate **palliative** surgery, aimed at achieving adequate mixing of oxygenated and unoxygenated blood, can enable the child to survive until corrective surgery can be performed.

Arrhythmias

An **arrhythmia** is any deviation from the normal pattern of the heartbeat. The following is a list of some of the more common arrhythmias.

atrial flutter (**AY**-tree-al flutter)	Condition in which the contractions of the atria become extremely rapid, at the rate of between 250 and 350 beats per minute.

An important characteristic of **atrial flutter** is that a therapeutic block occurs at the AV node, preventing some impulse transmission. This, in turn, prevents the rapid firing of the impulses to the ventricles, which could result in ventricular fibrillation, a life-threatening **arrhythmia**.

Treatment for **atrial flutter** is medication given to slow and strengthen the heartbeat. If drug therapy is unsuccessful, **atrial flutter** will often respond to electrical cardioversion (electrical shock), which will slow the heart rate and restore the heart's normal rhythm.

fibrillation (atrial/ventricular) (**fih**-brill-**AY**-shun)	Atrial fibrillation is extremely rapid, incomplete contractions of the atria resulting in disorganized and uncoordinated twitching of the atria.

The rate of contractions for the atria may be as high as 350 to 600 beats per minute, with a ventricular response rate of contraction being between 120 to 200 beats per minute. At these rates, the ventricles cannot contract efficiently or recover adequately between contractions. These inefficient contractions of the heart reduce the blood flow, leading to angina and **congestive heart failure**. Treatment involves medication directed at decreasing the atrial contraction rate and the ventricular response rate.

Ventricular fibrillation is a condition similar to atrial fibrillation, which results in rapid, tremulous (quivering like a bowl of gelatin), and ineffectual contractions of the ventricles. The patient has no audible heartbeat, no palpable pulse, no respiration, and no blood circulation. If prolonged, this will lead to cardiac arrest.

Immediate treatment is necessary, consisting of cardiopulmonary resuscitation (CPR) and defibrillation (electrical countershock using defibrillation paddles). Ventricular fibrillation will result in death if an effective rhythm is not reestablished within three to four minutes.

| **heart block (AV)** | **Heart block** is an interference with the normal conduction of electric impulses that control activity of the heart muscle. |

In first-degree AV block, the impulse initiated by the **SA node** is conducted normally through the atria but is slowed when passing through the AV node (i.e., AV block). After the impulse passes through the AV node, it continues normally through the ventricles.

AV block may be a result of organic heart disease or the effect of digitalis. It may also be a complication of a **myocardial infarction** or **rheumatic fever**. There is no specific treatment for first-degree AV block, but it should be watched because it may precede higher degrees of block.

ventricular tachycardia
(ven-**TRIK**-yoo-lar **tak**-ee-**CAR**-dee-ah)
   ventricul/o = ventricles of the heart or brain
   -ar = pertaining to
   tachy- = rapid
   cardi/o = heart
   -ia = condition

Ventricular tachycardia is a condition in which the ventricles of the heart beat at a rate greater than 100 beats per minute; characterized by three or more consecutive premature ventricular contractions (PVCs). It is also known as "V-tach" (VT).

Ventricular tachycardia may be non-sustained (lasting less than 30 seconds) or sustained (lasting more than 30 seconds) and may occur in either ventricle. When the ventricles of the heart beat so rapidly, they do not have time to fill with blood before the next beat. This causes the heart to pump less blood than the body needs, thus creating the symptoms: palpitations, light-headedness or dizziness, fainting, **dyspnea**, or angina. Causes of ventricular tachycardia include but may not be limited to ischemic heart disease, cardiomyopathy, **myocardial infarction**, and valvular disease.

Treatment varies according to the symptoms and the underlying cardiac problem. It may become an emergency situation and require cardiopulmonary resuscitation (CPR), electrical defibrillation, or cardioversion (electric shock). Long-term treatment may include the use of antiarrhythmic medications or surgically inserting an **implantable cardioverter defibrillator** (ICD). The ICD is discussed in the section on diagnostic techniques and procedures.

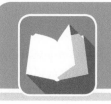

Review Checkpoint

Check your understanding of this section by completing the **Pathological Conditions** exercises in your workbook.

Diagnostic Techniques, Treatments, and Procedures

angiography (**an**-jee-**OG**-rah-fee) angi/o = vessel -graphy = process of recording	X-ray visualization of the internal anatomy of the heart and blood vessels after introducing a radiopaque substance (contrast medium) that promotes the imaging (makes them visible) of internal structures that are otherwise difficult to see on X-ray film. This substance is injected into an artery or a vein.

It is important to perform a hypersensitivity test before the radiographic material is used because the iodine in the contrast material has been known to cause severe allergic reactions in some patients. **Angiography** is used to diagnose conditions such as **myocardial infarction**, occlusion of blood vessels, calcified atherosclerotic plaques, stroke (cerebrovascular accident), **hypertension** of the vessels leading to the liver (portal hypertension), and narrowing of the renal artery.

cardiac catheterization (**CAR**-dee-ak **cath**-eh-ter-ih-**ZAY**-shun) cardi/o = heart -ac = pertaining to	A diagnostic procedure in which a catheter (a hollow, flexible tube) is introduced into a large vein or artery (usually of an arm or a leg) and then threaded through the circulatory system to the heart. **Cardiac catheterization** is used to obtain detailed information about the structure and function of the heart chambers, valves, and the great vessels.

In the case of **coronary artery disease**, the patient may undergo a **cardiac catheterization** to determine the amount of **occlusion** of his or her coronary arteries for the physician to determine the most appropriate treatment. Treatment may consist of coronary artery bypass surgery or percutaneous transluminal coronary angioplasty.

cardiac enzymes test (**CAR**-dee-ak **EN**-zyms test) cardi/o = heart -ac = pertaining to	**Cardiac enzymes tests** are performed on samples of blood obtained by venipuncture to determine the presence of damage to the myocardial muscle.

Cardiac enzymes are present in high concentrations in the myocardial tissue. Tissue damage causes the release of the cardiac enzymes from their normal intracellular area and creates an elevation of serum cardiac enzyme levels. In addition to indicating the presence of damage to the myocardial muscle, the elevated enzyme levels can disclose the timing of the acute cardiac event.

For example, the enzymes most commonly used to detect **myocardial infarction** (heart attack) are creatine kinase (CK) and lactic acid dehydrogenase (LDH). These enzyme levels are elevated after a **myocardial infarction**. Another enzyme level, CK-MB, determines muscle damage to the heart. An elevated CK-MB would indicate that there was myocardial muscle damage. (This particular enzyme level would elevate within 4 to 6 hours after the acute attack and would peak within 18 to 24 hours after the attack.)

computed axial tomography (CAT)

(computed **AK**-see-al toh-**MOG**-rah-fee)

tom/o = to cut
-graphy = process of recording

Computed axial tomography (CAT) is a diagnostic X-ray technique that uses ionizing radiation to produce a cross-sectional image of the body. It is often used to detect aneurysms of the aorta. X-ray signals are fed into a computer, which then turns them into a cross-sectional picture of the section of the body being scanned; called CAT scan.

CAT scans are helpful in evaluating areas of the body difficult to assess using standard X-ray procedures. As is true with **magnetic resonance imaging (MRI)**, patients should be informed that the CAT is a very confining procedure because they are placed within a tubelike structure and should be asked if they are claustrophobic (fear enclosed spaces).

echocardiography

(**ek**-oh-**car**-dee-**OG**-rah-fee)

echo- = sound
cardi/o = heart
-graphy = process of recording

Echocardiography is a diagnostic procedure for studying the structure and motion of the heart. It is useful in evaluating structural and functional changes in a variety of heart disorders. See *Figure 10-19*.

Ultrasound waves pass through the heart (via a transducer), bounce off tissues of varying densities, and are reflected backward (or echoed) to the transducer, creating an image on the graph. Uses for **echocardiography** include (but are not limited to) assessing and detecting atrial tumors, determining the measurement of the ventricular septa and ventricular chambers, and determining the presence of mitral valve motion abnormalities.

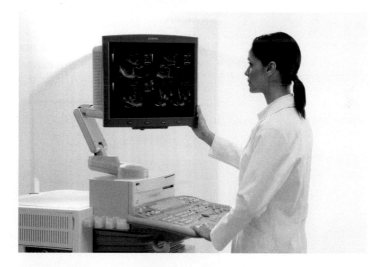

Figure 10-19 An example of an echocardiograph machine
Courtesy of Siemens Medical Solutions USA Inc.

electrocardiogram

(ee-**lek**-troh-**CAR**-dee-oh-**gram**)

electr/o = electrical; electricity
cardi/o = heart
-gram = record or picture

An **electrocardiogram** is a graphic record (visual representation) of the electrical action of the heart as reflected from various angles to the surface of the skin; known as an EKG or ECG.

An EKG is performed with an electrocardiograph, which is the machine that records the electrical activity of the heart to detect transmission of the cardiac impulse throughout the heart muscle. Electrodes are positioned on the chest wall in standardized anatomic positions that will provide the clearest EKG waveforms. See *Figure 10-20*.

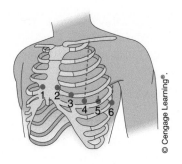

© Cengage Learning®.

The EKG is recorded as a tracing on a strip of graph paper that moves through the machine as the stylus (recording needle) records the impulses. Analysis of the EKG waveforms can assist the physician in identifying disorders of heart rate, rhythm, or conduction, presence of myocardial ischemia, or presence of a **myocardial infarction**.

Figure 10-20 Standard chest lead placements for EKG

event monitor

An **event monitor** is similar to the Holter monitor in that it also records the electrical activity of the heart while the patient goes about usual daily activities. A cardiac event monitor can be used for a longer period of time than a Holter monitor (usually a month).

The electrodes are attached to the chest in the same way as a Holter monitor. The monitor is always on, and when the patient feels any unusual symptoms (such as chest pain, shortness of breath, or palpitations), he or she presses a button on the monitor to record the heart rhythm. Once the recording is made, it can be transmitted over the phone to the doctor for interpretation.

exercise stress testing

A means of assessing cardiac function by subjecting the patient to carefully controlled amounts of physical stress (e.g., using the treadmill). See *Figure 10-21*.

A stress test may be ordered for many reasons, some of which include the following: to determine the cause of chest pain; to screen for ischemic heart problems; to identify any disorders of cardiac rate, rhythm, or conduction; to determine the functional ability of the heart after a **myocardial infarction**; and to identify any heart irregularities that may occur during physical exercise.

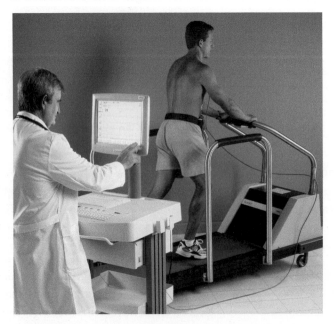

Figure 10-21 A cardiac stress test
Courtesy of Quinton Cardiology, Inc.

During **exercise stress testing**, the patient may walk on a treadmill, climb a set of stairs, or pedal a stationary bicycle. The exercise speed is increased as the patient can tolerate it. EKGs are recorded throughout the procedure. The patient is closely monitored throughout the test, and the procedure is discontinued if the patient shows any signs of distress.

Holter monitoring	A small, portable monitoring device that makes prolonged electrocardiograph recordings on a portable tape recorder. The continuous EKG (ambulatory EKG) is recorded on a magnetic tape recording while the patient conducts normal daily activities. See *Figure 10-22*.

The Holter monitor (not halter) is used to detect heart **dysrhythmias** or evidence of myocardial **ischemia**. It weighs about 2 pounds and can be carried over the shoulder, using the shoulder strap.

The patient usually maintains a diary of his or her daily activities, being careful to note the particular time of any unusual activities performed, any symptoms, or any unusual experiences that occur during the day. The monitor is returned the next day and is examined with a special scanner, analyzed, and interpreted by the doctor.

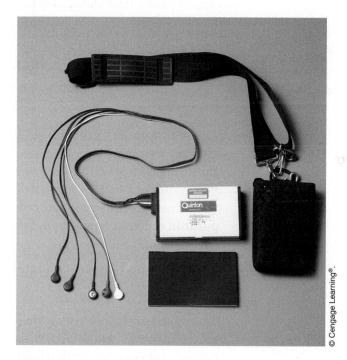

© Cengage Learning®.

Figure 10-22 One type of Holter monitor and supplies

implantable cardioverter defibrillator	An implantable cardioverter defibrillator (ICD) is a small, lightweight, electronic device placed under the skin or muscle in either the chest or abdomen to monitor the heart's rhythm. If an abnormal rhythm occurs, the ICD helps return the heart to its normal rhythm.

An incision is made in the chest wall just below the collarbone. A pocket is created to hold the ICD generator in place. Lead wires covered by soft, flexible plastic are guided (via X-ray monitors) through the vein into the heart. Once in place, the ICD generator is programmed to monitor the rhythm problem.

The capability of the ICD includes but is not limited to anti-tachycardia pacing (ATP), which involves sending a series of pulses to override a fast rhythm; cardioversion, which involves giving one or more small shocks to break up the fast rhythm; and defibrillation, which involves sending a strong shock to the heart to override a very fast, irregular rhythm.

magnetic resonance imaging (MRI) (mag-**NEH**-tic **REHZ**-oh-nans imaging)	**Magnetic resonance imaging (MRI)** involves the use of a strong magnetic field and radiofrequency waves to produce imaging that is valuable in providing images of the heart, large blood vessels, brain, and soft tissue.
	MRI is used to examine the aorta and to detect masses or possible tumors and pericardial disease. It can show the flowing of blood and the beating of the heart. The radiofrequency waves are directed at the heart and an image is produced on the screen.
	Patients with pacemakers, any recently implanted wires or clips, or prosthetic valves are not eligible for MRI because of the magnetic field. Patients should be informed that MRI is a very confining procedure because they are placed within a tubelike structure and should be asked if they are claustrophobic (fear enclosed spaces).

positron emission tomography (PET)
 	
(**PAHZ**-ih-tron *or* **PAWZ**-ih-tron ee-**MISH**-un toh-**MOG**-rah-fee)
   tom/o = to cut
   -graphy = process of recording
	A computerized X-ray technique that uses radioactive substances to examine the blood flow and the metabolic activity of various body structures such as the heart and blood vessels. The patient is given doses of strong radioactive tracers by injection or inhalation. The radiation emitted is measured by the PET camera.

	The PET scanner is helpful in detecting **coronary artery disease**, assessing the progression of narrowing of the coronary arteries (stenosis), and distinguishing between ischemic, infarcted, and normal cardiac tissue. PET is also used in the study and diagnosis of cancer and in the studies of the biochemical activity of the brain. One major disadvantage of the use of **positron emission tomography** is its high cost.

serum lipid test
 	
(**SEE**-rum **LIP**-id test)
   ser/o = blood serum
   lip/o = fat
	A **serum lipid test** measures the amount of fatty substances (cholesterol, triglycerides, and lipoproteins) in a sample of blood obtained by venipuncture.

	These fatty substances, which are insoluble in water, play a major role in the development of **atherosclerosis**. The lipid profile is used to assess the patient's degree of risk for developing **coronary artery disease**.
thallium stress test (**THAL**-ee-um stress test)	The **thallium stress test**, one of several nuclear stress tests, is a combination of exercise stress testing with thallium imaging (myocardial perfusion scan) to assess changes in coronary blood flow during exercise.
	Thallium imaging is used with exercise stress testing to determine if the coronary blood flow changes under stressed conditions such as increased activity. When injected intravenously, thallium concentrates in myocardial tissue in direct proportion to the blood flow to various regions of the myocardium. If severe coronary artery narrowing or decreased blood flow to an area (ischemia) is present, the concentration of thallium will be decreased. The area of decreased concentration of thallium is referred to as a "cold spot."

The thallium is injected intravenously one minute before the end of the exercise stress test. This allows enough time for adequate distribution of the thallium throughout the myocardium before the end of the test. Images of the myocardial tissue are taken immediately and are repeated three to four hours later to assess for any cold spots (areas of little or no concentration of thallium).

If a cold spot appears on the initial imaging but disappears on the repeated image, it is referred to as an ischemic area (area of decreased blood flow). If the cold spot continues to show on the repeated imaging, it indicates an area of no blood flow or an area of **infarction**.

In addition to thallium, other radioactive materials (such as Cardiolite) are used in nuclear stress testing. This is also injected intravenously, and images are taken to assess for any areas of little or no concentration of the radioactive material, which would indicate that the heart muscle does not have enough blood supply. Adenosine, another medication used for nuclear stress testing, increases blood flow to the heart to simulate exercise. This form of pharmacological (chemical) stress testing is used for patients who are unable to exercise on the treadmill. Although chemical stress testing is less physiologic than exercise testing, it is safer and more controllable.

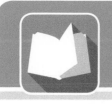

Review Checkpoint

Check your understanding of this section by completing the **Diagnostic Techniques, Treatments, and Procedures** exercises in your workbook.

COMMON ABBREVIATIONS

Abbreviation	Meaning	Abbreviation	Meaning
A Fib	atrial fibrillation	**CABG**	coronary artery bypass graft
AMI	acute myocardial infarction	**CAD**	coronary artery disease
AS	aortic stenosis	**Cath**	catheterization
ASD	atrial septal defect	**CC**	cardiac catheterization
ASHD	arteriosclerotic heart disease	**CCU**	coronary care unit
AV	atrioventricular	**CHD**	coronary heart disease
BBB	bundle branch block	**CHF**	congestive heart failure
BP	blood pressure	**CPR**	cardiopulmonary resuscitation

Abbreviation	Meaning	Abbreviation	Meaning
CT (scan) or CAT (scan)	computed axial tomography (scan)	MS	mitral stenosis
CVD	cardiovascular disease	MVP	mitral valve prolapse
DOE	dyspnea on exertion	PACs	premature atrial contractions
DVT	deep vein thrombosis	PAT	paroxysmal atrial tachycardia
ECG	electrocardiogram	PDA	patent ductus arteriosus
ECHO	echocardiogram	PET	positron emission tomography
EKG	electrocardiogram		
HCVD	hypertensive cardiovascular disease	PTCA	percutaneous transluminal coronary angioplasty
HDL	high-density lipoprotein	PVCs	premature ventricular contractions
ICD	implantable cardioversion defibrillator	SA	sinoatrial
LDL	low-density lipoprotein	V Fib	ventricular fibrillation
MI	myocardial infarction	VSD	ventricular septal defect
MRI	magnetic resonance imaging	VT, V Tach.	ventricular tachycardia

Review Checkpoint

Check your understanding of this section by completing the **Common Abbreviations** exercises in your workbook.

WRITTEN AND AUDIO TERMINOLOGY REVIEW

Review each of the following terms from this chapter. Study the spelling of each term and write the definition in the space provided. Check definitions by looking the term up in the glossary.

Term	Pronunciation	Definition
analgesic	☐ **an**-al-**JEE**-zik	_____
anastomosis	☐ ah-**nas**-toh-**MOH**-sis	_____
aneurysm	☐ **AN**-yoo-rizm	_____

Term	Pronunciation	Definition
aneurysmectomy	☐ **an**-yoo-riz-**MEK**-toh-mee	_____
angina pectoris	☐ **AN**-jih nah **PECK**-tor-is *or* an-**JYE**- nah **PECK**-tor-is	_____
angiography	☐ **an**-jee-**OG**-rah-fee	_____
anomaly	☐ ah-**NOM**-ah-lee	_____
anorexia	☐ **an**-oh-**REK**-see-ah	_____
anxiety	☐ ang-**ZIGH**-eh-tee	_____
aplastic	☐ ay-**PLAS**-tick	_____
arrhythmia	☐ ah-**RITH**-mee-ah	_____
arteriosclerosis	☐ ar-**tee**-ree-oh-skleh-**ROH**-sis	_____
arthralgia	☐ ar-**THRAL**-jee-ah	_____
ascites	☐ ah-**SIGH**-teez	_____
atherosclerosis	☐ **ath**-er-**oh**-skleh-**ROH**-sis	_____
atrial flutter	☐ **AY**-tree-al flutter	_____
benign	☐ bee-**NINE**	_____
bradycardia	☐ **brad**-ee-**KAR**-dee-ah	_____
bruit	☐ brew-**EE**	_____
cardiac catheretization	☐ **CAR**-dee-ak **cath**-eh-ter-ih-**ZAY**-shun	_____
cardiac enzymes test	☐ **CAR**-dee-ak **EN**-zyms test	_____
carditis	☐ car-**DYE**-tis	_____
carotid endarterectomy	☐ kah-**ROT**-id **end**-ar-ter-**ECK**-toh-mee	_____
claudication	☐ **klaw**-dih-**KAY**-shun	_____
computed axial tomography (CAT)	☐ computed **AK**-see-al toh-**MOG**-rah-fee	_____
congestive heart failure	☐ kon-**JESS**-tiv heart failure	_____
coronary artery	☐ **KOR**-ah-nair-ree **AR**-ter-ee	_____
coronary artery disease	☐ **KOR**-ah-nair-ree **AR**-ter-ee dih-**ZEEZ**	_____
cyanosis	☐ **sigh**-ah-**NO**-sis	_____
diastole	☐ dye-**ASS**-toh-lee	_____
dyspnea	☐ **DISP**-nee-ah	_____
dysrhythmia	☐ dis-**RITH**-mee-ah	_____
echocardiography	☐ **ek**-oh-**car**-dee-**OG**-rah-fee	_____
edema	☐ eh-**DEE**-mah	_____
electrocardiogram	☐ ee-**lek**-troh-**CAR**-dee-oh-**gram**	_____

Term	Pronunciation	Definition
embolus	☐ **EM**-boh-lus	_____
endocarditis	☐ **en**-doh-car-**DYE**-tis	_____
epicardium	☐ **ep**-ih-**CARD**-ee-um	_____
fatigue	☐ fah-**TEEG**	_____
fever	☐ **FEE**-ver	_____
fibrillation	☐ **fih**-brill-**AY**-shun	_____
hemostasis	☐ **hee**-moh-**STAY**-sis	_____
hepatomegaly	☐ **hep**-ah-toh-**MEG**-ah-lee	_____
hyperlipidemia	☐ **high**-per-lip-ih-**DEE**-mee-ah	_____
hypertension	☐ **high**-per-**TEN**-shun	_____
hypertensive heart disease	☐ **high**-per-**TEN**-siv heart dih-**ZEEZ**	_____
hypotension	☐ **high**-poh-**TEN**-shun	_____
infarction	☐ in-**FARC**-shun	_____
ischemia	☐ iss-**KEY**-mee-ah	_____
lesion	☐ **LEE**-zhun	_____
leukopenia	☐ **loo**-koh-**PEE**-nee-ah	_____
lipid	☐ **LIP**-id	_____
lumen	☐ **LOO**-men	_____
magnetic resonance imaging (MRI)	☐ mag-**NEH**-tic **REHZ**-oh-nance imaging (MRI)	_____
malaise	☐ mah-**LAYZ**	_____
mediastinum	☐ **mee**-dee-as-**TYE**-num	_____
megaloblastic anemia	☐ **MEG**-ah-loh-**blas**-tick ah-**NEE**-mee-ah	_____
mitral valve prolapse	☐ **MY**-tral valve **PROH**-laps	_____
myelodysplastic syndrome	☐ **my**-eh-loh-dis-**PLAS**-tick **SIN**-drohm	_____
myocardial infarction	☐ **my**-oh-**CAR**-dee-al in-**FARC**-shun	_____
myocarditis	☐ **my**-oh-car-**DYE**-tis	_____
myocardium	☐ **my**-oh-**CAR**-dee-um	_____
nausea	☐ **NAW**-see-ah	_____
nocturia	☐ nok-**TOO**-ree-ah	_____
occlusion	☐ ah-**KLOO**-shun	_____
orthopnea	☐ **or**-**THOP**-nee-ah	_____
pallor	☐ **PAL**-or	_____

Term	Pronunciation	Definition
palpable	☐ PAL-pah-bul	_____
palpitation	☐ pal-pih-TAY-shun	_____
patent ductus arteriosus	☐ PAY-tent DUCK-tus ar-tee-ree-OH-sis	_____
pericarditis	☐ pair-ih-car-DYE-tis	_____
pericardium	☐ pehr-ih-KAR-dee-um	_____
peripheral arterial occlusive disease	☐ per-IF-er-al ar-TEE-ree-al oh-KLOO-siv dih-ZEEZ	_____
petechiae	☐ pee-TEE-kee-ee	_____
phlebitis	☐ fleh-BYE-tis	_____
pitting edema	☐ pitting eh-DEE-mah	_____
prophylactic	☐ proh-fih-LAK-tik	_____
pulmonary artery	☐ PULL-mon-air-ee artery	_____
pulmonary vein	☐ PULL-mon-air-ee vein	_____
Raynaud's phenomenon	☐ ray-NOZ feh-NOM-eh-non	_____
rheumatic fever	☐ roo-MAT-ic fever	_____
septicemia	☐ sep-tih-SEE-mee-ah	_____
septum	☐ SEP-tum	_____
serum lipid test	☐ SEE-rum LIP-id test	_____
Sydenham's chorea	☐ SID-en-hamz koh-REE-ah	_____
systemic circulation	☐ sis-TEM-ik ser-kew-LAY-shun	_____
systole	☐ SIS-toh-lee	_____
tachycardia	☐ tak-ee-CAR-dee-ah	_____
tetralogy of Fallot	☐ teh-TRALL-oh-jee of fal-LOH	_____
thallium stress test	☐ THAL-ee-um stress test	_____
thrombophlebitis	☐ throm-boh-fleh-BY-tis	_____
thrombosis	☐ throm-BOH-sis	_____
varicose veins	☐ VAIR-ih-kohs veins	_____
vasoconstriction	☐ vass-oh-con-STRIK-shun	_____

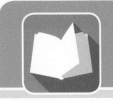

Review Checkpoint

Apply what you have learned in this chapter by completing the **Putting It All Together** exercise in your workbook.

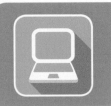

Online Resources

For additional study tools including PowerPoint® slides and animations go to the Student Companion Website.

Chapter Review Exercises

The following exercises provide a more in-depth review of the chapter material. Your goal in these exercises is to complete each section at a minimum 80% level of accuracy. A space has been provided for your score at the end of each section.

A. Labeling

Label the following structures of the heart by writing your answers in the spaces provided. Each correct answer is worth 10 points. When you have completed the exercise, record your score in the space provided.

1. _____
2. _____
3. _____
4. _____
5. _____
6. _____
7. _____
8. _____

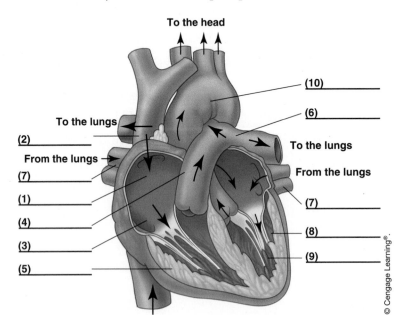

Number correct _____ × *10 points/correct answer: Your score* _____%

B. Follow the Flow

As you read the following review of the flow of blood through the heart, complete the statements below with the most appropriate answer. Each correct answer is worth 10 points. Record your score in the space provided at the end of this exercise.

As blood flows through the heart, deoxygenated blood enters the (1) _____ atrium from the (2) _____. It passes through the tricuspid valve into the right ventricle. From the right ventricle, the blood passes through the pulmonary valve into the (3) _____, which carries the blood to the lungs to receive oxygen. This propelling of the blood from the heart to the lungs and back to the heart is known as (4) _____ circulation. Oxygenated blood enters the (5) _____ atrium from the pulmonary veins. The blood passes from the atrium, through the (6) _____ valve, into the left ventricle. The freshly oxygenated blood then passes through the (7) _____ valve into the (8) _____, which branches into arteries and then into smaller vessels known as (9) _____, which then transport the blood throughout the body. This propelling of the blood from the heart to all parts of the body and back to the heart is known as (10) _____ circulation.

Number correct _____ **× 10 points/correct answer: Your score** _____**%**

C. Spelling

Circle the correctly spelled term in each pairing of words. Each correct answer is worth 10 points. Record your score in the space provided at the end of the exercise.

1. sistole	systole	6. rhumatic	rheumatic
2. diastole	dyastole	7. Fallot	Fallow
3. tachycardia	trachycardia	8. aneurism	aneurysm
4. palpatation	palpitation	9. ventriclar	ventricular
5. vomiting	vomiking	10. varicose	vericose

Number correct _____ **× 10 points/correct answer: Your score** _____**%**

D. Signs and Symptoms Review

Define each term by writing the definition in the space provided. Check the box if you are able to complete this exercise correctly the first time (without referring to the answers). Each correct answer is worth 10 points. Record your score in the space provided at the end of the exercise.

☐ 1. tachycardia _____
☐ 2. palpitation _____
☐ 3. pallor _____
☐ 4. cyanosis _____
☐ 5. edema _____
☐ 6. anorexia _____
☐ 7. nausea _____
☐ 8. vomiting _____

(*continued*)

☐ 9. anxiety _____

☐ 10. fatigue _____

Number correct _____ *× 10 points/correct answer: Your score* _____*%*

E. Matching Cardiovascular Conditions

Match the following cardiovascular conditions on the left with the applicable definitions on the right. Each correct answer is worth 10 points. Record your score in the space provided at the end of the exercise.

_____ 1. myocardial infarction

_____ 2. endocarditis

_____ 3. rheumatic fever

_____ 4. ventricular fibrillation

_____ 5. aneurysm

_____ 6. thrombophlebitis

_____ 7. varicose veins

_____ 8. Raynaud's phenomenon

_____ 9. hypertension

_____ 10. mitral valve prolapse

a. "click murmur syndrome"

b. a localized dilation of an artery that balloons out with each pulsation of the artery

c. an inflammatory disease that may develop as a delayed reaction to insufficiently treated group A beta-hemolytic streptococcal infection of the upper respiratory tract

d. severe pain and constriction about the heart

e. blood pressure persistently exceeding 140/90 mmHg

f. "heart attack"

g. inflammation of the inner lining of the heart

h. a condition that results in rapid, tremulous (quivering like a bowl of gelatin) and ineffectual contractions of this chamber of the heart

i. intermittent attacks of vasoconstriction of the arterioles, causing pallor of the fingers or toes

j. enlarged, superficial veins; a twisted, dilated vein with incompetent valves

k. inflammation of the outer lining of the heart

l. inflammation of a vein associated with the formation of a clot

Number correct _____ *× 10 points/correct answer: Your score* _____*%*

F. Proofreading Skills

Read the following Death Summary Report. For each bold term, provide a brief definition and indicate if the term is spelled correctly. If it is misspelled, provide the correct spelling. Each correct answer is worth 10 points. Record your score in the space provided at the end of the exercise.

Example:

> **cardiac** *pertaining to the heart* _____
>
> Spelled correctly? ☑ Yes   ☐ No _____

DEATH SUMMARY

Hillcrest
medical center

PATIENT NAME: Putul Barua

HOSPITAL NO: 135799

ROOM NO.: CCU-4

DATE OF ADMISSION
01/07/2014

DATE OF DEATH
01/15/2014 at 0041 hours

ADMITTING PHYSICIAN
Joshua Stephen Gatlin, MD

This 42-year-old gentleman was admitted on January 7 and died on January 15. He was admitted with progressive **cardiac palpatations**, hemoptysis, and **dyspnea**. Please see his admission history and physical exam for details.

HOSPITAL COURSE

Mr. Barua's hospital course was characterized by a progressively downhill course. He was initially hospitalized and found to be suffering from mild **hypoxemia**, which rapidly corrected with supplemental low-flow oxygen therapy; however, he gradually became more oxygen dependent on high-flow oxygen, eventually requiring intubation with mechanical ventilation to maintain his oxygenation.

He underwent an open-lung biopsy in an attempt to delineate the etiology of his pulmonary situation, and this was reported as idiopathic pulmonary fibrosis and alveolitis. The specimen was sent to the Mayo Clinic Pathology Department for further evaluation, and they were able to give no further help concerning the etiology of his pulmonary status. An **echocardiogram** showed left **ventriculer** wall motion hypokinesia and an ejection fraction of approximately 35%.

Dr. Cecil Burnett and other members of the **cardiology** department consulted on the patient. They felt that his hypoxemia and breathlessness were not secondary to his cardiac status. He had supraventricular cardiac **arrythmias** including **atrial fibrillation** and **atrial flutter**. The cardiology staff used intravenous medications that controlled the cardiac rate, adequately resolving these cardiac issues.

I managed the patient's ventilator and intensive care status along with my respiratory therapy team. Unfortunately the patient developed multiple infections, hospital acquired, including *Klebsiella pneumoniae* infection and probable fungemia. Multiple evaluations of the sputum and lungs for the presence of active pulmonary tuberculosis were negative.

The patient developed acute renal failure, managed by Dr. Rex Keating and the nephrologists via hemodialysis. A temporary tracheostomy, intravenous dialysis catheter, and gastrostomy tube were placed in an attempt to provide further support; however, the patient continued to deteriorate.

On January 15 at 0017 hours, he experienced **asistolee**. Code Blue was called. The patient underwent advanced cardiac life support with multiple medications. He failed to respond to the advanced cardiac life support and was pronounced dead at 0041 hours on January 15. Permission for autopsy was denied.

FINAL DIAGNOSES
1. Idiopathic pulmonary fibrosis with alveolitis.
2. History of tuberculosis.

(continued)

DEATH SUMMARY
Patient Name: Putul Barua
Hospital No.: 135799
Date of Death: 01/15/2014 at 0041 hours
Page 2

3. Acute renal failure.
4. Probable acute hepatic failure.
5. Hospital-acquired septicemia and fungemia secondary to multiple organisms.

_____

Joshua Stephen Gatlin, MD

JSG:xx

D:01/15/2014

T:01/20/2014

1. **palpatations** _____

_____

    Spelled Correctly? ☐ Yes ☐ No _____

2. **dyspnea** _____

    Spelled Correctly? ☐ Yes ☐ No _____

3. **hypoxemia** _____

    Spelled Correctly? ☐ Yes ☐ No _____

4. **echocardiogram** _____

    Spelled Correctly? ☐ Yes ☐ No _____

5. **ventriculer** _____

    Spelled Correctly? ☐ Yes ☐ No _____

6. **cardiology** _____

    Spelled Correctly? ☐ Yes ☐ No _____

7. **arrythmias** _____

    Spelled Correctly? ☐ Yes ☐ No _____

8. **atrial fibrillation** _____

    Spelled Correctly? ☐ Yes ☐ No _____

9. **atrial flutter** _____

_____

Spelled Correctly? ☐ Yes ☐ No _____

10. **asistolee** _____

_____

Spelled Correctly? ☐ Yes ☐ No _____

Number correct _____ **× 10 points/correct answer: Your score** _____ **%**

G. Abbreviations Identification

Read the following set of doctor's orders and define the highlighted abbreviations in the spaces provided. Each correct answer is worth 10 points. Record your score in the space provided at the end of this exercise.

John Peach was admitted to Fruitland Memorial Hospital on Saturday, March 31, 2014, with initial diagnoses of **CAD** and **HCVD**. He was placed in the **CCU** and was scheduled for an **MRI** the following morning. The doctor also ordered an **EKG**.

The results of the MRI revealed that Mr. Peach had greater than 60% blockage in two of his coronary arteries. The attending physician considered the treatment options of **PTCA** or directional coronary atherectomy versus surgery for Mr. Peach. Considering the fact that Mr. Peach was at increased risk for an **MI**, his **BP** was 240/120 mmHg, and he was experiencing **DOE**, the doctor opted for the **CABG** surgery as soon as all lab work had been completed.

On Tuesday, April 3, 2014, Mr. Peach went to surgery for the coronary artery bypass surgery. He tolerated the procedure well and was returned to CCU for the remainder of the week.

1. CAD: _____
2. HCVD: _____
3. CCU: _____
4. MRI: _____
5. EKG: _____
6. PTCA: _____
7. MI: _____
8. BP: _____
9. DOE: _____
10. CABG: _____

Number correct _____ **× 10 points/correct answer: Your score** _____ **%**

H. Matching Abbreviations

Match the abbreviations on the left with the correct definition on the right. Each correct answer is worth 10 points. Record your score in the space provided at the end of this exercise.

_____ 1. CHF   a. cardiopulmonary resuscitation

_____ 2. ECHO   b. arteriosclerotic heart disease

_____ 3. MVP   c. sinoatrial

(*continued*)

_____ 4. PET
_____ 5. PVCs
_____ 6. SA
_____ 7. PDA
_____ 8. ASHD
_____ 9. EKG
_____ 10. CPR

d. echocardiogram
e. bundle branch block
f. congestive heart failure
g. mitral valve prolapse
h. computerized tomography
i. positron emission tomography
j. premature ventricular contractions
k. patent ductus arteriosus
l. electrocardiogram
m. urinary tract infection

Number correct _____ **× 10 points/correct answer: Your score** _____ **%**

I. Crossword Puzzle

Each crossword answer is worth 10 points. When you have completed the crossword puzzle, total your points and enter your score in the space provided.

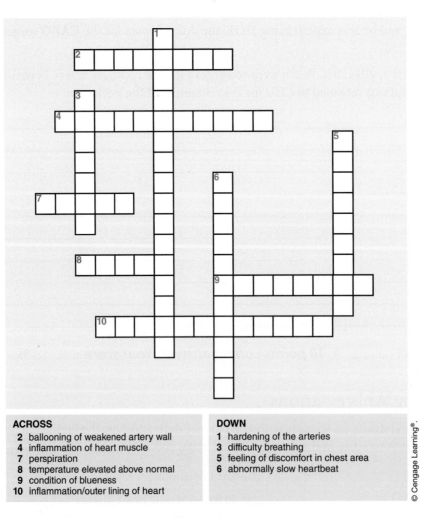

ACROSS
2 ballooning of weakened artery wall
4 inflammation of heart muscle
7 perspiration
8 temperature elevated above normal
9 condition of blueness
10 inflammation/outer lining of heart

DOWN
1 hardening of the arteries
3 difficulty breathing
5 feeling of discomfort in chest area
6 abnormally slow heartbeat

© Cengage Learning®.

Number correct _____ **× 10 points/correct answer: Your score** _____ **%**

J. Completion

Complete the statements below with the most appropriate answer. Each correct answer is worth 10 points. Record your score in the space provided at the end of this exercise.

1. An abnormal opening between the pulmonary artery and the aorta, caused by failure of the ductus arteriosus to close after birth, is known as:

   _____

2. A congenital heart anomaly that consists of four defects is known as:

   _____

3. The congenital heart disease in which the two major arteries of the heart are reversed in position, resulting in two noncommunicating circulatory systems, is known as:

   _____

4. A congenital heart disease characterized by a localized narrowing of the aorta, resulting in increased pressure in the upper extremities and decreased pressure in the lower extremities, is known as:

   _____

5. A condition that results in rapid, tremulous, and ineffective contractions of the ventricles; patient has no audible heartbeat, no palpable pulse, no respiration, and no blood circulation, known as:

   _____

6. An interference with the normal conduction of electric impulses that control activity of the heart muscle; the conduction time to the ventricles is abnormally prolonged, known as:

   _____

7. Extremely rapid, incomplete contractions of the atria resulting in disorganized and uncoordinated twitching of the atria is known as:

   _____

8. A form of treatment for varicose veins that involves the injection of a chemical irritant into the varicosed vein is:

   _____

9. A condition in which the contractions of the atria become extremely rapid, at the rate of between 250 to 400 beats per minute, is known as:

   _____

10. A condition in which the arteries of the leg are obstructed is known as:

    _____

Number correct _____ × *10 points/correct answer: Your score* _____ *%*

K. Word Search

Read each definition carefully and identify the applicable word from the list that follows. Enter the word in the space provided and then find it in the puzzle and circle it. The words may be read up, down, diagonally, across, or backward. Each correct answer is worth 10 points. Record your score in the space provided at the end of the exercise.

cyanosis	aneurysm	hypertension
bradycardia	angiography	atrial flutter
heart attack	pericarditis	endocarditis
tachycardia	thrombophlebitis	

Example: Condition of blueness; slightly bluish grayish, slatelike, or dark discoloration of the skin due to reduced hemoglobin in the blood.

cyanosis

1. The lay term for a myocardial infarction.

2. A slow heart rate characterized by a pulse rate less than 60 beats per minute.

3. An abnormally rapid heartbeat, usually defined as a heart rate greater than 100 beats per minute.

4. Inflammation of the membrane lining of the valves and chambers of the heart.

5. Inflammation of the saclike membrane that covers the heart muscle.

6. A localized dilation of an artery formed at a weak point in the vessel wall.

7. Inflammation of a vein associated with the formation of a thrombus (clot).

8. Another name for high blood pressure.

9. A condition in which the contractions of the atria become extremely rapid, at the rate of 250 to 400 beats per minute.

10. X-ray visualization of the internal anatomy of the heart and blood vessels after introducing a radiopaque substance into an artery or vein.

```
H  E  A  R  T  A  T  T  A  C  K  L  I  M  L
T  O  A  G  A  O  I  L  D  U  S  I  U  S  P
H  I  L  T ( C  Y  A  N  O  S  I  S ) V  L  E
R  A  F  Y  S  E  R  O  S  H  I  O  C  Y  R
O  L  S  A  N  E  U  R  Y  S  M  C  I  G  I
M  E  H  E  E  Y  T  S  O  I  E  Y  N  O  C
B  N  O  I  S  N  E  T  R  E  P  Y  H  L  A
O  R  R  T  S  L  N  E  I  R  R  E  A  O  R
P  A  B  R  A  D  Y  C  A  R  D  I  A  T  D
H  B  C  I  D  A  I  N  S  E  R  U  A  I
L  N  T  H  G  A  S  P  I  N  E  D  N  M  T
E  A  T  R  I  A  L  F  L  U  T  T  E  R  I
B  E  T  A  C  H  Y  C  A  R  D  I  A  E  S
I  L  E  N  N  P  A  L  E  A  S  Y  C  D  O
T  L  S  I  T  I  D  R  A  C  O  D  N  E  C
I  N  E  R  U  C  N  D  T  U  R  E  S  I  Y
S  I  S  S  L  R  E  A  S  I  E  M  N  I  S
Y  H  P  A  R  G  O  I  G  N  A  C  N  E  S
```

Number correct _____ × *10 points/correct answer: Your score* _____%

L. Medical Scenario

The following medical scenario presents information on one of the pathological conditions discussed in this chapter. Read the scenario carefully and select the most appropriate answer for each question that follows. Each correct answer is worth 20 points. Record your score in the space provided at the end of the exercise.

Grace Reddick is a 59-year-old retired schoolteacher and a patient of cardiologist, Dr. Patrick. Mrs. Reddick is three weeks post myocardial infarction and has a scheduled visit with Dr. Patrick this afternoon. Mrs. Reddick has a 10-year history of increased blood lipid levels, arteriosclerosis, and hypertension. She was diagnosed with diabetes mellitus and congestive heart failure about three months ago. The health care professional is preparing for the afternoon visit by reviewing information about Mrs. Reddick's medical diagnoses. He wants to be prepared for Mrs. Reddick's questions at her follow-up visit today.

1. The health care professional will base his responses to Mrs. Reddick's questions about myocardial infarctions on which of the following facts? A myocardial infarction is:

   a. an inflammatory disease that may develop as a delayed reaction to insufficiently treated group A beta-hemolytic streptococcal infection

   b. inflammation of the myocardium caused by viral, bacterial, or fungal infections or as a result of systemic diseases such as rheumatic fever

(continued)

    c. drooping of one or both cusps of the mitral valve back into the left atrium during ventricular systole, resulting in incomplete closure of the valve and mitral insufficiency

    d. a life-threatening condition resulting when myocardial tissue is destroyed in areas of the heart deprived of adequate blood supply due to occlusion of one or more of the coronary arteries

2. If Mrs. Reddick asks the health care professional about congestive heart failure, he will base this response on his knowledge that congestive heart failure would result in which of the following clinical manifestations?

    a. edema of the lower extremities and shortness of breath

    b. anemia, infection, and small bruises

    c. intermittent claudication and altered peripheral pulses

    d. one pale, cold, swollen extremity with a palpable cordlike vessel

3. Mrs. Reddick may be concerned about the mortality rate for myocardial infarctions. Which of the following responses by the health care professional would be correct? The mortality rate for myocardial infarctions is approximately:

    a. 10%, with most deaths occurring one to two weeks after the onset of the attack

    b. 20%, with most deaths occurring within the first 72 hours of the attack

    c. 35%, with most deaths occurring within the first 12 hours of the attack

    d. 50%, with the most deaths occurring within the first 3 hours of the attack

4. Mrs. Reddick may want the health care professional to explain what treatment was instituted when she first entered the hospital. After reviewing Mrs. Reddick's chart from the acute-care hospital, the health care professional would explain to her that the following are the priorities in treatment just after a patient experiences a myocardial infarction:

    a. completing blood cultures and then administering two different antibiotics intravenously to destroy the invading organisms

    b. administration of salicylates to reduce fever and joint pain and antibiotics to ensure that no traces of group A streptococci remain in the body

    c. administration of analgesics, complete bed rest with elevation of the affected extremity, and application of warm compresses

    d. minimizing damage to the heart muscle by relieving pain, providing rest, stabilizing the heart rhythm, and reducing the workload of the heart

5. The health care professional may ask Mrs. Reddick about the symptoms she remembers the night she went to the emergency room. Which of the following best describes the typical symptoms of a myocardial infarction?

    a. pain, swelling, and muscle cramps with a feeling of heaviness in the left leg along with palpable distended veins

    b. numbness, tingling, and pain (along with a pale color of the fingers on the left hand), followed by cyanosis and then redness

    c. prolonged heavy pressure or squeezing pain in the center of the chest sometimes radiating down the left shoulder to the fourth and fifth fingers

    d. lower extremities turn pale when elevated and cyanotic when allowed to dangle, along with unequal strength of pulses

Number correct _____ × *20 points/correct answer: Your score* _____ %

The Respiratory System

CHAPTER CONTENT

OBJECTIVES

Upon completing this chapter and the review exercises at the end of the chapter, the learner should be able to:

1. List two major functions of the respiratory system.

2. State the difference between external respiration and internal respiration.

3. Identify the pathway of air as it travels from the nose to the capillaries of the lungs.

4. Identify 10 structures related to the respiratory system.

5. Define 10 common respiratory signs and symptoms.

6. Identify at least 10 breath sounds.

7. Define 20 common pathological conditions of the respiratory system.

8. Identify at least 10 abbreviations common to the respiratory system.

9. Correctly spell and pronounce terms listed on the Written and Audio Terminology Review, using the phonetic pronunciations provided.

10. Correctly define at least 10 word elements relating to the respiratory system.

Overview

The respiratory system is responsible for the exchange of gases between the body and the air, a process called respiration. The respiratory system, along with the cardiovascular system, provides oxygen to the body cells for energy and removes carbon dioxide (a waste product of cellular metabolism) from the body cells. This is accomplished by two processes: external respiration and internal respiration.

In external respiration, oxygen is inhaled into the lungs (when you breathe in), passing through the **alveoli** of the lungs into the capillaries of the pulmonary bloodstream. Carbon dioxide passes from the blood through the same **capillaries** into the lungs and is exhaled (as you breathe out).

In internal respiration, the oxygen you inhale circulates from the pulmonary bloodstream, back through the heart, to the systemic bloodstream (which carries it all the way to the body cells). At the cellular level, the oxygen passes through the **capillaries** into the individual tissue cells (where it is used for energy). In exchange, carbon dioxide passes from the tissue cells into the **capillaries** and travels through the bloodstream for removal from the body via the lungs (from the tissues, via the bloodstream, to the heart, to the lungs). In addition to providing for the exchange of gases between the body and the air, the organs of the respiratory system also contribute to the production of sound and assist in the body's defense against foreign materials.

Anatomy and Physiology

The respiratory system consists of a series of tubes or airways that transport air into and out of the lungs. The respiratory system is divided into the upper respiratory tract (consisting of the nose, **pharynx**, and **larynx**) and the lower respiratory tract (consisting of the **trachea**, **bronchi**, and lungs). A discussion of these structures, and the processes of respiration they support, follows. See *Figure 11-1*.

Nose

Air enters the body through the **(1) nose** and mouth. The external portion of the nose is composed of cartilage and bone covered with skin. The entrance to the nose is known as the **nostrils** or **nares** (singular: naris). As the air enters through the nose,

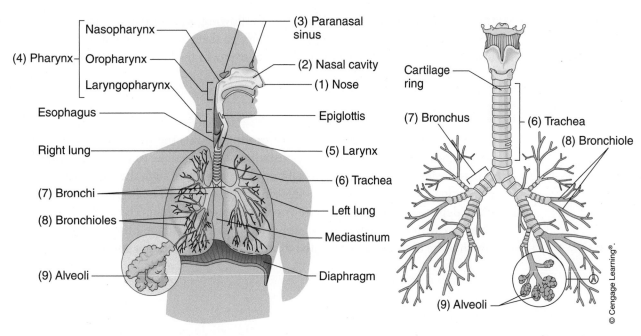

Figure 11-1 Pathway of air from nose to alveoli

it passes into the (**2**) **nasal cavity**, which is divided into left and right chambers by a dividing wall called the **septum**. Air passing through these chambers also passes through the (**3**) **paranasal sinuses**, which are hollow areas or cavities within the skull that communicate with the nasal cavity. The internal nose and the sinuses are lined with mucous membranes, which help warm and filter the air as it enters the respiratory system. Hairlike projections on the mucous membranes, called **cilia**, sweep dirt and foreign material toward the throat for elimination. Because the hollow cavities of the **paranasal sinuses** are air spaces and not solid bone, they also lighten the skull and enhance the sound of the voice.

Pharynx

Once the air passes through the nasal cavity and **paranasal sinuses**, it reaches the (**4**) **pharynx**. The **pharynx**, or throat, is the airway that connects the mouth and nose to the **larynx**. Although the **pharynx** is a single organ, it is commonly divided into three sections: the **nasopharynx**, the upper portion located behind the nose; the **oropharynx**, the middle portion located behind the mouth; and the **laryngopharynx** (also known as the hypopharynx), the lower portion located just behind the **larynx**.

Located in the **nasopharynx** are two rounded masses of lymphatic tissue known as the **adenoids** (also called the pharyngeal tonsils). The **adenoids** and the tonsils help filter out bacteria and other foreign matter that pass through the area. Hypertrophy (enlargement) of the **adenoids** in young children may be great enough to interfere with the child's breathing. The child will have a noisy, snoring sound when breathing. The **palatine tonsils** (more commonly called the tonsils) are located on either side of the soft palate in the **oropharynx**. The tonsils are normally enlarged in young children.

The **pharynx** is unique in that it serves as a common passageway for both air and food. As a result of this, there must be a mechanism to prevent food from accidentally entering the respiratory tract. During the act of swallowing, a small flap of cartilage called the **epiglottis** covers the opening of the **larynx** so that food cannot enter the **larynx** and lower airways while passing through the **pharynx** to the lower digestive structures.

Larynx

Also known as the voice box, the **(5) larynx** contains the structures that make vocal sounds possible: the vocal cords. Consisting of two reedlike folds of tissue that stretch across the **larynx**, the vocal cords vibrate as air passes through the space between them, producing sound. (This space is known as the **glottis**.) The high or low pitch of the voice depends on how tensely the vocal cords are stretched. The **larynx** connects the **pharynx** with the **trachea**. It is supported by nine cartilages, the most prominent of which is the thyroid cartilage at the front that forms the **Adam's apple**.

Trachea

The **(6) trachea** is commonly known as the windpipe. It extends into the chest and serves as a passageway for air to the **bronchi**. The **trachea** lies in front of the esophagus, the tube through which food passes on its way to the stomach. The **trachea** consists of muscular tissue embedded with 16 to 20 C-shaped rings of cartilage separated by fibrous connective tissue. These rings of cartilage provide rigidity to the **trachea**, which helps keep the tracheal tube open (you can feel these rings of cartilage if you press your fingers gently against the front of your throat). Without the structural rigidity, the long tracheal tube could collapse against the pressure of other internal tissues.

Bronchi

The **trachea** branches into two tubes called the **(7) bronchi** (singular: *bronchus*). Each bronchus leads to a separate lung and divides and subdivides into progressively smaller tubes called **(8) bronchioles**. The **bronchioles** terminate at the **(9) alveoli**, also known as air sacs. The **alveoli**, known as the **pulmonary parenchyma**, have very thin walls that allow for the exchange of gases between the lungs and the blood via the capillaries.

Lungs

The lungs are two cone-shaped spongy organs consisting of **alveoli**, blood vessels, elastic tissue, and nerves. Each of the two lungs consists of smaller divisions called lobes. The left lung has two lobes, whereas the right lung is divided into three lobes. The uppermost part of the lung is called the **apex**, and the lower part of the lung is called the **base**. The portion of the lung in the midline region where the blood vessels, nerves, and bronchial tubes enter and exit is known as the **hilum**. The lungs are surrounded by a double-folded membrane called the **pleura**. The outer layer of the **pleura**, which lines the thoracic cavity, is known as the **parietal pleura**. The inner layer of the **pleura**, which covers the lung, is known as the **visceral pleura**. The small space between these membranes, called the **pleural space**, is filled with a lubricating fluid that prevents friction when the two membranes slide against each other during respiration. The space between the lungs (called the **mediastinum**) contains the heart, aorta, **trachea**,

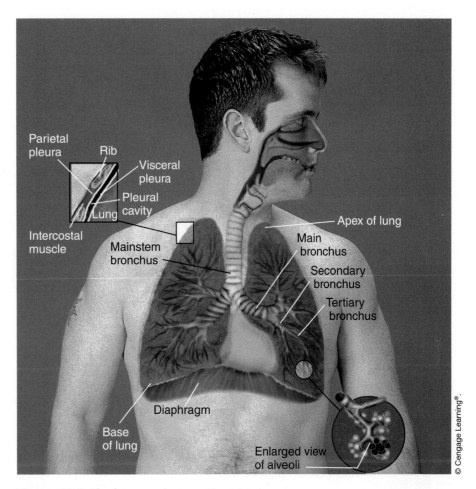

Figure 11-2 The lungs and supporting structures

esophagus, and **bronchi**. In the lungs, the **alveoli** are surrounded by a network of tiny blood vessels called **capillaries**. *Figure 11-2* shows the lungs and supporting structures.

Breathing Process

The lungs extend from the collarbone to the **diaphragm** in the thoracic cavity. The **diaphragm**, a muscular partition that separates the thoracic cavity from the abdominal cavity, aids in the process of breathing. The process of breathing is begun when the **phrenic nerve** stimulates the **diaphragm** to contract and flatten (descend), thus enlarging the chest cavity. This enlargement of the thoracic cavity creates a negative pressure within the **thorax**, which draws air into the lungs is called inhalation (inspiration). When the **diaphragm** relaxes, it rises back into the thoracic cavity, increasing the pressure within the **thorax**. This increase in pressure that causes the air to be forced out of the lungs is called exhalation (expiration). During quiet breathing, exhalation is more of a passive process due to the elastic recoil of the lungs in healthy individuals. *Figure 11-3* illustrates the increase and decrease of pressure within the thoracic cavity during the breathing process. (As you look at *Figure 11-3*, take a deep breath and hold it momentarily. Can you feel the enlargement of your chest cavity? As you release your breath, think about the process and how your chest cavity is now decreasing in size as it forces the air back out through the respiratory passages.)

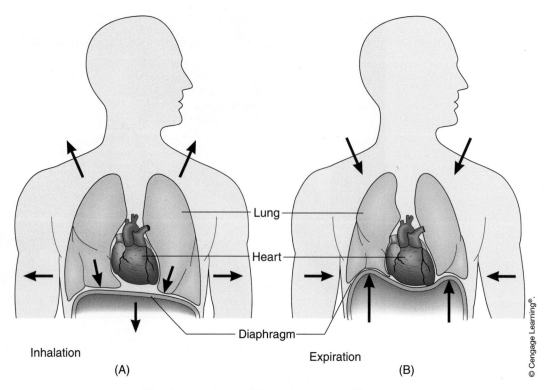

Figure 11-3 Position of diaphragm during (a) inhalation and (b) expiration

Media Link

Increase your understanding of the breathing process by viewing the **Respiration** animation on the Student Companion Website.

Physical Examination

The following terms relate to techniques used in the physical examination of the respiratory system.

inspection (in-**SPEK**-shun)	Visual examination of the external surface of the body as well as of its movements and posture.
palpation (pal-**PAY**-shun) 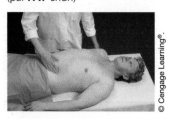	**Palpation** is the process of examining by application of the hands or fingers to the external surface of the body to detect evidence of disease or abnormalities in the various organs. See *Figure 11-4*.

Figure 11-4 Technique of light palpation

auscultation (oss-kull-**TAY**-shun) 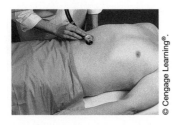	Process of listening for sounds within the body, usually to sounds of thoracic or abdominal viscera, to detect some abnormal condition or to detect fetal heart sounds. See *Figure 11-5*. **Auscultation** is performed with a stethoscope.

Figure 11-5 Auscultation with bell of stethoscope

percussion (per-**KUH**-shun) 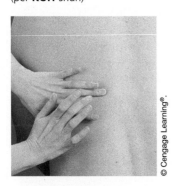	Use of the fingertips to tap the body lightly but sharply to determine position, size, and consistency of an underlying structure and the presence of fluid or pus in a cavity. See *Figure 11-6*. Tapping over a solid organ in the body produces a dull flat sound. Tapping over an air-filled structure (such as the lungs) produces a clear, hollow sound. If the lungs are filled with fluid (as in **pneumonia**), they will in turn take on a dull flat sound during **percussion**.

Figure 11-6 Percussion strike

Review Checkpoint

Check your understanding of this section by completing the **Anatomy and Physiology** exercises in your workbook.

VOCABULARY

The following vocabulary words are frequently used when discussing the respiratory system.

Word	Definition

adenoids
(**ADD**-eh-noydz)
  aden/o = gland
  -oid = resembling
	Lymphatic tissue forming a prominence on the wall of the recess of the **nasopharynx**.

alveoli (al-**VEE**-oh-lye)	Air cells of the lungs; known as the **pulmonary parenchyma** (functional units of the lungs).
apex (**AY**-peks)	The upper portion of the lung, rising about 2.5 to 5 cm above the collarbone.

Word	Definition

aphonia
(ah-**FOH**-nee-ah)
  a- = without, not, no
  phon/o = sound
  -ia = condition
	Without sound.

asymptomatic (ay-simp-toh-**MAT**-ik)	Without symptoms.

atelectasis
(**at**-ee-**LEK**-tah-sis)
  atel/o = imperfect or incomplete
  -ectasis = stretching or dilation
	Incomplete expansion of part or all of a lung.

base	The lowest part of the lung, resting on the **diaphragm**.

bronchi
(**BRONG**-kigh)
  bronch/o = bronchus
  -i = plural ending
	The two main branches leading from the **trachea** to the lungs, providing the passageway for air movement.

bronchiole
(**BRONG**-key-ohl)
  bronchi/o = bronchiole
  -ole = small or little
	One of the smaller subdivisions of the bronchial tubes.

bronchorrhea
(**brong**-koh-**REE**-ah)
  bronch/o = bronchus
  -rrhea = discharge or flow
	Discharge or drainage from the bronchial tubes.

capillaries (**CAP**-ih-**lair**-eez)	Any of the minute (tiny) blood vessels. The **capillaries** connect the ends of the smallest arteries (arterioles) with the beginnings of the smallest veins (venules).
diaphragm (**DYE**-ah-fram)	The musculomembranous wall separating the abdomen from the thoracic cavity.
epiglottis (ep-ih-**GLOT**-iss)	A thin, leaf-shaped structure located immediately posterior to the root of the tongue; covers the entrance of the **larynx** when the individual swallows.
glottis (**GLOT**-iss)	The sound-producing apparatus of the **larynx**, consisting of the two vocal folds and the intervening space (the **epiglottis** protects this opening).
laryngalgia (**lair**-ring-**GAL**-jee-ah)	Pain in the **larynx**.

laryngopharynx
(lah-**ring**-go-**FAIR**-inks)
  laryng/o = larynx
  pharyng/o = pharynx
	Lower portion of the **pharynx** that extends from the vestibule of the **larynx** (the portion just above the vocal cords) to the lowermost cartilage of the **larynx**.

Word	Definition
larynx (**LAIR**-inks) laryng/o = larynx	The enlarged upper end of the **trachea** below the root of the tongue; the voice box.
mediastinum (**mee**-dee-as-**TYE**-num)	The mass of organs and tissues separating the lungs. It contains the heart, aorta, **trachea**, esophagus, and **bronchi**.
nares (**NAIRZ**)	External nostrils.

nasopharynx
(**nay**-zoh-**FAIR**-inks)
  nas/o = nose
  pharyng/o = pharynx
	Part of the **pharynx** located above the soft palate (postnasal space).

oropharynx
(**or**-oh-**FAIR**-inks)
  or/o = mouth
  pharyng/o = pharynx
	Central portion of the **pharynx** lying between the soft palate and upper portion of the **epiglottis**.

palatine tonsils (**PAL**-ah-tyne **TON**-sills)	Lymphatic tissue located in the depression of the mucous membrane of fauces (the constricted opening leading from the mouth and the oral **pharynx**) and the **pharynx**.

paranasal sinuses
(pair-ah-**NAY**-sal **SIGH**-nuss-ez)
  para- = near, beside, beyond, two
          like parts
  nas/o = nose
  -al = pertaining to
  sinus/o = sinus
  -es = plural ending
	Hollow areas or cavities within the skull that communicate with the nasal cavity.

parietal pleura
(pah-**RYE**-eh-tal **PLOO**-rah)
  pleur/o = pleura
  -a = noun ending
	Portion of the **pleura** that is closest to the ribs.

pharynx (**FAIR**-inks) pharyng/o = pharynx	Passageway for air from nasal cavity to **larynx** and food from mouth to esophagus. Serves both the respiratory and digestive systems; the throat.

phrenic nerve
(**FREN-ic** nerve)
  phren/o = mind; also refers to the
          diaphragm
  -ic = pertaining to
	The nerve known as the motor nerve to the **diaphragm**.

pleura
(**PLOO**-rah)
  pleur/o = pleura
  -a = noun ending
	The double-folded membrane that lines the thoracic cavity.

Word	Definition
pleural space (**PLOO**-ral space) pleur/o = pleura -al = pertaining to	The space that separates the visceral and parietal pleurae, which contains a small amount of fluid that acts as a lubricant to the pleural surfaces during respiration.
pleurodynia (**ploor**-oh-**DIN**-ee-ah) pleur/o = pleura -dynia = pain	Pain in the pleura that occurs when the inflamed pleural membranes rub together during the breathing process.
pneumoconiosis (**new**-moh-**koh**-nee-**OH**-sis) pneum/o = lungs; air -osis = condition	A lung condition resulting from inhalation of dust; such as industrial dusts of iron ore or coal. For additional information refer to Chapter 11 (anthracosis).
pulmonary parenchyma (**PULL**-mon-air-ee par-**EN**-kih-mah) pulmon/o = lung -ary = pertaining to	The functional units of the lungs (for example, the **alveoli**) which have very thin walls that allow for the exchange of gases between the lungs and the blood.
septum (**SEP**-tum)	A wall dividing two cavities.
sputum (**SPEW**-tum)	Substance coughed up from the lungs, **bronchi**, and **trachea** that is expelled through the mouth; **sputum** is not the same as saliva, which is secreted by the salivary glands.
thoracotomy (**thoh**-rah-**KOT**-oh-mee) thorac/o = thorax; chest -otomy = incision into	A surgical incision into the chest wall, to open the chest, usually in order to gain access to the lungs or heart.
thorax (**THOH**-raks)	The chest; that part of the body between the base of the neck and the **diaphragm**.
trachea (**TRAY**-kee-ah) trache/o = trachea -a = noun ending	A cylinder-shaped tube lined with rings of cartilage (to keep it open) that is 4.5 inches long, from the **larynx** to the bronchial tubes; the windpipe.
visceral pleura (**VISS**-er-al **PLOO**-rah) viscer/o = internal organs -al = pertaining to pleur/o = pleura -a = noun ending	Portion of the **pleura** that is closest to the internal organs.

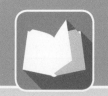

Review Checkpoint

Check your understanding of this section by completing the **Vocabulary** exercises in your workbook.

WORD ELEMENTS

The following word elements pertain to the respiratory system. As you review the list, pronounce each word element aloud twice and check the box after you "say it." Write the definition for the example term given for each word element. Use your medical dictionary to find the definitions of the example terms.

Word Element	Pronunciation	"Say It"	Meaning
alveol/o **alveol**ar	al-vee-**OHL**-oh al-**VEE**-oh-lar	☐	alveolus
atel/o **atel**ectasis	**AT**-ee-loh **at**-ee-**LEK**-tah-sis	☐	imperfect or incomplete
bronch/o **bronch**opneumonia	**BRONG**-koh **brong**-koh new-**MOH**-nee-ah	☐	bronchus
bronchiol/o **bronchiol**ar	brong-kee-**OH**-loh brong-kee-**OH**-lar	☐	bronchus
-dynia pleuro**dynia**	**DIN**-ee-ah **ploor**-oh-**DIN**-ee-ah	☐	pain
-ectasis gast**rectasis**	**EK**-tah-sis gas-**TREK**-tah-sis	☐	stretching or dilation
epiglott/o **epiglott**itis	ep-ih-**GLOT**-oh ep-ih-glot-**EYE**-tis	☐	**epiglottis**
laryng/o **laryng**ospasm	lair-**RING**-oh lair-**RING**-go-**spazm**	☐	**larynx**
nas/o **nas**al	**NAYZ**-oh **NAYZ**-al	☐	nose
orth/o **orth**opnea	**ORTH**-oh or-**THOP**-nee-ah	☐	straight
-otomy trache**otomy**	**OT**-oh-mee **tray**-kee-**OT**-oh-mee	☐	incision into
pector/o **pector**al	**PEK**-tor-oh **PEK**-toh-ral	☐	chest
pharyng/o **pharyng**itis	fair-**ING**-oh fair-in-**JYE**-tis	☐	**pharynx**
phon/o dys**phon**ia	**FOH**-noh diss-**FOH**-nee-ah	☐	sound
phren/o **phren**ic nerve	**FREN**-oh **FREN**-ic nerve	☐	mind; also refers to the **diaphragm**

Word Element	Pronunciation	"Say It"	Meaning
pleur/o **pleur**isy	**PLOO**-roh **PLOOR**-is-ee	☐	**pleura**
pne/o dys**pne**a	**NEE**-oh **DISP**-**nee**-ah	☐	breathing
pneum/o **pneum**othorax	**NEW**-moh new-moh-**THOH**-raks	☐	lungs; air
pneumon/o **pneumon**itis	new-**MOHN**-oh new-mohn-**EYE**-tis	☐	lungs; air
pulmon/o **pulmon**ary	pull-**MON**-oh **PULL**-mon-air-ee	☐	lungs
rhin/o **rhin**orrhea	**RYE**-noh rye-noh-**REE**-ah	☐	nose
-rrhea rhino**rrhea**	**REE**-ah	☐	discharge or flow
-scope naso**scope**	**SCOHP** **NAYZ**-oh-scohp	☐	an instrument used to view
sinus/o **sinus**itis	sigh-**NUS**-oh sigh-nus-**EYE**-tis	☐	sinus
thor/a **thor**acentesis	**THO**-rah **thoh**-rah-sen-**TEE**-sis	☐	chest
thorac/o **thorac**ic	thor-**AK**-oh tho-**RASS**-ik	☐	chest
trache/o **trache**obronchitis	**TRAY**-kee-oh tray-kee-oh-brong-**KIGH**-tis	☐	**trachea**

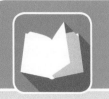

Review Checkpoint

Check your understanding of this section by completing the **Word Elements** exercises in your workbook.

Common Signs and Symptoms

Listening carefully to the signs and symptoms presented by the patient and reporting them accurately to the physician will help diagnose and treat the patient more effectively. Although many signs and symptoms are relatively nonspecific (i.e., they occur in several different respiratory conditions), they nevertheless point to certain types of abnormalities and thus provide clues about the patient's illness.

A knowledge of the signs and symptoms along with their definitions will enhance your skills as a history taker. The patient will not necessarily tell you the specific word but will describe the term in his or her own words. As you study the following terms, write each definition and word a minimum of three times, pronouncing the word aloud each time. Note that the word and the **basic definition** are in a green shaded box. A more detailed description follows most words. Once you have mastered each word to your satisfaction, check the box beside the word.

☐ **apnea**	**Apnea** is a temporary cessation of breathing; "without breathing."

(**AP**-nee-ah)
    a- = without, not
    -pnea = breathing
	Apnea may be a result of reduction in stimuli to the respiratory center, as in over-breathing (in which the carbon dioxide content of the blood is reduced), or from failure of the respiratory center to discharge impulses, as when the breath is held voluntarily. The following list includes, but is not limited to, conditions that contribute to apnea, such as sleep apnea (obstructive or central), heart conditions, metabolic disorders, and poisoning due to drug overdose.

☐ **bradypnea**	Abnormally slow breathing.

(**brad**-ip-**NEE**-ah)
    brady- = slow
    -pnea = breathing
	Bradypnea is evidenced by a respiratory rate slower than 12 respirations per minute. It could indicate neurological or electrolyte disturbance or infection; or it may indicate a protective response to pain, as in the pain of pleurisy. It may also indicate that the patient is in excellent physical fitness.

☐ **cough**	A forceful and sometimes violent expiratory effort preceded by a preliminary inspiration. The **glottis** is partially closed, the accessory muscles of expiration are brought into action, and the air is noisily expelled.

Most coughs are due to irritation of the airways (e.g., by dust, smoke, or mucus) or to infection. A cough may be described as brassy, bubbling, croupy, hacking, harsh, hollow, loose, metallic, nonproductive, productive, rasping, rattling, or wracking. The type of cough and the nature, color, and quantity of any **sputum** produced can be suggestive of the underlying cause.

Types of Coughs

- **Nonproductive, unproductive**: Not effective in bringing up **sputum** (no sputum is expectorated); also known as a "dry cough"

- **Productive**: Effective in bringing up **sputum**; "wet cough"

Types of **Sputum**

- **Mucoid**: resembling mucus

- **Mucopurulent**: containing mucus and pus

- **Purulent**: containing pus

- **Serous**: resembling serum; containing a thin, watery fluid

☐ **cyanosis**	Slightly bluish, grayish, slatelike, or dark discoloration of the skin due to presence of abnormal amounts of reduced hemoglobin in the blood.
(sigh-ah-**NOH**-sis)	Bluish discoloration of the skin and mucous membranes, especially the lips, tongue, and fingernail beds.
cyan/o = blue	
-osis = condition	

☐ **dysphonia**	Difficulty in speaking; hoarseness.
(diss-**FOH**-nee-ah)	May occur when the **larynx** becomes damaged as a result of infection, overuse, or tumor.
dys- = bad, difficult, painful, disordered	
phon/o = sound	
-ia = condition	

☐ **dyspnea**	Air hunger resulting in labored or difficult breathing, sometimes accompanied by pain.
(**DISP**-nee-ah)	Normal when due to vigorous work or athletic activity. Audible labored breathing, distressed anxious expression, dilated nostrils, protrusion of abdomen and expanded chest, gasping, and marked **cyanosis** are among the symptoms and signs of someone with **dyspnea**.
dys- = bad, difficult, painful, disordered	
-pnea = breathing	

| ☐ **epistaxis** | Hemorrhage from the nose; nosebleed. |
| (ep-ih-**STAKS**-is) | **Epistaxis** may be caused by a blow to the nose, fragile blood vessels, high blood pressure, or dislodging of crusted mucus or may be secondary to local infections or drying of the nasal mucous membrane. |

| ☐ **expectoration** | The act of spitting out saliva or coughing up materials from the air passageways leading to the lungs. |
| (ex-**pek**-toh-**RAY**-shun) | The expulsion of mucus or phlegm from the throat or lungs. |

☐ **hemoptysis**	**Hemoptysis** is **expectoration** of blood arising from the oral cavity, **larynx, trachea, bronchi**, or lungs.
(hee-**MOP**-tih-sis)	
hem/o = blood	
-ptysis = spitting	

☐ **hypercapnia**	Increased amount of carbon dioxide in the blood.
(**high**-per-**KAP**-nee-ah)	**Hypercapnia** results from inadequate ventilation or from great differences between ventilation and perfusion of the blood.
hyper- = excessive	
-capnia = (condition of) carbon dioxide content in the blood	

☐ **hypoxemia**	Insufficient oxygenation of arterial blood.
(**high**-pox-**EE**-mee-ah)	**Hypoxemia** is occasionally associated with decreased oxygen content.
hyp- = under, below, beneath, less than normal	
ox/o = oxygen	
-emia = blood condition	

☐ **hypoxia**	Deficiency of oxygen.
(**high**-POX-ee-ah) hyp- = under, below, beneath, less than normal ox/o = oxygen -ia = condition	**Hypoxia** is the state of having an inadequate supply of oxygen to the tissues, usually due to **hypoxemia**.
☐ **Kussmaul respirations** (**KOOS**-mowl)	**Kussmaul respirations** are a very deep, gasping type of respiration typically associated with severe diabetic acidosis. This hyperventilation (with very deep, but not labored, respirations) represents the body's attempt to decrease acidosis, counteracting the effect of the ketone buildup that occurs with diabetic acidosis.
☐ **orthopnea** (or-**THOP**-nee-ah) orth/o = straight -pnea = breathing	Respiratory condition in which there is difficulty in breathing in any but erect, sitting, or standing position. Symptoms of **orthopnea** include slow or rapid respiratory rate; sitting or standing posture necessary to breathe properly; muscles of respiration forcibly used; patients feel necessity of bracing themselves to breathe; anxious expression, cyanotic face; and struggle to inhale and exhale.
☐ **pleural rub** (**PLOO**-ral rub) pleur/o = pleura -al = pertaining to	Friction rub caused by inflammation of the **pleural space**. The sound is heard on **auscultation**.
☐ **rales** (**RALZ**)	An abnormal sound heard on **auscultation** of the chest, produced by passage of air through **bronchi** that contain secretion or exudate or that are constricted by spasm or a thickening of their walls; also known as crackles. The sound is a crackling sound similar to that of moisture crackling in a tube as air passes through it. The crackles are heard on **auscultation**, usually during inhalation. **Rales** may be described as bibasilar, bubbling, coarse, crackling, crepitant, post-tussive, moist, or sticky.
☐ **rhinorrhea** (**rye**-noh-**REE**-ah) rhin/o = nose -rrhea = discharge; flow	**Rhinorrhea** is thin, watery discharge from the nose.
☐ **rhonchi** (**RONG**-kigh)	Rattlings in the throat, especially when it resembles snoring. Loud, coarse, rattling sounds produced by passage of air through obstructed airways. The sounds are heard on **auscultation**. **Rhonchi** may be described as coarse, high-pitched, humming, low-pitched, musical, post-tussive, sibilant (hissing), sonorous (loud), or whistling.

| sneeze | To expel air forcibly through the nose and mouth by spasmodic contraction of muscles of expiration due to irritation of nasal mucosa. |
| | The sneeze reflex may be produced by a great number of stimuli. Placing a foot on a cold surface will provoke a sneeze in some people, whereas looking at a bright light or sunlight will cause it in others. Firm pressure applied to the middle of the upper lip and just under the nose will sometimes prevent a sneeze that is about to occur. |

| stridor (**STRIGH**-dor) | Harsh sound during respiration; high-pitched and resembling the blowing of wind, due to obstruction of air passages. |
| | **Stridor** is heard without the aid of a stethoscope, usually during inhalation. |

| tachypnea (**tak**-ip-**NEE**-ah) tachy- = rapid -pnea = breathing | Abnormal rapidity of breathing. |
| | One example of this is nervous **tachypnea**, evidenced by a respiratory rate of 40 or more respirations per minute. It occurs in hysteria and neurasthenia. If prolonged, it will cause excess loss of carbon dioxide, and the hyperventilation syndrome will develop (fall in blood pressure, vasoconstriction; sometimes fainting). Immediate treatment involves having the patient breathe into a paper bag until the carbon dioxide content of the blood has an opportunity to return to normal. It is important to keep the patient calm and reassured. |

| wheeze (**HWEEZ**) | A whistling sound or sighing sound resulting from narrowing of the lumen of a respiratory passageway. |
| | The **wheeze** is often heard without the aid of a stethoscope, usually during exhalation. Wheezing may occur in **asthma**, **croup**, hay fever, mitral stenosis, and **pleural effusion**. It may result from presence of tumors, foreign obstructions, bronchial spasm, **tuberculosis**, obstructive **emphysema**, or edema. |

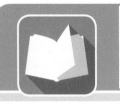

Review Checkpoint

Check your understanding of this section by completing the **Common Signs and Symptoms** exercises in your workbook.

Pathological Conditions

The pathological conditions are also divided into upper respiratory conditions and lower respiratory conditions. As you study the pathological conditions of the respiratory system, note that the **basic definition** is in a green shaded box, followed by a detailed description in regular print. The phonetic pronunciation is directly beneath each term, as well as a breakdown of the component parts of the term where applicable.

Upper Respiratory Conditions

coryza (kor-**RYE**-zuh)	**Coryza** is inflammation of the respiratory mucous membranes, known as rhinitis or the common cold. The term *common cold* is usually used when referring to symptoms of an upper respiratory tract infection.
	The patient may experience nasal discharge and obstruction, sore throat, sneezing, general malaise, fever, chills, headache, and muscle aches. A cough may also accompany a cold. The symptoms may last a week or more and usually occur without fever.
croup (**KROOP**)	A childhood disease characterized by a barking cough, hoarseness, **tachypnea**, inspiratory stridor, and laryngeal spasm.
	The symptoms of **croup** can be dramatic and anxiety-producing to the parent and the child. It is important to approach the child and parents in a calm manner to reduce fears and anxiety. Treatment includes providing a high-humidity atmosphere with cool moisture (cool mist vaporizer) and rest to relieve the symptoms. **Croup** may result from an acute obstruction of the **larynx** caused by an allergen, foreign body, infection, or new growth.
diphtheria (diff-**THEER**-ree-uh)	Serious infectious disease affecting the nose, **pharynx**, or **larynx**, usually resulting in sore throat, **dysphonia**, and fever. The disease is caused by the *Corynebacterium diphtheriae* bacterium, which forms a white coating over the affected airways as it multiplies.
	The bacterium releases a toxin into the bloodstream that can quickly damage the heart and nerves, resulting in heart failure, paralysis, and death. **Diphtheria** is uncommon in countries such as the United States, where a vaccine against the disease is routinely given to children. This immunization is one of the components of the DPT immunization.

laryngitis
(**lair**-in-**JYE**-tis)
  laryng/o = larynx
  -itis = inflammation
	Inflammation of the **larynx**, usually resulting in **dysphonia** (hoarseness), cough, and difficulty swallowing.

	Laryngitis commonly occurs as a result of abuse of the voice (as in **laryngitis** that often accompanies football games) and as part of an upper respiratory tract infection (but may also be the result of chronic **bronchitis** or chronic **sinusitis**). Acute **laryngitis** includes scratchy throat, hoarseness, or complete loss of voice (aphonia) as well as severe cough. Treatment for **laryngitis** includes resting the voice, avoiding irritants such as smoking, and using cool mist vaporizer.
pertussis (per-**TUH**-sis)	An acute upper respiratory infectious disease caused by the *Bordetella pertussis* bacterium; "whooping cough."
	Occurring mainly in children and infants, the early stages of **pertussis** are suggestive of the common cold (with slight elevation of fever, sneezing, **rhinitis**, dry cough, irritability, and loss of appetite). As the disease progresses (approximately two weeks later), the cough is more violent and

consists of a series of several short coughs followed by a long drawn inspiration during which the typical whoop is heard. The coughing episode may be severe enough to cause vomiting. If diagnosed early, **pertussis** can be treated with oral antibiotics. Otherwise, antibiotics are ineffective and treatment (when needed) consists of supportive care such as the administration of sedatives to reduce coughing and oxygen to facilitate respiration. **Pertussis** may be prevented by immunization of infants beginning at three months of age. This immunization is one of the components of the DPT immunization.

pharyngitis	Inflammation of the **pharynx**, usually resulting in sore throat. See *Figure 11-7*.

(fair-in-**JYE**-tis)

  pharyng/o = pharynx
  -itis = inflammation

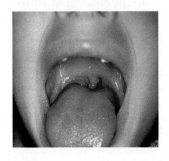

Pharyngitis is usually caused by viral infection but can also be caused by bacterial infection or other factors. In acute **pharyngitis**, the patient has fiery red pharyngeal membranes and swollen tonsils flecked with exudate, and the cervical lymph nodes are enlarged and tender. The patient usually experiences fever, malaise, and sore throat. When the causative organism is the group A streptococcus, the acute **pharyngitis** is termed *strep throat*.

Figure 11-7 Streptococcal pharyngitis
(Courtesy of the Centers for Disease Control and Prevention [CDC])

rhinitis	Inflammation of the mucous membranes of the nose, usually resulting in obstruction of the nasal passages, **rhinorrhea**, sneezing, and facial pressure or pain, also known as **coryza**.

(rye-NYE-tis)

  rhin/o = nose
  -itis = inflammation

Rhinitis is often caused by viral infection but can also be caused by allergy or other factors.

sinusitis	Inflammation of a sinus, especially a paranasal sinus.

(sigh-nus-**EYE**-tis)

  sinus/o = sinus
  -itis = inflammation

Sinusitis usually results in pain and a feeling of pressure in the affected sinuses. A purulent nasal discharge is also common. Acute **sinusitis** frequently develops as a result of a common cold, or allergy, or as a complication of an upper respiratory infection. Treatment of **sinusitis** includes antibiotics to control the infection, decongestants to decrease the swelling in the nasal mucosa, and analgesics to relieve the pain in the area.

tonsillitis	Inflammation of the **palatine tonsils**, located in the area of the **oropharynx**.

(ton-sill-**EYE**-tis)

  tonsill/o = tonsils
  -itis = inflammation

Symptoms include sore throat, fever, snoring, and difficulty in swallowing. The tonsils appear enlarged and red with yellowish exudate. Acute **tonsillitis** has a sudden onset accompanied by fever and chills. The patient may experience malaise and headache in addition to the general symptoms. Treatment includes bed rest, liquid diet, antipyretics, analgesics, and saline gargles. Antibiotic therapy may be indicated, depending on the causative organism.

Lower Respiratory Conditions

asthma (**AZ**-mah)	Paroxysmal dyspnea accompanied by wheezing caused by a spasm of the bronchial tubes or by swelling of their mucous membrane.

No age is exempt, but **asthma** occurs most frequently in childhood or early adulthood. **Asthma** differs from other obstructive lung diseases in that it is a reversible process. The attack may last from 30 minutes to several hours. In some circumstances the attack subsides spontaneously. The asthmatic attack starts suddenly with coughing and a sensation of tightness in the chest. Then slow, laborious, wheezy breathing begins. Expiration is much more strenuous and prolonged than inspiration, and the patient may assume a "hunched forward" position in an attempt to get more air. Recurrence and severity of attacks are greatly influenced by secondary factors, by mental or physical fatigue, by exposure to fumes, by endocrine changes at various periods in life, and by emotional situations. Acute attacks of **asthma** may be relieved by a number of drugs, such as epinephrine. Status asthmaticus is a severe **asthma** attack that is unresponsive to conventional therapy and lasts longer than 24 hours; it is considered a medical emergency.

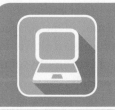

Media Link

Gain a better understanding of this condition by watching the **Asthma** animation on the Student Companion Website.

bronchiectasis
 	
(brong-key-**EK**-tah-sis)
  bronchi/o = bronchus
  -ectasis = stretching or dilation
	Chronic dilation of a bronchus or **bronchi**, with secondary infection that usually involves the lower portion of the lung.

The infection damages the bronchial wall, causing loss of its supporting structure and producing thick **sputum** that may ultimately obstruct the **bronchi**. The bronchial walls become permanently distended by severe coughing. Symptoms of **bronchiectasis** include chronic cough, the production of purulent **sputum** in copious amounts, **hemoptysis** in a high percentage of patients, and clubbing of the fingers. The patient is also subject to repeated pulmonary infections.

bronchitis
 	
(brong-**KIGH**-tis)
  bronch/o = bronchus
  -itis = inflammation
	Inflammation of the mucous membrane of the bronchial tubes. Infection is often preceded by the common cold.

The patient may experience a productive cough, sometimes accompanied by wheezing, **dyspnea**, and chest pain. Acute **bronchitis** is usually caused by viral infection but can also be caused by bacterial infection or airborne irritants such as smoke and pollution. In most cases, it resolves without treatment. If a bacterial infection is suspected, the patient may be treated with oral antibiotics, bed rest, increased intake of fluids, antipyretics and analgesics, and cool mist vaporizer.

Chronic **bronchitis** is primarily associated with cigarette smoking or exposure to pollution. The smoke irritates the airways, resulting in inflammation and hypersecretion of mucus. In chronic **bronchitis**, the productive cough is present for at least three months of two consecutive years. Treatment consists of having the patient who smokes stop smoking, prescribing bronchodilators, and treating with antibiotics as necessary.

bronchogenic carcinoma	A malignant lung tumor that originates in the **bronchi**; lung cancer.

(**brong**-koh-**JEN**-ic car-sin-**OH**-mah)
  bronch/o = bronchus
  -genic = pertaining to formation; producing
  carcin/o = cancer
  -oma = tumor

Bronchogenic carcinoma is usually associated with a history of cigarette smoking. It is increasing at a greater rate in women than in men and now exceeds breast cancer as the most common cause of cancer deaths in women. Symptoms of bronchogenic (lung) cancer include (but may not be limited to) a persistent cough, blood-streaked **sputum** (**hemoptysis**), chest pain, and voice change. Survival rate for lung cancer is low due to usually significant metastasis at the time of diagnosis. More than one-half of the tumors are advanced and inoperable when diagnosed.

emphysema	A chronic pulmonary disease characterized by increase beyond the normal in the size of air spaces distal to the terminal bronchiole, either from dilation of the **alveoli** or from destruction of their walls. See *Figure 11-8*.

(em-fih-**SEE**-mah)

This nonuniform pattern of abnormal permanent distention of the air spaces appears to be the end stage of a process that has progressed slowly for many years. By the time the patient develops the symptoms of **emphysema**, pulmonary function is often so impaired that it is irreversible.

The major cause of **emphysema** is cigarette smoking. The person with **emphysema** has a chronic obstruction (increase in airway resistance) to the inflow and outflow of air from the lungs. The lungs lose their elasticity and are in a chronic state of hyperexpansion, making expiration of air more difficult. The act of expiration then becomes one of active muscular movement to force the air out. The patient takes on a "barrel chest" appearance due to the loss of elasticity of lung tissue, becoming increasingly short of breath.

Treatment for **emphysema** is directed at smoking cessation, improving the quality of life for the patient and maximizing lung function. This may involve measures to improve the patient's ventilation (with the use of bronchodilators and medicine to thin the mucous secretions) as well as administration of medications to treat any infection present and the administration of oxygen to treat the **hypoxia** that may be present.

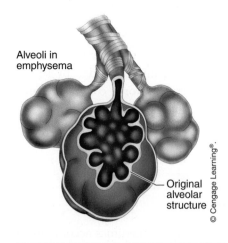

Alveoli in emphysema

Original alveolar structure

© Cengage Learning®.

Figure 11-8 Emphysema

empyema	Pus in a body cavity, especially in the pleural cavity (pyothorax); usually the result of a primary infection in the lungs.

(em-pye-**EE**-mah)

The patient has fever, night sweats, pleural pain, **dyspnea**, anorexia, and weight loss. **Empyema** is treated with antibiotic therapy and aspiration of **pleural** fluid.

hyaline membrane disease (**HIGH**-ah-lighn membrane dih-**ZEEZ**)	Also known as respiratory distress syndrome (RDS) of the premature infant, **hyaline membrane disease** is severe impairment of the function of respiration in the premature newborn. This condition is rarely present in a newborn of greater than 37 weeks' gestation or in one weighing at least 5 pounds.
	Shortly after birth, the premature infant will have a low Apgar score and will develop signs of acute respiratory distress due to atelectasis of the lung. **Tachypnea**, tachycardia, retraction of the rib cage during inspiration, **cyanosis**, and grunting during expiration will be present.
influenza (in-floo-**EN**-zah)	A highly contagious viral infection of the respiratory tract transmitted by airborne droplet infection; also known as the flu. Influenza can occur in isolated cases or can be epidemic. The incubation period is usually one to three days after exposure.
	Symptoms of the flu include sore throat, cough, fever, muscular pains, and generalized weakness. The onset is usually sudden, with the individual experiencing fever, chills, respiratory symptoms, headache, muscle pain, and extreme tiredness.
	Treatment for influenza is symptomatic and involves bed rest, plenty of fluids, and medications for pain. Recovery usually occurs within 3 to 10 days. Routine annual influenza vaccination of all persons aged 6 months and older continues to be recommended by the ACIP (Advisory Committee on Immunization Practices).
lung abscess (lung **AB**-sess)	A localized collection of pus formed by the destruction of lung tissue and microorganisms by white blood cells that have migrated to the area to fight infection.
	A **lung abscess** usually produces pneumonialike symptoms and a productive cough with blood and purulent or foul-smelling **sputum**. Most lung abscesses occur because of aspiration of nasopharyngeal or oropharyngeal material.

pleural effusion
 	
(PLOO-ral eh-FYOO-zhun)
  pleur/o = pleura
  -al = pertaining to
 	
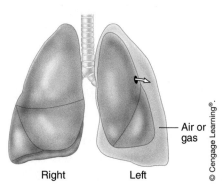
Right   Left
	Accumulation of fluid in the **pleural space**, resulting in compression of the underlying portion of the lung, with resultant **dyspnea**. See *Figure 11-9*.

	Pleural effusion is usually secondary to some other disease. Normally, the **pleural space** contains a small amount of fluid that acts as a lubricant to the pleural surfaces during respiration. With **pleural effusion**, a significant amount of fluid may accumulate in the **pleural space**. The presence of the fluid is confirmed by chest X-ray, ultrasound, physical examination, and **thoracentesis**. Treatment is designed to treat the cause, prevent fluid collection from recurring in the **pleural space**, and to relieve the discomfort and **dyspnea** experienced by the patient.

Air or gas

© Cengage Learning®.

Figure 11-9 Pleural effusion

pleuritis (pleurisy)	Inflammation of both the visceral and **parietal pleura**.
(ploor-**EYE**-tis) (**PLOOR**-ih-see) pleur/o = pleura -itis = inflammation	Remember that the **pleura** is the double-folded membrane that lines the thoracic cavity. The side of this membrane that is closest to the ribs is known as the **parietal pleura** and the side that is closest to the internal organs is known as the **visceral pleura**. The pleurae are moistened with a serous secretion that reduces friction during respiratory movements of the lungs. When these two membranes become inflamed (due to **pleurisy**) and rub together during respiration (particularly inspiration), the patient experiences a severe, sharp, "knifelike" pain. The pleural rub can be heard on **auscultation**. **Pleuritis** may be primary or secondary as a result of some other condition.

pneumonia	Inflammation of the lungs caused primarily by bacteria, viruses, and chemical irritants.
(new-**MOH**-nee-ah) pneumon/o = lungs, air -ia = condition	The most common bacterial **pneumonia**, **pneumococcal pneumonia**, is caused by the *Streptococcus pneumonia* bacterium. In certain situations, **pneumonia** is caused by other microorganisms or by other lung irritants. For example, people with severely impaired immune systems (e.g., those with acquired immune deficiency syndrome [AIDS] or certain types of cancer) are susceptible to **pneumocystis pneumonia**—a type of **pneumonia** caused by the protozoal parasite *Pneumocystis carinii*. Pneumocystis pneumonia is life-threatening in susceptible patients. Mild cases of **pneumonia** may resolve without treatment. Moderate cases are often treated with oral antibiotics, whereas severe cases often require hospitalization and treatment with intravenous antibiotics. If the patient has developed complications, these may need to be treated as well.

pneumothorax	A collection of air or gas in the **pleural** cavity. The air enters as the result of a perforation through the chest wall or the **pleura** covering the lung (**visceral pleura**), causing the lung to collapse. See *Figure 11-10*.
(new-moh-**THOH**-racks) pneum/o = lungs, air -thorax = chest	The symptoms of a spontaneous **pneumothorax** are sudden sharp pain, **dyspnea**, and cough. Pain may be referred to the shoulder. The majority of cases are mild and require only rest. A **pneumothorax**, if severe enough, can collapse the lung and shift the heart and the great vessels and **trachea** toward the unaffected side of the chest due to the pressure that builds up within the **pleural space** (tension pneumothorax). This type of **pneumothorax** would require immediate medical attention to increase the oxygen supply to the patient and to reexpand the lung.

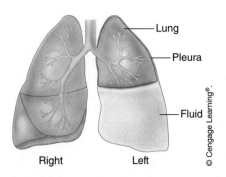

Figure 11-10 Pneumothorax

pulmonary edema	An abnormal accumulation of fluid in the lungs, either in the **alveoli** or the interstitial spaces.
(**PULL**-mon-air-ree eh-**DEE**-mah) pulmon/o = lung -ary = pertaining to	The most common cause of **pulmonary edema** is congestive heart failure. The pulmonary congestion occurs when the pulmonary vessels receive more blood from the right ventricle of the heart than the left ventricle can

accommodate and remove. This congestion (or backup of fluid) causes the fluid to leak through the capillary walls and permeate into the airways, creating breathlessness and a sense of suffocation. The patient's nail beds become cyanotic and the skin becomes gray. As the condition progresses, breathing is noisy and moist. The patient needs immediate medical attention—it is a medical emergency.

pulmonary embolism
 	
(**PULL**-mon-air-ree **EM**-boh-lizm)
  pulmon/o = lung
  -ary = pertaining to
  embol/i = to throw
  -ism = condition
	The obstruction of one or more pulmonary arteries by a thrombus (clot) that dislodges from another location and is carried through the venous system to the vessels of the lung.

The onset of a **pulmonary embolism** is sudden. The most common symptom is chest pain, followed by **dyspnea** and **tachypnea**. A massive embolism blocking the pulmonary artery can produce extreme **dyspnea**; sudden substernal pain; rapid, weak pulse; shock; fainting (syncope); and sudden death. Massive **pulmonary embolism** is a true medical emergency because the patient's condition tends to deteriorate rapidly. Most patients who die from a **pulmonary embolism** do so within the first two hours after the embolism.

pulmonary heart disease (cor pulmonale)
 	
(**PULL**-mon-air-ree heart dih-**ZEEZ**)
(cor pull-mon-**ALL**-ee)
  pulmon/o = lung
  -ary = pertaining to
	Pulmonary heart disease (cor pulmonale) is hypertrophy of the right ventricle of the heart (with or without failure) resulting from disorders of the lungs, pulmonary vessels, or chest wall; heart failure resulting from pulmonary disease.

The pulmonary disease reduces proper ventilation to the lungs, resulting in increased resistance in the pulmonary circulation. This, in turn, raises the pulmonary blood pressure. **Cor pulmonale** develops because of the pulmonary hypertension that causes the right side of the heart to work harder to pump the blood against the resistance of the pulmonary vascular circulation, thus creating hypertrophy of the right ventricle of the heart.

Chronic obstructive pulmonary disease (COPD), the most frequent cause of cor pulmonale, produces shortness of breath and cough. The patient develops edema of the feet and legs, distended neck veins, an enlarged liver, **pleural effusion**, ascites, and a heart murmur.

Treatment is related to treating the underlying cause of **cor pulmonale** and is often a long-term process. In the case of COPD, treatment involves improving the patient's ventilation (airways must be dilated to improve gas exchange within the lungs). The improved transport of oxygen to the blood and body tissues will reduce the strain on the pulmonary circulation, thus relieving the pulmonary hypertension that leads to **cor pulmonale**.

sudden infant death syndrome	The completely unexpected and unexplained death of an apparently well, or virtually well, infant. SIDS, also known as crib death, is the most common cause of death between the second week and first year of life.

In the United States, SIDS is responsible for the deaths of approximately 7,000 infants each year. This worldwide syndrome occurs more frequently in the third and fourth months of life, in premature infants, in males, and in infants living in poverty. The deaths usually occur during sleep and are more likely to happen in winter than in summer. Infants at risk for SIDS are monitored during their sleep and are sometimes placed on an **apnea** alarm mattress designed to sound an alarm when the infant lying on it ceases to breathe.

tuberculosis (too-**ber**-kyoo-**LOH**-sis)	An infectious disease caused by the *Mycobacterium tuberculosis* tubercle bacillus and characterized by inflammatory infiltrations, formation of tubercles, and caseous (cheeselike) necrosis in the tissues of the lungs. Other organ systems may also be infected.

This necrotic area of the lung, also known as a cavitation, usually appears in the **apex** of the lung. (It resembles an area shaded by a piece of chalk being rubbed on its side, in a circular motion on a chalkboard.)

In humans, the primary infection usually consists of a localized lesion and regional adenitis. From this state, lesions may heal by fibrosis and calcification and the disease exists in an arrested or inactive state.

Tuberculosis is spread by droplet infection. When organism-containing droplets sneezed or coughed into the air by an infected individual are inhaled by an uninfected individual, the *mycobacterium* usually settles in the lungs and lies dormant until the immune system is weakened. Then it multiplies, resulting in coughing (productive cough), chest pain, **dyspnea**, fever, night sweats, and poor appetite. The **sputum** may have a greenish tinge to it.

Sputum tests, tuberculin skin testing (PPD), and chest X-rays assist in the diagnosis of **tuberculosis**. A positive skin test will indicate the need for a diagnostic chest X-ray to determine the presence of active lesions. **Sputum** tests will also be performed to check for the presence of acid-fast bacillus. **Tuberculosis** is treated with a prolonged (9 to 12 months) course of antibacterial/antibiotic medications and vitamins. Resistance to prescribed medications can result if the treatment regimen is not completed and the patient is reinfected.

Work-Related Pathological Conditions

Lung diseases can occur in a variety of occupations as a result of exposure to dusts and gases. The effect of inhaling these materials depends on the nature of the material being inhaled and the length of exposure to the material as well as to the worker's susceptibility. In today's occupational environment, every effort is made by the employer to protect the employee from exposure to hazardous materials. Employees must be informed about all hazardous and toxic substances in their workplace. In addition, they must be educated as to the particular materials to which they will be exposed as well as to the proper methods of protection.

The Occupational Safety and Health Act (OSHA) provides guidelines for protecting the safety and health of individuals in industrial and medical settings. There are various other governmental agencies that enforce controls on the workplace for the protection of the employee. The following terms relate to occupational lung diseases.

anthracosis (an-thrah-**KOH**-sis) anthrac/o = coal -osis = condition	**Anthracosis** is the accumulation of carbon deposits in the lungs due to breathing smoke or coal dust (black lung disease); also called coal worker's pneumoconiosis.
	As the coal worker's pneumoconiosis progresses, the **bronchioles** and **alveoli** become clogged with coal dust, which leads to the formation of the "coal macule" (blackish dots on the lung). The macules enlarge, causing the weakened bronchiole to dilate, with subsequent development of a focal emphysema (a form of pulmonary emphysema associated with inhalation of environmental dusts, producing dilation of the terminal and respiratory **bronchioles**).
asbestosis (**as**-beh-**STOH**-sis)	**Asbestosis** is a lung disease resulting from inhalation of asbestos particles.
	Exposure to asbestos has been associated with the later development of cancer of the lung, especially mesothelioma. The latency period may be 20 years or more.
byssinosis (bis-ih-**NOH**-sis)	A lung disease resulting from inhalation of cotton, flax, and hemp; also known as brown lung disease.
	Byssinosis is characterized by wheezing and tightness in the chest. The disease does not occur in textile workers who work with cotton after it is bleached.
silicosis (sill-ih-**KOH**-sis)	**Silicosis** is a lung disease resulting from inhalation of silica (quartz) dust, characterized by formation of small nodules.
	With the passage of time and exposure, the nodules enlarge and grow together, forming dense masses. The lung eventually becomes unable to expand fully, and secondary **emphysema** may develop. Exposure to silica dust for 10 to 20 years is usually required before **silicosis** develops and shortness of breath is evident.

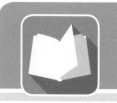

Review Checkpoint

Check your understanding of this section by completing the **Pathological Conditions** exercises in your workbook.

Diagnostic Techniques, Treatments, and Procedures

bronchoscopy (brong-**KOSS**-koh-pee) bronch/o = bronchus -scopy = process of viewing	**Bronchoscopy** is the examination of the interior of the **bronchi** using a lighted, flexible tube known as a bronchoscope (or endoscope).

The tube is inserted into the **bronchi** via the nose, **pharynx**, **larynx**, and **trachea** to visually examine the **trachea** and major **bronchi** with their branchings. A **bronchoscopy** may be performed to remove a foreign body, to improve air passage by suctioning out obstructions such as a mucus plug, to obtain a biopsy and/or secretions for examination, and to observe the air passages for signs of disease. As with most endoscopes, tiny forceps or other instruments can be passed through a laryngoscope or bronchoscope to obtain fluid/tissue specimens for laboratory analysis. See *Figure 11-11*.

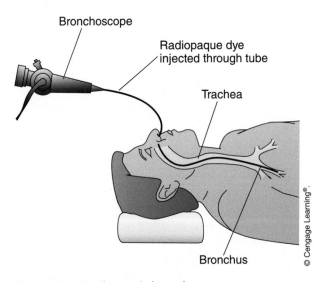

Figure 11-11 Fiberoptic bronchoscopy

chest X-ray	The use of high-energy electromagnetic waves passing through the body onto a photographic film to produce a picture of the internal structures of the body for diagnosis and therapy.

The chest X-ray allows the physician to visualize sites of abnormal density, such as collections of fluid or pus. *Figure 11-12* illustrates the normal posteroanterior (PA) view of the chest.

laryngoscopy (lar-in-**GOSS**-koh-pee) laryng/o = larynx -scopy = process of viewing	**Laryngoscopy** is the examination of the interior of the **larynx** using a lighted, flexible tube known as a laryngoscope (or endoscope).

The tube is inserted into the **larynx** via the mouth or nose to examine the **larynx** and associated structures visually.

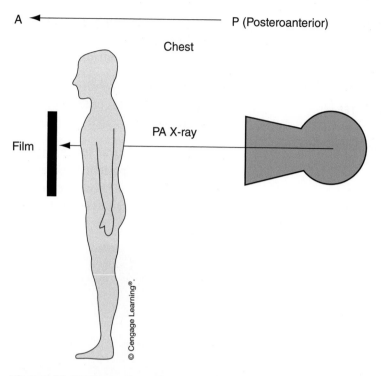

Figure 11-12 Posteroanterior view of chest

nuclear perfusion lung scan	The visual imaging of the distribution of ventilation or blood flow in the lungs by scanning the lungs after the patient has been injected with or has inhaled radioactive material.
	The scanning device records the pattern of pulmonary radioactivity after the patient has received the medication. This scan can show areas of the lungs that are not receiving enough blood.
pulmonary function tests	Physicians use this variety of tests to assess respiratory function.
putmon/o = lung -ary = pertaining to	One of the most common is the use of a measuring device called a **spirometer** to measure the patient's breathing capacity. Measurement of different portions of the patient's lung volume provides an indication of the nature of any breathing impairment, as does measurement of the volume of air a patient can expel during a rapid, vigorous exhalation.
sputum specimen (**SPEW**-tum specimen)	A specimen of material expectorated from the mouth. If produced after a cough, it may contain (in addition to saliva) material from the throat and **bronchi**.

The physical and bacterial character of the **sputum** depend on the disease process involved and the ability of the patient to cough up material. Some bronchial secretions are quite tenacious (adhere to bronchial walls) and are difficult to cough up. When requesting a **sputum** specimen from the patient, it is important that the patient understands the instructions. He or she should not be collecting saliva from the mouth only, as in spitting.

The patient should be instructed to collect a **sputum** specimen, preferably in the morning before eating or drinking. Encourage the patient to cough deeply (from as far down as possible). The **sputum** should be placed in the appropriate container and treated as infective until testing proves otherwise. **Sputum** may be described as blood streaked, foul tasting, frothy, gelatinous, green, purulent, putrid, stringy, rusty, viscid, viscous, watery, or yellow.

thoracentesis (**thoh**-rah-sen-**TEE**-sis) thor/a = chest -centesis = surgical puncture	**Thoracentesis** involves the use of a needle to collect pleural fluid for laboratory analysis or to remove excess pleural fluid or air from the **pleural space**.

To reach the **pleural space**, the needle is passed through the patient's skin and chest wall (puncturing these tissues). See *Figure 11-13*. The needle and syringe should be checked carefully to be certain that they fit snugly so that no air is permitted to enter the **pleural space**.

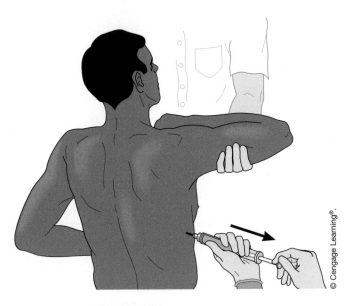

© Cengage Learning®.

Figure 11-13 Thoracentesis

tonsillectomy (ton-sill-**ECK**-toh-mee) tonsill/o = tonsils -ectomy = surgical removal	Surgical removal of the **palatine tonsils**.

A **tonsillectomy** is often combined with an adenoidectomy (surgical removal of the **adenoids**). When the tonsils and **adenoids** are removed at the same time, the procedure is called a tonsillectomy and adenoidectomy (T & A).

This procedure is among the most common surgical procedures performed on children in the United States. Indications for surgical removal of the tonsils include (but may not be limited to) the following:

- recurrent acute infections of the tonsils or chronic infections that have not responded to antibiotic therapy.
- enlarged tonsils that cause upper airway obstruction.
- abscess around the tonsils (peritonsillar abscess) that does not respond to antibiotic therapy.
- adults who have recurrent sore throats or ear pain or who snore due to enlarged adenoid or tonsillar tissue.

A tonsillectomy is usually performed under general anesthesia. The tonsillar tissue is dissected (cut away) and removed, and the bleeding areas are sutured and cauterized (burned) to control the bleeding.

During the first 12 to 24 hours following the procedure, the patient is closely monitored for signs of bleeding. The most serious complication following a tonsillectomy is hemorrhaging. Ice chips and cool clear liquids are encouraged following surgery, and the patient progresses to a bland (mild) diet as tolerated.

tuberculin skin test (TST) (too-**BER**-kew-lin skin test)	The tuberculin skin test is used to determine past or present **tuberculosis** infection present in the body. This is based on a positive skin reaction to the introduction of a purified protein derivative (PPD) of the tubercle bacilli, called tuberculin, into the skin.

The medication may be introduced into the skin by one of the following methods: intradermal injection, scratch test, or puncture. The reaction is noted as positive if the area around the area of administration of the PPD is raised or reddened, or if a hard area forms around the test site. Follow-up testing with chest X-ray and **sputum** testing is used to determine the presence of **tuberculosis** in the individual. A tuberculin skin test may also be called a PPD test, but recent changes with the CDC (Centers for Disease Control and Prevention) guidelines for **tuberculosis** have indicated a name change to TST. A negative reaction does not rule out a diagnosis of previous or active **tuberculosis**.

Review Checkpoint

Check your understanding of this section by completing the **Diagnostic Techniques, Treatments, and Procedures** exercises in your workbook.

COMMON ABBREVIATIONS

Abbreviation	Meaning	Abbreviation	Meaning
ABG(s)	arterial blood gas(es)	**ARD**	acute respiratory disease (or distress)
AFB	acid-fast bacilli (The only AFB of clinical significance are organisms of the genus *Mycobacterium*, which cause **tuberculosis** and leprosy.)	**ARDS**	adult respiratory distress syndrome
		ARF	acute respiratory failure
		CDC	Centers for Disease Control and Prevention
AP	anteroposterior (a directional term, used particularly in X-rays, meaning "from the front to the back"; i.e., anteroposterior view of the chest)	**CO$_2$**	carbon dioxide

Abbreviation	Meaning	Abbreviation	Meaning
COPD	chronic obstructive pulmonary disease (associated with chronic **bronchitis** and **emphysema**)	PCP	*Pneumocystis carinii* **pneumonia**
CPR	cardiopulmonary resuscitation	PFT(s)	pulmonary function test(s)
CXR	chest X-ray	PPD	purified protein derivative; substance used in intradermal test for **tuberculosis**; now called TST
DPT	diphtheria, **pertussis** (whooping cough), and tetanus; an immunization given in childhood to prevent these diseases by providing immunity	R	respiration
		RDS	respiratory distress syndrome
IPPB	intermittent positive pressure breathing	RLL	right lower lobe (of the lung)
		RML	right middle lobe (of the lung)
LLL	left lower lobe (of the lung)		
LUL	left upper lobe (of the lung)	RUL	right upper lobe (of the lung)
O_2	oxygen	SIDS	sudden infant death syndrome
PA	posteroanterior (a directional term, used particularly in X-rays, meaning "from the back to the front"; i.e., posteroanterior view of the chest)	SOB	shortness of breath
		T & A	tonsillectomy and adenoidectomy
		TB	**tuberculosis**
$PaCO_2$	partial pressure of carbon dioxide (CO_2) dissolved in the blood	TPR	temperature, pulse, and respiration
PaO_2	partial pressure of oxygen (O_2) dissolved in the blood	TST	tuberculin skin test
		URI	upper respiratory infection

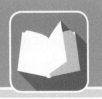

Review Checkpoint

Check your understanding of this section by completing the **Common Abbreviations** exercises in your workbook.

WRITTEN AND AUDIO TERMINOLOGY REVIEW

Review each of the following terms from the chapter. Study the spelling of each term and write the definition in the space provided. Check definitions by looking the term up in the glossary.

Term	Pronunciation	Definition
adenoids	☐ **ADD**-eh-noydz	_____
alveoli	☐ al-**VEE**-oh-lye	_____
anthracosis	☐ **an**-thrah-**KOH**-sis	_____
apex	☐ **AY**-peks	_____
aphonia	☐ ah-**FOH**-nee-ah	_____
apnea	☐ **AP**-nee-ah	_____
asbestosis	☐ **as**-beh-**STOH**-sis	_____
asthma	☐ **AZ**-mah	_____
atelectasis	☐ **at**-ee-**LEK**-tah-sis	_____
auscultation	☐ **oss**-kull-**TAY**-shun	_____
bradypnea	☐ **brad**-ip-**NEE**-ah	_____
bronchi	☐ **BRONG**-kigh	_____
bronchiectasis	☐ brong-key-**EK**-tah-sis	_____
bronchioles	☐ **BRONG**-key-ohlz	_____
bronchitis	☐ brong-**KIGH**-tis	_____
bronchogenic	☐ **brong**-koh-**JEN**-ic	_____
bronchorrhea	☐ **brong**-koh-**REE**-ah	_____
carcinoma	☐ **car**-sin-**OH**-mah	_____
bronchoscopy	☐ brong-**KOSS**-koh-pee	_____
byssinosis	☐ **bis**-ih-**NOH**-sis	_____
capillaries	☐ **CAP**-ih-**lair**-eez	_____
coryza	☐ kor-**RYE**-zuh	_____
croup	☐ **KROOP**	_____
cyanosis	☐ **sigh**-ah-**NOH**-sis	_____
diaphragm	☐ **DYE**-ah-fram	_____
dysphonia	☐ diss-**FOH**-nee-ah	_____

Term	Pronunciation	Definition
dyspnea	☐ **DISP**-nee-ah	_____
emphysema	☐ **em**-fih-**SEE**-mah	_____
empyema	☐ **em**-pye-**EE**-mah	_____
epiglottis	☐ **ep**-ih-**GLOT**-iss	_____
epistaxis	☐ **ep**-ih-**STAKS**-is	_____
expectoration	☐ ex-**pek**-toh-**RAY**-shun	_____
glottis	☐ **GLOT**-iss	_____
hemoptysis	☐ hee-**MOP**-tih-sis	_____
hyaline membrane disease	☐ **HIGH**-ah-lighn membrane dih-**ZEEZ**	_____
hypercapnia	☐ **high**-per-**KAP**-nee-ah	_____
hypoxemia	☐ **high**-pox-**EE**-mee-ah	_____
hypoxia	☐ **high**-**POX**-ee-ah	_____
Kussmaul respirations	☐ **KOOS**-mowl respirations	_____
laryngitis	☐ **lair**-in-**JYE**-tis	_____
laryngopharynx	☐ lair-**ring**-go-**FAIR**-inks	_____
laryngoscopy	☐ **lair**-in-**GOSS**-koh-pee	_____
larynx	☐ **LAIR**-inks	_____
lung abscess	☐ lung **AB**-sess	_____
mediastinum	☐ **mee**-dee-as-**TYE**-num	_____
nares	☐ **NAIRZ**	_____
nasopharynx	☐ **nay**-zoh-**FAIR**-inks	_____
oropharynx	☐ **or**-oh-**FAIR**-inks	_____
orthopnea	☐ **or**-**THOP**-nee-ah	_____
palatine tonsils	☐ **PAL**-ah-tyne **TON**-sills	_____
palpation	☐ pal-**PAY**-shun	_____
paranasal sinuses	☐ **pair**-ah-**NAY**-sal **SIGH**-nuss-ez	_____
parietal pleura	☐ pah-**RYE**-eh-tal **PLOO**-rah	_____
percussion	☐ per-**KUH**-shun	_____
pertussis	☐ per-**TUH**-sis	_____
pharyngitis	☐ **fair**-in-**JYE**-tis	_____
pharynx	☐ **FAIR**-inks	_____
phrenic nerve	☐ **FREN**-ic nerve	_____

Term	Pronunciation	Definition
pleura	☐ **PLOO**-rah	_____
pleural space	☐ **PLOO**-ral space	_____
pleural effusion	☐ **PLOO**-ral eh-**FYOO**-zhun	_____
pleuritis (pleurisy)	☐ ploor-**EYE**-tis (**PLOOR**-ih-see)	_____
pleurodynia	☐ **ploor**-oh-**DIN**-ee-ah	_____
pneumoconiosis	☐ **new**-moh-**koh**-nee-**OH**-sis	_____
pneumonia	☐ new-**MOH**-nee-ah	_____
pneumothorax	☐ new-moh-**THOH**-racks	_____
pulmonary edema	☐ **PULL**-mon-air-ree eh-**DEE**-mah	_____
pulmonary embolism	☐ **PULL**-mon-air-ee **EM**-boh-lizm	_____
pulmonary heart disease (cor pulmonale)	☐ **PULL**-mon-air-ree heart dih-**ZEEZ** (**cor** pull-mon-**ALL**-ee)	_____
pulmonary parenchyma	☐ **PULL**-mon-air-ee par-**EN**-kih-mah	_____
rales	☐ **RALZ**	_____
rhinitis	☐ rye-**NYE**-tis	_____
rhinorrhea	☐ **rye**-noh-**REE**-ah	_____
rhonchi	☐ **RONG**-kigh	_____
septum	☐ **SEP**-tum	_____
silicosis	☐ sill-ih-**KOH**-sis	_____
sinusitis	☐ sigh-nus-**EYE**-tis	_____
sputum	☐ **SPEW**-tum	_____
stridor	☐ **STRIGH**-dor	_____
tachypnea	☐ **tak**-ip-**NEE**-ah	_____
thoracentesis	☐ **thoh**-rah-sen-**TEE**-sis	_____
thoracotomy	☐ **thoh**-rah-**KOT**-oh-mee	_____
thorax	☐ **THOH**-raks	_____
tonsillitis	☐ ton-sill-**EYE**-tis	_____
trachea	☐ **TRAY**-kee-ah	_____
tuberculosis	☐ too-**ber**-kyoo-**LOH**-sis	_____
visceral pleura	☐ **VISS**-er-al **PLOO**-rah	_____
wheeze	☐ **HWEEZ**	_____

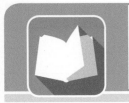

Review Checkpoint

Apply what you have learned in this chapter by completing the **Putting It All Together** exercise in your workbook.

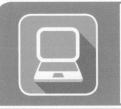

Online Resources

For additional study tools, including PowerPoint® slides and animations, go to the Student Companion Website.

Chapter Review Exercises

The following exercises provide a more in-depth review of the chapter material. Your goal in these exercises is to complete each section at a minimum 80% level of accuracy. A space has been provided for your score at the end of each section.

A. Spelling

Circle the correctly spelled term in each pairing of words. Each correct answer is worth 10 points. Record your score in the space provided at the end of the exercise.

1.	asthma	azthma	6.	tonsilitis	tonsillitis
2.	thoracentesis	throacentesis	7.	rales	rals
3.	emphysemia	emphysema	8.	apenea	apnea
4.	pluritis	pleuritis	9.	strydor	stridor
5.	diphtheria	diptheria	10.	epistaxis	epistacksis

Number correct _____ **× 10 points/correct answer: Your score** _____ **%**

B. Term to Definition: Signs and Symptoms

Define each term by writing the definition in the space provided. Check the box if you are able to complete this exercise correctly the first time (without referring to the answers). Each correct answer is worth 10 points. Record your score in the space provided at the end of the exercise.

1. rhinorrhea _____

2. hemoptysis _____

3. dysphonia _____

4. apnea _____

5. dyspnea _____

6. orthopnea _____

7. tachypnea _____

8. cyanosis _____

9. hypoxemia _____

10. hypoxia _____

Number correct _____ **× 10 points/correct answer: Your score** _____ **%**

C. Matching Breath Sounds

Match the following breath sounds on the left with the correct description on the right. Each correct answer is worth 10 points. Record your score in the space provided at the end of the exercise.

_____ 1. pleural rub

_____ 2. rales

_____ 3. rhonchi

_____ 4. stridor

_____ 5. wheeze

_____ 6. dyspnea

_____ 7. Kussmaul respirations

_____ 8. sneeze

_____ 9. cough

_____ 10. tachypnea

a. crackling sounds heard on auscultation, usually during inhalation

b. loud, coarse, rattling sounds heard on auscultation

c. abnormal rapidity of breathing

d. forceful, sometimes violent, expiratory effort preceded by a preliminary inspiration

e. harsh, high-pitched sound heard without a stethoscope (usually during inhalation)

f. to expel air forcibly through the nose and mouth by spasmodic contraction of muscles of expiration due to irritation of nasal mucosa

g. air hunger resulting in labored or difficult breathing

h. very deep gasping type of respiration associated with severe diabetic acidosis

i. whistling sound heard without a stethoscope, usually during exhalation

j. rubbing sound heard on auscultation

k. abnormally slow breathing

l. difficulty in speaking; hoarseness

Number correct _____ **× 10 points/correct answer: Your score** _____ **%**

D. Matching Respiratory Conditions

Match the following respiratory conditions on the left with the most appropriate definition on the right. Each correct answer is worth 10 points. Record your score in the space provided at the end of this exercise.

_____ 1. rhinitis

_____ 2. croup

_____ 3. sudden infant death syndrome

_____ 4. empyema

_____ 5. pleuritis

a. lung cancer

b. inflammation of the lungs caused primarily by viruses, bacteria, and chemical irritants

c. a childhood disease characterized by a barking cough, suffocative and difficult breathing, stridor, and laryngeal spasm

(*continued*)

_____ 6. pneumonia

_____ 7. asthma

_____ 8. emphysema

_____ 9. pneumothorax

_____ 10. bronchiogenic carcinoma

d. pus in a body cavity, especially in the pleural cavity

e. a collection of air or gas in the pleural cavity

f. inflammation of the mucous membrane of the nose

g. swelling of the lungs caused by an abnormal accumulation of fluid in the lungs

h. inflammation of both the visceral and parietal pleura; pleurisy

i. crib death

j. a chronic pulmonary disease characterized by increase beyond the normal in the size of the alveoli

k. paroxysmal dyspnea accompanied by wheezing caused by a spasm of the bronchial tubes

l. an infectious disease caused by the _Mycobacterium tuberculosis_ tubercle bacillus

Number correct _____ **× 10 points/correct answer: Your score** _____**%**

E. Proofreading Skills

Read the following Infectious Disease Consult Report. For each bold term, provide a brief definition and indicate if the term is spelled correctly. If it is misspelled, provide the correct spelling. Each correct answer is worth 10 points. Record your score in the space provided at the end of the exercise.

Example:

dyspnea _difficulty breathing_ _____

Spelled correctly? ☑ Yes ☐ No _____

INFECTIOUS DISEASE CONSULT

QUALI-CARE CLINIC

PATIENT NAME: Jorge Romero

PCP: Marie Aaron, DO

DATE OF BIRTH: 06/20/1957

AGE: 57

SEX: Male

DATE OF EXAM: 01/23/2014

REASON FOR CONSULT
Dr. Aaron referred this 57-year-old Latin American gentleman for evaluation of **pulmonary** cocci. At this point, I have tried to review the records from the hospital, speak with Dr. Aaron, and speak with the patient.

(continued)

INFECTIOUS DISEASE CONSULT
Patient Name: Jorge Romero
PCP: Marie Aaron, DO
Date of Exam: 01/23/2014
Page 2

HISTORY OF PRESENT ILLNESS
Our patient indicates that approximately 1 year ago, he apparently developed a right upper lobe lesion. At that point he was seen by Dr. Joshua Gatlin and actually underwent **bronchoscupy**. We pulled the results of those washings and cultures, and they demonstrated no fungus, no acid-fast bacilli. He had persistence of a nodule, so they opted to follow him as he was basically **asymptomatick**. Ultimately on a chest X-ray in October of last year, they thought the nodule was gradually increasing in size. Because of the history of non-Hodgkin lymphoma, they were concerned about recurrent cancer and decided to pursue evaluation. The patient underwent a needle aspiration in November, but no diagnosis was forthcoming. He underwent bone marrow aspiration and biopsy by Dr. Sharon Fisher, which was negative. He then saw Simon Williams, **thoracic** surgeon, who ultimately decided that the prudent thing would be to resect the lesion. The patient was taken to the operating room on December 19. Review of pathology showed a caseating granuloma and organisms consistent with coccidioidomycosis.

Based upon that, Dr. Williams spoke with me. I opted to place Mr. Romero on fluconazole 400 mg a day, which he started on December 23. In addition, we obtained urine cultures for cocci that are negative at this time. Our patient indicates he has tolerated the fluconazole well, although he is taking it q. 6 h.

Over the course of the last several months, the patient has experienced no fevers or chills. He did complain of anorexia, an 18-pound weight loss, and minimal sweats. He was unaware of a progressive cough, **sputim** production, hemoptysis, or progressive dyspnea. He relates that since his chemo, he has been a little bit short of breath, but he appreciates no major difference. As I stated, he has a history of non-Hodgkin lymphoma, although the last time it was active was 3½ years ago. No history of diabetes and no chronic use of steroids.

HABITS
A lifelong Florida resident, he is married with no children, enjoys traveling into northern Florida and Georgia, and goes hunting in Colorado.

PAST MEDICAL HISTORY
Non-Hodgkin lymphoma.

PAST SURGICAL HISTORY
1. Right upper lobe resection.
2. Bone spur, right shoulder.
3. Abdominal lymph node biopsies.

MEDICATION
Fluconazole 100 mg p.o. q. 6 h.

ALLERGIES
IODINE, which produces a rash. Some environmental allergies.

SOCIAL HISTORY
1. Smoking: One pack per day × 12 years, discontinued 19 years ago.
2. Ethanol: Three or four beers a month.

(continued)

INFECTIOUS DISEASE CONSULT
Patient Name: Jorge Romero
PCP: Marie Aaron, DO
Date of Exam: 01/23/2014
Page 3

3. IV drugs: None.
4. Occupation: Corrections officer for the state of Florida.

ASSESSMENT
Pulmonary coccidioidomycosis.

REVIEW OF SYSTEMS
At this point, no acute changes other than as mentioned above in the history of present illness.

PHYSICAL EXAMINATION
HEENT exam is basically unrevealing. Neck supple, good range of motion, no adenopathy. Back exam benign, no costovertebral angle (CVA) tenderness. Chest shows the right-sided incision to be well healed with no erythema, warmth, or drainage. Not fluctuant. Chest: Breath sounds good bilaterally. Cardiovascular: S1 and S2 without a significant rub or murmur. Abdomen: Bowel sounds present, soft, nontender; no guarding or rebound. Extremities: Motor 5/5 bilaterally. No unusual skin lesions or joint effusions. Neurologically he is awake, alert, and oriented x3, A nonfocal exam.

DISCUSSION
I truly believe that Mr. Romero currently has localized and limited disease. His antibody test was returned as negative. In general, if the titer is 1:8, this usually suggests the possibility of disseminated disease. At this point, I truly glean no history or physical findings suggestive of central nervous system (CNS) involvement, bone and joint involvement, or skin involvement. In light of the fact that he does have the underlying lymphoma, I feel the prudent thing is to pursue 6 months of fluconazole. In essence, I took this tactic because he had shown progression of this lesion over time.

In addition, his chest X-ray today shows some interstitial changes in the right midlung. This may be either postop or inflammatory in nature. I have taken the time to review with the patient the nature of this infection, its transmission, its clinical manifestations, and our planned therapy. I did review the toxicity of fluconazole, which is generally benign with only rare, occasional abnormal liver functions.

PLAN
1. Change fluconazole to 400 mg once a day.
2. Get CBC and liver function tests.
3. Assuming he remains stable, I will see him again in 6 weeks.

_____

Beth Brian, MD
Infectious Disease

BB:xx

D:01/23/2014

T:01/25/2014

C: Marie Aaron, DO, Joshua Stephen Gatlin, MD, Simon Williams, MD

1. **pulmonary** _____

_____

Spelled Correctly? ☐ Yes ☐ No _____

2. **bronchoscupy** _____

_____

Spelled Correctly? ☐ Yes ☐ No _____

3. **asymptomatick** _____

_____

Spelled Correctly? ☐ Yes ☐ No _____

4. **thoracic** _____

_____

Spelled Correctly? ☐ Yes ☐ No _____

5. **sputim** _____

_____

Spelled Correctly? ☐ Yes ☐ No _____

Number correct _____ × *20 points/correct answer: Your score* _____%

F. Matching Abbreviations

Match the abbreviations on the left with the correct definition on the right. Each correct answer is worth 10 points. When you have completed the exercise, record your score in the space provided at the end of the exercise.

_____	1. AFB	a. acute respiratory distress syndrome
_____	2. COPD	b. cardiopulmonary resuscitation
_____	3. LLL	c. pulmonary function tests
_____	4. URI	d. left upper lobe
_____	5. PFT(s)	e. left lower lobe
_____	6. SIDS	f. acid-fast bacilli
_____	7. SOB	g. chronic obstructive pulmonary disease
_____	8. IPPB	h. upper respiratory infection
_____	9. CPR	i. sudden infant death syndrome
_____	10. PA	j. shortness of breath
		k. intermittent positive pressure breathing
		l. posteroanterior
		m. urinary tract infection

Number correct _____ × *10 points/correct answer: Your score* _____%

G. Crossword Puzzle

Each crossword answer is worth 10 points. When you have completed the crossword puzzle, total your points and enter your score in the space provided.

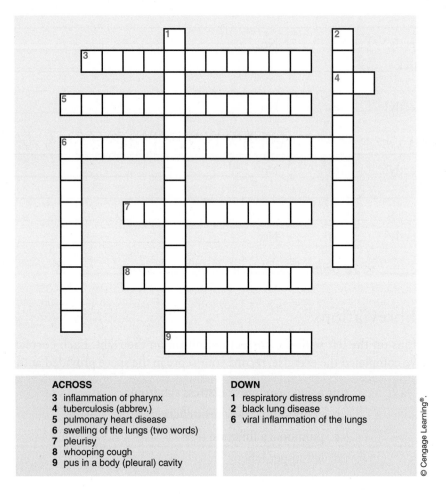

ACROSS
3 inflammation of pharynx
4 tuberculosis (abbrev.)
5 pulmonary heart disease
6 swelling of the lungs (two words)
7 pleurisy
8 whooping cough
9 pus in a body (pleural) cavity

DOWN
1 respiratory distress syndrome
2 black lung disease
6 viral inflammation of the lungs

© Cengage Learning®.

Number correct _____ × *10 points/correct answer: Your score* _____%

H. Word Element Review

The following words relate to the respiratory system. The prefixes and suffixes have been provided. Read the definition carefully and complete the word by filling in the blank, using the word elements provided in this chapter. If you have forgotten your word building rules, refer to Chapter 1. Each correct word is worth 10 points. Record your score in the space provided at the end of this exercise.

1. Inflammation of the lining of the chest cavity:

   _____ / itis

2. An instrument used to view the bronchi:

   _____ / o / scope

3. Inflammation of the nose:

   _____ / itis

4. Drainage or discharge from the nose:

   _____ / o / rrhea

5. Absence of breathing (without breathing):

a / _____ / a

6. Sitting up straight to breathe properly:

_____ / o / pne / a

7. Slow breathing:

brady / _____ / a

8. Rapid breathing:

tachy / _____ / a

9. Inflammation of the voice box:

_____ / itis

10. Pertaining to the air sacs in the lungs:

_____ / ar

Number correct _____ **× 10 points/correct answer: Your score** _____ **%**

I. Matching

Match the anatomical structures on the right with the most appropriate descriptions on the left. Each correct response is worth 10 points. When you have completed the exercise, record your score in the space provided at the end of the exercise.

_____ 1. hollow areas or cavities within the skull that communicate with the nasal cavity

_____ 2. hairlike projections on the mucous membranes that sweep dirt and foreign material toward the throat for elimination

_____ 3. another name for this structure is the throat

_____ 4. the two rounded masses of lymphatic tissue located in the nasopharynx are known as this

_____ 5. the two rounded masses of lymphatic tissue located on either side of the soft palate in the oropharynx are known as this

_____ 6. a small flap of cartilage that covers the opening of the larynx so that food cannot enter the larynx and lower airways while passing through the pharynx to the lower digestive structures

_____ 7. also known as the voice box

_____ 8. commonly known as the windpipe

_____ 9. these structures branch off from the trachea and lead into the lungs

_____ 10. the outer layer of the pleura that lines the thoracic cavity

a. epiglottis

b. pharynx

c. trachea

d. parietal pleura

e. paranasal sinuses

f. cilia

g. adenoids

h. palatine tonsils

i. larynx

j. bronchi

Number correct _____ **× 10 points/correct answer: Your score** _____ **%**

J. Word Search

Read each definition carefully and identify the applicable word from the list that follows. Enter the word in the space provided and then find it in the puzzle and circle it. The words may be read up, down, diagonally, across, or backward. Each correct answer is worth 10 points. Record your score in the space provided at the end of the exercise.

apex	tachypnea	diaphragm
pleura	rhinitis	apnea
epistaxis	rhinorrhea	nares
bradypnea	larynx	

Example: Inflammation of the mucous membranes of the nose.

rhinitis

1. The upper portion of the lung.

2. The musculomembranous wall separating the abdomen from the thoracic cavity.

3. The voice box.

4. The external nostrils.

5. The double-folded membrane that lines the thoracic cavity.

6. The medical term for nosebleed.

7. Thin, watery discharge from the nose.

8. Temporary cessation of breathing ("without breathing").

9. Abnormally slow breathing.

10. Abnormally rapid breathing.

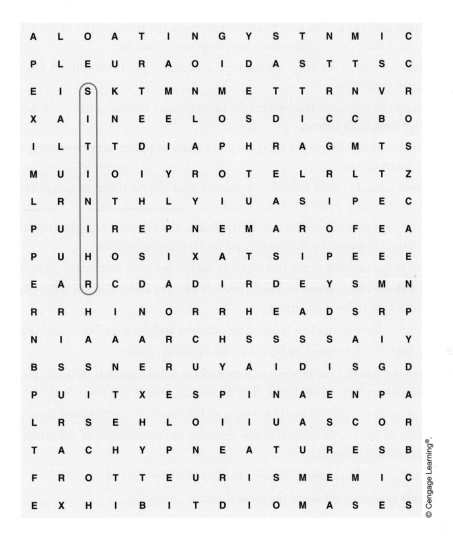

A	L	O	A	T	I	N	G	Y	S	T	N	M	I	C
P	L	E	U	R	A	O	I	D	A	S	T	T	S	C
E	I	S	K	T	M	N	M	E	T	T	R	N	V	R
X	A	I	N	E	E	L	O	S	D	I	C	C	B	O
I	L	T	T	D	I	A	P	H	R	A	G	M	T	S
M	U	I	O	I	Y	R	O	T	E	L	R	L	T	Z
L	R	N	T	H	L	Y	I	U	A	S	I	P	E	C
P	U	I	R	E	P	N	E	M	A	R	O	F	E	A
P	U	H	O	S	I	X	A	T	S	I	P	E	E	E
E	A	R	C	D	A	D	I	R	D	E	Y	S	M	N
R	R	H	I	N	O	R	R	H	E	A	D	S	R	P
N	I	A	A	A	R	C	H	S	S	S	S	A	I	Y
B	S	S	N	E	R	U	Y	A	I	D	I	S	G	D
P	U	I	T	X	E	S	P	I	N	A	E	N	P	A
L	R	S	E	H	L	O	I	I	U	A	S	C	O	R
T	A	C	H	Y	P	N	E	A	T	U	R	E	S	B
F	R	O	T	T	E	U	R	I	S	M	E	M	I	C
E	X	H	I	B	I	T	D	I	O	M	A	S	E	S

***Number correct* _____ × *10 points/correct answer: Your score* _____%**

K. Medical Scenario

The following medical scenario presents information on one of the pathological conditions discussed in this chapter. Read the scenario carefully and select the most appropriate answer for each question that follows. Each correct answer is worth 20 points. Record your score in the space provided at the end of the exercise.

George Burns is a 63-year-old retired Marine and a patient of the pneumonologist Dr. Garrett. Mr. Burns was diagnosed with COPD five years ago. Most recently, he was diagnosed with pulmonary heart disease. While the health care professional completed the health history on Mr. Burns, he had many questions about his diagnoses.

1. The health care professional will base her responses to Mr. Burns's questions about pulmonary heart disease on which of the following facts? Pulmonary heart disease is:

   a. an inflammatory disease of the lungs primarily caused by bacteria

   b. hypertrophy of the right ventricle resulting from pulmonary disease

   c. a collection of air, gas, or fluid in the pleural cavity

   d. an infection caused by the *Mycobacterium tuberculosis* tubercle bacillus

(*continued*)

2. When Mr. Burns asks the health care professional about the relationship of the COPD and pulmonary heart disease, the health care professional's best response would be:

    a. anemia and infection in the lungs are the typical causes of pulmonary heart disease and there is no relationship with COPD

    b. when the lung collapses and fluid enters the pleural space (usually after pneumonia), pulmonary heart disease frequently follows

    c. COPD (chronic bronchitis) is the most frequent cause of pulmonary hypertension that leads to pulmonary heart disease

    d. within a short period of time following a positive skin test for tuberculosis, pulmonary heart disease presents with shortness of breath and a cough

3. The health care professional reviews with Mr. Burns the clinical manifestations of pulmonary heart disease. The correct response by the health care professional would be:

    a. shortness of breath, edema of the feet and legs, distended neck veins, and pleural effusion

    b. chest pain followed by dyspnea and tachypnea, leading to sudden death if the clot and pleural effusion blocks the pulmonary artery

    c. weakness and pallor leading to a pulmonary effusion and the inability to ambulate independently

    d. tachypnea, high fever, elevated WBC count, and pleural effusion

4. Mr. Burns asks the health care professional to explain what a pleural effusion means. The health care professional would explain to him that a pleural effusion means that there is a(n):

    a. collection of air in the pleural cavity entering as the result of a perforation through the chest wall

    b. accumulation of fluid in the pleural space, resulting in compression of the underlying portion of the lung (with resultant dyspnea)

    c. bronchial inflammation causing chronic dilation of a bronchus or bronchi.

    d. pus in a body cavity, especially in the pleural cavity

5. The health care professional also explained to Mr. Burns the procedure used to resolve a pleural effusion, which is called a:

    a. lung scan

    b. bronchoscopy

    c. laryngoscopy

    d. thoracentesis

***Number correct* _____ × *20 points/correct answer: Your score* _____%**

The Digestive System

CHAPTER CONTENT

OBJECTIVES

Upon completing this chapter and the review exercises at the end of the chapter, the learner should be able to:

1. Identify and label the structures of the digestive system.

2. List five basic functions of the digestive system.

3. Identify and define at least 25 pathological conditions of the digestive system.

4. Identify at least 10 diagnostic techniques used in evaluating disorders of the digestive system.

5. Correctly spell and pronounce terms listed on the Written and Audio Terminology Review, using the phonetic pronunciations provided.

6. Create at least 10 medical terms related to the digestive system and identify the applicable combining form(s) for each term.

7. Identify at least 20 abbreviations common to the digestive system.

Overview

How many times a day do you eat? The American tradition is to have breakfast, lunch, and dinner (or supper, in the South). In addition to these three basic meals, count the number of snacks you consume each day and then answer the question as to how many times a day you eat. The answer could be surprising! Foods of little value or a well-balanced diet: What shall it be? The task of the digestive system will remain the same no matter what we choose.

The digestive system is also known as the **gastrointestinal tract**, **digestive tract**, or the **alimentary canal**. It is approximately 30 feet long, beginning with the mouth (oral cavity) and ending with the **anus**. The organs of the digestive system work together to prepare foods for **absorption** into the bloodstream and to prepare foods for use by the body cells. In addition to this vital function, the digestive system is also responsible for elimination of solid wastes from the body. Normal functioning of the human body depends on a properly functioning digestive system. Food ingested in a meal or snack must be modified both chemically and physically to be absorbed as nutrients that can be used by the body cells. As the ingested food passes through the **gastrointestinal tract**, it goes through the many changes necessary for it to be received into the bloodstream and distributed to the body cells as nutrients. The process of altering the chemical and physical composition of food is known as **digestion**.

The physician who specializes in the study of diseases affecting the **gastrointestinal tract** (including the **stomach**, intestines, **gallbladder**, and bile duct) is known as a **gastroenterologist**. The allied health professional who studies and applies the principles and science of nutrition is known as a **nutritionist**. A **dietitian** is an allied health professional trained to plan nutrition programs for sick as well as healthy people. This may involve planning meals for a hospital or large organization or individualized diet counseling with patients.

Anatomy and Physiology

The structures of the digestive system are divided into two sections: The **upper gastrointestinal tract** consists of the oral cavity, **pharynx**, **esophagus**, and **stomach**; the **lower gastrointestinal tract** consists of the large and small intestines. The related organs of the digestive system include the **salivary glands**, liver, **gallbladder**, and **pancreas**. Most of the digestive system organs lie within the abdominopelvic cavity (the space between the diaphragm and the groin). Remember that the abdominopelvic cavity is the largest of the ventral body cavities. The specific serous membrane that covers the entire abdominal wall of the body and is reflected over the contained organs is known as the **peritoneum**.

Oral Cavity

The oral cavity is the first part of the **digestive tract**. It is designed to receive food for ingestion. See *Figure 12-1*.

The oral cavity consists of the **(1) lips** (which surround the opening to the mouth) and the **(2) cheeks**, which form the walls of the oral cavity (and are continuous with the lips and lined with mucous membrane). The lips and cheeks help hold the food in the mouth and keep it in place for chewing. The oral cavity is also known as the **buccal cavity**. The **(3) hard palate**, which forms the anterior, upper roof of the mouth is supported by bone. It has irregular ridges or folds in its mucous membrane lining. These ridges are called **(4) rugae**. **Rugae** are also found in the **stomach**. The **(5) soft palate**, which forms the posterior portion of the upper roof of the mouth (closer to the throat), is composed of skeletal muscle and connective tissue. The soft palate ends in a small, cone-shaped projection called the **(6) uvula**. In addition to aiding in the digestive process, the **uvula** also helps in producing sounds and speech. The **(7) tongue** is a solid mass of very strong, flexible, skeletal muscle covered with mucous membrane. It is located in the floor of the mouth within the curve of the lower jaw bone (mandible). The tongue is the principal organ of the sense of taste and assists in the process of chewing (**mastication**) and swallowing (**deglutition**). The upper surface of the tongue is normally moist, pink, and covered with small, rough elevations known as **(8) papillae**. The **papillae** contain the

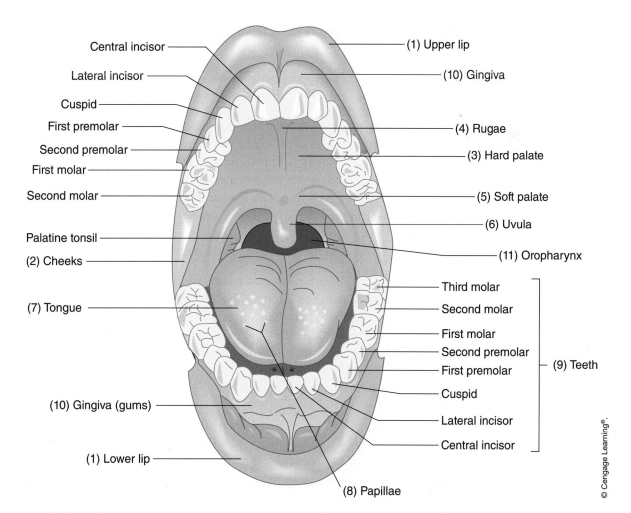

Figure 12-1 The oral cavity

taste buds that detect sweet, sour, salty, and bitter tastes of food or beverages. During the process of chewing the food, the tongue aids the digestive process by moving the food around to mix it with **saliva**, shaping it into a ball-like mass called a **bolus** and moving it toward the throat (**pharynx**) to be swallowed.

Salivary Glands

The three pairs of **salivary glands** (the parotids, the **submandibulars**, and the **sublinguals**) secrete most of the **saliva** produced each day. Saliva is mostly water but also contains mucus and digestive enzymes that aid in the digestive process. The water in the **saliva** helps liquefy the food as it is chewed. The mucus helps lubricate the food as it passes through the **gastrointestinal tract**. The digestive enzymes help break the food down into nutrients. Two enzymes contained in **saliva** are **amylase** (an **enzyme** that aids in the digestion of carbohydrates) and **lipase**, an **enzyme** that aids in the digestion of fats. The **salivary glands** are part of the accessory structures of the digestive system. They secrete **saliva** into the mouth by way of ducts.

The process of chewing is primarily the responsibility of the **(9) teeth**. When food enters the mouth, it is ground up by the teeth and softened by **saliva**. The process of chewing the food is known as **mastication**. The **(10) gums** surround the necks of the teeth. This fleshy tissue covers the upper and lower jaw bones and is lined with the same mucous membrane covering the interior of the oral cavity. The gums are also known as the **gingivae** (singular: **gingiva**). (A separate discussion of the teeth follows the section on accessory organs of digestion.)

Pharynx

The **pharynx**, also known as the throat, adjoins the oral cavity and is a passageway that serves both the respiratory and the digestive systems. The section of the **pharynx** leading away from the oral cavity is known as the **(11) oropharynx**. The portion of the **pharynx** behind the nasal cavity is known as the nasopharynx, and the lower portion of the **pharynx** (which opens into both the **esophagus** and the larynx) is known as the laryngopharynx. Near the base of the tongue, leading from the mouth into the **pharynx** (oropharyngeal area), are the tonsils. These masses of lymphatic tissue are located in the depressions of the mucous membrane of the oropharyngeal area.

During the act of swallowing, the soft palate and the **uvula** move upward to facilitate the movement of the food into the **pharynx** and to close off the nasal cavity. The tongue forces the food into the **pharynx**, and the epiglottis drops downward to cover the opening of the larynx, directing the food mass into the **esophagus**. The **bolus** of food is propelled through the **pharynx** into the **esophagus** by means of peristaltic movements.

Esophagus

The **esophagus** receives the food from the **pharynx** and propels it on to the **stomach**. This collapsible muscular tube, which is approximately 10 inches long, passes through an opening in the diaphragm into the abdominal cavity before connecting to the **stomach**. The passage of the food from the **esophagus** into the **stomach** is controlled by a muscular ring known as the lower esophageal sphincter (LES), or **cardiac sphincter**. When the lower esophageal sphincter relaxes, it opens to allow food to enter the **stomach**. When the LES contracts and closes, the **stomach** content is prevented from reentering the **esophagus**.

Stomach

The **stomach** is located in the upper left quadrant of the abdomen. It has three major divisions. See *Figure 12-2* for a visual reference of the structures and divisions of the **stomach**.

The upper rounded portion of the **stomach** is the **(1) fundus**. It rises to the left and above the level of the opening of the **esophagus** into the **stomach**. The **(2) body** is the central part of the **stomach** and curves to the right. The **(3) pylorus** is the lower tubular part of the **stomach** that angles to the right from the body of the **stomach** as it approaches the **duodenum** (the first part of the small intestines). This area is also referred to as the **gastric** antrum. The **(4) pyloric sphincter** regulates the passage of food from the **stomach** into the **duodenum**. The folds in the mucous membrane lining of the **stomach** are known as **(5) rugae**. These folds allow the **stomach** to expand to accommodate its content. The depressions between the **rugae** contain the gastric glands that secrete gastric juices containing digestive enzymes and **hydrochloric acid**. The gastric juices further the digestive process through the chemical breakdown of food, and the muscular action of the **stomach** causes churning (which mixes the food with the secretions). At this point in the digestive process, the liquidlike mixture of partially digested food and digestive secretions in the **stomach** is called **chyme**. It is released in small amounts through the **pyloric sphincter** into the small intestine. As we continue our discussion of the digestive process, *Figure 12-3* will provide a visual reference for the structures and divisions of the small and large intestine.

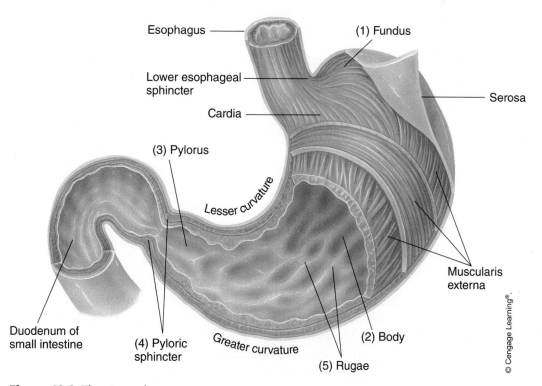

Esophagus

Lower esophageal sphincter

Cardia

(3) Pylorus

Lesser curvature

Duodenum of small intestine

(4) Pyloric sphincter

Greater curvature

(5) Rugae

(2) Body

(1) Fundus

Serosa

Muscularis externa

© Cengage Learning®.

Figure 12-2 The stomach

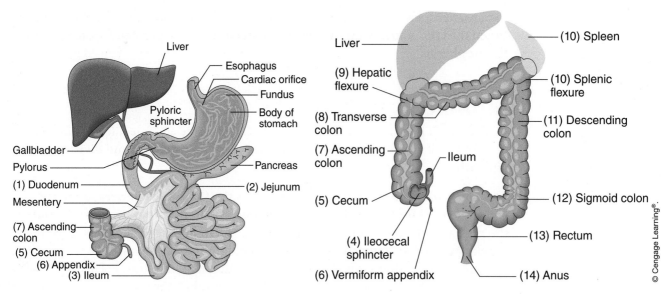

Figure 12-3 The small and large intestine

Small Intestine

The small intestine is approximately 20 feet long, coiling and looping as it fills most of the abdominal cavity. It is divided into three parts: the **duodenum**, the **jejunum**, and the **ileum**. The **(1) duodenum** is the first part of the small intestine (approximately 12 inches long), extending in a C-shaped curve from the pylorus of the **stomach** to the **jejunum**. The **duodenum** receives the **chyme** from the pylorus of the **stomach** along with secretions from the liver and the **pancreas** that further the digestive process. The second portion of the small intestine is the **(2) jejunum**, which connects the **duodenum** to the **ileum**. The **jejunum** is approximately 8 feet long. The third portion of the small intestine is the **(3) ileum**, which is approximately 12 feet long. The **ileum** is continuous with the **jejunum** and connects it to the large intestine at the ileocecal sphincter.

The small intestine, also known as the small **bowel**, completes the digestive process through **absorption** of the nutrients into the bloodstream and passage of the residue (waste products) on to the large intestine for excretion from the body. The mucous membrane lining the small intestine contains millions of tiny fingerlike projections known as **villi**. The **villi** surround blood capillaries, which function in the **absorption** of nutrients.

Large Intestine

The large intestine begins at the **ileocecal** junction and extends to the **anus**. The ileocecal junction contains a muscular ring called the **(4) ileocecal sphincter**, which prevents the backflow of wastes from the large intestine into the small intestine. The large intestine is divided into the **cecum**, the **colon**, and the **rectum**. The **(5) cecum** is a blind pouch, on the right side of the abdomen, that extends approximately 2 to 3 inches beyond the ileocecal junction to the beginning of the **colon**. At the lower portion of the **cecum** hangs a small wormlike structure known as the **(6) vermiform appendix**. It is approximately 3 to 6 inches in length and is less than 0.5 inch in diameter. The function of the appendix is uncertain, but it appears to serve no specific purpose in the digestive process. The longest portion of the large intestine is the **colon**. It is divided into four sections: the ascending, transverse, descending, and **sigmoid colon**. The **(7) ascending colon** begins at the ileocecal junction, curving upward toward the liver on the right side of the abdomen.

When it reaches the undersurface of the liver, it makes a horizontal turn to the left, becoming the **(8) transverse colon**. The point at which the ascending colon turns to the left (just below the liver) is known as the **(9) hepatic flexure**. The transverse colon advances horizontally across the abdomen, below the **stomach** toward the spleen. When it reaches the area below the spleen, the transverse colon takes a downward turn at a point known as the **(10) splenic flexure**. It then becomes the **(11) descending colon**, passing down toward the pelvis on the left side of the abdomen. At the pelvic brim (the curved top of the hip bones), the descending colon makes an S-shaped curve. This curved portion of the **colon** is known as the **(12) sigmoid colon**, which connects the descending colon to the **rectum**. The **(13) rectum**, which is the last 7 to 8 inches of the large intestine, connects the **sigmoid colon** to the **(14) anus**. The **anus** is the opening through which **feces** (the solid waste products of digestion) are eliminated from the body. The act of expelling **feces** from the body is called **defecation**. The anal sphincter controls the elimination of waste materials from the **rectum**.

Accessory Organs of Digestion

The accessory organs of digestion are the **salivary glands**, liver, **gallbladder**, and **pancreas**. The **salivary glands** have been discussed with the oral cavity. *Figure 12-4* provides a visual reference of the liver, **gallbladder**, and **pancreas**.

The **(1) liver** is located immediately under the diaphragm, slightly to the right. It is the largest gland in the body and weighs approximately 3 to 4 pounds. The only digestive function of the liver is the production of **bile** for the emulsification of fats in the small intestine. The liver cells, known as hepatocytes, produce a yellowish-green secretion

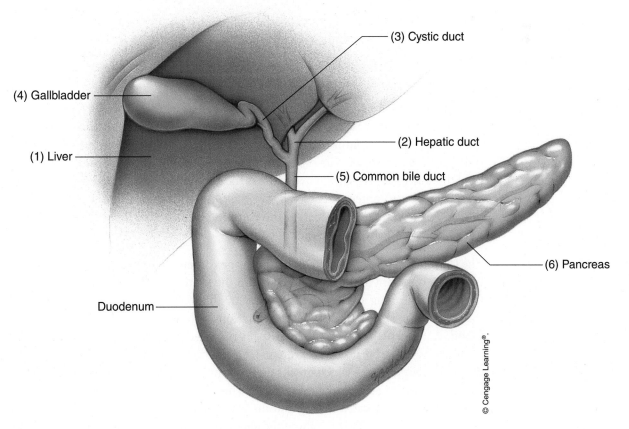

Figure 12-4 The liver, gallbladder, and pancreas

called **bile**. The main components of **bile** are bile salts, bile pigments, and cholesterol. **Bile** emulsifies (breaks apart) fats, preparing them for further digestion and **absorption** in the small intestine. Additional functions of the liver are as follows:

- Excretion of bile pigments into **bile**. The liver recycles the iron and converts the remaining portion into bile pigments, which are excreted with the **bile** as it is released from the liver. The **bile** travels down the **(2) hepatic duct** to the **(3) cystic duct**, which leads to the **gallbladder** (where the **bile** is stored). The primary bile pigment is **bilirubin**, which gives it the yellowish-green color. Bile pigments containing **bilirubin** are responsible for the color of urine and **feces**.

- Synthesis of vitamin K–dependent plasma proteins. Albumin, globulin carrier molecules, and the clotting factors.

- Amino acid metabolism.

- Carbohydrate metabolism (mainly **glycogenesis** and **glycogenolysis**). The liver converts the excess amounts of circulating blood **glucose** (simple sugar) into a complex form of sugar (starch) for storage in the liver cells, a process known as **glycogenesis**. This complex form of sugar, known as **glycogen**, is preserved in the liver cells for use when the blood sugar is extremely low. In response to dangerously low blood sugar levels, the liver breaks down the stored **glycogen** into **glucose**, releasing it into the circulating blood (a process known as **glycogenolysis**).

- Fat metabolism; synthesis of cholesterol, of lipoproteins for transport of fat to other tissues, and conversion of fatty acids to ketones to be used for energy production.

- Phagocytosis. Phagocytosis of old, worn-out red blood cells (erythrocytes). When the erythrocytes are destroyed in the spleen, they are broken down into heme, which contains iron and globin (a blood protein).

- Detoxification. The enzymes produced by the liver convert potentially harmful substances (such as ammonia, alcohol, and medications) into less toxic ones.

- Storage of vital nutrients. The liver is responsible for the storage of the vitamins, iron, and copper; fat-soluble vitamins A, D, E, and K; and vitamin B_{12}.

The **(4) gallbladder** is a pear-shaped sac located on the undersurface of the liver. Approximately 3 to 4 inches long, the **gallbladder** is connected to the liver via the cystic duct. The cystic duct joins the hepatic duct to form the **(5) common bile duct**, which leads to the **duodenum**. The main function of the **gallbladder** is to store and concentrate the **bile** produced by the liver. When food (**chyme**) enters the **duodenum** and the presence of fatty content is detected, the **gallbladder** is stimulated to release **bile**. The **bile** travels from the cystic duct, to the common bile duct, to the **duodenum** (where it serves its purpose as an emulsifier of fats).

The **(6) pancreas** is an elongated organ of approximately 6 to 9 inches. It is located in the upper left quadrant of the abdomen, behind the **stomach**. It extends horizontally across the body, beginning at the first part of the small intestines (**duodenum**) and ending at the edge of the spleen. The **pancreas** functions as both an exocrine and an **endocrine gland**. As an **exocrine gland**, the **pancreas** manufactures the digestive juices containing (1) trypsin (which breaks down proteins), (2) pancreatic lipase (which breaks down fats), (3) pancreatic amylase (which breaks down carbohydrates), and (4) sodium bicarbonate, which neutralizes acidic stomach content. These digestive juices are secreted into a network of tiny ducts located throughout the gland. The ducts merge into the main **pancreatic duct**, which extends throughout the length of the **pancreas**. The pancreatic duct joins the common bile duct just before it enters the **duodenum**. As an **endocrine gland**, the

pancreas manufactures **insulin**, which passes directly into the blood capillaries instead of being transported by way of ducts. The specialized group of cells known as the islets of Langerhans are scattered throughout the **pancreas**. The beta cells of the **pancreas** secrete **insulin**, a hormone that makes it possible for **glucose** to pass from the blood through the cell membranes to be used for energy. **Insulin** also promotes the conversion of excess **glucose** into **glycogen**. The alpha cells of the **pancreas** secrete **glucagon**, a hormone that stimulates the liver to convert **glycogen** into **glucose** in time of need.

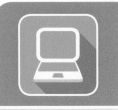

Media Link

Watch the **Pancreas animation** on the Student Companion Website to learn about the important role the pancreas plays in the digestive system.

Teeth

As mentioned, the process of chewing is the primary responsibility of the teeth. *Figures 12-5A* and *B* provide a visual reference for the teeth.

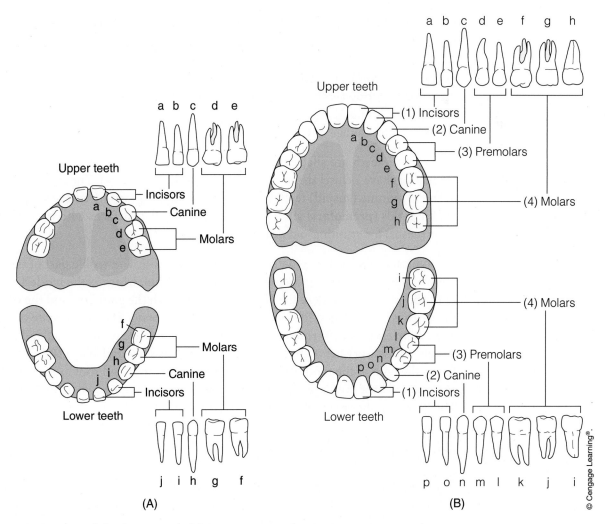

Figure 12-5 (A) Primary teeth (B) Permanent teeth

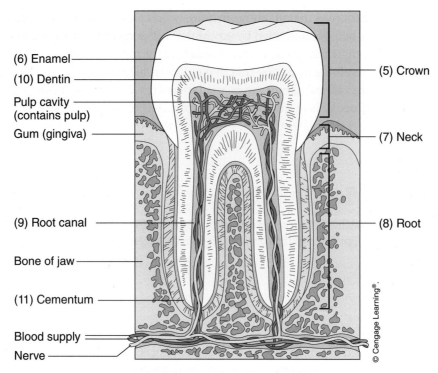

(6) Enamel
(10) Dentin
Pulp cavity
(contains pulp)
Gum (gingiva)

(9) Root canal

Bone of jaw

(11) Cementum

Blood supply
Nerve

(5) Crown

(7) Neck

(8) Root

© Cengage Learning®.

Figure 12-6 Layers of a tooth

Each individual has two sets of teeth that develop in the mouth during his or her life-time. The first set of teeth, or "baby teeth," are called the **primary** or **deciduous teeth**. This set of 20 teeth (10 in each jaw bone) begins to appear at approximately six months of age. The **secondary (permanent) teeth** begin to appear around the age of six, replacing the **deciduous teeth**. The set of permanent teeth consists of 32 teeth (16 in each jaw bone), with the last of the teeth, the third molars (wisdom teeth), usually erupting sometime after the age of 17.

The various teeth are shaped in different ways to aid in the digestion of food. The **(1)** incisors have a chisel shape with sharp edges for biting food. The single point (cusp) of the **(2)** canine (cuspid) teeth make them useful for grasping and tearing food. The **(3)** bicuspids (**premolars**) and the **(4)** molars have flat surfaces with multiple projections (cusps) for crushing and grinding food.

The typical tooth has three main parts. See *Figure 12-6*. The visible part of the tooth is known as the **(5)** **crown**. It is covered with **(6)** **enamel**, which is the hardest substance in the body. The **(7)** **neck** of the tooth lies just beneath the gum line, and the **(8)** **root** of the tooth is embedded in the bony socket of the jaw bone. The central core of the tooth is the **pulp** cavity, or **(9)** **root canal**. It contains connective tissue, blood and lymphatic vessels, and sensory nerve endings. The pulp cavity is surrounded by **(10)** **dentin**, which forms the bulk of the tooth shell. The **dentin** in the neck and root area of the tooth is surrounded by a thin layer of hardened connective tissue known as **(11)** **cementum**. The **dentin** in the crown of the tooth is covered by **enamel**.

The Process of Digestion

The **alimentary canal** begins with the mouth and ends with the **anus**. The process of digestion involves both physical and chemical processes. When food enters the mouth, the physical process of chewing (**mastication**) occurs when the teeth cut and grind the food. The **salivary glands** found in the mouth lubricate the food as it is chewed. The **enzyme amylase**, which is contained in **saliva**, begins the chemical breakdown of carbohydrates. During the process of chewing the food, the tongue aids the digestive process by moving the food around to mix it with **saliva**, shaping it into a ball-like mass called a **bolus** and moving it toward the throat (**pharynx**) to be swallowed. The process of swallowing is known as **deglutition**.

During the act of swallowing, the soft palate and the **uvula** move upward to facilitate the movement of the food into the **pharynx** and to close off the nasal cavity. The tongue forces the food into the **pharynx**, and the epiglottis drops downward to cover the opening of the larynx, directing the food mass into the **esophagus**. The **bolus** of food is propelled through the **pharynx** into the **esophagus** by means of **peristalsis**. The **esophagus** receives the food from the **pharynx** and propels it on to the **stomach**. When the lower esophageal sphincter (LES) relaxes, it opens to allow food to enter the **stomach**. When the LES contracts and closes, it prevents the **stomach** contents from reentering the **esophagus**. The **stomach** secretes gastric juices, which further the digestive process through the chemical breakdown of food. The muscular action of the **stomach** causes churning, which mixes the food with the secretions. At this point in the digestive process, the liquid-like mixture of partially digested food and digestive secretions in the **stomach** is called **chyme**. The **pyloric sphincter** releases this mixture into the small intestine.

The small intestine completes the digestive process through **absorption** of the **nutrients** into the bloodstream and passage of the residue (waste products) on to the large intestine for excretion from the body. As the digested food continues its passage through the large intestine, it moves through the ileocecal sphincter, which prevents the backflow of wastes from the large intestine into the small intestine. As the **chyme** moves through the large intestine, the process of **reabsorption** of water and electrolytes takes place. The remaining solid waste products of digestion (**feces**) are eliminated from the body through the **anus**. The act of expelling **feces** from the body is known as **defecation**.

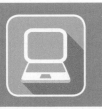

Media Link

Watch this process in 3D by viewing the **Digestion** animation on the Student Companion Website.

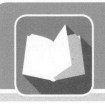

Review Checkpoint

Check your understanding of this section by completing the **Anatomy and Physiology** exercises in your workbook.

VOCABULARY

The following vocabulary words are frequently used when discussing the digestive system.

Word	Definition
abdomen (**AB**-dah-men)	The portion of the body between the thorax (chest) and the pelvis; the diaphragm separates the abdominal cavity from the thoracic cavity. The **stomach** is located in the upper left quadrant of the abdomen.
absorption (ab-**SORP**-shun)	The passage of substances across and into tissues, such as the passage of digested food molecules into intestinal cells or the passage of liquids into kidney tubules.

aerophagia
(**ay**-er-oh-**FAY**-jee-ah)
  aer/o = air; gas
  -phagia = to eat
	The swallowing of air; excessive swallowing of air while eating or drinking, which may result in belching and gas.

alimentary canal
(**al**-ih-**MEN**-tar-ee can-**NAL**)
  aliment/o = nutrition
  -ary = pertaining to
	A musculomembranous tube, about 30 feet long, extending from the mouth to the **anus** and lined with mucous membrane. Also called the **digestive tract** or the **gastrointestinal tract**.

amino acids (ah-**MEE**-noh acids)	An organic chemical compound composed of one or more basic amino groups and one or more acidic carboxyl groups.

amylase
(**AM**-ih-lays)
  amyl/o = starch
  -ase = enzyme
	An **enzyme** that breaks down starch into smaller carbohydrate molecules.

anastomosis (ah-nas-toh-**MOH**-sis)	A surgical joining of two ducts, blood vessels, or bowel segments to allow flow from one to the other. For additional information refer to Chapter 10 vocabulary list.

anus
(**AY**-nus)
  an/o = anus
  -us = noun ending
	The opening through which the solid wastes (**feces**) are eliminated from the body.

ascites (ah-**SIGH**-teez)	An abnormal intraperitoneal (within the peritoneal cavity) accumulation of a fluid containing large amounts of protein and electrolytes.
ascitic fluid (ah-**SIT**-ik fluid)	A watery fluid containing albumin, **glucose**, and electrolytes that accumulates in the peritoneal cavity in association with certain disease conditions (such as liver disease).

Word	Definition
bicuspid tooth (bye-**CUSS**-pid)	One of the two teeth between the molars and canines of the upper and lower jaw, the bicuspid teeth have a flat surface with multiple projections (cusps) for crushing and grinding food; also known as premolar tooth.
bile (**BYE**-al)	A bitter, yellow-green secretion of the liver.
bilirubin (bill-ih-**ROO**-bin)	The orange-yellow pigment of **bile**, formed principally by the breakdown of hemoglobin in red blood cells after termination of their normal life span.
bolus (**BOH**-lus)	A ball-like mass of chewed food (mixed with **saliva**) that is ready to be swallowed.
bowel (**BOW**-el)	The portion of the **alimentary canal** extending from the pyloric opening of the **stomach** to the **anus**.
cachexia (kah-**KEKS**-eeh-ah)	A condition of general ill health and malnutrition; physical wasting with loss of weight and muscle mass due to a disease.
canine tooth (**KAY**-nine)	Any one of the four teeth, two in each jaw, situated immediately lateral to the **incisor** teeth in the human dental arches; also called **cuspid tooth**.

cardiac sphincter
(**CAR**-dee-ak **SFINGK**-ter)
  cardi/o = heart
  -ac = pertaining to
	The muscular ring (**sphincter**) in the **stomach** that controls the passage of food from the **esophagus** into the **stomach**; also known as the lower esophageal sphincter.

cecum (**SEE**-kum)	A cul-de-sac containing the first part of the large intestine. It joins the **ileum**, the last segment of the small intestine.

cholangiogram
(koh-**LAN**-jee-oh-**gram**)
  chol/e = bile
  angi/o = vessel
  -gram = record or picture
	A record, or X-ray film, of the bile ducts following the injection of a radiopaque contrast medium.

choledocholithiasis
(koh-lee-**dock**-oh-lih-**THIGH**-ah-sis)
  choledoch/o = common bile duct
  lith/o = stone or calculus
  -iasis = presence of an abnormal
        condition
	The presence of a stone (calculus) in the common bile duct.

cholelithiasis
(**koh**-lee-lih-**THIGH**-ah-sis)
  chol/e = bile
  lith/o = stone; calculus
  -iasis = presence of an abnormal
        condition
	Abnormal presence of gallstones in the **gallbladder**.

Word	Definition
chyme (**KIGHM**)	The liquidlike material of partially digested food and digestive secretions found in the **stomach** just before it is released into the **duodenum**.
colon (**COH**-lon)	The portion of the large intestine extending from the **cecum** to the **rectum**.
common bile duct	The duct formed by the joining of the cystic duct and hepatic duct.
crown	The part of the tooth that is visible above the gum line.
cuspid tooth (**CUSS**-pid tooth)	See *canine tooth*.
deciduous teeth (dee-**SID**-you-us)	The first set or primary teeth; baby teeth.
defecation (deff-eh-**KAY**-shun)	The act of expelling **feces** from the **rectum** through the **anus**.
deglutition (**dee**-gloo-**TISH**-un)	Swallowing.
dentin (**DEN**-tin)	The chief material of teeth surrounding the pulp and situated inside of the **enamel** and cementum.
dietitian (**dye**-ah-**TIH**-shun)	An allied health professional trained to plan nutrition programs for sick as well as healthy people. This may involve planning meals for a hospital or large organization or individualized diet counseling with patients.
digestion (dye-**JEST**-shun)	The process of altering the chemical and physical composition of food so that it can be used by the body cells. This occurs in the **digestive tract**.
digestive tract (dye-**JESS**-tiv **TRAKT**)	See *alimentary canal*.
duodenum (doo-oh-**DEE**-num *or* do-**OD**-eh-num) duoden/o = duodenum -um = noun ending	The first portion of the small intestine. The **duodenum** is the shortest, widest, and most fixed portion of the small intestine, taking an almost circular course from the pyloric valve of the **stomach** so that its termination is close to its starting point.
emulsify (eh-**MULL**-sih-figh)	To disperse a liquid into another liquid, making a colloidal suspension. Bile is released from the gallbladder into the small intestine in response to the presence of fatty content; its purpose in the digestive process is to emulsify, or break down the fats into small droplets so the body can use them as nutrients.
enamel (en-**AM**-el)	A hard, white substance that covers the **dentin** of the crown of a tooth. **Enamel** is the hardest substance in the body.

Word	Definition
endocrine gland (**EN**-doh-krin) endo- = within -crine = secrete	A gland that secretes its enzymes directly into the blood capillaries instead of being transported by way of ducts.
enzyme (**EN**-zighm)	A protein produced by living cells that catalyzes chemical reactions in organic matter.
esophagogastroduodenoscopy (eh-**sof**-ah-goh-**gas**-troh-**dew**-oh-deh-**NOS**-koh-pee) esophagi/o = esophagus gastr/o = stomach duoden/o = duodenum -scopy = process of viewing	The process of direct visualization of the esophagus, stomach, and duodenum using a lighted fiberoptic endoscope; also known as an upper endoscopy.
esophagus (eh-**SOF**-ah-gus) esophag/o = esophagus -us = noun ending	A muscular canal, about 9.4 inches long, extending from the **pharynx** to the **stomach**.
exocrine gland (**EKS**-oh-krin) exo- = outward -crine = secrete	A gland that secretes its enzymes into a network of tiny ducts that transport it to the surface of an organ or tissue or into a vessel.
fatty acids	Any of several organic acids produced by the hydrolysis of neutral fats.
feces (**FEE**-seez)	Waste or excrement from the **digestive tract** that is formed in the intestine and expelled through the **rectum**.
gallbladder (**GALL**-blad-er)	A pear-shaped excretory sac lodged in a fossa on the visceral surface of the right lobe of the liver.
gastroenterologist (**gas**-troh-**en**-ter-**ALL**-oh-jist) gastr/o = stomach enter/o = small intestine -logist = one who specializes in the study of	A medical doctor who specializes in the study of the diseases and disorders affecting the **gastrointestinal tract** (including the **stomach**, intestines, **gallbladder**, and bile duct).
gastrointestinal tract (**gas**-troh-in-**TESS**-tih-nal **TRAKT**)	See *alimentary canal*.
gavage (gah-**VAZH**)	A procedure in which liquid or semiliquid food is introduced into the **stomach** through a tube.
gingiva (**JIN**-jih-vah *or* jin-**JYE**-vah) gingiv/o = gums -a = noun ending	Gum tissue (singular: *gingiva*; plural: *gingivae*).

Word	Definition

gingivitis
(jin-jih-**VIGH**-tis)
  gingiv/o = gums
  -itis = inflammation
	Inflammation of the gums.

glucagon (**GLOO**-kah-gon)	A hormone produced by the alpha cells of the **pancreas** that stimulates the liver to convert **glycogen** into **glucose** when the blood sugar level is dangerously low.

glucose
(**GLOO**-kohs)
  gluc/o = sugar, sweet
  -ose = carbohydrate
	A simple sugar found in certain foods, especially fruits, and major source of energy occurring in human and animal body fluids.

glycogen
(**GLIGH**-koh-jen)
  glyc/o = sugar, sweet
  -gen = that which generates
	A complex sugar (starch) that is the major carbohydrate stored in animal cells. It is formed from **glucose** and stored chiefly in the liver and, to a lesser extent, in muscle cells.

glycogenesis
(**gligh**-koh-**JEN**-eh-sis)
  glyc/o = sugar, sweet
  -genesis = the production of;
          formation of
	The conversion of simple sugar (**glucose**) into a complex form of sugar (starch) for storage in the liver.

glycogenolysis
(**gligh**-koh-jen-**ALL**-ih-sis)
  glyc/o = sugar, sweet
  gen/o = to produce
  -lysis = destruction or detachment
	The breakdown of **glycogen** into **glucose** by the liver, releasing it back into the circulating blood in response to a very low blood sugar level.

hematemesis
(**hee**-mah-**TEM**-eh-sis)
  hemat/o = blood
  -emesis = to vomit
	Vomiting of blood.

hepatocyte
(**HEP**-ah-toh-sight)
  hepat/o = liver
  -cyte = cell
	Liver cell.

hydrochloric acid (**high**-droh-**KLOH**-rik acid)	A compound consisting of hydrogen and chlorine.

ileum
(**ILL**-ee-um)
  ile/o = ileum
  -um = noun ending
	The distal portion of the small intestine extending from the **jejunum** to the **cecum**.

incisor (in-**SIGH**-zor)	One of the eight front teeth, four in each dental arch, that first appear as primary teeth during infancy are replaced by permanent incisors during childhood and last until old age.

Word	Definition
insulin (**IN**-soo-lin)	A naturally occurring hormone secreted by the beta cells of the islets of Langerhans in the **pancreas** in response to increased levels of **glucose** in the blood.
jejunum (jee-**JOO**-num) jejun/o = jejunum -um = noun ending	The intermediate or middle of the three portions of the small intestine, connecting proximally with the **duodenum** and distally with the **ileum**.
laparoscope (**LAP**-ah-rah-scope) lapar/o = abdominal wall -scope = instrument for viewing	A thin-walled, flexible tube with a telescopic lens and light that is inserted through an incision in the abdominal wall to examine or perform minor surgery within the abdominal or pelvic cavities.
lavage (lah-**VAZH**)	The process of irrigating (washing out) an organ—usually the bladder, **bowel**, paranasal sinuses, or **stomach**—for therapeutic purposes.
lipase (**LIH**-pays *or* **LIGH**-pays) lip/o = fat -ase = enzyme	An **enzyme** that aids in the digestion of fats.
liver	The largest gland of the body and one of its most complex organs.
lower esophageal sphincter (LES) (lower eh-**soff**-ah-**JEE**-al **SFINGK**-ter) esophag/o = esophagus -eal = pertaining to	See **cardiac sphincter**.
lower GI tract	The lower portion of the **gastrointestinal tract** consisting of the small and large intestines.
mastication (mass-tih-**KAY**-shun)	Chewing, tearing, or grinding food with the teeth while it becomes mixed with **saliva**.
McBurney's point	A point on the right side of the abdomen, about two-thirds of the distance between the umbilicus and the anterior bony prominence of the hip. When tenderness exists upon McBurney's point, a physician might suspect **appendicitis**.
molar tooth (**MOH**-lar)	Any of 12 molar teeth, 6 in each dental arch, located posterior to the premolar teeth. The molar teeth have a flat surface with multiple projections (cusps) for crushing and grinding food.
nutritionist (noo-**TRIH**-shun-ist)	An allied health professional who studies and applies the principles and science of nutrition.
oropharynx (or-oh-**FAIR**-inks) or/o = mouth	The section of the **pharynx** leading away from the oral cavity.

Word	Definition
palate (**PAL**-at)	A structure that forms the roof of the mouth.

palatoplasty
(**PAL**-ah-toh-**plas**-tee)
  palat/o = palate
  -plasty = surgical repair
	Surgical repair of the palate, usually to correct a cleft palate.

pancreas (**PAN**-kree-as)	An elongated organ approximately 6 to 9 inches long, located in the upper left quadrant of the abdomen that secretes various substances such as digestive enzymes, **insulin**, and glucagon.
papillae (pah-**PILL**-ay)	A small, nipple-shaped projection (such as the conoid papillae of the tongue and the **papillae** of the corium) that extend from collagen fibers, the capillary blood vessels, and sometimes the nerves of the dermis.
parotid gland (pah-**ROT**-id gland)	One of the largest pairs of **salivary glands** that lie at the side of the face just below and in front of the external ear.
peristalsis (pair-ih-**STALL**-sis)	The coordinated, rhythmic, serial contraction of smooth muscle that forces food through the **digestive tract, bile** through the bile duct, and urine through the ureters.

peritoneum
(pair-ih-toh-**NEE**-um)
  peritone/o = peritoneum
  -um = noun ending
	A specific serous membrane that covers the entire abdominal wall of the body and is reflected over the contained viscera.

peritonitis
(pair-ih-toh-**NIGH**-tis)
  peritone/o = peritoneum
  -itis = inflammation
	Inflammation of the **peritoneum.**

permanent teeth	The full set of teeth (32 teeth) that replace the deciduous or temporary teeth.
pharynx (**FAIR**-inks) pharyng/o = pharynx	The throat; a tubular structure about 5.1 inches long that extends from the base of the skull to the **esophagus** and is situated just in front of the cervical vertebrae.
premolars	See *bicuspid tooth*.
pulp	Any soft, spongy tissue such as that contained within the spleen, the pulp chamber of the tooth, or the distal phalanges of the fingers and the toes.
pyloric sphincter (pigh-**LOR**-ik **SFINGK**-ter)	A thickened muscular ring in the **stomach** that regulates the passage of food from the pylorus of the **stomach** into the **duodenum.**

pyorrhea
(pye-oh-**REE**-ah)
  py/o = pus
  -rrhea = discharge; flow
	Discharge or flow of pus.

Word	Definition
rebound tenderness	A sensation of severe pain experienced by the patient when the doctor applies deep pressure to the abdomen and releases it quickly. When this deep pressure is applied to the lower right quadrant of the abdomen at McBurney's point, and this type of pain is experienced, it is a strong indicator of **appendicitis**.
rectum (**REK**-tum) rect/o = rectum -um= noun ending	The portion of the large intestine, about 4.7 inches long, continuous with the descending **sigmoid colon** (just proximal to the anal canal).
rugae (**ROO**-gay)	A ridge or fold (such as the **rugae** of the **stomach**) that presents large folds in the mucous membrane of that organ.
saliva (sah-**LYE**-vah)	The clear, viscous fluid secreted by the salivary and mucous glands in the mouth.
salivary glands (**SAL**-ih-vair-ee glands)	One of the three pairs of glands secreting into the mouth, thus aiding the digestive process.
secondary teeth	See *permanent teeth*.
sigmoid colon (**SIG**-moyd colon)	The portion of the **colon** that extends from the end of the descending colon in the pelvis to the juncture of the **rectum**.
sphincter (**SFINGK**-ter)	A circular band of muscle fibers that constricts a passage or closes a natural opening in the body, such as the hepatic sphincter in the muscular coat of the hepatic veins near their union with the superior vena cava (and the external anal sphincter, which closes the **anus**).
stomach (**STUM**-ak)	The major organ of digestion located in the left upper quadrant of the abdomen and divided into a body and pylorus.
triglycerides (try-**GLISS**-er-eyeds)	A compound consisting of a fatty acid (oleic, palmitic, or stearic) and glycerol.
upper GI tract	The upper part of the **gastrointestinal tract** consisting of the mouth, **pharynx**, **esophagus**, and **stomach**.
uvula (**YOO**-vyoo-lah)	The small, cone-shaped process suspended in the mouth from the middle of the posterior border of the soft palate.
villi (**VIL**-eye)	One of the many tiny projections barely visible to the naked eye clustered over the entire mucous surface of the small intestine.
xerostomia (**zeer**-oh-**STOH**-mee-ah) xer/o = dry stom/o = mouth -ia = condition	A condition of dryness of the mouth caused by decreased secretions of the salivary glands. Some causes of xerostomia include, but may not be limited to, diabetes, adverse reaction to medications, hysteria, acute infections.

Review Checkpoint

Check your understanding of this section by completing the **Vocabulary** exercises in your workbook.

WORD ELEMENTS

The following word elements pertain to the digestive system. As you review the list, pronounce each word element aloud twice and check the box after you "say it." Write the definition for the example term given for each word element. Use your medical dictionary to find the definitions of the example terms.

Word Element	Pronunciation	"Say It"	Meaning
aer/o **aer**obic	**AYR**-oh **ayr**-**ROH**-bick	☐	air
amyl/o **amyl**ase	**AM**-ih-loh **AM**-ih-lays	☐	starch
append/o **append**ectomy	ah-**PEN**-doe ap-en-**DEK**-toh-mee	☐	appendix
appendic/o **appendic**itis	ah-**PEN**-dih-koh ap-**pen**-dih-**SIGH**-tis	☐	appendix
-ase lip**ase**	**AYS** **LYE**-pays	☐	**enzyme**
bil/i **bil**iary	**BILL**-ee **BILL**-ee-air-ee	☐	**bile**
bucc/o **bucc**al	**BUCK**-oh **BUCK**-al	☐	cheek
cec/o **cec**ostomy	**SEE**-koh see-**KOSS**-toh-mee	☐	**cecum**
celi/o **celi**ac rickets	**SEE**-lee-oh **SEE**-lee-ak **RICK**-ets	☐	pertaining to the abdomen
-centesis abdomino**centesis**	sen-**TEE**-sis ab-**dom**-ih-noh-sen-**TEE**-sis	☐	surgical puncture
cheil/o **cheil**osis	**KIGH**-loh kigh-**LOH**-sis	☐	lips
chol/e **chol**ecystogram	**KOH**-lee koh-lee-**SIS**-toh-gram	☐	**bile**

Word Element	Pronunciation	"Say It"	Meaning
cholecyst/o **cholecyst**itis	koh-lee-**SIS**-toh **koh**-lee-sis-**TYE**-tis	☐	**gallbladder**
choledoch/o **choledocho**lithiasis	koh-lee-**DOCK**-oh koh-lee-**dock**-oh-lih-**THIGH**-ah-sis	☐	common bile duct
cirrh/o **cirrh**osis	sih-**ROH** sih-**ROH**-sis	☐	yellow, tawny
col/o **col**orectal	**KOH**-loh **koh**-loh-**REK**-tal	☐	**colon**
colon/o **colon**oscopy	koh-**LON**-oh **koh**-lon-**OSS**-koh-pee	☐	**colon**
dent/o **dent**al hygienist	**DEN**-toh **DEN**-tahl high-**JEE**-nist	☐	tooth
duoden/o **duoden**ostomy	doo-**ODD**-en-oh **doo**-odd-eh-**NOSS**-toh-mee	☐	**duodenum** (first part of the small intestine)
-ectasia gastr**ectasia**	ek-**TAY**-zhe-ah gas-trek-**TAY**-zhe-ah	☐	stretching or dilation
-ectomy append**ectomy**	**EK**-toh-mee ap-en-**DEK**-toh-mee	☐	surgical removal
-emesis hemat**emesis**	**EM**-eh-sis **hee**-mah-**TEM**-eh-sis	☐	to **vomit**
enter/o **enter**itis	**EN**-ter-oh en-ter-**EYE**-tis	☐	intestine
esophag/o **esophag**itis	eh-**SOFF**-ah-go eh-soff-ah-**JIGH**-tis	☐	**esophagus**
gastr/o **gastr**ostomy	**GAS**-troh gas-**TROSS**-toh-mee	☐	**stomach**
gingiv/o **gingiv**itis	**JIN**-jih-voh jin-jih-**VIGH**-tis	☐	gums
gloss/o **gloss**itis	**GLOSS**-oh gloss-**SIGH**-tis	☐	tongue
gluc/o **gluc**ogenesis	**GLOO**-koh gloo-koh-**JEN**-eh-sis	☐	sugar, sweet
glyc/o **glyc**olysis	**GLIGH**-koh gligh-**KALL**-ih-sis	☐	sugar, sweet
hepat/o **hepat**omegaly	hep-**AH**-toh **hep**-ah-toh-**MEG**-ah-lee	☐	liver

Word Element	Pronunciation	"Say It"	Meaning
-iasis cholelith**iasis**	**EYE**-ah-sis koh-lee-lih-**THIGH**-ah-sis	☐	presence of an abnormal condition
ile/o **ile**ocecal	**ILL**-ee-oh **ILL**-ee-oh-**SEE**-kahl	☐	**ileum**
jejun/o **jejun**ostomy	jee-**JOO**-noh jee-joo-**NOSS**-toh-mee	☐	**jejunum**
lapar/o **lapar**oscopy	**LAP**-ah-roh lap-ar-**OSS**-koh-pee	☐	abdominal wall
lingu/o **lingu**al	**LING**-oo-oh **LING**-gwall	☐	tongue
lip/o **lip**oma	**LIH**-poh lih-**POH**-mah	☐	fat
lith/o **lith**ogenesis	**LITH**-oh **lith**-oh-**JEN**-eh-sis	☐	stone; calculus
-lysis lipo**lysis**	**LIH**-sis lip-**ALL**-ih-sis	☐	destruction or detachment
mandibul/o **mandibul**ar	man-**DIB**-yoo-loh man-**DIB**-yoo-lar	☐	mandible (lower jaw bone)
odont/o orth**odont**ist	oh-**DON**-toh or-thoh-**DON**-tist	☐	teeth
or/o **or**al	**OR**-oh **OR**-al	☐	mouth
palat/o **palat**itis	**PAL**-ah-toh **pal**-ah**TYE**-tis	☐	palate
pancreat/o **pancreat**itis	pan-kree-**AH**-toh pan-kree-ah-**TYE**-tis	☐	**pancreas**
-pepsia dys**pepsia**	**PEP**-see-ah diss-**PEP**-see-ah	☐	state of digestion
-phagia poly**phagia**	**FAY**-jee-ah pall-ee-**FAY**-jee-ah	☐	to eat
pharyng/o **pharyng**oscope	fair-**IN**-goh fair-**IN**-goh-skohp	☐	**pharynx**
peritone/o **peritone**al	**pair**-ih-toh-**NEE**-oh **pair**-ih-toh-**NEE**-al	☐	**peritoneum**

Word Element	Pronunciation	"Say It"	Meaning
-plasty stomato**plasty**	**PLASS**-tee **STOH**-mah-toh-**PLASS**-tee	☐	surgical repair
proct/o **proct**oscopy	**PROK**-toh prok-**TOSS**-koh-pee	☐	**anus** or **rectum**
rect/o **rect**ocele	**REK**-toh **REK**-toh-seel	☐	**rectum**
-rrhagia gastro**rrhagia**	**RAY**-jee-ah **gas**-troh-**RAY**-jee-ah	☐	excessive flow or discharge
-rrhaphy hepato**rrhaphy**	**RAH**-fee hep-ah-**TOR**-ah-fee	☐	suturing
sial/o **sial**ogram	sigh-**AL**-oh sigh-**AL**-oh-gram	☐	salivary gland; **saliva**
sigmoid/o **sigmoid**oscopy	sig-**MOYD**-oh **sig**-moyd-**OSS**-koh-pee	☐	**sigmoid colon**
-spasm gastro**spasm**	**SPAZM** **GAS**-troh-spazm	☐	twitching; involuntary contraction
splen/o **splen**omegaly	**SPLEE**-noh **splee**-noh-**MEG**-ah-lee	☐	spleen
steat/o **steat**orrhea	stee-**AH**-to stee-**AH**-toh-**REE**-ah	☐	fat
stomat/o **stomat**itis	stoh-**MAH**-toh stoh-mah-**TYE**-tis	☐	mouth
-tresia a**tresia**	**TREE**-zee-ah ah-**TREE**-zee-ah	☐	perforation
-tripsy litho**tripsy**	**TRIP**-see **LITH**-oh-**trip**-see	☐	intentional crushing
xer/o **xer**oderma	**ZEER**-oh **zeer**-oh-**DERM**-ah	☐	dry

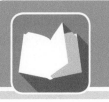

Review Checkpoint

Check your understanding of this section by completing the **Word Elements** exercises in your workbook.

Common Signs and Symptoms

Following are common complaints (signs and symptoms) that individuals with digestive system problems may experience, describe, or express when talking with the health professional. The observant health professional will listen carefully to all of the descriptions used by the patient. As you study the terms following, write each definition and word a minimum of three times, pronouncing the word aloud each time. Note that the word and the **basic definition** are in a green shaded box. Once you have mastered each word to your satisfaction, check the box provided beside the word.

☐ **achlorhydria**

(**ah**-klor-**HIGH**-dree-ah)

  a- = without, not
  chlor/o = green
  hydr/o = water
  -ia = condition

Achlorhydria is an abnormal condition characterized by the absence of **hydrochloric acid** in the gastric juice.

☐ **anorexia**

(an-oh-**REK**-see-ah)

  an- = without
  -orexia = appetite

Lack or loss of appetite, resulting in the inability to eat.

☐ **aphagia**

(ah-**FAY**-jee-ah)

  a- = without, not
  -phagia = to eat

Aphagia is a condition characterized by the loss of the ability to swallow as a result of organic or psychologic causes.

☐ **ascites**

(ah-**SIGH**-teez)

An abnormal accumulation of fluid within the peritoneal cavity. The fluid contains large amounts of protein and electrolytes.

☐ **borborygmus**

(bor-boh-**RIG**-mus)

Borborygmus is an audible abdominal sound produced by hyperactive intestinal **peristalsis**. Borborygmi are rumbling, gurgling, and tinkling noises heard when listening with a stethoscope.

☐ **constipation**

(**kon**-stih-**PAY**-shun)

Constipation is difficulty in passing stools or an incomplete or infrequent passage of hard stools.

☐ **diarrhea**

(dye-ah-**REE**-ah)

  dia- = through
  -rrhea = discharge; flow

The frequent passage of loose, watery stools.

☐ **dyspepsia**

(dis-**PEP**-see-ah)

  dys- = bad, difficult, painful,
    disordered
  -pepsia = digestion

A vague feeling of epigastric discomfort after eating. **Dyspepsia** involves an uncomfortable feeling of fullness, heartburn, bloating, and **nausea**.

☐ **dysphagia**	**Dysphagia** is difficulty in swallowing, commonly associated with obstructive or motor disorders of the **esophagus**.
(dis-**FAY**-jee-ah)	
dys- = bad, difficult, painful, disordered	
-phagia = to eat	

☐ **emaciation**	Excessive leanness caused by disease or lack of nutrition is **emaciation**.
(ee-**may**-she-**AY**-shun)	

☐ **emesis**	The material expelled from the **stomach** during vomiting; **vomitus**.
(**EM**-eh-sis)	

☐ **eructation**	**Eructation** is the act of bringing up air from the **stomach** with a characteristic sound through the mouth; belching.
(eh-ruk-**TAY**-shun)	

☐ **flatus; flatulence**	**Flatus** or **flatulence** is air or gas in the intestine that is passed through the **rectum**.
(**FLAY**-tus; **FLAT**-yoo-lens)	

☐ **gastroesophageal reflux**	**Gastroesophageal reflux** is a backflow of the content of the **stomach** into the **esophagus** that is often the result of incompetence of the lower esophageal sphincter.
(gas-troh-eh-soff-ah-**JEE**-al **REE**-flucks)	
gastr/o = stomach	
esophag/o = esophagus	
-eal = pertaining to	

☐ **icterus**	A yellow discoloration of the skin, mucous membranes, and sclera of the eyes caused by greater than normal amounts of **bilirubin** in the blood; also called **jaundice**.
(**ICK**-ter-us)	

☐ **jaundice**	See *icterus*.
(**JAWN**-diss)	

☐ **melena**	**Melena** is an abnormal, black, tarry stool containing digested blood.
(**MELL**-eh-nah)	

☐ **nausea**	An unpleasant sensation often leading to the urge to **vomit**.
(**NAW**-zee-ah)	

☐ **pruritus ani**	**Pruritus ani** is a common chronic condition of itching of the skin around the **anus**.
(proo-**RIGH**-tus **AN**-eye)	

☐ **steatorrhea**	Greater than normal amounts of fat in the **feces**, characterized by frothy, foul-smelling fecal matter that floats (as in **celiac disease**, some malabsorption syndromes, and any condition in which fats are poorly absorbed by the small intestine).
(stee-ah-toh-**REE**-ah)	
steat/o = fat	
-rrhea = discharge, flow	

☐ **vomit** (**VOM**-it)	To expel the content of the **stomach** through the **esophagus** and out of the mouth.

☐ **vomitus** (**VOM**-ih-tus)	See *emesis*.

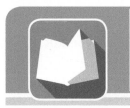

Review Checkpoint

Check your understanding of this section by completing the **Common Signs and Symptoms** exercises in your workbook.

Pathological Conditions

As you study the pathological conditions of the digestive system, note that the **basic definition** is in a green shaded box, followed by a detailed description in regular print. The phonetic pronunciation is directly beneath each term, as well as a breakdown of the component parts of the term where applicable.

achalasia (ak-al-**LAY**-zee-ah)	Decreased mobility of the lower two-thirds of the **esophagus** along with constriction of the lower esophageal sphincter.
	Because of the lack of nerve impulses and the absence of sympathetic receptors, the relaxation of the lower esophageal sphincter (LES) fails to happen with swallowing. Food and fluid accumulate in the lower esophagus due to the decreased mobility in the lower esophagus and its constriction. Among the diagnostic tests used to diagnose **achalasia** are the barium swallow and endoscopy studies.

anal fistula
(**AY**-nal **FISS**-tyoo-lah)
  an/o = anus
  -al = pertaining to
	An abnormal passageway in the skin surface near the **anus** usually connecting with the **rectum**.

	The **anal fistula** may occur as the result of a draining abscess.

aphthous stomatitis
(**AFF**-thus stoh-mah-**TYE**-tis)
  stomat/o = mouth
  -itis = inflammation
	Small, inflammatory, noninfectious, ulcerated lesions occurring on the lips, tongue, and inside the cheeks of the mouth; also called canker sores.

	There is no known cause for **aphthous stomatitis**. However, some of the possible causes are emotional stress, food and drug allergies, endocrine imbalances, viral infections, and vitamin deficiency. The lesions are painful but usually heal within 7 to 14 days. See *Figure 12-7*.

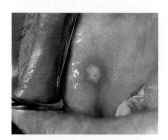

Figure 12-7 Aphthous stomatitis
(Courtesy of Dr. Joseph Konzelman, School of Dentistry, Medical College of Georgia)

appendicitis	**Appendicitis** is the inflammation of the vermiform appendix.
(ap-**pen**-dih-**SIGH**-tis) appendic/o = appendix -itis = inflammation	This is usually an acute condition that can lead to rupture (perforation) with resultant inflammation of the **peritoneum** (**peritonitis**).
	Inflammation of the appendix is caused by an obstruction of the opening of the appendix. If the opening becomes blocked with fecal material, the bacteria multiply and an infection develops in the appendix with pus formation. If the inflamed appendix ruptures, the content spills out into the abdominal cavity (causing peritonitis).
	Abdominal pain is usually the initial symptom with **appendicitis**. It may begin in the epigastric area or around the umbilicus (navel). The pain can, however, exist anywhere in the abdomen. After a few hours following the onset, the pain shifts to the right lower quadrant of the abdomen. The patient usually experiences **anorexia** and **nausea** following the onset of pain.
	Upon examination of the abdomen, the physician may apply deep pressure over **McBurney's point** and release the pressure quickly. If the patient experiences a sensation of severe pain, it is usually a strong indication of an inflamed appendix. This sensation of severe pain when deep pressure is applied and released quickly is known as **rebound tenderness**.
	The patient is admitted to the hospital for testing to confirm the diagnosis of **appendicitis**. Treatment involves surgical removal of the inflamed appendix and antibiotic therapy.
celiac disease	Nutrient malabsorption due to damaged small-bowel mucosa.
(**SEE**-lee-ak dih-**ZEEZ**)	The damage to the small-bowel mucosa occurs because of the ingestion of gluten-containing foods such as barley, rye, wheat, and oats. Fat digestion is affected, as is vitamin and carbohydrate **absorption**.
	Clinical manifestations of this gluten-sensitive disease of the small intestine (when untreated) include **steatorrhea** (large, foul-smelling stools with unabsorbed fat), abdominal distension, and a malnourished appearance. These symptoms typically begin after the infant begins to ingest cereals about six months of age. This disease may also affect adults.
	Effective treatment is dietary control of gluten ingestion. The person with **celiac disease** must remain on a gluten-free diet for life.
cirrhosis	A disease of the liver that is chronic and degenerative, causing injury to the hepatocytes (functional cells of the liver).
(sih-**ROH**-sis) cirrh/o = yellow, tawny -osis = condition	Fat infiltrates the lobules of the liver, the tissue covering the lobes becomes fibrous, and the functions of the liver eventually deteriorate. Multisystem problems result from the liver's obstructed blood flow and inability to metabolize. **Cirrhosis** is a final common course for numerous liver diseases. It also is a result of malnutrition, alcoholism, infection, or poisons. **Cirrhosis** ultimately results in portal hypertension and liver failure.

Diagnosis is made through a biopsy of the liver, results of blood tests, and physical examination. Treatment of **cirrhosis** is to eliminate the cause. When it is possible to eliminate the cause, liver cells will slowly regenerate. If the cause cannot be removed, hepatic failure will occur, leading to death due to the multisystem devastation. Liver transplantation becomes a viable option when an individual's liver is damaged to the point that liver failure is impending and/or the symptoms cannot be otherwise treated. Most liver transplants in adults are performed due to **cirrhosis** brought about by a variety of causes.

colorectal cancer	The presence of a malignant neoplasm in the large intestine.
(koh-loh-**REK**-tal **CAN**-sir) col/o = colon rect/o = rectum -al = pertaining to	Most neoplasms in the large intestine are adenocarcinomas, and at least 50% originate in the **rectum**, causing bleeding and pain. Although the cause of **colorectal cancer** is unknown, a number of known risk factors have been identified. These risk factors include the ingestion of a high-fat, low-residue diet that is high in refined foods or a history of **Crohn's disease**, **ulcerative colitis**, or familial polyposis. Along with the rectal examination, a **barium enema**, **sigmoidoscopy** and/or **colonoscopy**, and stool examination for occult blood are used for diagnosis.
constipation	A state in which the individual's pattern of **bowel** elimination is characterized by a decrease in the frequency of **bowel** movements and the passage of hard, dry stools. The individual experiences difficult **defecation**.
(kon-stih-**PAY**-shun)	**Constipation** is a common complaint among the older person. Contributing factors include decreased **peristalsis** in the intestinal tract, decreased appetite, inadequate fluid intake, and lack of exercise. Repeated overuse or abuse of laxatives over the years worsens the problem. Dietary concerns are important in preventing **constipation** in the elderly adult. The individual should be encouraged to eat small frequent meals, increase dietary fiber, and to drink plenty of fluids daily.
Crohn's disease	**Digestive tract** inflammation of a chronic nature, causing fever, cramping, **diarrhea**, weight loss, and **anorexia**.
(**KROHNZ** dih-**ZEEZ**)	The inflammation of the **bowel** wall results in extreme swelling, which can lead to an obstruction causing a tender, distended abdomen. The stools and/or **vomitus** may have blood. With this chronic disease, the individual may experience signs of malnutrition. The exact etiology of **Crohn's disease** is unknown. However, there have been various implications such as allergies, dietary factors, and immunological factors. A **colonoscopy** is used to diagnose this chronic inflammation of the **digestive tract**. Also known as regional enteritis.
dental caries	Tooth decay caused by acid-forming microorganisms.
(**DEN**-tal **KAIR**-eez) dent/o = tooth -al = pertaining to	These microorganisms are maintained in the mouth by fermentable carbohydrates (most commonly sugars), which create decalcification of the tooth's **enamel** and **dentin**. These fermentable carbohydrates and bacteria

are prone to accumulate in the form of plaque between the teeth and on the grooves of the chewing surfaces of the teeth. This is where **dental caries** are likely to form.

Prevention is the treatment of choice. The topical application or ingestion of fluoride helps the tooth **enamel** become more resistant to the acids and thus the formation of **dental caries**. Flossing and brushing will also aid in the removal of the plaque that leads to **dental caries**.

diverticular disease (**dye**-ver-**TIK**-yoo-lar dih-**ZEEZ**) 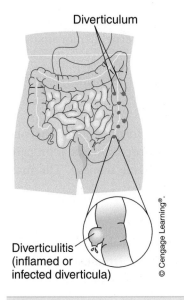 Diverticulum Diverticulitis (inflamed or infected diverticula) © Cengage Learning®.	An expression used to characterize both diverticulosis and diverticulitis. Diverticulosis describes the noninflamed outpouchings or herniations of the muscular layer of the intestine, typically the **sigmoid colon**. Inflammation of these outpouchings (called diverticula) is referred to as diverticulitis. See *Figure 12-8*. **Diverticular disease** is an increasingly common occurrence in persons over 45 years of age. Persons eating diets low in fiber predispose themselves to the formation of diverticula. Inflammation of a diverticulum (diverticulitis) results in cramping pain, fever, increased **flatus**, and elevated white blood cell count (leukocytosis). **Proctoscopy** and barium enemas are used in the diagnostic process. **Figure 12-8** Diverticulitis

dysentery
 	
(**DISS**-en-**ter**-ee)
 	
  dys- = bad, difficult, painful,
    disordered
  enter/o = intestine
  -y = noun ending
	A term used to describe painful intestinal inflammation typically caused by ingesting water or food containing bacteria, protozoa, parasites, or chemical irritants.
	
	The person suffering from **dysentery** has frequent stools that often contain blood. Other symptoms include abdominal pain and intestinal cramping. **Dysentery** often occurs as a result of unsanitary conditions.

esophageal varices
 	
(eh-soff-ah-**JEE**-al **VAIR**-ih-seez)
 	
  esophag/o = esophagus
  -eal = pertaining to
	Swollen, twisted (tortuous) veins located in the distal end of the **esophagus**.
	
	Esophageal varices is usually caused by portal hypertension, which occurs as a result of liver disease (in particular, **cirrhosis** of the liver). Portal hypertension causes the pressure in the veins to increase, making the vessels especially susceptible to hemorrhage.

gallstones (cholelithiasis)
 	
(koh-lee-lih-**THIGH**-ah-sis)
 	
  chol/e = bile
  lith/o = stone
  -iasis = presence of an abnormal
    condition
	Pigmented or hardened cholesterol stones formed as a result of **bile** crystallization.
	
	When the gallstones obstruct the common bile duct or the cystic duct, epigastric and/or upper right quadrant pain develops, sometimes radiating to the upper right back area. This discomfort is generally accompanied by **nausea** and vomiting.

The person's history along with an ultrasound of the **gallbladder** are usually reliable in diagnosing **cholelithiasis**. With recurring pain, surgical intervention is indicated. When removing a **gallbladder**, a laparoscopic cholecystectomy may be performed, resulting in a much quicker recovery. Gallstones may be removed through an endoscopic procedure. The medication, chenodiol, is used to disintegrate existing stones and reduce the liver's cholesterol synthesis.

hemorrhoids (**HEM**-oh-roydz)	A hemorrhoid is an unnaturally distended or swollen vein (called a varicosity) in the distal rectum or **anus**.

Hemorrhoids arising above the internal sphincter are classified as internal, and those emerging outside the **sphincter** are external hemorrhoids. Internal hemorrhoids become constricted and very painful and may bleed when they enlarge and extrude from the **anus**. External hemorrhoids do not typically bleed or cause pain.

hepatitis (**hep**-ah-**TYE**-tis) hepat/o = liver -itis = inflammation	Acute or chronic inflammation of the liver due to a viral or bacterial infection, drugs, alcohol, toxins, or parasites.

The resultant inflammation presents itself in the form of abdominal and **gastric** discomfort; enlarged, tender liver; **jaundice**; **anorexia**; joint pain; and elevated liver enzymes indicative of liver tissue damage. The most common type of **hepatitis** is viral hepatitis.

Viral hepatitis begins in the acute form as a result of:

1. Hepatitis A virus, frequently transmitted by the fecal–**oral** route or due to poor hygiene, contaminated water, or shellfish. (In most cases, there is a complete recovery.)

2. Hepatitis B virus, which is transmitted from the blood or body fluid of an infected individual to another individual and has the potential of leading to excessive destruction of liver cells, **cirrhosis**, or death.

3. Hepatitis C virus, which is transmitted through the intravenous route in blood transfusions or when persons share needles, and progresses in about one-half of the cases to a chronic form of **hepatitis**.

hernia (**HER**-nee-ah)	An irregular protrusion of tissue, organ, or a portion of an organ through an abnormal break in the surrounding cavity's muscular wall.

Weakness in the muscle walls may be inherited or obtained due to the aging process, heavy lifting, obesity, coughing, or pregnancy. The **hernia** associated with the digestive system is known as a hiatal hernia. Also called a diaphragmatic hernia, this condition occurs as a result of an upward protrusion of the **stomach** through the diaphragm due to an enlarged **cardiac sphincter**. See *Figure 12-9*. Individuals with a hiatal hernia may be completely free of symptoms (asymptomatic) or may experience daily symptoms that are usually similar to those of gastroesophageal reflux, the backflow of the acid content of the stomach into the **esophagus**.

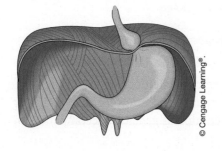

© Cengage Learning®.

Figure 12-9 Hiatal hernia

Diagnosis of a hiatal hernia can be made via X-ray films. Treatment is usually directed at relieving the discomfort associated with the reflux through the use of medications such as antacids and histamine receptor antagonists, diet, and proper positioning to decrease pain. Surgical intervention is usually necessary.

herpetic stomatitis
(her-**PEH**-tic stoh-mah-**TYE**-tis)
  stomat/o = mouth
  -itis = inflammation
	Inflammatory infectious lesions in or on the oral cavity occurring as a primary or a secondary viral infection caused by herpes simplex.

The primary infection usually occurs during early childhood and is often asymptomatic. Other times it appears in the form of ulcerations in the mouth. Secondary **herpetic stomatitis** is a recurrent viral infection believed to lie dormant until it is reactivated by a fever, an upper respiratory infection, or exposure to sunlight. These clear vesicular lesions appear on the lips, palate, tongue, and **gingiva** of the mouth and are often called "cold sores" or fever blisters.

The lesions from **herpetic stomatitis** are painful and contagious but heal without scarring in approximately seven days. There is no known preventive measure. The treatment includes use of analgesics, local ointments, and anesthetics for the relief of discomfort caused by the lesions. In immunocompromised persons, acyclovir is administered intravenously.

Hirschsprung's disease (congenital megacolon) (**HIRSH**-sprungz dih-**ZEEZ**) (kon-**JEN**-ih-tal meg-ah-**KOH**-lon)	Absence at birth of the autonomic ganglia in a segment of the intestinal smooth muscle wall that normally stimulates **peristalsis**.

With the absence of these autonomic ganglia, the intestinal peristalsis is poor or absent in the aganglionic segment, which results in a buildup of **feces** and thus the distention of the **bowel**. This enlarged **bowel** is sometimes called a megacolon.

Hirschsprung's disease is typically diagnosed during infancy and is often due to the failure of the newborn to have the first stool (called a meconium ileus). The diagnosis is confirmed with a **barium enema**, and the extent of the affected tissue is determined with biopsies. According to the extent and exact location of the aganglionic segment, surgical repair is done to remove the aganglionic portion.

ileus
(**ILL**-ee-us)
  ile/o = ileum
  -us = noun ending
	A term used to describe an obstruction of the intestine.

There are several reasons an **ileus** may occur (such as twisting of the **bowel**, absence of **peristalsis**, or presence of adhesions or tumor). An **ileus** may resolve with medical treatment or require surgical intervention such as an intestinal resection.

intestinal obstruction (in-**TESS**-tin-al ob-**STRUCK**-shun)	Complete or partial alteration in the forward flow of the content in the small or large intestines.

An obstruction in the small intestine constitutes a surgical emergency. All intestinal obstructions require rapid diagnosis and treatment within a 24-hour period to prevent death. There are numerous causes of an **intestinal obstruction**, such as:

1. Inflammation causes decreased diameter of the intestinal lumen.

2. Adhesions form after abdominal surgery as bands of fibrous scar tissue, which can become looped over or around the intestine.

3. Tumors may cause an obstruction in the small or large intestine.

4. Hernias may become incarcerated and thus cause an obstruction.

5. **Volvulus** occurs when the **bowel** becomes twisted or rotated on itself.

6. **Intussusception** occurs when the proximal bowel telescopes into the distal bowel.

7. Neurogenic factors result in lack of **peristalsis** after abdominal surgery.

The clinical manifestations of an **intestinal obstruction** include abdominal pain and distension, **nausea** and vomiting, and altered **bowel** sounds. Diagnostic tests used to evaluate an **intestinal obstruction** are flat plate X-ray, barium follow-through, **barium enema**, CBC, and blood chemistry studies.

The insertion of an intestinal tube is the primary medical treatment for an **intestinal obstruction**. If the intestinal tube is ineffective in relieving the obstruction, surgery is indicated.

intussusception (**in**-tuh-suh-**SEP**-shun)	Telescoping of a portion of proximal intestine into distal intestine, usually in the **ileocecal** region (causing an obstruction).

Intussusception typically occurs in infants and young children. Clinical manifestations include intermittent severe abdominal pain, vomiting, and a "currant jelly stool" (which indicates the presence of bloody mucus). See *Figure 12-10*.

Intussusception is diagnosed and medically treated with a **barium enema**. During the examination, the telescoping is often reduced with the pressure created with a **barium enema**. When the obstruction is not reduced with the **barium enema**, immediate surgical intervention is necessary.

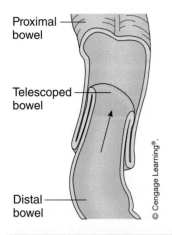

Proximal bowel

Telescoped bowel

Distal bowel

© Cengage Learning®.

Figure 12-10 Intussusception

irritable bowel syndrome (IBS); spastic colon (**EAR**-ih-tah-bul-**BOW**-el **SIN**-drom) (**SPAS**-tik **KOH**-lon)	Increased motility of the small or large intestinal wall, resulting in abdominal pain, **flatulence**, **nausea**, **anorexia**, and the trapping of gas throughout the intestines.

Diarrhea, more often than **constipation**, may occur. This increased motility is distinctively in response to emotional stress. There are no diagnostic tests to confirm **irritable bowel syndrome (IBS)** or **spastic colon**, and thus all other possible causes of the symptoms must be ruled out.

oral leukoplakia	A precancerous lesion occurring anywhere in the mouth.

(**OR**-al **loo**-koh-**PLAY**-kee-ah)

   or/o = mouth

   -al = pertaining to

   leuk/o = white

   -plakia = a plate; flat plane

These elevated gray-white or yellow-white, leathery-surfaced lesions have clearly defined borders. See *Figure 12-11*. Etiological factors of **oral leukoplakia** include chronic oral mucosal irritation, which occurs with the use of tobacco and alcohol.

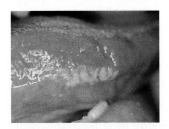

Figure 12-11 Oral leukoplakia
(Courtesy of Dr. Joseph Konzelman, School of Dentistry, Medical College of Georgia)

pancreatitis	An acute or chronic destructive inflammatory condition of the **pancreas**.

(pan-kree-ah-**TYE**-tis)

   pancreat/o = pancreas

   -itis = inflammation

Acute **pancreatitis** presents itself quickly and creates symptoms, which vary from mild, self-limiting pancreatic edema to massive necrotizing hemorrhagic **pancreatitis**. The initial outstanding symptom is severe continuous epigastric and abdominal pain that radiates to the back and follows the ingestion of excessive alcohol or a fatty meal. Other symptoms include rigid abdominal distension, decreased **bowel** sounds, **nausea** and vomiting, hypotension, elevated temperature, and clammy cold skin. After 24 hours, mild **jaundice** may appear. In addition to alcoholism, other causes of acute pancreatitis include trauma, surgery, metabolic disorders, drugs, infections, or ruptured **peptic ulcers**.

Serious complications may include development of abscesses or pseudocysts, diabetes mellitus, renal failure, heart failure, hypovolemic shock, multiple organ failure, ascites, and adult respiratory distress syndrome. Treatment is aimed at resolving the immediate problems, relief of pain, and avoiding any further GI irritation (NG tube and NPO status), and prevention of serious, life-threatening complications.

Chronic pancreatitis is a permanent, progressive destruction of the pancreatic cells identified with fibrosis, atrophy, fatty degeneration, and calcification. The causes of chronic pancreatitis include alcoholism, malnutrition, surgery, or neoplasm. Clinical manifestations include abdominal pain, large fatty stools, weight loss, and signs and symptoms of diabetes mellitus. Treatment includes the administration of pancreatic enzymes, antiemetics, antacids, and **insulin** if its production is stopped or decreased.

peptic ulcers (gastric, duodenal, perforated)	A break in the continuity of the mucous membrane lining of the **gastrointestinal tract** as a result of hyperacidity or the bacterium *Helicobacter pylori*.

(**PEP**-tik **ULL**-sirz)

(**GAS**-tric, doo-**OD**-en-al, **PER**-foh-ray-ted)

Peptic ulcers are acute or chronic, singular or clustered, and shallow or deep. Acute ulcers are typically multiple and shallow, therefore causing few symptoms, and heal without scarring. On the other hand, chronic ulcers are typically singular, deep, symptomatic, and persistent (and cause scarring). If an ulcer invades to the point of creating a hole through the complete depth of the **stomach** or **duodenum**, it is called a perforating ulcer (which will likely require surgical intervention).

Diagnosis is based on the client's history, upper GI barium studies, and endoscopy. Clinical manifestations of a peptic ulcer include some or all of the following: gnawing epigastric pain, heartburn or indigestion, **nausea** and vomiting, and bloated feeling after eating. Treatment includes therapy with agents that inhibit gastric acid secretion, lifestyle and diet changes (abstaining from tobacco and alcohol), and antibiotics if the ulcer is due to the *Helicobacter pylori (H. pylori)* bacterium.

periodontal disease
 	
(pair-ee-oh-**DON**-tal dih-**ZEEZ**)
 	
  peri- = around
  odont/o = teeth
  -al = pertaining to
	A term used to describe a group of inflammatory gum disorders, which may lead to degeneration of teeth, gums, and sometimes surrounding bones.
	
	Periodontal diseases are very common, occurring in at least 90% of the population. The formation and accumulation of plaque due to fermentable carbohydrates and bacteria is the primary cause of **periodontal disease**.
	
	In the early stages of **periodontal disease**, minor inflammation of the gums (**gingivitis**) occurs, causing discoloration and bleeding. As **periodontal disease** progresses to the late stages, purulent inflammation of the gums (pyorrhea) develops (causing pus to drain from the gum tissue).

polyps, colorectal
 	
(**POL**-ips, koh-loh-**REK**-tal)
 	
  polyp/o = polyps
  col/o = colon
  rect/o = rectum
  -al = pertaining to
	Colorectal polyps are small growths projecting from the mucous membrane of the **colon** or **rectum**.
	
	They may be sessile (attached by a base) or pedunculated (attached by a stalk) and may vary in size. Polyps may be benign or precancerous.
	
	Polyps are usually asymptomatic (without symptoms) and are discovered during routine physical examinations that include diagnostic testing or tests for blood in the stool. They can, however, cause rectal bleeding and intestinal bleeding. When polyps are detected, a **colonoscopy** may be ordered to rule out cancer. A biopsy of the polyp may be obtained, or the polyp may be completely removed during the procedure.

thrush (**THRUSH**) 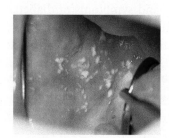	A fungal infection in the mouth and throat, producing sore, creamy white, slightly raised curdlike patches on the tongue and other oral mucosal surfaces. **Thrush** is caused by *Candida albicans*. **Thrush** is common in infants or persons who are debilitated, immunosuppressed, or receiving long-term antibiotic, corticosteroid, and antineoplastic therapy. Treatment consists of an antifungal medication for two weeks. See *Figure 12-12.* **Figure 12-12** Thrush *(Courtesy of Dr. Joseph Konzelman, School of Dentistry, Medical College of Georgia)*

ulcerative colitis (**ULL**-sir-ah-tiv koh-**LYE**-tis) col/o = colon -itis = inflammation	A chronic inflammatory condition resulting in a break in the continuity of the mucous membrane lining of the **colon** in the form of ulcers. **Ulcerative colitis** is characterized by large watery diarrheal stools containing mucus, pus, or blood. The **diarrhea** is accompanied by severe abdominal discomfort and spasms of the intestines. The person will likely experience fever, chills, weight loss, and anemia. Treatment for **ulcerative colitis** usually includes corticosteroids or other anti-inflammatory medications. In severe cases that do not respond to medical treatment, surgical intervention is implicated. **Ulcerative colitis** bears an increased risk of acquiring colon cancer.
volvulus (**VOL**-vyoo-lus)	A rotation of loops of **bowel**, causing a twisting on itself that results in an **intestinal obstruction** (see *intestinal obstruction*). See *Figure 12-13*.

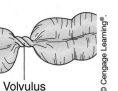

Volvulus

© Cengage Learning®.

Figure 12-13 Volvulus

Review Checkpoint

Check your understanding of this section by completing the **Pathological Conditions** exercises in your workbook.

Diagnostic Techniques, Treatments, and Procedures

abdominal ultrasound (ab-**DOM**-ih-nal **ULL**-trah-sound)	The use of very-high-frequency sound waves to provide visualization of the internal organs of the abdomen (liver, **gallbladder**, bile ducts, **pancreas**, kidneys, bladder, and ureters); also known as an abdominal sonogram. The **abdominal ultrasound** is a noninvasive diagnostic procedure that demonstrates normal or abnormal findings of the abdominal organs.
abdominocentesis (paracentesis) (ab-**dom**-ih-noh-sen-**TEE**-sis, **pair**-ah-sen-**TEE**-sis) abdomin/o = abdomen -centesis = surgical puncture para- = near, beside, beyond, two like parts -centesis = surgical puncture	**Abdominocentesis** involves insertion of a needle or trocar into the abdominal cavity to remove excess fluid, with the person in a sitting position. The trocar is attached to a tube and collection bottle. This invasive procedure is typically done to remove large amounts of **ascitic fluid** from the distended abdomen to reduce pressure, which sometimes keeps the person from being able to breathe effectively. A specimen of the **peritoneal** fluid will likely be tested in the laboratory. Increased levels of **amylase** in the peritoneal fluid are indicative of acute **pancreatitis**.

After the needle is withdrawn, a small dressing is secured over the puncture site. A physician's order may follow for the administration of salt-poor albumin to replace the lost protein.

alanine aminotransferase (ALT) (**AL**-ah-neen ah-mee-no-**TRANS**-fer-ays)	**Alanine aminotransferase** is a hepatocellular enzyme released in elevated amounts due to liver dysfunction; also known as serum glutamic pyruvic transaminase (SGPT).
	The normal serum level of ALT/SGPT is 5 to 35 IU/L. Abnormally high levels occur in **hepatitis**, **cirrhosis**, hepatic necrosis, hepatic ischemia, hepatic tumor, hepatotoxic drugs, obstructive jaundice, myositis, and **pancreatitis**.
alkaline phosphatase (ALP) (**AL**-kah-line **FOSS**-fah-tays)	**Alkaline phosphatase** enzyme is found in the highest concentrations in the liver, biliary tract, and bone.
	The mucosa of the intestine also contains ALP. A normal level of ALP is 30 to 85 ImU/mL (international milliunits/milliliter). Increased levels of ALP are found in **cirrhosis**, intrahepatic or extrahepatic biliary obstruction, liver tumors, and intestinal ischemia or infarction. Decreased levels are seen in malnutrition, **celiac disease**, and excess vitamin B ingestion. The serum ALP level is elevated in obstructive hepatitis or **jaundice**.
amylase (**AM**-ih-lays)	An **enzyme** secreted normally from the pancreatic cells that travels to the **duodenum** by way of the pancreatic duct and aids in digestion.
	When the pancreatic duct is blocked or there is damage to the pancreatic cells that secrete **amylase**, the **enzyme** pours into the free **peritoneum** and intrapancreatic lymph system (where blood vessels absorb the excess **amylase**). A normal blood amylase level is 56 to 190 IU/L. Abnormally increased levels are found in acute **pancreatitis**, penetrating or perforated **peptic ulcers**, perforated **bowel**, necrotic bowel, **duodenal** obstruction, and acute **cholecystitis**.
appendectomy (ap-en-**DEK**-toh-mee) appendic/o = appendix -ectomy = surgical removal	An **appendectomy** is the surgical removal of an inflamed appendix.
	If no rupture has occurred, a laparoscopic appendectomy may be performed. This involves removing the appendix through a scope (laparoscope), which would require only a small incision into the abdomen.
barium enema (BE) **(lower GI series)** (**BAH**-ree-um **EN**-eh-mah)	Infusion of a radiopaque contrast medium, barium sulfate, into the **rectum** and held in the lower intestinal tract while X-ray films are obtained of the lower GI tract.
	For the most definitive results, the **colon** should be empty of fecal material. Along with the use of a laxative and/or a cleansing enema, the person having a **barium enema** would be without food or drink from the midnight before the procedure. Abnormal findings include malignant tumors, colonic stenosis, colonic fistula, perforated colon, diverticula, and polyps.
barium swallow **(UGI) (upper GI series)** (**BAH**-ree-um swallow)	**Barium swallow** involves oral administration of a radiopaque contrast medium, barium sulfate, which flows into the **esophagus** as the person swallows.
	X-ray films are obtained of the **esophagus** and borders of the heart in which varices can be identified as well as strictures, tumors, obstructions,

achalasia, or abnormal motility of the **esophagus**. As the barium sulfate continues to flow into the upper GI tract (lower esophagus, **stomach**, and **duodenum**), X-ray films are taken to reveal ulcerations, tumors, hiatal hernias, or obstruction. Additional information and photos are found in Chapter 20.

capsule endoscopy
 	
(**CAP**-sool en-**DOSS**-koh-pee)
  endo- = within
  -scopy = the process of viewing
	Capsule endoscopy is the process of viewing the entire length of the small intestine by using an ingestible video camera with a light source, which is enclosed in a capsule (about the size of a large vitamin pill). This tiny video camera, known as the **camera pill**, produces digital images of the entire length of the small intestine and can visualize areas that other diagnostic techniques cannot. Use of the camera pill is not disruptive to the normal activities of the **digestive tract**; also known as wireless endoscopy.

The patient's physician will determine the specific preparation for the exam. At the beginning of the procedure, the patient swallows the camera pill with a glass of water. As the camera pill moves through the **alimentary canal**, digital images are continuously transmitted to a small recording device worn on a belt around the patient's waist. The patient will wear the apparatus for approximately eight hours. After removal of the belt, the physician transfers the information from the recording device to a computer to review the color images. The camera pill capsule leaves the body naturally via a bowel movement.

The use of computed tomography in combination with the camera pill provides a good global view of the body and assists in pinpointing abnormalities. The camera pill provides images that are useful in diagnosing ulcers, tumors, unexplained bleeding, and inflammatory bowel conditions. However, this procedure does not replace a standard upper gastrointestinal study (**barium swallow**) or **colonoscopy**. The capsule endoscopy is not advisable for patients with problems swallowing, intestinal narrowing, history of prior gastrointestinal surgery or bowel obstruction, or individuals with a pacemaker.

cheiloplasty
 	
(**KYE**-loh-plas-tee)
  cheil/o = lip
  -plasty = surgical repair
	Surgically correcting a defect of the lip is known as **cheiloplasty**.

cholecystectomy
 	
(**koh**-lee-sis-**TEK**-toh-mee)
  cholecyst/o = gallbladder
  -ectomy = removal of
	The surgical removal of the **gallbladder**.

The specific technique is based on the location of the stone and the severity of the individual's complications. A simple **cholecystectomy** is performed when the stones are found only in the **gallbladder**. This simple **cholecystectomy** may be done through laparascopic laser surgery or conventional surgical methods. When the stones are located or lodged within the ducts, a common bile duct exploration will be needed during surgery and there may also be placement of a T-tube in the duct (which allows the drainage of the **bile** until the edema of the duct has decreased).

cholecystography (oral) (**koh**-lee-sis-**TOG**-rah-fee) 　chol/e = bile 　cyst/o = bladder, sac, or cyst 　-graphy = process of recording	Visualization of the **gallbladder** through X-ray following the **oral** ingestion of pills containing a radiopaque iodinated dye.
	The oral **cholecystography** is not as accurate as the gallbladder ultrasound. Abnormal findings would include gallstones, gallbladder polyps, gallbladder cancer, or cystic duct obstruction, The radiographic image of the gallbladder that is obtained during the cholecystography is known as a cholecystogram.
colonoscopy (**koh**-lon-**OSS**-koh-pee) 　colon/o = colon 　-scopy = the process of viewing	The direct visualization of the lining of the large intestine using a fiberoptic colonoscope.
	A **colonoscopy** is indicated for individuals with a history of undiagnosed **constipation** and **diarrhea**, loss of appetite (**anorexia**), persistent rectal bleeding, or lower abdominal pain. The procedure is also used to check for colonic polyps or possible malignant tumors.
colostomy (koh-**LAHS**-toh-mee) 　col/o = colon 　-stomy = the surgical creation of a 　　　new opening	The surgical creation of a new opening on the abdominal wall through which the **feces** will be expelled (an abdominal-wall anus) by bringing the incised colon out to the abdominal surface.
	The **colostomy** may be needed temporarily for the **bowel** to heal from injury (traumatic or surgical) or inflammation, or it may be needed permanently as the only opening for elimination of **feces**.
CT of the abdomen (**CT** of the **AB**-doh-men)	A painless, noninvasive X-ray procedure that produces an image created by the computer representing a detailed cross section of the tissue structure within the abdomen, for example, computerized tomography **(CT) of the abdomen**.
	The CT scan of the abdomen aids in the diagnosis of tumors, abscesses, cysts, inflammation, obstructions, perforation, bleeding, aneurysms, and obstruction. For more information on CT scans, see Chapter 20.
CT colonography **(virtual colonoscopy)** (CT **koh**-lon-**OG**-rah-fee) 　colon/o = colon 　-graphy = process of recording (Virtual **koh**-lon-**OSS**-koh-pee) 　colon/o = colon 　-scopy = process of viewing with a 　　　scope	CT colonography uses CT scanning (or MRI) to obtain an interior view of the **colon** that is usually seen using an endoscope inserted into the **rectum**. This non-invasive, painless procedure provides two- and three-dimensional images that can show polyps and other lesions as clearly as when they are seen with direct visual colonoscopy. Use of the CT colonography allows these growths to be detected in their early stages; also called a virtual colonoscopy.
	Prior to the exam, the patient must follow a bowel-cleansing regimen to remove stool from the **colon**. The patient will be advised as to the specific preparation and diet prior to the exam. For the exam, the patient is placed on the CT exam table (may begin in a side-lying position). A very small, flexible tube is inserted approximately 2 inches into the patient's **rectum** to allow air to be gently pumped into the **colon**, using a handheld squeeze bulb; or an electronic pump may be used to administer carbon dioxide gas into the **colon**. The air or gas is inserted into the colon to distend the walls slightly to eliminate any folds and wrinkles that may obscure the visibility of polyps.

The table then moves through the scanner, and the patient is asked to hold his/her breath for about 15 seconds before turning over and lying on his/her back. The table then moves through the scanner for a second time. When the scan is completed; the tube is removed from the patient's **rectum**. CT colonography is an alternative to, not a substitute for, conventional **colonoscopy**.

endoscopic retrograde cholangiopancreatography (ERCP)	A procedure that examines the size of and the filling of the pancreatic and biliary ducts through direct radiographic visualization with a fiberoptic endoscope. See *Figure 12-14*.

(en-doh-**SKOP**-ic **RET**-roh-grayd koh-**lan**-jee-oh-**pan**-kree-ah-**TOG**-rah-fee)

endo- = within
scop/o = to view
-ic = pertaining to
chol/e = bile
angi/o = vessel
pancreat/o = pancreas
-graphy = process of recording

During the ERCP procedure, a fiberoptic scope (flexible tube with a lens and a light source) is passed through the patient's **esophagus** and **stomach** into the **duodenum**. Passage of the tube is observed on a fluoroscopic screen that makes it possible to view the procedure in action. The doctor locates the ampulla of Vater, a common passageway that connects the common bile duct and the pancreatic duct to the **duodenum**. Digestive enzymes can be removed from this area for analysis before a contrast medium is injected into the area for visualization upon X-ray.

This procedure requires the person to lie very still during the process. The patient is kept NPO (nothing by mouth) before the procedure and is mildly sedated during the procedure. Abnormal findings include strictures (narrowing) of the common bile duct, tumors, gallstones, cysts, and anatomic variations of the biliary or pancreatic ducts.

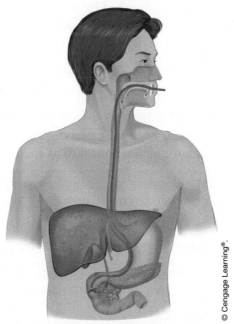

© Cengage Learning®.

Figure 12-14 Endoscopic retrograde cholangiopancreatography (ERCP)

esophagogastroduodenoscopy (EGD)	Esophagogastroduodenoscopy is the process of direct visualization of the **esophagus**, **stomach**, and **duodenum**, using a lighted fiberoptic endoscope; also known as an upper endoscopy.

(eh-**soff**-ah-goh-gass-troh-**doo**-oh-den-**OSS**-koh-pee)

esophag/o = esophagus
gastr/o = stomach

An endoscope can also be used for aspirating fluid, performing a biopsy, and coagulating areas of bleeding. In addition, a laser beam can be passed through the endoscope, which permits endoscopic surgery. Abnormal

duoden/o = duodenum -scopy = process of viewing	findings include tumors (malignant and benign), **esophagitis**, gastroesophageal varices, **peptic ulcers**, and the source of upper GI bleeding.

extracorporeal shock wave lithotripsy (ESWL)
 	
(**eks**-trah-kor-**POR**-ee-al shock wave **LITH**-oh-**trip**-see)
 	
  extra- = outside, beyond
  corpor/o = body
  -eal = pertaining to
  lith/o = stone
  -tripsy = intentional crushing
	An alternative treatment for gallstones by using ultrasound to align the computerized lithotripter and source of shock waves with the stones to crush the gallstones and thus enable the contraction of the **gallbladder** to remove stone fragments; also used to crush renal calculi (kidney stones).
	
	This contraction of the **gallbladder** will likely cause discomfort, **nausea**, and transient hematuria.

fluoroscopy
 	
(**floo**-or-**OS**-koh-pee)
 	
  fluor/o = luminous
  -scopy = the process of viewing
	Fluoroscopy is a radiological technique used to examine the function of an organ or a body part by using a fluoroscope.
	
	There are immediate serial images that are essential in many clinical procedures. For more information, see Chapter 20.

gastric analysis
 	
(**GAS**-trik analysis)
 	
  gastr/o = stomach
  -ic = pertaining to
	Study of the **stomach** content to determine the acid content and to detect the presence of blood, bacteria, **bile**, and abnormal cells.
	
	The **gastric** sample is typically obtained through a nasogastric tube and examined. An alternate tubeless method uses the ingestion of Diagnex Blue, a resin dye. The **hydrochloric acid** in the **stomach** displaces the dye, which is absorbed by the bowel and excreted in about two hours in the urine. The lack of blue color in the urine typically signifies the absence of **hydrochloric acid** in the **stomach**.

gastric lavage
 	
(**GAS**-trik lavage)
 	
  gastr/o = stomach
  -ic = pertaining to
	The irrigation, or washing out, of the **stomach** with sterile water or a saline solution.
	
	A gastric lavage is usually performed before and after surgery to remove irritants or toxic substances from the **stomach**. It may also be performed before examinations such as endoscopy or gastroscopy.

herniorrhaphy (her-nee-**OR**-ah-fee) -rrhaphy = suturing	**Herniorrhaphy** is the surgical repair of a **hernia** by closing the defect, using sutures, mesh, or wire. The person has activity restriction—no heavy labor or lifting for at least three weeks after surgery.

liver biopsy (**LIV**-er **BYE**-op-see)	A piece of liver tissue is obtained for examination by inserting a specially designed needle into the liver through the abdominal wall. Abnormal findings include **hepatitis**, abscess, cyst, or infiltrative diseases. There are specific procedures before, during, and after a **liver biopsy**.

liver scan (**LIV**-er **SCAN**)	A noninvasive scanning technique, which enables the visualization of the shape, size, and consistency of the liver after the IV injection of a radioactive compound. This compound is readily taken up by the liver's Kupffer cells and later the distribution is recorded by a radiation detector. The **liver scan** can detect cysts, abscesses, tumors, granulomas, or diffuse infiltrative processes affecting the liver.

magnetic resonance imaging (MRI)	A noninvasive scanning procedure that provides visualization of fluid, soft tissue, and bony structures without the use of radiation.
(mag-**NEH**-tic **REZ**-oh-nans **IM**-ij-ing)	The person is placed inside a large electromagnetic, tubelike machine where specific radio frequency signals change the alignment of hydrogen atoms in the body. The absorbed radio frequency energy is analyzed by a computer and an image is projected on the screen.

A strong magnetic field is used and radio frequency waves produce the imaging valuable in providing images of the heart, large blood vessels, brain, and soft tissue. MRI is also used to examine the aorta and to detect masses (or possible tumors) and pericardial disease. It can show the flowing of blood and the beating of the heart. The MRI provides far more precision and accuracy than most diagnostic tools.

Those persons with implanted metal devices cannot undergo an MRI due to the strong magnetic field and the possibility of dislodging a chip or rod. Thus, persons with pacemakers, any recently implanted wires or clips, or prosthetic valves are not eligible for MRI. Persons should be informed that MRI is a very confining procedure because they are placed within a tubelike structure, and they should be asked if they are claustrophobic (fearful of enclosed spaces).

nasogastric intubation	**Nasogastric intubation** involves tube placement through the nose into the **stomach** for the purpose of relieving gastric distension by removing gastric secretions, gas, or food.
(nay-zoh-**GAS**-trik **in**-too-**BAY**-shun) nas/o = nose gastr/o = stomach -ic = pertaining to	

The nasogastric tube may be the route for instilling medications, fluids, and/or food.

percutaneous transhepatic cholangiography (PTC)	An examination of the bile duct structure by using a needle to pass directly into an intrahepatic bile duct to inject a contrast medium; also abbreviated as PTHC.
(**per**-kyoo-**TAY**-nee-us trans-heh-**PAT**-ik koh-**lan**-jee-**OG**-rah-fee) per- = through cutane/o = skin -ous = pertaining to trans- = across hepat/o = liver -ic = pertaining to chol/e = bile angi/o = vessel -graphy = process of recording	

The bile duct structure can be observed for obstruction, strictures, anatomic variations, malignant tumors, and congenital cysts. If the cause is found to be extrahepatic in persons who are jaundiced, a catheter may be used for external drainage by leaving it in the bile duct. Abnormal findings include the following:

1. Tumors, gallstones, or strictures of the common bile or hepatic duct
2. **Biliary** sclerosis
3. Cysts of the common bile duct
4. Tumors, inflammation, or pseudocysts of the pancreatic duct
5. Anatomic biliary or pancreatic duct abnormalities

Although the complication rate after this invasive procedure is low, the patient must be observed closely for symptoms of bleeding, peritonitis (due to leakage of **bile**), and septicemia. Any signs of these complications and/or pain should be reported to the physician immediately.

48-hour pH study	The 48-hour pH study is a procedure used to measure and monitor the amount of gastric acid reflux into the **esophagus** during the specified period. The monitoring system will determine how often **stomach** contents reflux into the **esophagus**, how long the acid stays in the **esophagus**, and how much reflux occurs at nighttime. This test is used to determine if the patient has GERD (gastroesophageal reflux disease) and if so, the severity of the GERD; also known as 48-hour wireless esophageal pH monitoring.

A small, thin catheter containing a radio-transmitting capsule (about the size of a medication gel cap) is placed through the nose into the **esophagus**. Using a small amount of suction, the capsule attaches to the inside of the **esophagus**, and the catheter is removed. During the testing period, the patient is instructed to eat, drink, work and exercise as he or she normally would and is advised to avoid taking any antacid products unless instructed to by his or her physician.

The capsule collects pH data and transmits it via radio-frequency telemetry to an ambulatory miniaturized data recorder (about the size of a pager) worn on the patient's wrist, or belt, for 48 hours. The patient will maintain a diary of activities, meals, and snacks during the testing period. If any symptoms occur, such as heartburn, regurgitation, or chest pain, a button on the recording device is pressed to denote the time, and the incident is recorded in the diary. At the end of the 48 hours, the patient will return the recorder to the endoscopy lab for the data to be evaluated. The capsule naturally sloughs or falls off the esophageal wall in 5–7 days and passes through the digestive tract.

serum bilirubin (**SEE**-rum bill-ih-**ROO**-bin)	A measurement of the **bilirubin** level in the serum. **Serum bilirubin** levels are a result of the breakdown of red blood cells.

Jaundice is the yellow discoloration of body tissues caused by abnormally high levels of **bilirubin**. The normal levels of **bilirubin** in the blood are:

1. Total bilirubin = 0.1 to 1.0 mg/dL
2. Indirect bilirubin = 0.2 to 0.8 mg/dL
3. Direct bilirubin = 0.1 to 0.3 mg/dL

An elevated indirect bilirubin level is seen with hepatic damage, **hepatitis**, and **cirrhosis**. An elevated direct bilirubin level is seen with gallstones, extensive liver metastasis, and extrahepatic duct obstruction.

serum glutamic-oxaloacetic transaminase (SGOT) (**SEE**-rum gloo-**TAM**-ik **oks**-ah-loh-ah-**SEE**-tik trans-**AM**-in-ays)	An **enzyme** that has very high concentrations in liver cells; also known as aspartate aminotransferase (AST).

An AST/SGOT level, measured in the blood, that is elevated indicates the extent of disease on the liver cells. AST/SGOT enzyme levels are elevated with damaged hepatocytes. The normal adult level is 8 to 20 U/L. Abnormally increased levels of AST/SGOT are found in **hepatitis**, hepatic cirrhosis, drug-induced liver injury, hepatic metastasis, acute **pancreatitis**, hepatic necrosis, and hepatic infiltrative process (tumor).

small bowel follow-through	**Oral** administration of a radiopaque contrast medium, barium sulfate, which flows through the GI system. X-ray films are obtained at timed intervals to observe the progression of the barium through the small intestine.

Notable delays in the time for transit may occur with both malignant and benign forms of obstruction or diminished intestinal motility. In hyper-motility state, and in malabsorption, the flow of barium is much quicker. Small bowel tumors, obstructions, inflammatory disease, malabsorption syndrome, congenital defects, or perforation may be identified with a small bowel follow-through study.

stool analysis for occult blood (stool analysis for uh-**CULT** blood)	The analysis of a stool sample to determine the presence of blood not visible to the naked eye (i.e., hidden or occult blood).

A positive result of blood in the stool would indicate the need for a more thorough gastrointestinal examination. There is normally no occult blood in the stool. Benign and malignant tumors, inflammatory bowel disease, diverticulosis, and ulcers can cause occult blood.

stool culture (**STOOL KULL**-chir)	**Stool culture** involves collection of a stool specimen placed on one or more culture mediums and allowed to grow colonies of microorganisms to identify specific pathogen(s).

The collector of the specimen should be very careful not to mix the stool specimen with urine because it may inhibit the growth of the bacteria. Abnormal findings include parasitic enterocolitis, protozoan enterocolitis, and bacterial enterocolitis.

stool guaiac (**STOOL GWEE**-ak *or* **GWY**-ak)	**Stool guaiac** is a test on a stool specimen using guaiac as a reagent, which identifies the presence of blood in the stool.

Also called stool for occult blood or Hemoccult test. Abnormal findings that may cause blood to be identified in the stool include GI tumor, polyps, varices, inflammatory bowel disease, ulcer, GI trauma, ischemic bowel disease, **hemorrhoids**, gastritis, **esophagitis**, and diverticulosis. See *Figure 12-15*.

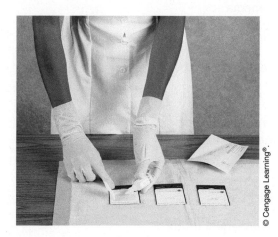

Figure 12-15 Hemoccult test

urinary bilirubin	A test performed on urine to check for conjugated or direct bilirubin in a urine specimen.
(**YOO**-rih-nair-ee bill-ih-**ROO**-bin)	
urin/o = urine	
-ary = pertaining to	

There should normally be no **bilirubin** in the urine. Presence of or increased levels of direct bilirubin found in the urine along with the other symptoms specific for the disorders following may be indicative of gallstones, extensive liver metastasis, or extrahepatic duct obstruction.

Review Checkpoint

Check your understanding of this section by completing the **Diagnostic Techniques, Treatments, and Procedures** exercises in your workbook.

COMMON ABBREVIATIONS

Abbreviation	Meaning	Abbreviation	Meaning
a.c.	before meals (ante cibum)	GI	gastrointestinal
ALT	alanine aminotransferase	GI series	gastrointestinal series
AST	aspartate aminotransferase (formerly called **serum glutamic-oxaloacetic transaminase [SGOT]**)	GTT	glucose tolerance test
		HAV	hepatitis A virus
		HBV	hepatitis B virus
Ba	barium	HCl	**hydrochloric acid**
BE	**barium enema**	HCV	hepatitis C virus
b.i.d.	twice a day	IBS	**irritable bowel syndrome**
CT SCAN	computed tomography (scan)	IVC	intravenous cholangiography
EGD	esophagogastroduodenoscopy	LES	lower esophageal sphincter (also known as the **cardiac sphincter**)
ERCP	**endoscopic retrograde cholangiopancreatography**		
		LFT	liver function test
GB	**gallbladder**	MRI	**magnetic resonance imaging**
GBS	gallbladder series	N&V	**nausea** and vomiting
GER	**gastroesophageal reflux**		
GERD	gastroesophageal reflux disease	NG	nasogastric

Abbreviation	Meaning	Abbreviation	Meaning
NPO, n.p.o.	nothing by mouth	SBS	small bowel series
OCG	oral cholecystogram	SGOT	**serum glutamic oxaloacetic transaminase**; now called aspartate aminotransferase (AST)
p.c.	after meals (post cibum)		
PP, pp	postprandial		
PPBS	postprandial blood sugar	SGPT	serum glutamic pyruvic transaminase
PPG	postprandial glucose		
PTC, PTHC	percutaneous transhepatic cholangiogram	TPN	total parenteral nutrition
		UGI series	upper gastrointestinal series
SBFT	small bowel follow-through		

Review Checkpoint

Check your understanding of this section by completing the **Common Abbreviations** exercises in your workbook.

WRITTEN AND AUDIO TERMINOLOGY REVIEW

Review each of the following terms from the chapter. Study the spelling of each term and write the definition in the space provided. Check definitions by looking the term up in the glossary.

Term	Pronunciation	Definition
abdominal ultrasound	☐ ab-**DOM**-ih-nal **ULL**-trah-sound	_____
abdominocentesis	☐ ab-**dom**-ih-noh-sen-**TEE**-sis	_____
absorption	☐ ab-**SORP**-shun	_____
achalasia	☐ **ack**-al-**LAY**-zee-ah	_____
achlorhydria	☐ **ah**-klor-**HIGH**-dree-ah	_____
aerophagia	☐ **ay**-er-oh-**FAY**-jee-ah	_____
alanine aminotransferase	☐ **AL**-ah-neen ah-mee-noh-**TRANS**-fer-ays	_____
alimentary canal	☐ **al**-ih-**MEN**-tar-ee can-**NAL**	_____
alkaline phosphatase (ALP)	☐ **AL**-kah-line **FOSS**-fah-tays	_____
amino acids	☐ ah-**MEE**-noh acids	_____

Term	Pronunciation	Definition
amylase	☐ **AM**-ih-lays	_____
anastomosis	☐ **ah**-nas-toh-**MOH**-sis	_____
anal fistula	☐ **AY**-nal **FISS**-tyoo-lah	_____
anorexia	☐ an-oh-**REK**-see-ah	_____
anus	☐ **AY**-nus	_____
aphagia	☐ ah-**FAY**-jee-ah	_____
aphthous stomatitis	☐ **AFF**-thus stoh-mah-**TYE**-tis	_____
appendectomy	☐ ap-en-**DEK**-toh-mee	_____
appendicitis	☐ ap-**pen**-dih-**SIGH**-tis	_____
ascites	☐ ah-**SIGH**-teez	_____
ascitic fluid	☐ ah-**SIT**-ik fluid	_____
atresia	☐ ah-**TREE**-zee-ah	_____
barium enema (BE)	☐ **BAH**-ree-um **EN**-eh-mah	_____
barium swallow	☐ **BAH**-ree-um swallow	_____
bicuspid tooth	☐ bye-**CUSS**-pid tooth	_____
bile	☐ **BYE**-al	_____
biliary	☐ **BILL**-ee-air-ee	_____
bilirubin	☐ bill-ih-**ROO**-bin	_____
bolus	☐ **BOH**-lus	_____
borborygmus	☐ **bor**-boh-**RIG**-mus	_____
bowel	☐ **BOW**-el	_____
buccal	☐ **BUCK**-al	_____
cachexia	☐ kah-**KEKS**-eeh-ah	_____
canine tooth	☐ **KAY**-nine tooth	_____
cardiac sphincter	☐ **CAR**-dee-ak **SFINGK**-ter	_____
cecostomy	☐ see-**KOSS**-tah-mee	_____
cecum	☐ **SEE**-kum	_____
celiac disease	☐ **SEE**-lee-ak dih-**ZEEZ**	_____
celiac rickets	☐ **SEE**-lee-ak **RICK**-ets	_____
cheiloplasty	☐ **KYE**-loh-**plas**-tee	_____
cheilosis	☐ kigh-**LOH**-sis	_____
cholecystectomy	☐ **koh**-lee-sis-**TEK**-toh-mee	_____
cholecystitis	☐ **koh**-lee-sis-**TYE**-tis	_____
cholecystogram	☐ **koh**-lee-**SIS**-toh-gram	_____
cholecystography	☐ **koh**-lee-sis-**TOG**-rah-fee	_____
cholelithiasis	☐ **koh**-lee-lih-**THIGH**-ah-sis	_____
chyme	☐ **KIGHM**	_____

Term	Pronunciation	Definition
cirrhosis	☐ sih-**ROH**-sis	_____
colon	☐ **COH**-lon	_____
colonoscopy	☐ **koh**-lon-**OSS**-koh-pee	_____
colorectal	☐ **koh**-loh-**REK**-tal	_____
colorectal cancer	☐ **koh**-loh-**REK**-tal **CAN**-sir	_____
colostomy	☐ koh-**LAHS**-toh-mee	_____
constipation	☐ **kon**-stih-**PAY**-shun	_____
Crohn's disease	☐ **KROHNZ** dih-**ZEEZ**	_____
CT of the abdomen	☐ **CT** of the **AB**-doh-men	_____
cuspid tooth	☐ **CUSS**-pid tooth	_____
deciduous teeth	☐ dee-**SID**-yoo-us teeth	_____
defecation	☐ deff-eh-**KAY**-shun	_____
deglutition	☐ **dee**-gloo-**TISH**-un	_____
dental caries	☐ **DEN**-tal **KAIR**-eez	_____
dentin	☐ **DEN**-tin	_____
diarrhea	☐ dye-ah-**REE**-ah	_____
digestive tract	☐ dye-**JESS**-tiv **TRAKT**	_____
diverticular disease	☐ **dye**-ver-**TIK**-yoo-lar dih-**ZEEZ**	_____
duodenal	☐ doo-**OD**-en-al	_____
duodenostomy	☐ **doo**-oh-den-**OSS**-toh-mee	_____
duodenum	☐ doo-**OD**-en-um _or_ doo-oh-**DEE**-num	_____
dysentery	☐ **DISS**-en-**ter**-ee	_____
dyspepsia	☐ dis-**PEP**-see-ah	_____
dysphagia	☐ dis-**FAY**-jee-ah	_____
emaciation	☐ ee-**may**-she-**AY**-shun	_____
emesis	☐ **EM**-eh-sis	_____
emulsify	☐ eh-**MULL**-sih-figh	_____
enamel	☐ en-**AM**-el	_____
endocrine gland	☐ **EN**-doh-krin gland	_____
endoscopic retrograde cholangiopancreatography (ERCP)	☐ en-doh-**SKOP**-ic **RET**-roh-grayd koh-**lan**-jee-oh-**pan**-kree-ah-**TOG**-rah-fee	_____
enteritis	☐ **en**-ter-**EYE**-tis	_____
enzyme	☐ **EN**-zighm	_____
eructation	☐ eh-ruk-**TAY**-shun	_____

Term	Pronunciation	Definition
esophageal varices	☐ eh-**soff**-ah-**JEE**-al **VAIR**-ih-seez	_____
esophagitis	☐ eh-soff-ah-**JIGH**-tis	_____
esophagogastroduodenos-copy	☐ eh-**sof**-ah-goh-**gas**-troh-**dew**-oh-deh-**NOS**-koh-pee	_____
esophagus	☐ eh-**SOFF**-ah-gus	_____
exocrine gland	☐ **EKS**-oh-krin gland	_____
extracorporeal shock wave lithotripsy (ESWL)	☐ **eks**-trah-kor-**POR**-ee-al shock wave **LITH**-oh-**trip**-see	_____
feces	☐ **FEE**-seez	_____
flatulence	☐ **FLAT**-yoo-lens	_____
flatus	☐ **FLAY**-tus	_____
fluoroscopy	☐ **floo**-or-**OS**-koh-pee	_____
gallbladder	☐ **GALL**-blad-er	_____
gastrectasia	☐ **gas**-trek-**TAY**-zhe-ah	_____
gastric	☐ **GAS**-trik	_____
gastroenterologist	☐ **gas**-troh-**en**-ter-**ALL**-oh-jist	_____
gastroesophageal reflux	☐ **gas**-troh-eh-**soff**-ah-**JEE**-al **REE**-flucks	_____
gastrointestinal tract	☐ **gas**-troh-in-**TESS**-tih-nal **TRAKT**	_____
gastrointestinal endoscopy	☐ **gas**-troh-in-**TESS**-tih-nal en-**DOSS**-koh-pee	_____
gastrorrhagia	☐ **gas**-troh-**RAY**-jee-ah	_____
gastrospasm	☐ **GAS**-troh-spazm	_____
gastrostomy	☐ gas-**TROSS**-toh-mee	_____
gavage	☐ gah-**VAZH**	_____
gingival	☐ **JIN**-jih-vah _or_ jin-**JYE**-vah	_____
gingivitis	☐ **jin**-jih-**VIGH**-tis	_____
gingivoplasty	☐ **JIN**-jih-voh-**plass**-tee	_____
glossitis	☐ gloss-**SIGH**-tis	_____
glucagon	☐ **GLOO**-kah-gon	_____
glucogenesis	☐ **gloo**-koh-**JEN**-eh-sis	_____
glucose	☐ **GLOO**-kohs	_____
glycogen	☐ **GLIGH**-koh-jen	_____
glycogenesis	☐ **gligh**-koh-**JEN**-eh-sis	_____
glycogenolysis	☐ **gligh**-koh-jen-**ALL**-ih-sis	_____
glycolysis	☐ gligh-**KALL**-ih-sis	_____
hematemesis	☐ **hee**-mah-**TEM**-eh-sis	_____
hemorrhoids	☐ **HEM**-oh-roydz	_____

Term	Pronunciation	Definition
hepatitis	☐ **hep**-ah-**TYE**-tis	_____
hepatocyte	☐ **hep**-**PAT**-oh-sight	_____
hepatomegaly	☐ **hep**-ah-toh-**MEG**-ah-lee	_____
hepatorrhaphy	☐ hep-ah-**TOR**-ah-fee	_____
hernia	☐ **HER**-nee-ah	_____
herniorrhaphy	☐ her-nee-**OR**-ah-fee	_____
herpetic stomatitis	☐ her-**PEH**-tic stoh-mah-**TYE**-tis	_____
Hirschsprung's disease	☐ **HIRSH**-sprungz dih-**ZEEZ**	_____
hydrochloric acid	☐ **high**-droh-**KLOH**-rik acid	_____
icterus	☐ **ICK**-ter-us	_____
ileocecal	☐ **ill**-ee-oh-**SEE**-kahl	_____
ileum	☐ **ILL**-ee-um	_____
ileus	☐ **ILL**-ee-us	_____
incisor	☐ in-**SIGH**-zor	_____
insulin	☐ **IN**-soo-lin	_____
intestinal obstruction	☐ in-**TESS**-tih-nal ob-**STRUCK**-shun	_____
intussusception	☐ **in**-tuh-suh-**SEP**-shun	_____
irritable bowel syndrome (IBS)	☐ **EAR**-ih-tah-bul **BOW**-el **SIN**-drom	_____
jaundice	☐ **JAWN**-diss	_____
jejunostomy	☐ **jee**-joo-**NOSS**-toh-mee	_____
jejunum	☐ jee-**JOO**-num	_____
laparoscopy	☐ **lap**-ar-**OSS**-koh-pee	_____
lingual	☐ **LING**-gwall	_____
lipase	☐ **LIH**-pays or **LIGH**-pays	_____
lipolysis	☐ lip-**ALL**-ih-sis	_____
lipoma	☐ lih-**POH**-mah	_____
lithogenesis	☐ **lith**-oh-**JEN**-eh-sis	_____
lithotripsy	☐ **LITH**-oh-**trip**-see	_____
liver biopsy	☐ **LIV**-er **BYE**-op-see	_____
liver scan	☐ **LIV**-er **SCAN**	_____
magnetic resonance imaging (MRI)	☐ mag-**NEH**-tic **REZ**-oh-nans **IM**-ij-ing	_____
mandibular	☐ man-**DIB**-yoo-lar	_____
mastication	☐ mas-tih-**KAY**-shun	_____
melena	☐ **MELL**-eh-nah	_____
molar tooth	☐ **MOH**-lar tooth	_____

Term	Pronunciation	Definition
nasogastric intubation	☐ nay-zoh-**GAS**-trik **in**-too-**BAY**-shun	_____
nausea	☐ **NAW**-zee-ah	_____
nutritionist	☐ noo-**TRIH**-shun-ist	_____
oral	☐ **OR**-al	_____
oral leukoplakia	☐ **OR**-al **loo**-koh-**PLAY**-kee-ah	_____
oropharynx	☐ **or**-oh-**FAIR**-inks	_____
orthodontist	☐ **or**-thoh-**DON**-tist	_____
palatoplasty	☐ **PAL**-ah-toh-**plas**-tee	_____
pancreas	☐ **PAN**-kree-as	_____
pancreatitis	☐ **pan**-kree-ah-**TYE**-tis	_____
papillae	☐ pah-**PILL**-ay	_____
paracentesis	☐ **pair**-ah-sen-**TEE**-sis	_____
parotid gland	☐ pah-**ROT**-id gland	_____
peptic ulcers	☐ **PEP**-tik **ULL**-sirz	_____
percutaneous transhepatic cholangiography (PTC)	☐ **per**-kyoo-**TAY**-nee-us trans-heh-**PAT**-ik koh-**lan**-jee-**OG**-rah-fee	_____
periodontal disease	☐ pair-ee-oh-**DON**-tal dih-**ZEEZ**	_____
peristalsis	☐ pair-ih-**STALL**-sis	_____
peritoneum	☐ **pair**-ih-toh-**NEE**-um	_____
pharyngoscope	☐ fair-**IN**-goh-skohp	_____
pharynx	☐ **FAIR**-inks	_____
polyphagia	☐ **pall**-ee-**FAY**-jee-ah	_____
proctoscopy	☐ prok-**TOSS**-koh-pee	_____
pruritus ani	☐ proo-**RIGH**-tus **AN**-eye	_____
pyloric sphincter	☐ pye-**LOR**-ik **SFINGK**-ter	_____
rectocele	☐ **REK**-toh-seel	_____
rectum	☐ **REK**-tum	_____
rugae	☐ **ROO**-gay	_____
saliva	☐ sah-**LYE**-vah	_____
salivary glands	☐ **SAL**-ih-vair-ee glands	_____
serum bilirubin	☐ **SEE**-rum bill-ih-**ROO**-bin	_____
serum glutamic-oxaloacetic transaminase (SGOT)	☐ **SEE**-rum gloo-**TAM**-ik **oks**-ah-loh-ah-**SEE**-tik trans-**AM**-in-ays	_____
sialogram	☐ sigh-**AL**-oh-gram	_____
sigmoid colon	☐ **SIG**-moyd colon	_____

Term	Pronunciation	Definition
sigmoidoscopy	☐ **sig**-moyd-**OSS**-koh-pee	_____
spastic colon	☐ **SPAS**-tik **COH**-lon	_____
sphincter	☐ **SFINGK**-ter	_____
steatorrhea	☐ **stee**-ah-toh-**REE**-ah	_____
stomach	☐ **STUM**-ak	_____
stomatitis	☐ stoh-mah-**TYE**-tis	_____
stomatoplasty	☐ **STOH**-mah-toh-**plass**-tee	_____
stool culture	☐ **STOOL KULL**-chir	_____
stool guaiac	☐ **STOOL GWEE**-ak *or* **GWY**-ak	_____
thrush	☐ **THRUSH**	_____
triglycerides	☐ try-**GLISS**-er-eyeds	_____
ulcerative colitis	☐ **ULL**-sir-ah-tiv koh-**LYE**-tis	_____
urinary bilirubin	☐ **YOO**-rih-nair-ee bill-ih-**ROO**-bin	_____
uvula	☐ **YOO**-vyoo-lah	_____
villi	☐ **VIL**-eye	_____
volvulus	☐ **VOL**-vyoo-lus	_____
vomit	☐ **VOM**-it	_____
vomitus	☐ **VOM**-ih-tus	_____
xerostomia	☐ **zeer**-oh-**STOH**-mee-ah	_____

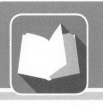

Review Checkpoint

Apply what you have learned in this chapter by completing the **Putting It All Together** exercise in your workbook.

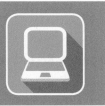

Online Resources

For additional study tools, including PowerPoint® slides and animations, go to the Student Companion Website.

Chapter Review Exercises

The following exercises provide a more in-depth review of the chapter material. Your goal in these exercises is to complete each section at a minimum 80% level of accuracy. A place has been provided for your score at the end of each section.

A. Crossword Puzzle

Read the clues carefully and complete the puzzle. Each crossword answer is worth 10 points. When you have completed the crossword puzzle, total your points and enter your score in the space provided at the end of the exercise.

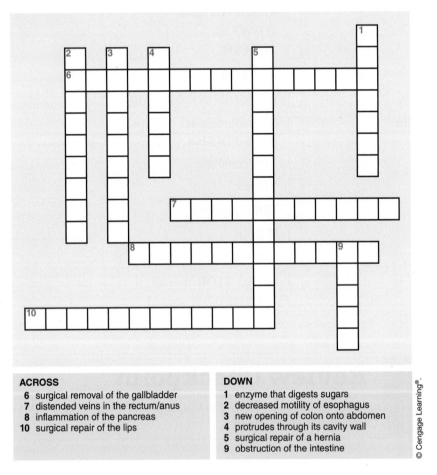

ACROSS
6 surgical removal of the gallbladder
7 distended veins in the rectum/anus
8 inflammation of the pancreas
10 surgical repair of the lips

DOWN
1 enzyme that digests sugars
2 decreased motility of esophagus
3 new opening of colon onto abdomen
4 protrudes through its cavity wall
5 surgical repair of a hernia
9 obstruction of the intestine

© Cengage Learning®.

Number correct _____ *× 10 points/correct answer: Your score* _____ *%*

B. Spelling

Circle the correctly spelled term in each pairing of words. Each correct answer is worth 10 points. Record your score in the space provided at the end of the exercise.

1. chyme   chime
2. decidious   deciduous
3. defication   defecation
6. peristaltsis   peristalsis
7. sphincter   spincter
8. uvula   uvala

4.	gavage	gevage	9. pharynx	pharynix
5.	jejenum	jejunum	10. lipase	lypase

Number correct _____ **× 10 points/correct answer: Your score** _____ **%**

C. Term to Definition

Define each diagnosis or procedure listed by writing the definition in the space provided. Check the box if you are able to complete this exercise correctly the first time (without referring to the answers). Each correct answer is worth 10 points. Record your score in the space provided at the end of the exercise.

☐ 1. dental caries _____

☐ 2. herpetic stomatitis _____

☐ 3. cirrhosis _____

☐ 4. intussusception _____

☐ 5. paracentesis _____

☐ 6. gastric analysis _____

☐ 7. small bowel follow-through _____

☐ 8. irritable bowel syndrome _____

☐ 9. ERCP _____

☐ 10. oral leukoplakia _____

Number correct _____ **× 10 points/correct answer: Your score** _____ **%**

D. Matching Pathological Conditions

Match the definitions on the right with the appropriate pathological condition on the left. Each correct answer is worth 10 points. Record your score in the space provided at the end of the exercise.

_____ 1. cholelithiasis

_____ 2. aphthous stomatitis

_____ 3. periodontal disease

_____ 4. celiac disease

_____ 5. achalasia

_____ 6. dysentery

_____ 7. hepatitis

_____ 8. Hirschsprung's disease

_____ 9. peptic ulcer

_____ 10. volvulus

a. a term used to describe a group of inflammatory gum disorders that may lead to degeneration of teeth, gums, and sometimes surrounding bones

b. nutrient malabsorption due to damaged small-bowel mucosa because of gluten sensitivity

c. a rotation of loops of bowel causing a twisting on itself, which results in an intestinal obstruction

d. pigmented or hardened cholesterol stones formed as a result of bile crystallization

e. acute or chronic inflammation of the liver due to a viral or bacterial infection, drugs, alcohol, toxins, or parasites

f. absence at birth of the autonomic ganglia in a segment of the intestinal smooth muscle wall that normally stimulates peristalsis

g. a term used to describe painful intestinal inflammation typically caused by ingesting water or food containing bacteria, protozoa, parasites, or chemical irritants

(continued)

h. small, inflammatory, noninfectious, ulcerated lesions occurring on the lips, tongue, and inside the cheeks of the mouth; also called canker sores

i. decreased mobility of the lower two-thirds of the esophagus along with constriction of the lower esophageal sphincter

j. a break in the continuity of the mucous membrane lining of the GI tract as a result of hyperacidity and/or the *Helicobacter pylori* bacterium

Number correct _____ × *10 points/correct answer: Your score* _____ *%*

E. Definition to Term

Using the following definitions, identify and provide the medical term to match the definition. Each correct answer is worth 10 points. Record your score in the space provided at the end of the exercise.

1. Complete or partial alteration in the forward flow of the content in the small or large intestines:

   _____

2. Noninflamed outpouchings or herniations through the muscular layer of the intestine, typically the sigmoid colon:

   _____

3. Inflammatory infectious lesions in or on the oral cavity occurring as a primary or a secondary viral infection caused by herpes simplex:

   _____

4. An abnormal passageway in the skin surface near the anus usually connecting with the rectum:

   _____

5. Digestive tract inflammation of a chronic nature causing fever, cramping, diarrhea, weight loss, and anorexia:

   _____

6. The presence of small growths projecting from the mucous membrane of the colon or rectum:

   _____

7. The presence of a malignant neoplasm in the large intestine:

   _____

8. An expression used to characterize both diverticulosis and diverticulitis:

   _____

9. Swollen, extended veins located in the esophagus at the distal end in a winding structure. Usually caused by portal hypertension, which occurs as a result of liver disease:

   _____

10. Absence at birth of the autonomic ganglia in a segment of the intestinal smooth muscle wall that normally stimulates peristalsis:

    _____

Number correct _____ × *10 points/correct answer: Your score* _____ *%*

F. Word Search

Read each definition carefully and identify the applicable word from the list that follows. Enter the word in the space provided and then find it in the puzzle and circle it. The words may be read up, down, diagonally, across, or backward. Each correct answer is worth 10 points. Record your score in the space provided at the end of the exercise.

cirrhosis	colostomy	hernia
hemorrhoid	hepatitis	pancreatitis
abdominocentesis	urinary bilirubin	thrush
intussusception	gastric analysis	

Example: A test for conjugated or direct bilirubin in a urine specimen:

urinary bilirubin _____

1. An unnaturally distended or swollen vein (called a varicosity) in the distal rectum or anus:

    _____

2. Acute or chronic inflammation of the liver due to a viral or bacterial infection, drugs, alcohol, toxins, or parasites:

    _____

3. An irregular protrusion of tissue, organ, or a portion of an organ through an abnormal break in the enveloping cavity's muscular wall:

    _____

4. Surgical creation of an artificial abdominal-wall anus by bringing the incised colon out to the abdominal surface:

    _____

5. Study of the stomach content to determine the acid content and to detect the presence of blood, bacteria, bile, and abnormal cells:

    _____

6. Insertion of a needle or trocar into the peritoneal cavity to remove ascitic fluid with the person in a sitting position:

    _____

7. A disease of the liver that is chronic and degenerative causing injury to the hepatocytes:

    _____

8. Telescoping of a portion of proximal intestine into distal intestine, usually in the ileocecal region, causing an obstruction:

    _____

9. A fungal infection in the mouth and throat, producing sore, pale yellow, slightly raised lesions or patches:

    _____

10. An acute or chronic destructive inflammatory condition of the pancreas:

    _____

(continued)

U	L	E	X	I	O	N	O	A	T	T	S	I	S	L
R	O	I	R	E	T	S	O	P	O	R	E	T	N	A
I	A	D	Y	A	H	U	T	E	A	A	G	R	Y	S
N	O	I	T	P	E	C	S	U	S	S	U	T	N	I
A	S	O	I	R	P	I	I	L	E	I	I	H	A	S
R	I	H	Y	O	A	T	H	R	U	S	H	P	D	Y
Y	T	R	D	E	T	H	I	M	B	E	I	A	I	L
B	I	R	E	U	I	O	E	X	R	T	N	R	O	A
I	V	O	C	V	T	N	G	N	T	N	P	G	P	N
L	N	M	C	I	I	N	I	I	I	E	N	O	A	A
R	C	H	O	L	Y	M	A	J	I	O	V	D	U	I
U	S	I	T	I	T	A	E	R	C	N	A	P	E	R
B	U	I	A	I	A	S	R	M	L	I	S	R	P	T
I	J	O	L	S	Y	H	S	H	C	M	S	Y	A	S
N	N	N	U	C	O	L	O	S	T	O	M	Y	R	A
S	O	O	S	S	R	S	L	F	D	E	P	X	G
P	C	A	I	M	I	G	A	I	U	B	H	P	Y	A
T	Q	S	D	A	R	E	P	Y	M	A	K	L	T	R

© Cengage Learning®.

***Number correct* _____ × *10 points/correct answer: Your score* _____ %**

G. Matching Abbreviations

Match the abbreviations on the left with the correct definition on the right. Each correct answer is worth 5 points. Record your score in the space provided at the end of the exercise.

_____ 1. a.c. a. total parenteral nutrition

_____ 2. BE b. small-bowel series

_____ 3. GBS c. postprandial

_____ 4. GERD d. percutaneous transhepatic cholangiogram

_____ 5. GTT e. after meals

_____ 6. IBS f. nasogastric

_____ 7. LES g. interbowel sphincter

_____ 8. NG h. nausea and vomiting

_____ 9. PTC i. magnetic resonance imaging

_____ 10. pp j. liver function tests

_____ 11. MRI k. motionless rugae internicus

_____ 12. IVC l. intravenous colostomy

_____ 13. GI   m. irritable bowel syndrome
_____ 14. HBV   n. intravenous cholangiography
_____ 15. HCl   o. before meals
_____ 16. LFTs   p. hepatitis B virus
_____ 17. N&V   q. hydrochloric acid
_____ 18. p.c.   r. barium enema
_____ 19. SBS   s. gallbladder series
_____ 20. TPN   t. gastroesophageal reflux disease
                                      u. gastrointestinal
                                      v. glucose tolerance test
                                      w. gastric endoscopic retrograde dissection
                                      x. neck and vein
                                      y. lower esophageal sphincter

Number correct _____ **× 5 points/correct answer: Your score** _____ **%**

H. Identify the Structures

Identify the structures of the oral cavity by writing your answers in the spaces provided. Each correct response is worth 10 points. Record your score in the space provided at the end of the exercise.

1. _____
2. _____
3. _____
4. _____
5. _____
6. _____
7. _____
8. _____
9. _____
10. _____

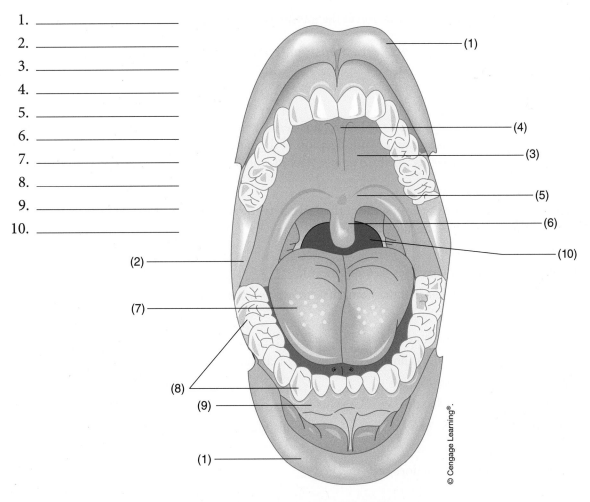

© Cengage Learning®.

Number correct _____ **× 10 points/correct answer: Your score** _____ **%**

I. Completion

The following sentences relate to the digestive system. Complete each sentence with the most appropriate word. Each correct answer is worth 10 points. Record your score in the space provided at the end of the exercise.

1. An abnormal condition characterized by the absence of hydrochloric acid in the gastric juice is known as _____.

2. A yellow discoloration of the skin, mucous membranes, and sclera of the eyes caused by greater than normal amounts of bilirubin in the blood is known as jaundice or _____.

3. The material expelled from the stomach during vomiting is known as vomitus or _____.

4. An abnormal accumulation of fluid within the peritoneal cavity (the fluid contains large amounts of protein and electrolytes) is known as _____.

5. An unpleasant sensation (often leading to the urge to vomit) is known as _____.

6. Decreased mobility of the lower two-thirds of the esophagus along with constriction of the lower esophageal sphincter is called _____.

7. A condition known as aphthous stomatitis (in which there are small, inflammatory, noninfectious, ulcerated lesions occurring on the lips, tongue, and inside the cheeks of the mouth) is called _____ _____ (two words).

8. Greater than normal amounts of fat in the feces (characterized by frothy, foul-smelling fecal matter that floats) is known as _____.

9. A permanently distended vein, called a varicosity, in the distal rectum or anus is known as a _____.

10. A term used to describe an obstruction of the intestine is _____.

Number correct _____ × 10 points/correct answer. Your score _____ %

J. True or False

Read each statement carefully and circle the correct answer as true or false. **HINT**: Pay close attention to the word elements written in bold as you make your decision. If the statement is false, identify the meaning of that word element. Each correct answer is worth 10 points. Record your score in the space provided at the end of the exercise.

1. Insertion of a needle or trocar into the peritoneal cavity to remove excess fluid, with the person in a sitting position, is known as an abdomino**centesis**.

    True   False

    If your answer is false, what does -*centesis* mean? _____

2. Surgically correcting a defect of the stomach is known as a **cheil**oplasty.

    True   False

    If your answer is false, what does *cheil/o* mean? _____

3. The surgical removal of the gallbladder is known as a **chol**ecystectomy.

    True   False

    If your answer is false, what does *chol/e* mean? _____

4. The surgical creation of a new opening into the gallbladder is known as a **col**ostomy.

    True   False

    If your answer is false, what does *col/o* mean? _____

5. The surgical removal of a hernia is known as a hernio**rrhaphy**.

   True   False

   If your answer is false, what does -**rrhaphy** mean? _____

6. The term **gingiv**ae is another name for the gums.

   True   False

   If your answer is false, what does **gingiv/o** mean? _____

7. The conversion of simple sugar (glucose) into a complex form of sugar (starch) for storage in the liver is known as glycogeno**lysis**.

   True   False

   If your answer is false, what does -**lysis** mean? _____

8. A backflow of content of the duodenum into the esophagus is known as **gastr**oesophageal reflux.

   True   False

   If your answer is false, what does **gastr/o** mean? _____

9. A condition characterized by the loss of the ability to swallow as a result of organic or psychologic causes is known as a**phag**ia.

   True   False

   If your answer is false, what does **phag/o** mean? _____

10. The frequent passage of loose, watery stools is known as dia**rrhea**.

   True   False

   If your answer is false, what does -**rrhea** mean? _____

Number correct _____ **× 10 points/correct answer: Your score** _____ **%**

K. Medical Scenario

The following medical scenario presents information on one of the pathological conditions discussed in this chapter. Read the scenario carefully and select the most appropriate answer for each question that follows. Each correct answer is worth 20 points. Record your score in the space provided at the end of the exercise.

Sam Smith is a 48-year-old firefighter and a patient of gastroenterologist Dr. Dreke. Sam has been bothered with heartburn and abdominal discomfort for years, thinking that it was just part of the job and his irregular eating patterns. He has recently been experiencing nausea and vomiting accompanied by a bloating feeling after eating and continuous, gnawing, epigastric pain. Sam had an appointment with Dr. Dreke this morning. While he was checking out, Sam asked the health care professional numerous questions about Dr. Dreke's suggestion that he may have a peptic ulcer.

1. The health care professional will base her responses to Mr. Smith's questions about peptic ulcers on which of the following facts? A peptic ulcer is a(n):

   a. inflammatory disease of the digestive tract resulting in a tender, distended abdomen with extreme swelling of the bowel walls

   b. fungal infection producing sore, creamy white, slightly raised curd-like patches on the mucosa of the gastrointestinal tract

   c. chronic inflammatory disease of the liver due to viral or bacterial infection, drugs, alcohol, toxins, or parasites

   d. break in the continuity of the mucous membrane lining of the gastrointestinal tract

(continued)

2. Mr. Smith is very curious about what can cause a peptic ulcer. The health care professional responds that a peptic ulcer occurs as a result of hyperacidity or the pathogen:

   a. *Candida albicans*

   b. *Staphylococcus aureus*

   c. *Helicobacter pylori*

   d. *Mycobacterium tuberculosis*

3. Mr. Smith is scheduled for an esophagogastroduodenoscopy next Tuesday. He asks the health care professional to explain this diagnostic procedure. The best response from the health care professional would be that an esophagogastroduodenoscopy, or upper endoscopy:

   a. visualizes the gallbladder through X-ray following the oral ingestion of pills containing a radiopaque iodinated dye

   b. is the surgical creation of a new opening on the abdominal wall through which the feces will be expelled

   c. is the irrigation, or washing out, of the stomach, with saline or sterile water

   d. involves direct visualization of the esophagus, stomach, and duodenum

4. When Mr. Smith asks the health care professional about confirming the diagnosis of a peptic ulcer, the health care professional's best response would be that the diagnosis is based on the endoscopy along with the:

   a. client's history and upper GI barium studies

   b. cholecystography and colonoscopy

   c. percutaneous transhepatic cholangiography and stool culture

   d. serum bilirubin and liver scan

5. The health care professional reviews with Mr. Smith the treatment for peptic ulcers. She includes that the treatment is based on the cause and includes antacids, frequent small meals, and medications. Examples of these are medications to:

   a. increase pancreatic enzymes and antibiotics to eradicate the organism

   b. eradicate the fungus and provide for pain relief

   c. decrease hyperacidity and antibiotics to eradicate the bacteria

   d. reduce inflammation such as an anti-inflammatory and corticosteroids

Number correct _____ × *20 points/correct answer: Your score* _____ %

L. Follow That Bite

The following completion exercise follows the passage of food through the alimentary canal during the digestive process. As you read the discussion, complete the blank spaces with the most appropriate word. Each correct response is worth 10 points. When you have completed the exercise, record your score in the space provided at the end of the exercise.

When food enters the mouth the, physical process of chewing, known as (1) _____, occurs when the teeth cut and grind the food. The salivary glands, found in the mouth, lubricate the food as it is chewed. During the process of chewing the food, the tongue aids the digestive process by moving the food around to mix it with saliva, shaping it into a ball-like mass called a (2) _____ and moving it toward the throat (pharynx) to be swallowed. The process of swallowing is known as (3) _____.

During the act of swallowing, the soft palate and the uvula move upward to facilitate the movement of the food into the pharynx and to close off the nasal cavity. The tongue forces the food into the pharynx, and the epiglottis drops downward to cover the opening of the larynx, directing the food mass into the esophagus. The bolus of food is propelled through the pharynx into the esophagus by means of wave-like movements called (4) _____. The esophagus receives the food from the pharynx and propels it on to the stomach. When the lower esophageal sphincter (LES) relaxes, it opens to allow food to enter the (5) _____ . When the LES contracts and closes, it prevents the stomach contents from reentering the esophagus. The stomach secretes gastric juices, which further the digestive process through the chemical breakdown of food. The muscular action of the stomach causes churning, which mixes the food with the secretions. At this point in the digestive process, the liquid-like mixture of partially digested food and digestive secretions in the stomach is called (6) _____. The pyloric sphincter releases this mixture into the small intestine.

The small intestine completes the digestive process through absorption of (7)_____ into the bloodstream and passage of the residue (waste products) on to the large intestine for excretion from the body. As the digested food continues its passage through the large intestine, it moves through the ileocecal sphincter, which prevents the backflow of wastes from the large intestine into the small intestine. As the chyme moves through the large intestine, the process of (8)_____ of water and electrolytes takes place. The remaining solid waste products of digestion, known as (9)_____, are eliminated from the body through the anus. The act of expelling feces from the body is known as (10)_____.

Number correct _____ × *10 points/correct answer: Your score* _____ %

M. Proofreading Skills

Read the following Request for Consultation. For each bold term, provide a brief definition and indicate if the term is spelled correctly. If it is misspelled, provide the correct spelling. Each correct answer is worth 10 points. Record your score in the space provided at the end of the exercise.

Example:

hepatosplenomegaly *enlargement of the liver and the spleen* _____

Spelled correctly? ☑ Yes ☐ No _____

REQUEST FOR CONSULTATION

Hillcrest medical center

PATIENT NAME: Janice McClure

PATIENT ID: 11049

CONSULTANT
Bernard Kester, MD, Surgical Services

REQUESTING PHYSICIAN
Kenneth Shaker, MD, Primary Care Physician

DATE
3-12-2014

(*continued*)

REQUEST FOR CONSULTATION
Patient: Janice McClure
Patient ID: 11049
Date of Consult: 03/12/14
Page 2

REASON FOR CONSULTATION
Please evaluate acute abdominal pain for possible surgical intervention.

I am asked to see this 62-year-old Caucasian female who was admitted with abdominal pain, **nausia**, and vomiting. No **melena** or **hematemisis**. Pain is in the right epigastrium and right upper quadrant. She has a prior history of similar bouts but not as bad. She was evaluated in the ER, and an obstruction series and sonogram were ordered by her PCP, Dr. Shaker. X-rays showed calcification in the right upper quadrant consistent with **cholelithiasis**. She had a low-grade fever and some chills. No apparent **jaundiss**. She had a uterine and bladder suspension in 1992. She is multiparous. She had an **appendectomy** at the age of 18. No history of **pancreatitis**, alcohol abuse, ulcers, liver disease, or **hepetitis**.

PHYSICAL EXAMINATION
Physical examination reveals a woman who appears her stated age. She appears to be in considerable discomfort. Temperature 99 degrees Fahrenheit. No apparent jaundice. Neck is normal. Abdomen shows tenderness and guarding in the epigastrium and right upper quadrant. No other mass, **hepatosplenomegaly**, or hernias noted. Pelvic and rectal unremarkable.

DIAGNOSTIC DATA
White blood cell count 10.1 with 79% segs. PTT is normal. SMA shows elevated bilirubin at 1.54 with alkaline phosphatase at 442. Sonography reveals multiple gallstones with a stone in the common bile duct. These were reviewed by Dr. Singh, radiologist. Chest x-ray was unremarkable.

IMPRESSION
Cholelithiasis, **choledoctolithiasis**, and early obstructive jaundice.

RECOMMENDATION
This patient is currently n.p.o. on IV fluids and antibiotics. She had initially shown interest in laparoscopic **cholecystecktomy**; however, in view of her common duct stone, I talked with the patient and her family at length. The options are (1) ERCP followed by laparoscopic cholecystectomy and (2) open cholecystectomy with common duct exploration.

It appears that with the weekend approaching, the ERCP may not be available until next week. The patient is at risk for pancreatitis and/or sepsis in the meantime. The patient is unwilling to wait, and she is in favor of open surgery as soon as possible. We plan to do the procedure later today. The nature of the surgery and the possible complications and problems, including stone recurrence, were explained to the patient and her family. Consent for open surgery was obtained.

Thank you for allowing me to share in the care of this patient.

Bernard Kester, MD

BK:BJ

D:03/12/14

T:03/14/14

1. **nausia** _____

_____

Spelled Correctly? ☐ Yes ☐ No _____

2. **melena** _____

_____

Spelled Correctly? ☐ Yes ☐ No _____

3. **hematemisis** _____

_____

Spelled Correctly? ☐ Yes ☐ No _____

4. **cholelithiasis** _____

_____

Spelled Correctly? ☐ Yes ☐ No _____

5. **jaundiss** _____

_____

Spelled Correctly? ☐ Yes ☐ No _____

6. **appendectomy** _____

_____

Spelled Correctly? ☐ Yes ☐ No _____

7. **pancreatitis** _____

_____

Spelled Correctly? ☐ Yes ☐ No _____

8. **hepetitis** _____

_____

Spelled Correctly? ☐ Yes ☐ No _____

9. **choledoctolithiasis** _____

_____

Spelled Correctly? ☐ Yes ☐ No _____

10. **cholecystecktomy** _____

_____

Spelled Correctly? ☐ Yes ☐ No _____

Number correct _____ × *10 points/correct answer: Your score* _____ *%*

The Endocrine System

CHAPTER CONTENT

OBJECTIVES

Upon completing this chapter and the review exercises at the end of the chapter, the learner should be able to:

1. Define diabetes mellitus, gestational diabetes, and diabetes insipidus, and identify the differences among the three conditions.

2. List the nine endocrine glands identified in this chapter.

3. Identify and define at least 20 pathological conditions of the endocrine system.

4. Correctly spell and pronounce terms listed on the Written and Audio Terminology Review, using the phonetic pronunciations provided.

5. Create at least 10 medical terms related to the endocrine system, and identify the correct combining form for each word.

6. Identify and define at least 10 abbreviations common to the endocrine system.

7. Identify and define at least 10 hormones secreted by the endocrine glands and the gland that secretes each of the hormones.

8. Identify and define at least 20 medical terms defined in the vocabulary section of this chapter.

Overview

The endocrine system consists of a network of ductless glands that secrete chemicals (called hormones) that affect the function of specific organs within the body, thus regulating many of the intricate functions of the body itself. These ductless glands secrete their hormones directly into the bloodstream as opposed to releasing them externally through ducts (as do the sweat glands and the oil glands).

The field of medicine that deals with the study of the endocrine system and the treatment of the diseases and disorders of the endocrine system is known as **endocrinology**. The physician who specializes in the medical practice of **endocrinology** is known as an **endocrinologist**.

This chapter concentrates on the following endocrine glands: the pituitary, pineal, **thyroid**, parathyroid, thymus, adrenal, pancreas, ovaries, and testes. The discussion of each gland will begin with an anatomical description followed by the physiology, or function, of that particular gland and the hormone(s) it secretes.

Anatomy and Physiology

Refer to *Figure 13-1* for a full body view of the endocrine glands discussed (as well as other body organs) to help identify the location of the glands in the body.

Pituitary Gland

The pituitary gland is a pea-sized gland of minute weight but important responsibility—so much so that it is often referred to as the "master gland." It secretes hormones that control the functions of other glands. It is located beneath the brain in the pituitary fossa (depression) of the sphenoid bone, which is behind and slightly above the nose and throat. Also known as the **hypophysis**, the pituitary gland is connected to the hypothalamus of the brain by a stalklike projection call the **infundibulum**. Although the pituitary gland appears as one gland, it has two distinct lobes: the anterior pituitary gland and the posterior pituitary gland, each with very different functions. *Figure 13-2* shows the pituitary gland.

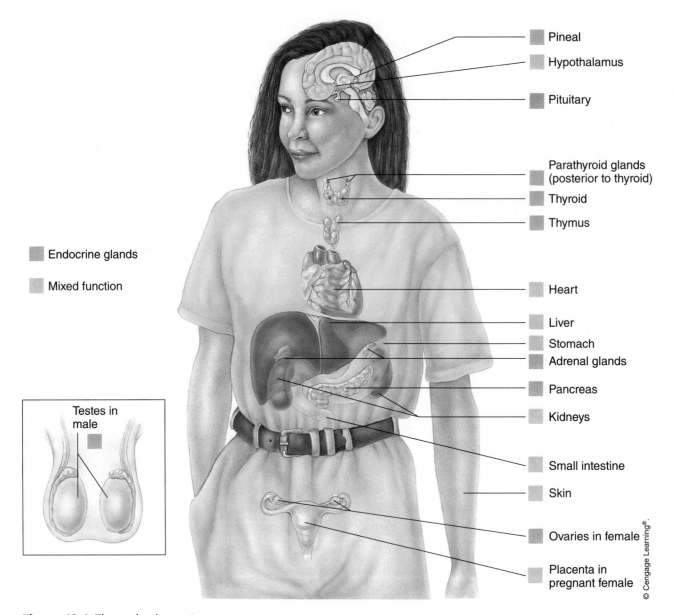

Endocrine glands

Mixed function

Pineal
Hypothalamus
Pituitary

Parathyroid glands
(posterior to thyroid)
Thyroid
Thymus

Heart

Liver
Stomach
Adrenal glands

Pancreas

Kidneys

Small intestine

Skin

Ovaries in female

Placenta in
pregnant female

Testes in
male

© Cengage Learning®.

Figure 13-1 The endocrine system

The **anterior pituitary gland**, also known as the **adenohypophysis**, develops from an upward projection of the pharynx in the embryo and is composed of regular endocrine tissue. The anterior pituitary gland secretes the following hormones:

1. **Growth hormone (GH)**, also known as **somatotropic hormone (STH)**, regulates the growth of bone, muscle, and other body tissues.

2. **Adrenocorticotropic hormone (ACTH)** stimulates the normal growth and development of the adrenal cortex and the secretion of corticosteroids (primarily **cortisol**, corticosterone, and **aldosterone**).

3. **Thyroid-stimulating hormone (TSH)** promotes and maintains the normal growth and development of the **thyroid** gland and stimulates the secretions of the **thyroid** hormones.

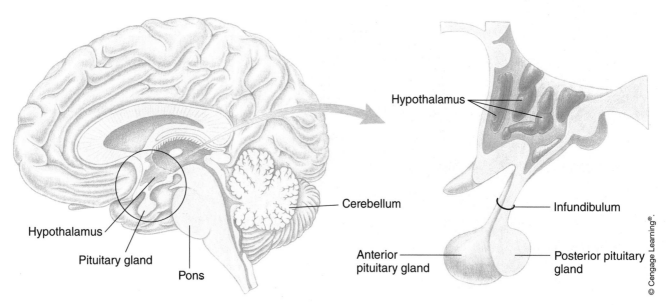

Figure 13-2 Pituitary gland

4. **Lactogenic hormone (LTH)**, also known as **prolactin**, promotes the development of the breasts during pregnancy and stimulates the secretion of milk from the breasts after delivery of the baby.

5. **Follicle-stimulating hormone (FSH)** stimulates the secretion of **estrogen** and the production of eggs (ova) in the female ovaries; also stimulates the production of sperm in the male testes.

6. **Luteinizing hormone (LH)** stimulates female ovulation and the secretion of testosterone (male sex hormone) in the male.

7. **Melanocyte-stimulating hormone (MSH)** controls the intensity of pigmentation in pigmented cells of the skin.

The **posterior pituitary gland**, also known as the **neurohypophysis**, develops from a downward projection of the base of the brain. The posterior pituitary gland stores and releases the following hormones:

1. **Antidiuretic hormone (ADH)**, also called **vasopressin**, decreases the excretion of large amounts of urine from the body by increasing the reabsorption of water by the renal tubules (thus helping maintain the body's water balance).

2. **Oxytocin (OT)** stimulates the contractions of the uterus during childbirth and stimulates the release of milk from the breasts of lactating women (women who breastfeed) in response to the suckling reflex of the infant.

Pineal Gland

The pineal gland is a tiny, pine cone–shaped gland located on the dorsal aspect of the midbrain region. See *Figure 13-3*.

Its exact function is not completely known, but the pineal gland does seem to play a part in supporting the body's "biological clock," that is, the regulation of our patterns of eating, sleeping, and reproduction. The pineal gland is responsible for secreting the hormone, **melatonin**, which is thought to induce sleep.

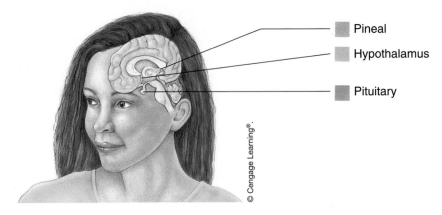

Figure 13-3 Pineal gland

Thyroid Gland

The **thyroid** gland is located in the front of the neck just below the larynx, on either side of the trachea. It consists of a right and left lobe connected across the front of the trachea by a narrow, island-shaped piece called the isthmus. Refer to *Figure 13-4* for a visual reference.

The **thyroid** gland secretes the following hormones:

1. **Triiodothyronine (T_3)** helps regulate growth and development of the body and control **metabolism** and body temperature.

2. **Thyroxine (T_4)** helps maintain normal body **metabolism**.

3. **Calcitonin** regulates the level of calcium in the blood.

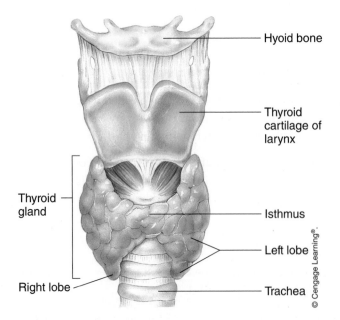

Figure 13-4 Thyroid gland

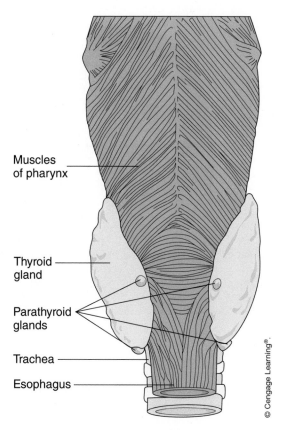

Muscles
of pharynx

Thyroid
gland

Parathyroid
glands

Trachea

Esophagus

© Cengage Learning®.

Figure 13-5 Parathyroid glands

Parathyroid Glands

The parathyroid glands consist of four tiny rounded bodies located on the dorsal aspect of the **thyroid** gland. See *Figure 13-5*.

The parathyroid glands are responsible for secreting the **parathyroid hormone (PTH)**, also known as **parathormone**, which regulates the level of calcium in the blood. Calcium is stored in the bones. If the blood calcium level falls too low (**hypocalcemia**), the parathyroid glands are triggered to secrete more PTH, which will draw the calcium from the bones into the bloodstream, restoring the blood calcium level to a normal level. On the other hand, if the blood calcium level is too high (**hypercalcemia**), the parathyroid glands secrete less PTH, which allows the excess calcium to be drawn from the bloodstream into storage in the bones, thus returning the blood calcium back to a normal level.

Thymus

The thymus is a single gland located in the mediastinum near the middle of the chest, just beneath the sternum. See *Figure 13-6* for a visual reference.

The thymus is large in the fetus and infants and shrinks with increasing age until there is merely a trace of active thymus tissue in older adults. Although it is a gland of the lymphatic system, the thymus is considered to be an **endocrine gland** because it secretes

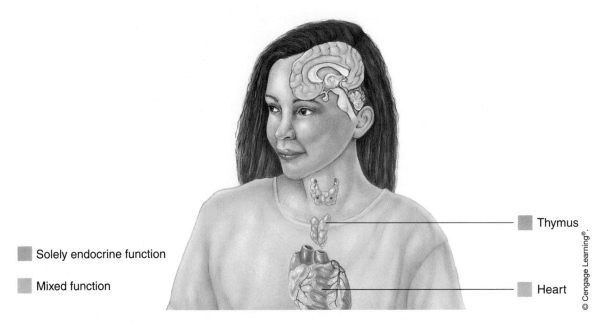

Solely endocrine function

Mixed function

Thymus

Heart

© Cengage Learning®.

Figure 13-6 Thymus

hormones directly into the bloodstream. The thymus hormones have a critical role in the development of the immune system. The hormones secreted by the thymus are:

1. **Thymosin** is thought to stimulate the production of specialized lymphocytes called T-cells (which are involved in the immune response).

2. **Thymopoietin** is also thought to stimulate the production of T-cells that are involved in the immune response.

Adrenal Glands

The adrenal glands consist of two small glands, with one being positioned atop each kidney. Each adrenal gland consists of an **adrenal cortex** (outer portion) and an **adrenal medulla** (inner portion), each part having independent functions. The adrenal glands are also known as the **suprarenal glands**. *Figure 13-7* provides a visual reference of the adrenal glands.

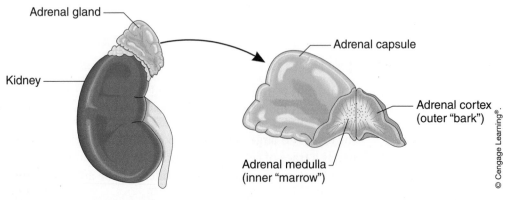

Adrenal gland

Kidney

Adrenal capsule

Adrenal cortex (outer "bark")

Adrenal medulla (inner "marrow")

© Cengage Learning®.

Figure 13-7 Adrenal glands

The adrenal **cortex** is the outer, greater portion of the adrenal gland. It secretes steroid hormones known as corticosteroids. The adrenal **cortex** secretes the following **corticosteroid** hormones:

1. **Mineralocorticoids** regulate how mineral salts are processed in the body. Mineral salts are also known as **electrolytes**. The primary mineralocorticoid hormone secreted by the body is **aldosterone**, which is responsible for regulating fluid and electrolyte balance by promoting sodium retention (which promotes water retention) and potassium excretion.

2. **Glucocorticoids** influence the **metabolism** of carbohydrates, fats, and proteins in the body. In addition, glucocorticoids are necessary in the body for maintaining a normal blood pressure level. They have an anti-inflammatory effect on the body, and during times of stress the increased secretion of glucocorticoids increases the **glucose** available for skeletal muscles needed in "fight-or-flight" responses by the body. The main glucocorticoid secreted in the human body is **cortisol**, or **hydrocortisone**.

3. **Gonadocorticoids** are sex hormones released from the adrenal **cortex** instead of the **gonads**. Although these sex hormones are produced primarily by the male testes and the female ovaries, they are secreted in small amounts by the adrenal **cortex** and contribute to secondary sex characteristics in males and females.

The adrenal **medulla** is the inner portion of the adrenal gland. It secretes nonsteroid hormones called **catecholamines**. The adrenal **medulla** secretes the following nonsteroid hormones:

1. **Epinephrine** (**adrenaline**) increases the heart rate and the force of the heart muscle contraction, dilates the bronchioles in the lungs, decreases peristalsis (wavelike movement) in the intestines, and raises blood **glucose** levels by causing the liver to convert glycogen into **glucose**. This hormone plays an important role in the body's response to stress by mimicking the actions of the sympathetic nervous system (i.e., increasing the heart rate, dilating the bronchioles, releasing **glucose** into the bloodstream). **Epinephrine** is therefore known as a **sympathomimetic agent**.

2. **Norepinephrine** (**noradrenaline**) produces a vasoconstrictor effect on the blood vessels, thereby raising the blood pressure. This hormone also plays an important role in the body's response to stress by mimicking the actions of the sympathetic nervous system (i.e., raising the blood pressure). **Norepinephrine** is also known as a sympathomimetic agent.

Pancreas

The **pancreas** is an elongated gland located in the upper left quadrant of the abdomen, behind the stomach. It extends horizontally across the body, beginning at the first part of the small intestines (duodenum) and ending at the edge of the spleen. See *Figure 13-8*.

The pancreas contains specialized groups of cells (known as the **islets of Langerhans**) that produce important hormones for the body. The islets of Langerhans of the pancreas produce the following hormones:

1. **Glucagon**, produced by the alpha cells of the islets of Langerhans, increases blood **glucose** levels by stimulating the liver to convert glycogen into **glucose**. Glycogen is the major carbohydrate stored by the body. It is formed from **glucose** and is

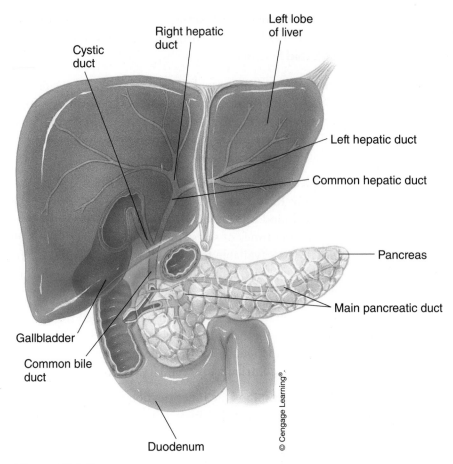

Cystic duct

Right hepatic duct

Left lobe of liver

Left hepatic duct

Common hepatic duct

Pancreas

Main pancreatic duct

Gallbladder

Common bile duct

Duodenum

© Cengage Learning®.

Figure 13-8 Pancreas

stored chiefly in the liver to be used as needed. When the blood sugar level is extremely low (**hypoglycemia**), the pancreas is stimulated to release **glucagon** into the bloodstream, thereby stimulating the liver to convert glycogen to **glucose**. **Glucose** is then released into the bloodstream, thereby raising the overall blood **glucose** level. This process is known as **glycogenolysis**.

2. **Insulin**, produced by the beta cells of the islets of Langerhans, makes it possible for **glucose** to pass from the blood through the cell membranes to be used for energy. **Insulin** also promotes the conversion of excess **glucose** into glycogen for storage in the liver for later use as needed, a process known as **glycogenesis**. When the blood sugar level is high (**hyperglycemia**), the pancreas is stimulated to release **insulin** into the bloodstream, thereby allowing the cells to use the **glucose** for energy and converting the excess **glucose** into a storable form (reducing the overall blood **glucose** level).

Ovaries

The **ovaries** are the female sex glands, also known as the female **gonads**. Each of the paired ovaries is almond shaped and is held in place by ligaments. The ovaries are located in the upper pelvic cavity, on either side of the lateral wall of the uterus, near the fimbriated (fringed) ends of the fallopian tubes. See *Figure 13-9*.

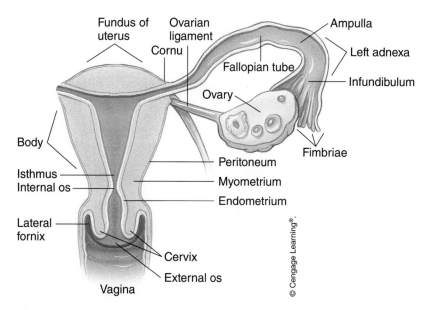

Figure 13-9 Ovaries

The ovaries are responsible for producing mature ova and releasing them at monthly intervals during ovulation. They are also responsible for producing hormones necessary to the normal growth and development of the female and to the maintenance of pregnancy. The hormones produced by the ovaries are as follows:

1. **Estrogen** promotes the maturation of the ovum (egg) in the ovary and stimulates the vascularization of the uterine lining each month in preparation for implantation of a fertilized egg. **Estrogen** also contributes to the secondary sex characteristic changes that occur in the female with the onset of puberty. These changes include development of the glandular tissue in the breasts and deposition of fat in the breasts that give them the characteristic rounded female look; deposition of fat in the buttocks and thighs, creating the rounded adult female curvatures; widening of the pelvis into a more rounded, basinlike shape that is more appropriate for childbirth; growth of pubic and axillary hair; a general skeletal growth spurt; and a general increase in size of the female reproductive organs. The most evident change during puberty is the onset of menstruation.

2. **Progesterone** is primarily responsible for the changes that occur within the uterus in anticipation of a fertilized ovum and for development of the maternal placenta after implantation of a fertilized ovum.

Testes

The **testes** (**male gonads**, also known as the **testicles**) are two ovoid glands that begin their development high in the abdominal cavity, near the kidneys (retroperitoneal cavity), during the gestational period. One to two months before, or shortly after birth, the testicles descend through the inguinal canal into the **scrotum** (where they remain). See *Figure 13-10*.

The testes are the primary organs of the male reproductive system. They are responsible for production of sperm (the male germ cell) and for the secretion of androgens, which

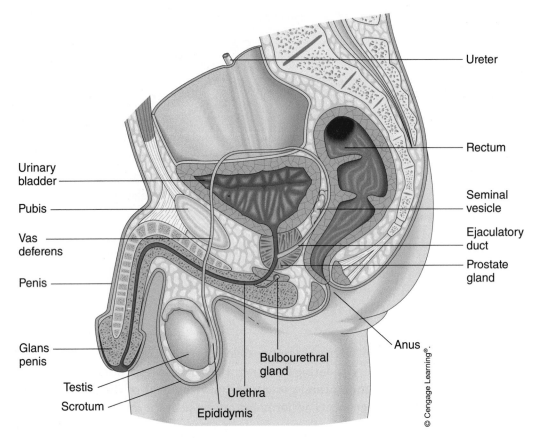

Figure 13-10 Testes

are male steroid hormones. The testes produce the male hormone, **testosterone**, which is responsible for the secondary sex characteristic changes that occur in the male with the onset of puberty. These changes include growth of facial hair (beard), growth of pubic hair, deepening of the voice, growth of skeletal muscles, and enlargement of the penis, scrotum, and testes. Testosterone is also responsible for the maturation of sperm.

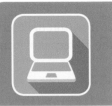

Media Link

For a review of the endocrine system structures you have just learned, go to the Student Companion Website and watch the **Endocrine System** animation.

Review Checkpoint

Check your understanding of this section by completing the **Anatomy and Physiology** exercises in your workbook.

VOCABULARY

The following vocabulary words are frequently used when discussing the endocrine system.

Word	Definition

acromegaly
(**ak**-roh-**MEG**-ah-lee)
  acr/o = extremities
  -megaly = enlargement
	A chronic metabolic condition characterized by gradual, noticeable enlargement and elongation of the bones of the face, jaw, and extremities due to oversecretion of the pituitary gland after puberty.

adenohypophysis (ad-eh-noh-high-**POFF**-ih-sis)	The anterior pituitary gland.

adenoma
(**ad**-eh-**NOH**-mah)
  aden/o = gland
  -oma = tumor
	A glandular tumor.

adenopathy
(ad-eh-**NOP**-ah-thee)
  aden/o = gland
  -pathy = disease
	Any disease of a gland, characterized by enlargement.

adrenalectomy
(ad-ree-nal-**ECK**-toh-mee)
  adren/o = adrenal gland
  -ectomy = surgical removal
	Surgical removal of one or both of the adrenal glands.

adrenalitis
(**ah**-dree-nal-**EYE**-tis)
  adrenal/o = adrenal gland
  -itis = inflammation
	Inflammation of the adrenal glands.

adrenocortical
(ad-ree-noh-**KOR**-tih-kal)
  adren/o = adrenal gland
  cortic/o = cortex
  -al = pertaining to
	Pertaining to the **cortex** of the adrenal gland(s).

aldosterone (al-**DOSS**-ter-ohn)	A hormone secreted by the adrenal **cortex** that regulates sodium and potassium balance in the blood.
androgen (**AN**-droh-jen)	Any steroid hormone (e.g., testosterone) that increases male characteristics.

antidiuretic
(an-tye-dye-yoo-**RET**-ik)
  anti- = against
  di/a = through
  ur/o = urine
  -etic = pertaining to
	Pertaining to the suppression of urine production; an agent given to suppress the production of urine.

Word	Definition
cortex (**COR**-tex)	Pertaining to the outer region of an organ or structure.
cortisol (**COR**-tih-sal)	A steroid hormone occurring naturally in the body; also called hydrocortisone.
cretinism (**KREE**-tin-izm)	A congenital condition (one that occurs at birth) caused by a lack of **thyroid** secretion. This condition is characterized by **dwarfism**, slowed mental development, puffy facial features, dry skin, and large tongue.
diabetes, gestational (**dye**-ah-**BEE**-teez, jess-**TAY**-shun-al)	A condition occurring in pregnancy characterized by the signs and symptoms of **diabetes mellitus** (such as impaired ability to metabolize carbohydrates due to **insulin** deficiency, and elevated blood sugar level). These symptoms usually disappear after delivery of the baby.
diabetes insipidus (**dye**-ah-**BEE**-teez in-**SIP**-id-us)	A metabolic disorder characterized by extreme **polydipsia** (excessive thirst) and **polyuria** (excessive urination). This is a disorder of the pituitary gland due to a deficiency in secretion of the **antidiuretic** hormone.
diabetes mellitus (**dye**-ah-**BEE**-teez **MELL**-ih-tus)	A disorder of the pancreas in which the beta cells of the islets of Langerhans of the pancreas fail to produce an adequate amount of **insulin**, resulting in the body's inability to metabolize carbohydrates, fats, and proteins appropriately.
diabetic ketoacidosis (**dye**-ah-**BEH**-tik kee-toh-ass-ih-**DOH**-sis)	A dangerous condition that occurs as a result of severe lack of **insulin**, causing the body to break down body fats instead of **glucose** for energy. The stored fat is broken down into fatty acids and glycerol. The liver changes the fatty acids into ketone bodies (acids), which leads to an increase in acidity of the blood (acidosis) called **diabetic ketoacidosis** (DKA). Also known as diabetic coma.
dwarfism (**DWARF**-ism)	A condition in which there is an abnormal underdevelopment of the body. This condition is characterized by extremely short height and is usually caused by undersecretion of the pituitary gland (growth hormone).

endocrine gland
(**EN**-doh-krin)
  endo- = within
  -crine = secrete
	A ductless gland that produces a chemical substance called a hormone, which is secreted directly into the bloodstream instead of exiting the body through ducts.

endocrinologist
(en-doh-krin-**OL**-oh-jist)
  endo- = within
  crin/o = secrete
  -logist = one who specializes in the
        study of
	A physician who specializes in the medical practice of treating the diseases and disorders of the endocrine system.

Word	Definition
endocrinology (en-doh-krin-**OL**-oh-jee) endo- = within crin/o = secrete -logy = the study of	The field of medicine that deals with the study of the endocrine system and of the treatment of the diseases and disorders of the endocrine system.
epinephrine (**ep**-ih-**NEF**-rin)	A hormone produced by the adrenal **medulla**. This hormone plays an important role in the body's response to stress by increasing the heart rate, dilating the bronchioles, and releasing **glucose** into the bloodstream.
estrogen (**ESS**-troh-jen)	One of the female hormones that promotes the development of female secondary sex characteristics.
euthyroid (yoo-**THIGH**-royd) eu- = well, easily, good, normal thyroid/o = thyroid gland	Pertaining to a normally functioning **thyroid** gland.
exocrine gland (**ECK**-soh-krin) exo- = outward -crine = secrete	A gland that opens onto the surface of the skin through ducts in the epithelium, such as an oil gland or a sweat gland.
exophthalmia (eck-sof-**THAL**-mee-ah) ex- = outward ophthalm/o = eye -ia = condition	An abnormal condition characterized by a marked outward protrusion of the eyeballs.
exophthalmos (eck-sof-**THAL**-mos) ex- = outward ophthalm/o = eye -os = a suffix indicating a singular noun	See *exophthalmia*.
gigantism (**JYE**-gan-tism)	An abnormal condition characterized by excessive size and height. This condition is usually due to an oversecretion of the pituitary gland (growth hormone).
glucagon (**GLOO**-kah-gon)	A hormone secreted by the islets of Langerhans of the pancreas that stimulates the liver to convert glycogen into **glucose**.
glucogenesis (gloo-koh-**JEN**-eh-sis) gluc/o = sugar, sweet -genesis = production of; formation	The formation of glycogen from fatty acids and proteins instead of from carbohydrates.
glucose (**GLOO**-kohs)	The simplest form of sugar in the body; a simple sugar found in certain foods, especially fruits; also a major source of energy for the human body.

Word	Definition
glycogenesis (glye-koh-**JEN**-eh-sis) glyc/o = sugar, sweet -genesis = production of; formation	The conversion of excess **glucose** into glycogen for storage in the liver for later use as needed.
glycosuria (glye-kohs-**YOO**-ree-ah) glycos/o = sugar, sweet -uria = urine condition	The presence of sugar in the urine.
goiter (**GOY**-ter)	Enlargement of the **thyroid** gland due to excessive growth (hyperplasia).
gonads (**GOH**-nadz)	A term used to refer to the female sex glands (ovaries) and the male sex glands (testes).
Graves' disease	**Hyperthyroidism.**
growth hormone	See *somatotropic hormone.*
gynecomastia (**gigh**-neh-koh-**MASS**-tee-ah) gynec/o = woman mast/o = breast -ia = condition	An abnormal enlargement of the breasts in men; may involve one or both.
hirsutism (**HER**-soot-izm)	A condition in which there is excessive body hair in a male distribution pattern.
hypercalcemia (**high**-per-kal-**SEE**-mee-ah) hyper- = excessive calc/o = calcium -emia = blood condition	Elevated blood calcium level.
hyperglycemia (**high**-per-glye-**SEE**-mee-ah) hyper- = excessive glyc/o = sugar, sweet -emia = blood condition	Elevated blood sugar level.
hypergonadism (**high**-per-**GOH**-nad-izm)	Excessive activity of the ovaries or testes.
hyperinsulinism (**high**-per-**IN**-soo-lin-izm)	An excessive amount of **insulin** in the body.
hyperkalemia (**high**-per-kal-**EE**-mee-ah) hyper- = excessive kal/i = potassium -emia = blood condition	An elevated blood potassium level.

Word	Definition
hypernatremia (**high**-per-nah-**TREE**-mee-ah) hyper- = excessive natr/i = sodium -emia = blood condition	An elevated blood sodium level.
hyperparathyroidism (**high**-per-pair-ah-**THIGH**-roy-dizm) hyper- = excessive parathyroid/o = parathyroid glands -ism = condition	Hyperactivity of any of the four parathyroid glands, resulting in an oversecretion of parathyroid hormone.
hyperpituitarism (**high**-per-pih-**TOO**-ih-tair-izm) hyper- = excessive	Overactivity of the anterior lobe of the pituitary gland.
hyperthyroidism (**high**-per-**THIGH**-roy-dizm) hyper- = excessive thyroid/o = thyroid gland -ism = condition	Overactivity of the **thyroid** gland; also called Graves' disease.
hypocalcemia (**high**-poh-kal-**SEE**-mee-ah) hypo- = under, below, beneath, less than normal calc/o = calcium -emia = blood condition	Less than normal blood calcium level.
hypoglycemia (**high**-poh-glye-**SEE**-mee-ah) hypo- = under, below, beneath, less than normal glyc/o = sugar, sweet -emia = blood condition	Less than normal blood sugar level.
hypokalemia (**high**-poh-kal-**EE**-mee-ah) hypo- = under, below, beneath, less than normal kal/i = potassium -emia = blood condition	Less than normal blood potassium level.
hyponatremia (**high**-poh-nah-**TREE**-mee-ah) hypo- = under, below, beneath, less than normal natr/i = sodium -emia = blood condition	Less than normal blood sodium level.

Word	Definition
hypophysectomy (**high**-poff-ih-**SEK**-toh-mee)	Surgical removal of the pituitary gland.

hypothyroidism (**high**-poh-**THIGH**-roy-dizm)
    hypo- = under, below, beneath, less
        than normal
    thyroid/o = thyroid gland
    -ism = condition
	Less than normal activity of the **thyroid** gland.

insulin shock (**IN**-soo-lin)	A state of shock due to extremely low blood sugar level caused by an overdose of **insulin**, a decreased intake of food, or excessive exercise by a patient who is diabetic and **insulin** dependent. Severe **hypoglycemia** is a medical emergency.
medulla (meh-**DULL**-lah)	The internal part of a structure or organ.
metabolism (meh-**TAB**-oh-lizm)	The sum of all physical and chemical processes that take place within the body.
myxedema (miks-eh-**DEE**-mah)	The most severe form of **hypothyroidism** in the adult. This condition is characterized by puffiness of the hands and face; coarse, thickened edematous skin; an enlarged tongue; slow speech; loss of and dryness of the hair; sensitivity to cold; drowsiness; and mental apathy.
norepinephrine (**nor**-ep-ih-**NEH**-frin)	A hormone produced by the adrenal **medulla**. This hormone plays an important role in the body's response to stress by raising the blood pressure.

oxytocin (ok-see-**TOH**-sin)
    oxy- = rapid, sharp
    toc/o = childbirth
    -in = enzyme
	A hormone secreted by the posterior pituitary gland. This hormone stimulates the contractions of the uterus during childbirth and stimulates the release of milk from the breasts of lactating women (women who breastfeed) in response to the suckling reflex of the infant.

polydipsia (**pol**-ee-**DIP**-see-ah)
    poly- = many, much, excessive
    -dipsia = thirst
	Excessive thirst.

polyphagia (**pol**-ee-**FAY**-jee-ah)
    poly- = many, much, excessive
    -phagia = eating condition
	Excessive eating.

polyuria (**pol**-ee-**YOO**-ree-ah)
    poly- = many, much, excessive
    -uria = urine condition
	The excretion of excessively large amounts of urine.

Word	Definition
progesterone (proh-**JESS**-ter-ohn)	A female hormone secreted by the ovaries. This hormone is primarily responsible for the changes that occur in the endometrium in anticipation of a fertilized ovum and for development of the maternal placenta after implantation of a fertilized ovum.
somatotropic hormone (soh-mat-oh-**TROH**-pik)	A hormone secreted by the anterior pituitary gland that regulates the cellular processes necessary for normal body growth; also called the growth hormone.
syndrome (**SIN**-drohm) syn- = joined, together -drome = that which runs together	A group of symptoms occurring together, indicative of a particular disease or abnormality.
T-cells	Specialized lymphocytes that are involved in the immune response.
tetany (**TET**-ah-nee)	A condition characterized by severe cramping and twitching of the muscles and sharp flexion of the wrist and ankle joints; a complication of **hypocalcemia**.
thymopoietin (thigh-moh-**POY**-eh-tin)	A hormone secreted by the thymus, thought to stimulate the production of T-cells (which are involved in the immune response).
thymosin (thigh-**MOH**-sin)	A hormone secreted by the thymus. This hormone is thought to stimulate the production of specialized lymphocytes, called T-cells, which are involved in the immune response.
thyroiditis (**thigh**-royd-**EYE**-tis) thyroid/o = thyroid gland -itis = inflammation	Inflammation of the **thyroid** gland.
thyroxine (thigh-**ROKS**-in)	A hormone secreted by the **thyroid** gland. This hormone helps maintain normal body **metabolism** (abbreviated as T_4).
triiodothyronine (**try**-eye-oh-doh-**THIGH**-roh-neen)	A hormone secreted by the **thyroid** gland. This hormone helps regulate growth and development of the body and control **metabolism** and body temperature (abbreviated as T_3).
virilism (**VEER**-il-izm)	The development of masculine physical traits in the female (such as growth of facial and body hair, increased secretion of the sebaceous glands, deepening of the voice, and enlargement of the clitoris); also called masculinization. This condition may be due to an abnormality or dysfunction of the adrenal gland, as in adrenal virilism.

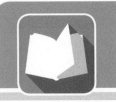

Review Checkpoint

Check your understanding of this section by completing the **Vocabulary** exercises in your workbook.

WORD ELEMENTS

The following word elements pertain to the endocrine system. As you review the list, pronounce each word element aloud twice and check the box after you "say it." Write the definition for the example term given for each word element. Use your medical dictionary to find the definitions of the example terms.

Word Element	Pronunciation	"Say It"	Meaning
acr/o **acr**omegaly	**AK**-roh ak-roh-**MEG**-ah-lee	☐	extremities
aden/o **aden**opathy	**AD**-en-noh ad-eh-**NOP**-ah-thee	☐	gland
adren/o **adren**omegaly	ad-**REE**-noh ad-ree-noh-**MEG**-ah-lee	☐	adrenal glands
adrenal/o **adrenal**ectomy	ad-**REE**-nal-oh ad-ree-nal-**ECK**-toh-mee	☐	adrenal glands
andr/o **andr**ogen	**AN**-droh **AN**-droh-jen	☐	man, male
calc/o hyper**calc**emia	**KAL**-koh high-per-kal-**SEE**-mee-ah	☐	calcium
cortic/o **cortic**osteroid	**KOR**-tih-koh kor-tih-koh-**STAIR**-oyd	☐	**cortex**
crin/o endo**crin**ology	**KRIN**-oh en-doh-krin-**OL**-oh-jee	☐	secrete
-crine endo**crine**	**KRIN** **EN**-doh-krin	☐	secrete
dips/o **dips**osis	**DIP**-soh dip-**SOH**-sis	☐	thirst
-dipsia poly**dipsia**	**DIP**-see-ah pol-ee-**DIP**-see-ah	☐	thirst
gonad/o **gonad**otropic	goh-**NAD**-oh goh-nad-oh-**TROH**-pik	☐	sex glands

Word Element	Pronunciation	"Say It"	Meaning
gluc/o **gluc**oneogenesis	**GLOO**-koh gloo-koh-nee-oh-**JEN**-eh-sis	☐	sugar, sweet
glyc/o **glyc**ogenolysis	**GLYE**-koh glye-koh-jen-**ALL**-eh-sis	☐	sugar, sweet
gynec/o **gynec**ologist	**GIGH**-neh-koh **gigh**-neh-**KOL**-oh-jist	☐	woman
-itis pancreat**itis**	**EYE**-tis **pan**-kree-ah-**TYE**-tis	☐	inflammation
kal/i hyper**kal**emia	**KAL**-ee high-per-kal-**EE**-mee-ah	☐	potassium
lact/o **lact**ogen	**LAK**-toh **LAK**-toh-jen	☐	milk
mastitis **mast**itis	**MASS**-toh mass-**TYE**-tis	☐	breast
myx/o **myx**edema	**MIKS**-oh miks-eh-**DEE**-mah	☐	relating to mucus
natr/i hyper**natr**emia	**NAH**-tree high-per-nah-**TREE**-mee-ah	☐	sodium
oxy- **oxy**tocin	**OK**-see ok-see-**TOH**-sin	☐	sharp, quick
pancreat/o **pancreat**itis	pan-kree-**AH**-toh pan-kree-ah-**TYE**-tis	☐	pancreas
parathyroid/o **parathyroid**ectomy	pair-ah-**THIGH**-royd-oh pair-ah-**thigh**-royd-**ECK**-toh-mee	☐	parathyroid glands
somat/o **somat**otropic hormone	soh-**MAT**-oh soh-mat-oh-**TROH**-pik hormone	☐	body
thym/o **thym**oma	**THIGH**-moh thigh-**MOH**-mah	☐	thymus gland
thyr/o **thyr**oxine	**THIGH**-roh thigh-**ROKS**-in	☐	**thyroid** gland
thyroid/o hyper**thyroid**ism	**THIGH**-royd-oh high-per-**THIGH**-royd-izm	☐	**thyroid** gland
toxic/o **toxic**ology	**TOKS**-ih-koh toks-ih-**KOL**-ih-jee	☐	poisons

Word Element	Pronunciation	"Say It"	Meaning
-tropin gonado**tropin**	**TROH**-pin goh-nad-oh-**TROH**-pin	☐	stimulating effect of a hormone
-uria poly**uria**	**YOO**-ree-ah pol-ee-**YOO**-ree-ah	☐	urine condition

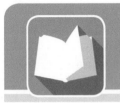

Review Checkpoint

Check your understanding of this section by completing the **Word Elements** exercises in your workbook.

Pathological Conditions

As you study the pathological conditions of the endocrine system, note that the **basic definition** is in a green shaded box followed by a detailed description in regular print. The phonetic pronunciation is directly beneath each term, as well as a breakdown of the component parts of the term where applicable.

The pathological conditions are presented in the same order as the discussion of the endocrine glands, with the exception of the ovaries and testes (which are discussed in detail in the chapters on female and male reproductive systems, respectively). Beneath each **endocrine gland** heading, the pathological conditions are alphabetized for ease of location.

Pituitary Gland

acromegaly (**ak**-roh-**MEG**-ah-lee) acr/o = extremities -megaly = enlarged	A chronic metabolic condition characterized by the gradual noticeable enlargement and elongation of the bones of the face, jaw, and extremities due to hypersecretion of the human growth hormone after puberty.
	The cause of oversecretion of the human growth hormone is most often due to a tumor of the pituitary gland. Treatment for **acromegaly** is aimed at reducing the size of the pituitary gland through surgery or radiation.
diabetes insipidus (**dye**-ah-**BEE**-teez in-**SIP**-ih-dus)	A condition caused by a deficiency in the secretion of **antidiuretic** hormone (ADH) by the posterior pituitary gland, characterized by large amounts of urine and sodium being excreted from the body.
	The person experiencing **diabetes insipidus** will complain of excessive thirst and will drink large volumes of water. The urine is very dilute, with a low specific gravity. ADH (vasopressin) is administered as treatment for **diabetes insipidus**.

dwarfism	Generalized growth retardation of the body due to the deficiency of the human growth hormone before puberty; also known as congenital hypopituitarism (or **hypopituitarism**). See *Figure 13-11*.
(**DWARF**-ism)	

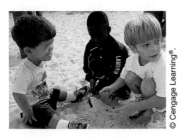

Figure 13-11 Dwarfism

The abnormal underdevelopment leaves the child extremely short with a small body. There is an absence of secondary sex characteristics. The condition may have a connection with other defects or varying degrees of mental retardation.

Treatment may include administration of human growth hormone or somatotropin until a height of 5 feet is reached. These children may need replacement of other hormones, especially just before and during puberty.

gigantism	A proportional overgrowth of the body's tissue due to the hypersecretion of the human growth hormone before puberty.
(**JYE**-gan-tizm)	

The child experiences accelerated abnormal growth chiefly in the long bones. The cause of oversecretion of the human growth hormone is most often due to an **adenoma** of the anterior pituitary. Treatment of **gigantism** is aimed at reducing the size of the pituitary gland through surgery or radiation.

hypopituitarism	A complex **syndrome** resulting from the absence or deficiency of the pituitary hormone(s).
(**high**-poh-pih-**TOO**-ih-tah-rizm)	

Metabolic dysfunction, growth retardation, and sexual immaturity are symptoms of **hypopituitarism**.

Thyroid Gland

cancer, thyroid gland	Malignant tumor of the **thyroid** gland, which leads to dysfunction of the gland and thus inadequate or excessive secretion of the **thyroid** hormone.

The presence of a palpable nodule or lump may be the first indication of **thyroid** cancer. A needle aspiration biopsy is used to confirm the diagnosis. A malignant tumor of the **thyroid** is classified and staged according to the site of origin, size of tumor, amount of lymph node involvement, and the presence of metastasis.

Treatment typically consists of partial or complete removal of the **thyroid** gland. Lifelong **thyroid** hormone replacement is required.

goiter (simple; nontoxic)	Hyperplasia of the **thyroid** gland.
(**GOY**-ter)	

This condition results from a deficient amount of iodine in the diet, required for the synthesis of T_3 and T_4 **thyroid** hormones produced by the **thyroid** gland.

When the body identifies the low levels of thyroid hormone, the anterior pituitary gland secretes the hormone thyrotropin, which continually stimulates the **thyroid** gland to produce T_3 and T_4. Consequently, the overstimulation increases the number of cells in the **thyroid** gland and a **goiter** is produced.

As the **goiter** increases in size, the person (typically a female) will notice a mass in the anterior aspect of the neck. As this mass or enlarged **thyroid** gland continuously increases in size, it begins to exert pressure on the trachea and esophagus (causing breathing and swallowing difficulties). Eventually, the **goiter** may cause the person to experience dizziness and fainting spells.

A **goiter** is noted on physical examination of the neck and confirmed with blood studies with evidence of decreased T_3 and T_4 levels and elevated thyrotropin levels. Simple goiters are usually responsive to the administration of potassium iodide. If the **goiter** is nonresponsive, a subtotal thyroidectomy may be needed. Maintaining iodine in the diet prevents the development of **goiter**.

Graves' disease (hyperthyroidism) (**high**-per-**THIGH**-royd-izm) hyper- = excessive thyroid/o = thyroid gland -ism = condition	Hypertrophy of the **thyroid** gland resulting in an excessive secretion of the **thyroid** hormone that causes an extremely high body **metabolism**, thus creating multisystem changes.

Hyperthyroidism occurs most often in the form of **Graves' disease**, which has three distinguishing characteristics:

1. **Hyperthyroidism**

2. **Thyroid** gland enlargement (**goiter**)

3. **Exophthalmia** (unnatural protrusion of the eyes)

The symptoms of Graves' disease are the result of **hyperthyroidism** and thus of hypermetabolism (which affects all body systems). **Hyperthyroidism** causes a rapid heartbeat, nervousness, inability to sleep, excitability, increased appetite, weight loss, nausea, vomiting, excessive thirst, and profuse sweating. The speeding up of physical and mental responses result in varied emotional responses from extreme happiness to hyperactivity or delirium. The **goiter** results from hyperactivity of the **thyroid** gland, which leads to an increase in the size of the **thyroid** gland (hypertrophy) and an increase in the number of **thyroid** cells (hyperplasia). The gland may enlarge up to three to four times the original size. The person with **hyperthyroidism** will have decreased levels of serum cholesterol.

Diagnosis is confirmed on the basis of the individual's physical appearance and lack of composure, restlessness, and agitation. The serum levels of T_3 and T_4 are elevated, and there is increased uptake of radioiodine in the **thyroid** scan. Other blood test results may expose elevated levels of particular antithyroid immunoglobulins, thus leaning toward an autoimmune response as a possible cause. The cause is uncertain.

Treatment includes the following therapies: antithyroid medication, radioiodine, and surgery (subtotal thyroidectomy). Graves' disease has three significant complications: (1) **exophthalmia**, (2) thyroid storm (see *thyrotoxicosis*), and (3) heart disease.

hypothyroidism

(**high**-poh-**THIGH**-royd-izm)

hypo- = under, below, beneath, less than normal

thyroid/o = thyroid gland

-ism = condition

A condition in which there is a shortage of **thyroid** hormone, causing an extremely low body **metabolism** due to a reduced usage of oxygen; also called **myxedema** in the most severe form.

Hypothyroidism may be the result of:

1. Congenital **thyroid** defects (**cretinism**)
2. Faulty hormone synthesis
3. **Thyroiditis** or iodine deficiency
4. Use of antithyroid medications
5. Loss of **thyroid** tissue due to surgery or radioactivity
6. **Thyroid** gland atrophy

Hypothyroidism has a sluggish onset with symptoms developing over months or years. The severity of the disorder varies from mild to severe. In the mild form of **hypothyroidism**, the person may demonstrate no symptoms or only vague symptoms.

In the more severe cases, symptoms include slowed physical and mental function, an obvious apathetic fatigued appearance, bradycardia, anemia, difficulty breathing, decreased urinary output, decreased peristalsis, constipation, transient musculoskeletal pain, dry scaly skin, loss of hair, expressionless face, cold intolerance, and slow movement. A **goiter** may be a manifestation of **hypothyroidism**.

The person with **hypothyroidism** will have increased levels of serum cholesterol and triglycerides as a result of the effect on lipid **metabolism**. **Myxedema** is the most severe form of **hypothyroidism**, identified by water retention all over the body in the connective tissues. The person with **myxedema** has a puffy appearance and a thick tongue. **Myxedema** coma occurs with an extreme reduction in metabolic rate and is manifested by hypoventilation, hypotension, and hypothermia.

Diagnosis of **hypothyroidism** is confirmed with the clinical presentation of the person and an elevated serum TSH level due to the attempt to compensate for the levels of T_3 and T_4, which are low. With **thyroid** hormone replacement therapy, the physical and mental symptoms will reverse. To maintain reversal permanently, a **thyroid** hormone preparation will be needed throughout life. **Hypothyroidism** occurs more frequently in females, with the highest incidence between 30 and 60 years of age.

thyroiditis, chronic

(thigh-royd-**EYE**-tis)

(Hashimoto's)

(**HASH**-ee-moh-**TOZ**)

thyroid/o = thyroid gland

-itis = inflammation

Chronic inflammation of the **thyroid** gland, leading to enlargement of the **thyroid** gland.

This is a disease of the immune system in which the gland tissue is destroyed by antibodies and replaced with fibrous tissue. Chronic inflammation causes massive infiltration of the **thyroid** gland with plasma cells and lymphocytes. **Thyroiditis** can also be acute or subacute. The body recognizes a decrease in the level of **thyroid** hormone and stimulates the anterior pituitary to secrete thyrotropin, which continually stimulates the **thyroid** gland to produce T_3 and T_4. Consequently, the stimulation increases the number of cells in the **thyroid** gland in an attempt to compensate, and a **goiter** is produced. Hashimoto's **thyroiditis** is a common form of primary **hypothyroidism** (see *hypothyroidism*).

To confirm the diagnosis, the blood is evaluated for autoantibodies and the function of the thyroid gland is measured with a **radioactive iodine uptake (RAIU) test**. A needle biopsy in a person with Hashimoto's disease will usually show characteristic changes in the gland tissue.

Treatment is **thyroid** hormone replacement for life. The replacement will prevent further growth of the **goiter**.

thyrotoxicosis (thyroid storm)	An acute, sometimes fatal, incident of overactivity of the **thyroid** gland resulting in excessive secretion of **thyroid** hormone.

(**thigh**-roh-toks-ih-**KOH**-sis)
(**THIGH**-royd storm)
  thyr/o = thyroid gland
  toxic/o = poisons
  -osis = condition

Thyroid storm is characterized by a critically high fever and pulse rate, dehydration, extreme irritability, and delirium. A thyroid storm is a medical emergency typically precipitated by infection, surgery, trauma, labor and delivery, a myocardial infarction, medication overdosage, or undiagnosed or untreated **hyperthyroidism**. Diagnosis is made on the clinical picture of the person. Also known as thyroid crisis.

Parathyroid Gland

hyperparathyroidism	Overactivity of any one of the parathyroid glands, which leads to high levels of calcium in the blood and low levels of calcium in the bones.

(**high**-per-pair-ah-**THIGH**-royd-izm)
(**hypercalcemia**)
(**high**-per-kal-**SEE**-mee-ah)
  hyper- = excessive
  parathyroid/o = parathyroid gland
  -ism = condition
  hyper- = excessive
  calc/i = calcium
  -emia = blood condition

The accelerated activity of the parathyroid gland in primary **hyperparathyroidism** is due to the effects of a parathyroid tumor or hyperplasia of the parathyroid gland (excessive increase in the number of cells). Secondary **hyperparathyroidism** is usually related to renal disease or endocrine disorders.

Symptoms of **hyperparathyroidism** are due to **hypercalcemia** and include muscle weakness and atrophy; nausea, vomiting, and gastrointestinal pain; increased irritability of the heart muscle (leading to arrhythmias); bone tenderness and fragility leading to bone fractures; and deposits of calcium in soft tissue leading to renal calculi and low back pain.

Diagnostic laboratory results will demonstrate a high level of PTH on the radioimmunoassay and elevated blood levels of calcium, alkaline phosphatase, and chloride. The blood phosphorus levels will be reduced. The extent of demineralization of the bones can be evaluated on X-ray film.

Treatment for **hyperparathyroidism** will vary but will be directly related to the cause. Surgical intervention involves removal of the gland or glands causing the hypersecretion of PTH.

hypoparathyroidism	Decreased production of parathyroid hormone, resulting in **hypocalcemia**, characterized by nerve and muscle weakness with muscle spasms or **tetany** (a state of continual contraction of the muscles).

(**high**-poh-pair-ah-**THIGH**-royd-izm)
  hypo- = under, below, beneath, less than normal
  parathyroid/o = parathyroid glands
  -ism = condition

Symptoms include hair loss, brittle nails, malabsorption, arrhythmias, mood disorders, and hyperactive reflexes. Blood phosphate levels are elevated.

Treatment of **hypoparathyroidism** is aimed at increasing calcium levels. Immediate administration of intravenous calcium will aid in decreasing **tetany**. Long-term calcium supplements, an increase of calcium in the diet, and vitamin D therapy are usually helpful to raise the blood calcium level.

Adrenal Glands

Addison's disease (**Ad**-ih-son's)	A life-threatening disease process due to failure of the adrenal **cortex** to secrete adequate mineralocorticoids and glucocorticoids resulting from an autoimmune process, a neoplasm, an infection, or a hemorrhage in the gland.

Symptoms include low blood **glucose**, low blood sodium, weight loss, dehydration, generalized weakness, gastrointestinal disturbances, increased pigmentation of the skin and mucous membranes, cold intolerance, anxiety, and depression.

Diagnosis is confirmed through an ACTH stimulation test. Treatment for **Addison's disease** is replacement of natural hormones with mineralocorticoid and glucocorticoid drugs, to continue for life, and dietary modifications.

Conn's disease **(primary aldosteronism)** (al-**DOSS**-ter-ohn-izm)	A condition characterized by excretion of excessive amounts of **aldosterone**, the most influential of the mineralocorticoids, which causes the body to retain extra sodium and excrete extra potassium, leading to an increased volume of blood (hypervolemia) and hypertension.

Other symptoms include headache, nocturia (excessive urination during the night), fatigue, ventricular arrhythmias, **tetany**, and muscular weakness. **Conn's disease** is caused by an aldosteronoma, a benign aldosterone-secreting **adenoma** or adrenal hyperplasia.

Surgical removal of one or both adrenal glands is the preferred treatment for **primary aldosteronism**. Medical treatment involves the administration of the medication Aldactone. Early diagnosis and treatment will aid in preventing progressive renal complications and hypertension.

Cushing's syndrome (**CUSH**-ings **SIN**-drom)	A condition of the adrenal gland in which a cluster of symptoms occur as a result of an excessive amount of **cortisol** or ACTH circulating in the blood.

The high levels of circulating **cortisol** have been either secreted from the adrenal **cortex** or are present because of the administration of very large doses of glucocorticoids for some time. A benign or malignant adrenal tumor is the cause of primary **Cushing's syndrome**, causing the excessive production of **cortisol**. Secondary **Cushing's syndrome** occurs as a result of Cushing's disease, a disorder of the pituitary or hypothalamus (which results in the increased release of ACTH). The increased ACTH stimulation leads to hyperplasia of the adrenal **cortex** and thus increased production of **cortisol**.

Symptoms of **Cushing's syndrome** are central obesity, round "moon" face, edema, hypertension, supraclavicular fat pads (buffalo hump), muscular weakness and wasting, skin infection, poor wound healing, low potassium level, and emotional changes. See *Figures 13-12A* and *B*.

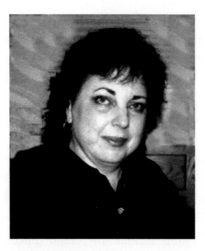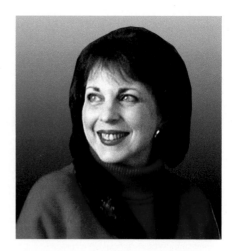

Figure 13-12 Cushing's syndrome (A) before treatment, (B) after treatment
(Courtesy of R. Jones)

Treatment varies according to the cause. When a tumor is the cause, surgical excision and/or radiation will be used. Drug therapy can be used to suppress ACTH secretions.

pheochromocytoma
 	
(fee-oh-**kroh**-moh-sigh-**TOH**-mah)
 	
  phe/o = dusky
 	
  chrom/o = color
 	
  cyt/o = cell
 	
  -oma = tumor
	A vascular tumor of the adrenal **medulla** that produces extra **epinephrine** and **norepinephrine**, leading to persistent or intermittent hypertension and heart palpitations.

Other symptoms include flushing of the face, sweating, severe headaches, muscle spasms, and high blood **glucose**. Possible complications of **pheochromocytoma** consist of weight loss, cardiac dysrhythmia, and heart failure. With surgical excision of one or both adrenal glands, depending on the tumor involvement, the person can be cured if cardiovascular damage has not become permanent. Early diagnosis and treatment is essential to prevent long-term complications.

virilism (**VEER**-il-izm)	Development of male secondary sex characteristics in the female due to the excessive secretion of **adrenocortical** androgens from the adrenal **cortex**.

The overactivity of the adrenal gland may be caused by an adrenal tumor or hyperplasia. **Virilism** typically occurs in adult women 30 to 40 years of age.

Symptoms include excessive hair on the body and face (**hirsutism**), absence of menstruation (amenorrhea), deepening of the voice, acne, oily skin, muscular hypertrophy, atrophy of the breasts and uterus, and ovarian changes. Treatment consists of tumor resection, **adrenalectomy**, and administration of **cortisol** to suppress **androgen** production.

Pancreas

diabetes mellitus (**dye**-ah-**BEE**-teez **MELL**-ih-tus)	A disorder of the pancreas in which the beta cells of the islets of Langerhans of the pancreas fail to produce an adequate amount of **insulin**, or to use **insulin** appropriately, resulting in the body's inability to metabolize carbohydrates, fats, and proteins appropriately.

The classic characteristic of the disease is **hyperglycemia**. First, the individual will experience abnormally elevated blood **glucose** levels (known as hyperglycemia) due to the body's inability to use **glucose** for energy. **Insulin** is necessary for the body cells to use **glucose** for energy. Second, when the body cannot use **glucose** for energy, the cells begin to break down fats and proteins for energy. This breakdown of fats and proteins releases waste products known as **ketones** into the bloodstream, which spill over into the urine as a result of abnormal accumulations.

The classic symptoms of **diabetes mellitus** are **glycosuria** (sugar in the urine), **polydipsia** (excessive thirst), and **polyuria** (excessive urine output). Other symptoms include increased eating (**polyphagia**) and weight loss, presence of ketones in the urine, itching (pruritus), muscle weakness, and fatigue.

Diabetes mellitus is classified as either type 1 diabetes (formerly known as insulin-dependent diabetes) or type 2 diabetes (formerly known as non-insulin-dependent diabetes). **Type 1 diabetes** is an autoimmune disorder that usually occurs before the age of 30, having a sudden onset (usually following a viral infection or other severe stressor). Individuals with type 1 diabetes usually have no pancreatic activity and require administration of **insulin** injections to control the disease. These individuals are prone to developing **diabetic ketoacidosis** (DKA).

Type 2 diabetes usually has a gradual onset and appears in adults after the age of 30. The majority of these individuals are obese. The age of onset has dropped dramatically in the past decade with the rise in the incidence of obesity in children, adolescents, and young adults. Individuals with type 2 diabetes usually have some pancreatic activity but experience **insulin** resistance (reduced ability of most cells to respond to **insulin**) followed by impaired **insulin** secretion. For these individuals, losing weight and gaining muscle helps the body use **insulin** more efficiently. Sometimes oral antidiabetic drugs are used in addition to dietary changes and exercise to control blood sugar levels. Approximately 90% of all people with diabetes have type 2 diabetes. Some people with type 2 diabetes, however, become **insulin** dependent. Type 2 diabetes is a progressive disease that is often present for 3 to 12 years prior to diagnosis. Although these individuals are usually able to control their diabetes with diet and exercise in the beginning, they eventually have to convert to the administration of **insulin** injections for proper control when the body is unable to get enough **glucose** because of **insulin** resistance or decreased ability to produce **insulin**. The individual with type 2 diabetes who does require **insulin** injections to control the disease may experience all of the symptoms and problems that accompany type 1 diabetes. They are not as likely to develop DKA early in the disease as are those with type 1 diabetes, due to the small amount of **insulin** they continue to secrete. However, later in the disease, if they become completely dependent on **insulin**, they have just as great a likelihood.

Treatment for type 1 diabetes consists of a balance among diet, exercise, and **insulin**. These individuals may take **insulin** injections several times a day to control their blood sugar level. **Insulin** is administered to mimic the activity of the normal pancreas as it secretes **insulin** throughout the day. The amount of **insulin** administered each time depends on the blood sugar reading at that time. There are various approaches to administering **insulin** to control diabetes. Control may be achieved by administering fast-acting

insulin approximately 5 to 15 minutes before meals (provides the greatest amount of **insulin** during the greatest need for **insulin** = bolus dose) and long-acting **insulin** once daily, usually at night (provides a steady control of the blood sugar level throughout the day and night = basal dose). Examples of types of **insulin** used are NovoLog® (fast-acting) and Lantus® (long-acting).

Another option to administering injections several times a day to control the blood sugar level is the use of the **insulin pump**. Today there are multiple brands of insulin pumps, such as t:slim®, OmniPod®, and Dexcom®. The insulin pump is a small computerized device (about the size of a pager or smaller) worn on the outside of the body (attached to a belt or slipped into a pocket). The pump reservoir administers **insulin** into the body via an infusion set that consists of a small, flexible plastic tube inserted with a small needle. The tubing connects the pump to the small, flexible tube that is inserted just beneath the skin in one of several acceptable sites for subcutaneous injections. The computer-driven pump administers specific amounts of fast-acting **insulin** on a continuous basis, 24 hours/day. This is known as the basal rate (i.e., amount of insulin/hour × 24 hours a day). This continuous subcutaneous infusion of a basal dose of **insulin** is designed to keep the blood sugar in the desired range between meals and during the night. The pump does not eliminate the need to check the blood sugar throughout the day or the need to administer additional **insulin** based on blood sugar readings. At mealtimes, the individual calculates the amount of **insulin** needed for that meal (usually based on carbohydrate content of the meal) and programs the pump to administer the required amount. This is known as the bolus dose.

The infusion set stays in place for two to three days or more and is then changed and repositioned to a new subcutaneous site. Most individuals who use the insulin pump do so because they feel it gives them better control and more flexibility. See *Figures 13-13A* and *13-13B*.

A newer option for administration of insulin for control of type-2 diabetes is the disposable insulin delivery device. The V-Go® is an example of this device. It mimics the insulin pattern of the body. The small device is placed

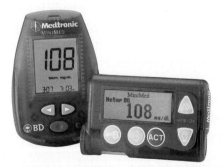 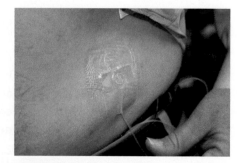

Figure 13-13 (A) Insulin pump, (B) Insulin pump attached to abdomen

(A: Courtesy of Medtronic MiniMed, Inc.; B: Courtesy of Fred Caldwell)

on the skin with an adhesive backing. Once attached, a button is pressed to insert the small needle into the skin. The device provides a continuous preset basal rate of insulin over 24 hours and an on-demand bolus at mealtimes (the bolus at mealtimes is administered by pressing a button on the device). The device has to be changed daily—at the same time each day to be most effective. Patch pumps are becoming popular: instead of having your pump connected to your body via an infusion set and tubing, the patch pump is worn directly on the body.

It is important for people with type 1 or type 2 diabetes to monitor their blood sugar on a regular basis. Frequent self-monitoring of blood **glucose** levels enables individuals with diabetes to obtain optimal blood **glucose** control. Self-monitoring is achieved by using one of many types of blood **glucose** monitors. Most monitoring systems involve obtaining a drop of blood from the fingertip, applying it to the strip specifically designed for the monitor being used, and leaving it on the strip for the specified time. The meter will then display a digital reading of the individual's blood sugar level at that time. Many blood **glucose** meters available today can store readings in a computer memory together with the date and time the reading was measured.

Blood **glucose** readings are used for making changes to the patient's treatment plan, including dietary changes; changes in type, amount, and timing of exercise; and in medications prescribed. The amount of **insulin** to be given is based on the patient's blood **glucose** level before a given meal.

A test that will determine the overall effectiveness of the plan for blood **glucose** control is called the glycohemoglobin A1c or the HbA1c. This blood test reflects the average blood **glucose** levels over a period of approximately three months. If the blood **glucose** levels are consistently high, the test results will be elevated. However, if the blood **glucose** levels are maintained at near-normal levels, the test results will not be greatly elevated. The American Diabetes Association (ADA) recommends that the HbA1c level should be maintained at 7% or below. The goal of achieving these near-normal blood **glucose** levels is made easier by self-monitoring of blood **glucose** levels.

An abnormally high blood **glucose** level is the main criterion for a diagnosis of **diabetes mellitus**. Diagnosis of diabetes is made in one of two ways: (a) a random blood **glucose** drawn in a lab with results greater than 200 mg/dL or (b) fasting blood **glucose** results of 126 mg/dL or more on two separate dates.

Complications of **diabetes mellitus** vary according to the individual and the type of diabetes. The most common acute complication for the person with insulin-dependent diabetes is **insulin shock**, which is the result of a drastic drop in the blood sugar level (severe **hypoglycemia**) due to an overdose of **insulin**, a decreased intake of food, or excessive exercise. Insulin shock is characterized by cool moist skin (damp skin that is cool to the touch), sweatiness (the clothing will be damp or wet), chilliness (the individual will begin to shiver in response to the shocklike symptoms), nervousness, and irritability, which may lead to disorientation and coma if left untreated.

Treatment for insulin shock requires an immediate dose of **glucose** orally if the individual is still alert. If the individual is stuporous and beyond the point of ingesting food or liquid by mouth, treatment (if readily available) would include the injection of the hormone **glucagon** to stimulate the liver to release **glucose** into the bloodstream (raising the blood **glucose** level to a normal level within 15 minutes and maintaining that level for approximately 45 minutes). The individual should then ingest a complex carbohydrate and protein snack to maintain the normal blood sugar level. If the individual is unresponsive, and a **glucagon** emergency kit is not available, emergency help will be necessary.

The individual with type 2 diabetes may also experience a low blood **glucose** level. An appropriate treatment for this would be to drink about 4 ounces of fruit juice, wait 15 minutes, and recheck the blood **glucose** to see if it is over 70 mg/dL. If the blood **glucose** is still too low, the individual should eat another serving of a quick-fix food. These steps should be repeated until the blood **glucose** level is 70 mg/dL or above. Once the blood **glucose** level is 70 mg/dL or above, the individual should eat a meal within the next 30 minutes or a snack if the next meal is an hour or more away.

Other complications of long-term diabetes include poor circulation in the extremities, especially the lower legs and feet; infections that heal poorly due to the decreased circulation; kidney disease and renal failure; **diabetic retinopathy**, which is a leading cause of blindness; involvement of the nervous system (diabetic neuropathy) characterized by numbness (decreased sensitivity of the fingers to touch and grasp); and intermittent but severe episodes of pain in the extremities. People with diabetes who maintain near-normal blood **glucose** levels can reasonably expect to live for many years without major complications.

It was estimated in 2007 (for all ages) that a total of 23.6 million people, or 7.8% of the population, have diabetes. Of that number, 17.9 million people were diagnosed and 5.7 million were undiagnosed. In adults, type 1 diabetes accounts for 5% to 10% of all diagnosed cases of diabetes, and type 2 diabetes accounts for about 90% to 95% of all diagnosed cases of diabetes. Each year, more than 1 million people, aged 20 or older, are diagnosed with diabetes.

diabetic retinopathy
(dye-ah-**BET**-ik ret-in-**OP**-ah-thee)
  retin/o = retina
  -pathy = disease
	A disorder of the blood vessels of the retina of the eye, in which the capillaries of the retina experience localized *areas of bulging* (microaneurysms), hemorrhages, leakage, and scarring.

This disorder occurs as a consequence of an 8- to 10-year duration of **diabetes mellitus**. The scarring, along with the leakage of blood, causes a permanent decline in the sharpness of vision. The inability to get the oxygen and nutrients needed for good vision to the retina will eventually lead to permanent loss of vision. In the United States, **diabetic retinopathy** is the leading cause of blindness.

gestational diabetes (jess-**TAY**-shun-al dye-ah-**BEE**-teez)	A disorder in which women who are not diabetic before pregnancy develop symptoms of diabetes during the pregnancy; that is, they develop an inability to metabolize carbohydrates (**glucose** intolerance) with resultant **hyperglycemia**.

This disorder develops during the latter part of pregnancy, with symptoms usually disappearing at the end of the pregnancy. Women who have **gestational diabetes** have a higher possibility of developing it with subsequent pregnancies. They are also at higher risk of developing type 2 diabetes later in life. Factors that increase the risk of developing **gestational diabetes** include, but are not limited to, the following:

1. Obesity
2. Maternal age over 30 years of age
3. History of birthing large babies (usually over 10 pounds)
4. Family history of diabetes
5. Previous, unexplained, stillborn birth
6. Previous birth with congenital anomalies (defects)

Symptoms vary from classic symptoms of diabetes (such as excessive thirst, hunger, and frequent urination) to being asymptomatic (no symptoms present). Because a high number of pregnant women have **gestational diabetes** without obvious symptoms, all pregnant women are routinely screened for diabetes with a blood test. This usually occurs between weeks 24 and 28 of the pregnancy.

pancreatic cancer
 	
(**pan**-kree-**AT**-ik **CAN**-sir)
  pancreat/o = pancreas
  -ic = pertaining to
	A life-threatening primary malignant neoplasm typically found in the head of the pancreas.

Of those diagnosed with **pancreatic cancer**, 95% lose their lives one to three years after diagnosis. The occurrence of **pancreatic cancer** for smokers is twice that for nonsmokers. Other related risk factors include high-fat diet, **pancreatitis**, exposure to chemicals and toxins, and **diabetes mellitus**.

With a slow onset, **pancreatic cancer** causes nonspecific symptoms such as nausea, anorexia, dull epigastric pain, weight loss, and flatulence. As the tumor grows, the pain worsens. If there is an early diagnosis, surgical removal of the tumor may be possible.

pancreatitis
 	
(**pan**-kree-ah-**TYE**-tis)
  pancreat/o = pancreas
  -itis = inflammation
	An acute or chronic destructive inflammatory condition of the pancreas.

Acute **pancreatitis** presents itself quickly and creates symptoms that vary from mild, self-limiting pancreatic edema to massive necrotizing hemorrhagic **pancreatitis**.

The initial outstanding symptom is severe, continuous epigastric and abdominal pain, which radiates to the back and follows the ingestion of excessive alcohol or a fatty meal. Other symptoms include rigid abdominal distension, decreased bowel sounds, nausea and vomiting, hypotension, elevated temperature, and clammy cold skin. After 24 hours, mild jaundice may appear.

In addition to alcohol abuse, other causes of acute **pancreatitis** include trauma, surgery, metabolic disorders, drugs, infections, or ruptured peptic ulcers. Serious complications may occur, including the development of abscesses or pseudocysts, **diabetes mellitus**, renal failure, heart failure, hypovolemic shock, multiple organ failure, accumulation of fluid within the abdomen (ascites), and adult respiratory distress **syndrome**. Treatment is aimed at resolving the immediate problems, relieving pain and avoiding any further GI irritation, and preventing serious life-threatening complications.

Chronic pancreatitis is a permanent, progressive destruction of pancreatic cells identified with fibrosis, atrophy, fatty degeneration, and calcification. The causes of chronic pancreatitis include alcoholism, malnutrition, surgery, and neoplasm. Symptoms include abdominal pain, large fatty stools, weight loss, and signs and symptoms of **diabetes mellitus**. Treatment includes the administration of pancreatic enzymes, antiemetics, antacids, and **insulin** if its production is stopped or decreased.

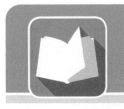

Review Checkpoint

Check your understanding of this section by completing the **Pathological Conditions** exercises in your workbook.

Diagnostic Techniques, Treatments, and Procedures

fasting blood sugar (FBS)	Blood **glucose** sample taken usually early in the morning after the person has been without food or drink since midnight.
	FBS is a more accurate evaluation of the blood **glucose** level because of the fasting state of the body.
glucose tolerance test (GTT) (**GLOO**-kohs **TOL**-er-ans) gluc/o = sugar, sweet -ose = carbohydrate	A test that evaluates the person's ability to tolerate a concentrated oral **glucose** load by measuring the **glucose** levels: 1. Prior to **glucose** administration 2. 30 minutes after **glucose** administration 3. One hour after **glucose** administration 4. Two hours after **glucose** administration 5. Three hours after **glucose** administration In persons with **diabetes mellitus**, the serum **glucose** levels at two hours will be equal to or greater than 200 mg/dL. The person whose **insulin** response is appropriate will have only a minimal elevation in serum **glucose** levels during the first hour.

hemoglobin A1c test (HbA1c)	The **hemoglobin A1c test** is a blood test that shows the average level of **glucose** in an individual's blood during the past 3 months. A small sample of blood is collected from a vein (usually an arm vein) and is sent to the lab for analysis.
	Glucose binds chemically to the hemoglobin molecules in the red blood cells. Therefore, if the blood **glucose** level is elevated, the HbA1c will be elevated. In adults who have poorly controlled diabetes, the HbA1c level may be 8.0% or higher. (Eight percent correlates to an average blood sugar level of 183 mg/dL over the past two to three months.) The American Diabetes Association (ADA) recommends an HbA1c level of less than 7.0%. (Seven percent correlates to an average blood sugar level of 154 mg/dL over the past two to three months.) At a level of less than 7%, the individual can significantly reduce his or her risk for serious complications from diabetes. HbA1c levels for children and teens are different from those of adults.
radioactive iodine uptake (RAIU) test (**ray**-dee-o-**AK**-tiv **EYE**-oh-dine **UP**-tayk)	A **thyroid** function test that evaluates the function of the **thyroid** gland by administering a known amount of radioactive iodine and later placing a gamma ray detector over the **thyroid** gland to determine the percentage or quantity of radioactive iodine absorbed by the gland over specific time periods. It is used in the diagnosis of thyroid problems, particularly hyperthyroidism.
	Persons in hyperthyroid states will have an increased uptake of the iodine. A decreased radioiodine uptake could be an indicator of acute thyroiditis (which can be treated with a course of oral antibiotics).
serum glucose test (**SEE**-rum **GLOO**-kohs) gluc/o = sugar, sweet	A **serum glucose test** measures the amount of **glucose** in the blood at the time the sample was drawn.
	True serum **glucose** elevations are indicative of **diabetes mellitus**. However, the value must be evaluated according to the time of day and the last time the person has eaten. A **glucose** level can be collected in a tube or evaluated with a finger stick.
thyroid echogram (**ultrasound**) (**THIGH**-royd **ECK**-oh-gram) thyr/o = thyroid gland -oid = resembling echo- = sound -gram = record or picture	An ultrasound examination important in distinguishing solid **thyroid** nodules from cystic nodules.
	The type of nodule will provide information for treatment. In addition to differentiating the type of nodule, the **thyroid echogram** can be used to measure the size and shape of the thyroid gland, nodule, and/or goiter.
thyroid function tests (**THIGH**-royd) (T_3, T_4, TSH) thyr/o = thyroid gland -oid = resembling	Laboratory tests that measure the blood levels of the T_3, T_4, and TSH hormones. These blood tests indicate how well the thyroid gland is working.
	The **thyroid** hormones aid in maintaining the body's metabolic rate and tissue growth and development. Hormones T_3 and T_4 are secreted in response to TSH.

thyroid panel	A laboratory blood test that produces an enhanced thyroid profile.
(**THIGH**-royd)	It includes evaluation of the following hormone levels:

thyr/o = thyroid gland
-oid = resembling

- TSH (thyroid-stimulating hormone): evaluates the overall function of the thyroid gland.

- T_4 level (total thyroxine): indicates the total amount of T_4 hormone produced by the thyroid gland.

- Free T_3 (free triiodothyronine): indicates the amount of T_3 present in the cells and tissues, an indication of hormonal balance.

- Free T4 levels (free thyroxine): indicates the total amount of T_4 hormone immediately available for use by the body cells.

thyroid scan	A test that determines the position, size, shape, and physiological function of the **thyroid** gland through the use of radionuclear scanning.
(**THIGH**-royd)	

thyr/o = thyroid gland
-oid = resembling

An image of the **thyroid** is recorded and visualized after the patient receives a radioactive substance. The scan can reveal specific regions in the thyroid that are using either too much or too little radioactive iodine. The **thyroid scan** is helpful in the diagnosis of the following cases:

1. Neck or substernal masses

2. **Thyroid** nodules or goiter

3. Cause of **hyperthyroidism**

thyroid-stimulating hormone (TSH) blood test	A test that measures the concentration of TSH in the blood.

thyr/o = thyroid gland
-oid = resembling

This test is used in differentiating primary **hypothyroidism** (due to a defect in the structure or function of the **thyroid** gland) from secondary **hypothyroidism** (due to insufficient stimulation of the normal **thyroid** gland).

In addition to differentiating primary and secondary **hypothyroidism**, the serum level of TSH is used to monitor **thyroid** hormone replacement. It is important to remember that TSH levels are decreased in persons with a severe illness.

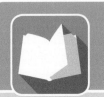

Review Checkpoint

Check your understanding of this section by completing the **Diagnostic Techniques, Treatments, and Procedures** exercises in your workbook.

COMMON ABBREVIATIONS

Abbreviation	Meaning	Abbreviation	Meaning
ACTH	adrenocorticotropic hormone	LTH	lactogenic hormone
ADH	antidiuretic hormone	MSH	melanocyte-stimulating hormone
BMR	basal metabolic rate	Na	sodium
Ca	calcium	NIDDM	non-insulin-dependent diabetes mellitus; also known as type 2 diabetes
DI	**diabetes insipidus**		
DKA	diabetic ketoacidosis		
DM	**diabetes mellitus**	OT	**oxytocin**
FBS	fasting blood sugar	PBI	protein-bound iodine
FSH	follicle-stimulating hormone	PTH	parathyroid hormone
GH	growth hormone	RAI	radioactive iodine
GTT	**glucose tolerance test**	RAIU	radioactive iodine uptake
HDL	high-density lipoprotein	T3	**triiodothyronine** (**thyroid** hormone)
HbA1c	hemoglobin A1c		
IDDM	insulin-dependent diabetes mellitus; also known as type 1 diabetes	T4	**thyroxine** (**thyroid** hormone)
		TFT	thyroid function test
		TSH	thyroid-stimulating hormone
K	potassium	VLDL	very-low-density lipoprotein
LH	luteinizing hormone		

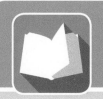

Review Checkpoint

Check your understanding of this section by completing the **Common Abbreviations** exercises in your workbook.

WRITTEN AND AUDIO TERMINOLOGY REVIEW

Review each of the following terms from this chapter. Study the spelling of each term and write the definition in the space provided. Check definitions by looking the term up in the glossary.

Term	Pronunciation	Definition
acromegaly	☐ **ak**-roh-**MEG**-ah-lee	_____
Addison's disease	☐ **AD**-ih-sons dih-**ZEEZ**	_____
adenohypophysis	☐ ad-eh-noh-high-**POFF**-ih-sis	_____
adenoma	☐ **ad**-eh-**NOH**-mah	_____
adenopathy	☐ **ad**-eh-**NOP**-ah-thee	_____
adrenalectomy	☐ ad-**ree**-nal-**ECK**-toh-mee	_____
adrenalitis	☐ **ah**-dree-nal-**EYE**-tis	_____
adrenocortical	☐ ad-**ree**-noh-**KOR**-tih-kal	_____
adrenomegaly	☐ ad-**ree**-noh-**MEG**-ah-lee	_____
aldosterone	☐ al-**DOSS**-te-rohn	_____
androgen	☐ **AN**-droh-jen	_____
antidiuretic	☐ **an**-tye-**dye**-yoo-**RET**-ik	_____
Conn's disease	☐ **KONZ** disease	_____
cortex	☐ **COR**-tex	_____
corticosteroid	☐ **kor**-tih-koh-**STAIR**-oyd	_____
cortisol	☐ **COR**-tih-sal	_____
cretinism	☐ **KREE**-tin-izm	_____
Cushing's syndrome	☐ **CUSH**-ings **SIN**-drom	_____
diabetes insipidus	☐ **dye**-ah-**BEE**-teez in-**SIP**-ih-dus	_____
diabetes mellitus	☐ **dye**-ah-**BEE**-teez **MELL**-ih-tus	_____
diabetic retinopathy	☐ **dye**-ah-**BET**-ik ret-in-**OP**-ah-thee	_____
dipsosis	☐ dip-**SOH**-sis	_____
dwarfism	☐ **DWARF**-ism	_____

Term	Pronunciation	Definition
endocrine gland	☐ **EN**-doh-krin gland	_____
endocrinologist	☐ **en**-doh-krin-**OL**-oh-jist	_____
endocrinology	☐ **en**-doh-krin-**OL**-oh-jee	_____
epinephrine	☐ **ep**-ih-**NEF**-rin	_____
estrogen	☐ **ESS**-troh-jen	_____
euthyroid	☐ yoo-**THIGH**-royd	_____
exocrine gland	☐ **ECK**-soh-krin gland	_____
exophthalmia	☐ eck-sof-**THAL**-mee-ah	_____
exophthalmos	☐ eck-sof-**THAL**-mohs	_____
gestational diabetes	☐ jess-**TAY**-shun-al **dye**-ah-**BEE**-teez	_____
gigantism	☐ **JYE**-gan-tizm	_____
glucagon	☐ **GLOO**-kuh-gon	_____
glucogenesis	☐ **gloo**-koh-**JEN**-eh-sis	_____
gluconeogenesis	☐ **gloo**-koh-**nee**-oh-**JEN**-eh-sis	_____
glucose	☐ **GLOO**-kohs	_____
glucose tolerance test (GTT)	☐ **GLOO**-kohs **TOL**-er-ans test	_____
glycogenesis	☐ **glye**-koh-**JEN**-eh-sis	_____
glycogenolysis	☐ **glye**-koh-jen-**OL**-eh-sis	_____
glycosuria	☐ **glye**-kohs-**YOO**-ree-ah	_____
goiter	☐ **GOY**-ter	_____
gonadotropic	☐ goh-**nad**-oh-**TROH**-pik	_____
gonadotropin	☐ goh-**nad**-oh-**TROH**-pin	_____
gonads	☐ **GOH**-nadz	_____
gynecomastia	☐ **gigh**-neh-koh-**MASS**-tee-ah	_____
hirsutism	☐ **HER**-soot-izm	_____
hypercalcemia	☐ **high**-per-kal-**SEE**-mee-ah	_____
hyperglycemia	☐ **high**-per-glye-**SEE**-mee-ah	_____
hypergonadism	☐ **high**-per-**GOH**-nad-izm	_____
hyperinsulinism	☐ **high**-per-**IN**-soo-lin-izm	_____
hyperkalemia	☐ **high**-per-kal-**EE**-mee-ah	_____
hypernatremia	☐ **high**-per-nah-**TREE**-mee-ah	_____

Term	Pronunciation	Definition
hyperparathyroidism (hypercalcemia)	☐ **high**-per-pair-ah-**THIGH**-royd-izm (**high**-per-kal-**SEE**-mee-ah)	_____
hyperpituitarism	☐ **high**-per-pih-**TOO**-ih-tair-izm	_____
hyperthyroidism	☐ **high**-per-**THIGH**-royd-izm	_____
hypocalcemia	☐ **high**-poh-kal-**SEE**-mee-ah	_____
hypoglycemia	☐ **high**-poh-glye-**SEE**-mee-ah	_____
hypokalemia	☐ **high**-poh-kal-**EE**-mee-ah	_____
hyponatremia	☐ **high**-poh-nah-**TREE**-mee-ah	_____
hypoparathyroidism	☐ **high**-poh-**pair**-ah-**THIGH**-royd-izm	_____
hypophysectomy	☐ **high**-poff-ih-**SEK**-toh-mee	_____
hypopituitarism	☐ **high**-poh-pih-**TOO**-ih-tah-rizm	_____
hypothyroidism	☐ **high**-poh-**THIGH**-royd-izm	_____
insulin	☐ **IN**-soo-lin	_____
lactogen	☐ **LAK**-toh-jen	_____
medulla	☐ meh-**DULL**-lah	_____
metabolism	☐ meh-**TAB**-oh-lizm	_____
myxedema	☐ **miks**-eh-**DEE**-mah	_____
norepinephrine	☐ nor-**EP**-ih-**neh**-frin	_____
oxytocin	☐ **ok**-see-**TOH**-sin	_____
pancreatic cancer	☐ **pan**-kree-**AT**-ik **CAN**-sir	_____
pancreatitis	☐ **pan**-kree-ah-**TYE**-tis	_____
parathyroidectomy	☐ **pair**-ah-**thigh**-royd-**ECK**-toh-mee	_____
pheochromocytoma	☐ **fee**-oh-**kroh**-moh-sigh-**TOH**-mah	_____
polydipsia	☐ **pol**-ee-**DIP**-see-ah	_____
polyuria	☐ **pol**-ee-**YOO**-ree-ah	_____
primary aldosteronism	☐ primary al-**DOSS**-ter-ohn-izm	_____
progesterone	☐ proh-**JESS**-ter-ohn	_____
radioactive iodine uptake test (RAIU)	☐ **ray**-dee-oh-**AK**-tiv **EYE**-oh-dine **UP**-take test	_____
serum glucose test	☐ **SEE**-rum **GLOO**-kohs test	_____

Term	Pronunciation	Definition
somatotropic hormone	☐ soh-**mat**-oh-**TROH**-pik hormone	_____
syndrome	☐ **SIN**-drom	_____
tetany	☐ **TET**-ah-nee	_____
thymoma	☐ thigh-**MOH**-mah	_____
thymopoietin	☐ **thigh**-moh-**POY**-eh-tin	_____
thymosin	☐ thigh-**MOH**-sin	_____
thyroid	☐ **THIGH**-royd	_____
thyroid echogram	☐ **THIGH**-royd **ECK**-oh-gram	_____
thyroiditis	☐ **thigh**-royd-**EYE**-tis	_____
thyroiditis (Hashimoto's)	☐ **thigh**-royd-**EYE**-tis (**HASH**-ee-**moh**-toz)	_____
thyrotoxicosis	☐ **thigh**-roh-**toks**-ih-**KOH**-sis	_____
thyroxine	☐ thigh-**ROKS**-in	_____
toxicology	☐ **toks**-ih-**KOL**-oh-jee	_____
triiodothyronine	☐ **try**-eye-**oh**-doh-**THIGH**-roh-neen	_____
Virilism	☐ **VEER**-il-izm	_____

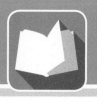

Review Checkpoint

Apply what you have learned in this chapter by completing the **Putting It All Together** exercise in your workbook.

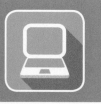

Online Resources

For additional study tools, including PowerPoint® slides and animations, go to the Student Companion Website.

Chapter Review Exercises

The following exercises provide a more in-depth review of the chapter material. Your goal in these exercises is to complete each section at a minimum 80% level of accuracy. A space has been provided for your score at the end of each section.

A. Term to Definition

Define each term by writing the definition in the space provided. Check the box if you are able to complete this exercise correctly the first time (without referring to the answers). Each correct answer is worth 10 points. Record your score in the space provided at the end of the exercise.

☐ 1. acromegaly _____

☐ 2. endocrinologist _____

☐ 3. exophthalmia _____

☐ 4. glucagon _____

☐ 5. glycogenesis _____

☐ 6. hirsutism _____

☐ 7. polydipsia _____

☐ 8. polyuria _____

☐ 9. tetany _____

☐ 10. virilism _____

Number correct _____ × 10 points/correct answer: Your score _____%

B. Spelling

Circle the correctly spelled term in each pairing of words. Each correct answer is worth 10 points. Record your score in the space provided at the end of the exercise.

1. acromegally	acromegaly
2. luteinizing	leutenizing
3. islets (of Langerhans)	ilets (of Langerhans)
4. cretanism	cretinism
5. uthyroid	euthyroid
6. hirsutism	hirtsutism
7. myxedema	mixedema
8. virelism	virilism
9. pancreatitis	pancretitis
10. thyroidectomy	throidectomy

Number correct _____ × 10 points/correct answer: Your score _____%

C. Matching Abbreviations

Match the abbreviations on the left with the appropriate definition on the right. Each correct response is worth 10 points. Record your score in the space provided at the end of the exercise.

_____ 1. ACTH   a. thyroid-stimulating hormone

_____ 2. BMR   b. protein-bound iodine

_____ 3. FBS   c. non-insulin-dependent diabetes mellitus (type 2)

_____ 4. GTT   d. adrenocorticotropic hormone

_____ 5. HDL   e. basal metabolic rate

_____ 6. K   f. hyperdiabetic lipidemia

_____ 7. Na   g. calcium

_____ 8. NIDDM   h. sodium

_____ 9. PBI   i. fasting blood sugar

_____ 10. TSH   j. glucose tolerance test

     k. high-density lipoprotein

     l. potassium

Number correct _____ **× 10 points/correct answer: Your score** _____%

D. Definition to Term

Using the following definitions, identify and provide the medical word to match the definition. Write the word in the first space and the appropriate combining form for the word in the second space. Each correct answer is worth 5 points. Record your score in the space provided at the end.

1. Enlargement of the extremities.

   _____   _____
   (word)   (combining from)

2. Surgical removal of one or both adrenal glands.

   _____   _____
   (word)   (combining from)

3. More than normal blood calcium level.

   _____   _____
   (word)   (combining from)

4. The study of the endocrine system.

   _____   _____
   (word)   (combining from)

5. More than normal blood potassium level.

   _____   _____
   (word)   (combining from)

6. Inflammation of the pancreas.

   _____   _____
   (word)   (combining from)

(continued)

7. Condition of an overactive thyroid gland.

_____   _____
(word)   (combining from)

8. The study of poisons and their antidotes.

_____   _____
(word)   (combining from)

9. More than normal blood sodium level.

_____   _____
(word)   (combining from)

10. Any disease of a gland.

_____   _____
(word)   (combining from)

Number correct _____ × 5 points/correct answer: Your score _____ %

E. Crossword Puzzle

Read the clues carefully and complete the puzzle. Each crossword answer is worth 10 points. When you have completed the crossword puzzle, total your points and enter your score in the space provided.

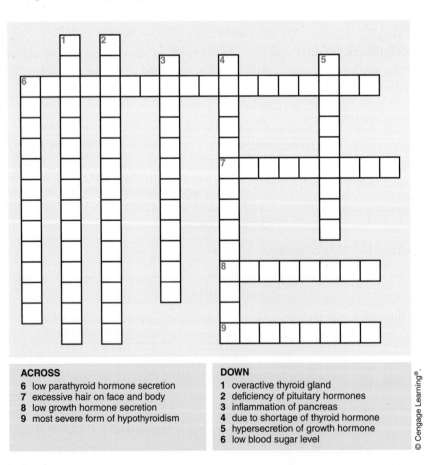

ACROSS
6 low parathyroid hormone secretion
7 excessive hair on face and body
8 low growth hormone secretion
9 most severe form of hypothyroidism

DOWN
1 overactive thyroid gland
2 deficiency of pituitary hormones
3 inflammation of pancreas
4 due to shortage of thyroid hormone
5 hypersecretion of growth hormone
6 low blood sugar level

© Cengage Learning®.

Number correct _____ × 10 points/correct answer: Your score _____%

F. Matching Hormones

Match the hormones on the left with the principal endocrine gland that secretes them on the right. Each correct answer is worth 10 points. Record your score in the space provided at the end of the exercise.

_____	1. growth hormone	a. pancreas
_____	2. antidiuretic hormone	b. adrenal cortex
_____	3. thyroxine	c. anterior pituitary gland
_____	4. parathormone	d. ovaries
_____	5. thymosin	e. testes
_____	6. hydrocortisone	f. thymus gland
_____	7. epinephrine (adrenaline)	g. parathyroid glands
_____	8. testosterone	h. thyroid gland
_____	9. estrogen	i. posterior pituitary gland
_____	10. insulin	j. adrenal medulla

Number correct _____ **× 10 points/correct answer: Your score** _____%

G. Proofreading Skills

Read the following portion of a history and physical report. For each boldface term, provide a brief definition and indicate if the term is spelled correctly. If it is misspelled, provide the correct spelling. Each correct answer is worth 10 points. Record your score in the space provided at the end of the exercise.

Example:

Polyphagia _excessive eating_ _____

Spelled correctly? ✔ Yes   ☐ No _____

HISTORY AND PHYSICAL EXAMINATION

Hillcrest
medical center

PATIENT NAME: Jane M. Smith

ROOM NO: 1256

HOSPITAL NO: 65231

ATTENDING PHYSICIAN
Richard Wright, MD

ADMISSION DATE: 06/22/2014

CHIEF COMPLAINT
Tiredness, headaches, increased thirst and hunger, frequency of urination, nervousness, irritability, sleepiness, vague pains, general malaise.

(continued)

HISTORY AND PHYSICAL EXAMINATION
Patient Name: Jane M. Smith
Room No: 1256
Hospital No: 65231
Admission Date: 06/22/2014
Page 2

HISTORY OF PRESENT ILLNESS
This 42-year-old female was admitted to the hospital because of a 3-week history of **polyuria**, **polydispia**, and **polyphagia**. She has been very nervous, irritable, and very sensitive emotionally and cries easily. During this time period, she has had frequent headaches, has become very sleepy and tired after eating, and has had leg pains. She was seen in my office 5 days ago and found then to have a blood pressure of 198/98 mmHg and **glycasuria** (4+). Lab tests revealed **hyperglycemia**.

MEDICATIONS
She takes Zyrtec for seasonal allergies.

ALLERGIES
Expresses allergies to dust, mold, and pollen but has not been tested.

FAMILY AND SOCIAL HISTORY
She has had the common childhood diseases. She states that when she was in college (approximately 17 years ago), she had bouts of **hypoglycemia** that were pretty severe at times. She found that adding protein snacks throughout the day seemed to help the situation. Nine years ago, when she was pregnant, she was found to have **gestational diabetes**, but this disappeared after delivery. She has no history of surgeries.

There is a strong family history of diabetes. Father and 2 sisters have **diabetes mellitis**. Mother has **hyperthroidism** with somewhat noticeable **exopthalmia**, but this is somewhat controlled with **thyroxine**. One brother was thought to have diabetes as a child, but GTT revealed that his blood glucose levels were normal.

PHYSICAL EXAMINATION
GENERAL APPEARANCE: This is a chronically ill-appearing female, alert, oriented, and cooperative. She moves with some difficulty because of fatigue and malaise.

VITAL SIGNS: Blood pressure 180/90, heart rate 100 and regular, respirations 22.

HEENT: Normocephalic. No scalp lesions. Dry eyes with conjunctival injection. Dry nasal mucosa.

SKIN: She has an area of mild ecchymosis on her skin and some erythema; she has some scales located on the flexor surfaces of the arms, but no obvious skin breakdown. No vesicles noted on the skin. One small skin laceration noted on the left forearm.

PULMONARY: Clear to percussion and auscultation.

CARDIOVASCULAR: No murmurs or gallops noted.

ABDOMEN: Protuberant, no organomegaly, and positive bowel sounds.

NEUROLOGIC: Cranial nerves II through XII are grossly intact. Diffuse hyporeflexia.

MUSCULOSKELETAL: Pulses present distally in both legs.

(continued)

HISTORY AND PHYSICAL EXAMINATION
Patient Name: Jane M. Smith
Room No: 1256
Hospital No: 65231
Admission Date: 06/22/2014
Page 3

PROBLEMS:
1. Possible diabetes mellitus
2. Hypertension

PLAN
Admit patient for laboratory testing for diabetes mellitus. If results are positive, as suspected, will begin patient on diet and insulin regimen (Novolog insulin). Will refer patient to diabetic education services. Will prescribe medication to control hypertension.

_____

Richard Wright, MD

RW:xx

D:06/22/2014

T:06/23/2014

1. **polyuria** _____
   Spelled Correctly?   ☐ Yes   ☐ No _____

2. **polydispia** _____
   Spelled Correctly?   ☐ Yes   ☐ No _____

3. **glycasuria** _____
   Spelled Correctly?   ☐ Yes   ☐ No _____

4. **hyperglycemia** _____
   Spelled Correctly?   ☐ Yes   ☐ No _____

5. **hypoglycemia** _____
   Spelled Correctly?   ☐ Yes   ☐ No _____

6. **gestational diabetes** _____
   Spelled Correctly?   ☐ Yes   ☐ No _____

7. **diabetes mellitis** _____
   Spelled Correctly?   ☐ Yes   ☐ No _____

8. **hyperthroidism** _____
   Spelled Correctly?   ☐ Yes   ☐ No _____

9. **exopthalmia** _____
   Spelled Correctly?   ☐ Yes   ☐ No _____

10. **thyroxine** _____
    Spelled Correctly?   ☐ Yes   ☐ No _____

Number correct _____ × *10 points/correct answer: Your score* _____%

H. Completion

Complete each sentence with the most appropriate pathological condition. Each correct answer is worth 10 points. Record your score in the space provided at the end of the exercise.

1. An abnormal overgrowth of the bones in the feet, hands, and face with onset occurring after puberty and epiphyseal closure is known as:

   _____

2. A disease in which chronic thyroiditis leads to enlargement of the thyroid. This disease of the immune system in which the gland tissue is destroyed by antibodies and replaced with fibrous tissue is known as:

   _____

3. Hypertrophy of the thyroid gland resulting in an excessive secretion of the thyroid hormone, causing an extremely high body metabolism, is known as:

   _____

4. An acute, sometimes fatal, incident of overactivity of the thyroid gland resulting in excessive secretion of thyroid hormone is known as:

   _____

5. A cluster of symptoms occurring due to an excessive amount of circulating cortisol or ACTH is termed:

   _____

6. A vascular tumor of the adrenal medulla that produces extra epinephrine and norepinephrine leading to persistent or intermittent hypertension and heart palpitations is known as:

   _____

7. A condition that occurs as a consequence of an 8- to 10-year duration of diabetes mellitus in which the capillaries of the retina experience scarring is known as:

   _____

8. A life-threatening primary malignant neoplasm typically found in the head of the pancreas is known as:

   _____

9. Thyroid function is evaluated by administering a known amount of radioactive iodine and later placing a gamma ray detector over the thyroid gland to determine the percentage or quantity of radioactive iodine absorbed by the gland over specific time. This diagnostic test is called:

   _____

10. An ultrasound examination important in distinguishing solid thyroid nodules from cystic nodules is a:

    _____

Number correct _____ × 10 points/correct answer: Your score _____%

I. Matching Conditions

Read the descriptions on the right and match them with the appropriate pathological conditions on the left. Each correct answer is worth 10 points. Record your score in the space provided at the end of the exercise.

_____ 1. diabetes mellitus

_____ 2. simple goiter

_____ 3. Addison's disease

_____ 4. hyperparathyroidism

a. occurs as a consequence of an 8- to 10-year duration of diabetes mellitus in which the capillaries of the retina experience scarring

b. excretion of excessive amounts of aldosterone, the most influential of the mineralocorticoids

_____ 5. primary aldosteronism

_____ 6. diabetic retinopathy

_____ 7. virilism

_____ 8. thyroid cancer

_____ 9. diabetes insipidus

_____ 10. thyrotoxicosis

c. output of extreme amounts of adrenocortical androgens caused by an adrenal tumor or hyperplasia typically in adult women (30 to 40 years)

d. an acute, sometimes fatal, incident of overactivity of the thyroid gland, resulting in excessive secretion of thyroid hormone

e. a life-threatening disease process caused from failure of the adrenal cortex to secrete adequate mineralocorticoids and glucocorticoids resulting from an autoimmune process, a neoplasm, an infection, or a hemorrhage in the gland

f. escalated activity of the parathyroid that leads to high levels of calcium in the blood and low levels of calcium in the bones as a result of demineralization, the breakdown of bone

g. a deficiency in the secretion of antidiuretic hormone (ADH) by the posterior pituitary gland

h. a disorder of the pancreas in which the beta cells of the islets of Langerhans of the pancreas fail to produce an adequate amount of insulin

i. hyperplasia, an elevation in the amount of cells of the thyroid gland

j. malignant tumors of the thyroid gland lead to dysfunction of the gland and thus inadequate or excessive secretion of the thyroid hormone

_**Number correct** _____ × **10 points/correct answer: Your score** _____%_

J. Definition to Term

Using the following definitions, identify and provide the word for the pathological condition to match the definition. (A clue has been provided for the number of words needed in your answer.) Each correct answer is worth 10 points. Record your score in the space provided at the end of the exercise.

1. congenital hypopituitarism

_____

(one word)

2. thyroid gland hyperplasia

_____

(three words)

3. chronic enlargement of the thyroid gland

_____

(two words)

4. causes an extremely high body metabolism

_____

(one word)

5. unnatural protruding of the eyes

_____

(one word)

(_continued_)

6. results in low levels of calcium in the blood

_____

(one word)

7. occurs when large doses of glucocorticoids are given over a period of time

_____

(two words)

8. excess secretion of the human growth hormone before puberty

_____

(one word)

9. causes an extremely low body metabolism

_____

(one word)

10. a result of demineralization in the bones

_____

(one word)

Number correct _____ × *10 points/correct answer: Your score* _____%

K. Word Search

Read each definition carefully and identify the applicable word from the list that follows. Enter the word in the space provided, and then find it in the puzzle and circle it. The words may be read up, down, diagonally, across, or backward. Each correct answer is worth 10 points. Record your score in the space provided at the end of the exercise.

hypoglycemia	virilism	myxedema
thyrotoxicosis	aldosteronism	Cushings
acromegaly	cretinism	goiter
parathyroidism	hyperthyroidism	

Example: Low blood sugar

hypoglycemia _____

1. Excretion of excessive amounts of aldosterone, the most influential of the mineralocorticoids, is known as primary:

_____

2. This adrenal gland syndrome is characterized by central obesity, round "moon" face, edema, hypertension, and supraclavicular fat pads (buffalo hump).

_____

3. Hyperplasia of the thyroid gland.

_____

4. An acute, sometimes fatal, incident of overactivity of the thyroid gland resulting in excessive secretion of thyroid hormones; also known as thyroid storm.

_____

5. An abnormal overgrowth of the bones of the feet, hands, and face with the onset occurring after puberty.

_____

6. Congenital hypothyroidism.

_____

7. The most severe form of hypothyroidism.

_____

8. Increased activity of this gland leads to high levels of calcium in the blood and low levels of calcium in the bones.

_____

9. The development of masculine physical traits in the female such as growth of facial and body hair, increased secretion of the sebaceous glands, deepening of the voice, and enlargement of the clitoris.

_____

10. Excessive secretion of the thyroid hormone, causing extremely high body metabolism.

_____

Number correct _____ × *10 points/correct answer: Your score* _____%

P	E	H	Y	P	O	G	L	Y	C	E	M	I	A	G
A	E	Y	D	A	B	N	I	A	L	L	I	U	G	S
R	D	P	Y	D	C	U	A	E	I	C	G	E	N	S
A	A	E	S	C	I	H	C	D	I	R	E	G	N	E
T	A	R	H	U	S	S	R	L	E	E	I	O	N	A
H	C	T	Y	S	I	T	O	N	O	T	S	I	D	M
Y	C	H	O	H	H	R	M	N	O	I	Y	T	O	M
R	N	Y	R	I	P	L	E	X	D	N	E	E	U	X
O	A	R	E	N	I	N	G	D	T	I	P	R	R	L
I	T	O	C	G	B	N	A	X	T	S	N	M	I	A
D	I	I	E	S	I	R	L	R	L	M	A	E	I	T
I	E	D	P	A	L	N	Y	E	A	D	D	R	C	I
S	N	I	M	S	I	L	I	R	I	V	R	S	N	O
M	S	S	A	I	E	S	U	S	P	O	S	U	P	N
H	O	M	M	Y	X	E	D	E	M	A	S	Y	A	T
T	H	Y	R	O	T	O	X	I	C	O	S	I	S	L
S	M	S	I	N	O	R	E	T	S	O	D	L	A	N

L. Medical Scenario

The following medical scenario presents information on one of the pathological conditions discussed in this chapter. Read the scenario carefully and select the most appropriate answer for each question that follows. Each correct answer is worth 20 points. Record your score in the space provided at the end of the exercise.

Marie Gonzales, a 47-year-old mother of four, has just returned to the physician's office for the first time after receiving the medical diagnosis of type 2 diabetes mellitus. She speaks English as a second langsuage and has much uncertainty about her new diagnosis. She has numerous questions for the health care professional.

1. The health care professional will base her responses to Mrs. Gonzales' questions about type 2 diabetes mellitus on which of the following facts? In clients with diabetes mellitus type 2, there is a(n):

   a. decreased production of parathyroid hormone, resulting in hypocalcemia

   b. excessive amount of cortisol or ACTH circulating in the blood

   c. cellular resistance to insulin and/or decreased production of insulin from the pancreatic beta cells

   d. absolute deficiency of insulin due to destruction of all pancreatic beta cells, requiring dependence on external insulin

2. Mrs. Gonzales was very curious about how her physician knew for sure that she had diabetes mellitus. She asked the health care professional if there could be a mistake, because she rarely ate anything with high sugar content. The best explanation by the health care professional would include the criteria for diagnosing diabetes mellitus, which may include (select all that apply):

   1. fasting blood glucose of more than 126 mg/dL

   2. random blood glucose of more than 200 mg/dL

   3. fasting blood glucose of less than 100 mg/dL

   4. HbA1c of 6% or more times 3 months

      a. 1, 2

      b. 2, 3

      c. 3, 4

      d. 2, 4

3. Mrs. Gonzales is taught about the acute complications of diabetes mellitus. When the health care professional explains that she may feel nervous and irritable and have cool, sweaty skin, she is describing which of the following?

   a. hyperglycemia

   b. hypoglycemia

   c. diabetic ketoacidosis

   d. thyrotoxicosis

4. The health care professional explains that when Mrs. Gonzales's blood glucose level is very low, the first thing she should do is:

   a. administer insulin

   b. administer glucagon

   c. wait until the next regular mealtime before eating more food

   d. drink about 4 oz. of fruit juice, wait 15 minutes, and recheck the blood glucose level to see if it is over 70 mg/dL

5. Mrs. Gonzales asks the health care professional about gestational diabetes. She wants to clarify if these two types of diabetes are the same. The health care professional explains that gestational diabetes is a(n):

   a. disorder of the blood vessels of the retina of the eye in which the capillaries of the retina experience localized areas of bulging, hemorrhages, and scarring

   b. disorder in which women develop diabetes during pregnancy, with symptoms typically disappearing at the end of pregnancy

   c. a condition of the adrenal gland in which a cluster of symptoms occur as a result of excessive cortisol or ACTH circulating in the blood

   d. excessive secretion of the thyroid hormone that causes an extremely high body metabolism, hypertrophy of the thyroid gland, and multisystem changes

Number correct _____ × *20 points/correct answer: Your score* _____ *%*

The Special Senses

CHAPTER CONTENT

OBJECTIVES

Upon completing this chapter and the review exercises at the end of the chapter, the learner should be able to:

1. Correctly identify and label the structures of the eye.

2. Identify and define 20 pathological conditions of the eye and ear.

3. Identify at least 10 diagnostic techniques used in treating disorders of the eye and ear.

4. Correctly spell and pronounce terms listed on the Written and Audio Terminology Review, using the phonetic pronunciations provided.

5. Create at least 10 medical terms related to the eye and ear and identify the appropriate combining form(s) for each term.

6. Identify at least 20 abbreviations common to the eye and ear.

7. Identify the pathway of sound from the external auditory canal to the cerebral cortex.

Overview of the Eye

Remember the saying "A picture is worth a thousand words." What a true statement! If you were a camera, you could capture the moment in a photograph by aiming in the right direction, adjusting the lens to bring the object into clear focus, and opening the shutter to allow just the right amount of light to enter upon the sensitive film layer to capture the picture. The processing of the picture, however, would be up to your owner!

You, however, are not a camera; but you do possess the ability to capture the moment with your eyes! As you observe a scene, the lens of your eye will adjust to bring the object into clear focus. The pupil of your eye will constrict to allow less light to enter in a bright setting or will dilate to allow more light to enter in a darker setting. Through several processes of bending the light rays, the image finally reaches the sensitive nerve cell layer of the eye (called the retina). From the retina, the image is transmitted to the brain for interpretation (or processing)—and so you have your picture.

As we discuss the eye, you will gain an understanding of the structure and function of this vital organ we take for granted but depend on so completely. We will also discuss the corrections for errors of refraction (inability to focus clearly), pathological conditions of the eye, and treatments and procedures common to the eye. As you read, you will see things more clearly!

Anatomy and Physiology (Eye)

The eyes are housed in bony orbits located within the facial bones, at the front of the skull. Embedded in a mass of orbital fat for protection and insulation, each eye is supplied by one of a pair of **optic** nerves. Most of the eye is contained within the bony orbit, with

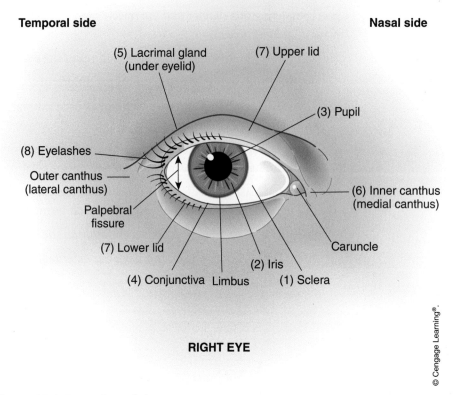

Temporal side　　　　　　　　　　　　　　　　　　　Nasal side

(5) Lacrimal gland
(under eyelid)

(7) Upper lid

(3) Pupil

(8) Eyelashes

Outer canthus
(lateral canthus)

Palpebral
fissure

(6) Inner canthus
(medial canthus)

(7) Lower lid

Caruncle

(4) Conjunctiva　Limbus

(2) Iris

(1) Sclera

RIGHT EYE

© Cengage Learning®.

Figure 14-1 Front view of the eye

only the anterior portion of the eye being exposed to view. We begin the description of the eye structures based on the frontal view of the eye shown in *Figure 14-1*.

The **(1) sclera** is the tough, white outer covering that surrounds the eyeball except at the front of the eye. It maintains the shape of the eyeball and serves as a protective covering for the eye. The colored portion of the eye is known as the **(2) iris**, which may appear to be blue, green, brown, or hazel (yellowish brown). In the center of the iris is an opening called the **(3) pupil**. The pupil controls the amount of light entering the eye, and its diameter is regulated by relaxation and contraction of the iris. The **(4) conjunctiva** is the thin, transparent tissue that covers the outer surface of the eye. It begins at the outer edge of the **cornea**, covering the visible part of the **sclera** and lining the inside of the eyelids.

The conjunctiva is colorless but appears white because it covers the **sclera**. If the blood vessels beneath the conjunctiva become dilated due to irritation, it will have a reddish ("bloodshot") appearance. Crying, smoke, dust, and other eye irritants can cause the blood vessels of the eyes to dilate and give the reddened appearance.

Located at the upper outer edge of each eye (under the upper eyelid) is the **(5) lacrimal gland**, which produces tears. The tears flow constantly across the conjunctival surfaces to cleanse and lubricate them. Tears help prevent bacterial infections in the eye due to the presence of an antibacterial enzyme called lysozyme, which destroys microorganisms. Tears drain from the eye through the **lacrimal duct**, located at the **(6) inner canthus** (also called the medial canthus) of the eye. In addition to the body's natural production

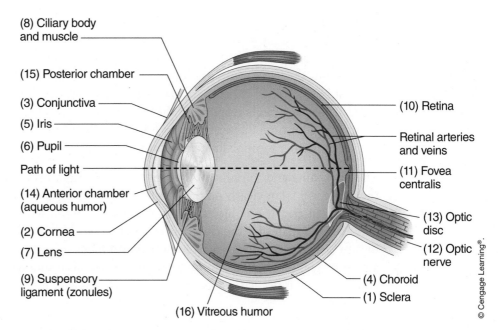

(8) Ciliary body and muscle

(15) Posterior chamber

(3) Conjunctiva

(5) Iris

(6) Pupil

Path of light

(14) Anterior chamber (aqueous humor)

(2) Cornea

(7) Lens

(9) Suspensory ligament (zonules)

(10) Retina

Retinal arteries and veins

(11) Fovea centralis

(13) Optic disc

(12) Optic nerve

(4) Choroid

(1) Sclera

(16) Vitreous humor

© Cengage Learning®.

Figure 14-2 Lateral cross section of the eye

of tears for functional purposes, the human eye also produces tears in response to an emotional upset in the form of crying.

The upper and lower **(7) eyelids** are continuous with the skin and cover the eyeball, keeping the surface of the eyeball lubricated and protected from dust and debris through their blinking motion. The eyelid skin is very thin. The **(8) eyelashes** are located along the edges of the eyelids. They help further protect the eyeball by preventing foreign materials and/or insects from coming in contact with the surface of the eyeball.

The lateral cross section of the eye, illustrated in *Figure 14-2*, shows the structures of the eye from front to back. This figure serves as a visual reference as the discussion of the eye continues.

The **(1) sclera**, also known as the "white of the eye," is thinnest near the anterior surface of the eye (at the insertion point of muscles that move the eye) and thickest at the back of the eye (near the opening for the entrance of the **optic** nerve). Continuous with the anterior portion of the **sclera** is the **(2) cornea** (protected by corneal epithelium), which is a transparent, nonvascular layer covering the colored part of the eye, known as the iris. The **(3) conjunctiva** covers the outer surface of the eye, beginning at the outer edge of the cornea.

The vascular middle layer of the eye (known as the uvea) contains the **(4) choroid**, a layer just beneath the **sclera**, which contains extensive capillaries that provide the blood supply and nutrients to the eye; the iris; and the ciliary body. The **(5) iris**, which is the colored portion of the eye, can be seen through the transparent corneal layer. In the center of the iris is a round opening called the **(6) pupil**.

The pupil controls the amount of light entering the eye by contracting or dilating. This action is actually controlled by two sets of muscles within the iris: the radial muscles within the iris (that dilate the pupil in dim light to allow more light to enter the eye) and the circular muscles within the iris, which constrict the pupil in bright light to allow less light to enter the eye.

Posterior to the iris is the **(7) lens**, a colorless biconvex structure that aids in focusing the images clearly on the sensitive nerve cell layer called the retina. On each side of the lens is the **(8) ciliary body**, which secretes **aqueous humor** and contains muscles responsible for adjusting the lens to view near objects. Radiating from the ciliary body are numerous straight fibrils (called **(9) suspensory ligaments**) that attach to the lens and hold it in place. These ligaments respond to the contraction and relaxation of the ciliary body muscles to adjust the shape of the lens for proper focusing of the eye. The lens becomes thicker or thinner through the relaxation and contraction of these sets of muscles.

The thickening and thinning of the lens causes the light rays to bend appropriately so the image will focus clearly on the sensitive nerve cell layer of the eye. The ability of the lens to focus clearly on objects at various distances is known as **accommodation**. The lens accommodates for the closeness of an object by increasing its curvature (or bulging) to bend the rays more sharply so they will focus directly on the retina, producing a clear image. As one ages, the ability of the lens to accommodate to near vision is lost and correction is needed. This condition is discussed later in the section on pathological conditions.

The third innermost layer of the eye is the **(10) retina**. This sensitive nerve cell layer changes the energy of the light rays into nerve impulses. The nerve impulses are transmitted via the **optic** nerve to the brain for interpretation of the image seen by the eye. These nerve cells, which are highly specialized for stimulation by light rays, are called **rods** and **cones**. The cones are responsible for visualizing colors, central vision, and vision in bright light. The highest concentration of cones is in the **(11) fovea centralis**, a small depression located within the **macula lutea**. The macula lutea is an oval, yellowish spot near the center of the retina. When the image focuses directly on the fovea centralis, the sharpest image is obtained. This is known as central vision. The rods (with the highest concentration in the periphery of the retina) are responsible for vision in dim light and for peripheral vision.

The impulses from the retina are transmitted through the **(12) optic nerve** to the brain, where they are interpreted as vision. The only part of the retina insensitive to light is the **(13) optic disc** because it contains no rods or cones (thus also known as the "blind spot" of the eye). The center of the **optic** disc serves as a point of entry for the artery that supplies the retina.

The lens separates the interior of the eye into two cavities: the anterior cavity and the posterior cavity. The anterior cavity contains two chambers: the **(14) anterior chamber** (located in front of the lens and iris and behind the **cornea**) and the **(15) posterior chamber**, located between the iris and the suspensory ligaments. These chambers are filled with a clear watery fluid known as **aqueous humor**, which flows freely between them. It is constantly produced by the ciliary body and is reabsorbed into the venous circulation. The balance between production and absorption of the **aqueous humor** maintains the proper pressure within the eye.

The posterior cavity is posterior to the lens and is filled with **(16) vitreous humor**, a clear jellylike substance that gives shape to the eyeball. The **vitreous** humor is not constantly reproduced. The loss of vitreous humor during an eye injury has a poor visual prognosis mainly because of the associated retinal damage. Vitreous humor can be removed in a surgical procedure called a vitrectomy and replaced by clear fluid without a problem. Both the **aqueous humor** and the **vitreous** humor aid in the refracting, or bending, of light rays as they pass through these chambers on their way to the retina.

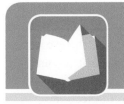

Review Checkpoint

Check your understanding of this section by completing the **Anatomy and Physiology** exercises in your workbook.

The Process of Vision

When light rays enter the eye, they are transmitted through the **cornea**, **aqueous humor**, pupil, lens, and the **vitreous** humor to the retina (where the sensitive nerve cells transmit the image through the **optic** nerve to the brain, where it is interpreted as vision). As the light rays pass through these various structures and fluids, a process of bending occurs that eventually allows the image to focus clearly on the retina, producing a clearly focused image needed for sharp vision. This bending of the light rays as they pass through the various structures of the eye to produce a clear image on the retina is known as **refraction**. If the eye is abnormally shaped or the lens has lost its ability to accommodate to near vision, the individual will have difficulty forming a clear image and will experience blurred vision. These errors of refraction can be adjusted by placing the lenses of glasses in front of the lens of the eye to further refract the light rays, bringing them into focus on the retina. Four errors of refraction are discussed in the section on pathological conditions: **astigmatism**, **hyperopia**, **myopia**, and **presbyopia**.

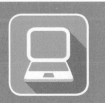

Media Link

Increase your understanding of how we see. Go to the Student Companion Website and watch the **Vision** animation.

VOCABULARY (EYE)

The following vocabulary words are frequently used when discussing the eye.

Word	Definition
ambiopia (am-bee-**OH**-pee-ah) ambi- = both sides -opia = visual condition	Double vision caused by each eye focusing separately; also known as **diplopia**.
amblyopia (am-blee-**OH**-pee-ah) ambly/o = dull, dim -opia = visual condition	Reduced vision that is not correctable with lenses and with no obvious pathological or structural cause ("dullness or dimness of vision").

Word	Definition
ametropia (**am**-eh-**TROH**-pee-ah) -tropia = to turn	A condition in which there is an error of refraction, causing the eye not to focus parallel rays of light on the retina. The word "ametropia" can be used interchangeably with "refractive error." A discussion of four errors of refraction can be found in this chapter (14) in the section on pathological conditions. For more information refer to the discussion on astigmatism, hyperopia, myopia, and presbyopia.
anisocoria (**an**-eye-soh-**KOH**-ree-ah) aniso- = unequal cor/o = pupil -ia = condition	Inequality in the diameter of the pupils of the eyes.
aphakia (ah-**FAY**-kee-ah) a- = without, not phak/o = lens -ia = condition	Absence of the lens of the eye.
aqueous (**AY**-kwee-us) aque/o = water -ous = pertaining to	Watery.
Argyll-Robertson pupil (ar-**GILL ROB**-ert-son pupil)	A pupil that constricts upon accommodation but not in response to light. This can be due to **miosis** or advanced neurosyphilis.
biomicroscopy (**BYE**-oh-mye-**kros**-koh-pee) bio- = life micr/o = small -scopy = process of viewing	Ophthalmic examination of the eye by use of a slit lamp and a magnifying lens; also known as a slit-lamp exam.
blepharochalasis (blef-ah-roh-**KAL**-ah-sis) blephar/o = eyelid	Relaxation of the skin of the eyelid (usually the upper eyelid). The skin may droop over the edge of the eyelid when the eyes are open; also known as dermatochalasis.
blepharoptosis (blef-ah-roh-**TOH**-sis) blephar/o = eyelid -ptosis = drooping or prolapse	Drooping of the upper eyelid.
blepharospasm (blef-ah-roh-**SPAZM**) blephar/o = eyelid -spasm = twitching, involuntary contraction	A twitching of the eyelid muscles; may be due to eyestrain or nervous irritability.
conjunctivitis (kon-junk-tih-**VYE**-tis) conjunctiv/o = conjunctiva -itis = inflammation	Inflammation of the conjunctiva of the eye; may be caused by a bacterial infection, a viral infection, allergy, or a response to the environment.

Word	Definition
corneal (**COR**-nee-al) corne/o = cornea -al = pertaining to	Pertaining to the **cornea**.
cycloplegia (sigh-kloh-**PLEE**-jee-ah) cycl/o = ciliary body -plegia = paralysis	Paralysis of the ciliary muscle of the eye.
dacryoadenitis (dak-ree-oh-ad-en-**EYE**-tis) dacry/o = tears aden/o = gland -itis = inflammation	Inflammation of the **lacrimal** (tear) gland.
dacryorrhea (dak-ree-oh-**REE**-ah) dacry/o = tears -rrhea = discharge, flow	Excessive flow of tears.
diplopia (dip-**LOH**-pee-ah) dipl/o = double -opia = vision	Double vision caused by each eye focusing separately. See *ambiopia*.
ectropion (eck-**TROH**-pee-on)	Eversion (turning outward) of the edge of the eyelid.
emmetropia (em-eh-**TROH**-pee-ah)	A state of normal vision. The eye is at rest and the image is focused directly on the retina.
entropion (en-**TROH**-pee-on)	Inversion (turning inward) of the edge of the eyelid.
episcleritis (ep-ih-skleh-**RYE**-tis) epi- = upon scler/o = hard; also refers to sclera of the eye -itis = inflammation	Inflammation of the outermost layers of the **sclera**.
esotropia (**ess**-oh-**TROH**-pee-ah) eso- = within -tropia = to turn	An obvious inward turning of one eye in relation to the other eye; also called crosseyes.
exotropia (**eck**-soh-**TROH**-pee-ah) exo- = outward -tropia = to turn	An obvious outward turning of one eye in relation to the other eye; also called walleye.

Word	Definition
extraocular (eks-trah-**OCK**-yoo-lar) extra- = outside, beyond ocul/o = eye -ar = pertaining to	Pertaining to outside the eye.
floaters	One or more spots that appear to drift, or "float," across the visual field.
funduscopy (fund-**DUSS**-koh-pee)	The examination of the fundus of the eye, the base or the deepest part of the eye, with an instrument called an **ophthalmoscope** through a procedure called **ophthalmoscopy**.
hemianopsia (**hem**-ee-ah-**NOP**-see-ah) hemi- = half an- = without -opsia = visual condition	Loss of vision, or blindness, in one-half of the visual field; also known as *hemianopia*.
iridocyclitis (ir-id-oh-sigh-**KLEYE**-tis) irid/o = iris cycl/o = ciliary body -itis = inflammation	Inflammation of the iris and ciliary body of the eye.
iritis (ih-**RYE**-tis) ir/o = iris -itis = inflammation	Inflammation of the iris.
keratoconjunctivitis (kair-ah-toh-kon-junk-tih-**VYE**-tis) kerat/o = hard, horny; also refers to cornea of the eye conjunctiv/o = conjunctiva -itis = inflammation	Inflammation of the **cornea** and the conjunctiva of the eye.
keratoconus (kair-ah-toh-**KOH**-nus) kerat/o = hard, horny; also refers to cornea of the eye	A cone-shaped protrusion (bulging) of the center of the **cornea**, not accompanied by inflammation, usually associated with thinning of the cornea. The bulging results in distorted vision.
keratomycosis (kair-ah-toh-my-**KOH**-sis) kerat/o = hard, horny; also refers to cornea of the eye myc/o = fungus -osis = condition	A fungal growth present on the **cornea**.

Word	Definition

lacrimal
(**LAK**-rim-al)
  lacrim/o = tears
  -al = pertaining to
	Pertaining to tears.

lacrimation (lak-rih-**MAY**-shun)	The secretion of tears from the **lacrimal** glands.

miosis
(my-**OH**-sis)
  mi/o = smaller
  -sis = condition
	Abnormal constriction of the pupil of the eye.

miotic
(my-**OT**-ik)
  mi/o = smaller
  -tic = pertaining to
	An agent that causes the pupil of the eye to constrict.

mydriasis
(mid-**RYE**-ah-sis)
  mydr/o = widen
  -iasis = presence of an abnormal
       condition
	Abnormal dilation of the pupil of the eye.

mydriatic
(mid-ree-**AT**-ik)
  mydr/o = widen
  -iatic = pertaining to a condition
	An agent that causes the pupil of the eye to dilate.

nasolacrimal
(nay-zoh-**LAK**-rim-al)
  nas/o = nose
  lacrim/o = tears
  -al = pertaining to
	Pertaining to the nose and the **lacrimal** (tear) ducts.

nystagmus (niss-**TAG**-mus)	Involuntary, rhythmic jerking movements of the eye. These "quivering" movements may be from side to side, up and down, or a combination of both.

ophthalmologist
(**off**-thal-**MOL**-oh-jist)
  ophthalm/o = eye
  -logist = one who specializes in
       the study of
	A medical doctor (M.D.) who specializes in the comprehensive care of the eyes and visual system in the prevention and treatment of eye disease and injury. The **ophthalmologist** is the medically trained specialist who can deliver total eye care and diagnose general diseases of the body affecting the eye.

ophthalmology
(off-thal-**MOL**-oh-jee)
  ophthalm/o = eyes
  -logy = the study of
	The branch of medicine that specializes in the study of the diseases and disorders of the eye.

Word	Definition
ophthalmopathy (off-thal-**MOP**-ah-thee) ophthalm/o = eye -pathy = disease	Any disease of the eye.
optic (**OP**-tik) opt/o = eye, vision -ic = pertaining to	Pertaining to the eyes or to sight.
optician (op-**TISH**-an) optic/o = eye, vision -ian = specialist in a field of study	A health professional (not an M.D.) who specializes in filling prescriptions for corrective lenses for glasses or for contact lenses.
optometrist (op-**TOM**-eh-trist) opt/o = eye, vision metr/o = to measure -ist = practitioner	The **optometrist**, or doctor of optometry (O.D.) is responsible for examination of the eye, and associated structures—to determine vision problems. He or she can also prescribe lenses or optical aids.
palpebral (**PAL**-peh-brahl)	Pertaining to the eyelid.
papilledema (pap-ill-eh-**DEE**-mah)	Swelling of the **optic** disc, visible upon ophthalmoscopic examination of the interior of the eye.
photophobia (foh-toh-**FOH**-bee-ah) phot/o = light -phobia = abnormal fear	Abnormal sensitivity to light, especially by the eyes.
presbyopia (**prez**-bee-**OH**-pee-ah) presby/o = old age -opia = vision	Loss of accommodation for near vision; poor near-vision due to the natural aging process.
pupillary (**PEW**-pih-lair-ee)	Pertaining to the pupil of the eye.
retinopathy (**ret**-in-**OP**-ah-thee) retin/o = retina -pathy = disease	Any disease of the retina.
sclerectomy (skleh-**REK**-toh-mee) scler/o = hard; also refers to sclera of the eye -ectomy = surgical removal	Excision, or removal, of a portion of the **sclera** of the eye.

Word	Definition
scotoma (skoh-**TOH**-mah) scot/o = darkness -oma = tumor	An area of depressed vision (blindness) within the usual visual field, surrounded by an area of normal vision; an abnormal "blind spot."
uveitis (yoo-vee-**EYE**-tis)	Inflammation of the uveal tract of the eye, which includes the iris, ciliary body, and choroid.
vitreous (**VIT**-ree-us) vitre/o = glassy -ous = pertaining to	Pertaining to the vitreous body of the eye.

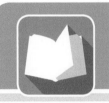

Review Checkpoint

Check your understanding of this section by completing the **Vocabulary** exercises in your workbook.

WORD ELEMENTS (EYE)

The following word elements pertain to the diseases, disorders, signs, symptoms, and diagnostic techniques associated with the eye. As you review the list, pronounce each word element aloud twice and check the box after you "say it." Write the definition for the example term given for each word element. Use your medical dictionary to find the definitions of the example terms.

Word Element	Pronunciation	"Say It"	Meaning
ambi- **ambi**opia	**AM**-bee am-bee-**OH**-pee-ah	☐	both, both sides
ambly/o **ambly**opia	**AM**-blee-oh am-blee-**OH**-pee-ah	☐	dull
aque/o **aque**ous humor	**AY**-kwee-oh **AY**-kwee-us humor	☐	watery
blephar/o **blephar**itis	**BLEF**-ah-roh blef-ah-**RYE**-tis	☐	eyelid
conjunctiv/o **conjunctiv**itis	kon-junk-tih-**VOH** kon-junk-tih-**VYE**-tis	☐	conjunctiva

Word Element	Pronunciation	"Say It"	Meaning
cor/o aniso**cor**ia	**KOH**-roh **an**-eye-soh-**KOH**-ree-ah	☐	pupil
corne/o **corne**al	**COR**-nee-oh **COR**-nee-al	☐	**cornea**
dacry/o **dacry**oadenitis	**DAK**-ree-oh dak-ree-oh-ad-en-**EYE**-tis	☐	tears
dacryocyst/o **dacryocyst**ectomy	dak-ree-oh-**SISS**-toh dak-ree-oh-siss-**TEK**-toh-mee	☐	tear sac
dipl/o **dipl**opia	dip-**LOH** dip-**LOH**-pee-ah	☐	double
epi- **epi**scleritis	**EP**-ih ep-ih-skleh-**RYE**-tis	☐	upon, over
eso- **eso**tropia	**ESS**-oh ess-oh-**TROH**-pee-ah	☐	within
exo- **exo**tropia	**EKS**-oh eck-soh-**TROH**-pee-ah	☐	outward
extra- **extra**ocular	**EKS**-trah eks-trah-**OCK**-yoo-lar	☐	outside, beyond
glauc/o **glauc**oma	**GLAW**-koh glaw-**KOH**-mah	☐	gray, silver
hemi- **hemi**anopsia	**HEM**-ee hem-ee-ah-**NOP**-see-ah	☐	half
ir/o **ir**itis	**IH**-roh ih-**RYE**-tis	☐	iris
irid/o **irid**oplegia	**IR**-id-oh ir-id-oh-**PLEE**-jee-ah	☐	iris
kerat/o **kerat**itis	kair-**AH**-toh kair-ah-**TYE**-tis	☐	hard, horny; also refers to **cornea** of the eye
lacrim/o **lacrim**al	**LAK**-rim-oh **LAK**-rim-al	☐	tears
mi/o **mi**osis	**MY**-oh my-**OH**-sis	☐	smaller
nas/o **nas**olacrimal	**NAY**-zoh nay-zoh-**LAK**-rim-al	☐	nose

Word Element	Pronunciation	"Say It"	Meaning
nyct/o, nyctal/o **nyctal**opia	**NIK**-toh, nik-**TAH**-loh nik-tah-**LOH**-pee-ah	☐	night
ocul/o **ocul**omotor	**OK**-yoo-loh **ok**-yoo-loh-**MOH**-tor	☐	eye
ophthalm/o **ophthalm**oscope	off-**THAL**-moh off-**THAL**-moh-scohp	☐	eye
-opia dipl**opia**	**OH**-pee-ah dip-**LOH**-pee-ah	☐	visual condition
-opsia hemian**opsia**	**OP**-see-ah hem-ee-ah-**NOP**-see-ah	☐	visual condition
opt/o **opt**ic	**OP**-toh **OP**-tik	☐	eye, vision
optic/o **optic**ian	**OP**-tik-oh op-**TISH**-an	☐	eye, vision
palpebr/o **palpebr**al	**PAL**-peh-broh **PAL**-peh-brahl	☐	eyelid
phot/o **phot**ophobia	**FOH**-toh foh-toh-**FOH**-bee-ah	☐	light
-ptosis blepharo**ptosis**	**TOH**-sis blef-ah-roh-**TOH**-sis	☐	drooping or prolapse
pupill/o **pupill**ary	**PEW**-pill-oh **PEW**-pill-air-ee	☐	pupil
retin/o **retin**itis	**RET**-in-oh ret-in-**EYE**-tis	☐	retina
scler/o **scler**a	**SKLAIR**-oh **SKLAIR**-ah	☐	hard; also refers to **sclera** of the eye
scot/o **scot**oma	**SKOH**-toh skoh-**TOH**-mah	☐	darkness
ton/o **ton**ometry	**TOHN**-oh tohn-**OM**-eh-tree	☐	tension
-tropia exo**tropia**	**TROH**-pee-ah Eks-oh-**TROH**-pee-ah	☐	to turn
vitre/o **vitre**ous humor	**VIT**-ree-oh **VIT**-ree-us humor	☐	glassy
xer/o **xer**ophthalmia	**ZEE**-roh zee-roff-**THAL**-mee-ah	☐	dry

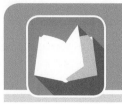

Pathological Conditions (Eye)

As you study the pathological conditions of the eye, note that the **basic definition** is in a green shaded box, followed by a detailed description in regular print. The phonetic pronunciation is directly beneath each term as well as a breakdown of the component parts of the term where applicable.

astigmatism (ah-**STIG**-mah-tizm)	A refractive error causing light rays entering the eye to be focused irregularly on the retina due to an abnormally shaped **cornea** or lens.
	Astigmatism causes blurred vision. The individual also may complain of headaches and squinting. The diagnosis of **astigmatism** may be verified through retinoscopy or an automatic refraction test to determine the person's refractive error. Correction can usually be obtained through contact lenses or eyeglasses, which neutralize the condition.
blepharitis (blef-ah-**RYE**-tis) blephar/o = eyelid -itis = inflammation	Acute or chronic inflammation of the eyelid margins stemming from seborrheic, allergic, or bacterial origin.
	Blepharitis is characterized by redness, swelling, burning, and itching of the margin of the eyelid. There is also usually a mucous drainage and sometimes a buildup of scaling, granulation, or crusting on the eyelid margin. In some cases of **blepharitis**, ulcerations form and eyelashes fall out. Treatment includes cleansing the eyelid gently with a damp cotton applicator to remove scales, crusts, and granules at least daily; applying warm compresses; and applying an antibiotic or topical steroid ointment to the eyelid margins.
blepharoptosis (ptosis) (blef-ah-roh-**TOH**-sis) blephar/o = eyelid -ptosis = drooping	Occurs when the eyelid partially or entirely covers the eye as a result of a weakened muscle. See *Figure 14-3*.
	Ptosis most commonly affects both eyes, but often one eye is more severely affected than the other. Typically only one eye is affected, although both eyes may be involved. This weakened muscle (causing drooping of the upper eyelid) is most commonly seen in older adults (acquired blepharoptosis). Congenital, traumatic, or neurological causes may also occur. If severe, **blepharoptosis** can completely obstruct vision. Ptosis may occur at any age and often follows a familial pattern.
	There may be an underlying disease process (such as myasthenia gravis, muscular dystrophy, diabetes mellitus, or a brain tumor) that has caused the weakened eyelid muscle. When treating this condition, an underlying

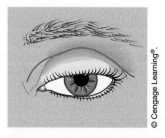

© Cengage Learning®.

Figure 14-3 Blepharoptosis

disease must be ruled out so that if one is present, treatment can be started. **Blepharoptosis** is often corrected with successful treatment of the underlying disease. Other treatment options include surgery to strengthen the eyelid muscle or application of a support device into the individual's glasses, which will keep the eyelid raised.

blindness	Loss of the sense of sight, or extreme visual limitations.

The term *blindness* may refer to total blindness (in which there is total loss of vision), to no light perception, or to particular visual limitations. Legal blindness is present when the visual acuity of the better eye is evaluated with the correction of contact lenses or glasses to be at best 20/200, or when the visual field (the total area that can be seen with one fixed eye) is less than 20 degrees. Causes of blindness include trauma, cataracts, **glaucoma**, nutritional deficiencies, **trachoma**, and onchocerciasis.

color blindness	An inability to perceive visual colors sharply.

One of the more common forms of color blindness is red-green. This is an inherited sex-linked disorder, with females being the carriers and males being affected. Approximately 8% of males are color blind. Color blindness can range from mild to extreme, with the most severe form, which is rare, being evidenced by the inability to see any color: only white, gray, and black.

cataract (**KAT**-ah-rakt)	The lens in the eye becomes progressively cloudy, losing its normal transparency and thus altering the perception of images due to the interference of light transmission to the retina.

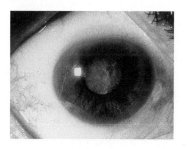

Figure 14-4 Cataract
(Courtesy of the National Eye Institute, NIH)

The occurrence of a **cataract** can be classified as senile or secondary on the basis of etiology. See *Figure 14-4.*

Senile cataracts typically begin after the age of 50, at which time degenerative changes occur, resulting in the gradual clouding of the crystalline lens due to wear and tear and the change in fibers and protein as it ages. Senile cataracts are common and can be found in an estimated 95% of persons over 65 years of age. Secondary cataracts result from trauma, radiation injury, inflammation, taking certain medications such as corticosteroids, or metabolic diseases such as diabetes mellitus. Congenital cataracts, seen in infants, are usually caused by maternal infection during pregnancy and are considered secondary cataracts.

Immature cataracts, those in which only a portion of the lens is affected, are diagnosed through **biomicroscopy** and the person's history. Mature cataracts, those in which the entire lens is clouded, can be visualized with the naked eye and appear as a gray-white area behind the pupil. A loss of the red reflex is noted as the **cataract** matures.

Treatment includes surgical intervention to remove the **cataract**. **Phacoemulsification** and **extracapsular cataract extraction (ECCE)**, the two primary ways to remove a **cataract**, are discussed in the section on diagnostic procedures and techniques at the end of the chapter. Surgery is indicated when the vision loss handicaps the person in the accomplishment of daily activities or when **glaucoma** or another secondary condition occurs. Surgical intervention for **cataract** removal is typically completed on an outpatient basis. There is no medical treatment available for cataracts at present other than surgical removal.

chalazion (kah-**LAY**-zee-on)	A cyst or nodule on the eyelid, resulting from an obstruction of a meibomian gland, which is responsible for lubricating the margin of the eyelid.

A **chalazion** is diagnosed through a visual examination and the person's history. It may vary in size and will usually disappear spontaneously within one to two months. When a **chalazion** does not spontaneously disappear, it can easily be removed through minor surgery in the ophthalmologist's office or on an outpatient basis.

conjunctivitis, acute (kon-junk-tih-**VYE**-tis) conjunctiv/o = conjunctiva -itis = inflammation	Inflammation of the mucous membrane lining the eyelids and covering the front part of the eyeball; often called "pink eye." Three types of conjunctivitis are viral, bacterial, and allergic. Viral and bacterial conjunctivitis are highly contagious, with viral conjunctivitis being the most common. Allergic conjunctivitis is caused by the body's response to allergens or irritants and is not contagious.

The clinical manifestations of acute **conjunctivitis** include redness, tearing, drainage (especially with the contagious type), and itching (primarily with the allergic type). The drainage from viral or bacterial **conjunctivitis** is highly contagious, and precautions must be taken to prevent spread, such as using separate tissues and cloths for each eye, washing hands thoroughly after contact with infected eye(s) (specifically the drainage), and seeking prompt medical treatment. These precautions are especially important when dealing with children because of their close contact with one another and their lack of understanding about the spread of infections.

Diagnosis is made upon the visual examination of the eye, and the cause is determined through the person's history and/or a culture and sensitivity of the drainage. Treatment will vary somewhat according to the cause. However, it may include cool compresses to the eye(s) several times a day, antibiotics for bacterial infections, ophthalmic ointments or drops, and antihistamines for allergic **conjunctivitis**.

corneal abrasion (**COR**-nee-al ah-**BRAY**-zhun) corne/o = cornea -al = pertaining to	A disruption of the cornea's surface epithelium commonly caused by an eyelash, a small foreign body, contact lenses, or a scratch from a fingernail.

A **corneal abrasion** may also occur as a result of a chemical irritant and/or dryness of the eye. Clinical manifestations other than pain include redness, tearing, sensitivity to light, and occasionally visual impairment. Diagnosis of a **corneal abrasion** is identified by the individual's history and by visual examination, which is confirmed with **fluorescein staining** (which readily detects abrasions on the **cornea**).

Word	Definition
serous (**SEER**-us) ser/o = blood serum -ous = pertaining to	Pertaining to producing serum.
stapedectomy (stay-pee-**DEK**-toh-mee) staped/o = stapes -ectomy = surgical removal	Surgical removal of the stapes (middle ear) and insertion of a graft and prosthesis.
tinnitus (tin-**EYE**-tus)	A ringing or tinkling noise heard in the ears; may be a sign of injury to the ear, some disease process, or toxic levels of some medications from prolonged use (such as aspirin).
tympanoplasty (tim-pan-oh-**PLASS**-tee) tympan/o = eardrum -plasty = surgical repair	See *myringoplasty*. A tympanoplasty may also involve surgical repair of the bones in the middle ear (ossicles).
tympanometry (**tim**-pah-**NOM**-eh-tree) tympan/o = eardrum -metry = the process of measuring	The process of measuring middle ear function. This test measures the ear's responses to sound and different pressures by creating variations of air pressure in the ear canal.
tympanotomy (tim-pan-**OT**-oh-mee) tympan/o = eardrum -tomy = incision into	See *myringotomy*.
vertigo (**VER**-tih-goh)	A sensation of spinning around or of having things in the room or area spinning around the person; a result of disturbance of the equilibrium.

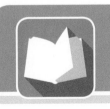

Review Checkpoint

Check your understanding of this section by completing the **Vocabulary** exercises in your workbook.

WORD ELEMENTS (EAR)

The following word elements pertain to the diseases, disorders, signs, symptoms, and diagnostic procedures associated with the ear. As you review the list, pronounce each word element aloud twice and check the box after you "say it." Write the definition for the example term given for each word element. Use your medical dictionary to find the definitions of the example terms.

Word Element	Pronunciation	"Say It"	Meaning
acous/o **acous**tic	ah-**KOOS**-oh ah-**KOOS**-tik	☐	hearing
audi/o **audi**ogram	**AW**-dee-oh **AW**-dee-oh-gram	☐	hearing
audit/o **audit**ory	**AW**-dih-toh **AW**-dih-tor-ee	☐	hearing
labyrinth/o **labyrinth**itis	lab-ih-**RIN**-tho lab-ih-rin-**THIGH**-tis	☐	inner ear
-metry audio**metry**	**MEE**-tree aw-dee-**OM**-eh-tree	☐	the process of measuring
myring/o **myring**otomy	mir-**IN**-goh mir-in-**GOT**-oh-mee	☐	eardrum
ot/o **ot**itis media	**OH**-toh oh-**TYE**-tis **MEE**-dee-ah	☐	ear
tympan/o **tympan**oplasty	tim-**PAN**-oh tim-pan-oh-**PLASS**-tee	☐	eardrum

Review Checkpoint

Check your understanding of this section by completing the **Word Elements** exercises in your workbook.

Pathological Conditions (Ear)

As you study the pathological conditions of the ear, note that the **basic definition** is in a green shaded box, followed by a detailed description in regular print. The phonetic pronunciation is directly beneath each term as well as a breakdown of the component parts of the term where applicable.

cholesteatoma	A slow-growing cystic mass made up of epithelial cell debris in the middle ear.

(koh-lee-stee-ah-**TOH**-mah)
  chol/e = bile
  steat/o = fat
  -oma = tumor

A **cholesteatoma** occurs as an attic retraction pocket (sac or recessed area within the middle ear), a congenital defect, or as a result of chronic **otitis media**. With chronic **otitis media**, the epithelial cell debris is formed largely due to marginal tympanic membrane perforations.

The scaly epithelial cells migrate into the middle ear from the ear canal, where they accumulate to form a pocket of skin cells (which can become an infected, cystlike mass). The **cholesteatoma** can lead to conductive hearing loss, occlusion of the middle ear, and destruction of the ossicles. Rarely, it can expand into the inner ear or intracranial cavity. It can become infected, causing the ear to drain. Other symptoms include hearing loss and earache. Very serious late symptoms include **vertigo** and facial weakness.

Diagnosis is confirmed through the person's history, **audiometry**, otoscopy, and X-ray studies. If drainage is present, the culture results will be helpful in choosing the most effective antibiotic(s).

Treatment is surgical removal of the **cholesteatoma**. If deterioration of the lining has not begun, the **cholesteatoma** can be extracted by thoroughly cleaning the middle ear cavity. The removal becomes much more difficult when the **cholesteatoma** is in advanced stages. Without surgical intervention, the **cholesteatoma** will deteriorate the roof of the middle ear cavity, providing an opportunity for the formation of an abscess or for meningitis to develop.

deafness, conductive	Hearing loss caused by the breakdown of the transmission of sound waves through the middle and/or external ear.

(kon-**DUK**-tiv)

This conductive hearing loss generally occurs when there is a mechanical abnormality in one of the following structures: oval or round windows, tympanic membrane, eustachian tube, ear ossicles, external **auditory** canal, and/or pinna. These mechanical defects may occur because of **otosclerosis**, **otitis media**, ruptured tympanic membrane, or impacted **cerumen**.

Audiometry is used to assess for and evaluate the extent of conductive hearing loss. Treatment is based on the causative factor or mechanical abnormality. Correcting the mechanical defect should be the beginning point. If the underlying defect cannot be fixed, hearing aids are helpful because of their ability to amplify sound. Hearing aids will improve hearing as long as the inner ear and sound perception organs are functioning normally.

deafness, sensorineural	Hearing loss caused by the inability of nerve stimuli to be delivered to the brain from the inner ear due to damage to the **auditory** nerve or the cochlea or to lesions of the 8th cranial nerve (**auditory**).

(sen-soh-ree-**NOO**-ral)
  neur/o = nerve
  -al = pertaining to

The results vary from a mild hearing loss to a profound hearing loss. **Sensorineural deafness** can occur because of the aging process or damaged hair cells of the organ of Corti, which may result from loud machinery noise, loud music, or medication side effects. Other causes of sensorineural hearing loss include genetic predisposition, tumors, infections (such as bacterial meningitis), trauma altering the central **auditory** pathways, vascular disorders, and degenerative or demyelinating diseases. Sensorineural hearing loss makes speech discrimination difficult primarily in noisy surroundings.

Diagnosis is based on the person's history and the results of the **audiometry** test. The best treatment is prevention when possible, which is accomplished by avoiding exposure to loud noises and being aware of medication with ototoxic effects. If the person cannot totally avoid the loud noises, wearing earplugs will be helpful in preventing or escaping further damage. Hearing aids are helpful in some cases. However, the person with profound sensorineural hearing loss may require a **cochlear** implant to have sound perception restored.

impacted cerumen (seh-**ROO**-men)	An excessive accumulation of the waxlike secretions from the glands of the external ear canal.

Excessive hair or dry and scaly skin in the ear canal, or a narrow ear canal, may lead to the accumulation of earwax (causing the ear canal to become impacted). The accumulation may cause a hearing loss or an earache. The person may also complain of the ear being "plugged" or **tinnitus** (ringing noise in the ear).

When an ear is found to have **impacted cerumen**, it can be removed various ways. This condition may recur; thus regular ear examinations should be performed .

labyrinthitis (**lab**-ih-rin-**THIGH**-tis) labyrinth/o = labyrinth -itis = inflammation	Infection or inflammation of the labyrinth or the inner ear—specifically, the three semicircular canals in the inner ear, which are fluid-filled chambers and control balance.

The primary symptom is **vertigo** (dizziness) with altered balance. Other symptoms include **nystagmus** (rapid involuntary movements of the eye) and sometimes sensorineural hearing loss. A virus is typically the cause, and more rarely, bacteria.

The diagnosis of **labyrinthitis** is usually based on a complete physical and neurological exam. Persons suffering from **labyrinthitis** are placed on bed rest for several days. Medications may be given to lessen symptoms of vertigo. **Labyrinthitis** should clear up in one to three weeks when therapy is carried out properly.

mastoiditis (mass-toyd-**EYE**-tis) mastoid/o = mastoid process -itis = inflammation	Inflammation of the mastoid process, which is usually an acute expansion of an infection in the middle ear (**otitis media**).

Chronic **mastoiditis** may occur and is sometimes associated with **cholesteatoma**. The mastoid process is a round portion of the skull's temporal bone located adjacent to the middle ear and can be felt just behind both ears. The mastoid process is filled with air cavities or mastoid sinuses.

Infections of the middle ear may extend into the mastoid sinuses. These infections are eliminated when the middle ear infection is effectively treated with antibiotics. If the **otitis media** is not treated effectively with the appropriate antibiotics, the mastoid sinuses remain filled with **purulent** material, resulting in a bacterial infection of the mastoid process or acute **mastoiditis**.

The symptoms of acute **mastoiditis** occur approximately two to three weeks after the onset of acute **otitis media**. Symptoms include hearing loss and earache on the affected side, tenderness and swelling over the mastoid process, and constant throbbing pain. The swelling is often so severe that the pinna is displaced interiorly and anteriorly. The affected individual may also have a fever and complain of **tinnitus**. There is often a profuse drainage from the affected ear.

Diagnosis is confirmed through the person's history, X-ray studies of the mastoid, **audiometry**, otoscopy, and results of culture studies and blood work. The treatment of acute **mastoiditis** includes aggressive intravenous antibiotics for a two-week period. **Mastoiditis** not responding to the antibiotic treatment may necessitate a surgical procedure to remove the severe infection due to its close proximity to the brain and the possibility of a brain abscess.

Ménière's disease (may-nee-**ARYZ**)	Chronic inner ear disease in which there is an overaccumulation of endolymph (fluid in the labyrinth) characterized by recurring episodes of **vertigo** (dizziness), hearing loss, feeling of pressure or fullness in the affected ear, and **tinnitus**; usually unilateral, but occurs bilaterally in about 10% to 20% of patients.

Episodes may last for hours or days. Other symptoms include nausea, vomiting, loss of balance, and sweating. Usually, only one ear is involved. However, over time both ears may become affected.

The cause of **Ménière's disease** is unknown, but exacerbating factors include, but may not be limited to, stress, excessive salt intake, or menstrual periods. Diagnosis is usually based on the four major symptoms: **vertigo**, progressive hearing loss, **tinnitus**, and a feeling of pressure or fullness in the ear. If these symptoms are not present or are too vague, additional testing with X-ray studies and **audiometry** will likely be done.

To treat **Ménière's disease** for the long term, the person may be instructed to modify his or her lifestyle with such details as eating a low-sodium diet, and using mild sedatives, antihistamines, and diuretics. Antiemetics are usually prescribed for the acute attacks of **Ménière's disease**.

otitis externa (OE)
 	
(oh-**TYE**-tis eks-**TER**-nah)
(swimmer's ear)
  ot/o = ear
  -itis = inflammation
	Inflammation of the outer or external ear canal; also called "swimmer's ear." This inflammation is produced from the growth of bacteria or fungi in the external ear. In addition to the occurrence after swimming, **otitis externa** can develop due to conditions such as psoriasis or seborrhea, injury to the ear canal when trying to scratch or clean it with a foreign object, and frequent use of earphones or earplugs.

The major symptom is pain, especially when the ear is tugged on, along with a red, swollen ear canal. Treatment includes the use of steroid or antibiotic eardrops.

otitis media, acute (AOM) (oh-**TYE**-tis **MEE**-dee-ah) ot/o = ear -itis = inflammation medi/o = middle -a = noun ending	A middle ear infection, which predominantly affects infants, toddlers, and preschoolers. The air-filled middle ear is inflamed, causing an accumulation of fluid behind the tympanic membrane. Upper respiratory infections and dysfunction of the **auditory** tube are associated with both types of **otitis media**. The two types are **serous otitis media** and **suppurative otitis media**. A discussion of each type follows.
serous otitis media (SOM) (**SEER**-us oh-**TYE**-tis **MEE**-dee-ah) ot/o = ear -itis = inflammation ser/o = blood serum -ous = pertaining to medi/o = middle -a = noun ending	A collection of clear fluid in the middle ear that may follow acute **otitis media** or be due to an obstruction of the eustachian tube. Symptoms of **serous otitis media** include complaints of a feeling of fullness in the ear, "popping" or "snapping" in the ear, and diminished mobility of the tympanic membrane. When examined, the eardrum or tympanic membrane appears dull and will look retracted, sometimes with air bubbles or fluid visible behind the membrane.
suppurative otitis media (**SOO**-per-ah-tiv oh-**TYE**-tis **MEE**-dee-ah) ot/o = ear -itis = inflammation medi/o = middle -a = noun ending	A **purulent** collection of fluid in the middle ear, causing the person to experience pain (possibly severe), an elevation in temperature, dizziness, decreased hearing, **vertigo**, and **tinnitus**; also called acute **otitis media**. A concern with **suppurative otitis media** is the potential of a spontaneous rupture of the tympanic membrane as the pressure inside the middle ear rises.
otosclerosis (oh-toh-sklair-**OH**-sis) ot/o = ear scler/o = hard; also refers to the sclera of the eye -osis = condition	A condition in which the footplate of the stapes becomes immobile and secured to the oval window, resulting in a hearing loss. The hearing loss is due to the inability of the stapes to rock the oval window and thus transmit sound to the inner ear. **Otosclerosis** typically results in conductive hearing loss. Occasionally, individuals experience sensorineural hearing loss or a mixed hearing loss if neural components are involved. **Otosclerosis** occurs most commonly in females and Caucasians, resulting in progressive hearing loss. Its onset typically begins between the ages of 11 and 30, with the person having problems with **tinnitus** and inability to hear soft-spoken tones. Treatment for **otosclerosis** includes the use of hearing aids and surgical intervention such as a **stapedectomy**.
perforation of the tympanic membrane (per-for-**AY**-shun of the tim-**PAN**-ik) tympan/o = eardrum -ic = pertaining to	Rupture of the tympanic membrane or eardrum. This condition may be due to middle ear trauma such as a severe middle ear infection, direct injury from a sharp object, barotrauma caused by an explosion, or explosive **acoustic** trauma. The person experiencing the rupture of the eardrum typically complains of partial hearing loss and pain. If infection is present, there may be severe pain. The pain is usually relieved when rupture occurs. With some perforations of the tympanic membrane, there is drainage from the ear.

The rupture makes a direct opening into the middle ear, and the risk for an infection is present until the perforation is closed through the healing process (which requires about one to two weeks). If needed, a patch can be applied to the eardrum to improve hearing and aid in healing.

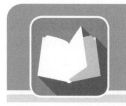

Review Checkpoint

Check your understanding of this section by completing the **Pathological Conditions** exercises in your workbook.

Diagnostic Techniques, Treatments, and Procedures (Ear)

audiometry (aw-dee-**OM**-eh-tree) audi/o = hearing -metry = the process of measuring	The process of measuring how well an individual hears various frequencies of sound waves.
	Audiometry is more specific than the bone conduction hearing tests (Rinne and Weber) because it provides information on the extent of hearing loss and on which frequencies are involved. One form of **audiometry** frequently used to assess hearing acuity is the pure tone **audiometry**, which uses pure tones that are almost completely free of extraneous noises. The person is placed in a soundproof cubicle with earphones and is instructed to signal or indicate when the sounds are first heard and when the sounds can no longer be heard as the decibels (loudness of the sound) are lowered gradually. The audiometer delivers a single frequency at a time, beginning with low-frequency tones and going up to high-frequency tones. Each ear is assessed separately, and the results are recorded on a graph known as an **audiogram**.
nasal endoscopy (**NAY**-sal en-**DOSS**-koh-pee) nas/o = nose -al = pertaining to endo- = within -scopy = process of viewing	A nasal endoscopy is the process of viewing the inside of the nose and sinuses using a thin, usually flexible, fiberoptic tube with a telescopic lens. The endoscope is attached to a light source and a video camera to project the images on a monitor. This diagnostic procedure allows a detailed examination of the nasal and sinus cavities.
	The nasal endoscopy is used to evaluate problems such as nasal stuffiness and obstruction, chronic sinusitis, nasal polyps, and nasal tumors. Before the nasal endoscope is inserted, the inside of the nose is sprayed with a topical anesthetic to temporarily numb the area and a topical decongestant to reduce any swelling present. The endoscope is then passed through the nostril to examine the nasal passages, structures, and sinuses. This procedure is usually performed by an ear, nose, and throat doctor (otolaryngologist).
otoscopy (oh-**TOSS**-koh-pee) ot/o = ear -scopy = process of viewing	The use of an otoscope to view and examine the tympanic membrane and various parts of the outer ear.
	The external ear is examined for lesions, **cerumen**, color, and intactness.

tuning fork test (Rinne test) (**RIN**-nee test)	An examination that compares bone conduction and air conduction. See *Figure 14-15*.

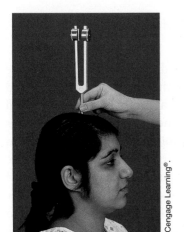

When performing the **Rinne test**, the base of a vibrating tuning fork is placed on the person's mastoid bone and held there until sound can no longer be heard, at which time, it is quickly moved in front of the ear near the ear canal. At this time, it is determined if the person continues to hear the sound at the ear canal. The person with normal hearing will hear the sound vibrating through the air longer than through bone.

With conduction hearing loss, the sound will be heard longer through bone. With sensorineural hearing loss, air conduction is longer, as is the normal hearing pattern.

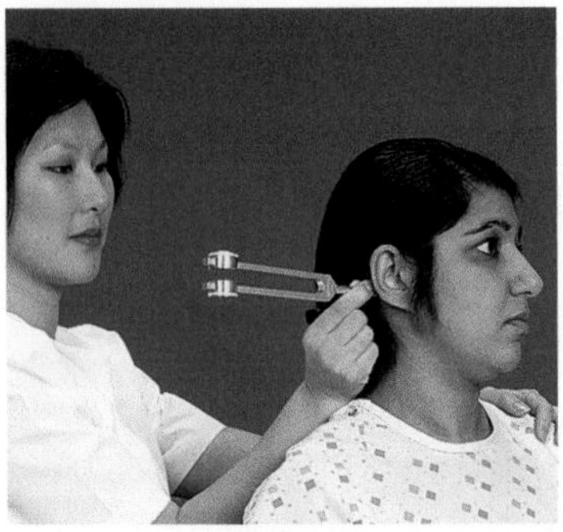

Figure 14-15 Rinne tuning fork test

tuning fork test (Weber test)	An examination used to evaluate **auditory** acuity and to discover whether a hearing deficit is a conductive loss or a sensorineural loss. See *Figure 14-16*.

After placing the base of a vibrating tuning fork on the center of the person's forehead, the person is instructed to evaluate the loudness of the sound heard in each ear. Normally, the loudness of sound heard is identical in both ears. Hearing the sound more in one ear than in the other is an abnormal finding.

If conductive hearing loss is present, the sound will be heard louder in the affected ear due to the inability to hear normal background sounds conducted through the air. If sensorineural loss is present in one ear, the sound is heard louder in the unaffected ear.

Figure 14-16 Weber tuning fork test

otoplasty
(**OH**-toh-plass-tee)
  ot/o = ear
  -plasty = surgical repair
	Removal of a portion of ear cartilage to bring the pinna and auricle nearer the head.
	
	Otoplasty is accomplished typically for cosmetic purposes through reconstructive plastic surgery.

stapedectomy
(stay-pee-**DEK**-toh-mee)
  staped/o = stapes
  -ectomy = surgical removal
	Microsurgical removal of the stapes diseased by **otosclerosis**, typically under local anesthesia.

The stapes removal is followed by placement of a tissue graft and prosthesis to reestablish a pathway for vibrations to deliver sound waves through the oval window and to the inner ear. The prosthesis is attached to the incus on one end and to a graft on the oval window on the other end.

The person experiencing hearing loss due to **otosclerosis** has improved hearing immediately after the **stapedectomy**. This improved hearing is temporarily diminished after the onset of postoperative swelling and ear packing.

hearing aids

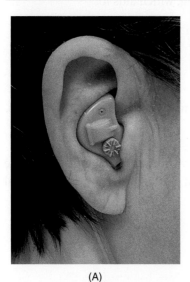

(A)

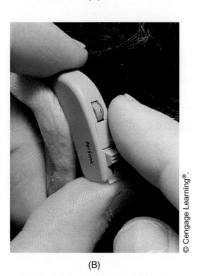

(B)

© Cengage Learning®.

Figure 14-17 (A) In-ear style hearing aid; (B) Behind-ear style hearing aid

Devices that amplify sound to provide more precise perception and interpretation of words communicated to the individual with a hearing deficit. They may be analog (makes continuous sound waves louder) or digital (amplifies the sound, but also filters out unwanted sounds like feedback and background noise).

Most hearing aids consist of several components: a microphone that picks up the sound, an amplifier that makes the sound louder, a receiver (miniature loudspeaker) that sends the amplified sound into the ear canal, and batteries that provide the operating power.

Hearing aids are accessible in an assortment of styles. Selection of the particular hearing aid is usually based on the type and severity of the hearing loss, and the needs and lifestyle of the patient. A discussion of the different styles of hearing aids follows:

1. The **"in-the-canal style" hearing aid** is the least conspicuous of the devices, fitting completely into the ear canal. This type of hearing aid fits comfortably since the shell of the aid is custom-made to fit the individual's ear canal. The disadvantages of using this style of hearing aid occur for those individuals who do not have good dexterity with their hands. Because of the size of the hearing aid, the handling, cleaning, and changing of batteries require good manual dexterity (which is difficult for many older individuals). Cleaning is important because of the possible accumulation of earwax, which will plug the small portals and disrupt sound transmission.

2. The **"in-the-ear style" hearing aid** is worn in the external ear and is larger and more noticeable than the in-canal style. The care of the in-ear style also requires manual dexterity, often a concern for the older individual. Advantages of the in-ear style include a greater degree of amplification and toggle switches that allow for usage of the telephone. Cleaning is important because of the possible accumulation of earwax, which will plug the small portals and disrupt sound transmission. See *Figure 14-17A*.

3. The **"behind-the-ear style" hearing aid** allows for even greater amplification of sound than the in-ear style and is much easier to manipulate manually for care and control. See *Figure 14-17B*. Wearing glasses with the behind-ear style hearing aid is no longer problematic, due to the newer, smaller size and models.

4. A **"body hearing aid"** is used by individuals with profound hearing loss. Sound is delivered to the ear canal by way of a microphone and amplifier clipped on the clothing in a pocket-size container connected to a receiver, which is clipped to the ear mold.

myringotomy with tubes

(mir-in-**GOT**-oh-mee)

myring/o = eardrum

-tomy = incision into

A surgical procedure with insertion of a small ventilation tube introduced into the inferior segment of the tympanic membrane.

These small tubes provide ventilation and drainage of the middle ear when there is a problem with persistent ear infection not responding to antibiotics or persistent severe negative middle ear pressure. A myringotomy allows drainage of fluid by way of a surgical opening, which aids to:

1. Avoid a potential spontaneous rupture of the tympanic membrane.
2. Relieve pain.
3. Restore hearing.
4. Improve speech problems and learning deficits associated with hearing loss.
5. Equalize pressure in the middle ear.

The small tubes usually fall out spontaneously within a few months. While the tubes are in place, the individual must avoid getting water into the ear canal and potentially into the middle ear.

tympanotomy	See *myringotomy*.
(tim-pan-**OT**-oh-mee) **tympan/o** = eardrum, tympanic membrane **-tomy** = incision into	

myringoplasty	Surgical repair of the tympanic membrane with a tissue graft after a spontaneous rupture that results in hearing loss; also called a **tympanoplasty**.
(mir-**IN**-goh-**plas**-tee) **myring/o** = eardrum **-plasty** = surgical repair	The surgical procedure is performed under local or general anesthesia. Topical antibiotics and an absorbable packing are applied to the graft site to secure its position.

tympanoplasty	See *myringoplasty*. A tympanoplasty may also involve surgical repair of the bones in the middle ear (ossicles).
(tim-pan-oh-**PLASS**-tee) **tympan/o** = eardrum **-plasty** = surgical repair	

Review Checkpoint

Check your understanding of this section by completing the **Diagnostic Techniques, Treatments, and Procedures** exercises in your workbook.

COMMON ABBREVIATIONS (EAR)

Abbreviation	Meaning	Abbreviation	Meaning
ABLB	alternate binaural loudness balance	**AC**	air conduction
ABR	**auditory** brain stem response	**AD**	right ear (auris dextra)

Abbreviation	Meaning	Abbreviation	Meaning
AS	left ear (auris sinistra)	EENT	ears, eyes, nose, and throat
AOM	acute **otitis media**	ENT	ears, nose, and throat
AU	each ear (auris unitas)	OE	**otitis externa**
BC	bone conduction	PTS	permanent threshold shift
BOM	bilateral **otitis media**	SOM	**serous otitis media**
COM	chronic **otitis media**	TM	tympanic membrane
db	decibel	TTS	temporary threshold shift

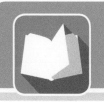

Review Checkpoint

Check your understanding of this section by completing the **Common Abbreviations** exercises in your workbook.

WRITTEN AND AUDIO TERMINOLOGY REVIEW

Review each of the following terms from this chapter. Study the spelling of each term and write the definition in the space provided. Check definitions by looking the term up in the glossary.

Term	Pronunciation	Definition
acoustic	☐ ah-**KOOS**-tik	_____
ambiopia	☐ am-bee-**OH**-pee-ah	_____
amblyopia	☐ am-blee-**OH**-pee-ah	_____
ametropia	☐ **am**-eh-**TROH**-pee-ah	_____
anisocoria	☐ **an**-eye-soh-**KOH**-ree-ah	_____
aphakia	☐ ah-**FAY**-kee-ah	_____
aqueous	☐ **AY**-kwee-us	_____
aqueous humor	☐ **AY**-kwee-us humor	_____
Argyll-Robertson pupil	☐ ar-**GILL ROB**-ert-son pupil	_____
astigmatism	☐ ah-**STIG**-mah-tizm	_____
audiogram	☐ **AW**-dee-oh-gram	_____

Term	Pronunciation	Definition
audiometry	☐ aw-dee-**OM**-eh-tree	_____
auditory	☐ **AW**-dih-tor-ee	_____
aural	☐ **AW**-ral	_____
auriculotemporal	☐ aw-**rik**-yoo-loh-**TEM**-poh-ral	_____
barotitis media	☐ **bar**-oh-**TYE**-tis **MEE**-dee-ah	_____
blepharitis	☐ **blef**-ah-**RYE**-tis	_____
blepharochalasis	☐ **blef**-ah-roh-**KAL**-ah-sis	_____
blepharoptosis	☐ **blef**-ah-roh-**TOH**-sis	_____
cataract	☐ **KAT**-ah-rakt	_____
cerumen	☐ seh-**ROO**-men	_____
chalazion	☐ kah-**LAY**-zee-on	_____
cholesteatoma	☐ **koh**-lee-**stee**-ah-**TOH**-mah	_____
cochlear	☐ **COCK**-lee-ar(**KOH**-klee-ar)	_____
conjunctivitis	☐ kon-**junk**-tih-**VYE**-tis	_____
cornea	☐ **COR**-nee-a	_____
corneal abrasion	☐ **COR**-nee-al ay-**BRAY**-zhun	_____
corneal transplant	☐ **COR**-nee-al transplant	_____
cycloplegia	☐ **sigh**-kloh-**PLEE**-jee-ah	_____
dacryoadenitis	☐ **dak**-ree-oh-ad-en-**EYE**-tis	_____
dacryocystectomy	☐ **dak**-ree-oh-sis-**TEK**-toh-mee	_____
dacryorrhea	☐ **dak**-ree-oh-**REE**-ah	_____
diabetic retinopathy	☐ dye-ah-**BET**-ik reh-tin-**OP**-ah-thee	_____
diplopia	☐ dip-**PLOH**-pee-ah	_____
ectropion	☐ ek-**TROH**-pee-on	_____
electronystagmography	☐ ee-**lek**-troh-niss-tag-**MOG**-rah-fee	_____
electroretinogram (ERG)	☐ ee-**lek**-troh-**RET**-ih-noh-gram	_____
emmetropia	☐ **em**-eh-**TROH**-pee-ah	_____
entropion	☐ en-**TROH**-pee-on	_____
episcleritis	☐ **ep**-ih-skleh-**RYE**-tis	_____
esotropia	☐ **ess**-oh-**TROH**-pee-ah	_____
exophthalmia	☐ **eck**-soff-**THAL**-mee-ah	_____

Term	Pronunciation	Definition
extracapsular cataract extraction (ECCE)	☐ ecks-trah-**KAP**-syoo-lar **KAT**-ah-rakt eks-**TRAK**-shun	_____
extraocular	☐ ecks-trah-**OCK**-yoo-lar	_____
fluorescein staining	☐ floo-oh-**RESS**-ee-in staining	_____
funduscopy	☐ fun-**DUSS**-koh-pee	_____
glaucoma	☐ glah-**KOH**-mah	_____
gonioscopy	☐ gah-nee-**OSS**-kah-pee	_____
hemianopsia	☐ hem-ee-ah-**NOP**-see-ah	_____
hordeolum	☐ hor-**DEE**-oh-lum	_____
hyperopia	☐ high-per-**OH**-pee-ah	_____
hyphema	☐ high-**FEE**-mah	_____
intraocular	☐ in-trah-**OCK**-yoo-lar	_____
iridectomy	☐ ir-ih-**DECK**-toh-mee	_____
iridocyclitis	☐ ir-id-oh-sigh-**KLEYE**-tis	_____
iridoplegia	☐ ir-id-oh-**PLEE**-jee-ah	_____
iritis	☐ ih-**RYE**-tis	_____
keratitis	☐ kair-ah-**TYE**-tis	_____
keratoconjunctivitis	☐ kair-ah-toh-kon-**junk**-tih-**VYE**-tis	_____
keratoconus	☐ kair-ah-toh-**KOH**-nus	_____
keratomycosis	☐ kair-ah-toh-my-**KOH**-sis	_____
keratoplasty	☐ **KAIR**-ah-toh-**plass**-tee	_____
labyrinthitis	☐ **lab**-ih-rin-**THIGH**-tis	_____
lacrimal	☐ **LAK**-rim-al	_____
lacrimation	☐ **lak**-rih-**MAY**-shun	_____
mastoiditis	☐ **mass**-toyd-**EYE**-tis	_____
Ménière's disease	☐ may-nee-**AIRZ** dih-**ZEEZ**	_____
miosis	☐ my-**OH**-sis	_____
miotic	☐ my-**OT**-ik	_____
monochromatism	☐ **mon**-oh-**KROH**-mah-tizm	_____
mydriasis	☐ mid-**RYE**-ah-sis	_____
mydriatic	☐ **mid**-ree-**AT**-ik	_____
myopia	☐ my-**OH**-pee-ah	_____
myringoplasty	☐ mir-**IN**-goh-**plass**-tee	_____

Term	Pronunciation	Definition
nasolacrimal	☐ **nay**-zoh-**LAK**-rim-al	_____
nyctalopia	☐ **nik**-tah-**LOH**-pee-ah	_____
nystagmus	☐ niss-**TAG**-mus	_____
oculomotor	☐ **ock**-yoo-loh-**MOH**-tor	_____
ophthalmia neonatorum	☐ off-**THAL**-mee-ah nee-oh-nay-**TOR**-um	_____
ophthalmologist	☐ **off**-thal-**MOL**-oh-jist	_____
ophthalmology	☐ **off**-thal-**MOL**-oh-jee	_____
ophthalmoscope	☐ off-**THAL**-moh-scohp	_____
ophthalmoscopy	☐ off-thal-**MOS**-koh-pee	_____
optic	☐ **OP**-tik	_____
optician	☐ op-**TISH**-an	_____
optometrist	☐ op-**TOM**-eh-trist	_____
otalgia	☐ oh-**TAL**-jee-ah	_____
otitis externa	☐ oh-**TYE**-tis eks-**TER**-nah	_____
otitis media	☐ oh-**TYE**-tis **MEE**-dee-ah	_____
otodynia	☐ **oh**-toh-**DIN**-ee-ah	_____
otomycosis	☐ **oh**-toh-my-**KOH**-sis	_____
otoplasty	☐ **oh**-toh-**PLASS**-tee	_____
otorrhea	☐ **oh**-toh-**REE**-ah	_____
otosclerosis	☐ **oh**-toh-sklair-**OH**-sis	_____
palpebral	☐ **PAL**-peh-brahl	_____
papilledema	☐ **pap**-ill-eh-**DEE**-mah	_____
phacoemulsification	☐ **fak**-oh-ee-**MULL**-sih-fih-**kay**-shun	_____
phacomalacia	☐ **fak**-oh-mah-**LAY**-shee-ah	_____
photo-refractive keratectomy	☐ **FOH**-toh-ree-**FRAK**-tive **kair**-ah-**TEK**-toh-mee	_____
photophobia	☐ **foh**-toh-**FOH**-bee-ah	_____
presbycusis	☐ **prez**-bee-**KOO**-sis	_____
presbyopia	☐ **prez**-bee-**OH**-pee-ah	_____
pterygium	☐ ter-**IJ**-ee-um	_____
pupillary	☐ **PEW**-pih-lair-ee	_____

Term	Pronunciation	Definition
purulent	☐ **PYOO**-roo-lent	_____
retinal tear	☐ **RET**-in-al tair	_____
retinal photocoagulation	☐ **RET**-in-al **foh**-toh-coh-**ag**-yoo-**LAY**-shun	_____
retinitis	☐ ret-in-**EYE**-tis	_____
retinopathy	☐ **ret**-in-**OP**-ah-thee	_____
Rinne test	☐ **RIN**-nee test	_____
sclera	☐ **SKLAIR**-ah	_____
sclerectomy	☐ skleh-**REK**-toh-mee	_____
scleritis	☐ skleh-**RYE**-tis	_____
scotoma	☐ skoh-**TOH**-mah	_____
sensorineural deafness	☐ **sen**-soh-ree-**NOO**-ral deafness	_____
serous	☐ **SEER**-us	_____
serous otitis media	☐ **SEER**-us oh-**TYE**-tis **MEE**-dee-ah	_____
stapedectomy	☐ **stay**-pee-**DEK**-toh-mee	_____
strabismus	☐ strah-**BIZ**-mus	_____
suppurative otitis media	☐ **SOO**-per-ah-tiv oh-**TYE**-tis **MEE**-dee-ah	_____
synechia	☐ sin-**ECK**-ee-ah	_____
tinnitus	☐ tin-**EYE**-tus	_____
tonometry	☐ tohn-**OM**-eh-tree	_____
trabeculectomy	☐ trah-**bek**-yool-**ECK**-toh-mee	_____
trabeculoplasty	☐ trah-**BEK**-yoo-loh-**plass**-tee	_____
trachoma	☐ tray-**KOH**-mah	_____
tympanometry	☐ **tim**-pah-**NOM**-eh-tree	_____
tympanoplasty	☐ **tim**-pan-oh-**PLASS**-tee	_____
tympanotomy	☐ **tim**-pan-**OT**-oh-mee	_____
uveitis	☐ **yoo**-vee-**EYE**-tis	_____
vertigo	☐ **VER**-tih-goh	_____
vitreous	☐ **VIT**-ree-us	_____
xerophthalmia	☐ **zeer**-off-**THAL**-mee-ah	_____

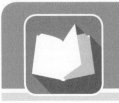

Review Checkpoint

Apply what you have learned in this chapter by completing the **Putting It All Together** exercise in your workbook.

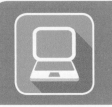

Online Resources

For additional study tools, including PowerPoint® slides and animations, go to the Student Companion Website.

Chapter Review Exercises

The following exercises provide a more in-depth review of the chapter material. Your goal in these exercises is to complete each section at a minimum 80% level of accuracy. A space has been provided for your score at the end of each section.

A. Spelling

Circle the correctly spelled term in each pairing of words. Each correct answer is worth 10 points. Record your score in the space provided at the end of the exercise.

1. ophthalmoscope   opthalmoscope
2. ambyopia   ambiopia
3. blepharoptosis   blephroptosis
4. corneitis   corniitis
5. nistagmus   nystagmus
6. cochlear   coclear
7. otorrhea   otorrea
8. serus   serous
9. tinnitus   tinnitis
10. tympanotomy   tempanotomy

Number correct _____ **× 10 points/correct answer: Your score** _____%

B. Term to Definition

Define each term by writing the definition in the space provided. Check the box if you are able to complete this exercise correctly the first time (without referring to the answers). Each correct answer is worth 10 points. Record your score in the space provided at the end of the exercise.

☐ 1. tinnitus _____

☐ 2. vertigo _____

☐ 3. presbycusis _____

☐ 4. myringoplasty _____

☐ 5. labyrinthitis _____

☐ 6. blepharoptosis _____

☐ 7. optician _____

☐ 8. conjunctivitis _____

☐ 9. ophthalmologist _____

☐ 10. glaucoma _____

Number correct _____ × 10 points/correct answer: Your score _____%

C. Matching Abbreviations

Match the abbreviations on the left with the applicable definition on the right. Each correct answer is worth 10 points. Record your score in the space provided at the end of the exercise.

_____ 1. EOM	a. visual acuity
_____ 2. OD	b. air conduction
_____ 3. PEARL	c. ears, nose, and throat
_____ 4. REM	d. pupils equal and reactive to light
_____ 5. VA	e. blister on middle ear
_____ 6. AC	f. decibel
_____ 7. ENT	g. right eye
_____ 8. BOM	h. left ear
_____ 9. AS	i. rapid eye movement
_____ 10. dB	j. extraocular movement
	k. pupils equal and reactive lens
	l. extraorbital mass
	m. bilateral otitis media

Number correct _____ × 10 points/correct answer: Your score _____%

D. Crossword Puzzle

Read the clues carefully and complete the puzzle. Each crossword answer is worth 10 points. When you have completed the crossword puzzle, total your points and enter your score in the space provided.

(continued)

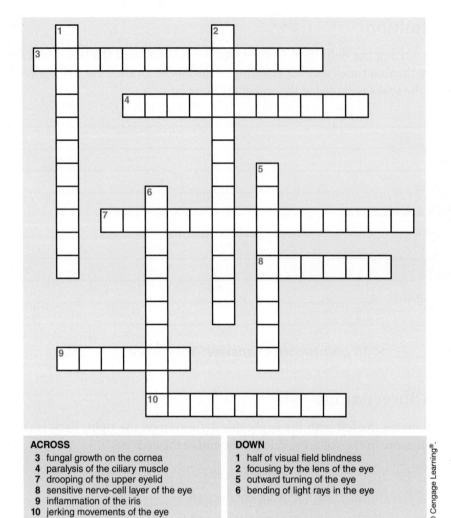

ACROSS
3 fungal growth on the cornea
4 paralysis of the ciliary muscle
7 drooping of the upper eyelid
8 sensitive nerve-cell layer of the eye
9 inflammation of the iris
10 jerking movements of the eye

DOWN
1 half of visual field blindness
2 focusing by the lens of the eye
5 outward turning of the eye
6 bending of light rays in the eye

© Cengage Learning®.

Number correct _____ × *10 points/correct answer: Your score* _____%

E. Definition to Term

Using the following definitions, identify and provide the medical term to match the definition. Write the word in the first space and the applicable combining form for the word in the second space. Each correct answer is worth 5 points. Record your score in the space provided at the end of the exercise.

1. drooping of the eyelid

_____   _____
(word)   (combining form)

2. double vision

_____   _____
(word)   (combining form)

3. paralysis of the ciliary muscle of the eye

_____   _____
(word)   (combining form)

4. excessive flow of tears

_____   _____
(word)   (combining form)

5. inflammation of the conjunctiva of the eye

_____   _____

(word)   (combining form)

6. recording of the faintest sounds an individual is able to hear

_____   _____

(word)   (combining form)

7. inflammation of the inner ear

_____   _____

(word)   (combining form)

8. incision into the eardrum

_____   _____

(word)   (combining form)

9. pertaining to the ear

_____   _____

(word)   (combining form)

10. pain in the ear

_____   _____

(word)   (combining form)

Number correct _____ × 5 points/correct answer: Your score _____%

F. Labeling

Label the following diagrams by identifying the structures indicated. Place your answers in the spaces provided. Each correct answer is worth 10 points. Record your score in the space provided at the end of the exercise.

1. _____
2. _____
3. _____
4. _____
5. _____

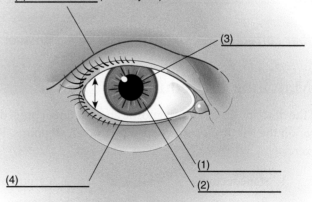

Temporal side   **Nasal side**

(5) _____ (under eyelid)

(3)

(1) _____

(2) _____

(4) _____

RIGHT EYE

(continued)

6. _____ (8) _____
7. _____
8. _____
9. _____ (9) _____
10. _____

Path of light ——— - - - - - (10) _____

(6) _____

(7) _____

© Cengage Learning®.

Number correct _____ × 10 points/correct answer: Your score _____%

G. Trace That Sound!

The following completion exercise traces sound vibrations through the ear. As you read the discussion, complete the blank spaces with the most appropriate word. Each correct response is worth 10 points. When you have completed the exercise, record your score in the space provided at the end of the exercise.

The process of hearing begins with the outer ear. The sound vibrations are received by the pinna and are funneled through the (1) _____ to the (2) _____. The sound waves strike the area just mentioned and cause it to vibrate. These vibrations move the three small bones of the middle ear: the (3) _____, the (4) _____, and the (5) _____ (each of which is attached to the other). As the last of the three small bones in the middle ear vibrates, it causes the (6) _____ to vibrate, setting in motion a "ripple effect" in the fluids within the (7) _____. As these fluids fluctuate, they transmit the stimulus on to the tiny hair cells of the (8) _____. The stimulation is picked up by the (9) _____ that lie close to these tiny hair cells, and the stimulation is transmitted on to the (10) _____ of the brain (where the impulses are interpreted as hearing).

Number correct _____ × 10 points/correct answer: Your score _____%

H. Matching Procedures

Read the descriptions of the diagnostic and treatment procedures on the right and match them with the applicable answer on the left. Each correct answer is worth 10 points. Record your score in the space provided at the end of the exercise.

_____ 1. stapedectomy

_____ 2. Rinne test

_____ 3. electroretinogram

_____ 4. myringotomy

_____ 5. electronystagmography

a. a group of tests used in evaluating the vestibulo-ocular reflex

b. determines the intraocular pressure by calculating the resistance of the eyeball to an applied force causing indentation

c. a recording of the changes in the electrical potential of the retina after the stimulation of light

d. examination of the fundus of the eye

_____ 6. myringoplasty

_____ 7. tonometry

_____ 8. funduscopy

_____ 9. laser iridectomy

_____ 10. photo-refractive keratectomy

e. creating several small openings in the iris to allow aqueous humor to flow to the anterior chamber from the posterior chamber

f. shaving off a few layers of the corneal surface to reduce myopia

g. an examination that compares bone conduction and air conduction in an individual

h. microsurgical removal of the stapes

i. insertion of a small ventilation tube into the inferior segment of the tympanic membrane through surgery

j. surgical repair of the tympanic membrane with a tissue graft

Number correct _____ **× 10 points/correct answer: Your score** _____ **%**

I. Completion

The following statements describe various pathological conditions of the eye and ear. Read each statement carefully and complete the sentences with the most appropriate pathological condition. Each correct answer is worth 10 points. Record your score in the space provided at the end of the exercise.

1. The accumulation of waxlike secretions in the external ear canal that may cause a hearing loss is called:

   _____

2. An inflammatory process that is typically an acute expansion of a middle ear infection is called:

   _____

3. A refractive error resulting in impaired close vision due to the eyeball being shorter than normal is known as:

   _____

4. A refractive error resulting in impaired distant vision due to the eyeball being longer than normal is known as:

   _____

5. A condition in which the eyelid partially or completely covers the eye as a result of a weakened muscle is known as:

   _____

6. Progressive vision loss due to clouding of the lens is:

   _____

7. A condition in which there is scarring of the retinal capillaries and leakage of blood, which result in a decline in the sharpness of vision, is known as:

   _____

8. Inversion (turning inward) of the edge of the eyelid is called:

   _____

9. An ocular disorder characterized by an increase in intraocular pressure is known as:

   _____

10. Inflammation of the cornea is called:

    _____

Number correct _____ **× 10 points/correct answer: Your score** _____ **%**

J. Word Search

Read each definition carefully and identify the applicable word from the list that follows. Enter the word in the space provided and then find it in the puzzle and circle it. The words may be read up, down, diagonally, across, or backward. Each correct answer is worth 10 points. Record your score in the space provided at the end of the exercise.

blepharoptosis	chalazion	ectropion
conjunctivitis	keratitis	astigmatism
Ménière's	nystagmus	otosclerosis
hordeolum	blepharitis	

Example: Drooping of the upper eyelid:
blepharoptosis _____

1. A chronic disease of the inner ear characterized by vertigo, hearing loss, a feeling of fullness in the affected ear, and tinnitus:

   _____

2. Causes a hearing loss due to the footplate of the stapes becoming immobile and secured to the oval window:

   _____

3. A refractive error causing the light rays entering the eye to be focused irregularly due to an abnormally shaped cornea:

   _____

4. Inflammation of the eyelid margins:

   _____

5. A cyst or nodule on the eyelid due to an obstruction of a meibomian gland:

   _____

6. Inflammation of the mucous membrane lining the eyelids and covering the front of the eyeball:

   _____

7. "Turning out" of the eyelashes:

   _____

8. Bacterial infection of an eyelash follicle or sebaceous gland:

   _____

9. Inflammation of the cornea:

   _____

10. Involuntary movements of the eyes; may be vertical, horizontal, rotary, or mixed movements:

    _____

Number correct _____ **× 10 points/correct answer: Your score** _____ **%**

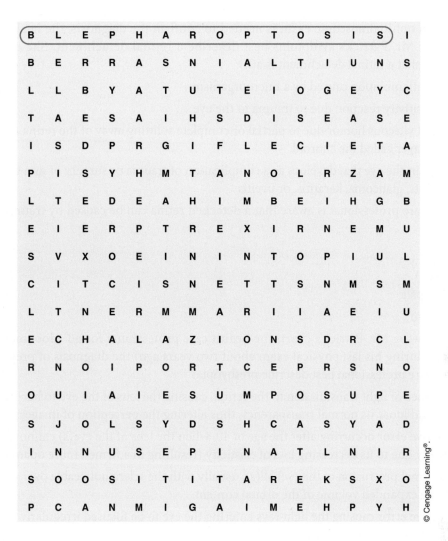

B	L	E	P	H	A	R	O	P	T	O	S	I	S	I
B	E	R	R	A	S	N	I	A	L	T	I	U	N	S
L	L	B	Y	A	T	U	T	E	I	O	G	E	Y	C
T	A	E	S	A	I	H	S	D	I	S	E	A	S	E
I	S	D	P	R	G	I	F	L	E	C	I	E	T	A
P	I	S	Y	H	M	T	A	N	O	L	R	Z	A	M
L	T	E	D	E	A	H	I	M	B	E	I	H	G	B
E	I	E	R	P	T	R	E	X	I	R	N	E	M	U
S	V	X	O	E	I	N	I	N	T	O	P	I	U	L
C	I	T	C	I	S	N	E	T	T	S	N	M	S	M
L	T	N	E	R	M	M	A	R	I	I	A	E	I	U
E	C	H	A	L	A	Z	I	O	N	S	D	R	C	L
R	N	O	I	P	O	R	T	C	E	P	R	S	N	O
O	U	I	A	I	E	S	U	M	P	O	S	U	P	E
S	J	O	L	S	Y	D	S	H	C	A	S	Y	A	D
I	N	N	U	S	E	P	I	N	A	T	L	N	I	R
S	O	O	S	I	T	I	T	A	R	E	K	S	X	O
P	C	A	N	M	I	G	A	I	M	E	H	P	Y	H

K. Medical Scenario

The following medical scenario presents information on one of the pathological conditions discussed in this chapter. Read the scenario carefully and select the most appropriate answer for each question that follows. Each correct answer is worth 20 points. Record your score in the space provided at the end of the exercise.

Charles Patrick, a 55-year-old construction worker, has just called his primary physician for advice about an accident in which he received a blow to his left eye. The accident occurred about two hours ago, at which time Charles had some blurred vision. He explained to the physician that now he is seeing light flashes and floating spots, and his eye seems to have a blind area beginning at the top moving downward. Charles's primary physician immediately refers him to an ophthalmologist.

1. The health care professional calls the ophthalmologist's office about the referral for a suspected retinal detachment and expects that he will be seen:

    a. as soon as possible

    b. within 72 hours

    c. within a week

    d. within two weeks

(continued)

2. Although an ophthalmoscopic exam is needed to confirm the diagnosis, the health care professional realizes that Mr. Patrick's symptoms best describe a retinal detachment. She explains to Mr. and Mrs. Patrick that a retinal detachment is a(n):

    a. corneal inflammation caused by a microorganism

    b. hypersensitivity reaction due to trauma to the eye

    c. leakage of vitreous humor due to partial or complete splitting away of the retina from the pigmented vascular layer called the choroid

    d. adhesion in the eye that develops as a complication of trauma or surgery or as a secondary condition of cataracts, glaucoma, keratitis, or uveitis

3. The health care professional is aware that a detached retina can be caused by trauma to the eye as well as by:

    a. aging

    b. tonometry

    c. hemianopsia

    d. hordeolum

4. While reviewing Mr. Patrick's chart, the health care professional found (documented under vision assessment during his last physical exam about two years ago) the diagnosis of presbyopia. How could the health care professional best describe presbyopia?

    a. interference of light transmission to the retina, causing the lens of the eye to become progressively cloudy and loose its normal transparency, thus altering the perception of images.

    b. a refractive error occurring after the age of 40, when the lens of the eye(s) cannot focus on an image accurately due to its decreasing loss of elasticity (resulting in a firmer, more opaque lens).

    c. an abnormal protrusion of the eyeball(s), usually with the sclera noticeable over the iris—typically due to an expanded volume of the orbital content.

    d. a refractive error causing the light rays entering the eye to be focused irregularly on the retina due to an abnormally shaped cornea.

5. The health care professional explains that if the ophthalmologist diagnoses Mr. Patrick with a retinal detachment, the treatment will include:

    a. medications

    b. bed rest

    c. surgical intervention

    d. ice packs

***Number correct* _____ × *20 points/correct answer: Your score* _____%**

L. Proofreading Skills

Read the following Ophthalmology Operative Report. For each bold term, provide a brief definition and indicate if the term is spelled correctly. If it is misspelled, provide the correct spelling. Each correct answer is worth 10 points. Record your score in the space provided at the end of the exercise.

Example:

    phacoemulsification _____

    Spelled correctly? ☑ Yes ☐ No _____

OPERATIVE REPORT

Hillcrest
medical center

PATIENT NAME: Rhian, Gretchen

PATIENT ID: 9672587

ADMITTING PHYSICIAN
Carla Nowell, MD

DATE OF ADMISSION
January 21, 2014

PREOPERATIVE DIAGNOSIS
Catarac, right eye.

POSTOPERATIVE DIAGNOSIS
Cataract, right eye.

SURGEON
Carla Nowell, MD

OPERATION
Extracapsular cataract extraction with implantation of **posterier chamber** intraocular lens, right eye.

ANESTHESIA
Local, CRNA standby.

PROCEDURE
The eye was prepped and draped in the usual sterile manner. A lid speculum was inserted. The fornices were cleaned with Weck-Cel® and balanced salt solution (BSS).

A peritomy was performed from 10 to 2 o'clock. Adequate hemostasis was obtained. A grooved incision was undertaken and reflected down in a wide flap to the **corneea**. Stab incisions into the anterior chamber were undertaken at 10 and 2 o'clock.

An anterior capsulotomy in a can-opener manner was undertaken, using a bent needle, and the nucleus was loosened and prolapsed from the superior pole into the **anterier chamber**. The incision was then enlarged to allow the nucleus to be prolapsed. Using irrigation and gentle pressure, the nucleus was gently prolapsed from the anterior chamber. The wound was closed with two interrupted postplaced 9–0 Vicryl sutures at 10 and 2 o'clock, following which the irrigating and aspirating device cleaned the remaining cortex.

Viscoelastic was inserted into the anterior chamber. The 10 o'clock postplaced suture was removed; an intraocular lens was inserted into place. Irrigation and aspiration removed the remaining viscoelastic.

The 10 o'clock Vicryl suture, which had been removed, was replaced. The wound was closed with a shoelace 10–0 nylon suture. Periocular medication was used. Patient tolerated the procedure well and returned to the holding room in satisfactory condition.

Carla Nowell, MD

CN:WO

D:1/21/2014

T:1/22/2014

1. **catarac** _____

_____

Spelled Correctly? ☐ Yes   ☐ No _____

2. **extracapsular cataract extraction** _____

_____

Spelled Correctly? ☐ Yes   ☐ No _____

3. **posterier chamber** _____

_____

Spelled Correctly? ☐ Yes   ☐ No _____

4. **corneea** _____

_____

Spelled Correctly? ☐ Yes   ☐ No _____

5. **anterier chamber** _____

_____

Spelled Correctly? ☐ Yes   ☐ No _____

Number correct _____ × *5 points/correct answer: Your score* _____%

The Urinary System

CHAPTER CONTENT

OBJECTIVES

Upon completing this chapter and the review exercises at the end of the chapter, the learner should be able to:

1. Identify and label the internal structure of the kidney.

2. List four major functions of the urinary system.

3. Using a flow chart, identify the appropriate structures involved in the process of forming and expelling urine.

4. Define at least 15 common signs and symptoms that indicate possible urinary system problems.

5. Correctly spell and pronounce terms listed on the Written and Audio Terminology Review, using the phonetic pronunciations provided.

6. Define 10 urinary system conditions.

7. Proof and correct the transcription exercise relative to the urinary system.

8. Identify at least 10 abbreviations common to the urinary system.

9. Identify the characteristics of normal urine.

Overview

The **urinary** system plays a major role in the elimination of waste from the body. In addition to removing waste products from the blood, the kidneys perform the vital function of regulating the volume and chemical composition of blood by selectively adjusting the amounts of water and electrolytes in the body. Whereas some substances are eliminated into the urine, other needed substances are retained in the bloodstream.

When the blood passes through the kidneys, waste products such as urea, uric acid, and creatinine are filtered out, whereas appropriate amounts of water and other dissolved substances (solutes) are reabsorbed into the bloodstream. Excess amounts of water and solutes are excreted as urine. This filtering–reabsorption process is necessary to maintain the balance of substances required for a relatively stable internal body environment. This stable internal body environment is known as homeostasis (*home/o* = same; *stasis* = control) and is necessary for the cells of the body to survive and carry out their functions effectively.

If the kidneys fail, there is no way the substances they excrete can be eliminated from the body. Consequently, the substances accumulate in the blood to **toxic** (poisonous) levels, upsetting the internal environment of the body to the point where the cells can no longer function. Death will ultimately follow unless the nonfunctioning kidney is replaced with a healthy kidney through kidney transplant or the impurities are filtered out of the blood by means of an artificial kidney known as kidney **dialysis**. Kidney transplant and kidney **dialysis** (artificial kidney) are discussed later in this chapter.

In addition to producing and eliminating urine, the kidneys act as endocrine glands by secreting substances into the bloodstream that produce specific effects on the body. Erythropoietin (EPO), a hormone that stimulates the production of red blood cells within the bone marrow, is produced by the kidneys. Renin, an enzyme that aids in raising the blood pressure by causing the constriction of blood vessels, is also produced by the kidneys.

Anatomy and Physiology

The **urinary** system (**urinary** tract) consists of two kidneys, two ureters, one bladder, and one **urethra**. See *Figure 15-1*.

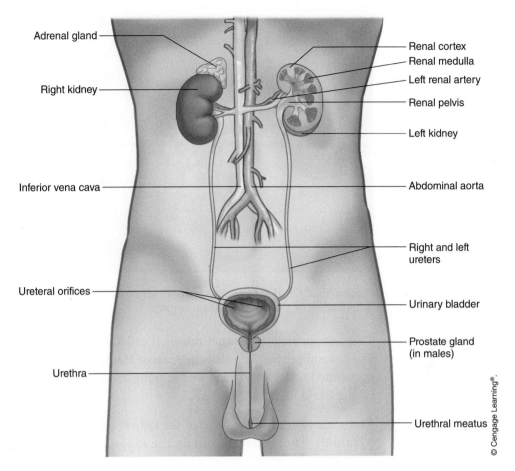

Figure 15-1 The urinary system

Kidneys

The **kidneys** are reddish-brown, bean-shaped organs located on either side of the vertebral column at the back of the upper abdominal cavity. The kidneys lie **retroperitoneal** (behind) the peritoneal membrane, resting between the muscles of the back and the peritoneal cavity. If you place your hand just above your waistline on your back, to either side of your spine, you will be touching the general vicinity of the kidneys within the abdominal cavity.

Each kidney is surrounded by a thick cushion of fatty tissues (adipose tissue), which is covered with a fibrous connective tissue layer. These tissue layers offer protection and support to the kidney and anchor it to the body wall. See *Figure 15-2*.

The adult kidney measures approximately 4 inches (10 cm) long, 2.2 inches (5.5 cm) wide, and 1.2 inches (3 cm) thick—weighing approximately 5.5 ounces (150 g). The size of the adult kidney varies little with differences in body build and weight.

The outer layer, or **cortex**, of the kidney contains millions of microscopic units called **nephrons**. The nephrons are the functional units of the kidneys, carrying on the essential work of forming urine by the process of filtration, reabsorption, and secretion. Each nephron consists of (**1**) a **glomerulus** (a ball-shaped collection of very tiny, coiled, and intertwined capillaries), (**2**) a **renal capsule**, or **Bowman's capsule** (a double-walled cup surrounding the **glomerulus**), (**3**) the **renal tubule**, and (**4**) the **peritubular capillaries**.

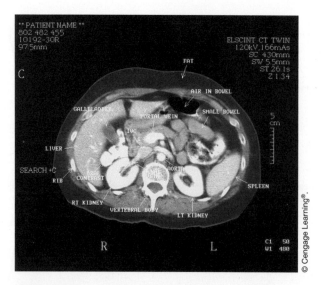

Figure 15-2 CT of the renal system, which shows the location of the urinary system organs

The first portion of the **renal tubule** is called the proximal convoluted (coiled) tubule. The second portion is called the loop of Henle. The third portion is called the distal convoluted tubule, which empties into the collecting tubule and leads to the inner portion of the kidney. See *Figure 15-3*.

The inner region, or **medulla**, of the kidney consists of triangular tissues called **renal pyramids**. The pyramids contain the loops and collecting tubules of the nephron.

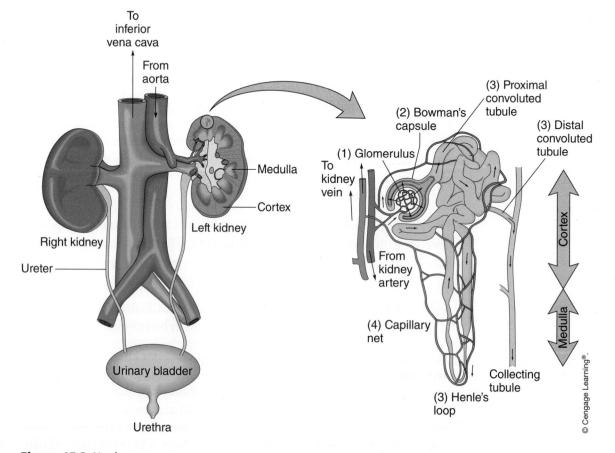

Figure 15-3 Nephron

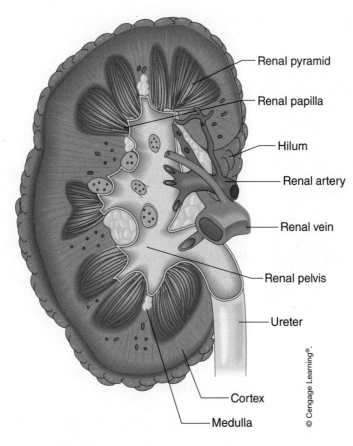

Renal pyramid

Renal papilla

Hilum

Renal artery

Renal vein

Renal pelvis

Ureter

Cortex

Medulla

© Cengage Learning®.

Figure 15-4 Internal anatomy of the kidney

The tip of each pyramid extends into a cuplike urine collection cavity called the minor **calyx**, with several of the minor calyces merging to form a major **calyx**. The major calyces, in turn, merge to form the central collecting area of the kidney (known as the **renal pelvis**). The urine secreted by the nephrons finally collects in this basinlike structure before entering the ureters. See *Figure 15-4*.

Ureters

The ureters are muscular tubes lined with mucous membrane, one leading from each kidney down to the urinary bladder. Each **ureter** is approximately 12 inches (30 cm) in length. Urine is propelled through the ureters by wavelike contractions known as peristalsis. The paths taken by the ureters in men and women are somewhat different because of variations in the nature, size, and position of the reproductive organs.

Bladder

The **urinary bladder** is a hollow muscular sac in the pelvic cavity that serves as a temporary reservoir for the urine. The dimensions of the bladder vary, depending on the amount of urine present, but a full urinary bladder can hold approximately a liter (L) of urine (about 1 quart). When full, the bladder is spherical in shape (egg shaped). When empty, it resembles an inverted pyramid.

The bladder lies between the pubic symphysis and the rectum in men. In women, the bladder lies between the pubic symphysis and the uterus and vagina. See *Figure 15-5*.

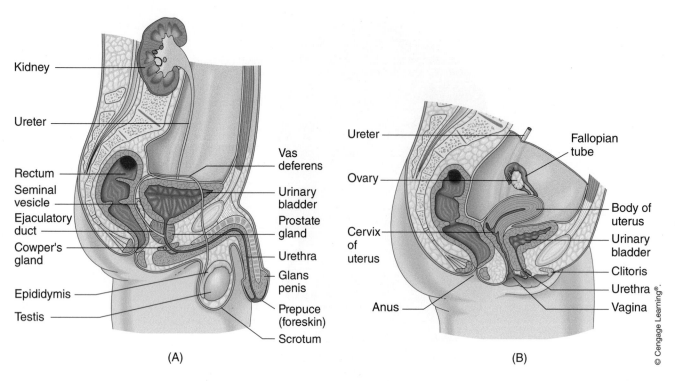

Figure 15-5 Location of urinary bladder: (A) male and (B) female

Urethra

The urine exits the bladder through the **urethra**. The **urethra** is a mucous membrane–lined tube that leads from the bladder to the exterior of the body. The external opening of the **urethra** is called the **urinary meatus**. The external sphincter, located below the neck of the bladder, controls the release of urine from the bladder. When the sphincter contracts, it closes the **urethra** and sends a message to the bladder to relax (releasing no urine). See *Figure 15-6A*. To void, or urinate, the sphincter relaxes and sends a message to the bladder to contract (opening the bladder neck and releasing urine from the body). See *Figure 15-6B*.

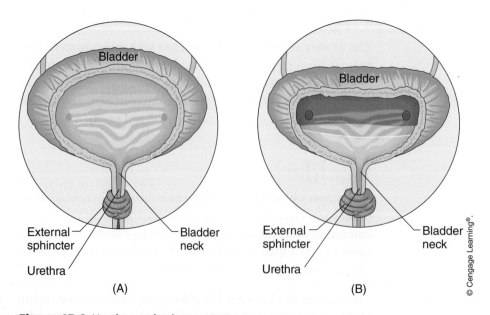

Figure 15-6 Urethra and urinary meatus

The female **urethra** carries only urine and is approximately 1 to 2 inches (3 to 5 cm) long. The male **urethra** is approximately 7 to 8 inches (18 to 20 cm) long and serves both the **urinary** and male reproductive systems. It transports urine and carries semen during ejaculation. The relationship of the male **urethra** to the male reproductive system is discussed in Chapter 16.

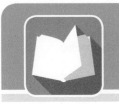

Review Checkpoint

Check your understanding of this section by completing the **Anatomy and Physiology** exercises in your workbook.

The Formation of Urine

The formation of urine consists of three distinct processes: glomerular filtration, tubular reabsorption, and tubular secretion. Blood enters the kidneys by way of the left and right renal arteries and leaves the kidneys by way of the left and right renal veins. The blood entering the kidneys comes directly from the abdominal aorta, passing through the renal arteries into the **hilum** of the kidney. The **hilum** is the depression, or pit, of the kidney where the vessels and nerves enter. See *Figure 15-4.*

After entering the kidney, the renal arteries branch out into smaller vessels throughout the kidney tissue until the smallest arteries (arterioles) reach the **cortex** of the kidney. Each **arteriole** leads to a **glomerulus.** It is here, in the **glomerulus**, that the formation of urine begins. See *Figure 15-7.*

As blood slowly but constantly passes through the thousands of glomeruli within the **cortex** of the kidneys, the blood pressure forces materials through the glomerular walls and into the **Bowman's capsule.** This process is known as **glomerular filtration.** Water, sugar, salts, and nitrogenous waste products (such as urea, creatinine, and uric acid) filter out of the blood through the thin walls of the glomeruli. These filtered products are called **glomerular filtrate.** Larger substances, such as proteins and blood cells, cannot press through the glomerular walls; they remain in the blood.

The filtered waste products and toxins (**glomerular filtrate**) are collected in the cup-shaped **Bowman's capsule** to be eliminated through the urine. Most of the water, electrolytes, and nutrients will be returned to the blood to maintain the balance of substances required for a relatively stable internal body environment.

The **glomerular filtrate** passes through the **Bowman's capsule** into the **renal tubule** (kidney tubule). As the **glomerular filtrate** passes through the renal tubules, the water, sugar, and salts are returned to the bloodstream through the network of capillaries that surround them. This process is known as **tubular reabsorption.** If it were not for this process of reabsorption, the body would be depleted of its fluid. Approximately 180 liters of **glomerular filtrate** pass through the tubules daily. As the filtrate passes through, some acids (such as potassium and uric acid) are secreted into the tubules directly from the bloodstream.

Tubular secretion occurs in the renal tubules when materials are selectively transferred from the blood into the filtrate to be excreted in the urine. These materials include substances that were unable to pass through the filtering tissues of the **glomerulus** as well as substances that may be present in the blood in excessive amounts. Examples of

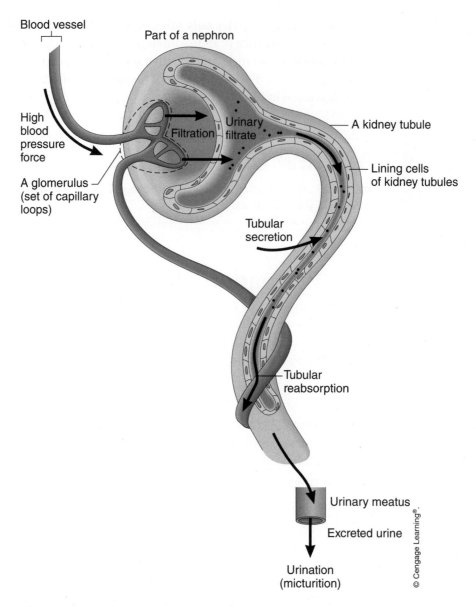

Figure 15-7 Major processes of urine formation

substances that may be secreted into the tubules for excretion through the urine include potassium, hydrogen, and certain drugs.

By the time the **glomerular filtrate** reaches the end of its journey through the renal tubules, the reabsorption of the essential components has been completed and only the remaining waste products, some water, some salts (electrolytes), and some acids are left to be excreted as **urine**. Normally, only 1% of the **glomerular filtrate** is excreted as urine. Urine, therefore, consists of water and other materials that were filtered or secreted into the tubules but were not reabsorbed. If a person has a normal daily fluid intake of 2 liters of fluid, the kidneys will filter that volume multiple times, producing a much larger glomerular filtrate of about 180 liters. Normally functioning kidneys will reabsorb 99% of the filtrate. Considering the fact that only 1% of the 180 liters of **glomerular filtrate** passing through the renal tubules is actually excreted as urine, the subsequent amount of urine excreted daily by healthy kidneys is approximately 1.8 liters (2 quarts), consisting of 95% water and 5% urea, creatinine, acids, and salts.

From the renal tubules, the urine is emptied into the **renal pelvis**. See *Figure 15-4*. Each **renal pelvis** narrows into the large upper end of the **ureter**. The urine passes down the ureters into the urinary bladder, a temporary reservoir for the urine. Urine is stored in the bladder until fullness stimulates a reflex contraction of the bladder muscle and the urine is expelled through the **urethra**. The release of urine is called **urination** or **micturition**. It is regulated by the sphincters (circular muscles) that surround the **urethra**. A flow chart depicting the formation of urine to the expelling of urine is shown in *Figure 15-8*. The illustrations in the figure are numbered to match those in the flow chart for better visual reference.

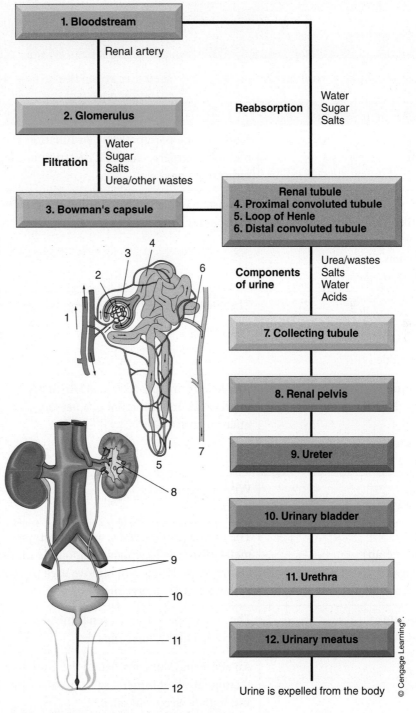

Figure 15-8 Flow chart of urine formation

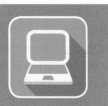

Media Link

Watch how urine is formed by viewing the **Urine Formation** animation on the Student Companion Website.

VOCABULARY

The following vocabulary words are frequently used when discussing the urinary system.

Word	Definition
ablation (ab-**LAY**-shun)	Removal of a part, pathway, or function by one of the following methods: surgery, chemical destruction, electrocautery, or radiofrequency.
antiseptic (**an**-tih-**SEP**-tik) anti- = against sept/o = infection -ic = pertaining to	A substance that tends to inhibit the growth and reproduction of microorganisms.
arteriole (ar-**TEE**-ree-ohl) arteri/o = artery -ole = small or little	The smallest branch of an artery.
aseptic technique (ay-**SEP**-tic tek-**NEEK**) a- = without, not sept/o = infection -ic = pertaining to	Any health care procedure in which precautions are taken to prevent contamination of a person, object, or area by microorganisms.
asymptomatic (ay-sim-toh-**MAT**-ic)	Without symptoms.
azotemia (**azz**-oh-**TEE**-mee-ah) azot/o = nitrogen -emia = blood condition	The presence of excessive amounts of waste products of metabolism (nitrogenous compounds) in the blood caused by failure of the kidneys to remove urea from the blood. **Azotemia** is characteristic of **uremia**.
Bowman's capsule (**BOW**-manz **CAP**-sool)	The cup-shaped end of a **renal tubule** containing a **glomerulus**; also called glomerular capsule.
calculus (**KAL**-kew-lus)	An abnormal stone formed in the body tissues by an accumulation of mineral salts; usually formed in the gallbladder and kidney. See *renal calculus*.

Word	Definition
calyx (**KAY**-liks) **calyces (plural)** (**KAL**-ih seez)	The cup-shaped division of the **renal pelvis** through which urine passes from the renal tubules.
catheter (**CATH**-eh-ter)	A hollow, flexible tube that can be inserted into a body cavity or vessel for the purpose of instilling or withdrawing fluid.
cortex (**KOR**-teks)	The outer layer of a body organ or structure.
cystocele (**SIS**-toh-seel) cyst/o = bladder -cele = swelling or herniation	Herniation or downward protrusion of the urinary bladder through the wall of the vagina.
cystometer (siss-**TOM**-eh-ter) cyst/o = bladder, sac, or cyst -meter = an instrument used to measure	An instrument that measures bladder capacity in relation to changing pressure.
cystopexy (**SIS**-toh-**peck**-see) cyst/o = bladder -pexy = surgical fixation	Surgical fixation of the bladder to the abdominal wall
cystoscope (**SISS**-toh-skohp) cyst/o = bladder, sac, or cyst -scope = instrument for viewing	An instrument used to view the interior of the bladder. It consists of an outer sheath with a lighting system, a scope for viewing, and a passage for catheters and devices used in surgical procedures; may also be referred to as a "cysto."
dialysate (dye-**AL**-ih-**SAYT**) dia- = through lys/o = breakdown or destruction -ate = something that . . .	Solution that contains water and electrolytes that passes through the artificial kidney to remove excess fluids and wastes from the blood; also called "bath."
dialysis (dye-**AL**-ih-sis) dia- = through -lysis = breakdown or destruction	The process of removing waste products from the blood when the kidneys are unable to do so. **Hemodialysis** involves passing the blood through an artificial kidney for filtering out impurities. **Peritoneal dialysis** involves introducing fluid into the abdomen through a **catheter**. Through the process of osmosis, this fluid draws waste products out of the capillaries into the abdominal cavity. It is then removed from the abdomen via a **catheter**.
dwell time	Length of time the **dialysis** solution stays in the peritoneal cavity during **peritoneal dialysis**.
epispadias (**ep**-ih-**SPAY**-dee-as) epi- = upon, over	A congenital defect (birth defect) in which the urethra opens on the upper side of the penis at some point near the glans.

Word	Definition
fossa (**FOSS**-ah)	A hollow or depression, especially on the surface of the end of a bone. In kidney transplantation, the donor kidney is surgically placed in the iliac **fossa** of the recipient.
glomerular filtrate (glom-**AIR**-yoo-lar **FILL**-trayt) glomerul/o = glomerulus -ar = pertaining to	Substances that filter out of the blood through the thin walls of the glomeruli (e.g., water, sugar, salts, and nitrogenous waste products such as urea, creatinine, and uric acid).
glomerulus (glom-**AIR**-yoo-lus) glomerul/o = glomerulus -us = noun ending	A ball-shaped collection of very tiny coiled and intertwined capillaries, located in the **cortex** of the kidney.
hilum (**HIGH**-lum)	The depression, or pit, of an organ where the vessels and nerves enter.
hydrostatic pressure	The pressure exerted by a liquid.
hydroureter (**high**-droh-yoo-**REE**-ter)	The distension of the **ureter** with urine due to blockage from an obstruction.
meatus (mee-**AY**-tus)	An opening or tunnel through any part of the body, as in the urinary **meatus**, which is the external opening of the **urethra**.
medulla (meh-**DULL**-ah)	The most internal part of a structure or organ.
micturition	The act of eliminating urine from the bladder; also called *voiding* or *urination*.
nephrolith (**NEF**-roh-lith) nephr/o = kidney -lith = stone	A kidney stone; also called a **renal calculus**.
nephrolithiasis (**nef**-roh-lith-**EYE**-ah-sis) nephr/o = kidney lith/o = stone, calculus -iasis = presence of an abnormal condition	A condition of kidney stones; also known as *renal calculi*.
neurogenic bladder (**new**-roh-**JEN**-ick **BLAD**-er) neur/o = nerve -genic = pertaining to formation, producing	A bladder dysfunction that results from interference with the normal nerve pathways associated with urination; may be due to disease of the central nervous system or peripheral nerves involved in the control of urination.
palpable (**PAL**-pah-bul)	Distinguishable by touch.

Word	Definition
peritoneum (pair-ih-toh-**NEE**-um) peritone/o = peritoneum -um = noun ending	A specific serous membrane that covers the entire abdominal wall of the body and is reflected over the contained viscera; the inner lining of the abdominal cavity.
peritonitis (**pair**-ih-ton-**EYE**-tis) peritone/o = peritoneum -itis = inflammation	Inflammation of the **peritoneum** (the membrane lining the abdominal cavity).
pyelitis (pye-eh-**LYE**-tis) pyel/o = renal pelvis -itis = inflammation	Inflammation of the **renal pelvis.**
radiopaque (ray-dee-oh-**PAYK**)	Not permitting the passage of X-rays or other radiant energy. **Radiopaque** areas appear white on an exposed X-ray film.
renal artery (**REE**-nal **AR**-teh-ree) ren/o = kidney -al = pertaining to arter/o = artery -y = noun ending	One of a pair of large arteries, branching from the abdominal aorta, that supplies blood to the kidneys, adrenal glands, and ureters.
renal calculus	A stone formation in the kidney (plural: *renal calculi*); also called a **nephrolith**.
renal pelvis (**REE**-nal **PELL**-viss) ren/o = kidney -al = pertaining to pelv/i = pelvis -is = noun ending	The central collecting part of the kidney that narrows into the large upper end of the **ureter**. It receives urine through the calyces and drains it into the ureters.
renal tubule (**REE**-nal **TOOB**-yool) ren/o = kidney -al = pertaining to	A long, twisted tube that leads away from the **glomerulus** of the kidney to the collecting tubules. As the **glomerular filtrate** passes through the renal tubules, the water, sugar, and salts are reabsorbed into the bloodstream through the network of capillaries that surround them.
renal vein (**REE**-nal **VAYN**) ren/o = kidney -al = pertaining to	One of two vessels that carries blood away from the kidney.
residual urine (rih-**ZID**-yoo-al **YOO**-rin)	Urine that remains in the bladder after **urination**.

Word	Definition
solute (**SOL**-yoot)	A substance dissolved in a solution, as in the waste products filtered out of the kidney into the urine.
specific gravity (speh-**SIH**-fik **GRAV**-ih-tee)	The weight of a substance compared with an equal volume of water, which is considered to be the standard. Water is considered to have a specific gravity of 1.000 (one). Therefore, a substance with a specific gravity of 2.000 would be twice as dense as water.
toxic (**TOKS**-ik) tox/o = poison -ic = pertaining to	Poisonous.
turbid (**TER**-bid)	Cloudy.
uremia (yoo-**REE**-mee-ah) ur/o = urine -emia = blood condition	The presence of excessive amounts of urea and other nitrogenous waste products in the blood; also called *azotemia*.
ureter (**YOO**-reh-ter) ureter/o = ureter	One of a pair of tubes that carries urine from the kidney to the bladder.
ureterectasis (**you**-ree-ter-**ECK**-tah-sis) ureter/o = ureter -ectasis = stretching or dilation	Stretching or dilation of a ureter.
ureterorrhagia (you-**ree**-ter-oh-**RAY**-jee-ah) ureter/o = ureter -rrhagia = excessive flow or discharge	Excessive flow or discharge of blood from the ureter.
urethra (yoo-**REE**-thrah) urethr/o = urethra -a = noun ending	A small tubular structure that drains urine from the bladder to the outside of the body.
urethritis (yoo-ree-**THRIGH**-tis) urethr/o = urethra -itis = inflammation	Inflammation of the **urethra. Urethritis**, characterized by **dysuria**, is usually the result of an infection of the bladder or kidneys.
urethropexy (you-**REE**-throh-**peck**-see) urethr/o = urethra -pexy = surgical fixation	Surgical fixation of the urethra.

Word	Definition
urethrostenosis (you-**ree**-thro-steh-**NOH**-sis) urethr/o = urethra -stenosis = tightening or narrowing	Narrowing of the urethra.
urinary incontinence (**YOO**-rih-**nair**-ee in-**CON**-tin-ens) urin/o = urine -ary = pertaining to	Inability to control **urination**; the inability to retain urine in the bladder.
urinary retention (**YOO**-rih-**nair**-ee ree-**TEN**-shun) urin/o = urine -ary = pertaining to	An abnormal involuntary accumulation of urine in the bladder; the inability to empty the bladder.
urination (**YOO**-rih-**NAY**-shun) urin/o = urine	The act of eliminating urine from the body; also called *micturition* or *voiding*.
urine (**YOO**-rin)	The fluid released by the kidneys, transported by the ureters, retained in the bladder, and eliminated through the **urethra**. Normal urine is clear, straw colored, and slightly acid.
vesicocele (**VESS**-ih-koh-**seel**) vesic/o = urinary bladder -cele = swelling or herniation	Herniation or downward protrusion of the urinary bladder through the wall of the vagina; also called a *cystocele*.
vesicovaginal fistula (**vess**-ih-koh-**VAJ**-ih-nahl **FIS**-chuh-lah) vesic/o = bladder vagin/o = vagina -al = pertaining to	An abnormal opening between the urinary bladder and the vagina.
voiding (**VOYD**-ing)	The act of eliminating urine from the body; also called *micturition* or **urination**.

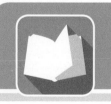

Review Checkpoint

Check your understanding of this section by completing the **Vocabulary** exercises in your workbook.

WORD ELEMENTS

The following word elements pertain to the urinary system. As you review the list, pronounce each word element aloud twice and check the box after you "say it." Write the definition for the example term given for each word element. Use your medical dictionary to find the definitions of the example terms.

Word Element	Pronunciation	"Say It"	Meaning
albumin/o **albumin**uria	al-**BYOO**-min-oh al-byoo-min-**YOO**-ree-ah	☐	albumin, protein
azot/o **azot**emia	azz-**OH**-toh **azz**-oh-**TEE**-mee-ah	☐	nitrogen
bacteri/o **bacteri**uria	bak-**TEE**-ree-oh bak-**tee**-ree-**YOO**-ree-ah	☐	bacteria
cali/o, calic/o **cali**ceal	**KAL**-ih-oh, kah-**LICK**-oh **kal**-ih-**SEE**-al	☐	**calyx**, calyces
-cele vesico**cele**	**SEEL** **VESS**-ih-koh **SEEL**	☐	Swelling or herniation
cyst/o **cyst**oscope	**SISS**-toh **SISS**-toh-skohp	☐	bladder, sac, or cyst
dips/o poly**dips**ia	**DIP**-soh pol-ee-**DIP**-see-ah	☐	thirst
epi- **epi**spadias	**EH**-pee eh-pih-**SPAY**-dee-as	☐	upon, over
-genic pyo**genic**	**JEN**-ick **pye**-oh-**JEN**-ick	☐	pertaining to formation, producing
glomerul/o **glomerul**ar	glom-**AIR**-yoo-loh glom-**AIR**-yoo-lar	☐	**glomerulus**
ket/o, keton/o **keton**uria	**KEE**-toh, kee-**TOH**-noh kee-toh-**NOO**-ree-ah	☐	ketone bodies
meat/o **meat**otomy	mee-**AH**-toh mee-ah-**TOT**-oh-mee	☐	**meatus**
nephr/o **nephr**itis	**NEH**-froh neh-**FRY**-tis	☐	kidney

Word Element	Pronunciation	"Say It"	Meaning
neur/o **neur**ogenic	**NEW**-roh **new**-roh-**JEN**-ick	☐	nerve
noct/i **noct**uria	**NOK**-tih nok-**TOO**-ree-ah	☐	night
olig/o **olig**uria	ol-**IG**-oh ol-ig-**YOO**-ree-ah	☐	few, little, scanty
-pexy cysto**pexy**	**PECK-see** **SIS**-toh-**peck**-see	☐	surgical fixation
pyel/o **pyel**itis	**PYE**-eh-loh **pye**-eh-**LYE**-tis	☐	**renal pelvis**
py/o **py**uria	**PYE**-yoh pye-**YOO**-ree-ah	☐	pus
ren/o **ren**al	**REE**-noh **REE**-nal	☐	kidney
-rrhagia cysto**rrhagia**	**RAY**-jee-ah sis-toh-**RAY**-jee-ah	☐	excessive flow or discharge
-stenosis urethro**stenosis**	steh-**NOH**-sis you-**ree**-throh-steh-**NOH**-sis	☐	tightening or narrowing
ureter/o **ureter**ostenosis	yoo-**REE**-ter-oh yoo-**ree**-ter-oh-sten-**OH**-sis	☐	**ureter**
urethr/o **urethr**itis	yoo-**REE**-throh yoo-ree-**THRIGH**-tis	☐	**urethra**
ur/o, urin/o **urin**ometer	**YOO**-roh, yoo-**RIN**-oh **yoo**-rih-**NOM**-eh-ter	☐	urine
-uria hemat**uria**	**YOO**-ree-ah hee-mah-**TOO**-ree-ah	☐	urine condition
vesic/o **vesic**ocele	**VESS**-ih-koh **VESS**-ih-koh-**seel**	☐	urinary bladder

Review Checkpoint

Check your understanding of this section by completing the **Word Elements** exercises in your workbook.

Characteristics of Urine

The examination of urine is an important screening test that provides valuable information about the status of the **urinary** system. The routine **urinalysis** is a test that involves the collection of a random sample of urine. The urine is examined to determine the presence of any abnormal elements that might indicate various pathological (disease-producing) conditions. The following characteristics of urine are determined by observation of the specimen (known as physical examination of urine) and by chemical examination, using a reagent strip.

Color

Normal urine varies in color from pale yellow to a deep golden color, depending on the concentration of the urine. The darker the urine, the greater the concentration. A very pale (almost colorless) urine indicates a large amount of water in the urine and less concentration. Certain medications and foods can change the color of urine. For example, certain foods (such as beets) can produce red hues in the urine, and certain medications (such as vitamin B complex) can produce a lemon yellow hue to the urine. The presence of blood in the urine (**hematuria**) can range from a reddish hue, to a cherry red, to a smoky red or brown color. The latter two colors would indicate a large amount of blood in the urine.

Clarity

Normal urine is clear. A cloudy (**turbid**) appearance to the urine may be due to the presence of pus (**pyuria**), bacteria (**bacteriuria**), or a specimen that has been standing for more than an hour. The cloudy urine may also indicate the presence of a bladder or kidney infection.

Odor

Normal urine is aromatic; that is, it has a strong but agreeable odor. A foul or putrid odor is common in some infections. Urine specimens that are not refrigerated may develop a foul odor after standing for a long period of time. A fruity odor to the urine is found in diabetes mellitus, starvation, or dehydration. Certain medications and foods can also cause a change in the odor of urine.

Specific Gravity

Normal urine has a **specific gravity** of 1.003 to 1.030. The **specific gravity** is the measurement of the amount of solids in the urine. The lower the **specific gravity**, the fewer solids; the higher the **specific gravity**, the more solids present in the urine. Distilled water is used as the standard of comparison for liquids when measuring the **specific gravity**. A low **specific gravity** can be found in kidney diseases, indicating that the urine has a greater concentration of water than solids. The water was not reabsorbed into the bloodstream as usual. Thus the urine has been greatly diluted, resembling the **specific gravity** of water more than that of normal urine. A high **specific gravity** can be found in diabetes mellitus due to the presence of sugar in the urine.

pH

Normal urine has a pH range of 4.5 to 8.0, with the slightly acid reading of 6.0 being the norm. The pH represents the relative acidity (or alkalinity) of a solution in which a value of 7.0 is neutral, below 7.0 is acid, and above 7.0 is alkaline (base). The urine pH may be alkaline when a urinary tract infection is present.

Protein

Normal urine may have small amounts of protein present, but only in insignificant amounts, that is, in amounts too small to be detected by the reagent strip method. Albumin is the major protein present in **renal** (kidney) diseases. Because albumin does not normally filter out through the glomerular membrane, the presence of large amounts of protein in the urine (proteinuria or **albuminuria**) may indicate a leak in the glomerular membrane.

Glucose

Normal urine does not contain glucose. There are some normal conditions that can cause glucose to appear in the urine, such as having eaten a high-carbohydrate meal, pregnancy, emotional stress, or ingestion of certain medications. If glucose does appear in the urine, the cause must be determined by further studies because the appearance of sugar in the urine can be an indicator of diabetes mellitus. In diabetes mellitus, the hyperglycemia (high blood sugar level) leads to the presence of sugar in the urine because the renal tubules are unable to reabsorb the total quantity of sugar filtered through the glomerular membrane.

Ketones

Normal urine does not contain ketone bodies. Ketones result from the breakdown of fats. In poorly controlled diabetes mellitus, the body is unable to use sugar for energy. Therefore, fat is broken down and used as energy for the body cells. When this happens, ketones accumulate in large quantities in the blood and the urine. It is important to note that the presence of ketones in the urine may also be a result of starvation, dehydration, or excessive ingestion of aspirin. Therefore, the cause of ketones in the urine must be determined by further testing.

Common Signs and Symptoms

The following is a list of common signs and symptoms that indicate possible **urinary** system problems. The patient may actually complain of these symptoms, or the results of the physical, chemical, or microscopic **urinalysis** may reveal the signs of **urinary** system problems. As your experience grows in listening carefully to the patient's description of his or her reasons for coming to the doctor, you will become more perceptive in determining which medical term the patient is describing. As you study the following terms, write each definition and word a minimum of three times (use a separate sheet of paper), pronouncing the word aloud each time. Note that the word and the basic definition are in a green shaded box, if you choose to learn only the abbreviated form of the definition. A more detailed description follows most words. Once you have mastered each word to your satisfaction, check the box provided beside the word.

☐ **albuminuria**

(**al**-byoo-min-**YOO**-ree-ah)

　albumin/o = albumin, protein

　-uria = urine condition

The presence in the urine of abnormally large quantities of protein, usually albumin. (**Albuminuria** is the same thing as proteinuria.) Healthy adults excrete less than 250 mg of protein per day. Persistent proteinuria is usually a sign of **renal** (kidney) disease or **renal** complications of another disease such as hypertension or heart failure.

☐ **anuria**

(an-**YOO**-ree-ah)

　an- = without, not

　-uria = urine condition

The cessation (stopping) of urine production or a **urinary** output of less than 100 mL per day.

Anuria may be caused by kidney failure or dysfunction, a decline in blood pressure below that required to maintain filtration pressure in the kidney, or an obstruction in the **urinary** passages.

☐ **bacteriuria**

(back-**tee**-ree-**YOO**-ree-ah)

　bacteri/o = bacteria

　-uria = urine condition

The presence of bacteria in the urine.

The presence of more than 100,000 pathogenic (disease-producing) bacteria per milliliter of urine is usually considered significant and diagnostic of urinary tract infection.

☐ **dysuria**

(diss-**YOO**-ree-ah)

　dys- = bad, difficult, painful, disordered

　-uria = urine condition

Painful **urination.**

Dysuria is usually the result of a bacterial infection or obstructive condition in the **urinary** tract. The patient will complain of a burning sensation when passing urine. Lab results may reveal the presence of blood, bacteria, or white blood cells.

☐ **enuresis**

(en-yoo-**REE**-sis)

　ur/o = urine

　-esis = condition of

A condition of **urinary incontinence**, especially at night in bed; bed-wetting.

☐ **fatigue**

(fah-**TEEG**)

A state of exhaustion or loss of strength or endurance such as may follow strenuous physical activity.

Fatigue may be indicative of emotional conflicts, boredom, the result of excessive activity, or a sign of some underlying physical cause.

☐ **frequency**

The number of repetitions of any phenomenon within a fixed period of time such as the number of heartbeats per minute; in the case of **urinary** frequency, **urination** at short intervals (frequently) without increase in the daily volume of **urinary** output, due to reduced bladder capacity.

Urinary frequency can be a sign of bladder infection.

☐ **glycosuria**

(**glye**-kohs-**YOO**-ree-ah)

　glyc/o = sugar, sweet

　-uria = urine condition

Abnormal presence of a sugar, especially glucose, in the urine.

Glycosuria can result from the ingestion of large amounts of carbohydrates, or it may be the result of endocrine or **renal** disorders. It is a finding most routinely associated with diabetes mellitus.

☐ **hematuria**	Abnormal presence of blood in the urine.
(hee-mah-**TOO**-ree-ah)	
hemat/o = blood	**Hematuria** is symptomatic of many **renal** diseases and disorders of the genitourinary system.
-uria = urine condition	

☐ **ketonuria**	Presence of excessive amounts of ketone bodies in the urine.
(kee-toh-**NOO**-ree-ah)	
keton/o = ketone bodies	**Ketonuria** occurs as a result of uncontrolled diabetes mellitus, starvation, or any other metabolic condition in which fats are rapidly broken down; also called ketoaciduria.
-uria = urine condition	

| ☐ **lethargy** | The state or quality of being indifferent, apathetic (without emotion), or sluggish. |
| (**LETH**-ar-jee) | |

| ☐ **malaise** | A vague feeling of bodily weakness or discomfort, often marking the onset of disease or infection. |
| (mah-**LAYZ**) | |

☐ **nocturia**	**Urination**, especially excessive, at night; also called nycturia.
(nok-**TOO**-ree-ah)	
noct/o = night	**Nocturia** may be a symptom of **renal** disease. It may also occur in the absence of disease in people who drink large amounts of fluids, particularly alcohol or coffee, before bedtime or in people with prostatic disease.
-uria = urine condition	

☐ **oliguria**	Secretion of a diminished amount of urine in relation to the fluid intake; scanty urine output.
(ol-ig-**YOO**-ree-ah)	
olig/o = few, little, scanty	The individual excretes less than 500 mL of urine in every 24 hours. Thus the end products of metabolism cannot be excreted efficiently. **Oliguria** is usually caused by imbalances in bodily fluids and electrolytes, by **renal** lesions, or by **urinary** tract obstruction.
-uria = urine condition	

☐ **polydipsia**	Excessive thirst.
(pol-ee-**DIP**-see-ah)	
poly- = many, much, excessive	**Polydipsia** may be indicative of **renal** problems. It is also characteristic of diabetes mellitus and diabetes insipidus, which are endocrine gland problems.
-dipsia = thirst	

☐ **polyuria**	Excretion of abnormally large amounts of urine.
(pol-ee-**YOO**-ree-ah)	
poly- = many, much, excessive	Several liters in excess of normal may be excreted each day. **Polyuria** occurs in conditions such as diabetes mellitus, diabetes insipidus, and chronic kidney infections.
-uria = urine condition	

☐ **pyuria**	The presence of an excessive number of white blood cells in the urine, usually a sign of an infection of the **urinary** tract; pus in the urine.
(pye-**YOO**-ree-ah)	
py/o = pus	
-uria = urine condition	

☐ **urgency**	A feeling of the need to void urine immediately.
(**ER**-jen-see)	
	Urgency may accompany a bladder infection.

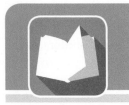

Review Checkpoint

Check your understanding of this section by completing the **Common Signs and Symptoms** exercises in your workbook.

Pathological Conditions

As you study the pathological conditions of the **urinary** system, note that the **basic definition** is in a green shaded box, followed by a more detailed description in regular print. The phonetic pronunciation is directly beneath each term, as well as a breakdown of the component parts of the term where applicable.

cystitis	Inflammation of the urinary bladder.
(siss-**TYE**-tis) cyst/o = bladder, sac, or cyst -itis = inflammation	**Cystitis** is characterized by **urgency** and frequency of **urination** and by **hematuria**. It may be caused by a bacterial infection, kidney stone, or tumor. Treatment for **cystitis** may include antibiotics, increased fluid intake (particularly water), bed rest, and medications to control the bladder spasms. If the cause is due to a stone or tumor, surgery may be necessary.
glomerulonephritis (acute)	An inflammation of the **glomerulus** of the kidneys.
(gloh-**mair**-yoo-loh-neh-**FRYE**-tis) glomerul/o = glomerulus nephr/o = kidney -itis = inflammation	This condition, primarily a disease of children, is characterized by proteinuria, **hematuria**, and decreased urine production. The **specific gravity** of the urine will be elevated because of scanty urine output, and the urine may appear as dark as the color of a cola beverage (i.e., dark and smoky). The patient frequently experiences headaches, moderate to severe hypertension, and generalized edema, particularly facial and periorbital (around the eye socket) swelling. **Glomerulonephritis** (acute) is usually caused by a beta-hemolytic streptococcal infection elsewhere in the body. It may also be caused by other microorganisms or the result of some other systemic disorder. Poststreptococcal **glomerulonephritis** typically occurs about three weeks after a streptococcal infection. Treatment includes the use of antibiotics, such as penicillin, to protect against the recurrence of infection. Sodium and fluid intake are restricted to control the hypertension and general fluid overload. Bed rest is continued until the clinical signs of nephritis have disappeared. Most patients with acute **glomerulonephritis** recover within a few weeks of the onset of symptoms. Approximately 90% of the children recover fully from this illness. About 30% of adults acquire this illness, progressing to chronic **glomerulonephritis**.

hydronephrosis

(high-droh-neh-**FROH**-sis)

hydro- = water
nephr/o = kidney
-osis = condition

Distension of the pelvis and calyces of the kidney caused by urine that cannot flow past an obstruction in a **ureter**. See *Figure 15-9*.

Urine production continues, but the urine is trapped at the point of the obstruction in the **ureter**. This distended **ureter** is known as a **hydroureter**. Obstruction in a single **ureter** will affect only one kidney. However, if the obstruction is in the bladder or **urethra**, both kidneys will be affected. The primary cause of obstruction in adults is kidney stones (renal calculi).

The patient with **hydronephrosis** may complain of intense flank pain, nausea, vomiting, scanty or no urine output, and the presence of blood in the urine (**hematuria**). Treatment is directed at removing the obstruction to urine flow and preventing infection.

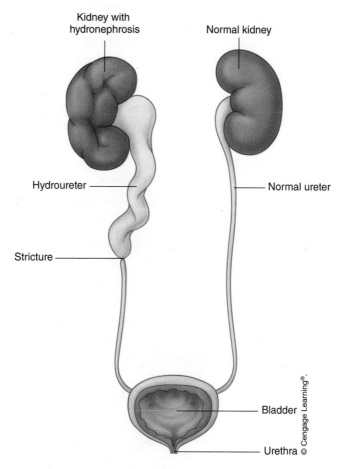

Figure 15-9 Hydronephrosis

nephrotic syndrome

(neh-**FROT**-ic **SIN**-drohm)

nephr/o = kidney
-tic = pertaining to
syn- = together, joined
drom/o = running
-y = noun ending

A group of clinical symptoms occurring when damage to the **glomerulus** of the kidney is present and large quantities of protein are lost through the glomerular membrane into the urine, resulting in severe proteinuria (presence of large amounts of protein in the urine); also called nephrosis.

The excessive loss of protein (albumin) results in a low blood albumin level. These changes create the resultant edema that accompanies the **nephrotic syndrome**. The patient will experience massive generalized edema.

Most cases of **nephrotic syndrome** result from some form of **glomerulo-nephritis**. The syndrome may also occur as a result of systemic diseases such as diabetes mellitus. Medical treatment for **nephrotic syndrome** is directed at controlling the edema and reducing the **albuminuria** as well as treating the underlying cause.

| **polycystic kidney disease** | A hereditary disorder of the kidneys in which grapelike, fluid-filled sacs or cysts replace normal kidney tissue. See *Figure 15-10*. |

(pol-ee-**SISS**-tik kidney disease)

poly- = many, much, excessive
cyst/o = bladder, sac, or cyst
-ic = pertaining to

The kidneys are larger than normal and are filled with cysts of various sizes. As the cysts continue to develop, the pressure from the expanding cysts slowly destroys the healthy kidney tissue, and **renal** function deteriorates.

This disease is usually symptom-free until midlife. Once symptoms begin to appear, the patient may complain of pain in one or both kidneys, described as a dull aching, a stabbing-type pain, or a vague sense of heaviness in the area of the kidneys. **Hematuria** is present in about half the cases, and hypertension is common.

Polycystic kidney disease is a slowly progressive disease that ultimately leads to **uremia** (kidney failure), a process that may take 15 to 30 years from the onset of symptoms. Treatment is directed at preventing **urinary** tract infections and controlling the secondary hypertension.

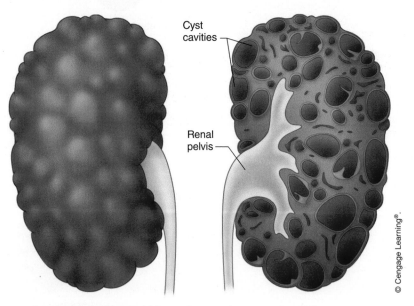

Cyst cavities

Renal pelvis

© Cengage Learning®.

Figure 15-10 Polycystic kidney disease

| **pyelonephritis (acute)** | A bacterial infection of the **renal pelvis** of the kidney. |

(pye-eh-loh-neh-**FRYE**-tis)

pyel/o = renal pelvis
nephr/o = kidney
-itis = inflammation

Pyelonephritis is one of the more common diseases of the kidney and usually occurs because of an ascending **urinary** tract infection, that is, one that begins in the bladder and travels up (ascends) the ureters to the **renal pelvis**. Acute **pyelonephritis** often occurs after bacterial contamination of the **urethra** or after some instrumentation procedure such as **cystoscopy** or **catheterization**. It is characterized by fever, chills, nausea, flank pain on the affected side, headache, and muscular pain. The urine may be cloudy or bloody, have a marked increase in white blood cells and white cell casts, and have a foul-smelling odor. Treatment includes the use of antibiotics.

renal calculi	Stone formations in the kidney.

(**REE**-nal **KAL**-kew-lye)

If the stone is large enough to lodge in the **ureter**, the individual experiences a sudden severe attack of pain in the region of one kidney and toward the thigh (known as renal colic). This may be accompanied by chills, fever, **hematuria** (blood in the urine), and frequency of **urination**.

Conservative treatment of renal calculi is directed at relief of pain and passage of the stone. Fluids are forced unless the **ureter** is completely blocked by the **calculus**. Smooth-muscle relaxants and pain relievers are administered. If the stone is completely blocking the ureter and cannot be passed by conservative means, surgery is indicated to remove the stone, or the stone may be disintegrated by ultrasound or other forms of energy.

renal cell carcinoma	A malignant tumor of the kidney occurring in adulthood.

(**REE**-nal **SELL** car-sin-**OH**-mah)
  ren/o = kidney
  -al = pertaining to
  carcin/o = cancer
  -oma = tumor

The patient is **asymptomatic** (symptom free) until the latter stages of the disease. The most common symptom of **renal cell carcinoma** is painless **hematuria** with later development of flank pain, a **palpable** mass, and intermittent fever. Once the diagnosis is confirmed, the treatment of choice is surgery to remove the tumor before it can invade adjacent tissue (metastasize). Chemotherapy and radiation treatment may also follow surgery.

renal failure, chronic	Progressively slow development of kidney failure occurring over a period of years. The late stages of **chronic renal failure** are known as end-stage renal disease (ESRD).

(**REE**-nal **FAIL**-yoor, **KRON**-ik) (uremia)
(yoo-**REE**-mee-ah)
  ren/o = kidney
  -al = pertaining to
  ur/o = urine
  -emia = blood condition

In **chronic renal failure**, there is a progressive irreversible deterioration in **renal** function in which the body's ability to maintain metabolic, fluid, and electrolyte balance fails. A gradual progression toward **uremia** occurs. Waste products of metabolism (urea and creatinine) that would normally filter out of the kidney into the urine remain in the bloodstream; that is, urine constituents are present in the blood. The accumulation of these end products of protein metabolism in the blood is known as **azotemia**. The most common causes of **chronic renal failure** are hypertension and diabetes.

The numerous symptoms of end-stage renal failure include nausea, vomiting, anorexia, and hiccups. Numbness and burning sensations in both legs and feet are common, with prickly sensations being more intense at night. Anemia is present due to the kidney's suppressed secretion of erythropoietin, which stimulates the production of red blood cells in the bone marrow. Hypertension is usually present and may require antihypertensive therapy to control the blood pressure. The patient may also experience pruritus (itching of the skin), **polyuria**, weight loss, lack of energy, pale skin with a sallow or brownish hue, and mental confusion. The point at which the patient displays obvious signs of **renal** failure occurs when approximately 80% to 90% of the **renal** function has been lost.

Initial treatment is directed at controlling or relieving the symptoms to prevent further complications. Medications may be given to relieve the nausea and the hypertension. The patient may be placed on a protein-, sodium-, and potassium-restricted diet due to the impaired kidney function. Injectable erythropoietin (Epogen) may be administered three times per week to improve the anemic state. As the patient's condition deteriorates, **dialysis** may be used to take over as a functioning artificial kidney, prolonging the patient's life until a kidney transplant becomes available.

vesicoureteral reflux	An abnormal backflow (reflux) of urine from the bladder to the **ureter**.

(**vess**-ih-koh-yoo-**REE**-ter-al **REE**-fluks)
  vesic/o = urinary bladder
  ureter/o = ureter
  -al = pertaining to

Vesicoureteral reflux may result from a congenital defect, a **urinary** tract infection, or obstruction of the outlet of the bladder. The reflux of urine may result in bacterial infection of the upper **urinary** tract and damage to the ureters and kidney due to increased **hydrostatic pressure**.

Symptoms include abdominal or flank pain, recurrent **urinary** tract infections, **dysuria**, frequency, and **urgency**. **Pyuria**, **hematuria**, proteinuria, and **bacteriuria** may also be present. Treatment is directed at correcting the underlying cause of the reflux.

Wilms' tumor	A malignant tumor of the kidney occurring predominantly in childhood.

The most frequent finding is a **palpable** mass in the abdomen and hypertension. The child may also be experiencing abdominal pain, fever, anorexia, nausea, vomiting, and **hematuria**. Once diagnosis is confirmed, the treatment of choice is surgery to remove the tumor, followed by chemotherapy and radiation. With treatment and no evidence of spreading to other areas, the cure rate is high for patients with Wilms' tumors.

Treatment of Renal Failure

The following is a discussion of the various methods of treatment for **renal** failure.

peritoneal dialysis	**Dialysis** is a mechanical filtering process used to cleanse the blood of waste products, draw off excess fluids, and regulate body chemistry when the kidneys fail to function properly. Instead of using the **hemodialysis** machine as a filter, the peritoneal membrane (also called the peritoneum) is used as the filter in **peritoneal dialysis**.

(**pair**-ih-toh-**NEE**-al dye-**AL**-ih-sis)
  peritone/o = peritoneum
  -al = pertaining to
  dia- = through
  -lysis = breakdown or destruction

The peritoneal membrane is a thin membrane that lines the abdominal cavity. It is richly supplied with tiny blood vessels, thus providing a continuous supply of blood to be filtered.

Prior to the first **peritoneal dialysis** exchange, an **access tube** (catheter, known as a Tenckhoff peritoneal catheter) is surgically placed in the lower abdomen. See *Figure 15-11.*

The access tube is used for the infusion of the **dialysate** solution and draining of the fluid from the abdomen. The **dialysate** solution is a mixture of water and electrolytes that will draw the excess fluid and toxins from the blood, across the peritoneal membrane, into the abdominal cavity.

This process of draining and infusing of **dialysate** solution is called an exchange cycle. There are two types of **peritoneal dialysis** exchange that can be performed at home: continuous ambulatory peritoneal dialysis (CAPD) or continuous cycling peritoneal dialysis (CCPD).

CAPD can be performed by the patient and does not require a machine. Sterile plastic tubing, called a transfer set, is connected to a bag of approximately

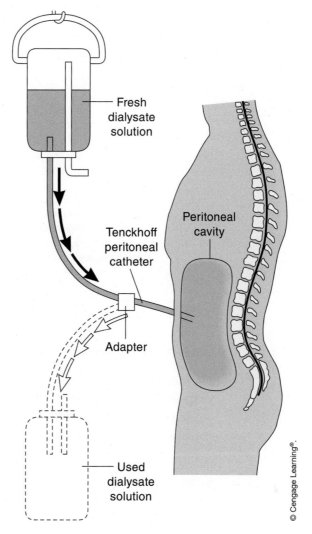

Figure 15-11 Peritoneal dialysis

2 liters of slightly warmed **dialysate** solution. After the proper connections are made with the tubing and the patient's access tube, the **dialysate** bag is raised above the shoulder and the solution slowly flows into the abdomen.

During a **peritoneal dialysis** exchange, the **dialysate** solution remains in the abdomen for approximately four hours. This process is repeated three to five times every day, with the residual fluid from the previous exchange being drained first, followed by the infusion of the **dialysate**. The last exchange of the day is performed just before bedtime, and the **dialysate** is left in the abdomen overnight.

Training for continuous CAPD procedures takes approximately one to two weeks. Patients are taught the procedure, the signs and symptoms of infection, and how to make decisions about using the appropriate **dialysate** solution strength to obtain optimal results. The advantage of CAPD is that a machine is not used and the procedure is convenient for traveling.

CCPD, on the other hand, uses a machine that warms the solution and cycles it in and out of the peritoneal cavity at evenly spaced intervals at night while the patient sleeps. This process takes 8 to 10 hours.

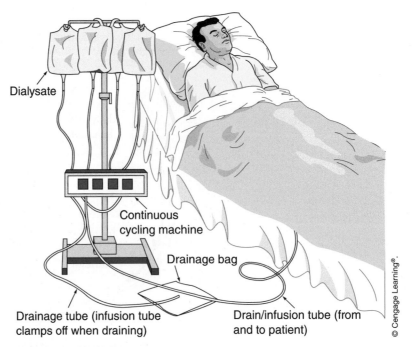

Dialysate

Continuous cycling machine

Drainage bag

Drainage tube (infusion tube clamps off when draining)

Drain/infusion tube (from and to patient)

© Cengage Learning®.

Figure 15-12 Continuous cyclic peritoneal dialysis

The initial exchange begins with the infusion of a prescribed amount of **dialysate** into the abdominal cavity. Upon completion, the patient's access tube is clamped and removed from the infusion tubing. The **dialysate** fluid then remains in the abdomen during the day for approximately 12 to 15 hours.

Before the patient goes to sleep at night, the access **catheter** is reconnected to the **dialysis** machine and the residual fluid is drained out of the abdomen. This is followed by the nighttime exchanges: a series of four or more cycles of infusion of **dialysate**, retention of the solution in the abdominal cavity (known as **dwell time**), and draining of the fluid from the abdomen. The cyclic exchanges are controlled by the machine as the patient sleeps. See *Figure 15-12*.

When the final cycle of draining is completed, the abdomen is once again infused with **dialysate** solution that will remain in the abdomen throughout the day. This process is repeated daily. The advantage of CCPD is that exchanges are done at night by the machine instead of several times throughout the day by the patient (as in ambulatory **dialysis**).

The major concern with the **peritoneal dialysis** is the possibility of the patient developing **peritonitis** (inflammation of the peritoneum). Patients are instructed to report any signs of fever, tenderness around the access site, nausea, weakness, or cloudy appearance of the **dialysate** solution that drains from the abdominal cavity. If **peritonitis** develops, it is treated with antibiotics.

hemodialysis	The process of removing excess fluids and toxins from the blood by continually shunting the patient's blood from the body into a **dialysis** machine for filtering and then returning the clean blood to the patient's bloodstream.
(**hee**-moh-dye-**AL**-ih-sis)	
hem/o = blood	
dia- = through	
-lysis = breakdown or destruction	

While the patient's blood flows through the dialyzer, the toxins and excess fluid are drawn across the semipermeable membrane into the **dialysate**

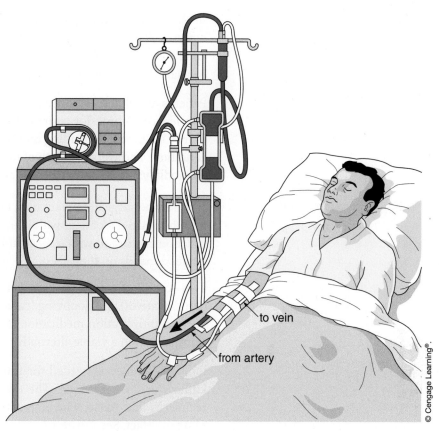

Figure 15-13 Hemodialysis

solution (which is circulating on the other side of the membrane). The fil-tered blood is then routed back into the body while the waste products are channeled out of the machine via the **dialysate**. See *Figure 15-13*.

To be able to shunt blood from the body to the hemodialyzer and back, a large vessel with a good blood flow is necessary. Therefore, an "access" vessel is created. The access of choice for chronic **hemodialysis** is the inter-nal **arteriovenous fistula** in which an opening, or fistula, has been created between an artery and a vein in the forearm. See *Figure 15-14*.

The flow of the arterial blood into the venous system at the point of the fistula causes the vein to become distended, providing a large enough vessel with a strong blood flow for the **hemodialysis** connection. The arteriovenous fistula needs approximately two to six weeks to "mature"

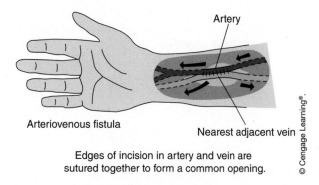

Arteriovenous fistula

Artery

Nearest adjacent vein

Edges of incision in artery and vein are sutured together to form a common opening.

Figure 15-14 Arteriovenous fistula for hemodialysis

so that it is strong enough and large enough for needle insertion during **dialysis**. The mix of arterial and venous blood, created by the arteriovenous fistula, is so insignificant that it does not cause a problem with the oxygen concentration of the blood.

Patients usually receive **hemodialysis** treatments three times a week. The length of time for a single **hemodialysis** treatment may vary from four to six hours, depending on the type of dialyzer used and the patient's condition. The average length of time for treatments is three to four hours. **Hemodialysis** may be performed at home or at the **dialysis** center.

kidney transplantation (kidney tranz-plan-**TAY**-shun)	Involves the surgical implantation of a healthy human donor kidney into the body of a patient with irreversible **renal** failure. Kidney function is restored with a successful transplant, and the patient no longer depends on **dialysis**.

Two sources are used in kidney transplantation: living donors (usually blood relatives) and nonliving (cadaver) donors. Advances in tissue matching and antirejection medications (immunosuppressive drugs) have made transplantation a viable alternative for treating end-stage renal failure.

Only one kidney is needed for transplantation. Generally, the recipient's kidneys are not removed. The donor kidney is surgically placed in the recipient's iliac **fossa**. The blood supply to the recipient's natural kidneys remains intact. See *Figure 15-15*.

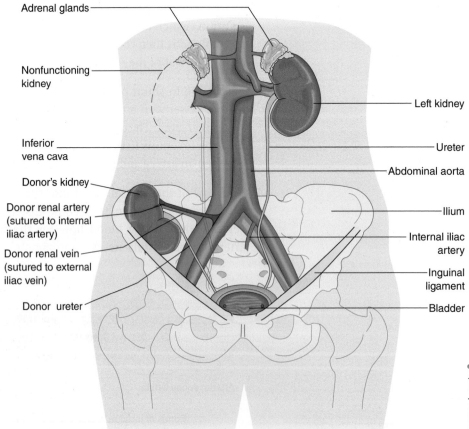

© Cengage Learning®.

Figure 15-15 Kidney placement for renal transplant

The **renal artery** of the donor kidney is connected to the recipient's iliac artery, and the iliac vein of the donor kidney is connected to the recipient's iliac vein. Once the transplanted kidney is in place, it usually begins to function immediately. If adequate function is delayed for a few days, a return to **dialysis** may be necessary until good kidney function is established.

Survival rates (i.e., kidney not being rejected) one year after transplantation are 80% to 90% for living related donor transplants and 70% to 90% for cadaver donor transplants.

Review Checkpoint

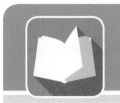

Check your understanding of this section by completing the **Pathological Conditions** exercises in your workbook.

Diagnostic Techniques, Treatments, and Procedures

blood urea nitrogen (BUN) (blud yoo-**REE**-ah **NIGH**-troh-jen)	A blood test performed to determine the amount of urea and nitrogen (waste products normally excreted by the kidney) present in the blood. The **blood urea nitrogen** level is usually increased with impaired glomerular filtration.
catheterization (**cath**-eh-ter-**EYE**-zay-shun)	The introduction of a **catheter** (flexible hollow tube) into a body cavity or organ to instill a substance or to remove a fluid. The most common type of **catheterization** is the insertion of a **catheter** into the urinary bladder for the purpose of removing urine. A urinary **catheterization** may be performed to obtain a sterile specimen of urine for testing, to provide relief for **urinary retention**, to empty the bladder completely before surgery, or to instill a contrast medium into the bladder for the purpose of visualizing the structures of the **urinary** system on X-ray.
creatinine clearance test (kree-**AT**-in-in clearance test)	A diagnostic test for kidney function that measures the filtration rate of creatinine, a waste product (of muscle metabolism) normally removed by the kidney. Creatinine levels are determined on a 24-hour urine specimen collection and on a sample of blood drawn during the same 24-hour period. Impaired glomerular function will result in a decrease in creatinine clearance rate and an increase in serum creatinine levels.
cystometrography (**siss**-toh-meh-**TROG**-rah-fee) **cyst/o** = bladder, sac, or cyst **metr/o** = measure **-graphy** = process of recording	An examination performed to evaluate bladder tone; measuring bladder pressure during filling and **voiding**. At the beginning of the **cystometrography**, the patient is asked to empty his or her bladder. A **catheter** is then inserted through the **urethra** into the

bladder. Any **residual urine** present is removed through the **catheter** and the amount is recorded.

Saline solution or water is then instilled into the bladder, at a constant rate, through the **catheter**. The patient is asked to report when the urge to urinate is first felt, when the bladder feels full, and when it is impossible to hold any more fluid in the bladder without **voiding**.

Bladder pressure is measured with the **cystometer** that is attached to the **catheter**. The measurement of the pressure the bladder musculature exerts on the fluid being instilled is recorded after the instillation of every 50 mL of solution.

cystoscopy	The process of viewing the interior of the bladder, using a **cystoscope**.

(siss-**TOSS**-koh-pee)
   cyst/o = bladder, sac, or cyst
   -scopy = process of viewing

The **cystoscope** is a hollow metal or flexible tube introduced into the bladder through the urinary meatus. Visualization of the inside of the bladder is made possible by a light source and magnifying lenses, which are a part of the **cystoscope**. See *Figure 15-16*.

Cystoscopy is useful in detecting tumors, inflammation, renal calculi, and structural irregularities. It can also be used as a means of obtaining biopsy specimens.

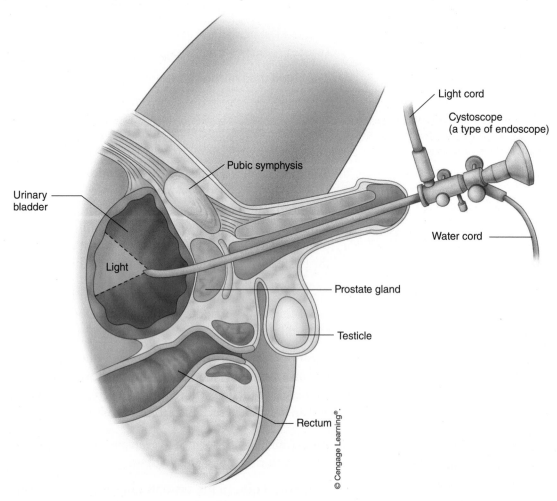

© Cengage Learning®.

Figure 15-16 Cystoscopy

extracorporeal lithotripsy (**ex**-trah-cor-**POR**-ee-al **LITH**-oh-trip-see) extra- = outside, beyond corpor/o = body -eal = pertaining to lith/o = stone, calculus -tripsy = intentional crushing	Also known as extracorporeal shock-wave lithotripsy. This is a noninvasive mechanical procedure for using sound waves to break up renal calculi so that they can pass through the ureters.
intravenous pyelogram (IVP) (in-trah-**VEE**-nus **PYE**-eh-loh-gram) intra- = within ven/o = vein -ous = pertaining to pyel/o = renal pelvis -gram = record or picture	Also known as intravenous pyelography or excretory urogram. This radiographic procedure provides visualization of the entire **urinary** tract: kidneys, ureters, bladder, and **urethra**. A contrast dye is injected intravenously, and multiple X-ray films are taken as the medium is cleared from the blood by the glomerular filtration of the kidney. **Intravenous pyelogram (IVP)** is useful in diagnosing **renal** tumors, cysts, stones, structural or functional abnormalities of the bladder, and ureteral obstruction.
KUB (kidneys, ureters, bladder)	An X-ray of the lower abdomen that defines the size, shape, and location of the kidneys, ureters, and bladder. A contrast medium is not used with this X-ray. The KUB is useful in identifying malformations of the kidney, soft tissue masses, and **calculi** (stones).
renal angiography (**REE**-nal **an**-jee-**OG**-rah-fee) ren/o = kidney -al = pertaining to angi/o = vessel -graphy = process of recording	X-ray visualization of the internal anatomy of the **renal** blood vessels after injection of a contrast medium. A radiopaque catheter is inserted into the femoral artery. Using fluoroscopy, the **catheter** is guided up the aorta to the level of the renal arteries. A contrast dye is then injected, and a series of X-rays is taken to visualize the renal vessels. **Renal angiography** is used to detect narrowing of the renal vessels, vascular damage, renal vein thrombosis (clots), cysts, or tumors.
renal scan (**REE**-nal scan) ren/o = kidney -al = pertaining to	A procedure in which a radioactive isotope (tracer) is injected intravenously, and the radioactivity over each kidney is measured as the tracer passes through the kidney. A **renal scan** procedure is useful in evaluating **renal** function and shape of the kidney. The radioactivity emitted from the tracer rises rapidly as the material concentrates in the kidney and then declines as it leaves the kidney. This produces a characteristic curve. The information is recorded in graph form, with various patterns in the curve being associated with specific conditions. The patient should be reassured that only a small amount of the radioactive tracer will be administered and that the material is completely excreted from the body within 24 hours.
retrograde pyelogram (RP) (**RET**-roh-grayd **PYE**-eh-loh-gram) retro- = backward, behind pyel/o = renal pelvis -gram = a record or picture	A radiographic procedure in which small-caliber catheters are passed through a **cystoscope** into the ureters to visualize the ureters and the **renal pelvis**. A contrast medium is injected through the catheters into the ureters and **renal pelvis**, and X-ray pictures are taken to define the structures of the

collecting system of the kidneys. X-ray pictures are taken to record the outline of these structures.

The **retrograde pyelogram** is useful in determining the degree of ureteral obstruction and is used when the IVP does not satisfactorily visualize the **renal** collecting system and the ureters. It is also used when patients are allergic to the intravenous dye used in the IVP, because the contrast medium is not absorbed through the mucous membranes.

---

ultrasonography

(ul-trah-son-**OG**-rah-fee)
  ultra- = beyond, excess
  son/o = sound
  -graphy = process of recording

Also called ultrasound. This is a procedure in which sound waves are transmitted into the body structures as a small transducer is passed over the patient's skin.

The area to be examined is lubricated before applying the transducer. As the sound waves are reflected back into the transducer, they are interpreted by a computer, which in turn presents the composite in a picture form.

An ultrasound of the kidneys is useful in distinguishing between fluid-filled cysts and solid masses, detecting renal calculi, identifying obstructions, and evaluating transplanted kidneys. **Ultrasonography** is a noninvasive procedure that requires no contrast medium.

---

urinalysis

(**yoo**-rih-**NAL**-ih-sis)
  urin/o = urine
  -lysis = breakdown or destruction

Urinalysis is a physical, chemical, or microscopic examination of urine.

The physical examination of urine includes examining the specimen for color, turbidity (cloudiness), **specific gravity**, and pH. Chemical analysis of urine may involve checking the specimen for presence of sugar, ketones, protein, or blood. This may be accomplished with reagent tablets or reagent strips. See *Figure 15-17.*

Microscopic examination of urine involves examining the urine specimen for the presence of blood cells, casts, crystals, pus, and bacteria. A microscopic examination is performed after the urine specimen has been spun in a centrifuge to allow for collection of a small amount of sediment (which is placed on the microscope slide for examination).

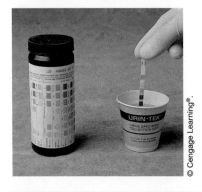

© Cengage Learning®.

Figure 15-17 Reagent strip immersed in urine sample

---

urine culture

(**YOO**-rin)
  urin/o = urine
  -e = noun ending

A procedure used to cultivate the growth of bacteria present in a urine specimen for proper microscopic identification of the specific pathogen (disease-producing microorganism).

A sample of the urine specimen is swabbed onto a culture medium plate and placed into an incubator for 24 to 72 hours. The plate is then examined for growth on the culture medium. A sample is obtained from any colony of growth and examined under the microscope to identify the name and quantity of the specific organism present.

Once the bacterium has been identified, sensitivity testing is performed. This test involves exposing the identified organism to various antibiotics to determine which specific antibiotic will most effectively destroy the pathogen. Identifying the most effective antibiotic for optimum results through **urine culture** and sensitivity will avoid longer than necessary treatment with a less effective medication.

Urine culture and sensitivity (C & S) testing has become more and more important as the number of resistant organisms increases. It is best to use the first voided specimen of the day for the urine culture because the bacteria will be more numerous in this specimen. A clean-catch urine specimen is usually collected, although a **catheterized specimen** may be obtained. The specimen should be cultured within 30 minutes because bacteria will multiply more rapidly at room temperature. If this is not possible, the specimen should be refrigerated.

24-hour urine specimen (24-hour **YOO**-rin **SPEH**-sih-men)	A collection of all of the urine excreted by the individual over a 24-hour period. The urine is collected in one large container. This urine specimen is also called composite urine specimen.

When the 24-hour urine collection begins, the individual should void and discard the first specimen. Each time after that, during the next 24 hours, all of the urine voided should be collected and placed in the container. The large container should be refrigerated. At the end of the 24-hour period (24 hours after the first **voiding**), the individual should void one last time, adding this urine to the specimen in the large container.

Composite urine specimens, such as the **24-hour urine specimen**, provide information on the ability of the kidneys to excrete and/or retain various solutes such as creatinine, sodium, urea, or phosphorus. The amount of these solutes excreted in the urine during a 24-hour period will be compared with their concentration in a blood sample taken at the end of the 24-hour period. The comparisons of urine level to blood concentration will be disproportionate in the presence of kidney disorders.

voiding cystourethrography (**VOY**-ding **siss**-toh-yoo-ree-**THROG**-rah-fee) cyst/o = bladder, sac, or cyst urethr/o = urethra -graphy = process of recording	X-ray visualization of the bladder and **urethra** during the **voiding** process, after the bladder has been filled with a contrast material.

A **radiopaque** dye is instilled into the bladder via a urethral **catheter**. The **catheter** is then removed and the patient is asked to void. X-ray pictures are taken as the patient is expelling the urine. The **voiding cystourethrography** is helpful in diagnosing urethral lesions, bladder and urethral obstructions, and **vesicoureteral reflux**.

Urine Specimen Collections

In addition to the 24-hour urine specimen collection, there are other methods of obtaining urine specimens for laboratory testing. It is important that the urine is collected and stored properly for optimum testing results. If a specimen will not be tested immediately, it must be refrigerated to lessen the potential for growth of bacteria. The usual amount of urine collected is 50 mL. The following methods for collecting a urine specimen are defined for your convenience and understanding: **catheterized specimen**, **clean-catch specimen** (midstream), **first-voided specimen**, random specimen, and **residual urine specimen**.

catheterized specimen (**CATH**-eh-ter-eyezd **SPEH**-sih-men) (**sterile specimen**)	Using aseptic techniques, a very small straight **catheter** is inserted into the bladder via the **urethra** to withdraw a urine specimen. The urine flows through the **catheter** into a sterile specimen container.

This specimen may be obtained for a urine culture.

clean-catch specimen (**CLEAN-CATCH SPEH**-sih-men) (**midstream specimen**)	This collection is used to avoid contamination of the urine specimen from the microorganisms normally present on the external genitalia.
	The patient cleanses the external genitalia with an **antiseptic** wipe. After expelling a small amount of urine into the toilet, the patient collects a specimen in a sterile container. The remaining amount of urine is expelled in the toilet. This specimen may be obtained for a urine culture or to determine the presence of a **urinary** tract infection.
first-voided specimen (**FIRST-VOYD**-ed **SPEH**-sih-men) (**early-morning specimen**)	The patient is instructed to collect the first-voided specimen of the morning and to refrigerate it until it can be taken to the medical office or laboratory.
	This specimen may be obtained for pregnancy testing or for any other test that requires more concentrated urine because it contains the greatest concentration of dissolved substances.
random specimen (**RAN**-dom **SPEH**-sih-men)	A urine specimen that is collected at any time.
	Freshly voided urine, which is a **random specimen**, is most often used for testing in the medical office. After the patient collects the urine specimen, it is tested immediately.
residual urine specimen (ree-**ZID**-yoo-ahl)	A residual urine specimen is obtained by **catheterization** after the patient empties the bladder by **voiding**. The amount of urine remaining in the bladder after **voiding** is noted as the residual amount.

Review Checkpoint

Check your understanding of this section by completing the **Diagnostic Techniques, Treatments, and Procedures** exercises in your workbook.

COMMON ABBREVIATIONS

Abbreviation	Meaning	Abbreviation	Meaning
ADH	antidiuretic hormone	**CCPD**	continuous cycling peritoneal dialysis
AGN	acute glomerular nephritis		
ARF	acute **renal** failure	**CRF**	**chronic renal failure**
BUN	**blood urea nitrogen**	**C & S**	culture and sensitivity
CAPD	continuous ambulatory peritoneal dialysis	**Cysto**	**cystoscopy**
		EPO	erythropoietin

Abbreviation	Meaning	Abbreviation	Meaning
ESRD	end-stage renal disease	pH	abbreviation for the degree of acidity or alkalinity of a solution; pH means potential hydrogen
ESWL	extracorporeal shock-wave lithotripsy	RP	retrograde pyelogram
GFR	glomerular filtration rate	sp.gr.	specific gravity
HD	hemodialysis	UA	urinalysis
IVP	intravenous pyelogram	UTI	urinary tract infection
KUB	kidneys, ureters, bladder	VCUG	voiding cystourethrogram

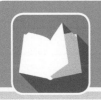

Review Checkpoint

Check your understanding of this section by completing the **Common Abbreviations** exercises in your workbook.

WRITTEN AND AUDIO TERMINOLOGY REVIEW

Review each of the following terms from this chapter. Study the spelling of each term and write the definition in the space provided. Check definitions by looking the term up in the glossary.

Term	Pronunciation	Definition
ablation	☐ ab-**LAY**-shun	_____
albuminuria	☐ al-byoo-min-**YOO**-ree-ah	_____
antiseptic	☐ **an**-tih-**SEP**-tik	_____
anuria	☐ an-**YOO**-ree-ah	_____
arteriole	☐ ar-**TEE**-ree-ohl	_____
aseptic technique	☐ ay-**SEP**-tik tek-**NEEK**	_____
asymptomatic	☐ ay-sim-toh-**MAT**-ik	_____
azotemia	☐ azz-oh-**TEE**-mee-ah	_____
bacteriuria	☐ back-**tee**-ree-**YOO**-ree-ah	_____
blood urea nitrogen	☐ blud-yoo-**REE**-ah **NIGH**-tro-jen	_____

Term	Pronunciation	Definition
Bowman's capsule	☐ **BOW**-manz **CAP**-sool	_____
calculi	☐ **KAL**-kew-lye	_____
calyx	☐ **KAY**-liks	_____
catheter	☐ **CATH**-eh-ter	_____
catheterization	☐ cath-eh-ter-ih-**ZAY**-shun	_____
catheterized specimen	☐ **CATH**-eh-ter-eyezd **SPEH**-sih-men	_____
chronic renal failure (uremia)	☐ **KRON**-ik **REE**-nal **FAIL**-yoor (yoo-**REE**-mee-ah)	_____
cortex	☐ **KOR**-teks	_____
creatinine clearance test	☐ kree-**AT**-in-in clearance test	_____
cystitis	☐ siss-**TYE**-tis	_____
cystocele	☐ **SIS**-toh-seel	_____
cystometer	☐ siss-**TOM**-eh-ter	_____
cystometrography	☐ **siss**-toh-meh-**TROG**-rah-fee	_____
cystopexy	☐ **SIS**-toh-**peck**-see	_____
cystoscope	☐ **SISS**-toh-skohp	_____
cystoscopy	☐ siss-**TOSS**-koh-pee	_____
dialysate	☐ dye-**AL**-ih-sayt	_____
dialysis	☐ dye-**AL**-ih-sis	_____
dysuria	☐ diss-**YOO**-ree-ah	_____
epispadias	☐ **ep**-ih-**SPAY**-dee-as	_____
extracorporeal lithotripsy	☐ **ex**-trah-cor-**POR**-ee-al **LITH**-oh-trip-see	_____
fatigue	☐ fah-**TEEG**	_____
fossa	☐ **FOSS**-ah	_____
glomerular filtrate	☐ glom-**AIR**-yoo-lar **FILL**-trayt	_____
glomerulonephritis	☐ glom-**air**-yoo-loh-neh-**FRYE**-tis	_____
glomerulus	☐ glom-**AIR**-yoo-lus	_____
glycosuria	☐ **glye**-kohs-**YOO**-ree-ah	_____
hematuria	☐ hee-mah-**TOO**-ree-ah	_____
hemodialysis	☐ **hee**-moh-dye-**AL**-ih-sis	_____
hilum	☐ **HIGH**-lum	_____
hydronephrosis	☐ **high**-droh-neh-**FROH**-sis	_____

Term	Pronunciation	Definition
intravenous pyelogram (IVP)	☐ **in**-trah-**VEE**-nus **PYE**-eh-loh-gram	_____
ketonuria	☐ **kee**-toh-**NOO**-ree-ah	_____
lethargy	☐ **LETH**-ar-jee	_____
malaise	☐ mah-**LAYZ**	_____
meatotomy	☐ **mee**-ah-**TOT**-oh-mee	_____
meatus	☐ mee-**AY**-tus	_____
nephrolithiasis	☐ **nef**-roh-lith-**EYE**-ah-sis	_____
nephrotic syndrome	☐ neh-**FROT**-ik **SIN**-drohm	_____
neurogenic bladder	☐ **new**-roh-**JEN**-ick **BLAD**-er	_____
nocturia	☐ nok-**TOO**-ree-ah	_____
oliguria	☐ **ol**-ig-**YOO**-ree-ah	_____
palpable	☐ **PAL**-pah-bul	_____
peritoneal dialysis	☐ **pair**-ih-**TOH**-nee-al dye-**AL**-ih-sis	_____
peritonitis	☐ **pair**-ih-ton-**EYE**-tis	_____
polycystic kidney disease	☐ **pol**-ee-**SISS**-tik kidney dih-**ZEEZ**	_____
polydipsia	☐ **pol**-ee-**DIP**-see-ah	_____
polyuria	☐ **pol**-ee-**YOO**-ree-ah	_____
pyelitis	☐ **pye**-eh-**LYE**-tis	_____
pyelonephritis	☐ **pye**-eh-loh-neh-**FRYE**-tis	_____
pyuria	☐ pye-**YOO**-ree-ah	_____
radiopaque	☐ **ray**-dee-oh-**PAYK**	_____
renal	☐ **REE**-nal	_____
renal angiography	☐ **REE**-nal an-jee-**OG**-rah-fee	_____
renal artery	☐ **REE**-nal **AR**-teh-ree	_____
renal cell carcinoma	☐ **REE**-nal sell car-sin-**OH**-mah	_____
renal pelvis	☐ **REE**-nal **PELL**-viss	_____
renal scan	☐ **REE**-nal scan	_____
renal tubule	☐ **REE**-nal **TOOB**-yool	_____
renal vein	☐ **REE**-nal **VAYN**	_____
residual urine	☐ rih-**ZID**-yoo-al **YOO**-rin	_____
retrograde pyelogram (RP)	☐ **RET**-roh-grayd **PYE**-eh-loh-gram	_____

Term	Pronunciation	Definition
solute	☐ **SOL**-yoot	_____
specific gravity	☐ speh-si-**FIK GRAV**-ih-tee	_____
toxic	☐ **TOKS**-ik	_____
turbid	☐ **TER**-bid	_____
ultrasonography	☐ ul-trah-son-**OG**-rah-fee	_____
uremia	☐ yoo-**REE**-mee-ah	_____
ureter	☐ **YOO**-reh-ter	_____
ureterectasis	☐ **you**-ree-ter-**ECK**-tah-sis	_____
ureterorrhagia	☐ you-**ree**-ter-oh-**RAY**-jee-ah	_____
ureterostenosis	☐ yoo-**ree**-ter-oh-sten-**OH**-sis	_____
urethra	☐ yoo-**REE**-thrah	_____
urethritis	☐ yoo-ree-**THRIGH**-tis	_____
urethropexy	☐ you-**REE**-throh-**peck**-see	_____
urethrostenosis	☐ you-**ree**-thro-steh-**NOH**-sis	_____
urgency	☐ **ER**-jen-see	_____
urinalysis	☐ **yoo**-rih-**NAL**-ih-sis	_____
urinary	☐ **YOO**-rih-nair-ee	_____
urination	☐ yoo-rih-**NAY**-shun	_____
urinometer	☐ y**oo**-rih-**NOM**-eh-ter	_____
vesicocele	☐ **VESS**-ih-koh-**seel**	_____
vesicoureteral reflux	☐ **vess**-ih-koh-yoo-**REE**-ter-al **REE**-fluks	_____
vesicovaginal fistula	☐ **ves**-ih-koh-**VAJ**-ih-nahl **FIS**-chuh-lah	_____
voiding	☐ **VOYD**-ing	_____
voiding cystourethrography	☐ **VOYD**-ing **siss**-toh-yoo-ree-**THROG**-rah-fee	_____

Review Checkpoint

Apply what you have learned in this chapter by completing the **Putting It All Together** exercise in your workbook.

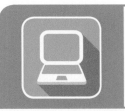

Online Resources

For additional study tools, including PowerPoint® slides and animations, go to the Student Companion Website.

Chapter Review Exercises

The following exercises provide a more in-depth review of the chapter material. Your goal in these exercises is to complete each section at a minimum 80% level of accuracy. If you score below 80% in any area, return to the applicable section in the chapter and read the material again. A place has been provided for your score at the end of each section.

A. Trace the Flow

As you trace the flow of urine from the kidney to the urethra, fill in the missing word(s). Each correct answer is worth 10 points. When you have completed this exercise, record your score in the space provided at the end of the exercise.

Blood flows into the kidney via the (1) _____ _____ and leaves the kidneys via the (2) _____ _____. After entering the kidney, the renal arteries branch out into smaller vessels throughout the kidney until the smallest arteries—known as (3) _____—reach the cortex of the kidney. Each of these small arteries leads to a ball-shaped collection of very tiny coiled capillaries known as the (4) _____. It is here that the formation of urine begins. As blood slowly, but constantly, passes through the thousands of glomeruli within the cortex of the kidney, the blood pressure forces water, salts, sugar, and nitrogenous waste products through the glomeruli walls into the (5) _____. This process is known as (6) _____. The glomerular filtrate, as it is now called, passes from the Bowman's capsule into a long, twisted tube called the (7) _____ _____. It is here in these tubules that water, sugar, and salts are returned to the bloodstream through the network of capillaries that surround them. This process is known as (8) _____ _____.

From the renal tubules, the urine is emptied into the central part of the kidney known as the (9) _____ _____. The central part of the kidney narrows into the large upper end of a tubular structure known as the (10) _____, which transports the urine from the kidney to the bladder. Urine is stored in the bladder until fullness stimulates its expulsion through the urethra.

Number correct _____ × *10 points/correct answer: Your score* _____%

B. Spelling

Circle the correctly spelled term in each pairing of words. Each correct answer is worth 10 points. Record your score in the space provided at the end of the exercise.

1. hilum	hylum	6.	urether	urethra
2. olyguria	oliguria	7.	urinary	uronary
3. micturition	micturation	8.	dysuria	disuria
4. palpable	palpitable	9.	hemeturia	hematuria
5. residule	residual	10.	hydronephrosis	hidronephrosis

Number correct _____ *× 10 points/correct answer: Your score* _____ *%*

C. Crossword Puzzle

Read the clues carefully and complete the puzzle. Each crossword answer is worth 10 points. When you have completed the crossword puzzle, total your points and enter your score in the space provided.

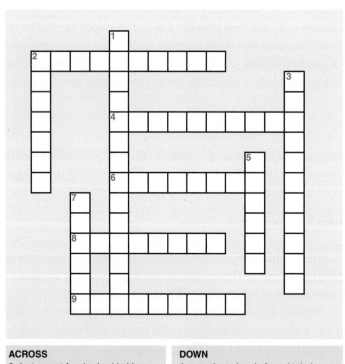

ACROSS
2 instrument for viewing bladder
4 inhibits growth of microorganisms
6 hollow, flexible tube
8 amount remaining; what is left over
9 time solution stays in body cavity

DOWN
1 cup-shaped end of renal tubule
2 abnormal stones formed in body
3 urination; voiding
5 connects the kidneys to the bladder
7 cloudy

© Cengage Learning®.

Number correct _____ *× 10 points/correct answer: Your score* _____ *%*

D. Term to Definition

Define each of the following sign and symptom terms by writing the definition in the space provided. Check the space provided if you are able to complete this exercise correctly the first time (without referring to the answers). Each correct answer is worth 10 points. Record your score in the space provided at the end of the exercise.

☐   1. albuminuria _____

☐   2. polyuria _____

☐   3. anuria _____

☐   4. urgency _____

☐   5. dysuria _____

☐   6. pyuria _____

☐   7. frequency _____

☐   8. glycosuria _____

☐   9. nocturia _____

☐   10. oliguria _____

Number correct _____ **× 10 points/correct answer: Your score** _____ **%**

E. Is It Normal?

In this exercise, you will read descriptions of urine samples. Decide whether the description indicates if the urine is normal or abnormal. If it is normal, check the applicable area. If it is abnormal, identify the condition. Each correct answer is worth 10 points. Record your score in the space provided at the end of this exercise.

Specimen Sample Number	Description of Urine Sample	Check (✓) if Normal Findings	Abnormal findings: Identify Possible Condition
1.	Pale yellow color		
2.	Smoky red color		
3.	Cloudy appearance		
4.	Specific gravity of 1.020		
5.	pH of 7.4		
6.	Reagent strip negative for protein		
7.	Reagent strip negative for glucose		
8.	Reagent strip negative for ketones		
9.	Reagent strip 4+ for glucose		
10.	Reagent strip 3+ for ketones		

Number correct _____ **× 10 points/correct answer: Your score** _____ **%**

F. Matching Conditions

Match the following urinary system conditions on the left with the most appropriate definitions on the right. Each correct answer is worth 10 points. Record your score in the space provided at the end of the exercise.

_____ 1. cystitis

_____ 2. pyelonephritis

_____ 3. hydronephrosis

_____ 4. glomerulonephritis

_____ 5. polycystic kidney

_____ 6. vesicoureteral reflux

_____ 7. Wilms' tumor

_____ 8. renal cell carcinoma

_____ 9. renal failure

_____ 10. nephrotic syndrome

a. large amounts of protein are lost through glomerular membrane into the urine, resulting in severe proteinuria; patient experiences massive generalized edema

b. abnormal backflow of urine from the bladder to the ureter

c. malignant tumor of the kidney, occurring in adulthood

d. distention of the pelvis and calyces of the kidney caused by urine that cannot flow past an obstruction in a ureter

e. malignant tumor of the kidney, occurring in childhood

f. uremia

g. a hereditary disorder of the kidneys in which grapelike fluid-filled sacs replace normal kidney tissue

h. an inflammation of the glomerulus of the kidneys

i. inflammation of the urinary bladder

j. a bacterial infection of the renal pelvis of the kidney

Number correct _____ **× 10 points/correct answer: Your score** _____ **%**

G. Proofreading Skills

Read the following History and Physical Examination Report. For each bold term, provide a brief definition and indicate if the term is spelled correctly. If it is misspelled, provide the correct spelling. Each correct answer is worth 10 points. Record your score in the space provided at the end of the exercise.

Example:

kidney _reddish-brown, bean-shaped organ located in the retroperitoneal area of the abdominal cavity._

Spelled correctly? ☑ Yes ☐ No _____

HISTORY AND PHYSICAL EXAMINATION

Hillcrest medical center

PATIENT NAME: Carlos Lopez

HOSPITAL NO.: 11546

ROOM NO.: 498

DATE OF ADMISSION
08/15/2014

ADMITTING PHYSICIAN
Nancy Lawrence, MD

ADMITTING DIAGNOSIS
Difficulty voiding

(continued)

HISTORY AND PHYSICAL EXAMINATION
Patient Name: Carlos Lopez
Hospital No.: 11546
Admission Date: 08/15/2014
Page 2

CHIEF COMPLAINT
"It is hard to pass my water."

HISTORY OF PRESENT ILLNESS
This 67-year-old Hispanic male is admitted for an elective transurethral resection of the prostate gland. He was referred by me in May to Dr. Mendez, complaining of nocturnal frequency of **urination** approximately every 2 hours. There had been no significant hesitancy, but he did notice slowing of the urinary stream and a feeling of incomplete emptying of the bladder. There had been no **hemeturia** or **disuria**. The patient was evaluated by Dr. Mendez and found to have a normal abdominal exam and normal external genitalia with a small, atrophic left testicle. The rectal examination showed normal sphincter tone and a 11 to 21 g enlarged prostate gland, which was clinically benign without induration. A cystourethroscopy was performed. The findings were enlarged prostate with bladder neck obstruction, 60% of the bladder volume being present as **residual urine**. There was a possible soft tissue mass in the right **kidney**. Because of this, a CT scan was performed, which showed benign findings. There was also a suggestion of splenomegaly. On review of the CT scan with the radiologist, both the radiologist and I felt that no splenomegaly was present. The patient was tried on Hytrin 2 mg at bedtime without improvement. Therefore, the patient is admitted for transurethral resection of the prostate gland.

PAST HISTORY
The patient has been treated by me since October 2002 for orthostatic hypotension, presumably on the basis of autonomic dysfunction. He has had a cholecystectomy, appendectomy, and renal **calculi** in the past.

SOCIAL HISTORY
The patient is a retired brick mason. He lives in Miami with his wife. He does not use tobacco or alcohol.

ALLERGIES
CODEINE, which causes nausea.

REVIEW OF SYSTEMS
Other than the urinary symptoms, review of systems is entirely negative. Specifically, head, eyes, ears, nose and throat, respiratory, heart, GI, endocrine, skin, and bones are all negative.

PHYSICAL EXAMINATION
GENERAL APPEARANCE: The patient is alert, cooperative, and oriented; appears healthy.

VITAL SIGNS: Blood pressure is 142/80 in the right arm sitting and 136/80 in the right arm standing.

HEENT: Head, eyes, ears, nose, and throat, including optic fundi, are normal.

NECK: Carotids are normal. There are no bruits. Jugular pulse is normal. Trachea is central. Thyroid is not enlarged. Lymphatics are not palpable.

CHEST: No dullness, no rales, rhonchi, or wheezes.

HEART: The heart tones are normal. There is no third or fourth heart sound. There is no murmur.

(continued)

HISTORY AND PHYSICAL EXAMINATION
Patient Name: Carlos Lopez
Hospital No.: 11546
Admission Date: 08/15/2014
Page 3

ABDOMEN: There are right upper quadrant and right lower quadrant scars. Bowel sounds are normal. There is no abdominal tenderness. There are no organs or masses palpable. There are no abnormal pulsations.

GENITALIA AND RECTAL: See history of present illness (HPI).

EXTREMITIES: Normal peripheral pulses.

DIAGNOSTIC DATA
Preoperative tests include a chest X-ray showing old granulomatous process evident but clear lung fields. Normal preoperative electrocardiogram and normal chemical profile. The urinalysis and CBC are likewise normal.

NOTE
The patient is an acceptable candidate for surgery. Anesthesia should be forewarned about his autonomic dysfunction with orthostatic hypotension, but other than this, I anticipate no complications or problems during surgery.

_____

Nancy Lawrence, MD

NL:bj

D:08/15/2014

T:08/15/2014

1. **urination** _____

_____

Spelled Correctly? ☐ Yes ☐ No _____

2. **hemeturia** _____

_____

Spelled Correctly? ☐ Yes ☐ No _____

3. **disuria** _____

_____

Spelled Correctly? ☐ Yes ☐ No _____

4. **residual urine** _____

_____

Spelled Correctly? ☐ Yes ☐ No _____

5. **calculi** _____

_____

Spelled Correctly? ☐ Yes ☐ No _____

Number correct _____ × *20 points/correct answer: Your score* _____%

H. Completion

Complete each sentence by identifying the appropriate diagnostic technique. Each correct answer is worth 10 points. Record your score in the space provided at the end of the exercise.

1. A physical, chemical, or microscopic examination of urine is known as a:

   _____

2. A procedure that uses sound waves to produce composite pictures is known as:

   _____

3. A procedure used to cultivate the growth of bacteria present in a urine specimen for proper microscopic identification of the specific pathogen is a:

   _____

4. An examination performed to evaluate bladder tone (measuring bladder pressure during filling and voiding) is known as a:

   _____

5. The introduction of a flexible, hollow tube into the bladder to instill a substance or to remove urine is known as a:

   _____

6. The radiographic procedure that provides visualization of the urinary tract by injecting a contrast dye intravenously into the body is called:

   _____

7. The X-ray visualization of the internal anatomy of the renal blood vessels after injection of a contrast medium is called a:

   _____

8. A collection of all of the urine excreted by the individual over a 24-hour period of time is called a:

   _____

9. X-ray visualization of the bladder and urethra during the voiding process after the bladder has been filled with a contrast medium is a:

   _____

10. The introduction of a radiopaque dye through a cystoscope into the ureters and renal pelvis for the purpose of taking X-ray pictures of the collecting structures is known as a:

    _____

Number correct _____ **× 10 points/correct answer: Your score** _____**%**

I. Matching Abbreviations

Match the abbreviations on the left with the correct definition on the right. Each correct answer is worth 10 points. Record your score in the space provided at the end of the exercise.

_____	1. KUB	a. blood urea nitrogen
_____	2. IVP	b. erythropoietin
_____	3. CCPD	c. continuous ambulatory peritoneal dialysis
_____	4. GFR	d. kidneys, ureters, bladder

(*continued*)

_____ 5. ESRD   e. urinalysis
_____ 6. EPO   f. voiding cystourethrogram
_____ 7. ADH   g. intravenous pyelogram
_____ 8. UA   h. glomerular filtration rate
_____ 9. VCUG   i. continuous cycling peritoneal dialysis
_____ 10. BUN   j. end-stage renal disease
                            k. antidiuretic hormone
                            l. cystoscopy

Number correct _____ × *10 points/correct answer: Your score* _____ *%*

J. Word Search

Read each definition carefully and identify the applicable word from the list that follows. Enter the word in the space provided and then find it in the puzzle and circle it. The words may be read up, down, diagonally, across, or backward. Each correct answer is worth 10 points. Record your score in the space provided at the end of the exercise.

arteriole	dialysis	peritonitis
hilum	ureter	toxic
incontinence	renal pelvis	turbid
residual	micturition	

Example: The smallest branch of an artery.
  *arteriole*_____

1. A mechanical filtering process used to cleanse the blood of waste products, draw off excess fluids, and regulate body chemistry when the kidneys fail to function properly.

   _____

2. The depression, or pit, of an organ where the vessels and nerves enter.

   _____

3. Another name for the act of eliminating urine from the bladder, other than voiding or urination.

   _____

4. Inflammation of the peritoneum (the membrane that lines the abdominal cavity).

   _____

5. The central collecting part of the kidney that narrows into the large upper end of the ureter.

   _____

6. Urine that remains in the bladder is known as _____ urine.
7. The medical term that means "cloudy."

   _____

8. One of a pair of tubes that carries urine from the kidney to the bladder.

   _____

9. Inability to control urination (the inability to retain urine in the bladder) is known as urinary

_____

10. The medical term for *poisonous* ("pertaining to poison").

_____

F	L	O	A	R	T	E	R	I	O	L	E	M	I	C
A	C	Y	N	G	E	S	M	S	I	D	A	S	T	T
M	I	H	T	T	M	N	S	I	S	Y	L	A	I	D
C	A	O	I	E	E	O	O	S	D	I	C	C	B	O
I	L	C	S	L	T	N	L	I	E	O	O	I	T	S
N	U	H	E	I	U	T	T	O	T	E	L	N	L	T
C	R	O	P	H	L	M	B	I	U	A	E	C	O	E
O	U	S	T	N	P	N	E	M	A	R	O	O	E	O
N	U	I	I	P	O	I	P	I	A	T	E	N	E	C
T	A	V	C	D	A	I	N	D	E	Y	T	M	Y
I	A	L	H	G	R	L	T	O	X	I	C	P	E	T
N	I	E	A	A	R	C	H	I	S	I	S	A	I	R
E	S	P	N	D	R	U	Y	A	R	D	I	S	G	S
N	U	L	T	I	R	E	S	I	D	U	A	L	D	T
C	R	A	E	B	L	O	I	I	U	A	T	C	O	A
E	E	N	R	R	H	C	S	U	T	U	R	C	S	A
F	R	E	T	U	U	R	I	S	M	E	M	N	I	C
P	E	R	I	T	O	N	I	T	I	S	A	S	E	M

© Cengage Learning®.

_Number correct _____ × 10 points/correct answer: Your score _____%_

K. Medical Scenario

The following medical scenario presents information on one of the pathological conditions discussed in this chapter. Read the scenario carefully and select the most appropriate answer for each question that follows. Each correct answer is worth 20 points. Record your score in the space provided at the end of the exercise.

Rob Ivey, a 25-year-old mechanic, has an appointment with his primary physician today because of seeing blood in his urine. The health care professional admits Mr. Ivey to the office, requesting a urine sample. Mr. Ivey had a difficult time getting a urine specimen. After the physician examined Mr. Ivey and assessed the results of his urine specimen, he was diagnosed with acute glomerulonephritis.

(continued)

1. The health care professional responds to Rob's questions about glomerulonephritis based on the fact that acute glomerulonephritis is a(n):

    a. distension of the pelvis and calyces of the kidney caused by urine that cannot flow past an obstruction in a ureter

    b. inflammation of the glomerulus of the kidney characterized by blood and protein in the urine

    c. group of clinical symptoms occurring due to damage to the glomerulus of the kidney resulting in large amounts of protein lost in the urine

    d. hereditary disorder of the kidneys in which grapelike, fluid-filled sacs or cysts replace normal kidney tissue.

2. While completing the initial assessment on Mr. Ivey, the health care professional is aware that the urine specific gravity measurement will most likely be:

    a. 1.003 to 1.030

    b. less than 1.003

    c. greater than 1.030

    d. unchanged

3. The health care professional expects Rob to demonstrate which characteristic symptoms of acute glomerulonephritis?

    a. complaints of headache and dark-colored, concentrated urine (containing bloods cells and protein)

    b. polyuria with accumulation of urine constituents moving into the bloodstream

    c. generalized edema, low blood pressure, and dilute urine

    d. hypotension with glycosuria and ketonuria

4. Rob questioned the health care professional about why he might have developed acute glomerulonephritis. He explained to her that he had never had any kidney problems before. The health care professional explained to Rob that acute glomerulonephritis is usually caused by:

    a. a sex-linked chromosome abnormality

    b. major trauma to the kidney area

    c. a beta-hemolytic streptococcal infection elsewhere in the body

    d. adhesion in the kidney that develops as a complication of surgery

5. The health care professional is aware that treatment for Rob's acute glomerulonephritis will likely include:

    1. chemotherapy and radiation

    2. restriction of sodium and fluids

    3. bed rest while clinical symptoms persist

    4. administration of antibiotics

        a. 1, 3

        b. 2, 4

        c. 2, 3, 4

        d. 1, 2, 4

Number correct _____ × 20 points/correct answer: Your score _____%

The Male Reproductive System

CHAPTER CONTENT

OBJECTIVES

Upon completing this chapter and the review exercises at the end of the chapter, the learner should be able to:

1. Correctly label the structures of the male reproductive system.

2. Correctly spell and pronounce terms listed on the Written and Audio Terminology Review, using the phonetic pronunciations provided.

3. Identify and define at least 10 pathological conditions of the male reproductive system.

4. Identify at least 10 diagnostic techniques used in treating disorders of the male reproductive system.

5. Proof and correct the transcription exercise relative to the male reproductive system provided at the end of this chapter.

6. Demonstrate the ability to correctly construct words relating to the male reproductive system by completing the appropriate exercise at the end of the chapter.

7. Identify three secondary sex characteristic changes that occur in the male body at the onset of puberty.

8. Identify six sexually transmitted diseases.

Overview

The male reproductive system functions to produce, sustain, and transport sperm; to propel the sperm from the penis into the female vagina during sexual intercourse (**copulation**); and to produce the male hormone, **testosterone**. The primary organs of the male reproductive system are the **gonads**, or male sex glands, which are called the **testes** (singular: *testis* or **testicle**). The **testes** are responsible for production of **spermatozoa** (the male germ cell) and for the secretion of **testosterone**. **Testosterone** is responsible for the secondary sex characteristic changes that occur in the male with the onset of puberty. These changes include growth of facial hair (beard), growth of pubic hair, and deepening of the voice.

The accessory organs of the male reproductive system are a series of ducts that transport the sperm to the outside of the body (i.e., the **epididymis, vas deferens, seminal vesicle**, ejaculatory duct, **urethra**, and **prostate gland**). The supporting structures of the male reproductive system are the **scrotum**, the penis, and a pair of spermatic cords. The learner will note that a section on male and female sexually transmitted diseases has been included in this chapter.

Anatomy and Physiology

As you study the anatomy and physiology of the male reproductive system, refer to *Figure 16-1* for a visual reference.

Primary Organs

The male gonads [(1) **testicles**] are small ovoid glands that begin their development high in the abdominal cavity, near the kidneys (retroperitoneal cavity), during the gestational period. A month or two before (or shortly after) birth, the testicles descend through the inguinal canal into the (2) **scrotum** (where they remain). The **scrotum** is a sac located posterior to the penis and suspended from the (3) **perineum**. The **perineum** is the area between the **scrotum** and the anus in the male. Each **testicle** remains suspended in the scrotal sac by a spermatic cord that contains blood and lymphatic vessels, nerves, and the **vas deferens**. If the testicles are to function normally, they must remain suspended in the scrotal sac.

The **scrotum** is divided into two compartments, or sacs. Each scrotal sac contains one **testicle**. Each **testicle** consists of specialized coils of tiny tubules responsible for

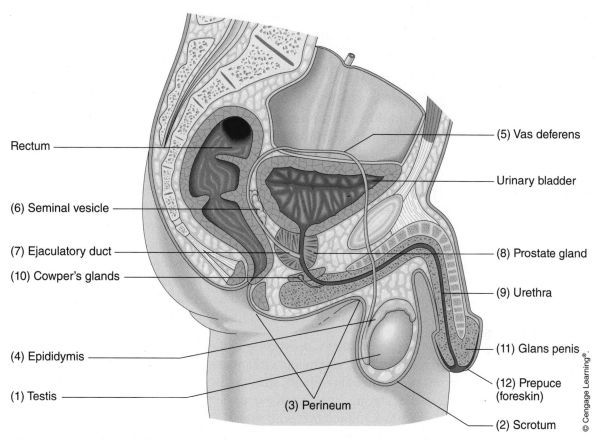

Rectum

(5) Vas deferens

(6) Seminal vesicle

Urinary bladder

(7) Ejaculatory duct

(10) Cowper's glands

(8) Prostate gland

(9) Urethra

(4) Epididymis

(11) Glans penis

(1) Testis

(12) Prepuce (foreskin)

(3) Perineum

(2) Scrotum

© Cengage Learning®

Figure 16-1 Male reproductive system

production of sperm. These tubules are known as the **seminiferous tubules**. The specialized interstitial tissue located between the tubules of the testes is responsible for secreting the male hormone, **testosterone**.

Accessory Organs

After being produced, sperm are transported through the network of tubules within the male reproductive system to reach the outside of the body. When they leave the **seminiferous tubules**, the sperm pass through the **(4) epididymis**, a tightly coiled tubule that resembles a comma. It is here in the **epididymis** that the sperm mature, becoming fertile and motile (capable of movement). Mature sperm are stored in the lower portion of the **epididymis**.

The **epididymis** leads to the **(5) vas deferens**, also called the ductus deferens. This straight tube, which is continuous with the **epididymis**, takes a sharp upward turn and ascends through the **scrotum** into the abdominopelvic cavity. Passing along the lateral pelvic wall, the **vas deferens** crosses over the top of the ureter and then descends along the posterior surface of the urinary bladder toward the **prostate gland**. At this location, just before the **prostate gland**, the **vas deferens** enlarges to form an **ampulla** (a saclike dilation). The **vas deferens** merges with the adjacent **(6) seminal vesicle** to form the **(7) ejaculatory duct**.

The **seminal vesicles** secrete a thick, yellowish fluid that is known as seminal fluid. This constitutes a large part of the volume of the **semen**. The **semen** is a combination of sperm and various secretions expelled from the body, through the **urethra**, during **ejaculation** (sexual intercourse). The process of ejecting, or expelling, the **semen** from the male **urethra** is known as **ejaculation**. Each ejaculatory duct (one from each side) passes through the **(8) prostate gland**.

The **prostate gland** lies just below the urinary bladder, where it surrounds the base of the **urethra** as it leaves the bladder. Ducts from the **prostate gland** transport its secretions to the **urethra**. These thin, milky-colored, alkaline secretions enhance the **motility** of the sperm and help neutralize the secretions within the vagina. The muscular action of the **prostate gland** also aids in expelling the **semen** from the body. The ducts from the **prostate gland** empty into the **(9) urethra**, which serves both the urinary system and the male reproductive system. The **urethra** transports urine from the bladder and the **semen** (when ejaculated) to the outside of the body. Just below the **prostate gland** are a pair of pea-sized glands called the **bulbourethral glands** or **(10) Cowper's glands**. The ducts from the bulbourethral glands empty into the **urethra** just before it extends through the penis. During sexual intercourse, the glands are stimulated to secrete an alkaline mucous-like fluid that provides lubrication during sexual intercourse.

The **seminal vesicles**, **prostate gland**, and bulbourethral glands each secrete fluids that nourish the sperm and enhance their motility. These fluids also make up the total volume of the **semen**, with the largest amount being secreted by the **seminal vesicles**. During sexual intercourse, the volume of **semen** in a single **ejaculation** may vary from 1.5 to 6.0 mL, with each milliliter of **semen** containing between 50 and 150 million sperm. Sperm counts below 10 to 20 million per milliliter may indicate fertility problems.

The **penis** is the male organ of copulation. It consists of a base that attaches it to the pubic arch, a body that is the visible pendant portion, and a tip called the **(11) glans penis**. The **glans penis** is covered by a loose retractable fold of skin called the **(12) prepuce (foreskin)**. Shortly after birth, the **foreskin** is sometimes removed. This procedure is known as a **circumcision**. The **urethra** extends the length of the penis and ends as an opening at the tip of the **glans penis**. This opening is called the **external urinary meatus**.

The penis is made of a sponge-like tissue containing many blood spaces that are relatively empty in the absence of sexual arousal, and the penis is **flaccid**. During sexual arousal, however, these spaces fill with blood, causing the penis to become rigid and enlarge in diameter and length. This process, known as **erection**, allows the penis to remain rigid enough to enter the female vagina during sexual intercourse. The **urethra** serves as a passageway for the exit of the **semen** following **ejaculation**, allowing deposit of sperm in the vagina.

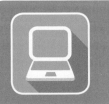

Media Link

For an overview of the male reproductive system and to learn how sperm are formed, watch the **Male Reproductive System** and **Sperm Formation** animations on the Student Companion Website.

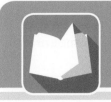

Review Checkpoint

Check your understanding of this section by completing the **Anatomy and Physiology** exercises in your workbook.

VOCABULARY

The following vocabulary words are frequently used when discussing the male reproductive system.

Word	Definition
andropause (**AN**-droh-pawz) andr/o = male	A change of life for men, occurring in their late forties or early fifties, in which there is a decrease in male hormone (androgen) levels.
asymptomatic (ay-simp-toh-**MAT**-ik)	Without symptoms.
bulbourethral glands (**buhl**-boh-yoo-**REE**-thral glands) urethr/o = urethra -al = pertaining to	A pair of pea-sized glands that empty into the **urethra** just before it extends through the penis; also known as **Cowper's glands**.
chancre (**SHANG**-ker)	A skin lesion, usually of primary **syphilis**, that begins at the site of infection as a small raised area and develops into a red painless ulcer with a scooped-out appearance; also known as a venereal sore.
Cowper's glands (**KOW**-perz)	See bulbourethral glands.
cryosurgery (**kry**-oh-**SER**-jer-ee) cry/o = cold	Use of subfreezing temperature to destroy tissue. The coolant is circulated through a metal probe, chilling it to as low as −160° C. When the probe touches the tissues of the body, the moist tissues adhere to the cold metal of the probe and freeze.
debridement (day-breed-**MENT**)	The removal of dirt, damaged tissue, and cellular debris from a wound or a burn to prevent infection and promote healing.
dormant (**DOOR**-mant)	Inactive.
dysuria (dis-**YOO**-ree-ah) dys = bad, difficult, painful, disordered -uria = urine condition	Painful urination.

Word	Definition
ejaculation (ee-**jack**-yoo-**LAY**-shun)	The process of ejecting, or expelling, the **semen** from the male **urethra**.

epididymectomy
(**ep**-ih-**did**-ih-**MEK**-toh-mee)
  epididym/o = epididymis
  -ectomy = surgical removal
	Surgical removal of the **epididymis**.

epididymis
(**ep**-ih-**DID**-ih-mis)
  epididym/o = epididymis
  -is = noun ending
	A tightly coiled tubule that resembles a comma. Its purpose is that of housing the sperm until they mature, becoming fertile and motile. Mature sperm are stored in the lower portion of the **epididymis**.

epididymitis
(**ep**-ih-**did**-ih-**MY**-tis)
  epididym/o = epididymis
  -itis = inflammation
	Acute or chronic inflammation of the **epididymis**. This condition can be the result of a urinary tract infection, prolonged use of indwelling catheters, or venereal disease in the male.

exudate (**EKS**-yoo-dayt)	Fluid, pus, or serum slowly discharged from cells or blood vessels through small pores or breaks in cell membranes.
flaccid (**FLAK**-sid)	Weak; lacking normal muscle tone.
foreskin (**FOR**-skin)	A loose, retractable fold of skin covering the tip of the penis; also called the **prepuce**.
glans penis (**GLANS PEE**-nis)	The tip of the penis.
gonad (**GOH**-nad)	The male sex glands, which are called the testes (singular: *testis* or **testicle**). These are the primary organs of the male reproductive system.

hematospermia
(**hee**-mah-toh-**SPER**-mee-ah)
  hemat/o = relating to blood
  sperm = sperm
  -ia = abnormal condition
	The presence of blood in the seminal fluid.

Kaposi's sarcoma (**KAP**-oh-seez sar-**KOH**-mah)	A malignant growth that begins as soft, brownish or purple raised areas on the feet and slowly spreads in the skin, spreading to the lymph nodes and internal organs. It occurs most often in men and is associated with AIDS.
malaise (mah-**LAYZ**)	A vague feeling of bodily weakness or discomfort, often marking the onset of disease.
malodorous (mal-**OH**-dor-us)	Foul smelling; having a bad odor.

Word	Definition
motility (moh-**TILL**-ih-tee)	The ability to move spontaneously.
mucopurulent (**mew**-koh-**PEWR**-yoo-lent) muc/o = mucus	Characteristic of a combination of mucus and pus.
opportunistic infection (**op**-or-**TOON**-is-tik in-**FEK**-shuns)	An infection caused by normally nondisease-producing organisms that set up in a host whose resistance has been decreased by surgery, illnesses, and disorders such as AIDS.
orchidopexy (**OR**-kid-oh-**peck**-see) orchid/o = testicle -pexy = surgical fixation	Surgical fixation of an undescended **testicle**.
orchiopexy (**OR**-kee-oh-**peck**-see) orchi/o = testicle -pexy = surgical fixation	See **orchidopexy**.
palpation (pal-**PAY**-shun)	A technique used in physical examinations that involves feeling parts of the body with the hands.
pelvic inflammatory disease (**PELL**-vik in-**FLAM**-mah-tor-ee)	Inflammation of the upper female genital tract (cervix, uterus, ovaries and fallopian tubes [also known as **salpingitis**]); may be associated with sexually transmitted diseases.
perineum (pair-ih-**NEE**-um)	The area between the **scrotum** and the anus in the male and between the vulva and anus in the female.
prepuce (**PRE**-pus)	See **foreskin**.
prophylactic (**proh**-fih-**LAK**-tik)	Any agent or regimen that contributes to the prevention of infection and disease.
prostate gland (**PROSS**-tayt gland) prostat/o = prostate gland -e = noun ending	A gland that surrounds the base of the **urethra**, which secretes a milky-colored secretion into the **urethra** during **ejaculation**. This secretion enhances the motility of the sperm and helps to neutralize the secretions within the vagina.
prostatectomy (**pross**-tah-**TEK**-toh-mee) prostat/o = prostate gland -ectomy = surgical removal	Removal of all or part of the **prostate gland**. A discussion of two approaches to removing the **prostate gland** is presented in the section on diagnostic techniques.
purulent (**PEWR**-yoo-lent)	Producing or containing pus.

Word	Definition

rectoscope
(**REK**-toh-skohp)
  rect/o = rectum
  -scope = instrument for viewing
	An instrument used to view the rectum that has a cutting and cauterizing (burning) loop. Also known as proctoscope.

resectoscope (ree-**SEK**-toh-skohp)	An instrument used to remove tissue surgically from the body. It has a light source and lens attached for viewing the area.
residual urine (rih-**ZID**-yoo-al **YOO**-rin)	Urine that remains in the bladder after urination.
residual urine test	Obtaining a catheterized specimen after the patient has emptied the bladder by voiding, to determine the amount of urine remaining in the bladder; also known as a residual specimen. **Residual urine** may also be determined by ultrasound and bladder scan.

salpingitis
(sal-pin-**JYE**-tis)
  salping/o = eustachian tubes; also refers
          to fallopian tubes
  -itis = inflammation
	Inflammation of the fallopian tubes; also known as **pelvic inflammatory disease** (included in this section because it is associated with sexually transmitted diseases).

scrotum (**SKROH**-tum)	An external sac that houses the testicles. It is located posterior to the penis and is suspended from the **perineum**.
semen (**SEE**-men)	A combination of sperm and various secretions that is expelled from the body through the **urethra** during sexual intercourse.
seminal vesicles (**SEM**-in-al **VESS**-ih-kulz)	Glands that secrete a thick, yellowish fluid (known as seminal fluid) into the **vas deferens**.
seminiferous tubules (**SEM**-in-**IF**-er-us **TOO**-byools)	Specialized coils of tiny tubules responsible for production of sperm; located in the testes.
spermatozoan (**sper**-mat-oh-**ZOH**-ahn)	A mature male germ cell; also known as **spermatozoon** (plural: *spermatozoa*).
spermatozoon (**sper**-mat-oh-**ZOH**-on)	See **spermatozoan**.
testicles (**TESS**-tih-kuls) (**testes**)	The male gonads, or male sex glands, responsible for production of spermatozoa (the male germ cell) and for the secretion of the male hormone **testosterone**.
testosterone (tess-**TOSS**-ter-own)	A male hormone secreted by the testes, responsible for the secondary sex characteristic changes that occur in the male with the onset of puberty. These changes include growth of facial hair (beard), growth of pubic hair, and deepening of the voice.
truss	An apparatus worn to prevent or block the herniation of the intestines or other organ through an opening in the abdominal wall.

Word	Definition
urethra (yoo-**REE**-thrah) urethr/o = urethra -a = noun ending	A small, tubular structure extending the length of the penis that transports urine from the bladder (and **semen**, when ejaculated) to the outside of the body.
urethritis (yoo-ree-**THRYE**-tis) urethr/o = urethra -itis = inflammation	Inflammation of the **urethra**.
vas deferens (vas **DEF**-er-enz)	The narrow, straight tube that transports sperm from the **epididymis** to the ejaculatory duct.
vesicles (**VESS**-ih-kulz)	Blisters; small, raised skin lesions containing clear fluid.

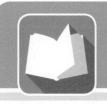

Review Checkpoint

Check your understanding of this section by completing the **Vocabulary** exercises in your workbook.

WORD ELEMENTS

The following word elements pertain to the male reproductive system. As you review the list, pronounce each word element aloud twice and check the box after you "say it." Write the definition for the example term given for each word element. Use your medical dictionary to find the definitions of the example terms.

Word Element	Pronunciation	"Say It"	Meaning
andr/o **andr**oid	**AN**-droh **AN**-droyd	☐	man, male
balan/o **balan**itis	bal-**AH**-noh bal-ah-**NYE**-tis	☐	**glans penis**
cry/o **cry**osurgery	**KRY**-oh kry-oh-**SIR**-jeer-ee	☐	cold
crypt/o **crypt**orchidism	**KRIPT**-oh kript-**OR**-kid-izm	☐	hidden
epididym/o **epididym**itis	ep-ih-**DID**-ih-moh **ep**-ih-**did**-ih-**MY**-tis	☐	**epididymis**

Word Element	Pronunciation	"Say It"	Meaning
hemat/o **hemat**ospermia	hee-**MAT**-oh	☐	blood
hydro- **hydr**ocele	**HIGH**-droh **HIGH**-droh-seel	☐	water
orch/o **orch**itis	**OR**-koh or-**KIGH**-tis	☐	**testicle**
orchi/o **orchio**pexy	**OR**-kee-oh **OR**-kee-oh **peck**-see	☐	**testicle**
orchid/o **orchid**oplasty	**OR**-kid-oh **OR**-kid-oh-**plass**-tee	☐	**testicle**
prostat/o **prostat**itis	pross-**TAH**-toh pross-tah-**TYE**-tis	☐	**prostate gland**
semin/i **semin**al vesicles	**SEM**-ih-neye **SEM**-ih-nal **VESS**-ih-kulz	☐	**semen**
sperm/o **sperm**olysis	**SPERM**-oh sperm-**ALL**-ih-sis	☐	sperm
spermat/o **spermat**ogenesis	sper-**MAT**-oh **sper**-mat-oh-**JEN**-eh-sis	☐	sperm
test/o **test**icular	**TESS**-toh tess-**TIK**-yoo-lar	☐	testis, testes
vas/o **vas**ectomy	**VAS**-oh vas-**EK**-toh-mee	☐	vessel; also refers to **vas deferens**
zo/o a**zo**ospermia	**ZOH**-oh ah-zoh-oh-**SPER**-mee-ah	☐	animal (man)

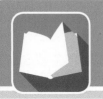

Review Checkpoint

Check your understanding of this section by completing the **Word Elements** exercises in your workbook.

Pathological Conditions

As you study the pathological conditions of the male reproductive system, note that the **basic definition** is in a green shaded box, followed by a more detailed description in regular print. The phonetic pronunciation is directly beneath each term, as well as a breakdown of the component parts of the term where applicable.

---

anorchism

(an-**OR**-kizm)

  an- = without, not
  orch/o = testicle
  -ism = condition

Anorchism is the absence of one or both testicles.

---

balanitis

(bal-ah-**NYE**-tis)

  balan/o = glans penis
  -itis = inflammation

Inflammation of the **glans penis** and the mucous membrane beneath it.

Balanitis is caused by irritation and invasion of microorganisms. Treatment with antibiotics will help control the localized infection. Good hygiene and thorough drying of the penis when bathing are important preventive measures.

---

benign prostatic hypertrophy

(bee-**NINE** pross-**TAT**-ik
high-**PER**-troh-fee)

  prostat/o = prostate gland
  -ic = pertaining to
  hyper- = excessive
  -trophy = development, growth

A benign (noncancerous) enlargement of the **prostate gland**, creating pressure on the upper part of the **urethra** or neck of the bladder (causing obstruction of the flow of urine).

Benign prostatic hypertrophy is a common condition occurring in men over the age of 50. Men with hypertrophy of the **prostate gland** may complain of symptoms such as difficulty in starting urination, a weak stream of urine (not being able to maintain a constant stream), the inability to empty the bladder completely, or "dribbling" at the end of voiding.

Diagnosis is usually confirmed by thorough patient history and a rectal examination by the physician to confirm prostatic enlargement. The physician may order a urinalysis and culture of the urine to check for urinary tract infection or any abnormalities in the urine, such as blood. Other diagnostic tests may be a **cystourethroscopy** to visualize the interior of the bladder and the **urethra**, a **KUB** (kidneys, ureters, bladder) **X-ray** to visualize the urinary tract, or a **residual urine test** to check for incomplete emptying of the bladder. If a malignancy (cancer) is suspected, a biopsy of the prostatic tissue may be ordered.

Treatment for **benign prostatic hypertrophy** depends on the degree of urinary obstruction noted. For patients with mild cases of prostatic enlargement (which is normal as the male ages), the condition may simply be monitored. For patients with recurrent and obstructive problems due to hyperplasia of the **prostate gland**, surgery is usually indicated to remove the **prostate gland**. Two types of surgery used are **transurethral resection of the prostate** (TURP) and **suprapubic prostatectomy**, each of which is discussed in the diagnostic procedures section of this chapter.

carcinoma of the prostate

(**kar**-sih-**NOH**-mah of the **PROSS**-tayt)

    carcin/o = cancer
    -oma = tumor
    prostat/o = prostate gland
    -e = noun ending

Malignant growth within the **prostate gland**, creating pressure on the upper part of the **urethra**.

Cancer of the prostate is the most common cause of cancer among men and the most common cause of death due to cancer in men over the age of 55. Unfortunately, symptoms are not usually present in the early stages of cancer of the prostate. By the time symptoms are evident, the cancer may have already metastasized (spread) to other areas of the body. When symptoms of prostate cancer do occur, they may include any of the following:

1. A need to urinate frequently (i.e., urinary frequency), especially at night

2. Difficulty starting or stopping urine flow

3. Inability to urinate

4. Weak or interrupted flow of urine when urinating (patient may complain of "dribbling" instead of having a steady stream of urine)

5. Pain or burning when urinating

6. Pain or stiffness in the lower back, hips, or thighs

7. Painful **ejaculation**

Because the presence of symptoms usually means that the disease is more advanced, early detection of cancer of the prostate is essential to successful treatment. All men over the age of 40 should have a yearly physical examination that includes a digital rectal examination of the **prostate gland**. The rectal examination can reveal a cancerous growth before symptoms appear. A prostate-specific antigen (PSA) blood test may be performed during the examination to detect increased growth of the prostate (the growth could be benign or malignant). The PSA test measures the substance called prostate-specific antigen. The level of PSA in the blood may rise in men who have prostate cancer or **benign prostatic hypertrophy**. If the level is elevated, the physician will order additional tests to confirm a diagnosis of cancer of the prostate.

The most common surgical procedure used to treat cancer of the prostate is **radical prostatectomy**. Other treatment options include radiation therapy and hormonal therapy. Treatment depends on the patient's age and medical history and on the stage of the cancer.

Benign (noncancerous) growth of the **prostate gland** may be treated medically or surgically. Medical treatment is aimed at relieving the symptoms of an enlarged prostate. These symptoms include urinary difficulty, recurrent urinary tract infections, and hematuria. The most common form of surgery for this condition is the TURP (**transurethral resection of the prostate**).

carcinoma of the testes

(**kar**-sih-**NOH**-mah of the **TESS**-teez)

    carcin/o = cancer
    -oma = tumor

A malignant tumor of the **testicle** that appears as a painless lump in the **testicle**; also called **testicular** cancer.

This type of tumor is rare and usually occurs in men under the age of 40. The cause is unknown.

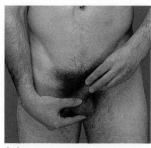

(A)

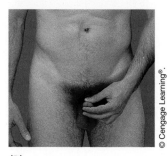

(B)

The diagnosis of **testicular** cancer is usually confirmed by biopsy after the physician has palpated the lump in the **testicle**. The treatment of choice is surgery to remove the diseased **testicle**, followed by radiation therapy and chemotherapy. Although male fertility requires only one **testicle**, many men who have had a **testicle** removed for cancer suffer from impaired fertility. This is thought to be due to the toxic effects of the cancer on the opposite **testicle** or from the treatment for the cancer (i.e., surgery and/or chemotherapy). Chances for complete recovery are excellent if the malignancy is detected in the early stages.

Testicular cancer can spread throughout the body via the lymphatic system if not treated in the early stages. Early treatment is essential for complete recovery. Therefore, it is recommended that all men perform monthly **testicular** self-examinations (TSE). See *Figure 16-2*. If a lump is discovered, it should be reported immediately to the man's personal physician.

Figure 16-2 (A) Palpating the testis; (B) Assessing for penile discharge

cryptorchidism	Condition of undescended **testicle(s)**; the absence of one or both testicles from the **scrotum**.
(kript-**OR**-kid-izm) crypt/o = hidden orchid/o = testicle -ism = condition	

In **cryptorchidism**, the **testicle** may be located in the abdominal cavity or in the inguinal canal. If the **testicle** does not descend on its own, surgery will be necessary to correct the position. The surgery (known as an **orchiopexy**) involves making an incision into the inguinal canal, locating the **testicle**, and bringing it back down into the scrotal sac. This surgery is usually done on an outpatient basis, with normal physical activity being restored within a few weeks to a month.

epispadias	A congenital defect (birth defect) in which the **urethra** opens on the upper side of the penis at some point near the glans. See *Figure 16-3*.
(ep-ih-**SPAY**-dee-as) epi- = upon, over	

The treatment for **epispadias** is surgical correction with redirection of the opening of the **urethra** to its normal position at the end of the penis.

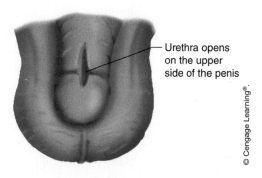

Urethra opens on the upper side of the penis

Figure 16-3 Epispadias

hydrocele
 (**HIGH**-droh-seel)
   hydro- = water
   -cele = swelling or herniation
	An accumulation of fluid in any saclike cavity or duct, particularly the scrotal sac or along the spermatic cord.
	
	 This condition is caused by inflammation of the **epididymis** or testis or by obstruction of lymphatic or venous flow within the spermatic cord. The treatment for a **hydrocele** is surgery to remove the fluid pouch.

hypospadias
 (high-poh-**SPAY**-dee-as)
   hypo- = under, below, beneath,
       less than normal
	A congenital defect in which the **urethra** opens on the underside of the penis instead of at the end. See *Figure 16-4*.
	
	 Treatment for **hypospadias** involves surgery to redirect the opening of the **urethra** to its normal location at the end of the penis.

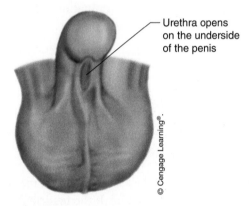

Urethra opens on the underside of the penis

© Cengage Learning®.

Figure 16-4 Hypospadias

impotence (**IM**-poh-tens)	The inability of a male to achieve or sustain an erection of the penis. The cause of **impotence** may be psychological (due to anxiety or depression) or physiological (due to some physical disorder such as diabetes, spinal cord injury, or a response to medications). Individuals who are experiencing **impotence** may be sexually aroused but with an inability to sustain an erection, or they may lose their sexual appetite. A thorough physical examination, along with a complete medical and sexual history, will help the physician determine the underlying cause of **impotence**. If the cause is determined to be psychological, counseling and/ or psychotherapy may be prescribed. If the cause of **impotence** is determined to be physiological in nature, treatment of the underlying condition may restore normal sexual function. If the underlying physiological cause of **impotence** is due to an untreatable condition (such as irreversible nerve and/or vascular problems), the patient may choose to have a penile prosthesis surgically implanted.

inguinal hernia (**ING**-gwih-nal **HER**-nee-ah)	A protrusion of a part of the intestine through a weakened spot in the muscles and membranes of the inguinal region of the abdomen. The intestine pushes into, and sometimes fills, the entire scrotal sac in the male. See *Figure 16-5*. The patient may notice a bulge in the inguinal area, particularly when standing. He may also experience a sharp, steady pain in the groin area.

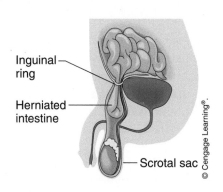

Inguinal ring

Herniated intestine

Scrotal sac

© Cengage Learning®.

Conservative treatment of an **inguinal hernia** may involve nonsurgical intervention. If the patient is able to press the hernia back into the abdomen, it may be treated with a type of support (called a **truss**) until the muscle wall strengthens again. If the bulge cannot be gently pressed back into the abdomen, there is a possibility of the herniated intestine being trapped (strangulated). In this case, surgery will be necessary to return the herniated intestine to its normal environment and to correct the weakened muscle wall. The surgery for a hernia repair is called a herniorrhaphy.

Figure 16-5 Indirect inguinal hernia

orchitis	Inflammation of the testes due to a virus, bacterial infection, or injury. The condition may affect one or both testes. **Orchitis** typically results from the mumps virus.
(or-**KIGH**-tis)	
orch/o = testicle	
-itis = inflammation	

If the inflammation is severe enough it can result in atrophy (wasting away) of the affected **testicle**. If severe inflammation involves both testicles, sterility results.

The patient may experience swelling, tenderness, and acute pain in the area. He may also experience fever, chills, nausea, and vomiting and a general feeling of discomfort (**malaise**).

Treatment for **orchitis** due to bacterial invasion is antibiotics. There is no specific treatment for **orchitis** caused by the mumps virus other than bed rest and medications to reduce the swelling and fever. All adult men who have never had the mumps virus should take the mumps vaccine as a preventive measure.

phimosis	A tightness of the **foreskin** (**prepuce**) of the penis that prevents it from being pulled back. The opening of the **foreskin** narrows due to the tightness and may cause some difficulty with urination.
(fih-**MOH**-sis)	

Phimosis is usually congenital but may be the result of edema and inflammation. Parents of the uncircumcised male infant and adult males who have not been circumcised should understand the importance of proper cleansing of the **glans penis**. The **foreskin** should be gently pulled back from the **glans penis** to clean the area properly. Failure to do this may result in the accumulation of normal secretions and subsequent inflammation of the **glans penis** (**balanitis**). Treatment for **phimosis** is **circumcision** (surgery to remove the **foreskin**).

premature ejaculation	The discharge of seminal fluid prior to complete erection of the penis or immediately after the penis has been introduced into the vaginal canal.
(premature ee-**jack**-yoo-**LAY**-shun)	

The cause of **premature ejaculation** may be psychological (due to anxiety) or physiological (due to some physical disorder such as diabetes, **prostatitis**, or urethritis). A thorough physical examination, along with a complete medical and sexual history, will help the physician determine the underlying cause of **premature ejaculation**. If the cause is determined to be psychological, counseling and/or psychotherapy may be prescribed. If the cause of **premature ejaculation** is determined to be physiological in nature, treatment of the underlying condition may restore normal sexual function.

prostatitis	Inflammation of the **prostate gland**.

(pross-tah-**TYE**-tis)
   prostat/o = prostate gland
   -itis = inflammation
	Prostatitis may be acute (sudden flare-up) or chronic (recurring flare-ups) and may be due to bacterial invasion. The patient with **prostatitis** will usually complain of low back pain, fullness or pain in the perineal area, urinary frequency, and discharge from the **urethra**. An examination of the prostate gland by **palpation** will reveal an enlarged and tender **prostate gland**.
	
	 Diagnosis of **prostatitis** is confirmed with urinalysis, urine culture, and **palpation** of the **prostate gland** (via a rectal examination). Treatment involves the use of medications to destroy the bacteria (antimicrobial), medications for pain (analgesics), and medications for fever (antipyretics).

varicocele	An abnormal dilation of the veins of the spermatic cord leading to the **testicle**.
(**VAIR**-ih-koh-seel) **-cele** = swelling or herniation	Each **testicle** is suspended into the **scrotum** by a spermatic cord. This stringlike structure is located in the inguinal canal between the **scrotum** and the abdominal cavity. Each spermatic cord is composed of arteries, veins, lymphatics, nerves, and the **vas deferens** of the testis. A **varicocele** usually causes more discomfort than actual pain. The dilated veins cause some swelling around the **testicle**. See *Figure 16-6*. This condition is more common in men between the ages of 15 and 25 and more often affects the left spermatic cord than the right. A **varicocele** can lower the sperm count because the heat generated from the venous congestion near the **testicle** may significantly reduce the production of sperm by the **testicle**. Treatment for a **varicocele** consists of relieving the discomfort experienced because of the condition. The patient may be instructed to wear tight-fitting underwear or to use an athletic scrotal supporter until the swelling subsides. If the **varicocele** causes a great deal of pain, the treatment of choice would be a varicocelectomy to remove the **varicocele**.

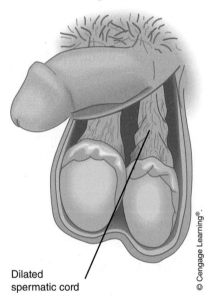

Dilated
spermatic cord

© Cengage Learning®.

Figure 16-6 Varicocele

Male and Female Sexually Transmitted Diseases

Sexually transmitted diseases (STDs) in the male are the same as those in the female. These contagious diseases are spread from one person to another through contact with body fluids such as blood, **semen**, and vaginal secretions. STDs may be spread during vaginal, anal, or oral sex, or they may be spread by direct contact with infected skin.

The incidence of sexually transmitted diseases is alarmingly high in the United States. It has greatly increased in recent years, especially among young people. The following section is a discussion of the more common sexually transmitted diseases.

| acquired immunodeficiency syndrome (AIDS) | AIDS is a deadly virus that destroys the body's immune system by invading the helper T lymphocytes (T cells), which play an important part in the body's immune response. The human immunodeficiency virus (HIV) replicates itself within the T cells, destroys the lymphocyte, and then invades other lymphocytes. |

HIV is transmitted from person to person through sexual contact, the sharing of HIV-contaminated needles and syringes, and transfusion of infected blood or its components. (The risks of receiving HIV-infected blood through transfusion have been greatly reduced since screening procedures have been improved.) The HIV virus can also be transmitted through the placenta of an infected mother to the baby (during the birth process) and through the breast milk of an infected mother to the baby (when nursing the baby).

Symptoms are not easily detectable in someone who has been infected with HIV. The condition may lie **dormant** for years, with the individual appearing to be in good health.

Within one to two weeks after exposure to HIV, the patient may experience a sore throat with fever and body aches. The time period from infection with HIV to the development of detectable antibodies in the blood is usually one to three months. HIV is transmissible (capable of being passed from one person to another) early after the onset of infection and continues throughout life.

As the disease progresses, the patient may experience enlargement of the lymph glands, fatigue, weight loss, diarrhea, and night sweats. With further progression, the body's immune system continues to deteriorate. The patient is susceptible to frequent infections, pneumonia, fever, and malignancies. The most common type of malignancy associated with AIDS is **Kaposi's sarcoma**, which is an aggressive malignancy of the blood vessels characterized by rapidly growing purple lesions appearing on the skin, in the mouth, or anywhere in the body.

The time from HIV infection to a diagnosis of AIDS ranges from 1 to 10 years or longer. About half of the HIV-infected adults develop AIDS within 10 years after infection. In the latter stages of AIDS, the patient will eventually die as a result of the repeated bouts of opportunistic infections and/or cancer.

The only sure way to avoid HIV infection through sex is to abstain from sexual intercourse or to engage in mutually monogamous (only one partner) sexual intercourse with someone known to be uninfected. Latex condoms with water-based lubricants have been shown to reduce the risk of sexual transmission of HIV. It is essential that latex condoms be used correctly each time individuals engage in vaginal, anal, or oral sex.

Both education of the public and health education classes in the schools should stress the facts that having multiple sexual partners and sharing drug paraphernalia increase the risk of infection with HIV. Health care professionals should use precautions, known as standard precautions, when caring for all patients. These precautions include wearing latex gloves, eye protection, and other personal protective equipment to avoid contact with blood and other fluids that are visibly bloody—and taking particular care in handling, using, and disposing of needles.

Selected antiviral agents may prolong life and reduce the risk of the AIDS patient developing opportunistic infections. Even though these drugs are used as part of the treatment for AIDS patients, there is no known cure for AIDS and no known treatment for the underlying immune deficiency.

chlamydia (klah-**MID**-ee-ah)	A sexually transmitted bacterial infection that causes inflammation of the cervix (cervicitis) in women and inflammation of the **urethra** (**urethritis**) and the **epididymis** (**epididymitis**) in men.

Symptoms of **chlamydia** in men appear one to three weeks after exposure. These symptoms include a discharge from the penis with burning and itching along with a burning sensation on urination.

Unfortunately, symptoms do not often appear in women until complications occur as a result of the chlamydial infection. Early symptoms, however, include a thick vaginal discharge consisting of a combination of mucus and pus (**mucopurulent**) accompanied by burning and itching. If left untreated, a chlamydial infection can result in **pelvic inflammatory disease** (which can lead to sterility in the female). Because infection is often **asymptomatic**, treatment of sex partners is important in eradicating infection and its consequences in women.

Preventive measures against the spread of chlamydial infections include the use of latex condoms during sexual intercourse. The infection is effectively treated with antibiotic therapy, and the patient should refrain from sexual intercourse until the treatment is completed.

genital herpes (**JEN**-ih-tal **HER**-peez)	A highly contagious viral infection of the male and female genitalia; also known as venereal herpes. Caused by the herpes simplex virus (usually HSV-2), **genital herpes** is transmitted by direct contact with infected body secretions (usually through sexual intercourse). **Genital herpes** differs from other sexually transmitted diseases in that it can recur spontaneously once the virus has been acquired.

This virus is characterized by two phases: the active phase and the **dormant** phase. The active phase is when the symptoms are present and the virus can be spread. The **dormant** phase is when the individual is free of symptoms. Unfortunately, some individuals can still transmit the virus during this stage.

Symptoms include multiple shallow ulcerations and/or reddened **vesicles** of the cervix and vulva in women, and ulcerations of the **glans penis**, **prepuce**, or scrotal sac in men. The ulcerations are similar to cold sores, can be very painful, and may be accompanied by itching. See *Figure 16-7*. In addition, the individual may experience flulike symptoms such as fever, headache, **malaise**, muscle pain (myalgia), swollen glands, and painful urination.

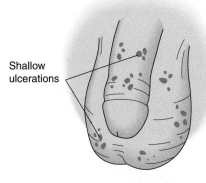
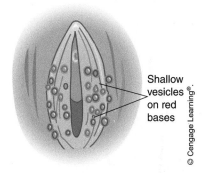

Shallow
ulcerations

Shallow
vesicles
on red
bases

© Cengage Learning®.

Figure 16-7 (A) Genital herpes in the male (B) Genital herpes in the female

Treatment for **genital herpes** is symptomatic (the symptoms are treated); that is, medications are given to reduce the swelling and pain. There is no cure for **genital herpes**. Women who have been diagnosed with **genital herpes** should be advised to have a Pap smear every six months, because the virus is known to be associated with cervical cancer.

genital warts (**JEN**-ih-tal warts)	Small, cauliflower-like, fleshy growths usually seen along the penis in the male and in or near the vagina in women. **Genital warts** are transmitted from person to person through sexual intercourse. They are caused by the human papillomavirus (HPV). The time span from initial contact with the virus to occurrence of symptoms can be from one to six months.

The characteristic appearance and location of the **genital warts** is usually significant enough for a diagnosis. A biopsy may be indicated in some cases for a definitive diagnosis.

Treatment for **genital warts** is not particularly effective because recurrence is common. However, treatment may include the application of a topical medication to destroy the warts or surgical removal (by **cryosurgery** or **debridement**). In some cases, the warts may disappear spontaneously. Although using latex condoms may reduce the transmission of **genital warts**, individuals are advised to avoid sexual contact with anyone who has the lesions.

gonorrhea (**gon**-oh-**REE**-ah)	A sexually transmitted bacterial infection of the mucous membrane of the genital tract in men and women. It is spread by sexual intercourse with an infected partner and can also be passed on from an infected mother to her infant during the birth process (as the baby passes through the vaginal canal). *Neisseria gonorrhoeae* is the causative organism.

Symptoms of **gonorrhea** differ in the male and female, being much more obvious in the male than in the female. The male may display symptoms such as a greenish-yellow drainage of pus from the **urethra** (**purulent** drainage), painful urination (**dysuria**), and frequent urination within two to seven days after becoming infected with **gonorrhea**.

The female infected with **gonorrhea** may be **asymptomatic** (without symptoms) or may display symptoms such as a greenish-yellow **purulent** vaginal discharge, **dysuria**, and urinary frequency. As the infection spreads in the female, inflammation of the fallopian tubes (**salpingitis**) may develop.

Diagnosis is confirmed by culturing the infected body secretions and by microscopic examination of a Gram-stained specimen of the **exudate** (drainage). Treatment with antibiotics is an effective cure for **gonorrhea**. Generally, patients with **gonorrhea** infections should be treated at the same time for presumed chlamydial infections because their symptoms are often similar and they can occur concurrently. Newborn infants routinely receive an instillation of erythromycin ophthalmic ointment in their eyes immediately after birth as a prophylaxis (prevention) against contracting a serious eye infection during the birthing process, due to the presence of **gonorrhea** or **chlamydia** in the vaginal canal.

syphilis (**SIF**-ih-lis)	A sexually transmitted disease characterized by lesions that may involve any organ or tissue. It is spread by sexual intercourse with an infected partner and can also be passed through the placenta from an infected mother to her unborn infant. The spirochete *Treponema pallidum* is the causative organism of this highly contagious disease. If left untreated, this disease progresses through three stages (each with characteristic signs and symptoms): primary **syphilis**, secondary **syphilis**, and tertiary **syphilis**.

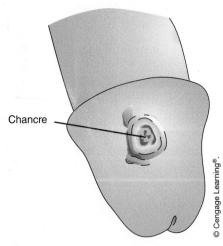

Chancre

Figure 16-8 Primary syphilis: Male

© Cengage Learning®.

1. Primary **syphilis** is characterized by the appearance of a small, painless, red pustule on the skin or mucous membrane. This highly contagious lesion, known as a **chancre**, appears within 10 days to a few weeks after exposure. The **chancre** usually develops on the penis of the male and on the labia of the vagina of the female. Primary **syphilis** can be treated effectively with antibiotics (penicillin G). See *Figure 16-8*.

2. Secondary **syphilis** occurs approximately two months later, if the primary phase of **syphilis** is left untreated (the spirochetes have had time to multiply and spread throughout the body). The dominant sign of secondary **syphilis** is the presence of a nonitching rash on the palms of the hands and the soles of the feet. The individual may also experience symptoms such as headache, sore throat, fever, a generally poor feeling (**malaise**), loss of appetite (anorexia), and bone and joint pain. The disease is still highly contagious during the secondary stage but can be treated effectively with penicillin. Following the secondary stage of **syphilis**, the disease (if left untreated) may lie **dormant** (inactive) for 5 to 20 years before reappearing in its final stage.

3. Tertiary **syphilis** is the final and most serious stage of the disease (in cases of untreated syphilis). Evidence of tertiary **syphilis** may appear from two to seven years after the initial infection. By this time, the lesions have invaded body organs and systems. The lesions of tertiary **syphilis** are not reversible, do not respond to treatment with penicillin, and can lead to life-threatening disorders of the brain, spinal cord, and heart.

Diagnosis of **syphilis** is confirmed with microscopic examination of a smear taken from the primary lesion and screening tests for the presence of antibodies in the individual's blood (such as the FTA-ABS or the VDRL). The treatment of choice for **syphilis** is administration of penicillin G in the early stages (primary or secondary) before irreversible damage to the body occurs. Following adequate treatment with penicillin, the individual is usually noncontagious within 48 hours. Individuals who are sexually active should be advised to use latex condoms during sexual intercourse to lessen the chances of contracting **syphilis**.

trichomoniasis (**trik**-oh-moh-**NYE**-ah-sis)	A sexually transmitted protozoal infection of the vagina, **urethra**, or prostate. It is usually spread by sexual intercourse and affects approximately 15% of all sexually active people. The causative organism is *Trichomonas vaginalis*.

Most men are **asymptomatic**, but some will experience **dysuria** (painful urination), urinary frequency, and **urethritis** (inflammation of the **urethra**). Women who have **trichomoniasis** will experience symptoms such as itching and burning and a strong-smelling (**malodorous**) vaginal discharge that is frothy and greenish-yellow. They may also complain of having to change underwear frequently throughout the day due to the drainage and odor.

Diagnosis of **trichomoniasis** is confirmed by microscopic examination of fresh vaginal secretions from the female or fresh urethral discharge from the male (**wet prep**). The treatment of choice for **trichomoniasis** is an anti-infective drug called Flagyl (metronidazole). It is important that both sexual partners be treated concurrently to prevent passing the infection back and forth.

Review Checkpoint

Check your understanding of this section by completing the **Pathological Conditions** exercises in your workbook.

Diagnostic Techniques, Treatments, and Procedures

castration (kass-**TRAY**-shun)	The surgical removal of the **testicles** in the male (or the ovaries in the female); also known as an **orchidectomy** or **orchiectomy** in the male and as an oophorectomy in the female.

Castration is usually performed to reduce the production and secretion of certain hormones that may encourage the growth of malignant (cancerous) cells in either the male or female. An individual who has been castrated is sterile.

circumcision (**sir**-kum-**SIH**-zhun)	A surgical procedure in which the **foreskin (prepuce)** of the penis is removed. A discussion of elective infant **circumcision** can be found in Chapter 19. Adult male **circumcision** is much less common than infant **circumcision** and more complicated.
	The most frequent medical indication for adult male **circumcision** is **phimosis** (discussed in this chapter). Other indications may be unreplaceable retraction of a narrow **foreskin** that causes a painful swelling of the **glans penis** (known as paraphimosis), patient complaint of pain with erection or during intercourse, or recurrent **balanitis** (inflammation of the **glans penis**).
	The simplest technique is the guided forceps method, in which the **foreskin** is pulled forward over the **glans penis** with a pair of forceps; using the forceps as a guide, the **foreskin** is then snipped. Other surgical methods are available depending on the causative need for the **circumcision**.
cystoscopy (sis-**TOSS**-koh-pee) cyst/o = bladder, sac, or cyst -scopy = process of viewing	**Cystoscopy** is the process of viewing the interior of the bladder by using a cystoscope.
	The cystoscope is a hollow metal or flexible tube introduced into the bladder through the urinary meatus. Visualization of the inside of the bladder is made possible by a light source and magnifying lenses, which are a part of the cystoscope. For a visual reference of **cystoscopy**, see Chapter 15 (*Figure 15-16*).
	Cystoscopy is useful in detecting tumors, inflammation, renal calculi, and structural irregularities. It can also be used as a means of obtaining biopsy specimens.
FTA-ABS test	A serological test for **syphilis** (performed on blood serum). The acronym stands for fluorescent treponemal antibody-absorption test.
	This test uses a fluorescent dye to stain antibodies (as in the treponemal antibody in **syphilis**) for identification in specimens. The dyed organisms glow visibly when examined under a fluorescent microscope, making identification of the causative organism easier. If the test is nonreactive, no fluorescence will be noted.
intravenous pyelogram (IVP) (**in**-trah-**VEE**-nuss **PYE**-el-oh-**gram**) intra- = within ven/o = vein -ous = pertaining to pyel/o = renal pelvis -gram = a record	Also known as intravenous pyelography or excretory urogram, this radiographic procedure provides visualization of the entire urinary tract (kidneys, ureters, bladder, and **urethra**). A contrast dye is injected intravenously, and multiple X-ray films are taken as the medium is cleared from the blood by the glomerular filtration of the kidney.
	Intravenous pyelogram is useful in diagnosing renal tumors, cysts, or stones; structural or functional abnormalities of the bladder; and ureteral obstruction.

orchidectomy	The surgical removal of a **testicle**.

(**or**-kid-**EK**-toh-mee)
(orchiectomy)
(**or**-kee-**EK**-toh-mee)
  orchi/o = testicle
  orchid/o = testicle
  -ectomy = surgical removal
	Orchidectomy may be performed when it is determined that an undescended **testicle** is no longer functional or as a palliative (relieves the intensity of the symptoms) surgery for cancer of the **prostate gland**. When used as a palliative surgery, the intent is not to cure the cancer but to halt its spread by removing the **testosterone** hormone (which is produced by the testicles).

orchidopexy	A surgical fixation of a **testicle**.

(**OR**-kid-oh-**peck**-see)
(orchiopexy)
(**OR**-kee-oh-**peck**-see)
  orchi/o = testicle
  orchid/o = testicle
  -pexy = surgical fixation
	This procedure involves making an incision into the inguinal canal, locating the **testicle**, and bringing it back down into the scrotal sac. The surgery is usually done on an outpatient basis, with normal physical activity being restored within a few weeks to a month.

radical prostatectomy	A radical prostatectomy is the surgical removal of the entire **prostate gland** as a treatment for cancer.

(**RAD**-ih-kal **pross**-tah-**TEK**-toh-mee)
  prostat/o = prostate gland
  -ectomy = surgical removal	

semen analysis	An assessment of a sample of **semen** for volume, viscosity, sperm count, sperm motility, and percentage of any abnormal sperm.
(**SEE**-men ah-**NAL**-ih-sis)	A **semen analysis** may be performed as part of the evaluation process in attempting to determine the cause of infertility in couples and is often the first test performed. A **semen analysis** is also performed after a **vasectomy** to confirm the success of the procedure (male sterility).
	A fresh specimen of **semen** should be collected after a period of abstaining from sexual intercourse for at least two to five days. The specimen should be delivered to the physician's office within two hours after **ejaculation** and should be protected from the cold.
	Examination of a fresh specimen of **semen** should reveal a very viscous, opaque, grayish-white substance. Examination of a **semen** specimen after a period of approximately 45 minutes should reveal a more translucent, turbid, and viscous (but more liquid) substance.
	The volume of a normal ejaculated specimen should be approximately 3 to 5 mL. A sperm count of more than 20 million sperm/milliliter of **semen** is considered normal. Approximately 70% of the sperm in a normal specimen should be motile (show movement). The normal **semen** specimen should contain no more than 25% abnormal sperm forms.
suprapubic prostatectomy	The surgical removal of the **prostate gland** by making an incision into the abdominal wall, just above the pubic bone.

(**soo**-prah-**PEW**-bik **pross**-tah-**TEK**-toh-mee)
  supra- = above, over
  pub/o = pubis
  -ic = pertaining to
  prostat/o = prostate gland
  -ectomy = surgical removal
	A small incision is then made into the bladder, which has been distended with fluid. The **prostate gland** is removed through the bladder cavity. **Suprapubic prostatectomy** is done when the surgeon believes the **prostate gland** is too enlarged to be removed through the **urethra**.

transurethral resection of the prostate (TUR or TURP)
 	
(**trans**-yoo-**REE**-thral **REE**-sek-shun of the **PROSS**-tayt)
  trans- = across, through
  urethr/o = urethra
  -al = pertaining to
	The surgical removal of a portion of the **prostate gland** by inserting a **resectoscope** (an instrument used to remove tissue from the body) through the **urethra** and into the bladder.

vasectomy
 	
(vas-**EK**-toh-mee)
  vas/o = vas deferens; vessel
  -ectomy = surgical removal
	A surgical cutting and tying of the **vas deferens** to prevent the passage of sperm, consequently preventing pregnancy; male sterilization. See *Figure 16-9*.

The **vas deferens** is the tube that carries the sperm from the testes to the penis. A **vasectomy** involves making an incision into each side of the scrotal sac, exposing the **vas deferens**, and cutting it. The ends are tied separately and may then be cauterized for additional blockage. Because sperm may remain in the **vas deferens** for a month or more after the **vasectomy**, it is important for the man and his sex partner to remember that additional protection during sexual intercourse will be necessary until his physician verifies that all of the sperm have been eliminated from the **vas deferens**. The man will have to submit periodic **semen** samples to be examined for the presence of sperm. When two separate **semen** samples show no evidence of sperm, the man is considered sterile.

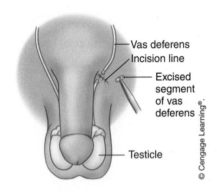

Vas deferens
Incision line
Excised segment of vas deferens
Testicle

© Cengage Learning®.

Figure 16-9 Vasectomy

VDRL test	A serological test for **syphilis** (test performed on blood serum); widely used to test for primary and secondary **syphilis**. The acronym stands for Venereal Disease Research Laboratory test.

The **VDRL test** generally becomes positive in one to three weeks after the appearance of a **chancre**. This test examines the patient's serum under the microscope (after it has been heat treated and mixed with the VDRL antigen) for the presence of clumping, which indicates a reaction. The results are reported as reactive (medium to large clumps present), weakly reactive (small clumps noted), or nonreactive (no clumping noted). Reactive and weakly reactive results on the VDRL test are considered positive for **syphilis**. If positive, further testing is done to confirm the presence of the *Treponema pallidum* spirochete. False-positive and false-negative results may occur.

wet mount; wet prep	The microscopic examination of fresh vaginal or male urethral secretions to test for the presence of living organisms.

A specimen of vaginal or urethral secretions is placed on two separate, clean microscopic slides, and a drop of normal saline is placed on top of one specimen (to check for the presence of **trichomoniasis**), whereas a drop of potassium hydroxide is placed on top of the other specimen (to check for yeast or fungi). After the specimen is mixed with the solution, a cover slip is placed on the slide, and the organisms are immediately observed under the microscope.

Review Checkpoint

Check your understanding of this section by completing the **Diagnostic Techniques, Treatments, and Procedures** exercises in your workbook.

COMMON ABBREVIATIONS

Abbreviation	Definition	Abbreviation	Definition
BPH	benign prostatic hypertrophy	KUP	kidneys, ureters, bladder; an X-ray of the urinary tract, using no contrast medium
DRE	digital rectal exam		
FTA-ABS	fluorescent treponemal antibody-absorption test; a serological test for **syphilis**	NGU	nongonococcal **urethritis**
		PSA	prostate-specific antigen
GC	**gonorrhea**; gonococcus	STS	serological test for **syphilis**
GU	genitourinary	TSE	**testicular** self-examination
HSV-2	herpes simplex virus, strain 2	TUR, TURP	transurethral resection of the **prostate gland**
IVP	**intravenous pyelogram**	VDRL	Venereal Disease Research Laboratory

Review Checkpoint

Check your understanding of this section by completing the **Common Abbreviations** exercises in your workbook.

WRITTEN AND AUDIO TERMINOLOGY REVIEW

Review each of the following terms from this chapter. Study the spelling of each term and write the definition in the space provided. Check definitions by looking the term up in the glossary.

Term	Pronunciation	Definition
android	☐ **AN**-droyd	_____
andropause	☐ **AN**-droh-pawz	_____
anorchism	☐ an-**OR**-kizm	_____
asymptomatic	☐ ay-simp-toh-**MAT**-ik	_____
azoospermia	☐ ah-zoh-oh-**SPER**-mee-ah	_____
balanitis	☐ bal-ah-**NYE**-tis	_____
benign prostatic hypertrophy	☐ bee-**NINE** pross-**TAT**-ik high-**PER**-troh-fee	_____
castration	☐ kass-**TRAY**-shun	_____
chancre	☐ **SHANG**-ker	_____
chlamydia	☐ klah-**MID**-ee-ah	_____
circumcision	☐ **sir**-kum-**SIH**-zhun	_____
Cowper's glands	☐ **KOW**-perz glands	_____
cryosurgery	☐ **kry**-oh-**SER**-jer-ee	_____
cryptorchidism	☐ kript-**OR**-kid-izm	_____
cystoscopy	☐ sis-**TOSS**-koh-pee	_____
debridement	☐ day-breed-**MENT**	_____
dormant	☐ **DOOR**-mant	_____
dysuria	☐ dis-**YOO**-ree-ah	_____
ejaculation	☐ ee-**jack**-yoo-**LAY**-shun	_____
epididymectomy	☐ **ep**-ih-**did**-ih-**MEK**-toh-mee	_____
epididymis	☐ **ep**-ih-**DID**-ih-mis	_____
epididymitis	☐ **ep**-ih-**did**-ih-**MYE**-tis	_____
epispadias	☐ **ep**-ih-**SPAY**-dee-as	_____
exudate	☐ **EKS**-yoo-dayt	_____
foreskin	☐ **FOR**-skin	_____

Term	Pronunciation	Definition
genital herpes	☐ JEN-ih-tal HER-peez	_____
genital warts	☐ JEN-ih-tal warts	_____
glans penis	☐ GLANS PEE-nis	_____
gonad	☐ GOH-nad	_____
gonorrhea	☐ gon-oh-REE-ah	_____
hematospermia	☐ hee-mah-toh-SPER-mee-ah	_____
hydrocele	☐ HIGH-droh-seel	_____
hypospadias	☐ high-poh-SPAY-dee-as	_____
impotence	☐ IM-poh-tens	_____
inguinal hernia	☐ ING-gwih-nal HER-nee-ah	_____
intravenous pyelogram (IVP)	☐ in-trah-VEE-nuss PYE-el-oh-gram	_____
malaise	☐ mah-LAYZ	_____
malodorous	☐ mal-OH-dor-us	_____
mucopurulent	☐ mew-koh-PEWR-yoo-lent	_____
opportunistic infection	☐ op-or-toon-IS-tik infection	_____
orchidectomy	☐ or-kid-EK-toh-mee	_____
orchiectomy	☐ or-kee-EK-toh-mee	_____
orchidoplasty	☐ OR-kid-oh-plass-tee	_____
orchidopexy	☐ OR-kid-oh-peck-see	_____
orchitis	☐ or-KIGH-tis	_____
palpation	☐ pal-PAY-shun	_____
pelvic inflammatory disease	☐ PELL-vik in-FLAM-mah-tor-ee dih-ZEEZ	_____
perineum	☐ pair-ih-NEE-um	_____
phimosis	☐ fih-MOH-sis	_____
premature ejaculation	☐ premature ee-jack-yoo-LAY-shun	_____
prepuce	☐ PRE-pus	_____
prophylactic	☐ proh-fih-LAK-tik	_____
prostate gland	☐ PROSS-tayt gland	_____
prostatectomy	☐ pross-tah-TEK-toh-mee	_____
prostatitis	☐ pross-tah-TYE-tis	_____

Term	Pronunciation	Definition
purulent	☐ **PEWR**-yoo-lent	_____
rectoscope	☐ **REK**-toh-skohp	_____
residual urine	☐ rih-**ZID**-yoo-al **YOO**-rin	_____
salpingitis	☐ **sal**-pin-**JYE**-tis	_____
scrotum	☐ **SKROH**-tum	_____
semen	☐ **SEE**-men	_____
semen analysis	☐ **SEE**-men ah-**NAL**-ih-sis	_____
seminal vesicles	☐ **SEM**-ih-nal **VESS**-ih-kulz	_____
seminiferous tubules	☐ **sem**-in-**IF**-er-us **TOO**-byools	_____
spermatogenesis	☐ **sper**-mat-oh-**JEN**-eh-sis	_____
spermatozoan	☐ **sper**-mat-oh-**ZOH**-ahn	_____
spermatozoon	☐ **sper**-mat-oh-**ZOH**-on	_____
spermolysis	☐ sperm-**OL**-ih-sis	_____
suprapubic prostatectomy	☐ **soo**-prah-**PEW**-bik **pross**-tah-**TEK**-toh-mee	_____
syphilis	☐ **SIF**-ih-lis	_____
testicle	☐ **TES**-tih-kul	_____
testicular	☐ tess-**TIK**-yoo-lar	_____
testosterone	☐ tess-**TOSS**-ter-own	_____
trichomoniasis	☐ **trik**-oh-moh-**NYE**-ah-sis	_____
urethra	☐ yoo-**REE**-thrah	_____
urethritis	☐ **yoo**-ree-**THRYE**-tis	_____
varicocele	☐ **VAIR**-ih-koh-seel	_____
vas deferens	☐ vas **DEF**-er-enz	_____
vasectomy	☐ vas-**EK**-toh-mee	_____
vesicles	☐ **VESS**-ih-kulz	_____

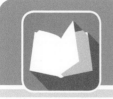

Review Checkpoint

Apply what you have learned in this chapter by completing the **Putting It All Together** exercise in your workbook.

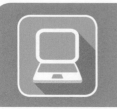

Online Resources

For additional study tools, including PowerPoint® slides and animations, go to the Student Companion Website.

Chapter Review Exercises

The following exercises provide a more in-depth review of the chapter material. Your goal in these exercises is to complete each section at a minimum 80% level of accuracy. If you score below 80% in any area, return to the applicable section in the chapter and read the material again. A place has been provided for your score at the end of each section.

A. Spelling

Circle the correctly spelled term in each pairing of words. Each correct answer is worth 10 points. Record your score in the space provided at the end of the exercise.

1. epididymis	epididymus	6. syphilis	syphillis
2. azospermia	azoospermia	7. variocele	varicocele
3. seminal	seminel	8. vas deferens	vas defrens
4. orchipexy	orchiopexy	9. epispadias	episapdius
5. prostatectomy	prostratectomy	10. impotent	imputent

Number correct _____ **× 10 points/correct answer: Your score** _____ **%**

B. Matching

Match the terms on the left with the applicable definition on the right. Each correct answer is worth 10 points. Record your score in the space provided at the end of the exercise.

_____ 1. balanitis

_____ 2. chancre

_____ 3. glans penis

_____ 4. prepuce

_____ 5. hypospadias

_____ 6. epispadias

a. blisters

b. the process of expelling the semen from the male urethra

c. congenital defect in which the urethra opens on the upper side of the penis at some point near the glans

d. a skin lesion, usually of primary syphilis, that begins at the site of infection as a small raised area and develops into a red, painless ulcer with a scooped-out appearance; also known as a venereal sore

(continued)

_____   7. spermatogenesis

_____   8. ejaculation

_____   9. scrotum

_____   10. vesicles

e. a loose, retractable fold of skin covering the tip of the penis

f. sac that houses the testicles

g. inflammation of the glans penis

h. the tip of the penis

i. the formation of sperm

j. a congenital defect in which the urethra opens on the underside of the penis instead of at the end

Number correct _____ × *10 points/correct answer: Your score* _____ %

C. Definition to Term

Using the following definitions, provide the medical term to match the definition. Each correct answer is worth 10 points. Record your score in the space provided at the end of this exercise.

Create a word that means:

1. Pertaining to male

   _____

2. Condition of undescended testicles

   _____

3. Inflammation of the testicles

   _____

4. Destruction of sperm

   _____

5. Surgical removal of the vas deferens

   _____

6. Inflammation of the glans penis

   _____

7. Formation of sperm

   _____

8. Surgical fixation of the testicles

   _____

9. Inflammation of the prostate gland

   _____

10. Surgery involving the rapid freezing of tissue

   _____

Number correct _____ × *10 points/correct answer: Your score* _____ %

D. Matching Procedures

Match the procedures on the left with the applicable description on the right. Each correct answer is worth 10 points. Record your score in the space provided at the end of the exercise.

_____ 1. cryosurgery

_____ 2. circumcision

_____ 3. semen analysis

_____ 4. castration

_____ 5. TURP

_____ 6. vasectomy

_____ 7. suprapubic prostatectomy

_____ 8. orchiopexy

_____ 9. VDRL

_____ 10. PSA test

a. a serological test for syphilis, performed on blood serum

b. a test in which elevated levels may indicate significant prostatic hypertrophy or cancer of the prostate

c. the surgical removal of the testicles in the male

d. a surgical procedure in which the foreskin of the penis is removed

e. the destruction of tissue by rapid freezing with substances such as liquid nitrogen

f. a surgical fixation of a testicle

g. assessment of a sample of semen for volume, viscosity, sperm count, motility, and percentage of any abnormal sperm

h. the surgical removal of the prostate gland by making an incision into the abdominal wall, just above the pubis

i. the surgical removal of the prostate gland by inserting a resectoscope through the urethra and into the bladder

j. surgically cutting and tying the vas deferens to prevent the passage of sperm

Number correct _____ **× 10 points/correct answer: Your score** _____**%**

E. Crossword Puzzle

Read the clues carefully and complete the puzzle. Each crossword answer is worth 10 points. When you have completed the crossword puzzle, total your points and enter your score in the space provided.

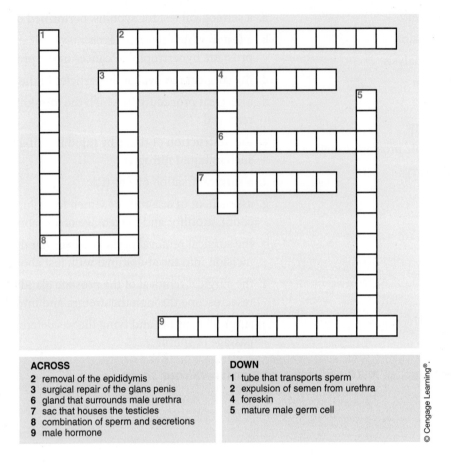

ACROSS
2 removal of the epididymis
3 surgical repair of the glans penis
6 gland that surrounds male urethra
7 sac that houses the testicles
8 combination of sperm and secretions
9 male hormone

DOWN
1 tube that transports sperm
2 expulsion of semen from urethra
4 foreskin
5 mature male germ cell

© Cengage Learning®.

Number correct _____ × *10 points/correct answer: Your score* _____%

F. Proofreading Skills

Read the following Operative Report. For each bold term, provide a brief definition and indicate if the term is spelled correctly. If it is misspelled, provide the correct spelling. Each correct answer is worth 10 points. Record your score in the space provided at the end of the exercise.

Example:

    ampulla   *a saclike dilation* _____

    Spelled correctly? ☑ Yes   ☐ No _____

OPERATIVE REPORT

Hillcrest
medical center

PATIENT NAME: Verberkmoes, Robert

PATIENT ID: 8620935

DATE OF ADMISSION
October 24, 2014

ADMITTING PHYSICIAN
Suzuki Watanabe, MD

SURGEON
Suzuki Watanabe, MD

ASSISTANT
Linda Walters, MD

PREOPERATIVE DIAGNOSIS
Prostate cancer

POSTOPERATIVE DIAGNOSIS
Prostate cancer

PROCEDURE
Bilateral pelvic lymphadenectomy, radical retropubic **prostatectomy**

ANESTHESIA
General endotracheal

ESTIMATED BLOOD LOSS
Approximately 600 mL

TRANSFUSIONS
Two autologous units of packed red blood cells during the procedure.

PROCEDURE IN DETAIL
The patient was premedicated adequately on the floor and brought to the operating room suite and placed on the operating table in the supine position. The patient was placed under general endotracheal anesthesia. On the operative field, the 24 French Foley catheter was inserted per **urethra** and placed within the bladder. Midline incision was made, extending from the symphysis up to the umbilicus. The incision was carried down using sharp dissection to the rectus fascia. The rectus fascia was incised the full length of the incision, and the rectus muscles were split apart. The transversalis fascia was incised, and the perivesical space was then developed, and a Bookwalter retractor was placed. Right pelvic lymphadenectomy was initially performed by using the nodes over the iliac vein. The extent of the dissection was carried inferiorly down to the circumflex iliac vein and superiorly up to the bifurcation of the iliac vessels. Dissection was carried down into the obturator fossa. This nodal bundle was sent for pathologic analysis. Lymphostasis was provided using hemoclip ligation. There were no grossly suspicious nodes. Care was taken to preserve the obturator nerve.

(continued)

OPERATIVE REPORT
Patient Name: Verberkmoes, Robert
Patient ID: 8620935
Admission Date: October 24, 2014
Page 2

The left pelvic lymphadenectomy was performed in a similar fashion, and again there were no grossly suspicious nodes. The endopelvic fascia was then incised on each side of the prostate, and the puboprostatic ligaments were incised. A right-angle retractor was passed around the dorsal venous complex, and a 0 Vicryl tie was used to tie off the dorsal venous complex. The dorsal venous complex was then incised. The periprostatic fascia was then incised to let the neurovascular bundles fall laterally. A right-angle retractor was then placed around the urethra with care taken to preserve the neurovascular bundles. A piece of umbilical tape was then used for traction on the urethra. The urethra was then incised, and the Foley was seen. The Foley was grasped with a Kelly clamp and brought out. The distal end of the Foley was then excised. The balloon was left inflated on this Foley to maintain traction on the prostatic urethra. Complete incision of the urethra was performed, and then, using blunt digital dissection, Denonvillier space was developed between the rectum and the prostate. The lateral vascular pedicles were ligated using hemoclips and incised. At this point, the bladder neck was then opened. The Foley balloon was seen, and the Foley balloon was drained. The Foley was then wrapped around the prostatic urethra to maintain traction on the prostatic urethra. The ureteral orifices were identified, and 5 French ureteral stents were placed up each ureteral orifice. Complete incision of the bladder neck was performed and carried posteriorly back to the **ampulla** of the base on each side. Each ampulla was ligated using hemoclip and then incised. The **seminal vesicles** were dissected free.

There was some question of induration, particularly on the patient's right seminal vesicle. Hemoclips were placed around the distal end of the seminal vesicles, and these were incised, and the entire specimen was removed to be sent for permanent section analysis. The bladder neck was then closed in tennis-racket fashion, closing the mucosal layer, using a running 3-0 chromic. The seromuscular layer was closed over this, using a running 2-0 Vicryl. A small opening was left large enough to accommodate a 22 French Foley.

The mucosa was everted to the serosa of this opening, using interrupted 4-0 chromic stitches. At this point, the 28 Roth-Greenwald retractor was inserted per urethra and proximal urethral stitches were placed using 3-0 PDS at the 12, 2, 4, 6, 8, and 10 o'clock positions. The Roth-Greenwald retractor was removed, and a 20 French silicone catheter was inserted per urethra and placed within the newly created bladder neck opening. The balloon was inflated, and proximal urethral stitch was then placed in the respective positions on the bladder neck.

The bladder neck was then pulled down on the proximal urethra. Each stitch was successively tied. The bladder was irrigated. There was no evidence of extravasation. It was irrigated through the Foley catheter, and there was no evidence of extravasation. It irrigated easily with return of clear irrigation. The wound was irrigated thoroughly with antibiotic solution. The ureteral stents had been removed prior to placing the Foley catheter. The flat Blake drain was then left in the perivesical space and brought out through a right **inguinal** stab incision. It was anchored to the skin, using a 2-0 silk tie.

The rectus muscles were reapproximated using interrupted 0 Vicryl ties. The rectus fascia was closed using a running #1 PDS. The subcutaneous tissue was closed using interrupted 3-0 Vicryl, and the skin was closed using staples. There were no complications to the procedure.

Suzuki Watanabe, MD

SW:BY

D:10/25/2014

T:10/27/2014

1. **prostate** _____

_____

Spelled Correctly? ☐ Yes ☐ No _____

2. **prostatectomy** _____

_____

Spelled Correctly? ☐ Yes ☐ No _____

3. **urethra** _____

_____

Spelled Correctly? ☐ Yes ☐ No _____

4. **seminal vesicles** _____

_____

Spelled Correctly? ☐ Yes ☐ No _____

5. **inguinal** _____

_____

Spelled Correctly? ☐ Yes ☐ No _____

Number correct _____ × *20 points/correct answer: Your score* _____%

G. Word Search

Read each definition carefully and identify the applicable word from the list that follows. Enter the word in the space provided and then find it in the puzzle and circle it. The words may be read up, down, diagonally, across, or backward. Each correct answer is worth 10 points. Record your score in the space provided at the end of the exercise.

AIDS	balanitis	chancre
genital warts	phimosis	epispadias
anorchism	orchitis	urethritis
vasectomy	cryptorchidism	

Example: Men who contract trichomoniasis may experience dysuria and inflammation of the urethra, which is known as:

urethritis _____

1. The abbreviation for acquired immunodeficiency syndrome:

_____

2. Inflammation of the glans penis and the mucous membrane beneath it:

_____

3. Absence of one or both testicles:

_____

4. Condition of undescended testicles:

_____

(*continued*)

5. Small, cauliflower-like, fleshy growths usually seen along the penis in the male and in or near the vagina in women; sexually transmitted:

_____

6. A tightness of the foreskin (prepuce) of the penis that prevents it from being pulled back:

_____

7. Inflammation of the testes due to a virus, bacterial infection, or injury:

_____

8. A congenital defect in which the urethra opens on the upper side of the penis at some point near the glans:

_____

9. A surgical cutting and tying of the vas deferens to prevent the passage of sperm:

_____

10. A highly contagious lesion that appears within 10 days to a few weeks after exposure to syphilis:

_____

H	E	A	R	G	A	T	T	A	I	D	S	I	M	L
T	O	A	G	E	O	A	N	O	R	C	H	I	S	M
H	B	L	T	N	Y	A	N	O	S	I	S	V	L	E
R	A	C	Y	I	S	A	I	D	A	P	S	I	P	E
O	L	S	H	T	E	U	R	Y	S	M	C	I	G	I
M	A	H	E	A	Y	T	S	O	I	E	Y	N	O	C
B	N	O	I	L	N	E	T	R	E	P	Y	R	L	A
O	I	R	T	W	L	C	E	I	R	R	C	A	O	R
P	T	B	R	A	D	Y	R	A	R	H	I	A	T	D
H	I	C	I	R	A	I	I	E	I	E	S	I	P	E
L	S	T	H	T	A	S	P	T	N	E	D	N	M	T
E	U	S	I	S	O	M	I	H	P	T	E	R	R	I
B	E	R	U	M	C	S	T	A	N	D	H	L	E	S
I	L	E	N	N	P	V	A	S	E	C	T	O	M	Y
U	R	E	T	H	R	I	T	I	S	O	D	N	E	C
I	N	E	R	U	C	N	D	T	U	R	E	S	I	T
S	I	S	S	L	R	E	A	S	I	E	M	N	I	S
Y	C	R	Y	P	T	O	R	C	H	I	D	I	S	M

Number correct _____ × *10 points/correct answer: Your score* _____%

H. Matching Conditions

Match the pathological conditions on the left with the applicable definition on the right. Each correct answer is worth 10 points. Record your score in the space provided at the end of the exercise.

_____ 1. phimosis

_____ 2. epispadias

_____ 3. cryptorchidism

_____ 4. anorchism

_____ 5. cancer of the prostate

_____ 6. hypospadias

_____ 7. impotence

_____ 8. cancer of the testes

_____ 9. inguinal hernia

_____ 10. orchitis

a. the absence of one or both testicles

b. malignant growth of the gland that surrounds the base of the urethra in the male

c. a congenital defect in which the urethra opens on the underside of the penis instead of at the end

d. inflammation of the testes due to a virus, bacterial infection, or injury

e. the inability of a male to achieve or sustain an erection of the penis

f. condition of undescended testicles

g. a congenital defect in which the urethra opens on the upper side of the penis at some point near the glans

h. a tightness of the foreskin of the penis of the male infant that prevents it from being pulled back

i. a protrusion of a part of the intestine through a weakened spot in the muscles and membranes of the inguinal region of the abdomen

j. a malignant tumor of the primary organs of the male reproductive system; malignancy of the male gonads

Number correct _____ × 10 points/correct answer: Your score _____%

I. Completion

Complete the following definitions by filling in the blanks with the most appropriate word. Each correct answer is worth 10 points. Record your score in the space provided at the end of the exercise.

1. Loss of appetite is known as _____.

2. A pair of pea-sized glands that empty into the urethra just before it extends through the penis (known as Cowper's glands) are called the _____ glands.

3. When a disease, such as syphilis, remains inactive for a period of time, it is said to be _____.

4. A tightly coiled tubule that houses the sperm until they mature is known as the _____.

5. A loose, retractable fold of skin covering the tip of the penis is the foreskin, or _____.

6. A vague feeling of bodily weakness or discomfort, often marking the onset of disease or illness, is known as _____.

7. An infection that sets up in a host whose resistance has been decreased is known as a(n) _____.

8. The area between the scrotum and the anus in the male is known as the _____.

(_continued_)

9. The specialized coils of tiny tubules that are responsible for production of sperm and are located in the testes are known as the _____.

10. A male hormone secreted by the testes, responsible for the secondary sex characteristic changes that occur in the male with the onset of puberty is _____.

Number correct _____ **× 10 points/correct answer: Your score** _____ **%**

J. Multiple Choice

Read each statement carefully and select the correct answer from the options listed. Each correct answer is worth 10 points. Record your score in the space provided at the end of the exercise.

1. The medical term for surgical repair of the glans penis is:
   a. balanoplasty
   b. debridement
   c. cryosurgery
   d. prostatectomy

2. Inflammation of the urethra is known as:
   a. ureteritis
   b. salpingitis
   c. balanoplasty
   d. urethritis

3. The medical term for painful urination is:
   a. pyuria
   b. dysuria
   c. hematuria
   d. oliguria

4. The area between the scrotum and the anus in the male is called the:
   a. prepuce
   b. peritoneum
   c. perineum
   d. truss

5. The absence of one or both testicles is termed:
   a. balanitis
   b. prostatitis
   c. orchitis
   d. anorchism

6. A congenital defect in which the urethra opens on the underside of the penis instead of at the end is known as:
   a. hypospadias
   b. epispadias
   c. cryptorchidism
   d. orchitis

7. The surgical removal of the testicles in the male is known as:

    a. circumcision

    b. castration

    c. orchidopexy

    d. vasectomy

8. A surgical procedure in which the foreskin (prepuce) of the penis is removed is known as:

    a. circumcision

    b. castration

    c. orchidopexy

    d. vasectomy

9. An X-ray of the urinary tract, using no contrast medium, is known as a:

    a. HSV-2

    b. VDRL

    c. KUB

    d. NGU

10. A male sterilization is called a:

    a. vasectomy

    b. circumcision

    c. orchidopexy

    d. semen analysis

***Number correct* _____ × *10 points/correct answer: Your score* _____%**

K. Medical Scenario

The following medical scenario presents information on one of the pathological conditions discussed in this chapter. Read the scenario carefully and select the most appropriate answer for each question that follows. Each correct answer is worth 20 points. Record your score in the space provided at the end of the exercise.

Edward Bain, a 61-year-old patient, visited his internist today for a physical exam. During the visit, Edward told the physician he was having difficulty when trying to start urination. He also complained that he was not able to maintain a constant stream. Edward's internist will follow up on this health history information by checking for benign prostatic hypertrophy (BPH) during the physical exam.

1. The health care professional explains to Edward that the physician will check his prostate by completing a:

    a. orchidectomy

    b. circumcision

    c. rectal exam

    d. cystoscopy

2. Edward has many questions about this possible diagnosis. The health care professional will describe BPH based on which of the following explanations?

    a. It is an accumulation of fluid in the scrotal sac and along the spermatic cord, creating pressure.

    b. It is a tightness of the foreskin of the penis that prevents it from being pulled back.

(continued)

    c. It is a protrusion of a part of the intestine through a weakened spot in the muscles and membranes of the inguinal region of the abdomen.

    d. It is a noncancerous enlargement of the prostate gland, creating pressure on the upper part of the urethra or neck of the bladder.

3. The health care professional explains to Edward that the following diagnostic tests may be ordered by the physician to check for infection or other abnormalities in the urine. The following tests will be ordered:

    1. urinalysis and residual urine

    2. urine culture and KUB X-ray

    3. vasectomy

    4. cystourethroscopy

        a. 1, 2

        b. 3, 4

        c. 1, 2, 4

        d. 1, 2, 3, 4

4. Edward asks the health care professional what treatment is typically ordered by the physician for patients with BPH. The health care professional explains that the treatment really depends on the degree of:

    a. urinary obstruction

    b. lymph node involvement

    c. infection in the scrotum

    d. inflammation in the fallopian tubes

5. The health care professional explains to Edward that for patients with recurrent problems due to hyperplasia of the prostate gland, surgery is usually indicated to remove the prostate. One type of surgery used is called a:

    a. epididymectomy

    b. circumcision

    b. orchidopexy

    d. transurethral resection

Number correct _____ *× 20 points/correct answer: Your score* _____ *%*

The Female Reproductive System

CHAPTER CONTENT

OBJECTIVES

Upon completing this chapter and the review exercises at the end of the chapter, the learner should be able to:

1. Identify the four phases of the menstrual cycle.
2. Correctly spell and pronounce terms listed on the Written and Audio Terminology Review, using the phonetic pronunciations provided.
3. Identify 10 abbreviations common to the female reproductive system.

4. Identify and define at least 10 pathological conditions of the female reproductive system.

5. Identify at least 10 diagnostic techniques used in evaluating disorders of the female reproductive system.

6. Demonstrate the ability to proof and correct a transcription exercise relative to the female reproductive system by completing the appropriate exercise at the end of the chapter.

7. Demonstrate the ability to correctly identify and label the internal genitalia of the female reproductive system using the diagram provided at the end of the chapter.

8. Identify five secondary sex characteristic changes that occur in the female body at the onset of puberty.

9. Identify and define four surgical approaches to removing a malignant growth from the female breast.

10. Identify the steps involved in breast self-examination.

Overview

To understand medical care basic to women and the childbearing process, the health care professional must be knowledgeable of the structures and function of the female reproductive system. The medical specialty that deals with diseases and disorders of the female reproductive system is known as **gynecology** (gynec/o = woman + logy = the study of). The physician who specializes in the field of **gynecology** is known as a **gynecologist** (gynec/o = woman + logist = one who specializes in the study of). This chapter is devoted to the study of the anatomy and physiology of the female reproductive system and **gynecology**. The study of obstetrics (childbirth) is covered in Chapter 18.

As complex as it may seem, the female reproductive system serves a very basic purpose: that of reproduction. After the onset of **puberty**, the female reproductive system begins the monthly repetition of providing an environment suitable for **fertilization** of the **ovum** (female egg) and then implantation of that **ovum**. **Puberty** is the period of life at which the ability to reproduce begins and the development of secondary sex characteristic changes (such as breast development, growth of pubic hair, and **menstruation**) occur.

The structures of the female reproductive system provide the environment for **coitus** (sexual intercourse), also known as copulation. If **fertilization** and implantation of the **ovum** occur, the female reproductive system then sustains the **pregnancy**, providing for the growth, development, and birth of the baby. If **fertilization** does not occur, the receptive environment changes with the shedding of the uterine lining through a bloody discharge (**menstruation**). This cyclic process repeats itself each month throughout the female's reproductive years. The end of the reproductive period is marked by the cessation, or stopping, of the menstrual cycles. This is known as **menopause**, or **climacteric**, and is characterized by a decrease in hormone production.

Anatomy and Physiology

In this section we discuss the external and internal genitalia of the female reproductive system, the breasts (accessory organs), and the shape of the female pelvis and its relationship to childbearing. The **mammary glands** are considered accessory organs of the female reproductive system because they play a part in the overall process by producing milk (lactation) for nourishing the infant.

External Genitalia

The **external genitalia** consist of the mons pubis, **labia majora**, **clitoris**, **labia minora**, vestibule, urinary **meatus**, vaginal **orifice**, **Bartholin's glands**, and the **perineum**. Collectively, the external genitalia are referred to as the **vulva** or **pudendum**. See *Figure 17-1*. As you continue to read about the external genitalia, refer to this figure for a visual reference.

The **(1) mons pubis** is the fatty tissue that covers and cushions the symphysis pubis. The triangular pattern of hair that covers the mons pubis appears after the onset of **puberty**. The **(2) labia majora** consists of two folds of skin containing fatty tissue and covered with hair that lie on either side of the vaginal opening, extending from the mons pubis to the **perineum**. The outer surface of the **labia majora** is covered by pubic hair; the inner surface is smooth and moist. The **(3) labia minora** consists of two thin folds of

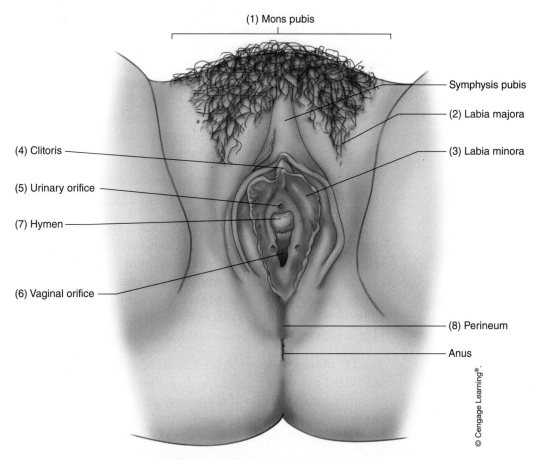

Figure 17-1 External genitalia, female reproductive system

tissue located within the folds of the **labia majora**. The **labia minora** extends from the **clitoris** downward toward the **perineum**. The point at which the **labia minora** comes together at the lower or posterior edge of the vaginal opening is known as the **fourchette**. The vestibule is an oval-shaped area between the **labia minora**, containing the urinary meatus, the vaginal orifice, and the **Bartholin's glands**. The **Bartholin's glands** are located one on each side of the vaginal orifice. They secrete a mucous substance that lubricates the **vagina**. The **labia minora** encloses the vestibule and its structures.

The **(4) clitoris** is a short, elongated organ composed of erectile tissue. It is located just behind the upper junction of the **labia minora** and is homologous to the penis in the male. The **(5) urinary orifice** is not a true part of the female reproductive system but is mentioned here because it is included as a part of the **vulva**. The urinary meatus is located just above the vaginal orifice. The **(6) vaginal orifice** is located in the lower portion of the vestibule, below the urinary meatus. The vaginal orifice (opening) is also known as the **vaginal introitus**.

A thin layer of elastic, connective tissue membrane known as the **(7) hymen** forms a border around the outer opening of the **vagina** and may partially cover the vaginal opening. The **hymen** may remain intact or may be stretched and torn during sexual intercourse or by other means, such as physical activity or using tampons. Therefore, although some cultures still believe that an intact **hymen** is proof of virginity, its presence does not prove or disprove virginity. If the **hymen** remains intact and completely covers the vaginal opening (termed an **imperforate hymen**), it must be surgically perforated (punctured) before **menstruation** begins, thus allowing the menstrual flow to escape.

The **(8) perineum** is the area between the vaginal orifice and the anus. It consists of muscular and fibrous tissue and serves as support for the pelvic structures. This thick muscular area thins out during the labor process and is sometimes torn during the stress of childbirth. The physician may choose to incise the area surgically to enlarge the vaginal opening for delivery. If this is done, the incision is called an episiotomy. This term is further discussed in Chapter 18.

Internal Genitalia

The **internal genitalia** of the female reproductive system consists of the **vagina, uterus, fallopian tubes,** and the ovaries. See *Figure 17-2.*

The **(1) vagina** is the muscular tube that connects the **uterus** with the **vulva**. It is approximately 3 inches in length and rests between the bladder (anteriorly) and the rectum (posteriorly). The folds of the inner lining of the **vagina** resemble corrugated cardboard. The stretchable folds are called **rugae**. The rugae allow the **vagina** to expand during childbirth to permit the passage of the baby's head without tearing the lining. In addition to functioning as part of the birth canal, the **vagina** is the female organ of copulation (**coitus**, sexual intercourse) and serves as the passageway for the menstrual flow.

The **(2) uterus** is a pear-shaped, hollow, muscular organ that houses the fertilized implanted **ovum** as it develops throughout **pregnancy**. It is also the source of the monthly menstrual flow if **pregnancy** does not occur. The **uterus** tilts forward over the urinary bladder and is anterior to the rectum. Also called the womb, the **uterus** has three identifiable portions: The **(2a) fundus** is the small, dome-shaped portion that rises above the area where the **fallopian tubes** enter the **uterus**; the **(2b) body of the**

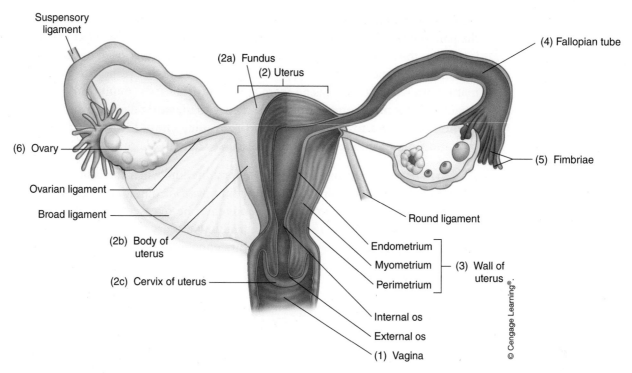

Figure 17-2 Internal genitalia, female reproductive system

uterus is the wider, central portion (near the bladder); and the **(2c) cervix of the uterus** is the narrower, necklike portion at the lower end of the **uterus**.

The **(3) wall of the uterus** consists of three layers: the **perimetrium**, which is the outermost serous membrane layer; the **myometrium**, which is the middle, muscular layer; and the **endometrium**, which is the innermost layer. The **endometrium** is the highly vascular layer that builds up each month in anticipation of receiving a fertilized egg. If **pregnancy** does not occur, this inner layer of the **uterus** is shed through a bloody discharge known as **menstruation**. Two lower segments of the **uterus** are strictures (or openings) known as the internal cervical os (or **internal os**), which separates the body of the **uterus** from the **cervix**, and the external cervical os (or **external os**) at the lower end of the cervical canal (which opens into the **vagina**).

The **(4) fallopian tubes**, also known as the uterine tubes or the oviducts, serve as a passageway for the ova (eggs) as they exit the **ovary** en route to the **uterus**. The tubes are approximately 5 inches in length and are lined with mucous membrane and **cilia** (small hairlike projections) that assist in propelling the **ovum** toward the **uterus**. One end of each tube is attached to either lateral side of the **fundus** of the **uterus**, and the other end of each tube ends in fingerlike projections called **(5) fimbriae**. The fimbriated ends, which open into the peritoneal cavity, do not actually connect with the ovaries but are able to draw the **ovum** into the tube through wavelike motions when the **ovum** is released from the **ovary**. Once the **ovum** is drawn into the fallopian tube, the sweeping motion of the cilia and the rhythmic contractions (peristalsis) of the tubes propel the **ovum** toward the **uterus**. It takes the **ovum** approximately five days to pass through the fallopian tube on its way to the **uterus**. It is in the **fallopian tubes** that **fertilization** takes place.

The **(6) ovaries** are the female sex cells, also known as the female **gonads**. Each of the paired ovaries is almond shaped and is held in place by ligaments. The ovaries are located in the upper pelvic cavity, on either side of the lateral wall of the **uterus**, near the fimbriated ends of the **fallopian tubes**. The ovaries are responsible for producing mature ova (eggs) and releasing them at monthly intervals (**ovulation**). They are also responsible for producing hormones necessary to the normal growth and development of the female and to maintenance of **pregnancy** should it occur. The process of **ovulation** and hormone production is discussed later in the chapter.

A woman has all of the ova she will have for a lifetime when she is born. At birth, the ovaries contain more than 700,000 immature ova. Throughout a woman's reproductive years, usually one **ovum** matures enough to be released from either **ovary** each month. Considering that a woman's reproductive years may span 30 or more years, approximately 400 ova may become mature enough to be fertilized during this time. The remaining ova reach various stages of development without reaching full maturity.

Mammary Glands (Breasts)

Although the **mammary glands** (breasts) do not actually play a part in the reproductive process, they are considered part of the female reproductive system because they are responsible for the production of milk (lactation). As we discuss the anatomy and physiology of the **mammary glands**, *Figure 17-3* and *Figure 17-4* will provide a visual reference of the breast appearance and structure. The breasts are located on the anterior chest wall, over the pectoral muscles. They consist of glandular tissue, with supporting adipose (fatty) tissue and fibrous connective tissue, and are covered with skin. Observation of the female breasts will reveal similarity in size and shape but not completely equal size and shape. Size and shape of the breast will also vary from individual to individual, depending on the amount of adipose tissue present in the breast. See *Figure 17-3*.

At the center of each breast is a **(1) nipple**, which consists of sensitive erectile tissue. The nipple can be stimulated, through touch, to become erect. The darker pigmented area surrounding the nipple is known as the **(2) areola**. The **areola** has a roughened

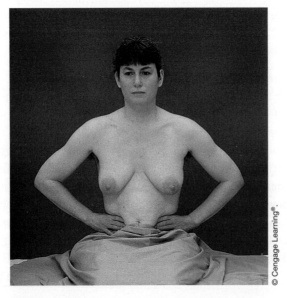

Figure 17-3 Visual appearance of the breast

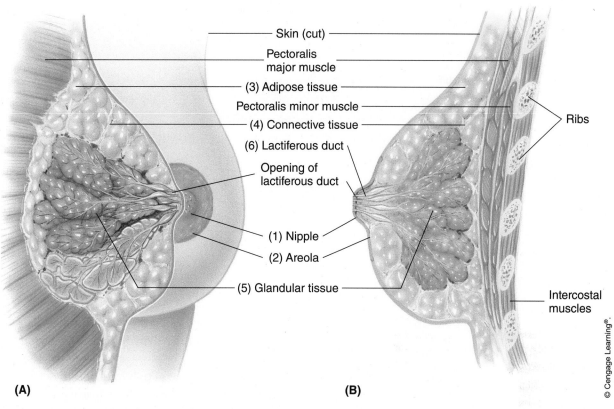

Figure 17-4 Structure of the breast: (A) anterior view; (B) sagittal view

appearance due to the presence of small sebaceous glands known as **Montgomery's tubercles** or **glands**. These glands are active only during **pregnancy** and lactation. Their purpose is to produce a substance (waxy secretion) during this time that will keep the nipple soft and prevent dryness and cracking of the nipple during nursing.

The internal structure of the breast reveals **(3) adipose tissue** located around the outer edges. The adipose tissue (fatty tissue) is supported by **(4) connective tissue**. The central portion of the breast contains **(5) glandular tissue** that radiates outward around the nipple, like beams of light shining outward all around a central point. There are 15 to 20 glandular lobes that are responsible for the production of milk during lactation. After these glands produce the milk, it travels through a network of passageways (or narrow tubular structures) called **(6) lactiferous ducts** to the nipple for breastfeeding the infant. The amount of glandular tissue is the same in all women. Therefore, breast size is not a factor in the ability to produce and secrete milk. The amount of adipose tissue present in the breast determines individual breast size.

The Female Pelvis

As you read about the female pelvis, refer to *Figure 17-5* for a visual reference. The female pelvis has a slightly oval pelvic inlet. The ischial spines are not prominent and the pubic arch is wide. The pelvic outlet has a well-rounded appearance.

Several landmarks of the pelvis play an important role in the successful passage of the fetus from the **uterus**, through the bony pelvic ring, to the outside of the body. These landmarks are found in the "true" pelvis. The boundaries of the true pelvis are defined

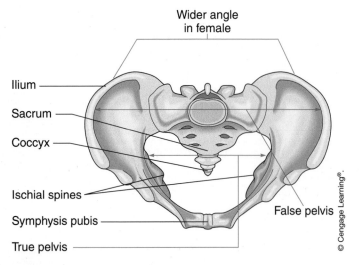

Figure 17-5 The female pelvis

by the sacrum, coccyx, and pubic bone as well as by the ischial spines. These bones serve as reference points for measuring across the pelvic outlet from varying angles to determine the size of the outlet and its adequacy for passage of the fetus. The measurement of the pelvis is known as **pelvimetry**. The goal of **pelvimetry** is to determine if the head of the fetus can pass through the bony pelvis during the delivery process. Measurement of the pelvis is usually determined by **pelvic ultrasound** during the early part of **pregnancy**. X-ray **pelvimetry** may be performed late in the **pregnancy** or during labor if more precise measurements are needed. The size of the pelvic outlet will determine if the baby is delivered vaginally or by cesarean section.

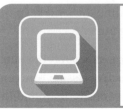

Media Link

For an overview of the female reproductive system, view the **Female Reproductive System**, animation on the Student Companion Website.

Puberty and the Menstrual Cycle

Puberty is defined as the period of life at which the ability to reproduce and secondary sex characteristics begin to develop. The onset of **puberty** marks the beginning of the reproductive years, which span some 30 or more years in the female.

In the female, some secondary sex characteristics change. These changes include development of the glandular tissue in the breasts and deposition of fat in the breasts that give them the characteristic rounded female look; deposition of fat in the buttocks and thighs, creating the rounded adult female curvatures; widening of the pelvis into a more rounded, basinlike shape that is more appropriate for childbirth; growth of pubic and axillary hair; a general skeletal growth spurt; and a general increase in size of the female reproductive organs. The most evident change during **puberty** is the onset of **menstruation**. The first menstrual period is called the **menarche**.

The **menstrual cycle** is also known as the female reproductive cycle. Influenced by hormones (**estrogen** and **progesterone**), the menstrual cycle is a regularly occurring set of changes that occur in the female body in preparation for **pregnancy**. If **pregnancy** does not occur, the nurturing environment that develops within the **uterus** in anticipation of a fertilized **ovum** is no longer needed. The hormone levels drop and the uterine lining is shed through the menstrual flow. Also known as **menses**, the menstrual flow lasts for approximately 3 to 5 days. The average menstrual cycle occurs every 28 days. The range, however, may vary from 24 to 35 days. The length of the cycle begins with the first day of the current menstrual period and ends with the first day of the menstrual period for the following month. **Ovulation** (the release of the mature **ovum** from the **ovary**) occurs approximately 14 days prior to the beginning of menses.

The menstrual cycle is divided into four time intervals, or phases, which comprise the complete cycle. These four phases consist of the menstrual phase (days 1 to 5), the postmenstrual phase (days 6 to 12), the ovulatory phase (days 13 to 14), and the premenstrual phase (days 15 to 28). A more complete description of each phase follows.

Menstrual Phase

The menstrual phase consists of days 1 to 5. The menstrual flow occurs on day 1 and lasts for 3 to 5 days.

Postmenstrual Phase

The postmenstrual phase, also called the proliferative phase, consists of days 6 to 12. This is the interval between the menses and **ovulation**. As the **estrogen** level rises, several ova begin to mature in the **graafian follicles** (with usually only one **ovum** reaching full maturity).

Ovulatory Phase

The ovulatory phase consists of days 13 to 14. This phase is known as **ovulation**. The **graafian follicle** ruptures, releasing the mature **ovum** into the pelvic cavity. The **ovum** is swept up into the **fallopian tubes** by the fimbriated ends of the tubes. **Ovulation** usually occurs on day 14 of a 28-day cycle.

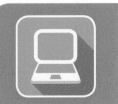

Media Link

Gain a deeper understanding of this concept by viewing the **Ovulation** animation on the Student Companion Website.

Premenstrual Phase

The premenstrual phase, also known as the secretory phase, consists of days 15 to 28. This phase occurs between the ovulatory phase and the onset of the menstrual flow. Following the rupture of the **graafian follicle** and the release of the **ovum**, the empty **graafian follicle** fills with a yellow substance called **lutein**, which is high in **progesterone**, with some **estrogen**. Thus the empty **graafian follicle** is transformed into the **corpus luteum**.

Functioning as an endocrine gland, the **corpus luteum** secretes high levels of **estrogen** and **progesterone**, preparing the uterine lining to receive a fertilized **ovum**. If **fertilization** does not occur, hormone levels decrease, the **corpus luteum** shrinks, and the uterine lining breaks down and sloughs off in the menstrual flow.

In some women, the drop in hormone levels creates a group of symptoms known as **premenstrual syndrome** (**PMS**). Symptoms include irritability, fluid retention, tenderness of the breasts, and a general feeling of depression.

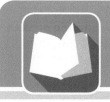

Review Checkpoint

Check your understanding of this section by completing the **Anatomy and Physiology** exercises in your workbook.

VOCABULARY

The following vocabulary words are frequently used when discussing the female reproductive system.

Word	Definition
adnexa (add-**NEK**-sah)	Tissues or structures in the body that are next to or near another. As in the **uterus**, the **adnexa** consists of the **fallopian tubes**, **ovaries**, and ligaments of the **uterus**.
areola (ah-**REE**-oh-lah)	The darker pigmented, circular area surrounding the nipple of each breast; also known as the **areola** mammae or the **areola** papillaris (plural: *areolae* [ah-**REE**-oh-lee]).
Bartholin's glands (**BAR**-toh-linz glands)	Two small, mucus-secreting glands located on the posterior and lateral aspects of the entrance to the **vagina**.

cervical dysplasia
(**SER**-vih-kal dis-**PLAY**-see-ah)
  cervic/o = cervix (neck of the uterus)
  -al = pertaining to
  dys- = bad, difficult, painful,
      disordered
  -plasia = formation or development
	The presence of abnormal tissue in the uterine cervix; this atypical tissue may be precancerous

Word	Definition
cervix (**SER**-viks)	The part of the **uterus** that protrudes into the cavity of the **vagina**; the neck of the **uterus**.
climacteric (kly-**MAK**-ter-ik)	The cessation of **menstruation**; see **menopause**.
clitoris (**KLIT**-oh-ris)	The vaginal erectile tissue (structure) corresponding to the male penis.
coitus (**KOH**-ih-tus)	The sexual union of two people of the opposite sex in which the penis is introduced into the **vagina**; also known as sexual intercourse or copulation.
colpopexy (**KOL**-poh-**peck**-see) colp/o = vagina -pexy = surgical fixation	Surgical fixation of a relaxed vaginal wall
corpus luteum (**KOR**-pus **LOO**-tee-um)	A yellowish mass that forms within the ruptured ovarian follicle after **ovulation**, containing high levels of **progesterone** and some **estrogen**. It functions as a temporary endocrine gland for the purpose of secreting **estrogen** and large amounts of **progesterone**, which will sustain **pregnancy** (should it occur) until the placenta forms. If **pregnancy** does not occur, the **corpus luteum** will degenerate approximately three days prior to the beginning of **menstruation**.
cul-de-sac (kull-dih-**SAK**)	A pouch located between the **uterus** and rectum within the peritoneal cavity. This pouch is formed by one of the ligaments that serves as support to the **uterus**. Because it is the lowest part of the abdominal cavity, blood, pus, and other drainage collect in the **cul-de-sac**.
diaphragm (**DYE**-ah-fram)	A term used in **gynecology** to represent a form of contraception.
ectopic pregnancy (eck-**TOP**-ick **PREG**-nan-see) ecto- = outside -ic = pertaining to	Abnormal implantation of a fertilized ovum outside the uterine cavity; also called a tubal pregnancy.
endometrium (en-doh-**MEE**-tree-um) endo- = within metri/o = uterus -um = noun ending	The inner lining of the **uterus**.
episiotomy (eh-**piz**-ee-**OT**-oh-mee) episi/o = vulva -otomy = incision into	A surgical procedure in which an incision is made into the woman's perineum to enlarge the vaginal opening for the delivery of the baby. This incision is usually made shortly before the baby's birth (second stage of labor) to prevent tearing of the perineum.
estrogen (**ESS**-troh-jen)	One of the female hormones that promotes the development of the female secondary sex characteristics.

Word	Definition
fallopian tubes (fah-**LOH**-pee-an **TOOBS**)	One of a pair of tubes opening at one end into the **uterus** and at the other end into the peritoneal cavity, over the **ovary**.
fertilization (fer-til-eye-**ZAY**-shun)	The union of a male **sperm** and a female **ovum**.
fimbriae (**FIM**-bree-ay)	The fringelike end of the fallopian tube.
fourchette (foor-**SHET**)	A tense band of mucous membranes at the posterior rim of the vaginal opening: the point at which the **labia minora** connect.
fundus (**FUN**-dus)	The dome-shaped central, upper portion of the **uterus** between the points of insertion of the **fallopian tubes**.
galactorrhea (gah-**lack**-toh-**REE**-ah) galact/o = milk -rrhea = discharge; flow	Discharge or flow of milk from the breasts of women who are not breastfeeding; not associated with childbirth or nursing of an infant.
gamete (**GAM**-eet)	A mature sperm or **ovum**.
gonads (**GOH**-nads)	A **gamete**-producing gland such as an **ovary** or a testis.
graafian follicles (**GRAF**-ee-an **FOL**-ik-kulz)	A mature, fully developed ovarian cyst containing the ripe **ovum**.
gynecologist (gigh-neh-**KOL**-oh-jist) gynec/o = woman -logist = one who specializes in the study of	A physician who specializes in the medical specialty that deals with diseases and disorders of the female reproductive system.
gynecology (gigh-neh-**KOL**-oh-jee) gynec/o = woman -logy = the study of	The branch of medicine that deals with the study of diseases and disorders of the female reproductive system.
hymen (**HIGH**-men)	A thin layer of elastic, connective tissue membrane that forms a border around the outer opening of the **vagina** and may partially cover the vaginal opening.
hysterosalpingography (**hiss**-ter-oh-**sal**-pin-**GOG**-rah-fee) hyster/o = uterus salping/o = fallopian tubes -graphy = process of recording	An X-ray of the uterus and the fallopian tubes by injecting a contrast material into these structures.

Word	Definition
labia majora (**LAY**-bee-ah mah-**JOR**-ah)	Two folds of skin containing fatty tissue and covered with hair that lie on either side of the vaginal opening, extending from the mons pubis to the **perineum**. The outer surface of the **labia majora** is covered by pubic hair; the inner surface is smooth and moist.
labia minora (**LAY**-bee-ah mih-**NOR**-ah)	Two folds of hairless skin located within the folds of the **labia majora**. The **labia minora** extend from the **clitoris** downward toward the **perineum**.
lumpectomy (lum-**PEK**-toh-mee)	Surgical removal of only the tumor and the immediate adjacent breast tissue; a method of treatment for breast cancer when detected in the early stage of the disease.
mammary glands (**MAM**-ah-ree glands) mamm/o = breast -ary = pertaining to	The female breasts.
mastectomy (mass-**TEK**-toh-mee) mast/o = breast -ectomy = surgical removal	Surgical removal of the breast as a treatment method for breast cancer; can be simple (breast only), modified radical (breast plus lymph nodes in axilla), or radical (breast, lymph nodes, and chest muscles on affected side).
mastitis (mass-**TYE**-tis) mast/o = breast -itis = inflammation	Inflammation of the breast.
meatus (mee-**AY**-tus)	An opening or tunnel through any part of the body.
menarche (meh-**NAR**-kee) men/o = menstruation -arche = beginning	Onset of **menstruation**; the first menstrual period.
menometrorrhagia (**men**-oh-**met**-roh-**RAY**-jee-ah) men/o = menstruation metr/o = uterus -rrhagia = excessive flow or discharge	Excessive flow of menstrual period and at times other than the menstrual period.
menopause (**MEN**-oh-pawz) men/o = menstruation	The permanent cessation (stopping) of the menstrual cycles.
menorrhea (men-oh-**REE**-ah) men/o = menstruation -rrhea = discharge; flow	Menstrual flow; **menstruation**.

Word	Definition
menses (**MEN**-seez)	Another name for **menstruation** or menstrual flow.
menstruation (men-stroo-**AY**-shun)	The periodic shedding of the lining of the nonpregnant **uterus** through a bloody discharge that passes through the **vagina** to the outside of the body. It occurs at monthly intervals and lasts for 3 to 5 days.
myometrium (**my**-oh-**MEE**-tree-um) 　my/o = muscle 　metri/o = uterus 　-um = noun ending	The muscular layer of the uterine wall.
nulligravida (null-ih-**GRAV**-ih-dah) 　nulli- = none 　-gravida = pregnancy	A woman who has never been pregnant.
nullipara (nuh-**LIP**-ah-rah) 　nulli- = none 　-para = to bear	A woman who has never completed a **pregnancy** beyond 20 weeks' gestation.
orifice (**OR**-ih-fis)	The entrance or outlet of any body cavity; as in the vaginal **orifice**.
ovariorrhexis (oh-**vay**-ree-oh-**RECK**-sis) 　ovari/o = ovary 　-rrhexis = rupture	Rupture of an ovary.
ovary (**OH**-vah-ree) 　ov/o = egg 　-ary = pertaining to	One of a pair of female **gonads** responsible for producing mature ova (eggs) and releasing them at monthly intervals (**ovulation**); also responsible for producing the female hormones, **estrogen** and **progesterone**.
ovulation (ov-yoo-**LAY**-shun) 　ov/o = egg	The release of the mature **ovum** from the **ovary**, occurring approximately 14 days prior to the beginning of menses.
ovum (**OH**-vum) 　ov/o = egg 　-um = noun ending	The female reproductive cell; female sex cell or egg.
perineum (pair-ih-**NEE**-um)	The area between the vaginal orifice and the anus that consists of muscular and fibrous tissue and serves as support for the pelvic structures.
pregnancy (**PREG**-nan-see)	The period of intrauterine development of the fetus from conception through birth. The average **pregnancy** lasts approximately 40 weeks; also known as the gestational period.

Word	Definition
premenstrual syndrome (pre-**MEN**-stroo-al **SIN**-drom)	A group of symptoms that include irritability, fluid retention, tenderness of the breasts, and a general feeling of depression occurring shortly before the onset of **menstruation**; also called PMS.
primigravida (**prye**-mih-**GRAV**-ih-dah) primi- = first -gravida = pregnancy	A woman who is pregnant for the first time
primipara (prye-**MIP**-ah-rah) primi- = first -para = to bear	A woman who has given birth for the first time, after a **pregnancy** of at least 20 weeks' gestation
progesterone (proh-**JESS**-ter-own)	One of the female hormones secreted by the **corpus luteum** and the placenta. It is primarily responsible for the changes that occur in the **endometrium** in anticipation of a fertilized **ovum** and for development of the maternal placenta after implantation of a fertilized **ovum**.
puberty (**PEW**-ber-tee)	The period of life at which the ability to reproduce begins; that is, in the female, it is the period when the female reproductive organs are fully developed.
sperm	A mature male germ cell; spermatozoon.
testes (**TESS**-teez)	The paired male **gonads** that produce sperm. They are suspended in the scrotal sac in the adult male.
uterus (**YOO**-ter-us)	The hollow, pear-shaped organ of the female reproductive system that houses the fertilized, implanted **ovum** as it develops throughout **pregnancy**; also the source of the monthly menstrual flow from the nonpregnant **uterus**.
vagina (vah-**JEYE**-nah)	The muscular tube that connects the **uterus** with the **vulva**. It is approximately 3 inches long and rests between the bladder (anteriorly) and the rectum (posteriorly).
vulva (**VULL**-vah)	The external genitalia that consists of the mons pubis, **labia majora**, **clitoris**, **labia minora**, vestibule, urinary meatus, vaginal **orifice**, **Bartholin's glands**, and the **perineum**; also known as the pudendum.

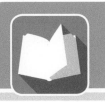

Review Checkpoint

Check your understanding of this section by completing the **Vocabulary** exercises in your workbook.

WORD ELEMENTS

The following word elements pertain to the female reproductive system. As you review the list, pronounce each word element aloud twice and check the box after you say it. Write the definition for the example word given for each word element. Use your medical dictionary to find the definitions of the example words.

Word Element	Pronunciation	"Say It"	Meaning
ante- **ante**flexion	**AN**-tee an-tee-**FLEK**-shun	☐	before; in front
-arche men**arche**	**AR**-kee meh-**NAR**-kee	☐	beginning
cervic/o **cervic**itis	**SER**-vih-koh ser-vih-**SIGH**-tis	☐	neck; **cervix**
colp/o **colp**odynia	**KOL**-poh kol-poh-**DIN**-ee-ah	☐	**vagina**
dys- **dys**menorrhea	**DIS** **dis**-men-oh-**REE**-ah	☐	bad, difficult, painful, disordered
ecto- **ecto**pic	**ECK**-toh eck-**TOP**-ick	☐	outside
endo- **endo**metrium	**EN**-doh en-doh-**MEE**-tree-um	☐	within
episi/o **episi**otomy	eh-**PIZ**-ee-oh eh-**piz**-ee-**OT**-oh-mee	☐	vulva
galact/o **galact**orrhea	gah-**LACK**-toh gah-**lack**-toh-**REE**-ah	☐	milk
-graphy mammo**graphy**	**GRAFF**-ee mam-**OG**-rah-fee	☐	process of recording
gynec/o **gynec**ologist	**GIGH**-neh-koh gigh-neh-**KOL**-oh-jist	☐	woman
hyster/o **hyster**ectomy	**HISS**-ter-oh hiss-ter-**EK**-toh-mee	☐	**uterus**
in- **in**competent cervix	**IN** in-**COMP**-eh-tent **SIR**-viks	☐	in, inside, within, not

Word Element	Pronunciation	"Say It"	Meaning
intra- **intra**uterine device	**IN**-trah in-trah-**YOO**-ter-in dee-**VICE**	☐	within
mamm/o **mamm**ography	**MAM**-oh mam-**OG**-rah-fee	☐	breast
mast/o **mast**ectomy	**MASS**-toh mass-**TEK**-toh-mee	☐	breast
men/o a**men**orrhea	**MEN**-oh ah-men-oh-**REE**-ah	☐	**menstruation**
metr/o **metr**orrhagia	**MET**-roh **met**-roh-**RAY**-jee-ah	☐	**uterus**
metri/o endo**metri**osis	**MEE**-tree-oh en-doh-**MEE**-tree-**OH**-sis	☐	**uterus**
my/o **my**ometrium	**MY**-oh my-oh-**MEE**-tree-um	☐	muscle
o/o **o**ogenesis	**OH**-oh oh-oh-**JEN**-eh-sis	☐	egg, **ovum**
oophor/o **oophor**itis	oh-**OFF**-oh-roh oh-off-oh-**RIGH**-tis	☐	ovary
ov/o **o**vulation	**OV**-oh **ov**-yoo-**LAY**-shun	☐	**ovum**, egg
ovari/o **ovari**opexy	oh-**VAIR**-ree-oh oh-vair-ree-oh-**PEK**-see	☐	ovary
-pexy hystero**pexy**	**PECK**-see **hiss**-ter-oh-**PECK**-see	☐	surgical fixation
-rrhea meno**rrhea**	**REE**-ah men-oh-**REE**-ah	☐	discharge, flow
retro- **retro**version	**RET**-roh ret-roh-**VER**-zhun	☐	backward, behind
-rrhagia meno**rrhagia**	**RAY**-jee-ah **men**-oh-**RAY**-jee-ah	☐	excessive flow or discharge
-rrhexis hystero**rrhexis**	**RECK**-sis **hiss**-ter-oh-**RECK**-sis	☐	rupture
salping/o **salping**itis	sal-**PING**-oh sal-pin-**JIGH**-tis	☐	eustachian tubes; also refers to **fallopian tubes**

Word Element	Pronunciation	"Say It"	Meaning
-tomy uterotomy	**TOH**-mee yoo-ter-**OT**-oh-mee	☐	incision into
uter/o **uter**otomy	**YOO**-ter-oh yoo-ter-**OTT**-oh-mee	☐	**uterus**
vagin/o **vagin**itis	**VAJ**-in-oh vaj-in-**EYE**-tis	☐	**vagina**
vulv/o **vulv**ovaginitis	**VULL**-voh **vull**-voh-**VAJ**-in-eye-tis	☐	**vulva**

Review Checkpoint

Check your understanding of this section by completing the **Word Elements** exercises in your workbook.

Common Signs and Symptoms

The following is a list of complaints or concerns the female patient might express or describe. These signs or symptoms may be the only reason she wishes to be seen by the physician. These symptoms may be easily treated, or they may be signs of more serious conditions. Be sure to gather your data carefully when interviewing the patient.

As you study the following terms, write each definition and word a minimum of three times (use a separate sheet of paper), pronouncing the word aloud each time. You will notice that the word and the **basic definition** are written in a green shaded box, if you choose to learn only the abbreviated form of the definition. A more detailed description follows most words. Once you have mastered each word to your satisfaction, check the box provided beside each word.

☐ **amenorrhea**

(ah-men-oh-**REE**-ah)
   a- = without, not
   men/o = menstruation
   -rrhea = discharge, flow

Absence of menstrual flow.

Amenorrhea is normal before **puberty**, during **pregnancy**, and after **menopause**. Some individuals experience temporary **amenorrhea** after discontinuing birth control pills. **Amenorrhea** can also be due to stress, strenuous exercising (as in competitive exercise), and eating disorders such as anorexia nervosa.

☐ **dysmenorrhea**

(**dis**-men-oh-**REE**-ah)
   dys- = bad, difficult, painful,
       disordered
   men/o = menstruation
   -rrhea = discharge, flow

Painful menstrual flow.

Dysmenorrhea is extremely common, occurring at least occasionally in all women. If the episode of pain during **menstruation** is brief and mild, it is considered normal and requires no particular treatment. In approximately 10% of all women, **dysmenorrhea** may be severe enough to disable them temporarily.

☐ **menorrhagia**	Abnormally long or very heavy menstrual periods.
(**men**-oh-**RAY**-jee-ah) men/o = menstruation -rrhagia = excessive flow or discharge	Chronic **menorrhagia** can result in anemia, due to recurrent excessive blood loss. **Menorrhagia** can also be caused by the presence of benign uterine fibroid tumors.

☐ **metrorrhagia**	Uterine bleeding at times other than the menstrual period.
(**met**-roh-**RAY**-jee-ah) metr/o = uterus -rrhagia = excessive flow or discharge	Abnormal uterine bleeding may be due to numerous causes, such as diseases of the thyroid gland, diabetes mellitus, cervical polyps, fibroid tumors of the **uterus**, excessive buildup of the inner lining of the **uterus**, and endometrial cancer. Any woman who experiences prolonged **metrorrhagia** that is not associated with normal menstrual periods should seek medical advice.

☐ **oligomenorrhea**	**Oligomenorrhea** is abnormally light or infrequent **menstruation**.
(ol-ih-goh-**men**-oh-**REE**-ah) olig/o = few, little, scanty men/o = menstruation -rrhea = discharge, flow	Other symptoms of possible female reproductive system disorders include, but are not limited to, the following: lower abdominal or pelvic pain, abnormal vaginal discharge or itching, breast changes such as pain and tenderness, abnormalities in the nipple, and feeling a mass or lump in the breast. If a female patient presents with any of these symptoms, they need to be brought to the attention of the physician during the visit.

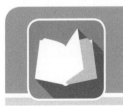

Review Checkpoint

Check your understanding of this section by completing the **Common Signs and Symptoms** exercises in your workbook.

Family Planning

The term *family planning* encompasses choosing *when to have* children and choosing *when not to have* children. It involves various forms of contraception to prevent **pregnancy** as well as methods that will help the couple achieve **pregnancy**. This section discusses **contraception**: methods used to prevent **pregnancy**. Methods used to achieve **pregnancy** are discussed in Chapter 18.

Considering the fact that the female reproductive years span some 30 or more years, the female may actually be faced with making decisions about which form of birth control she chooses to use for more than 30 years. If it is her choice to bear a limited number of children (the national average is two), effective contraceptive methods are essential. Most forms of contraception used by women can be terminated when **pregnancy** is desired and resumed after **pregnancy**.

The decision as to which form of contraception to use primarily rests with the female. The advantages and disadvantages of each type should be considered as she selects the particular form that best suits her body, her health, and her lifestyle. The number of sex partners she has will also affect the female's decision on birth control methods, particularly because of acquired immunodeficiency syndrome (AIDS) and other sexually transmitted diseases. If contraception is a planned decision and not a spontaneous one, the female may seek counsel from her physician as she determines her approach to family planning. Literature on the various methods of contraception should be available through her physician's office.

Forms of Contraception

Each form of contraception discussed in this chapter is defined as to how it is used, followed by a listing of the advantages and disadvantages of its use. Contraindications (reasons for not using) are listed, when applicable. Although many of these forms of contraception are 99% to 100% effective in preventing **pregnancy** when used correctly, it must be remembered that they do not protect the female against sexually transmitted diseases. Women who are sexually active should also have their sexual partner(s) use a condom for added protection.

abstinence	Abstinence means to abstain from having vaginal intercourse.
(**AB**-stih-nens)	**Abstinence** is 100% effective as a means of birth control. Various religious groups support **abstinence** among unmarried people. With the rise in AIDS and other sexually transmitted diseases, an increased push for **abstinence** among unmarried people is becoming more evident. Many television commercials may now be seen promoting the "I'm worth waiting for" concept among teenagers.

oral contraceptives	Oral contraceptives, or birth control pills, contain synthetic forms of the **estrogen** and **progesterone** hormones and are taken by mouth.
(**ORAL** con-trah-**SEP**-tivz)	

The hormonal influence of **oral contraceptives** prevents **ovulation** in the female. This can be reversed when the female ceases to take them. Birth control pills have a nearly 100% effectiveness rate when taken correctly. The advantages of taking birth control pills include but are not limited to the following:

1. Convenience of taking a pill by mouth

2. Decreased incidence of **dysmenorrhea** and **premenstrual syndrome** while taking birth control pills

3. Decreased menstrual flow, making iron-deficiency anemia less of a problem than in nonpill users

4. Regulation of **menorrhagia** and elimination of menstrual irregularity

The disadvantages of taking birth control pills include but are not limited to the following:

1. Nausea

2. Headaches

3. Weight gain

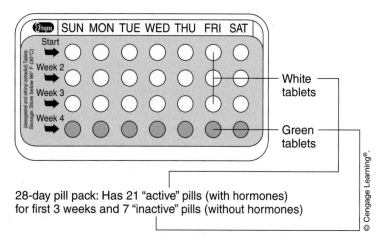

28-day pill pack: Has 21 "active" pills (with hormones)
for first 3 weeks and 7 "inactive" pills (without hormones)

Figure 17-6 Oral contraceptive packaging

4. Breakthrough bleeding (i.e., spotting between periods)

5. Mild hypertension

Contraindications (or reasons for not taking **oral contraceptives**) include but are not limited to the following:

1. History of thromboembolic disorders, breast cancer, **estrogen**-fed tumors, depression, or coronary artery disease

2. Migraine headaches

3. Women over the age of 35 who are heavy smokers

4. Women who are breastfeeding (the **estrogen** decreases the milk supply)

Birth control pills are packaged in convenient dispensers, making them easy to carry when traveling. See *Figure 17-6.* Most are packaged in 21- or 28-pill packs. Many women prefer the 28-day pill package because no days are skipped, making it easier to stay on schedule.

| **Depo-Provera injection** | **Depo-Provera injection** is a form of contraception administered intramuscularly, approximately once every 12 weeks. |
| (**DEP**-oh proh-**VAIR**-ah) | |

Depo-Provera acts by preventing **ovulation** and is considered about 99% effective. This injectable form of birth control is also reversible. The advantages of using Depo-Provera injections as a means of birth control are as follows:

1. The user does not have to remember to take pills daily or to insert a contraceptive just before intercourse.

2. The sexual act can be more spontaneous and more meaningful for some.

3. The medication is taken once every 12 weeks.

The disadvantages of using Depo-Provera injections include but are not limited to the following:

1. Menstrual spotting

2. Weight gain

3. Headaches

4. Decrease in bone mineral stored in the body

5. Women must return to their physician every 12 weeks for the injections.

Contraindications for use of Depo-Provera injections as a means of birth control include but are not limited to the following:

1. **Pregnancy**

2. Women who have or have had breast cancer

3. Women who have thromboembolic disease

4. Women who have liver disease

intrauterine device

(**in**-trah-**YOO**-ter-in)
  intra- = within
  uter/o = uterus

The **intrauterine device** is a small, plastic T-shaped object with strings attached to the leg of the T. It is inserted into the **uterus**, through the **vagina**, and remains in place in the **uterus**.

Also known as an IUD, the **intrauterine device** acts by preventing implantation of an **ovum** into the **uterus**. Although the exact action of the IUD is not understood, it is thought that the presence of the foreign body in the **uterus** prevents the implantation of the **ovum**. Some IUDs provide effective contraception for up to five to ten years. The advantages of using an IUD as a form of birth control include the following:

1. Once the IUD is inserted, the female only has to check periodically for the strings (which should be suspended in the **vagina**).

2. The user does not have to remember to take pills daily or to insert a contraceptive just before intercourse.

3. The sexual act can be more spontaneous and more meaningful for some.

4. The IUD can be removed at any time.

The disadvantages of the IUD include but are not limited to the following:

1. **Pelvic inflammatory disease**, the most serious complication of using an IUD

2. Spotting or uterine cramping for the first few weeks

3. Possible heavier than normal menstrual periods for the first few months after insertion of an IUD

4. Higher risk of tubal **pregnancy**

Contraindications for using the **intrauterine device** as a means of birth control include but are not limited to the following:

1. Women who have never been pregnant or who are known to have an abnormally shaped **uterus** (their small **uterus** could be punctured during insertion)

2. Women who have a history of **dysmenorrhea** or **metrorrhagia**

3. History of pelvic infections

4. History of ectopic **pregnancy**

birth control patch	A thin, flexible square patch that continuously delivers hormones through the skin and into the bloodstream for a full seven days to prevent **pregnancy**. The **birth control patch** contains hormones similar to those in birth control pills but must be changed every seven days.

The patch can be worn on the buttock, abdomen, upper torso (not the breast area), or on the outside of the upper arm. Remove the used patch before applying a new one in a different location. The new patch must be applied to clean, dry skin and held in place firmly for 10 seconds to make sure the entire patch adheres to the skin.

The birth control patch should be changed once a week on the same day of each week for three weeks in a row. On the fourth week, the female should not wear the patch to allow time for her regular menstrual period. After her menstrual period, the process of three weeks on the patch and one week off continues. The advantages of using the patch form of birth control include the following:

1. The patch is considered 99% effective in preventing **pregnancy** when used correctly.

2. The user does not have to remember to take pills daily or to insert a contraceptive just before intercourse.

3. The sexual act can be more spontaneous and more meaningful for some.

The disadvantages of using the patch form of birth control include but are not limited to the following:

1. If the patch is not applied on time each week or the patch becomes loose or falls off for more than 24 hours, backup contraception (such as a condom, **diaphragm**, or spermicide) must be used for one week.

2. Care should be taken to avoid putting creams, body lotions, oils, powders, or makeup near the patch.

Contraindications for using the patch as a means of birth control are similar to those of birth control pills. They include but are not limited to the following:

1. History of blood clots, breast cancer, **estrogen**-fed tumors, or coronary artery disease

2. Migraine headaches

3. Women over the age of 35 who are heavy smokers

| **contraceptive ring** | A flexible **contraceptive ring** (placed into the **vagina**) that slowly releases a low dose of hormones that prevent **pregnancy**. |

The contraceptive ring is approximately 2 inches in diameter and is placed in the **vagina** once a month. The muscles in the vaginal wall keep the ring in place. Contact with the vaginal wall activates the release of hormones similar to those of birth control pills. The contraceptive ring is left in place for three weeks, removed for one week (during which time the menstrual period occurs). Exactly one week after the contraceptive ring is removed, a new one is inserted. The advantages of using the contraceptive ring as a method of birth control include the following:

1. The contraceptive ring is easy to use and can be self-inserted.

2. The user does not have to remember to take pills daily or to insert a contraceptive just before intercourse.

3. The sexual act can be more spontaneous and more meaningful for some.

4. The contraceptive ring is changed monthly.

5. Fewer hormonal ups and downs than with pills or the patch.

The disadvantages of using the contraceptive ring as a method of birth control include but are not limited to the following:

1. If the contraceptive ring slips out of the **vagina** for more than three hours, backup contraception (such as a condom, **diaphragm**, or spermicide) must be used until the reinserted ring has been in place for one full week.

Contraindications for using the birth control ring as a means of birth control include but are not limited to the following:

1. Women over the age of 35 who are heavy smokers

2. Women who are breastfeeding

3. History of blood clots or coronary artery disease

| **barrier methods** | Methods of birth control that place physical barriers between the **cervix** and the sperm so that the sperm cannot pass the **cervix** and enter the **uterus** and thus the **fallopian tubes**. |

Barrier methods are used only during sexual intercourse. Because they function the same way, only three of the more commonly used barrier methods of birth control are discussed.

1. **Spermicidal** jellies and creams are inserted into the **vagina**. They increase the acidity of the vaginal secretions, causing the death of the sperm before they can reach the **cervix**. The advantages include the fact that they can be purchased without a prescription.

   The disadvantages include the inconvenience of having to insert the spermicide no more than 1 hour before sexual intercourse and having to leave it in for at least 6 hours after for optimal effect. The other disadvantage is the higher failure rate of the products. Contraindications for use of spermicidal jellies and creams as a means of birth control include women nearing **menopause** and those with inflammation of the **cervix**.

2. **Condoms** are thin latex sheaths worn on the penis of the male during sexual intercourse (male condoms), or loose-fitting latex sheaths that are inserted into the female **vagina** before sexual intercourse (female condoms). Both types of condoms are designed to collect semen that leaks or is expelled from the penis during ejaculation, and both are designed for one-time use only.

   The advantages of the male condom are that they are readily available without a prescription and they provide good protection against sexually transmitted diseases and the AIDS virus. The advantages of the female condom are the same as those for the male condom. In addition, they are less likely to break or tear than male condoms. The female condoms also allow vaginal penetration before the penis is completely erect.

   The disadvantages are limited mainly to the male condom and include the possibility of the condom becoming dislodged from the penis during sexual intercourse and the need for the penis to be erect to apply the condom. There are basically no contraindications for the use of condoms as a means of birth control.

3. Diaphragms are flexible, circular rubber discs that fit over the **cervix** after being inserted through the **vagina**. They prevent the sperm from entering the **uterus** and thus the **fallopian tubes**. They are primarily used in conjunction with spermicidal creams and jellies for added protection. Initial fitting of the **diaphragm** is performed by the physician to ensure a proper fit. The female inserts the **diaphragm** thereafter.

   Advantages include the fact that the **diaphragm** can be inserted up to 6 hours before intercourse and can be left in place for 24 hours. Disadvantages include **cervicitis** (inflamation of the **cervix**) and the possibility of increased incidence of urinary tract infections due to the pressure of the **diaphragm** on the urethra.

Permanent Methods of Birth Control

Permanent methods of birth control include surgical sterilization of either the female (**tubal ligation**) or the male (**vasectomy**). After having children, many people choose sterilization as a permanent means of birth control. Occasionally, they will decide to have the procedure reversed, but this is much more complicated than the sterilization itself and is not always successful. When individuals are considering permanent methods of birth control, they should weigh the pros and cons carefully. Even though they may not wish to do so, men and women who have children at a young age should consider the possibilities of divorce, remarriage, or even death of a spouse or a child before deciding on permanent means of birth control.

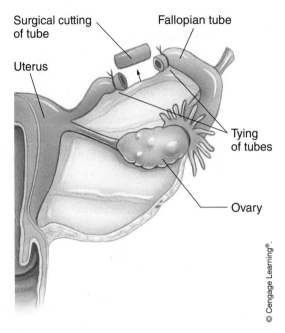

Figure 17-7 Tubal ligation

tubal ligation (**TOO**-bal lye-**GAY**-shun)	**Tubal ligation** is surgically cutting and tying the **fallopian tubes** to prevent passage of ova or sperm through the tubes, consequently preventing **pregnancy**; female sterilization. See *Figure 17-7*.
	The surgery for a **tubal ligation** may be performed the day after giving birth, or it may be scheduled as an outpatient procedure. One surgical method involves making a small incision into the abdomen (minilaparotomy) and bringing the tubes up through the incision. A piece of each tube is then cut away and the ends are tied separately.
micro-insert system	An alternative to **tubal ligation** that provides bilateral occlusion of the **fallopian tubes** by inserting a soft, flexible micro-insert into each fallopian tube.
	This procedure requires no incisions and can be performed without general anesthesia. The micro-inserts are made with the same materials that have been used for blood vessel grafts for years. Once the insert is in place, it works with the body to form a tissue barrier that prevents sperm from reaching the egg. It takes approximately three months for the tissue growth to block the **fallopian tubes**. During the first three months after insertion of the micro-inserts, backup methods of contraception (such as a condom, **diaphragm**, or spermicide) must be used.

vasectomy
 	
(vas-**EK**-toh-mee)
 	
  vas/o = vessel, vas deferens
  -ectomy = surgical removal
	Also known as a male sterilization, a vasectomy is surgically cutting and tying the vas deferens to prevent the passage of sperm, consequently preventing **pregnancy**. See *Chapter 16* for more detailed information on a vasectomy.

Pathological Conditions

As you study the pathological conditions of the female reproductive system, note that the **basic definition** is in a green shaded box (followed by a more detailed description in regular print). The phonetic pronunciation is directly beneath each term, as well as a breakdown of the component parts of the term where appropriate.

carcinoma of the breast

(**kar**-sih-**NOH**-mah)

  carcin/o = cancer

  -oma = tumor

A malignant (cancerous) tumor of the breast tissue. The most common type (ductal carcinoma) originates in the mammary ducts. This tumor has the ability to invade surrounding tissue if not detected early enough. Once the cancer cells penetrate the duct, they will metastasize (spread) through the surrounding breast tissue, eventually reaching the axillary lymph nodes. Through the lymph vessels, the cancer cells can spread to distant parts of the body.

Cancer of the breast is the second most common malignancy in women in the United States today. It is estimated that one in eight women in the United States will develop breast cancer during their lifetime, based on a 100-year life expectancy. Most breast lumps are discovered by the woman and are felt as a movable mass, generally in the upper outer quadrant of the breast. In some cases, the woman's husband or sexual partner will feel the lump in the breast first. Many women, however, fail to follow through with seeking medical attention when they discover a lump in their breast. Any lump, no matter how small, should be reported to a physician immediately!

Factors that place some women in a higher risk category than others include a family history of breast cancer, nulliparity (having borne no children), early **menarche**, late **menopause**, hypertension, obesity, diabetes, chronic cystic breast disease, exposure to radiation, age (increased risk after age 60), and possibly postmenopausal **estrogen** therapy.

Once a lump has been discovered in the female breast and has been palpated (felt) by the physician, a mammogram is ordered to confirm the presence of a suspicious mass. This is usually followed with a biopsy of the lump to confirm the diagnosis.

Most women with early-stage breast cancer are successfully treated. Treatment involves surgical removal of the lump and any diseased tissue surrounding it. If the lump is detected in the early stage of the disease, a **lumpectomy** may be the only surgery necessary. This involves removal of only the tumor and the immediate adjacent breast tissue. Other treatment options include a simple **mastectomy**, in which only the breast is removed; a modified radical **mastectomy**, in which the breast and the lymph nodes in the axilla (armpit) are removed; and a radical **mastectomy**, in which the breast, the chest muscles on the affected side, and the lymph nodes in the axilla are removed. Surgery is usually followed by a series of radiation treatments (radiation therapy), by chemotherapy, or sometimes by both.

Some women opt to have reconstructive breast surgery following a **mastectomy**. The types of material used to reconstruct the breast include implants and tissue transplanted from one part of the patient's body (such as the hips or thighs) to the breast. Patients considering breast reconstruction should discuss this thoroughly with the physician to ensure their understanding of breast reconstruction.

Women should be encouraged to perform breast self-examinations monthly, to have yearly physical examinations by their physicians, to have a baseline mammogram done at age 35, and to have mammograms as recommended by their physician. The procedure for **breast self-examination** appears in the section on diagnostic techniques.

cervical carcinoma (**SER**-vih-kal **kar**-sih-**NOH**-mah) cervic/o = cervix -al = pertaining to carcin/o = cancer -oma = tumor	A malignant tumor of the **cervix**. Cervical cancer is one of the most common malignancies of the female reproductive tract. Symptoms include an abnormal **Pap smear** and bleeding between menstrual periods, after sexual intercourse, or after **menopause**.

Cervical cancer appears to be most frequent in women aged 30 to 50. Factors that increase the risk of developing cervical cancer at a later age including the following:

1. First sexual intercourse before the age of 20

2. Having many sex partners

3. Having certain sexually transmitted diseases

4. History of smoking

In the earliest stage of cervical cancer, the cancer remains in place without spreading. This early stage is known as carcinoma in situ; that is, "it just sits there." The progression into a more advanced stage that can metastasize to other parts of the body is usually slow. This particular quality of cervical cancer makes the prognosis excellent if the disease is detected in its earliest stage.

The **Papanicolaou smear** (**Pap smear**) is used to detect early changes in the cervical tissue that may indicate cervical cancer. The Pap test consists of obtaining scrapings from the **cervix** and examining them under a microscope to detect any abnormalities in cervical tissue. Approximately 90% of the early changes in the cervical tissue are detected by this test. The diagnosis of cervical cancer is confirmed with a tissue biopsy.

Treatment for cervical cancer includes surgery to remove the diseased tissue and a margin of healthy tissue. This may involve removing the **cervix** or may be more extensive, involving removal of the **uterus**, **fallopian tubes**, and ovaries as well. Surgery may be followed with radiation therapy.

Studies now indicate that the human papilloma virus (HPV) has a strong correlation to risk for cervical cancer. The HPV is passed from one person to another through sexual contact. There are many types of HPVs. Some cause no harm, some cause genital warts, and others are associated with certain types of cancer ("high-risk" HPVs). When a woman becomes infected with certain high-risk types of HPV and the infection is not cleared by the body, abnormal cells can develop in the lining of the **cervix**. If this is not detected early and treated properly, the abnormal cells can lead to precancerous conditions and possibly to cancer. Most women are diagnosed with HPV as a result of an abnormal **Pap smear**.

The U.S. Food and Drug Administration (FDA) has approved a vaccine that is highly effective in preventing infections from two high-risk HPVs that cause approximately 70% of cervical cancers and two HPVs that cause approximately 90% of genital warts. This vaccine is given in three separate doses by injection over the course of six months. The vaccine, Gardasil, is recommended for 11- to 12-year-old girls (ideally before sexual activity begins) and can be given as early as 9 years of age through 26 years of age. Licensing the vaccine for use in women older than 26 (and possibly men) is being studied.

cervicitis
 	
(ser-vih-**SIGH**-tis)
  cervic/o = cervix
  -itis = inflammation
	An acute or chronic inflammation of the uterine **cervix**.

Symptoms may include a thick, foul-smelling vaginal discharge, pelvic pressure or pain, scant bleeding after sexual intercourse, and itching or burning of the external genitalia. Upon examination, the **cervix** will appear red and swollen. Bleeding may occur on contact.

Cervicitis is usually caused by the following microorganisms: *Trichomonas vaginalis, Candida albicans, Haemophilus vaginalis,* or *Chlamydia trachomatis.* Diagnosis is confirmed by a **Pap smear** culture of the area. A biopsy may be taken to rule out the possibility of cervical cancer. Once the causative organism is identified, medication specific to the organism is prescribed.

Cervicitis can also cause cervical erosion. Upon visual examination of the **cervix**, the cervical mucosa appears "raw" (ulcerated), with red patches on the mucosa. This abrasion, or ulceration, of the **cervix** is caused by irritation from the infection. It can also be a result of trauma, such as childbirth.

Symptoms of cervical erosion include a white or yellowish mucus discharge from the **vagina**. This is known as leukorrhea.

Once the diagnosis of cervical erosion is confirmed by **Pap smear** and tissue biopsy, the treatment of choice is **cryosurgery** or cryocautery. Each procedure involves freezing the eroded tissue. Antibiotic therapy may follow.

cystocele
 	
(**SIS**-toh-seel)
  cyst/o = bladder, sac, or cyst
  -cele = swelling or herniation
	Herniation or downward protrusion of the urinary bladder through the wall of the **vagina**. See *Figure 17-8.*

This condition develops over a period of years as a result of weakening of the anterior wall of the **vagina**, often after the woman has given birth to several babies. The weakened anterior wall of the **vagina** can no longer support the weight of the urine in the bladder, and thus the bladder protrudes downward into the **vagina**. Complete emptying of the bladder becomes a problem because the **cystocele** sags below the neck of the bladder when it protrudes into the **vagina**. Cystitis may also become a problem as a result of the incomplete emptying of the bladder.

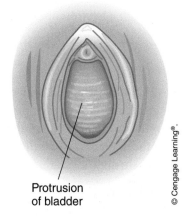

Protrusion
of bladder

© Cengage Learning®.

Figure 17-8 Cystocele

endometrial carcinoma (en-doh-**MEE**-tree-al **kar**-sih-**NOH**-mah) endo- = within metri/o = uterus -al = pertaining to carcin/o = cancer -oma = tumor	Malignant tumor of the inner lining of the **uterus**; also known as adenocarcinoma of the **uterus**.

This is the most common cancer of the female reproductive tract, occurring in women during or after **menopause** (peak incidence between the ages of 50 and 60).

The classic symptom of endometrial cancer is abnormal uterine bleeding. This includes any postmenopausal bleeding, recurrent **metrorrhagia**, or postcoital bleeding with **metrorrhagia** in the premenopausal patient. An abnormal discharge (mucoid or watery discharge) may precede the bleeding by weeks or months.

Diagnosis is usually confirmed with an **endometrial biopsy**, or **dilation and curettage** with microscopic examination of the tissue sample. Dilation involves enlarging the cervical opening, and curettage involves scraping tissue cells from the uterine lining for sampling.

Treatment involves a total abdominal **hysterectomy** (removal of the **uterus**, **fallopian tubes**, and ovaries), followed by radiation. A total abdominal **hysterectomy** (TAH) is also referred to as a complete **hysterectomy**.

endometriosis (en-doh-**mee**-tree-**OH**-sis) endo- = within metri/o = uterus -osis = condition	The presence and growth of endometrial tissue in areas outside the **endometrium** (lining of the **uterus**). See *Figure 17-9.*

The ectopic (out of place) endometrial tissue is generally found within the abdominal cavity. It may be found in the wall of the **uterus** or on its surface, in the peritoneum of the pelvis, on the small intestine, in or on the **fallopian tubes** and ovaries, on the surface of the bladder and in the bladder.

Symptoms of **endometriosis** include **dysmenorrhea** with constant pain and discomfort in the lower abdomen, back, and **vagina**. The pain may begin before **menstruation** and continue for several days after the end of **menstruation**. The woman with **endometriosis** may also experience heavy menstrual periods and pelvic pain during sexual intercourse. The pain and discomfort are due to the buildup of scar tissue and adhesions resulting from the endometrial tissue thickening and bleeding in unnatural places.

Diagnosis of **endometriosis** is usually confirmed by visualization of the endometrial deposits in the abdominal cavity through a laparoscope.

The physician may also note areas of tenderness within the pelvis while performing a bimanual examination.

There is no known cure for **endometriosis** other than the removal of the **uterus**, **fallopian tubes**, and ovaries. Treatment, therefore, is symptomatic, based on the severity of the condition, and can range from regular monitoring of the condition, to analgesics for mild pain and discomfort, to hormonal therapy (use of birth control pills) to shrink the endometrial tissue for those experiencing severe pain.

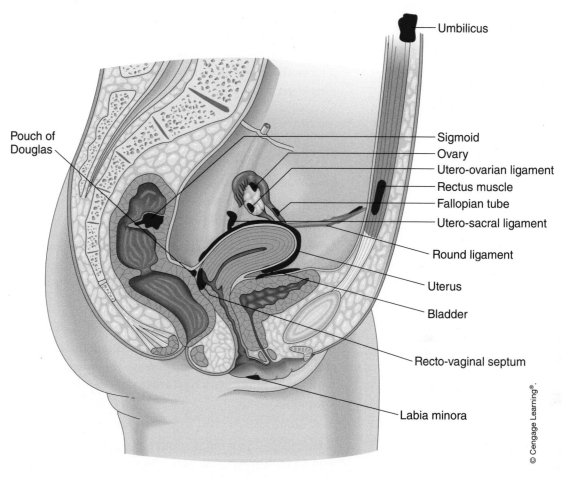

Umbilicus

Pouch of
Douglas

Sigmoid
Ovary
Utero-ovarian ligament
Rectus muscle
Fallopian tube
Utero-sacral ligament
Round ligament
Uterus
Bladder
Recto-vaginal septum
Labia minora

© Cengage Learning®.

Figure 17-9 Common sites of endometriosis

fibrocystic breast disease
 	
(figh-broh-**SIS**-tik)
 	
  fibr/o = fiber
  cyst/o = bladder, sac, or cyst
  -ic = pertaining to
	The presence of single or multiple fluid-filled cysts that are palpable in the breasts.

	The cysts are benign (not malignant) and they fluctuate in size with the menstrual period, becoming tender just before **menstruation**. Often, the woman will not experience any symptoms but will seek medical attention after she discovers a lump in her breast. Diagnosis is confirmed with a biopsy of the cyst, especially for deeper cysts that are indistinguishable by palpation from carcinoma. **Mammography** (coupled with the patient's symptoms of pain, fluctuation in size of the cysts, and lumpiness in the breast) is helpful but not conclusive. Treatment for **fibrocystic breast disease** includes use of a good support bra to lessen the pain, restriction of caffeine in the diet, and use of mild analgesics. Monthly breast self-examinations are advised because the cysts may continue to recur until **menopause**, after which time they will subside.

fibroid tumor
 	
(**FIGH**-broyd tumor)
  fibr/o = fiber
  -oid = resembling
	A benign, fibrous tumor of the **uterus**.

	This is one of the most common types of benign tumors of the female reproductive system. Fibroid tumors vary in number, size, and location within the **uterus**, occurring only in premenopausal women.

Symptoms range from none to pelvic pain and pressure accompanied by **menorrhagia** or **metrorrhagia**. Patient history and ultrasonography are used to confirm the diagnosis. Treatment usually ranges from surgery to remove the tumors to a **hysterectomy**, depending on the severity of the symptoms.

leiomyoma (**ligh**-oh-my-**OH**-mah) lei/o = smooth my/o = muscle -oma = tumor	A benign, smooth-muscle tumor of the **uterus**. Uterine leiomyomas are often mislabeled as **fibroid tumors**, when in fact they are not.

Leiomyomas do, however, present the same type of symptoms and are treated in the same manner as fibroid tumors. This may account for the interchangeable terminology.

Leiomyomas and fibroid tumors are the most common types of benign tumors of the female reproductive system. Leiomyomas also vary in number, size, and location within the **uterus** occurring only in premenopausal women.

Symptoms range from none to pelvic pain and pressure accompanied by **menorrhagia** or **metrorrhagia**. Patient history and ultrasonography are used to confirm the diagnosis. Treatment ranges from surgery to remove the tumors to a **hysterectomy**, depending on the severity of the symptoms.

ovarian carcinoma (oh-**VAIR**-ree-an **kar**-sih-**NOH**-mah) ovari/o = ovary -an = characteristic of carcin/o = cancer -oma = tumor	A malignant tumor of the ovaries, most commonly occurring in women in their 50s. It is rarely detected in the early stage and is usually far advanced when diagnosed.

Symptoms usually do not appear with ovarian cancer until the disease is well advanced. The earliest symptoms of ovarian cancer are swelling, bloating, or discomfort in the lower abdomen, and mild digestive complaints (loss of appetite, feeling of fullness, indigestion, nausea, and weight loss). As the tumor increases in size, it may create pressure on adjacent organs, such as the urinary bladder or the rectum, causing frequent urination and dysuria or constipation. Later developments in the course of the disease include an accumulation of fluid within the abdominal cavity (ascites), resulting in swelling and discomfort.

Diagnosis is confirmed with examination of a sample of the tumor tissue under a microscope. This is achieved through surgical removal of the affected **ovary**. If the **ovary** is diseased with cancer, the surgeon will then remove the other **ovary**, the **uterus**, and the **fallopian tubes**. A process called staging is important to determine the amount of metastasis, if any.

This process involves taking samples (biopsy) of nearby lymph nodes and the **diaphragm** and sampling the fluid from the abdomen.

Treatment involves the use of surgery, chemotherapy, or radiation therapy. It may involve one or a combination of the treatment choices, depending on the extent of the disease.

ovarian cysts
 	
(oh-**VAIR**-ree-an **SISTS**)
  ovari/o = ovary
  -an = characteristic of
	Benign, globular sacs (cysts) that form on or near the ovaries. These cysts may be fluid filled or may contain semisolid material.

An ovarian cyst may develop from an unruptured **graafian follicle** (follicular cyst), or it may develop when the **corpus luteum** fails to regress, becoming cystic (lutein cyst). Symptoms vary but may include the following: painless swelling in the lower abdomen that feels firm to touch; pain during sexual intercourse; pelvic pain; low back pain; and an acute, colicky abdominal pain.

A pelvic examination will usually detect an ovarian cyst. In some cases, however, a **pelvic ultrasound** is necessary to verify the ovarian cyst. Most **ovarian cysts** will disappear by themselves. If the cyst does not disappear within a few months, **laparoscopy** with direct visualization may be necessary to rule out the possibility of other causes, such as malignancy. The cyst may be removed surgically for biopsy.

pelvic inflammatory disease (PID)
 	
(**PELL**-vik in-**FLAM**-mah-toh-ree dih-**ZEEZ**)
salpingitis
(sal-pin-**JYE**-tis)
  salping/o = eustachian tubes; also
                  refers to fallopian tubes
  -itis = inflammation
	Infection of the **fallopian tubes**; also known as **salpingitis**.

PID occurs predominantly in women under the age of 35 who are sexually active. The most frequent causative organisms of **pelvic inflammatory disease** are *Chlamydia trachomatis* and *Neisseria gonorrhoeae*; both are sexually transmitted. There is also a higher incidence of PID in women who use IUDs (**intrauterine devices** used as a means of birth control). Current data indicates that some women may have a slightly increased risk of PID within the first few weeks only, after insertion of an IUD. That risk is reduced if fluid or tissue from the vaginal and cervical area is checked for possible infection prior to insertion of the IUD. **Pelvic inflammatory disease** begins with a cervical infection that spreads by surface invasion along the uterine lining (**endometrium**) and then out to the **fallopian tubes** and ovaries.

Symptoms of acute PID include fever, chills, malaise, abdomen tender to touch with sudden release (rebound), backache, and a foul-smelling vaginal discharge. As with any active infection, the white blood cell count will be elevated.

Diagnosis is confirmed by obtaining a specimen of the uterine secretions for culture and sensitivity. Once the causative organism is isolated, an antibiotic that is specific in action to the particular bacteria can be prescribed. Medications to relieve pain (analgesics) and bed rest are also prescribed. Early treatment is necessary to prevent complications, such as peritonitis, from the spread of the inflammation throughout the abdominal cavity. PID is a major cause of infertility in women.

stress incontinence, urinary (**STRESS** in-**CON**-tin-ens, **YOO**-rih-**nair**-ee)	The inability to hold urine when the bladder is stressed by sneezing, coughing, laughing, or lifting.

As women age, they may develop a decrease in urethral muscle support and experience decreased bladder sphincter control. This may also result from having had several babies. The involuntary loss of urine occurs when the sneezing, coughing, laughing, or lifting activities increase intra-abdominal pressure. The female is unable to tighten the urethra sufficiently to overcome the pressure placed on the bladder, and leakage of urine results.

Treatment may include teaching exercises to strengthen perineal muscle tone and minimize urinary leakage, use of perineal pads to absorb urine leakage, and reducing intake of caffeine to reduce urinary frequency. Medications may be prescribed to increase the resistance of the urethra. Surgery is usually a treatment of last resort.

vaginitis
(vaj-in-**EYE**-tis)
  vagin/o = vagina
  -itis = inflammation
	Inflammation of the **vagina** and the **vulva**.

This is a common disease that affects women when there is a disturbance in the normal flora or pH of the **vagina** that allows microorganisms to flourish. The three most common types of **vaginitis** are candidiasis, trichomoniasis, and bacterial vaginosis. While yeast infections are the most commonly discussed vaginal infections, bacterial vaginosis is actually the most common form of vaginitis in women of reproductive age.

1. Candidiasis is also known as moniliasis or as a yeast (fungal) infection. It is the most common form of **vaginitis**. It occurs when the normal vaginal flora and pH (environment) are disturbed and the conditions are right for accelerated growth of the causative organism, *Candida albicans*, commonly found on the skin and in the digestive tract. The use of certain antibiotics, diabetes, an impaired immune system, or **pregnancy** can cause a change in the environment of the **vagina** that promotes the growth of *Candida albicans*.

   Symptoms of candidiasis include itching and burning of the vagina and vulva, and soreness of the area. The discharge has a typical "cottage cheese" appearance and has no odor, and the vulvar and vaginal walls have a red, inflamed appearance. Diagnosis is confirmed with visual inspection through pelvic examination and microscopic examination of a wet mount of the vaginal secretions.

   Treatment consists of applications of vaginal creams designed to destroy yeast/fungal infections. These medications can now be purchased without a prescription. The female should seek medical attention if the symptoms do not disappear after treatment with a vaginal cream. If the discharge is yellow or green and has a bad odor, it may be indicative of another causative microorganism and will require medical attention.

2. Trichomoniasis is caused by the *Trichomonas vaginalis* protozoan, which thrives in an alkaline environment and is usually transmitted by sexual intercourse. In some cases, infection can be introduced through fecal material due to improper wiping after elimination.

   Symptoms include a greenish-yellow vaginal discharge that has a bad odor. Itching, swelling, and redness of the **vulva** are usually present. Diagnosis for trichomoniasis is confirmed by microscopic examination of the vaginal secretions by wet mount preparation.

   Treatment includes the use of an antibacterial/antiprotozoal medication. It is advisable to treat the female's sex partner to prevent reinfection because men often harbor the protozoan without symptoms.

3. Bacterial vaginosis (or Gardnerella **vaginitis**) is caused by the bacillus, *Gardnerella vaginalis*, which normally inhabits the **vagina**. It is not clear what causes the conditions that set the stage for the overgrowth of bacteria that occurs with bacterial vaginosis, but it does produce an extremely contagious **vaginitis**.

The main symptom is an increased vaginal discharge, which is usually thin, watery, and a grayish white or yellow color. The discharge usually has a strong fishy odor, which may be more noticeable after sexual intercourse. Redness and itching of the **vulva** are much more typical with yeast infections; however, itching, irritation, and burning may also be present with bacterial vaginosis. Diagnosis is confirmed by microscopic examination of the vaginal secretions by a saline wet mount preparation.

Treatment includes the use of antibiotics or antibacterial medications. Usually there is no need to treat the female's sex partner. If the woman has repeated infections, treatment may be extended over the course of a few months.

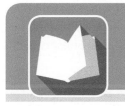

Review Checkpoint

Check your understanding of this section by completing the **Pathological Conditions** exercises in your workbook.

Diagnostic Techniques, Treatments, and Procedures

aspiration biopsy (as-pih-**RAY**-shun **BYE**-op-see)	An invasive procedure in which a needle is inserted into an area of the body, such as the breast, to withdraw a tissue or fluid sample for microscopic examination and diagnosis.

Aspiration biopsy is usually performed using a local anesthetic. After the area is anesthetized, a fine needle is inserted into the site to be aspirated. Suction is applied by pulling the plunger of the syringe back until the sample of fluid or tissue is drawn up into the syringe through the needle. The sample is then affixed to a slide and sent to the laboratory for diagnosis.

breast self-examination (BSE)	A procedure in which the woman examines her breasts and surrounding tissue for evidence of any changes that could indicate the possibility of malignancy.

By the age of 20, women should perform the breast self-examination every month. The best time for breast self- examination (BSE) is a few days after the end of the menstrual period. At this time of the month, the breasts are usually their softest, making the examination easier. Furthermore, women who are familiar with their own normal breast characteristics can notice the development of any abnormalities at an earlier point. They should also be taught the importance of breast self-examinations on a monthly basis and should understand that early detection, if a malignancy is found, increases the survival rate significantly. Women who are post-menopausal or post-hysterectomy should try to do the breast self-examination approximately the same time each month, for example, on the first day of the month.

A good time of day to perform a breast self-examination is just before taking a shower. The breast self-examination consists of inspecting and palpating both breasts in a consistent pattern to detect any abnormalities or lumps. If any abnormalities are detected, they should be reported to a physician immediately. The steps for breast self-examination follow. See *Figure 17-10*.

1. The woman should stand before a mirror to observe the appearance of her breasts. She should check both breasts for any abnormalities, that is, dimpling or puckering of the nipples, unusual scaling of the skin of the breasts, or any unusual discharge from the nipples. She should then observe the breasts for similarity in contour and shape by placing her hands on her hips and tightening her chest muscles as she observes the shape of her breasts. See *Figure 17-10A* and *B*.

2. The female should check the nipples for discharge by squeezing each nipple to see if discharge is present. See *Figure 17-10C*.

3. The female should palpate each breast for the presence of lumps, in an orderly pattern. Beginning at the armpit of the left breast, she should use three fingers of the right hand and firmly press a section at a time, in a circular motion. Continuing to press in the circular motion, she should move clockwise around the breast, progressing toward the nipple of the breast with each round. The same process should be repeated with the right breast, palpating with the fingers of the left hand. See *Figure 17-10D*.

4. The process of checking the breasts for lumps in a clockwise pattern and checking the nipples for discharge should now be performed while in the shower. The soap on the skin allows the fingers to glide more smoothly over the breasts. Check each breast in the careful manner previously described.

5. Following the shower or perhaps before the shower, the female should check both breasts while lying down. She should lie flat on her back, with her left arm over her head and a small pillow or folded towel under her left shoulder. This will flatten the breast, making it easier to examine. Using the same clockwise pattern and the same circular motion, she should examine her left breast carefully with the flat part of the fingers of her right hand. This process should be repeated with the right breast (using the left hand). See *Figure 17-10E*.

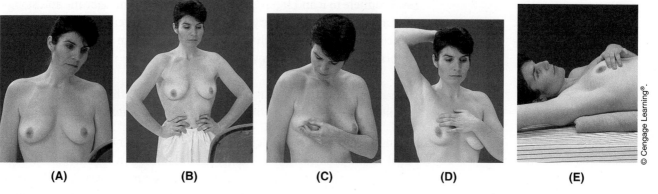

(A)   (B)   (C)   (D)   (E)

© Cengage Learning®.

Figure 17-10 Breast self-examination

colposcopy	Visual examination of the **vagina** and **cervix** with a colposcope.

(kol-**POSS**-koh-pee)
   colp/o = vagina
   -scopy = process of viewing

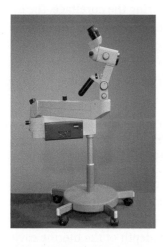

A colposcope is a lighted binocular microscope for direct examination of the surfaces of the **vagina** and **cervix**. The lenses of the microscope magnify the vaginal and cervical tissue for better viewing. See *Figure 17-11*. A **colposcopy** is advised for all women who have Pap smears showing dysplasia (abnormal cells).

After insertion of a speculum into the **vagina** and visualization of the **cervix**, the tissue is prepped by application of a 5% acetic acid (common household vinegar) solution. The solution is used to remove mucus and debris from the area and to slightly dehydrate the cells on the **cervix**, improving visibility of the cervical tissue. The physician observes the **cervix** and **vagina** with the colposcope, searching for any suspicious lesions. If a suspicious lesion or tissue is noted during the examination, a biopsy of the tissue will be obtained at that time.

Figure 17-11 Colposcope 150 EC
(Courtesy of Carl Zeiss Surgical, Inc.)

cone biopsy	Surgical removal of a cone-shaped segment of the **cervix** for diagnosis or treatment; also known as a **conization**.

(**KOHN BY**-op-see)

A **cone biopsy** (**conization**) may be ordered when a lesion is in the inner lining of the cervical canal (endocervix) or when a **Pap smear** shows abnormal cells in the **cervix**. A cone-shaped segment is removed from the **cervix** that contains the lesion or abnormal tissue, along with a margin of healthy tissue. The patient should be observed for any unusual bleeding following a cone biopsy. The patient should be instructed to not have sexual intercourse or participate in active sports for four to six weeks after the biopsy, to allow for adequate healing of the **cervix**.

cryosurgery	The destruction of tissue by rapid freezing with substances such as liquid nitrogen.

(**cry**-oh-**SER**-jer-ee)
   cry/o = cold

The coolant is circulated through a metal probe, chilling it to subfreezing temperatures. When the cold metal probe touches the tissues, the moist tissues adhere to it and freeze. The tissues then become necrotic and slough off in a few days. **Cryosurgery** can be used for treatment of abnormal tissue of the **cervix**. It is frequently used to remove benign and malignant skin tumors and growths such as warts.

culdocentesis (kull-doh-sen-**TEE**-sis) culd/o = cul-de-sac -centesis = surgical puncture	The surgical puncture through the posterior wall of the **vagina** into the **cul-de-sac** to withdraw intraperitoneal fluid for examination.

During a **culdocentesis**, a culdoscope is inserted into the **cul-de-sac** to visualize the area for any evidence of inflammation, purulent drainage, bleeding, **ovarian** cysts, ectopic **pregnancy**, or ovarian malignancy. A needle is then inserted into the **cul-de-sac** through the scope, and fluid is aspirated for examination.

dilation and curettage (dye-**LAY**-shun and **koo**-reh-**TAHZ**)	Dilation or widening of the cervical canal with a dilator, followed by scraping of the uterine lining with a curet; also termed D&C. See *Figure 17-12A*.

During the dilation, the **cervix** is expanded with a series of probes (increasing in diameter with each insertion). During the curettage, the lining of the uterine cavity is scraped with the cutting edge of a spoon-shaped metal loop (curet, *Figure 17-12B*) for the purpose of diagnosing uterine disease, correcting heavy or prolonged uterine bleeding, or emptying the uterine contents. The patient should be observed for excessive bleeding within the first few hours after this procedure.

endometrial biopsy (en-doh-**MEE**-tree-al **BYE**-op-see) endo- = within metri/o = uterus -al = pertaining to	**Endometrial biopsy** is an invasive test for obtaining a sample of endometrial tissue (with a small curet) for examination.

The endometrial tissue may be analyzed in cases of irregular bleeding, during infertility studies, and to examine tissue for possible endometrial cancer. During the procedure, the **cervix** is dilated and an instrument (uterine sound) is passed into the **uterus** to measure the depth of the uterine cavity

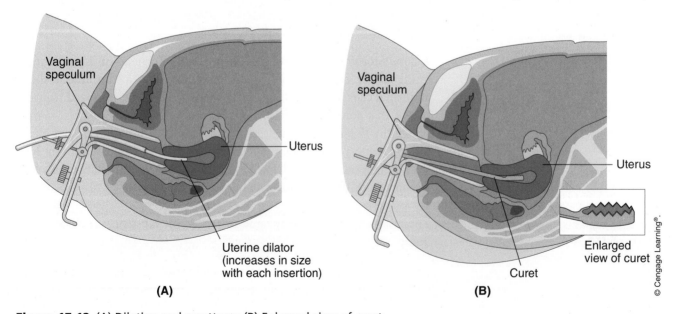

Figure 17-12 (A) Dilation and curettage; (B) Enlarged view of curet

© Cengage Learning®.

(measures from the cervical os to the uterine **fundus**). A curet, or aspiration needle, is then inserted into the **fundus** of the **uterus** and a sample of endometrial tissue is extracted.

The patient will experience a "pinching" sensation during the procedure, followed by a short period of cramping after the procedure. This should be relieved by mild analgesics (pain relievers). The patient should experience only light bleeding following the procedure but should be instructed to report any heavy bleeding.

hysterosalpingography	X-ray of the **uterus** and the **fallopian tubes** by injecting a contrast material into these structures.

(**hiss**-ter-oh-**sal**-pin-**GOG**-rah-fee)
   hyster/o = uterus
   salping/o = eustachian tubes; also
                    refers to fallopian tubes
   -graphy = process of recording

The contrast medium is injected through a cannula inserted into the **cervix**. As the material is slowly injected, the filling of the **uterus** and **fallopian tubes** is observed with a fluoroscope. **Hysterosalpingography** is performed to evaluate the **uterus** for any abnormalities in structure or the presence of possible tumors and to test for tubal obstructions. The patient may feel occasional menstrual-type cramping during the procedure and will have vaginal drainage for a couple of days after the procedure (from the drainage of the contrast material).

laparoscopy	The process of viewing the abdominal cavity with a laparoscope (a thin-walled flexible tube with a telescopic lens and light).

(lap-ar-**OS**-koh-pee)
   lapar/o = abdominal wall
   -scopy = process of viewing

A small incision is made into the abdominal wall near the umbilicus (navel) and the laparoscope is inserted. This procedure is used to visualize abdominal and pelvic organs. See *Figure 17-13*.

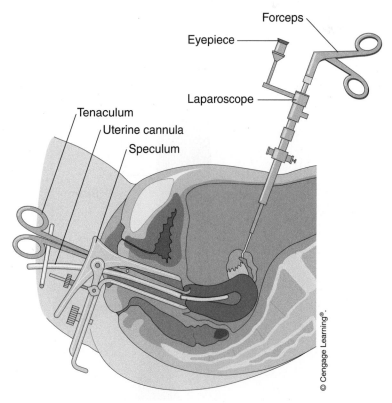

© Cengage Learning®.

Figure 17-13 Laparoscopy

The reasons for performing a **laparoscopy** include but are not limited to diagnosing unexplained pelvic or abdominal pain, confirming or ruling out suspected cases of tubal **pregnancy** or **endometriosis**, visualizing and assessing the female reproductive organs during various infertility studies, and performing therapeutic procedures such as **tubal ligations** and other types of minor surgery.

loop electrosurgical excision procedure (LEEP)	A procedure used to remove abnormal cells from the surface of the **cervix** using a thin wire loop that acts like a scalpel. A painless electrical current passes through the loop as it cuts away a thin layer of surface cells from the **cervix**.

The loop is inserted through the **vagina** to the **cervix**. A solution is applied to the **cervix** to reveal the abnormal cells, and the **cervix** will be numbed with a local anesthetic for the procedure. The tissue specimen is sent to a lab for evaluation and confirmation of a diagnosis.

The LEEP is an effective and simple way to treat cervical dysplasia. This in-office procedure can be completed in just a few minutes.

mammography
(mam-**OG**-rah-fee)
  mamm/o = breasts
  -graphy = process of recording
	The process of examining with X-ray the soft tissue of the breast to detect various benign and/or malignant growths before they can be felt. See *Figure 17-14*.

The American College of Radiology recognizes the use of X-ray **mammography** as the approved method of screening for breast cancer. This procedure takes approximately 15 to 30 minutes to complete and can be performed in an X-ray department of a hospital or in a private radiology facility. Each facility should have equipment designed and used exclusively for mammograms.

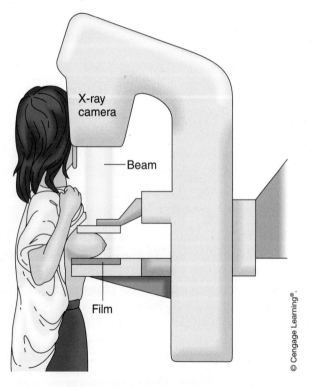

© Cengage Learning®.

Figure 17-14 Mammography

During the examination, the breast tissue is compressed between two clear disks for each X-ray view. The first view requires compressing the breast from top to bottom to take a top-to-bottom (craniocaudal) view.

The second view requires compressing the breast from side to side to take a mediolateral view. The patient may experience fleeting discomfort as the breast tissue is compressed between the plates, but this is necessary to facilitate maximum visualization of the breast tissue.

The American Cancer Society recommends that women have their first mammogram between ages 35 and 39. This will provide a baseline for reference with future mammograms. Between ages 40 and 49, mammograms are usually recommended every two years unless the woman is in a high-risk category. From age 50 and thereafter, mammograms are recommended annually.

| **Papanicolaou (Pap) smear** | A diagnostic test for cervical cancer; that is, a microscopic examination of cells scraped from within the **cervix** (endocervix), from around the **cervix** (ectocervix), and from the posterior part of the **vagina** (near the **cervix**) to test for cervical cancer; also called Pap test. |

(pap-ah-**NIK**-oh-low smear)

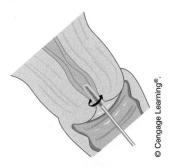

Figure 17-15 Endocervical smear

As part of the annual gynecological examination, the **Pap smear** consists of obtaining a small amount of secretions taken from the endocervix (see *Figure 17-15*) and from the posterior vaginal area (nearest the **cervix**). The health care professional will obtain the samples with a wooden or plastic scraper and a cervical brush.

In a conventional Pap test, the secretions are smeared onto separate clean microscope slides and "set" with a spray fixative. The slides are marked for their source as either "C" for cervical or "V" for vaginal. In an automated liquid-based Pap test, the cervical cells collected with a brush or other instrument are placed in a vial of liquid preservative. In either procedure, the specimens obtained will be sent to a laboratory for analysis.

Patients should be instructed not to douche or tub-bathe for at least 24 hours before a **Pap smear**, because this may cause cellular material to be washed away with the douching solution or the bath water. A lubricant is not used on the speculum for a **Pap smear**, because this can interfere with the accurate reading of the slide. Furthermore, the **Pap smear** should be performed during or close to the middle of the menstrual cycle because the presence of blood interferes with an accurate interpretation of the specimen and may camouflage atypical cells.

The **Pap smear** is up to 95% accurate in diagnosing early cervical cancer when the specimen sample is obtained correctly. When the Pap test is positive, additional tissue studies (that is, biopsy or even surgery) may be performed to confirm the diagnosis of cancer.

The current method of reporting cervical, endocervical, and vaginal cytology (**Pap smear**) specimens is the *Bethesda 2001 System*. The National Cancer Institute recommends use of this system for reporting laboratory findings. The classifications have been simplified from the previous

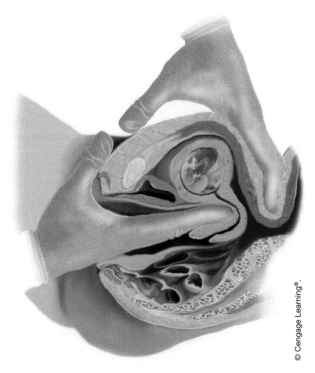

© Cengage Learning®.

Figure 17-16 Bimanual examination

multiple categories to two categories: *Negative for intraepithelial lesion or malignancy* and *Epithelial cell abnormality*. The standardized language used by the Bethesda System allows for more consistent communication among laboratories, clinicians, and patients. The American Cancer Society (ACS) recommends that all women should begin cervical cancer screening (**Pap smear**) and gynecological examination at age 21. They also recommend that women aged 21 to 29 should have a Pap test every three years. Additional guidelines have been introduced regarding the frequency of screening for women with normal results over the age of 30 and for women over the age of 70.

The annual exam will also include palpation of the female internal organs by bimanual examination (see *Figure 17-16*). When palpating the female pelvic organs by bimanual examination, the examiner places one hand on the abdomen and inserts one or two fingers of the other gloved hand into the **vagina**. This allows the examiner to feel the female organs between the two hands.

liquid-based Pap (LBP)	A process of collecting a tissue sample from the endocervix and the exocervix with a sampling device that is placed directly into a liquid fixative instead of being spread onto a glass slide. This process provides immediate fixation and improves specimen adequacy. The LBP is an increasingly popular alternative to conventional cervical cytology smears and has largely replaced the traditional **Pap smear** in the United States. Additionally, the liquid-based Pap test seems to reduce the likelihood of an unsatisfactory specimen.

When submitting the specimen for examination, both the endocervical and exocervical sampling devices are placed in the same container with appropriate fixative solution and are labeled with the patient's name.

pelvic ultrasound	A noninvasive procedure that uses high-frequency sound waves to examine the abdomen and pelvis.

(PELL-vik **ULL**-trah-sound)

pelv/i = pelvis
-ic = pertaining to
ultra- = beyond, excess

The sound waves pass through the abdominal wall from the transducer, which is moved back and forth across the abdomen. When the sound waves bounce from the internal organs in the abdominopelvic region, these waves are converted to electrical impulses eventually recorded on an oscilloscope screen. The oscilloscope transforms the electrical impulses into visual images. A photograph of the images is then taken for further study.

Pelvic ultrasound can be used to locate a pelvic mass, an ectopic **pregnancy**, or an **intrauterine device** as well as to inspect and assess the **uterus**, ovaries, and **fallopian tubes**. Clearer ultrasonic pictures of the pelvic organs can be obtained using **transvaginal ultrasonography**. This procedure produces the same type of picture as abdominal ultrasound but involves the use of a vaginal probe inserted into the **vagina** while the patient is in **lithotomy position**. The probes are encased in a sterile sheath and placed in the transducer before it is inserted into the **vagina**. The sound waves function in the same way as those for the abdominopelvic ultrasound, but the transvaginal ultrasonic image is much clearer.

pelvimetry	The process of measuring the female pelvis, manually or by X-ray, to determine its adequacy for childbearing.

(pell-**VIM**-eh-tree)

pelv/i = pelvis
-metry = the process of measuring

Clinical **pelvimetry** is an estimate of the size of the birth canal by vaginal palpation of bony landmarks in the pelvis and a mathematical estimate of the distance between them. This is performed during the early part of the **pregnancy** and is recorded as "adequate," "borderline," or "inadequate."

X-ray **pelvimetry** is an actual X-ray of the pelvis to determine the dimensions of the bony pelvis of a pregnant woman. It is performed when there is doubt that the head of the fetus can safely pass through the pelvis during the labor process. Measurements are actually made on the X-ray, and the true dimensions of the birth canal and the head of the fetus can be calculated to determine if the proportions are suitable.

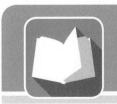

Review Checkpoint

Check your understanding of this section by completing the **Diagnostic Techniques, Treatments, and Procedures** exercises in your workbook.

Sexually Transmitted Diseases (Male and Female)

Sexually transmitted diseases (STDs) in the female are the same as those in the male. These contagious diseases are spread from one person to another through contact with body fluids such as blood, semen, and vaginal secretions. STDs may be spread during vaginal, anal, or oral sex or by direct contact with infected skin.

AIDS, a sexually transmitted disease, can also be transmitted through blood and blood products, sharing of needles (as in intravenous drug users), through the placenta of an infected mother to the baby (during the birth process), and through the breast milk of an infected mother to the baby (when nursing the baby). The incidence of STDs is alarmingly high in the United States. It has greatly increased in recent years, especially among young people. Discussion of the more common STDs can be found in Chapter 16.

COMMON ABBREVIATIONS

Abbreviation	Meaning	Abbreviation	Meaning
AB	abortion	LBP	**liquid-based Pap**
ACS	American Cancer Society	LEEP	**loop electrosurgical excision procedure**
BSE	breast self-examination		
CIS	carcinoma in situ	LH	luteinizing hormone
Cx	cervix	LMP	last menstrual period
D&C	**dilation and curettage**	LSO	left salpingo-oophorectomy
ECC	endocervical curettage	Pap	**Papanicolaou smear**
EMB	**endometrial biopsy**	Path	pathology
ERT	estrogen replacement therapy	PID	pelvic inflammatory disease
GYN	**gynecology**	PMS	**premenstrual syndrome**
HSG	**hysterosalpingography**	RSO	right salpingo-oophorectomy
HPV	human papilloma virus	TAH	total abdominal hysterectomy
IUD	intrauterine device; a particular type of contraceptive device	TVH	total vaginal hysterectomy

Review Checkpoint

Check your understanding of this section by completing the **Common Abbreviations** exercises in your workbook.

WRITTEN AND AUDIO TERMINOLOGY REVIEW

Review each of the following terms from this chapter. Study the spelling of each term and write the definition in the space provided. Check definitions by looking the term up in the glossary.

Term	Pronunciation	Definition
abstinence	☐ **AB**-stih-nens	_____
adnexa	☐ add-**NEK**-sah	_____
amenorrhea	☐ **ah**-men-oh-**REE**-ah	_____
andropause	☐ **AN**-droh-pawz	_____
anteflexion	☐ **an**-tee-**FLEK**-shun	_____
areola	☐ ah-**REE**-oh-lah	_____
aspiration biopsy	**as**-pih-**RAY**-shun	
	☐ **BYE**-op-see	_____
Bartholin's glands	☐ **BAR**-toh-linz glands	_____
cervical dysplasia	☐ **SER**-vih-kal dis-**PLAY**-see-ah	_____
cervicitis	☐ **ser**-vih-**SIGH**-tis	_____
cervix	☐ **SER**-viks	_____
climacteric	☐ kly-**MAK**-ter-ik	_____
clitoris	☐ **KLIT**-oh-ris	_____
coitus	☐ **KOH**-ih-tus	_____
colpodynia	☐ **kol**-poh-**DIN**-ee-ah	_____
colpopexy	☐ **KOL**-poh-**peck**-see	_____
colposcopy	☐ kol-**POSS**-koh-pee	_____
conization	☐ **kon**-ih-**ZAY**-shun	_____
corpus luteum	☐ **KOR**-pus **LOO**-tee-um	_____
cryosurgery	☐ **cry**-oh-**SER**-jer-ee	_____
cul-de-sac	☐ **KULL**-dih-**SAK**	_____
culdocentesis	☐ **kull**-doh-sen-**TEE**-sis	_____
cystocele	☐ **SIS**-toh-seel	_____
Depo-Provera injection	☐ **DEP**-oh proh-**VAIR**-ah injection	_____
diaphragm	☐ **DYE**-ah-fram	_____
dilation and curettage	☐ dye-**LAY**-shun and koo-reh-**TAHZ**	_____
dysmenorrhea	☐ **dis**-men-oh-**REE**-ah	

Term	Pronunciation	Definition
ectopic pregnancy	☐ eck-**TOP**-ick **PREG**-nan-see	_____
endometrial biopsy	☐ **en**-doh-**MEE**-tree-al **BYE**-op-see	_____
endometriosis	☐ **en**-doh-mee-tree-**OH**-sis	_____
endometrium	☐ **en**-doh-**MEE**-tree-um	_____
episiotomy	☐ eh-**piz**-ee-**OT**-oh-mee	_____
estrogen	☐ **ESS**-troh-jen	_____
fallopian tubes	☐ fah-**LOH**-pee-an **TOOBS**	_____
fertilization	☐ **fer**-til-eye-**ZAY**-shun	_____
fibrocystic breast disease	☐ **figh**-broh-**SIS**-tik breast dih-**ZEEZ**	_____
fibroid tumor	☐ **FIGH**-broyd **TOO**-mor	_____
fimbriae	☐ **FIM**-bree-ay	_____
fourchette	☐ foor-**SHET**	_____
fundus	☐ **FUN**-dus	_____
galactorrhea	☐ gah-**lack**-toh-**REE**-ah	_____
gamete	☐ **GAM**-eet	_____
gonads	☐ **GOH**-nads	_____
graafian follicles	☐ **GRAF**-ee-an **FOL**-ik-kulz	_____
gynecologist	☐ **gigh**-neh-**KOL**-oh-jist	_____
gynecology	☐ **gigh**-neh-**KOL**-oh-jee	_____
hymen	☐ **HIGH**-men	_____
hysterectomy	☐ **hiss**-ter-**EK**-toh-mee	_____
hysterosalpingography	☐ **hiss**-ter-oh-sal-pin-**GOG**-rah-fee	_____
incompetent cervix	☐ in-**COMP**-eh-tent **SIR**-viks	_____
intrauterine device	☐ **in**-trah-**YOO**-ter-in device	_____
labia majora	☐ **LAY**-bee-ah mah-**JOR**-ah	_____
labia minora	☐ **LAY**-bee-ah mih-**NOR**-ah	_____
laparoscopy	☐ **lap**-ar-**OS**-koh-pee	_____
leiomyoma	☐ **ligh**-oh-my-**OH**-mah	_____
mammary glands	☐ **MAM**-ah-ree glands	_____
mammography	☐ mam-**OG**-rah-fee	_____
mastectomy	☐ mass-**TEK**-toh-mee	_____
menarche	☐ meh-**NAR**-kee	_____
menometrorrhagia	☐ **men**-oh-**met**-roh-**RAY**-jee-ah	_____
menopause	☐ **MEN**-oh-pawz	_____
menorrhagia	☐ **men**-oh-**RAY**-jee-ah	_____

Term	Pronunciation	Definition
menorrhea	☐ **men**-oh-**REE**-ah	_____
menstruation	☐ **men**-stroo-**AY**-shun	_____
metrorrhagia	☐ **met**-roh-**RAY**-jee-ah	_____
myometrium	☐ **my**-oh-**MEE**-tree-um	_____
nulligravida	☐ null-ih-**GRAV**-ih-dah	_____
nullipara	☐ nuh-**LIP**-ah-rah	_____
oligomenorrhea	☐ **ol**-ih-goh-**men**-oh-**REE**-ah	_____
oogenesis	☐ **oh**-oh-**JEN**-eh-sis	_____
oophoritis	☐ oh-**off**-oh-**RIGH**-tis	_____
oral contraceptives	☐ **ORAL** con-trah-**SEP**-tivz	_____
ovarian cysts	☐ oh-**VAIR**-ree-an **SISTS**	_____
ovariopexy	☐ oh-vair-ree-oh-**PEK**-see	_____
ovariorrhexis	☐ oh-**vay**-ree-oh-**RECK**-sis	_____
ovary	☐ **OH**-vah-ree	_____
ovulation	☐ **ov**-yoo-**LAY**-shun	_____
ovum	☐ **OH**-vum	_____
Pap smear	☐ **PAP** smear	_____
Papanicolaou smear	☐ **pap**-ah-**NIK**-oh-low smear	_____
pelvic inflammatory disease	☐ **PELL**-vik in-**FLAM**-mah-**toh**-ree dih-**ZEEZ**	_____
pelvic ultrasound	☐ **PELL**-vik **ULL**-trah-sound	_____
pelvimetry	☐ pell-**VIM**-eh-tree	_____
perineum	☐ **pair**-ih-**NEE**-um	_____
pregnancy	☐ **PREG**-nan-see	_____
premenstrual syndrome	☐ pre-**MEN**-stroo-al **SIN**-drom	_____
primigravida	☐ **prye**-mih-**GRAV**-ih-dah	_____
primipara	☐ prye-**MIP**-ah-rah	_____
progesterone	☐ proh-**JES**-ter-own	_____
puberty	☐ **PEW**-ber-tee	_____
retroversion	☐ **ret**-roh-**VER**-zhun	_____
salpingitis	☐ sal-pin-**JYE**-tis	_____
tubal ligation	☐ **TOO**-bal lye-**GAY**-shun	_____
uterus	☐ **YOO**-ter-us	_____
vagina	☐ vah-**JEYE**-nah	_____
vaginitis	☐ vaj-in-**EYE**-tis	_____
vulva	☐ **VULL**-vah	_____
vulvovaginitis	☐ **vull**-voh-vaj-in-**EYE**-tis	_____

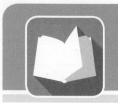

Review Checkpoint

Apply what you have learned in this chapter by completing the **Putting It All Together** exercise in your workbook.

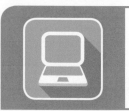

Online Resources

For additional study tools, including PowerPoint® slides and animations, go to the Student Companion Website.

Chapter Review Exercises

The following exercises provide a more in-depth review of the chapter material. Your goal in these exercises is to complete each section at a minimum 80% level of accuracy. If you score below 80% in any area, return to the applicable section in the chapter and read the material again. A space has been provided for your score at the end of each section.

A. Spelling

Circle the correctly spelled term in each pairing of words. Each correct answer is worth 10 points. Record your score in the space provided at the end of the exercise.

1. ministration   menstruation
2. meatus   meatis
3. clitoris   clitorus
4. menarkey   menarche
5. mammogram   mammagram
6. laproscope   laparoscope
7. colposcopy   culposcopy
8. coldocentesis   culdocentesis
9. diaphram   diaphragm
10. graffian follicles   graafian follicles

Number correct _____ × *10 points/correct answer: Your score* _____ %

B. Matching

Match the following terms on the left with the most appropriate definitions on the right. Each correct answer is worth 10 points. Record your score in the space provided at the end of the exercise.

_____ 1. menstrual phase   a. female reproductive organs are fully developed

_____ 2. premenstrual phase   b. absence of menstrual flow

_____ 3. postmenstrual phase   c. days 1 to 5; lasts for approximately 3 to 5 days

_____ 4. ovulatory phase   d. abnormally light or infrequent menstruation

_____ 5. oligomenorrhea

_____ 6. amenorrhea

_____ 7. dysmenorrhea

_____ 8. metrorrhagia

_____ 9. menorrhagia

_____ 10. puberty

e. abnormally long or very heavy menstrual periods

f. graafian follicle ruptures, releasing the mature ovum

g. painful menstruation

h. interval between the menses and ovulation; days 6 to 12

i. days 15 to 28; if pregnancy does not occur, hormone level drops, causing irritability, fluid retention, and breast tenderness

j. uterine bleeding at times other than the menstrual period

***Number correct* _____ × *10 points/correct answer: Your score* _____ %**

C. Crossword Puzzle

Read the clues carefully and complete the puzzle. Each crossword answer is worth 10 points. When you have completed the crossword puzzle, total your points and enter your score in the space provided at the end of the exercise.

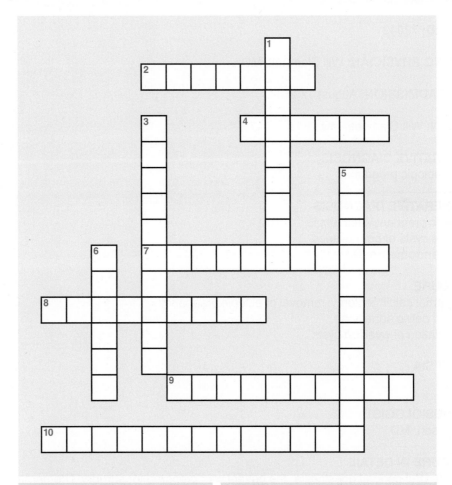

ACROSS

2 cancer, rarely detected early
4 _____ mastectomy; removal of only the breast
7 visual examination of the vagina and cervix with a colposcope
8 bladder protrudes into the vagina
9 inflammation of the uterine cervix
10 uterine lining tissue out of place

DOWN

1 inflammation of the vagina and vulva
3 removal of tumor only and some breast tissue
5 inflammation of the fallopian tubes
6 early-stage cancer; just sits there

***Number correct* _____ × *10 points/correct answer: Your score* _____ %**

D. Proofreading Skills

Read the following excerpt from an operative report. For each boldface term, provide a brief definition in the space provided and indicate if the term is spelled correctly. If it is misspelled, provide the correct spelling. Each correct answer is worth 10 points. Record your score in the space provided at the end of the exercise.

Example:

fimbriated *Having fingerlike projections*

Spelled Correctly? ☑ Yes   ☐ No

OPERATIVE REPORT

Hillcrest
medical center

PATIENT NAME: Luna, Sophia

PATIENT ID: 720431

ADMITTING PHYSICIAN: Will Clampett, MD

DATE OF ADMISSION: August 17, 2014

SURGEON: Will Clampett, MD

PREOPERATIVE DIAGNOSIS
Probable ectopic pregnancy

POSTOPERATIVE DIAGNOSIS
1. **Ectopic** pregnancy, left tubule
2. Multiple cysts of both ovaries
3. Pelvic **endometriosis**

PROCEDURE
1. Left partial salpingectomy; removal of ectopic pregnancy
2. Lysis of pelvic adhesions
3. Coagulation of **ovarion** cysts

ANESTHESIA
General.

ANESTHESIOLOGIST
Jack Johnson, MD

PROCEDURE IN DETAIL
After successful general anesthesia, the patient was prepared for surgery. The pelvic cavity was entered without incident. Upon opening the abdomen, one could see some old dark blood and a modest amount of bright red blood. The **uteris** was held back and downwards, somewhat, by a mass filling the left side of the **col-de-sac** and extending over to the left lateral wall of the **pelvis**. This material was quite friable. The bowel seemed looped about it. Careful dissection freed the mass and brought it into view, revealing a tubal pregnancy in the outer portion of the left tube.

(continued)

OPERATIVE REPORT
Patient Name: Luna, Sophia
Patient ID: 720431
Admitting Physician: Will Clampett, MD
Date of Admission: August 17, 2014
Page 2

The left **ovary** was small but contained multiple tiny **cysks**. The right tube appeared normal with the **fimbriated** ends being open and intact. A partial **salpinjectomy** was carried out on the left side, removing the outer portion of the tube including the ectopic pregnancy.

After suctioning the blood from the cul-de-sac area, it was noted that there were massive adhesions of friable necrotic tissue on the posterior wall of the **fundus** of the uterus.

The area was cleaned up as best as possible and tiny bleeders were coagulated. Fascia and peritoneum were closed together using running continuous interlocking sutures of 0 Vicryl. The skin was closed using a running subcuticular stitch of 3–0 Vicryl on a cutting needle. The wound was dressed, and the patient was taken to the recovery room. She was in good condition postprocedure with IV line in place. Sponge and lap count was reported as correct.

ESTIMATED BLOOD LOSS
Less than 5 mL.

COMPLICATIONS
None.

CONDITION
Stable postoperatively.

_____

Will Clampett, MD

WC:bj

D:8/17/2014

T:8/18/2014

1. **ectopic** _____
   Spelled Correctly? ☐ Yes ☐ No _____

2. **endometriosis** _____
   Spelled Correctly? ☐ Yes ☐ No _____

3. **ovarion** _____
   Spelled Correctly? ☐ Yes ☐ No _____

4. **uteris** _____
   Spelled Correctly? ☐ Yes ☐ No _____

5. **col-de-sac** _____
   Spelled Correctly? ☐ Yes ☐ No _____

6. **pelvis** _____
   Spelled Correctly? ☐ Yes ☐ No _____

(continued)

7. **ovary** _____

Spelled Correctly? ☐ Yes ☐ No _____

8. **cysks** _____

Spelled Correctly? ☐ Yes ☐ No _____

9. **salpinjectomy** _____

Spelled Correctly? ☐ Yes ☐ No _____

10. **fundus** _____

Spelled Correctly? ☐ Yes ☐ No _____

Number correct _____ × *10 points/correct answer: Your score* _____ %

E. Word Search

Read each definition carefully and identify the appropriate word from the list that follows. Enter the word in the space provided; then find it in the puzzle and circle it. The words may be read up, down, diagonally, across, or backward. Each correct answer is worth 10 points. Record your score in the space provided at the end of the exercise.

colposcopy	hysterosalpingography	conization
laparoscopy	culdocentesis	Pap smear
mammography	cryosurgery	pelvimetry
pelvic ultrasound	endometrial biopsy	

```
C O L P O S C O P Y A V E O L A R O S C O H
O R E E N D C M A N B R A D Y E V Y U S Q Y
N A Y C A R C I N O M E T F R I A B L U J S
I V Z O V A R I E N T E S I C P E L M I S T
Z I S I S E T N E C O D L U C I N V A S I E
A B C D E U S C O P I C A P E R Y A I P O R
T R I M E S R Y L T R A P S O U N D Y E A O
I A O M M A N G R U P H A C U L D H E L P S
O I N V A S I X E N T E R I E S P Y A V I A
N D I L A T I O X R S C O T Y A V E N I L L
C R Y O S U R G I N Y U S A R C O N I C U P
A S P I R A T U L V E M C G B I O L O U G I
S A L P Y I N G O S C E O R R H A P H L Y N
T Y P O G R A P I C U M P A R E O L U T E G
A D V E N T T U R E M S Y I N T M R M R L O
M E D I C A W E L A W O R D S W A T I A U G
R I G H E N D O M E T R I A L B I O P S Y R
Y O U R A N S W E I R I S C O R R U J O I A
T E R M I B O L O G V I N T R A U T E U R P
I N T R A V E N L P O L L A T E R O N N M H
C L A S S I F I C B R A E N D O S C O D U Y
P A P I N I (R A E M S P A P) A N I C O L A O
```

Example: A diagnostic test for cervical cancer

Pap smear _____

1. Visual examination of the vagina and cervix with a scope

_____

2. Surgical removal of a cone-shaped segment of the cervix for diagnosis or treatment

_____

3. The destruction of tissue by rapid freezing with substances such as liquid nitrogen

_____

4. The surgical puncture through the posterior wall of the vagina into the cul-de-sac to withdraw intraperitoneal fluid for examination

_____

5. An invasive test for obtaining a sample of endometrial tissue with a small curet for examination

_____

6. The process of X-raying the uterus and the fallopian tubes

_____

7. The process of viewing the abdominal cavity with a thin, flexible tube with a telescopic lens and light

_____

8. The process of X-raying the soft tissue of the breast

_____

9. The process of measuring the female pelvis manually or by X-ray

_____

10. A noninvasive procedure that uses high-frequency waves to examine the abdomen and pelvis

_____

Number correct _____ **× 10 points/correct answer: Your score** _____ **%**

F. Word Element Review

The following words relate to the female reproductive system. The word elements have been labeled (WR = word root, P = prefix, S = suffix, and V = combining vowel). Read the definition carefully and complete the word by filling in the blank, using the word elements provided in this chapter. If you have forgotten the word building rules, see Chapter 1. Each correct word is worth 10 points. Record your score in the space provided at the end of the exercise.

1. Surgical puncture of the amniotic sac:

   _____ / _____ / _____
        WR   V   S

2. Inflammation of the cervix:

   _____ / _____
        WR   S

3. One who specializes in treating diseases/disorders of women:

   _____ / _____ / _____
        WR   V   S

(continued)

4. Surgical removal of the uterus:

_____ / _____

          WR   S

5. Absence of menstrual flow:

_____ / _____ / _____ / _____

          P   WR   V   S

6. Condition of the inner lining of the uterus:

_____ / _____ / _____

          P   WR   S

7. Surgical removal of the breast:

_____ / _____

          WR   S

8. Inflammation of the fallopian tubes:

_____ / _____

          WR   S

9. Beginning of menses; first menstrual period:

_____ / _____

          WR   S

10. Painful menstruation:

_____ / _____ / _____ / _____

          P   WR   V   S

Number correct _____ × *10 points/correct answer: Your score* _____ %

G. Matching Abbreviations

Match the abbreviations on the left with the correct definition on the right. Each correct answer is worth 10 points. Record your score in the space provided at the end of the exercise.

_____ 1. D&C   a. last menstrual period

_____ 2. EMB   b. total abdominal hysterectomy

_____ 3. GYN   c. premenstrual syndrome

_____ 4. IUD   d. carcinoma in situ

_____ 5. Pap   e. dilation and curettage

_____ 6. PID   f. gynecology

_____ 7. PMS   g. Papanicolaou smear

_____ 8. TAH   h. intrauterine device

_____ 9. CIS   i. pelvic inflammatory disease

_____ 10. LMP   j. endometrial biopsy

Number correct _____ × *10 points/correct answer: Your score* _____ %

H. Completion

The following is a discussion of secondary sex characteristic changes experienced by the female during puberty and instructions for breast self-examination. Fill in the blanks with the most appropriate word(s). Each correct answer is worth 10 points. Record your score in the space provided at the end of the exercise.

Puberty is the time during which the female experiences some secondary sex characteristic changes. These changes include the following: changes in the breast, which include (1) _____ and deposition of (2) _____ in the buttocks and thighs, creating a more (3) _____ appearance; widening of the (4) _____, making it more appropriate for childbirth; and growth of (5) _____ and (6) _____ hair. The most evident change during puberty is the onset of menstruation, with the first menstrual period being called the (7) _____. By the time a young woman reaches the age of 20, she should perform the breast self-examination every month about 7 to 10 days after the menstrual period. She should begin the process by standing (8) _____ to observe the appearance of her breasts. As she palpates her breasts for the presence of any lumps, she should press firmly, moving in a circular motion, beginning at the armpit and progressing toward (9) _____. Each breast should be checked in the same manner. After palpating the breasts for lumps, the female should then check her breast while in the (10a*) _____ and while (10b*) _____. *Note*: 10a and 10b count as one answer.

Number correct _____ *× 10 points/correct answer: Your score* _____ *%*

I. Matching

Match the terms on the left with the appropriate descriptions on the right. Each correct answer is worth 10 points. Record your score in the space provided at the end of the exercise.

_____ 1. lumpectomy

_____ 2. simple mastectomy

_____ 3. modified radical mastectomy

_____ 4. radical mastectomy

_____ 5. aspiration biopsy

_____ 6. colposcopy

_____ 7. cryosurgery

_____ 8. mammography

_____ 9. conization

_____ 10. culdocentesis

a. the surgical puncture through the posterior wall of the vagina into the cul-de-sac to withdraw intraperitoneal fluid for examination

b. tissue or fluid sample is withdrawn for microscopic examination and diagnosis

c. visual examination of the vagina and cervix with a colposcope

d. removal of only the tumor and a small margin of breast tissue

e. the process of examining with X-ray the soft tissue of the breast to detect various benign and/or malignant growths before they can be felt

f. removal of the breast, chest muscles, and lymph nodes on the affected side

g. removal of the breast and lymph nodes on the affected side

h. the destruction of tissue by rapid freezing with substances such as liquid nitrogen

i. surgical removal of a cone-shaped segment of the cervix for diagnosis or treatment

j. only the breast is removed

Number correct _____ *× 10 points/correct answer: Your score* _____ *%*

J. Label

Using the following figure, label the internal genitalia of the female reproductive system. Each correct answer is worth 10 points. Record your score in the space provided at the end of the exercise.

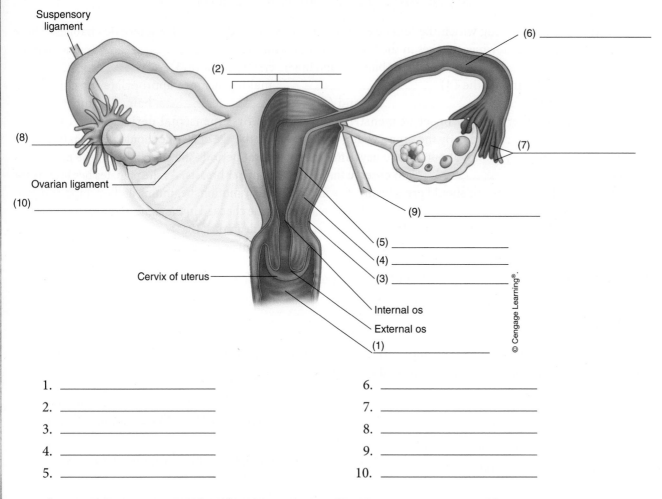

Number correct _____ × **10 points/correct answer: Your score** _____ **%**

K. Medical Scenario

The following medical scenario presents information on one of the pathological conditions discussed in this chapter. Read the scenario carefully and select the most appropriate answer for each question that follows. Each correct answer is worth 20 points. Record your score in the space provided at the end of the exercise.

Selena Bandaro, a 40-year-old patient, is visiting her gynecologist today because she felt a lump in her breast that became painful just before her menstrual period. Upon palpating the breast, the doctor detected the presence of a single fluid-filled cyst. Although he told Selena he believes she has fibrocystic breast disease, he has ordered a mammogram and a biopsy of the cyst. Selena's physician has also recommended the use of a good support bra to lessen the pain, restriction of caffeine in her diet, and mild analgesics for any discomfort.

1. Selena asks the health care professional to explain what fibrocystic breast disease means. The best explanation would be:

   a. the presence of single or multiple fluid-filled cysts that can be felt when examining the breasts

   b. a benign, smooth-muscle tumor of the breast often mistaken for fibroid tumors

   c. presence of multiple tumors varying in size and location within the uterus

   d. tenderness following adhesions (which are the result of endometrial thickening)

2. Selena's physician will most likely order which of the following diagnostic tests to confirm the diagnosis of fibrocystic breast disease and differentiate it from carcinoma?

   a. mammography

   b. biopsy of the cyst

   c. bimanual examination

   d. ultrasonography

3. To lessen the discomfort Selena is having from the fibrocystic breast disease, she will be instructed to:

   a. take narcotics

   b. apply warm compresses to the chest

   c. wear a bra with good support

   d. avoid wearing a bra to decrease the pressure on the breasts

4. When instructing Selena on dietary changes, the health care professional will include the importance of omitting:

   a. protein

   b. fats

   c. calcium

   d. caffeine

5. What other preventive measure do you think the physician will recommend to Selena in connection with her disorder?

   a. monthly breast self-examination because the cysts tend to recur

   b. no more breast self-examination, because this may irritate the area

   c. regular Pap smears

   b. checking the breasts monthly for equality of size

Number correct _____ *× 20 points/correct answer: Your score* _____*%*

CHAPTER 18

Obstetrics

CHAPTER CONTENT

OBJECTIVES

Upon completing this chapter and the review exercises at the end of the chapter, the learner should be able to:

1. State the difference between presumptive and probable signs of pregnancy.

2. Correctly spell and pronounce terms listed on the Written and Audio Terminology Review, using the phonetic pronunciations provided.

3. Define at least 20 abbreviations common to obstetrics.

4. Define 10 physiological changes that occur in the female during pregnancy.

5. List and define at least five diagnostic techniques used in treating obstetrical patients.

6. Demonstrate the ability to correctly construct words relating to the field of obstetrics by completing the word element review exercise at the end of the chapter.

7. List and define at least 10 complications of pregnancy.

8. Differentiate between the signs and symptoms of impending labor and those of false and/or true labor.

Overview

Obstetrics is the field of medicine that deals with **pregnancy (prenatal)**, delivery of the baby, and the first six weeks after delivery (the postpartum period). The physician who specializes in the care of women during pregnancy, the delivery of the baby, and the first six weeks following the delivery is known as an **obstetrician**. **Perinatology** is a subspecialty of **obstetrics**. Physicians specializing in this area are called **perinatologists**. These doctors have had extensive training in the field of high-risk **obstetrics** and are concerned with the care of the mother and **fetus** at higher than normal risk for complications. A perinatologist may also be described as a maternal-fetal medicine specialist. Pregnancy signifies the **fertilization** of the **ovum** by the **sperm**: the creation of another human being. With this creation comes many changes, physiological as well as psychological. The physiological changes occur in a certain order as the **fetus** develops. Many of the physiological changes are discussed later in this chapter.

The psychological changes will vary with individuals. For some, pregnancy is desired and is perceived as one of the most exciting times of a woman's life. For others, pregnancy is not desired and may be the result of poor timing, ineffective birth control practices, or possibly rape. The psychological responses to pregnancy may vary from wonder and excitement to anxiety or despair.

Pregnancy is calculated to last 9 calendar months, or 10 lunar months (40 weeks, or 280 days). For reference, it is divided into trimesters (three intervals of three months each). Meeting the needs of the pregnant female is of utmost importance during this period between **conception** and **labor**, known as the **gestational period**. The health care professional in the obstetrician's office needs to be knowledgeable in all areas of obstetrical care to assist in providing the safest possible care during pregnancy.

Pregnancy

The female reproductive system provides an environment suitable for **fertilization** of the **ovum** (the female sex cell) and implantation of the fertilized **ovum**. This cyclic process repeats itself on a monthly basis throughout the female's reproductive years. The male reproductive system, on the other hand, functions to produce, store, and transmit the sperm (the male sex cell) that will fertilize the mature **ovum**. **Fertilization**, or **conception**, occurs when a sperm comes in contact with and penetrates a mature **ovum**. The time frame during which **fertilization** can occur is usually brief because of the short life span of the **ovum**. However, it may be as long as five days each month. After **ovulation**, a mature **ovum** survives for up to 24 hours. Sperm have been known to survive for 24 to 72 hours after **ejaculation** into the area of the female **cervix**.

Fertilization takes place in the outer third of the fallopian tube (that part closest to the **ovary**). The fertilized **ovum**, now called a zygote, continues to travel down the fallopian tube and burrows into the receptive uterine lining, where it will remain throughout the pregnancy as it continues to grow and develop. As development continues, the fertilized **ovum** (product of **conception**) also changes; that is, it is called an **embryo** from the second through the eighth week of pregnancy and a **fetus** beginning with the ninth week of pregnancy through the duration of the gestational period.

During pregnancy, two major accessory structures develop simultaneously with the baby's development. These two structures sustain the pregnancy and promote normal **prenatal** development. The first accessory structure is the **amniotic sac**: a strong, thin-walled, membranous sac that envelops and protects the growing **fetus**. The amniotic sac is also known as the **fetal** membrane. The outer layer of the sac is called the **chorion** and the inner layer is called the **amnion**. See *Figure 18-1*. Within the amniotic sac is a fluid that cushions and protects the **fetus** during pregnancy. This fluid is called the **amniotic fluid**.

The second accessory structure is the **placenta**: a temporary organ of pregnancy that provides for fetal respiration, nutrition, and excretion. It also functions as an endocrine gland in that it produces several hormones necessary for normal pregnancy (**human chorionic gonadotropin [HCG]**, **estrogen**, **progesterone**) and human placental lactogen (HPL), also known as human chorionic somatomammotropin. The maternal side of the **placenta** is attached to the wall of the **uterus** and has a "beefy" red appearance. The fetal side of the **placenta** has a shiny, slightly grayish, appearance. It contains the arteries and veins that intertwine to form the **umbilical cord**. See *Figure 18-2*.

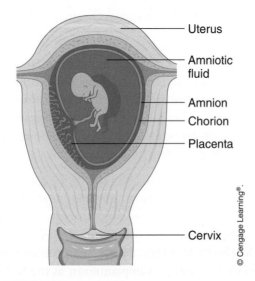

Figure 18-1 The amniotic sac

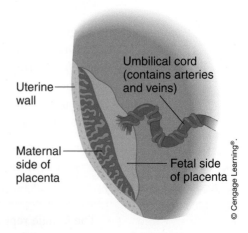

Figure 18-2 The placenta and umbilical cord

The **umbilical cord** arises from the center of the **placenta** and attaches to the umbilicus of the **fetus**. It serves as the lifeline between the mother and the **fetus**, becoming the means of transport for the nutrients and waste products to and from the developing baby. The maternal blood and the fetal blood do not mix during pregnancy. However, they do pass very close to each other within the **placenta**. These two independent circulatory networks are separated by a very thin layer of tissues known as the placental membrane, or placental barrier. Oxygen and nutrients transfer across this membrane from the maternal circulation into the fetal circulation, and waste materials transfer across the membrane from the fetal circulation into the maternal circulation to be excreted.

The amniotic sac remains intact until uterine contractions begin with regularity and enough strength to indicate true **labor**. Sometimes the amniotic sac ruptures at the onset of **labor**, during the early stages of **labor**, or occasionally it is punctured by the physician at some point during the **labor** process. When this happens spontaneously, you may hear the woman describe it as "my membranes ruptured" or "my water broke."

Barring any complications, the **placenta** remains intact and attached to the uterine lining until after the delivery of the baby. It then detaches from the **uterus** and is eliminated through the vaginal canal. Following childbirth, the **placenta** is known as the **afterbirth**.

Physiological Changes During Pregnancy

Pregnancy places increased demands on the expectant mother's body. Significant changes occur in her body that are necessary to support and nourish the **fetus**. These changes also prepare her body for childbirth and **lactation** (breastfeeding). The concept of being pregnant is often different from the reality of being pregnant. Some women find that they are psychologically unprepared for the physiological changes that occur during pregnancy. Each will need the support and guidance of a well-trained, perceptive staff within the obstetrician's office to understand better the changes her body is experiencing during this gestational period.

To provide the best care possible, the health care professional must understand the physiological changes that occur during pregnancy and the effect they may have on the pregnant woman. The most obvious physiological changes that occur within the female reproductive system during pregnancy are discussed in the following segment.

Amenorrhea

Amenorrhea, or absence of menstruation, is usually one of the first things women consider being a sign of pregnancy. Although **amenorrhea** can occur for other reasons, it usually is a strong suggestion of pregnancy in women who have regular menstrual periods. The menstruation stops as a result of hormonal influence during pregnancy. **Amenorrhea**, alone, is not significant enough to confirm pregnancy. Other **signs** and tests will be necessary for confirmation. These are discussed in the next section.

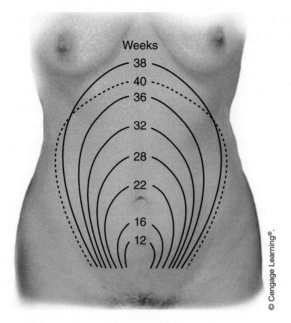

Figure 18-3 Changes in the uterus during pregnancy

Changes in the Uterus

Before pregnancy, the **uterus** is a small, pear-shaped organ that weighs approximately 2 ounces. During pregnancy, the woman's **uterus** grows large enough to accommodate the growing **fetus, placenta,** amniotic sac, and **amniotic fluid,** increasing in size to over 2 pounds. As the **uterus** grows, and the **fetus** develops, it rises up and out of the pelvic cavity. By the end of the pregnancy, the top of the **uterus** (**fundus**) can be palpated (felt) just under the xiphoid process. See *Figure 18-3.*

Changes in the Cervix

The most obvious changes in the uterine **cervix** are those of color and consistency. After approximately the sixth week of pregnancy, the **cervix** and **vagina** take on a bluish-violet hue as a result of the local venous congestion. This is known as **Chadwick's sign** and is an early sign of pregnancy. The changes in the **cervix** occur as a result of increased blood flow to the pregnant **uterus.** The increased fluid in this area also causes the **cervix** to soften in consistency in preparation for childbirth. This softening of the **cervix** is a probable sign of pregnancy and is known as **Goodell's sign.**

By the end of the pregnancy, the **cervix** has softened so significantly that it has a somewhat mushy feel to the examiner's touch. This marked softening of the **cervix** signifies that the **cervix** is ready for the dilation and thinning that is necessary for the birth of the baby. At this time, the **cervix** is said to be "ripe" for birth.

Changes in the Vagina

The hormones secreted during pregnancy also prepare the vaginal canal for the great distention it will undergo during **labor.** As mentioned, the **vagina** takes on the same bluish-violet hue of the **cervix** during pregnancy. The hormonal influences during pregnancy generate increasing amounts of **glycogen** in the vaginal cells, which causes **increased vaginal discharge** and heavy shedding of vaginal cells. This in turn creates a thick, white vaginal discharge known as **leukorrhea**. It should be noted that the increase in **glycogen** in the cells favors the growth of *Candida albicans*, a causative organism in yeast infections of the **vagina**. Persistent yeast infections are not uncommon in **pregnancy**.

Changes in the Breasts

During pregnancy, the breasts undergo characteristic changes. Hormonal influences result in an increase in size and shape of the breasts; the nipples increase in size and become more erect, and the **areola** become larger and more darkly pigmented. The sebaceous glands within the **areola** (Montgomery's tubercles) become more active during pregnancy and secrete a substance that lubricates the nipples. The pregnant woman will also notice a thin, yellowish discharge from the nipples throughout the pregnancy. This is normal, and the discharge is called **colostrum** (a forerunner of breast milk). If the woman does not plan to breastfeed after delivery, natural suppression of **lactation** can be achieved by use of a snug-fitting support bra worn around the clock (except when bathing) and ice packs several times a day to help reduce engorgement (swelling) of breasts. Pain medication may be necessary.

Changes in Blood Pressure

The blood pressure of a pregnant woman should remain within fairly normal limits. It is important to monitor the woman's blood pressure carefully throughout the pregnancy because a significant or continual increase in blood pressure may be indicative of complications of pregnancy such as **pregnancy-induced hypertension** (discussed in the next section). During the second and third trimesters (four to nine months), the expectant mother may experience **hypotension** when she is in the supine (lying on one's back) position. This is known as **supine hypotension**, supine hypotension syndrome, or vena cava syndrome. The drop in blood pressure occurs because the weight of the pregnant **uterus** presses against the descending aorta and the inferior vena cava in the abdominal cavity when the woman is lying on her back. This pressure on these major blood vessels partially blocks the blood flow, therefore reducing the maternal cardiac output and blood pressure. These responses in the mother can subsequently result in a decrease in the fetal heart rate and fetal bradycardia. The pregnant female may complain of faintness, lightheadedness, and dizziness. It is important to advise these women to use the side-lying position when resting to relieve the pressure on the abdominal blood vessels. See *Figure 18-4*.

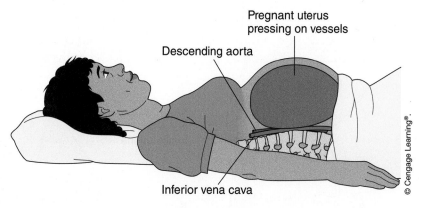

Figure 18-4 Example of supine hypotension

Changes in Urination

During the first three months of pregnancy (first **trimester**), the pregnant woman may experience urinary frequency due to the increasing size of the **uterus**, which creates pressure on the bladder. When the **uterus** rises up out of the pelvis during the second **trimester**, the pressure on the bladder is relieved. The urinary frequency will return during the last **trimester** due to the pressure of the baby's head on the bladder as it settles into the pelvis before delivery.

The increased demands placed on the urinary system during pregnancy can result in a minimal amount of spilling of glucose into the urine. Regular monitoring of the pregnant female's urine throughout the pregnancy is important because a finding of more than a trace of glucose in a routine sample of urine may be indicative of problems (in particular, **gestational diabetes**, discussed in the next section).

Changes in Posture

As the pregnancy progresses, changes in the posture of the pregnant female are observable beginning in the second **trimester**. The softening of the pelvic joints and relaxing of the pelvic ligaments may offset the pregnant woman's center of gravity due to the pelvic instability. To compensate for this, the woman assumes a wider stance and a **waddling gait** as she walks.

The increasing size of the **uterus** places stress on the abdominal muscles, particularly during the third **trimester** of pregnancy. During this time, one may observe that the pregnant female will stand straighter and taller (with her shoulders back and her abdomen forward). This stance is in an effort to adjust her center of gravity to the changes taking place within her body and to make ambulation easier. Standing this way, however, creates a forward curve of the lumbar spine (**lordosis**), which may lead to complaints of **backache**. See *Figure 18-5*.

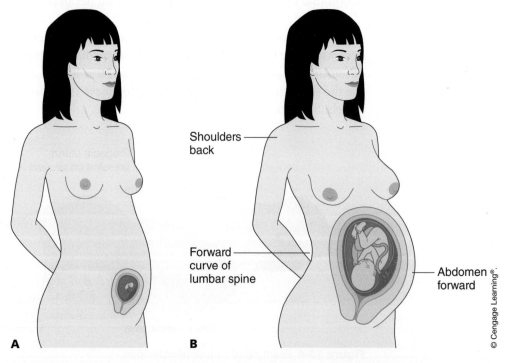

Shoulders back

Forward curve of lumbar spine

Abdomen forward

© Cengage Learning®

A   B

Figure 18-5 Changes in posture due to pregnancy: (A) 6 weeks; (B) 40 weeks

Changes in the Skin

During pregnancy, some women may experience an increased feeling of warmth and sweating due to the increased activity of the sweat glands. They may also experience problems with facial blemishes due to the increased activity of the sebaceous glands during pregnancy. These, however, are not the most noticeable changes in the skin of the pregnant woman. What comes to mind as probably one of the most obvious skin changes during pregnancy is the increased pigmentation of the skin **(hyperpigmentation)**.

The **hyperpigmentation** seen on the forehead, cheeks, and the bridge of the nose appears as brown patches called **chloasma**, or the "**mask of pregnancy**." Women who have brown hair or darker skin usually display more pigmentation than women who are fair skinned.

The **hyperpigmentation** that appears on the abdomen of the pregnant female is seen as a darkened vertical midline between the fundus and the symphysis pubis and is known as the **linea nigra**. See *Figure 18-6*. The **areola** of the breast (area surrounding the nipple) also becomes darker as pregnancy progresses.

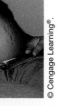

© Cengage Learning®.

Figure 18-6 Linea nigra with striae gravidarum

During the second half of pregnancy, a woman may experience stretch marks on the abdomen, thighs, and breasts (known as **striae gravidarum**). These linear tears in the connective tissue usually occur in the areas of greatest stretch during pregnancy. The marks appear as slightly depressed, pinkish-purple streaks in these areas. See *Figure 18-6*. After pregnancy, the stretch marks fade to silvery lines, but they do not disappear completely. Some women may complain of an itching sensation when these stretch marks appear and may require relief for this.

Changes in Weight

Over the years there have been many theories concerning the acceptable amount of weight that could be gained during pregnancy. In the 1970s the recommended weight gain was 15 to 25 pounds, with some physicians even placing their patients on low sodium diets for the duration of the pregnancy. The belief then was that by restricting the weight gain during pregnancy, the patient was less likely to develop pregnancy-induced hypertension.

Today, the recommended weight gain during pregnancy ranges from 25 to 30 pounds for women who begin pregnancy at or near their normal weight. The weight gain during pregnancy, no matter what the mother's prepregnant weight, should be at least 15 pounds to ensure adequate nutrition to the developing **fetus**.

The pattern of weight gain during pregnancy is just as important as the amount of weight gained. In the early months of pregnancy, there is very little weight gain; only 3 to 4 pounds is recommended. During the remainder of the pregnancy (fourth to ninth month), the expected weight gain is about 1 pound per week. It is critical that the pregnant woman's weight be monitored during each **prenatal** visit. Significant, unexplained weight gains from one visit to the next may be indicative of fluid retention or problems such as pregnancy-induced hypertension.

Review Checkpoint

Check your understanding of this section by completing the **Physiological Changes During Pregnancy** exercises in your workbook.

Signs and Symptoms of Pregnancy

Traditionally, the confirmation of pregnancy has been based on **symptoms** experienced by the mother-to-be, as well as signs observed by the physician or health practitioner. These signs and symptoms are grouped into three categories, based on likelihood of accuracy. They are presumptive signs, probable signs, and positive signs of pregnancy.

Presumptive Signs

Presumptive signs of pregnancy are those experienced by the expectant mother, which suggest pregnancy but are not necessarily positive. These early **symptoms** experienced by the expectant mother include **amenorrhea, nausea** and vomiting, **fatigue**, urinary disturbances, and breast changes. A detailed discussion of these signs has been presented in the section on physiological changes of pregnancy. Another presumptive sign of pregnancy is **quickening**, or movement of the **fetus** felt by the mother. This usually occurs about 18 to 20 weeks' **gestation** and may be described as a faint abdominal fluttering. Presumptive signs are slightly predictive of pregnancy as a group of **symptoms** but taken individually, they can be indicative of other conditions.

Probable Signs

Probable signs of pregnancy are those observable by the examiner. Even though they are much stronger indicators of pregnancy, they can be due to other pathological conditions and should not be used as the sole indicator of pregnancy. Probable signs that have already been discussed in the section on physiological changes of pregnancy include:

- Goodell's sign (softening of the **cervix** and **vagina**)

- Chadwick's sign (**cervix** and **vagina** take on a bluish-violet hue)

- Uterine enlargement

- **Hyperpigmentation** of the skin (mask of pregnancy)

- Abdominal stria (stretch marks)

- **Hegar's sign**, which is softening of the lower segment of the **uterus**

- **Braxton Hicks contractions** are irregular contractions of the **uterus** that may occur throughout the pregnancy and are relatively painless

- **Ballottement**, which is a technique of using the examiner's finger to tap against the **uterus**, through the **vagina**, to cause the **fetus** to "bounce" within the **amniotic fluid** and feeling it rebound quickly

- Fetal outline, which can be palpated by the examiner at approximately 24 weeks' **gestation**

- Pregnancy tests, which are commonly based on the presence of the hormone, human chorionic gonadotropin, secreted during pregnancy

To read the list of probable signs of pregnancy and then hear that they are not positive signs of pregnancy may sound a bit confusing to the individual just beginning in health care. It must be remembered that although the presumptive and probable signs of pregnancy are most often correct as indicators of pregnancy, they can be due to other causes. As you continue to read, we will discuss the positive signs of pregnancy.

Positive Signs

There are only three positive signs of pregnancy, which are the only absolute indicators of a developing **fetus**.

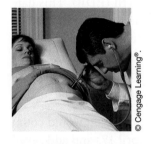

Figure 18-7 Fetoscope used to hear fetal heartbeat

1. Fetal heartbeat, which can be detected by ultrasound at approximately 10 weeks' **gestation** or by **fetoscope** at 18 to 20 weeks' **gestation**. (A **fetoscope** is a special stethoscope for hearing the fetal heartbeat through the mother's abdomen.) The fetal heart rate can vary from 120 to 180 beats per minute. See *Figure 18-7*.

2. Identification of an **embryo** or **fetus** by ultrasound, which can be detected as early as five to six weeks with 100% reliability, providing the earliest positive confirmation of a pregnancy.

   The **ultrasonography** is a noninvasive procedure that involves the use of reflected sound waves to detect the presence of the **embryo** or **fetus**. The waves reflected from the **fetus** are transmitted into a machine that converts them into an image produced on the screen.

3. Fetal movements felt by the examiner are palpable by the physician/ examiner by the second **trimester** of the pregnancy. Fetal movements can also be observed by ultrasound earlier in the pregnancy.

For the learner's convenience, the presumptive, probable, and positive signs of pregnancy are presented in *Table 18-1*.

Table 18-1 Signs of Pregnancy

Presumptive Signs	Probable Signs	Positive Signs
1. Amenorrhea	1. Goodell's sign	1. Fetal heartbeat
2. Nausea and vomiting	2. Chadwick's sign	2. Ultrasound identification of fetus
3. Fatigue	3. Uterine enlargement	3. Palpated fetal movements
4. Urinary disturbances	4. Hyperpigmentation of the skin	
5. Breast changes	5. Abdominal stria	
6. Quickening	6. Hegar's sign	
	7. Braxton Hicks contractions	
	8. Ballottement	
	9. Fetal outline palpated	
	10. Pregnancy tests	

Calculation of Date of Birth

Everyone wants to know, "When will the baby be born?" It is not possible to predict the exact date of birth with a high degree of accuracy. The birth date, or due date, is determined based on the average length of a normal pregnancy, with a two-week margin on either side of the date being considered within the normal limit.

The birth date for the baby is termed as the **expected date of confinement (EDC)**, the **expected date of delivery (EDD)**, or the **expected date of birth (EDB)**. This date is determined using a formula that calculates from the date of the first day of the **last menstrual period (LMP)**. The formula used to calculate the date of birth is known as **Nagele's rule,** named after the German **obstetrician,** Franz K. Nagele. *To calculate the estimated date of delivery, subtract three months from the beginning of the last normal menstrual period (LMP) and add one year and seven days to the date.*

Example: If the woman's last normal menstrual period began July 17, you would count back three months (which would be June . . . May . . . April . . . April 17) and add seven days to the date (which would be April 24). The EDD, or expected date of delivery, would be April 24.

VOCABULARY

The following vocabulary words are frequently used when discussing the field of obstetrics.

Word	Definition
afterbirth	The **placenta,** the **amnion,** the **chorion,** some **amniotic fluid,** blood, and blood clots expelled from the **uterus** after childbirth.

amenorrhea
(ah-men-oh-**REE**-ah)
  a- = without
  men/o = menstruation
  -rrhea = flow, drainage
	Absence of menstrual flow.

amnion (**AM**-nee-on) amni/o = amnion	The inner of the two membrane layers that surround and contain the **fetus** and the **amniotic fluid** during pregnancy.

amniotic fluid
(am-nee-**OT**-ik fluid)
  amni/o = amnion
  -tic = pertaining to
	A liquid produced by and contained within the fetal membranes during pregnancy. This fluid protects the **fetus** from trauma and temperature variations, helps maintain fetal oxygen supply, and allows for freedom of movement by the **fetus** during pregnancy.

amniotic sac
(am-nee-**OT**-ik sack)
  amni/o = amnion
  -tic = pertaining to
	The double layered sac that contains the **fetus** and the amniotic fluid during pregnancy.

Word	Definition
areola (ah-**REE**-oh-lah)	The darker pigmented, circular area surrounding the nipple of each breast; also known as the **areola** mammae or the **areola** papillaris.
ballottement (bah-**LOT**-ment)	A technique of using the examiner's finger to tap against the **uterus**, through the **vagina**, to cause the **fetus** to "bounce" within the **amniotic fluid** and feeling it rebound quickly.
Braxton Hicks contractions (**BRACKS**-ton **HICKS** con-**TRAK**-shuns)	Irregular, ineffective contractions of the **uterus** that occur throughout pregnancy.
cerclage (sair-**KLAZH**)	Suturing the **cervix** to keep it from dilating prematurely during the pregnancy. This procedure is sometimes referred to as a "purse string procedure." The sutures are removed near the end of the pregnancy.
cervix (**SER**-viks)	The part of the **uterus** that protrudes into the cavity of the **vagina**; the neck of the **uterus**.
cesarean section (see-**SAYR**-ee-an section)	A surgical procedure in which the abdomen and **uterus** are incised and a baby is delivered transabdominally. Also called cesarean birth or cesarean delivery.
Chadwick's sign	The bluish-violet hue of the **cervix** and **vagina** after approximately the sixth week of pregnancy.
chloasma (kloh-**AZ**-mah)	Patches of tan or brown pigmentation associated with pregnancy, occurring mostly on the forehead, cheeks, and nose; also called the "mask of pregnancy."
chorion (**KOH**-ree-on)	The outer of the two membrane layers that surround and contain the **fetus** and the **amniotic fluid** during pregnancy.
coitus (**KOH**-ih-tus)	**Sexual intercourse; copulation.**
colostrum (koh-**LOSS**-trum)	The thin, yellowish fluid secreted by the breasts during pregnancy and the first few days after birth, before **lactation** begins.
conception (con-**SEP**-shun)	The union of a male sperm and a female **ovum**; also termed **fertilization**.
copulation (kop-yoo-**LAY**-shun)	Sexual intercourse; **coitus**.
corpus luteum (**COR**-pus **LOO**-tee-um)	A mass of yellowish tissue that forms within the ruptured ovarian follicle after **ovulation**. It functions as a temporary endocrine gland for the purpose of secreting **estrogen** and large amounts of **progesterone**, which will sustain pregnancy, should it occur, until the **placenta** forms. If pregnancy does not occur, the **corpus luteum** will degenerate approximately three days before the beginning of menstruation.

Word	Definition
culdocentesis (kull-doh-sen-**TEE**-sis) culd/o = cul-de-sac -centesis = surgical puncture	Needle aspiration, through the **vagina**, into the cul-de-sac area (area in the peritoneal cavity immediately behind the **vagina**) for the purpose of removing fluid from the area for examination or diagnosis. Aspiration of unclotted blood from the cul-de-sac area may indicate bleeding from a ruptured fallopian tube. The aspiration of clear fluid from the area would rule out a ruptured fallopian tube.
dilation (of cervix) (dye-**LAY**-shun)	The enlargement of the diameter of the **cervix** during **labor**. The calculation of the amount of dilation is measured in centimeters (cm). When the **cervix** has dilated to 10 cm, it is said to be completely dilated.
Doppler © Cengage Learning®. **Figure 18-8** Doppler	A technique used in ultrasound imaging to monitor the behavior of a moving structure such as flowing blood or a beating heart. Fetal heart monitors operate on the **Doppler** sound wave principle to determine the fetal heart rate. See *Figure 18-8*.
eclampsia (eh-**KLAMP**-see-ah)	The most severe form of **hypertension** during pregnancy, evidenced by seizures (convulsions).
edema (eh-**DEE**-mah)	Swelling, with water retention.
effacement (eh-**FACE**-ment)	Thinning of the **cervix**, which allows it to enlarge the diameter of its opening in preparation for childbirth. This occurs during the normal processes of **labor**.
ejaculation (eh-jak-yoo-**LAY**-shun)	The sudden emission of semen from the male urethra, usually occurring during sexual intercourse or masturbation.
embryo (**EM**-bree-oh)	The name given to the product of **conception** from the second through the eighth week of pregnancy (through the second month).
endometrium (en-doh-**MEE**-tree-um) endo- = within metri/o = uterine lining -um = noun ending	The inner lining of the **uterus**.
episiotomy (eh-**piz**-ee-**OT**-oh-mee) episi/o = vulva -tomy = incision into	A surgical procedure in which an incision is made into the woman's **perineum** to enlarge the vaginal opening for delivery of the baby. This incision is usually made shortly before the baby's birth (second stage of **labor**) to prevent tearing of the **perineum**.

Word	Definition
estrogen (**ESS**-troh-jen)	One of the female hormones that promotes the development of the female secondary sex characteristics.
fallopian tubes (fah-**LOH**-pee-an tubes)	A pair of tubes opening at one end into the **uterus** and at the other end into the peritoneal cavity, over the **ovary**.
fertilization (fer-til-ih-**ZAY**-shun)	The union of a male sperm and a female **ovum**; also termed **conception**.
fetoscope (**FEET**-oh-skohp) fet/o = fetus -scope = instrument for viewing	A special stethoscope for hearing the fetal heartbeat through the mother's abdomen.
fetus (**FEE**-tus) fet/o = fetus -us = noun ending	The name given to the developing baby from approximately the ninth week after **conception** until birth.
fimbriae (**FIM**-bree-ay)	The fringelike end of the fallopian tube.
fundus	Superior aspect of the **uterus**.
gamete (**GAM**-eet)	A mature sperm or **ovum**.
gastroesophageal reflux (**gas**-troh-eh-soff-ah-**JEE**-al **REE**-flucks) gastr/o = stomach esophag/o = esophagus -eal = pertaining to	A return, or reflux, of gastric juices into the esophagus, resulting in a burning sensation.
gestation (jess-**TAY**-shun)	The term of pregnancy, which equals approximately 280 days from the onset of the last menstrual period. The period of intrauterine development of the **fetus** from **conception** through birth; also termed the gestational period.
gestational hypertension (jess-**TAY**-shun-al **high**-per-**TEN**-shun)	A complication of pregnancy in which the expectant mother develops high blood pressure after 20 weeks' **gestation**, with no signs of **proteinuria** or **edema**.
glycogen (**GLYE**-koh-jen) glyc/o = sugar	The form of sugar stored in body cells, primarily the liver.
gonads (**GO**-nads)	A **gamete**-producing gland such as an **ovary** or a testis.
Goodell's sign	The softening of the uterine **cervix**, a probable sign of pregnancy.

Word	Definition
graafian follicles (**GRAF**-ee-an-**FOL**-ik-kulz)	A mature, fully developed ovarian cyst containing the ripe **ovum**.
gravida	A woman who is pregnant. She may be identified as **gravida I** if this is her first pregnancy, **gravida II** for a second pregnancy, and so on.
Hegar's sign (**HAY**-garz sign)	Softening of the lower segment of the **uterus**; a probable sign of **pregnancy**.
hyperpigmentation (**high**-per-**pig**-men-**TAY**-shun) hyper- = excessive	An increase in the pigmentation of the skin.
hypertension (high-per-**TEN**-shun) hyper- = excessive tens/o = strain -ion = action; process	High blood pressure; a common, often asymptomatic, disorder in which the blood persistently exceeds 140/90 mmHg.
hypotension (**high**-poh-**TEN**-shun) hypo- = less than, low tens/o = strain -ion = action; process	Low blood pressure; an abnormal condition in which the blood pressure is not adequate for normal passage through the blood vessels or for normal oxygenation of the body cells.
hypovolemic shock (**high**-poh-voh-**LEE**-mik) hypo- = under, below, beneath, less than normal	A state of extreme physical collapse and exhaustion due to massive blood loss; "less than normal" blood volume.
labor (**LAY**-bor)	The time and the processes that occur during birth, from the beginning of cervical dilation to the delivery of the **placenta**.
lactation (lak-**TAY**-shun) lact/o = milk	The production and secretion of milk from the female breasts as nourishment for the infant. **Lactation** can be referred to as a process or as a period of time during which the female is breastfeeding.
lactiferous ducts (lak-**TIF**-er-us ducts) lact/o = milk	Channels or narrow tubular structures that carry milk from the lobes of each breast to the nipple.
laparoscopy (lap-ar-**OS**-koh-pee) lapar/o = abdominal wall -scopy = process of viewing	Visualization of the abdominal cavity with an instrument called a laparoscope through an incision into the abdominal wall.
leukorrhea (**loo**-koh-**REE**-ah) leuk/o = white -rrhea = discharge, flow	A white discharge from the **vagina**.

Word	Definition
lightening	The settling of the fetal head into the pelvis, occurring a few weeks prior to the onset of **labor**.
linea nigra (**LIN**-ee-ah **NIG**-rah)	A darkened vertical midline appearing on the abdomen of a pregnant woman, extending from the fundus to the symphysis pubis.
lithotomy position (lih-**THOT**-oh-mee position) 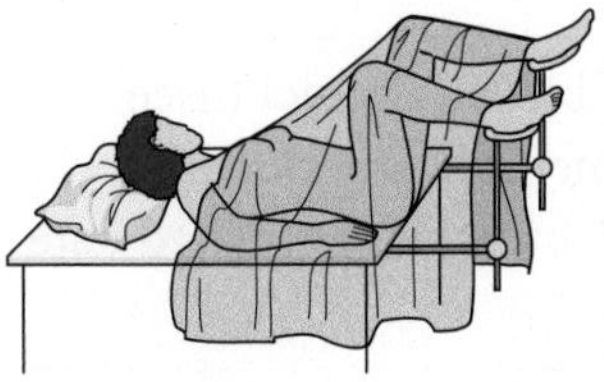 Figure 18-9 Lithotomy position	A position in which the patient lies on her back, buttocks even with the end of the table, with her knees bent back toward her abdomen and the heel of each foot resting in an elevated foot rest at the end of the examination table. See *Figure 18-9*.
lordosis (lor-**DOH**-sis) lord/o = bent -osis = condition 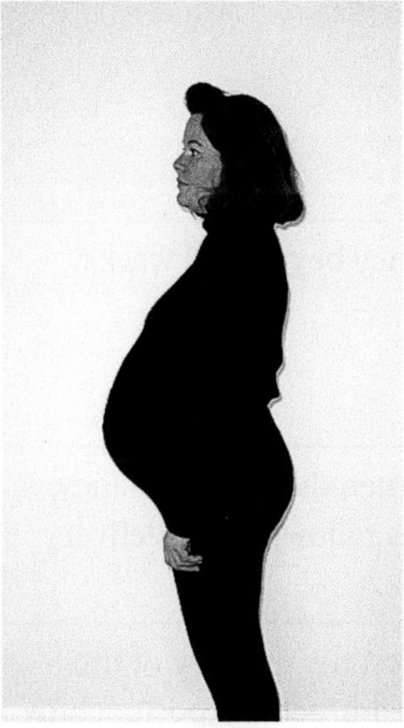 Figure 18-10 Lordosis	A forward curvature of the spine, noticeable if the person is observed from the side. See *Figure 18-10*.
lunar month (**LOON**-ar)	Four weeks or 28 days; approximately the amount of time it takes the moon to revolve around the earth.
mammary glands (**MAM**-ah-ree glands) mamm/o = breast -ary = pertaining to	The female breasts.
mask of pregnancy	Patches of tan or brown pigmentation associated with pregnancy, occurring mostly on the forehead, cheeks, and nose; also known as **chloasma**.

Word	Definition
multigravida (**mull**-tih-**GRAV**-ih-dah) multi- = many -gravida = pregnancy	A woman who has been pregnant more than once.
multipara (**mull**-**TIP**-ah-rah) multi- = many -para = to bear	A woman who has given birth two or more times after 20 weeks' **gestation**.
Nagele's rule (**NAY**-geh-leez)	A formula that is used to calculate the date of birth: Subtract three months from the first day of the last normal menstrual period and add one year and seven days to that date to arrive at the estimated date of birth.
neonatology (**nee**-oh-nay-**TOL**-oh-jee) neo- = new nat/o = birth -logy = the study of	The branch of medicine that specializes in the treatment and care of the diseases and disorders of the newborn through the first four weeks of life.
nulligravida (**null**-ih-**GRAV**-ih-dah) nulli = none -gravida = pregnancy	A woman who has never been pregnant.
nullipara (nuh-**LIP**-ah-rah) nulli- = none -para = to bear	A woman who has never completed a pregnancy beyond 20 weeks' **gestation**.
obstetrician (ob-steh-**TRISH**-an)	A physician who specializes in the care of women during pregnancy, the delivery of the baby, and the first six weeks following the delivery (known as the immediate postpartum period).
obstetrics (ob-**STET**-riks)	The field of medicine that deals with pregnancy, the delivery of the baby, and the first six weeks after delivery (the immediate postpartum period).
ovary (**OH**-vah-ree) ov/o = ovum -ary = pertaining to	One of a pair of female **gonads** responsible for producing mature ova (eggs) and releasing them at monthly intervals (**ovulation**); also responsible for producing the female hormones, **estrogen** and **progesterone**.
ovulation (**ov**-yoo-**LAY**-shun)	The release of the mature **ovum** from the **ovary**; occurs approximately 14 days prior to the beginning of menses.
ovum (**OH**-vum) ov/o = egg -um = noun ending	The female reproductive cell; female sex cell or egg.

Word	Definition
para	A woman who has produced an infant regardless of whether the infant was alive or stillborn. This term applies to any pregnancies carried to more than 20 weeks' **gestation**. The term may be written **para II**, **para III**, and so on, to indicate the number of pregnancies lasting more than 20 weeks' **gestation**, regardless of the number of offspring produced by the pregnancy. A woman who has had only one pregnancy resulting in multiple births is still a **para I**.
parturition (par-too-**RISH**-un)	The act of giving birth.
perineum (pair-ih-**NEE**-um)	The area between the vaginal orifice and the anus. It consists of muscular and fibrous tissue and serves as support for the pelvic structures.
placenta (plah-**SEN**-tah)	A highly vascular, disk-shaped organ that forms in the pregnant uterine wall for exchange of gases and nutrients between the mother and the **fetus**. The maternal side of the **placenta** attaches to the uterine wall, whereas the fetal side of the **placenta** gives rise to the **umbilical cord** (which connects directly to the baby). After the delivery of the baby, when the **placenta** is no longer needed, it separates from the uterine wall and passes to the outside of the body through the **vagina** (at which time it is called the afterbirth).
preeclampsia (**pre**-eh-**KLAMP**-see-ah)	A state during pregnancy in which the expectant mother develops high blood pressure, accompanied by **proteinuria** or **edema**, or both, after 20 weeks' **gestation**.
pregnancy (**PREG**-nan-see)	The period of intrauterine development of the **fetus** from **conception** through birth. The average pregnancy lasts approximately 40 weeks; also known as the gestational period.
prenatal (pre-**NAY**-tal) pre- = before, in front -natal = pertaining to birth	Pertaining to the period of time during pregnancy; that is, before the birth of the baby.
primigravida (**prye**-mih-**GRAV**-ih-dah) primi- = first -gravida = pregnancy	A woman who is pregnant for the first time.
primipara (prye-**MIP**-ah-rah) primi- = first -para = to bear	A woman who has given birth for the first time, after a pregnancy of at least 20 weeks' **gestation**.
progesterone (proh-**JES**-ter-on)	A female hormone secreted by the **corpus luteum** and the **placenta**. It is primarily responsible for the changes that occur in the **endometrium** in anticipation of a fertilized **ovum** and for development of the maternal **placenta** after implantation of a fertilized **ovum**. Also known as progestin.

Word	Definition
proteinuria (**proh**-teen-**YOO**-ree-ah) -uria = urine condition	The presence of protein (albumin) in the urine; also called albuminuria. This can be a sign of pregnancy-induced hypertension (PIH).
puberty (**PEW**-ber-tee)	The period of life at which the ability to reproduce begins; that is, in the female, it is the period when the female reproductive organs become fully developed and secondary sex characteristics appear.
pyrosis (pye-**ROH**-sis) pyr/o = fire, heat -osis = condition	**Heartburn;** indigestion.
quickening (**KWIK**-en-ing)	The first feeling of movement of the **fetus** felt by the expectant mother; usually occurs at about 16 to 20 weeks' **gestation**.
salpingectomy (**sal**-pin-**JEK**-toh-mee) salping/o = eustachian tubes; also refers to fallopian tubes -ectomy = surgical removal	Surgical removal of a fallopian tube.
sexual intercourse	The sexual union of two people of the opposite sex in which the penis is introduced into the **vagina**; also known as **copulation** or **coitus.**
signs	Objective findings as perceived by an examiner, such as the measurement of a fever on the thermometer, the observation of a rash on the skin, or the observation of a bluish-violet color of the **cervix**.
sperm	A mature male germ cell; spermatozoon.
striae gravidarum (**STRIGH**-ay grav-ih-**DAR**-um)	Stretch marks that occur during pregnancy due to the great amount of stretching that occurs. They appear as slightly depressed, pinkish-purple streaks in the areas of greatest stretch (which are the abdomen, the breasts and the thighs).
supine hypotension (soo-**PINE high**-poh-**TEN**-shen)	Low blood pressure that occurs in a pregnant woman when she is lying on her back. It is caused by the pressure of the pregnant **uterus** on the vena cava; also known as supine **hypotension** syndrome or vena cava syndrome.
symptoms (**SIM**-toms)	A subjective indication of a disease or a change in condition as perceived by the patient; something experienced or felt by the patient.
tachycardia (**tak**-eh-**CAR**-dee-ah) tachy- = rapid cardi/o = heart -a = noun ending	Rapid heartbeat, consistently over 100 beats per minute.

Word	Definition
testes (**TESS**-teez)	The paired male gonads that produce sperm. They are suspended in the scrotal sac in the adult male.
transvaginal ultrasonography (trans-**VAJ**-in-al ull-trah-son-**OG**-rah-fee) trans- = across, through vagin/o = vagina -al = pertaining to ultra- = beyond son/o = sound -graphy = process of recording	An ultrasound image that is produced by inserting a transvaginal probe into the **vagina**. The probe is encased in a disposable cover and is coated with a gel for easy insertion. The gel also promotes conductivity. This procedure allows clear visualization of the **uterus**, gestational sac, and **embryo** in the early stages of pregnancy. It also allows the examiner to visualize deeper pelvic structures such as the **ovaries** and **fallopian tubes**.
trimester (**TRY**-mes-ter)	One of the three periods of approximately three months into which pregnancy is divided. The first **trimester** consists of weeks 1 to 12, the second **trimester** consists of weeks 13 to 27, and the third **trimester** consists of weeks 28 to 40.
ultrasonography (ull-trah-son-**OG**-rah-fee) ultra- = beyond son/o = sound -graphy = recording	A noninvasive procedure that involves the use of reflected sound waves to detect the presence of the **embryo** or **fetus**.
umbilical cord (um-**BILL**-ih-kal cord)	A flexible structure connecting the umbilicus (navel) of the **fetus** with the **placenta** in the pregnant **uterus**. It serves as passage for the umbilical arteries and vein.
uterus (**YOO**-ter-us)	The hollow, pear-shaped organ of the female reproductive system that houses the fertilized, implanted **ovum** as it develops throughout pregnancy; also the source of the monthly menstrual flow from the nonpregnant **uterus**.
vagina (vah-**JIGH**-nah)	The muscular tube that connects the **uterus** with the vulva. It is approximately 3 inches in length and rests between the bladder (anteriorly) and the rectum (posteriorly).
varicose veins (**VAIR**-ih-kohs veins)	Twisted, swollen veins that occur as a result of the blood pooling in the legs.
waddling gait (**WOD**-ling **GATE**)	A manner of walking in which the feet are wide apart and the walk resembles that of a duck.

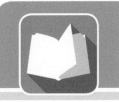

Review Checkpoint

Check your understanding of this section by completing the **Vocabulary** exercises in your workbook.

WORD ELEMENTS

The following word elements pertain to the field of **obstetrics**. As you review the list, pronounce each word element aloud twice and check the box after you "say it." Write the definition for the example term given for each word element. Use your medical dictionary to find the definitions of the example terms.

Word Element	Pronunciation	"Say It"	Meaning
amni/o **amni**ocentesis	**AM**-nee-oh am-nee-oh-sen-**TEE**-sis	☐	**amnion**
ante- **ante**flexion	**AN**-tee an-tee-**FLEK**-shun	☐	before; in front
culd/o **culd**ocentesis	**KULL**-doh **kull**-doh-sen-**TEE**-sis	☐	cul-de-sac
-cyesis pseudo**cyesis**	sigh-**EE**-sis **soo**-doh-sigh-**EE**-sis	☐	pregnancy
episi/o **episi**otomy	eh-**PEEZ**-ee-oh eh-peez-ee-**OT**-oh-mee	☐	vulva
fet/o **fet**oscope	**FEET**-oh **FEET**-oh-skohp	☐	**fetus**
-gravida primi**gravida**	**GRAV**-ih-dah **prye**-mih-**GRAV**-ih-dah	☐	pregnancy
hyper- **hyper**emesis	**HIGH**-per high-per-**EM**-eh-sis	☐	excessive
lact/o **lact**ation	**LAK**-toh lak-**TAY**-shun	☐	milk
multi- **multi**gravida	**MULL**-tih mull-tih-**GRAV**-ih-dah	☐	many
nat/o pre**nat**al	**NAY**-toh pre-**NAY**-tal	☐	birth
nulli- **nulli**para	**NULL**-ih nuh-**LIP**-ah-rah	☐	none
-para multi**para**	**PAIR**-ah mull-**TIP**-ah-rah	☐	to bear
primi- **primi**gravida	**PRYE**-mih prye-mih-**GRAV**-ih-dah	☐	first

Word Element	Pronunciation	"Say It"	Meaning
obstetr/o **obstetr**ics	ob-**STET**-roh ob-**STET**-riks	☐	midwife
pelv/i **pelv**imetry	**PELL**-vih pell-**VIM**-eh-tree	☐	pelvis
perine/o **perine**al	pair-ih-**NEE**-oh pair-ih-**NEE**-al	☐	**perineum**
salping/o **salping**ectomy	sal-**PIN**-goh **sal**-pin-**JEK**-toh-mee	☐	eustachian tubes; also refers to **fallopian tubes**
-tocia dys**tocia**	**TOH**-see-ah dis-**TOH**-see-ah	☐	**labor**
vagin/o trans**vagin**al	**VAJ**-in-oh trans-**VAJ**-in-al	☐	vagina

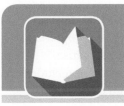

Review Checkpoint

Check your understanding of this section by completing the **Word Elements** exercises in your workbook.

Discomforts of Pregnancy

Throughout the pregnancy, the expectant mother will experience various discomforts. It is important that she realize these will be temporary discomforts and should subside after delivery. It is also important that the health care professional be aware of the difference between discomforts of pregnancy and signs of possible complications of pregnancy. The knowledgeable health care professional will have the responsibility of educating the patient regarding measures for relief of these temporary discomforts. The following list includes, but is not limited to, the more common discomforts of pregnancy.

backache	Backache is common during the second and third **trimesters** of pregnancy and is due to the body's adaptation to the stresses placed upon the back as the pregnancy progresses. Recommended treatment includes encouraging good posture, wearing comfortable shoes, getting adequate rest, and bending from the knees—not from the waist.
edema	**Edema**, or swelling, of the lower extremities is not uncommon in pregnancy (particularly as the pregnancy progresses). Recommended treatment includes elevating the feet and legs when sitting, lying down when resting, drinking plenty of water, and avoiding foods high in sodium. If the **edema** is present in the hands and face also, it should be reported immediately to the physician because this could be an indication of complications of pregnancy.

fatigue	Fatigue usually occurs during the first **trimester** of pregnancy, disappears during the second **trimester**, and returns toward the end of the pregnancy. This is due to the body's adjustment to the stresses of pregnancy. Recommended treatment includes encouraging at least 8 to 10 hours of sleep per night and allowing for short naps during the day.
heartburn	Heartburn is also known as **pyrosis** (pyr/o = fever, fire + osis = condition). This discomfort occurs mainly in the last few weeks of pregnancy due to the pressure exerted on the esophagus by the enlarged, pregnant **uterus**. This pressure may also cause a return, or reflux, of gastric juices into the esophagus, resulting in a burning sensation, a condition known as **gastroesophageal reflux**. Recommended treatment includes avoiding greasy or spicy foods, drinking plenty of water, avoiding coffee, eating several small meals instead of three larger meals, sitting upright for an hour after eating, and lying with head and shoulders elevated.
hemorrhoids	**Hemorrhoids** are swollen veins of the rectum and anus that develop as a result of the increasing pressure on the area due to the progressing pregnancy. They usually disappear after delivery but can cause discomfort in the pregnant female. Recommended treatment includes drinking plenty of fluids to avoid constipation (which causes hemorrhoids to become more severe), soaking in warm-water baths, and applying topical anesthetic ointments.
nausea	Nausea usually occurs during the first **trimester** of pregnancy and is known as "morning sickness," although it may occur during the morning, in the afternoon, or throughout the day. Recommended treatment includes eating dry toast or crackers, eating small frequent meals, eating something before taking **prenatal** vitamins, or drinking fluids between meals instead of with meals. Any prolonged nausea and vomiting should be reported to the physician immediately, that is, severe nausea that is preventing proper eating and hydration or severe vomiting that persists.
varicose veins	**Varicose veins** are twisted, swollen veins that occur as a result of the blood pooling in the legs due to the added weight (from the pregnancy) to the lower extremities of the body. Recommended treatment includes the use of support hosiery, encouraging the pregnant woman to avoid crossing her legs, regular exercise of walking to increase the blood flow to the legs, and elevation of the feet and legs when sitting.

Complications of Pregnancy

For most women, pregnancy is a time of anticipation and excitement. Most begin pregnancy in a state of seemingly good health. All women look forward to completing the pregnancy without any complications and to delivering a normal, healthy baby. For most women, this will happen; for others it will not. Unfortunately, deviations from the normal course of pregnancy do occur in some women. Even though the reasons may be unclear as to why the complication occurs during the pregnancy, the warning signs may appear early enough to take preventive action.

Early and regular **prenatal** visits are essential to the well-being of the **fetus** and the mother. The regular monitoring of the **fetus**, the expectant mother, and her body's response to the pregnancy will provide the opportunity for skilled health professionals to anticipate some of the problems associated with pregnancy. Keen observation and listening skills are vital in an obstetrical office because it may be *what the patient says* or *how the patient looks* that sets off the warning signal. Some complications of pregnancy can be made less severe if treated early enough. Some may even be prevented.

Whether by phone or in person, the health care professional is often the first person to hear the complaints and concerns of the expectant mother. It is critical that this individual be knowledgeable of the signs and **symptoms** of complications of pregnancy, listening carefully as the patient describes her **symptoms** and immediately reporting deviations from the norm to the physician.

The following is a discussion of pregnancy-related complications, that is, those that occur during pregnancy and are not seen at other times in the female. These complications of pregnancy are listed in alphabetical order for easy reference; they are not listed in the order in which they might occur during pregnancy. Preexisting conditions that complicate pregnancy are not discussed in this chapter.

abortion (ah-**BOR**-shun)	Termination of a pregnancy before the **fetus** has reached a viable age; that is, an age at which the **fetus** could live outside of the uterine environment.

The medical consensus is that a **fetus** has not reached a viable age if it is under 20 weeks' **gestation** or under 500 g in weight. The term **abortion** is a medical term used to denote any type of termination of pregnancy before the age of viability. Many laypeople use the term *miscarriage* to describe a spontaneous **abortion**.

A spontaneous **abortion** is one that occurs on its own as a result of abnormalities of the maternal environment or abnormalities of the **embryo** or **fetus**. Most spontaneous abortions occur within the first three months of pregnancy.

Symptoms include vaginal bleeding, rhythmic uterine cramping, continual backache, and a feeling of pressure in the pelvic area. Tissue may be passed through the **vagina**, depending on the type of **abortion**.

A spontaneous **abortion** may be a complete **abortion** in which all products of **conception** are expelled, an incomplete **abortion** in which some but not all products of **conception** are expelled, or a threatened **abortion** in which the **symptoms** of an impending **abortion** are present (but ultrasound indicates that a live **fetus** is present).

Under any circumstances, when vaginal bleeding is reported during pregnancy, the health care professional should obtain detailed information about the nature of the bleeding and the length of the pregnancy and should report this to the physician immediately.

abruptio placenta (ah-**BRUP**-she-oh plah-**SEN**-tah)	The premature separation of a normally implanted **placenta** from the uterine wall after the pregnancy has passed 20 weeks' **gestation** or during **labor** (the birthing process).

Abruptio placenta is a dangerous and potentially life-threatening condition for both the mother and the **fetus** due to the potential for hemorrhage. When bleeding occurs on the maternal side of the **placenta** (the side that attaches to the uterine lining), a clot (hematoma) forms in the area. This can lead to the premature separation of the **placenta** in the area. The severity of the complications from **abruptio placenta** depend on the amount of bleeding and the size of the clot that forms. The degree of separation may range from partial to complete, with bleeding being concealed or apparent.

Abruptio placenta does not usually occur alone but may accompany other complications of pregnancy. Some of the conditions that may increase the risk of **abruptio placenta** are **hypertension**, use of cocaine by the expectant mother, trauma to the abdomen while pregnant (as in injury or abuse), and the presence of a short **umbilical cord** (creating tension on the **placenta** during the birth process).

A classic symptom of **abruptio placenta** is uterine tenderness with a boardlike firmness to the abdomen. Additional **symptoms** include vaginal bleeding accompanied by abdominal or low back pain or frequent cramplike contractions of the **uterus** (uterine irritability). If the bleeding is concealed, the patient may display other signs indicative of this such as **tachycardia**, **hypotension**, and restlessness. Treatment for **abruptio placenta** usually involves immediate delivery of the **fetus** by **cesarean section** if there are signs of fetal distress or if the expectant mother displays signs of hemorrhaging.

ectopic pregnancy (eck-**TOP**-ick **PREG**-nan-see) ecto- = outside	Abnormal implantation of a fertilized **ovum** outside the uterine cavity; also called a tubal pregnancy.

Approximately 90% of all ectopic pregnancies occur in the **fallopian tubes**. Other sites for ectopic implantation are the **ovaries** and the abdomen. Rarely are abdominal pregnancies carried to full term. See *Figure 18-11.*

Possible causes of **ectopic pregnancy** include scarring of the **fallopian tubes** due to infections, inflammation, or surgery; adhesions due to endometriosis; congenital defects causing deformity of the tubes; **pregnancy**

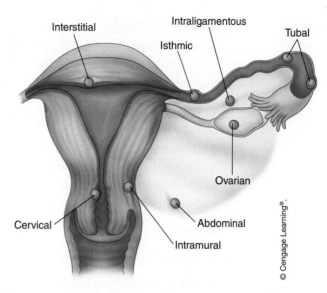

Figure 18-11 Potential sites for ectopic pregnancy

occurring while an IUD (intrauterine device) is in place; and maternal age over 35 years. Tubal pregnancies usually rupture between 6 and 12 weeks' **gestation**. Some women do not even realize that they are pregnant because the more common signs of pregnancy may not be present during the early stage of **gestation**. **Symptoms** include vaginal spotting (usually dark) and sharp abdominal pain (usually described as colicky or cramping).

Diagnosis of an **ectopic pregnancy** is often confirmed with a positive pregnancy test (ruling out other conditions) and **transvaginal ultrasonography,** which will reveal the absence of a gestational sac within the **uterus.** The physician may perform a culdocentesis to rule out a ruptured **ectopic pregnancy.** The aspiration of unclotted blood from the cul-de-sac area may indicate bleeding from a ruptured fallopian tube. The aspiration of clear fluid from the area would rule out a ruptured fallopian tube.

If ultrasound and **culdocentesis** are inconclusive and **symptoms** indicate the possibility of an **ectopic pregnancy, laparoscopy** may be necessary to confirm the diagnosis. For an unruptured **ectopic pregnancy** (tubal pregnancy), treatment usually includes surgery to remove the products of **conception** from the area. However, if the unruptured **ectopic pregnancy** is caught early enough, medications may be used instead of surgery to treat the ectopic pregnancy. *Methotrexate©* is the most commonly used medication to treat ectopic pregnancies that are caught early. The medication will stop the growth of the cells, ending the pregnancy, and the body will absorb it over time, thus saving the affected fallopian tube. A ruptured **ectopic pregnancy** is much more serious, with the potential being present for hemorrhage and **hypovolemic shock** (diminished blood volume). The affected tube is surgically removed **(salpingectomy)** and the bleeding is brought under control by tying (ligating) the bleeding vessels. Although the chances may decline, it is possible for a woman to have successful subsequent pregnancies with only one fallopian tube present.

gestational diabetes (jess-**TAY**-shun-al dye-ah-**BEE**-teez)	A disorder in which women who are not diabetic before pregnancy develop diabetes during the pregnancy; that is, they develop an inability to metabolize carbohydrates (glucose intolerance), with resultant hyperglycemia.

This disorder develops during the latter part of pregnancy, with **symptoms** usually disappearing at the end of the pregnancy. Women who have **gestational diabetes** have a higher possibility of developing it with subsequent pregnancies. They are also at higher risk of developing diabetes later in life. Factors that increase the risk of developing **gestational diabetes** include, but are not limited to, the following:

- Obesity

- Maternal age over 30 years

- History of birthing large babies (usually over 10 pounds)

- Family history of diabetes

- Previous, unexplained stillborn birth

- Previous birth with congenital anomalies (defects)

Symptoms vary from classic **symptoms** of diabetes—such as excessive thirst, hunger, and frequent urination—to being asymptomatic (no **symptoms** present). Because a high number of pregnant women have **gestational diabetes** without obvious **symptoms**, all pregnant women are routinely screened for diabetes with a blood test usually between weeks 24 and 28 of the pregnancy.

HELLP syndrome	The acronym HELLP stands for **H** (hemolysis: breaking down of red blood cells), **EL** (elevated liver enzymes), and **LP** (low platelet count).

HELLP syndrome is a group of **symptoms** that occur in approximately 10% of pregnant women with **preeclampsia** or **eclampsia**. However, many patients with HELLP syndrome may not have signs or **symptoms** of severe **preeclampsia**. They may have a normal blood pressure or only slight elevations, and **proteinuria** may be absent. Because the **symptoms** are present in other conditions, this serious obstetrical complication can be frequently misdiagnosed at first as cholecystitis, hepatitis, or idiopathic thrombocytopenia.

The diagnosis of HELLP syndrome can be frustrating to physicians due to the vague nature of the complaints expressed by the patient. Patients may present with any of the following **symptoms**: generalized malaise (most frequent), epigastric pain, nausea and vomiting, and headache. Physical examination may be normal, but right upper quadrant tenderness is often present. Most commonly, HELLP syndrome is seen in older Caucasian women who have had multiple births.

Early diagnosis is critical. Therefore, any woman who presents with malaise or a viral-type illness in the third **trimester** of pregnancy should be evaluated and should have a complete blood cell count and liver function tests. Laboratory diagnosis is necessary to confirm HELLP syndrome.

Treatment is usually based on the estimated gestational age and the condition of the mother and the **fetus**. If the pregnancy is close to term (34 weeks and beyond), delivery may be the treatment of choice. Delivery is usually by cesarean section. If the pregnancy is less than 34 weeks' gestation and the complications of HELLP are rapidly getting worse, premature delivery of the baby may still be necessary to prevent harmful effects to the mother and the baby. If the pregnancy is not close to term, conservative measures may be used. Bed rest may be ordered, and the patient is monitored closely to prevent further complications.

hydatidiform mole (high-dah-**TID**-ih-form mohl)	An abnormal condition that begins as a pregnancy and deviates from normal development very early. The diseased **ovum** deteriorates (not producing a **fetus**), and the chorionic villi of the **placenta** (small vessels protruding from the outer layer) change to a mass of cysts resembling a bunch of grapes.

The growth of this mass progresses much more rapidly than uterine growth with a normal pregnancy. A **hydatidiform mole** is known as a molar pregnancy; also called a hydatid mole.

Symptoms include, but are not limited to, extreme nausea, uterine bleeding, anemia, an unusually large **uterus** for the duration of pregnancy (at three months the uterus may be the size expected at five or six months), absence of fetal heart sounds, **edema**, and **hypertension**. Diagnosis is confirmed through the use of **ultrasonography** (no fetal skeleton will be visible) and laboratory findings (the human chronic gonadotropin [HCG] level will be extremely high).

Treatment options include evacuation of the **uterus**, followed by a **dilation** and curettage when the uterine wall has regained its firmness (a few days later) or a hysterectomy (in which the **uterus** is removed). The age of the woman and the condition of the **uterus** will be factors determining the need for a hysterectomy. The tissue from the mass will be tested for presence of malignant (cancerous) cells.

Follow-up treatment involves close medical supervision for about one year following a molar pregnancy. This will include careful monitoring of the HCG levels (until they return to normal) and avoidance of another pregnancy for at least a year after all tests are negative. If no malignancy is detected and the HCG levels decrease, the prognosis (prediction of the outcome) is favorable.

hyperemesis gravidarum
 	
(high-per-**EM**-eh-sis
grav-ih-**DAR**-um)
 	
  hyper- = excessive
  -emesis = to vomit
  gravid/o = pregnancy
	An abnormal condition of pregnancy characterized by severe vomiting that results in maternal dehydration and weight loss.

The nausea and vomiting associated with **hyperemesis gravidarum** persists beyond the first three months of pregnancy and persists throughout the day to the point that eventually nothing can be retained by mouth. The exact cause of this condition is unknown, but the incidence seems to be greater in younger mothers, first-time mothers, and those with increased body weight. Psychological factors have been considered as being instrumental in the development of **hyperemesis gravidarum** (such as stress over the pregnancy, ambivalent feelings toward the pregnancy, and conflicting feelings over becoming a mother). Physical factors may include hyperthyroidism, elevated levels of **estrogen**, a multiple pregnancy, and the presence of a **hydatidiform mole**.

Treatment includes control of the vomiting, replacement of lost fluids and electrolytes, and emotional support for the woman. In most women, **hyperemesis gravidarum** is self-limiting and health is restored.

incompetent cervix (in-**COMP**-eh-tent **SER**-viks)	A condition in which the cervical os (opening) dilates before the **fetus** reaches term, without **labor** or uterine contractions; usually occurring during the second **trimester** of pregnancy and resulting in a spontaneous **abortion** of the **fetus**.

Treatment for an **incompetent cervix** involves suturing the **cervix** to keep it from opening during the pregnancy. This is known as **cerclage**. If the woman is going to have a vaginal delivery, the sutures are removed near the end of the pregnancy. If she is to have a cesarean section delivery, the sutures may be left in place.

placenta previa (plah-**SEN**-tah **PRE**-vee-ah)	A condition of pregnancy in which the **placenta** is implanted in the lower part of the **uterus** and precedes the **fetus** during the birthing process.

The cause (etiology) is unknown. The degree of **placenta previa** may range from marginal previa—when the **placenta** barely comes to the edge of the cervical os (opening)—to partial previa (when the **placenta** partially covers the cervical os), to total previa when the **placenta** completely covers the cervical os. See *Figure 18-12*.

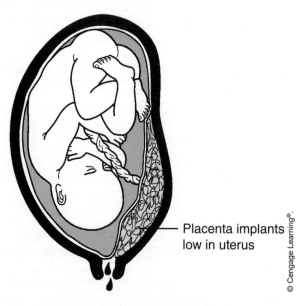

Placenta implants low in uterus

© Cengage Learning®.

Figure 18-12 Example of placenta previa

The classic symptom of **placenta previa** is painless bleeding during the third **trimester** of pregnancy. The bleeding is usually abrupt and bright red and very frightening to the expectant mother.

Diagnosis of **placenta previa** is confirmed by **ultrasonography**. Sometimes it is detected before **symptoms** occur, through routine use of **ultrasonography**.

Treatment ranges from conservative measures of bed rest to immediate delivery by cesarean section, depending on the condition of the expectant mother and the condition of the **fetus**, that is, maturity of **fetus** and whether fetal distress is detected.

pregnancy-induced hypertension	The development of **hypertension** (high blood pressure) during pregnancy in women who had normal blood pressure readings (normotensive) prior to pregnancy.

For ease in understanding, pregnancy-induced hypertension (PIH) is divided into three categories based on degree of severity.

1. **Gestational hypertension** is the development of **hypertension** after 20 weeks' gestation, with no signs of **edema** or **proteinuria**. A blood pressure reading of 140/90 mmHg or greater on more than one occasion or a blood pressure reading of 30 mm Hg systolic or 15 mm Hg diastolic over the patient's normal baseline readings are indicative of **gestational hypertension**. The **hypertension** usually subsides after pregnancy.

2. **Preeclampsia** is the development of **hypertension** (as defined previously) with the presence of **proteinuria** after 20 weeks' **gestation** in a woman who previously had normal blood pressure. The factor that distinguishes **preeclampsia** from **gestational hypertension** is the presence of **proteinuria**. The patient may also exhibit **edema** of the hands and face.

   Edema of the feet and legs is common during pregnancy. However, **edema** that occurs above the waist may be indicative of pregnancy-induced hypertension. One of the first signs of **edema** may be a sudden rapid weight gain of more than 4 pounds in a week. This may be followed by visible signs of **edema**, such as puffiness or swelling of the face and hands. The woman may remove the rings from her fingers as they seem increasingly tight on the fingers.

   It is important that the health care professional carefully monitor the pregnant woman's weight and vital signs during each **prenatal** visit and that any rise in blood pressure be taken seriously and considered a possible indication of impending complications. It is also important that early measures be taken to lower the blood pressure, reduce the **edema**, and correct the **proteinuria**.

   If the condition worsens, the patient with **preeclampsia** may experience blurred vision or see spots in front of the eyes and complain of severe headaches and epigastric pain. These **symptoms** are strong indicators of impending **eclampsia**, and medical treatment will be necessary.

3. **Eclampsia** is the most severe form of **hypertension** during pregnancy and is evidenced by the presence of seizures. An eclamptic seizure may jeopardize the life of the expectant mother and her **fetus**.

Delivery of the baby is the cure for pregnancy-induced hypertension. If it is determined that the **fetus** is mature enough for delivery, the pregnancy is ended by inducing **labor** or by performing a cesarean section. If the **fetus** is not mature enough for delivery, medical treatment will involve hospitalization of the expectant mother, bed rest, administration of medications to reduce her blood pressure, and administration of medications to prevent convulsions until the baby can be delivered.

Rh incompatibility	An incompatibility between an Rh negative mother's blood with her Rh positive baby's blood, causing the mother's body to develop antibodies that will destroy the Rh positive blood.

All blood types either have the Rh factor or they do not. Individuals who have the Rh factor present on their red blood cells are said to be Rh positive. Those who do not have it are said to be Rh negative. **Rh incompatibility** can occur if the father of the baby is Rh positive and the mother of the baby is Rh negative. It does not occur when the expectant mother is Rh positive.

An Rh negative mother will give birth to either an Rh negative baby or an Rh positive baby. If her baby is Rh negative, the two are compatible. If her baby is Rh positive, the potential for incompatibility in subsequent births is present. During the birth process, if there is a mixing of Rh negative maternal and Rh positive fetal blood (as the **placenta** separates from the uterine wall), the mother's blood will recognize this as foreign to her body and will respond by producing antibodies to destroy the Rh positive blood.

The first Rh positive baby born to an Rh negative mother will not be affected by an Rh incompatibility. However, the antibodies that develop in response to the first pregnancy will be present during subsequent pregnancies. If a subsequent pregnancy produces an Rh positive **fetus**, the antibody production will increase. These antibodies are small enough to cross the placental barrier into the fetal circulation and destroy the red blood cells of the **fetus**, which have been recognized as "foreign" to the mother's body.

Treatment for prevention of Rh incompatibility is to administer an injection of Rh immune globulin (RhoGAM) to the Rh negative, pregnant woman during week 28 of pregnancy. If she gives birth to an Rh positive baby, she will be administered another injection of RhoGAM within 72 hours after the birth. The administration of this Rh immune globulin will prevent the formation of the antibodies in the Rh negative mother's blood. It is important that an Rh negative woman realizes that if her first pregnancy ends in **abortion**, it is still counted as a pregnancy, and she should receive the injection of RhoGAM after the **abortion** to prevent the formation of antibodies that will affect future pregnancies, should the **fetus** be Rh positive.

Review Checkpoint

Check your understanding of this section by completing the **Complications of Pregnancy** exercises in your workbook.

Signs and Symptoms of Labor

The material listed in this segment is an elementary discussion of the signs and **symptoms** of impending **labor** and comparison of true **labor** and false **labor**.

bloody show	A vaginal discharge that is a mixture of thick mucus and pink or dark brown blood. It may begin a few weeks prior to the onset of **labor** and occurs as a result of the softening, **dilation**, and **effacement** (thinning) of the **cervix** in preparation for childbirth. The **bloody show** will continue and will increase during **labor** as the **cervix** continues to dilate and efface.
Braxton Hicks contractions	Mild, irregular contractions that occur throughout pregnancy. As full term approaches, these contractions intensify and are sometimes mistaken for true **labor**.
increased vaginal discharge	When the baby settles into the pelvis prior to the onset of **labor**, the pressure of the baby's head in the area creates congestion of the vaginal mucosa, which results in an increase in clear, nonirritating vaginal secretions.
lightening	The expectant mother will notice that she can breathe easier because the descent of the baby relieves some of the pressure from her diaphragm. When **lightening** occurs, most expectant mothers will refer to it by saying that the baby has "dropped." Lightening is more obvious in women who are having their first baby.
rupture of the amniotic sac	The **rupture of the amniotic sac** (membranes) may occur prior to the onset of **labor**, may occur during **labor**, or may not occur without assistance. Expectant mothers are usually advised to report to the hospital or birthing center for evaluation if the membranes rupture prior to the onset of **labor**. This is important because the amniotic sac serves as a barrier between the baby and the unsterile outside environment, and when broken the chance for infection is increased. Women often refer to the rupture of the amniotic sac by saying their "water broke," because there may be a sudden gush of **amniotic fluid** as the membranes rupture.
sudden burst of energy	This occurs in some women shortly before the onset of **labor**. These women may suddenly have the energy to do major housecleaning duties—things they have not had the energy to do previously.

They should be cautioned to save their energy during this time so they will not be fatigued when **labor** actually begins. The essential distinction between false **labor** and true **labor** is that true **labor** is characterized by progressive change in the **cervix**. For the baby to pass from the uterine cavity and descend through the vaginal canal to the outside of the body, the **cervix** must dilate (enlarge) and efface (thin) to allow passage. See *Figure 18-13*.

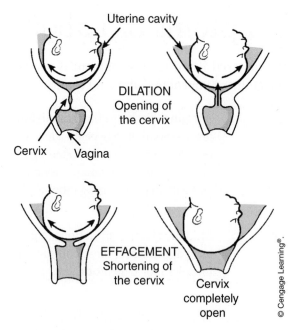

Figure 18-13 Dilation and effacement of the cervix

Preparations for childbirth should be discussed with the expectant mother regardless if she has attended **prenatal** classes. This will allow the health care professional the opportunity to review the signs and **symptoms** of impending **labor**, assist the expectant mother in distinguishing between false **labor** and true **labor**, and answer any questions that might follow the discussion. For the learner's convenience, the comparison of false **labor** to true **labor** is arranged in *Table 18-2*.

Table 18-2 Comparison of False Labor and True Labor

False Labor	True Labor
1. Contractions Irregular Not too frequent Shorter duration Not too intense	1. Contractions Regular More frequent Longer duration More intense
2. Discomfort Felt in abdomen Felt in groin area	2. Discomfort Felt in lower back Radiates to lower abdomen Feels like menstrual cramps
3. Walking May relieve or decrease contractions	3. Walking May strengthen contractions
4. Effacement/Dilation Dilation and effacement of cervix does not change	4. Effacement/Dilation Cervix progressively effaces (thins) and dilates (enlarges)

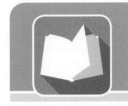

Review Checkpoint

Check your understanding of this section by completing the **Signs and Symptoms of Labor** exercises in your workbook.

Diagnostic Techniques, Treatments, and Procedures

AFP screening

AFP (**alpha-fetoprotein**) is a serum screening test that checks the level of AFP in a pregnant woman's blood. The amount of AFP in the pregnant woman's blood—along with her age and other factors—help the health care provider estimate the chance that the baby may have certain problems or birth defects, such as spina bifida (defective closure of the vertebrae of the spinal column), trisomy 21 (Down syndrome), and trisomy 18 (severe mental retardation and severe birth defects).

The test is offered to pregnant women between 15 and 21 weeks' **gestation**. The AFP offers enhanced **prenatal** screening for these birth defects and can detect approximately 80% of the cases of spina bifida, approximately 75% to 80% of the cases of Down syndrome, and approximately 60% of the cases of trisomy 18.

The AFP test does not confirm that the pregnant woman has these complications but indicates whether the individual might be at high risk for one of these conditions. Additional testing will be offered for positive results, such as ultrasound or **amniocentesis**. In addition, a negative test does not eliminate the possibility of having a child affected by one of these conditions but does greatly reduce the likelihood that the **fetus** has one of these conditions. In addition to AFP screening, multiple marker screenings are also offered between 15 and 21 weeks' gestation. These include Triple Screen Test and Quad Screen Test; both tests include AFP in addition to other markers. The Quad Screen Test is also known as AFP Tetra Maternal Screen Screening. One of the newest tests available is the *Free Fetal DNA Test*, which identifies pregnancies that may be at risk for trisomy 21, 18, and 13.

amniocentesis

am-nee-oh-sen-**TEE**-sis)

amni/o = amnion
-centesis = surgical puncture

A surgical puncture of the amniotic sac for the purpose of removing **amniotic fluid** for examination.

A needle is passed through the abdomen and **uterus** into the amniotic sac. Fluid is removed for laboratory analysis to detect fetal abnormalities and maternal–fetal blood incompatibilities and to determine fetal maturity. An amniocentesis may also be ordered to establish fetal lung maturity when early delivery of the baby is being considered for medical reasons. If necessary, an amniocentesis is usually performed between 16 and 20 weeks' **gestation**. See *Figure 18-14*.

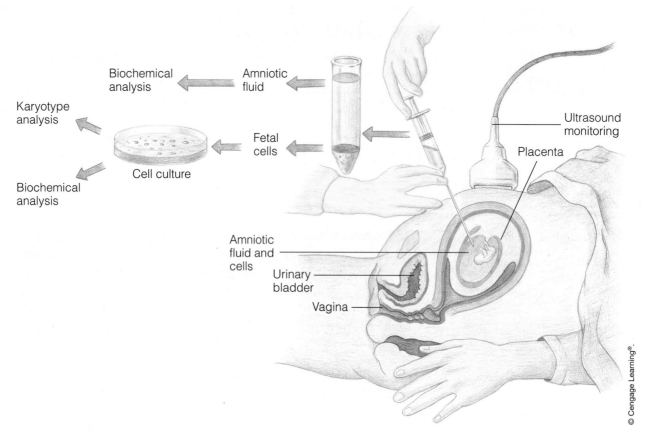

Figure 18-14 Amniocentesis

cesarean section (see-**SAYR**-ee-an section)	A surgical procedure in which the abdomen and **uterus** are incised and a baby is delivered transabdominally. Also known as cesarean delivery.
	It is performed when abnormal fetal or maternal conditions exist that are judged likely to make a vaginal delivery hazardous. See *Figure 18-15*.
chorionic villus sampling (**koh**-ree-**ON**-ik **VILL**-us sampling)	Chorionic villus sampling (CVS) is a prenatal diagnostic test performed in the first **trimester** of pregnancy to detect chromosomal abnormalities (such as Down syndrome) in an unborn child.
	The procedure involves removing a small amount of placental tissue during the 11th to 13th week of pregnancy for genetic testing. (Chorionic villi tissue originates from the same fertilized egg as the **fetus** and contains the same genetic data as the **fetus**.)
	During the procedure, a thin needle is inserted, either through the **cervix** or through the abdomen, into the **uterus** to remove the placental tissue. The tissue that is removed is analyzed for fetal genetic disorders. The patient may feel a slight cramping during the procedure. This invasive test has about a 1% risk of miscarriage.
contraction stress test	A stress test used to evaluate the ability of the **fetus** to tolerate the stress of **labor** and delivery (CST); also known as oxytocin challenge test.
	The hormone oxytocin is diluted in an IV solution and is administered intravenously to the expectant mother to stimulate uterine contractions. The

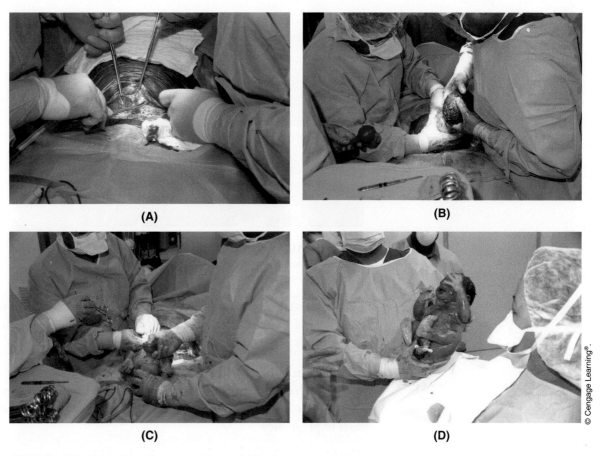

Figure 18-15 Cesarean section (A) The central muscle is retracted and dissected to access the fascia (B) The infant's head is delivered through the incision, followed by the remainder of his body (C) The infant's mouth and nose are suctioned immediately to remove amniotic fluid from the airway (D) The infant is handed to the nursery personnel, who receive him in a sterile blanket.

amount of oxytocin infused into the patient is monitored and is increased every 15 to 20 minutes until three uterine contractions, lasting approximately 30 to 40 seconds, are observed within a 10-minute period. The fetal heart rate (FHR) is then interpreted, and the infusion of oxytocin is discontinued.

The purpose of the oxytocin challenge test is to simulate **labor** for a measurable period of time to determine if the infant will tolerate **labor** well. During **labor**, uterine contractions decrease the oxygen supply to the **fetus**. If there is a significant decrease in the oxygen supply, it may cause a decrease in the fetal heart rate.

The maternal uterine activity and the fetal heart rate are monitored closely during this stress test. If it appears that the contractions of the **uterus** will endanger the **fetus** as **labor** progresses, an emergency cesarean section may be indicated.

fetal monitoring (electronic)	The use of an electronic device to monitor the fetal heart rate and the maternal uterine contractions. This procedure can be done with external or internal devices.
(**FEE**-tal **MON**-ih-tor-ing)	

This monitoring is valuable during **labor** to assess the quality of the uterine contractions and the effects of **labor** on the **fetus**. See *Figure 18-16*.

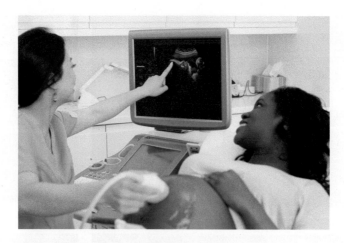

Figure 18-16 Fetal monitoring
(*© Monkey Business Images/Shutterstock.com*)

first trimester screening

First trimester screening consists of a blood test (maternal serum sample) and an ultrasound to identify pregnancies at risk for birth defects such as Down syndrome and trisomy 18.

The test can indicate whether the **fetus** has a higher or lower than average risk to have either condition. This screening can be performed as early as 11 weeks and one day of pregnancy but no later than 13 weeks and six days of pregnancy.

The blood test measures 2 proteins produced by the pregnancy, PAPP-A (pregnancy associated plasma protein-A) and beta HCG (beta human chorionic gonadotropin). The ultrasound measures the thickness of the skin on the back of the fetal neck (the nuchal translucency). Based on the results of the blood test and the nuchal translucency test, an analysis can be performed to estimate the risk for Down syndrome and trisomy 18 in the pregnancy. If the nuchal translucency (NT) measurement is significantly increased, the **fetus** is at increased risk for other birth defects, and a level II ultrasound would be recommended during the second **trimester** of pregnancy.

The first trimester screening is accurate for detecting over 90% of fetuses with Down syndrome and 98% with trisomy 18. A positive first trimester screen result does not mean that a **fetus** is definitely affected with Down syndrome but does indicate that the risk for this condition is increased.

First trimester screening is a noninvasive test and therefore causes no physical risk to the **fetus**. If abnormal test results are obtained, the mother is referred for diagnostic testing such as chorionic villus sampling (CVS) or amniocentesis.

nipple stimulation test

A noninvasive technique that produces basically the same results as the **contraction stress test** by having the pregnant woman stimulate the nipples of her breasts by rubbing them between her fingers.

This causes the natural release of oxytocin that causes contractions of the **uterus**. The nipple stimulation test is less stressing to the **uterus**.

obstetrical ultrasound

(ob-**STET**-rik-al **ULL**-trah-sound)

Ultrasound (also called **ultrasonography**) is a noninvasive procedure that uses high-frequency sound waves to examine internal structures of the body. In the field of **obstetrics**, **ultrasonography** is used to examine the internal structures and contents of the **uterus**. It can be used to detect very early pregnancy as well as the size and development of the **fetus**. It is also used to confirm complications of pregnancy such as **placenta previa**, breech presentation, and other abnormal positions of the **fetus**. **Ultrasonography** is also a valuable tool for diagnosis of multiple gestations.

When the transducer passes over the abdomen, the sound waves are transmitted into the **uterus** and are reflected back into the transducer (where they are interpreted by a computer). It is helpful if the pregnant woman has a full bladder at the time of the ultrasound, in that the full bladder provides an anatomical landmark for the sonographer to identify the **uterus** and surrounding structures such as the ovaries, **fallopian tubes**, and other significant structures. For a visual image of a three-dimensional ultrasound of a 28 weeks' **gestation fetus**, see *Figure 18-17*.

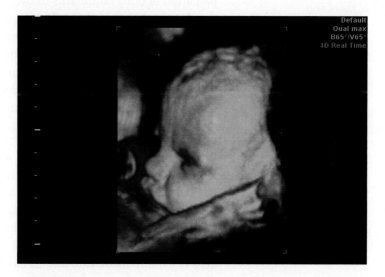

Figure 18-17 3-D ultrasound of 28 weeks' gestation fetus
(Courtesy of Ward Adcock, M.D., Gastonia, NC)

pelvic ultrasound

(**PELL**-vik **ULL**-trah-sound)

A noninvasive procedure that uses high-frequency sound waves to examine the pelvis.

The sound waves pass through the abdominal wall from the transducer, which is moved back and forth across the abdomen. When the sound waves bounce from the internal organs in the pelvic region, these waves are converted to electrical impulses eventually recorded on an oscilloscope screen. A photograph of the images is then taken for further study. See *Figure 18-18*.

Pelvic ultrasound can be used to locate a pelvic mass, an **ectopic pregnancy**, or an intrauterine device and to inspect and assess the **uterus**,

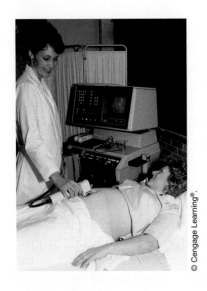

© Cengage Learning®.

ovaries, and **fallopian tubes**. Clearer ultrasonic pictures of the pelvic organs can be obtained by using **transvaginal ultrasonography**. This procedure produces the same type of picture as abdominal ultrasound but involves the use of a vaginal probe inserted into the **vagina** while the patient is in lithotomy position. The probes are encased in a sterile sheath and placed in the transducer before it is inserted into the **vagina**. The sound waves function in the same way as those for the abdominopelvic ultrasound, but the transvaginal ultrasonic image is much clearer.

Figure 18-18 Pelvic ultrasound

pelvimetry (pell-**VIM**-eh-tree) **pelv/i** = pelvis **-metry** = the process of measuring	The process of measuring the female pelvis, manually or by X-ray, to determine its adequacy for childbearing. Clinical **pelvimetry** is an estimate of the size of the birth canal by vaginal palpation of bony landmarks in the pelvis and a mathematical estimate of the distance between them. This is performed during the early part of the pregnancy and is recorded as "adequate," "borderline," or "inadequate." This measurement gives the examiner an impression of pelvic size, but is rarely used as criteria to skip labor and perform a cesarean section. A true test of pelvic adequacy for vaginal delivery is a "trial labor." The baby will or will not fit into the pelvic inlet, and the labor will or will not progress. X-ray **pelvimetry** is an actual X-ray of the pelvis to determine the dimensions of the bony pelvis of a pregnant woman. It is performed when there is doubt that the head of the **fetus** can safely pass through the pelvis during the **labor** process. Measurements are actually made on the X-ray, and the true dimensions of the birth canal and the head of the **fetus** can be calculated to determine if the proportions are suitable. Studies on pregnant women have indicated that X-ray pelvimetry is usually most valuable in cases of a normal pelvis or gross bony disproportion. It appears to be least effective in those with a "borderline" pelvis, in which the proper management of the patient would require an adequate trial of labor.
pregnancy testing	Tests performed on maternal urine and/or blood to determine the presence of the hormone HCG (human chorionic gonadotropin). HCG is detected shortly after the first missed menstrual period. Tests performed on blood are highly reliable and results are usually available in approximately one hour. Tests performed on urine are fairly accurate when done correctly and are very popular in the form of home testing kits. Results are available within minutes. Women using home testing kits should test the first voided urine specimen of the day because the level of HCG is highest at that time.

Review Checkpoint

Check your understanding of this section by completing the **Diagnostic Techniques, Treatments, and Procedures** exercises in your workbook.

COMMON ABBREVIATIONS

Abbreviation	Meaning	Abbreviation	Meaning
AFP	alpha-fetoprotein	HELLP	*Hemolysis*, *E*levated *L*iver enzymes, *Low P*latelet count
C-section	cesarean section	L & D	labor and delivery
CS	cesarean section	LMP	last menstrual period
CST	contraction stress test	LNMP	last normal menstrual period
EDB	expected date of birth	Multip	multipara
EDC	expected date of confinement; estimated date of confinement (i.e., estimated date for birth of baby)	NSD	normal spontaneous delivery
		NST	non-stress test
EDD	expected date of delivery	OB	obstetrics
EFM	electronic fetal monitoring	Primip	primipara
FHR	fetal heart rate	SVD	spontaneous vaginal delivery
FHS, FHT	fetal heart sound; fetal heart tone	TPAL	term, preterm, abortions, living (this is used on obstetrical history forms to obtain patient data)
FSH	follicle-stimulating hormone		
G	gravida (pregnant)		
GPA	gravida, para, **abortion**	UC	uterine contractions
HCG	human chorionic gonadotropin		

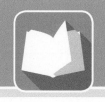

Review Checkpoint

Check your understanding of this section by completing the **Common Abbreviations** exercises in your workbook.

WRITTEN AND AUDIO TERMINOLOGY REVIEW

Review each of the following terms from this chapter. Study the spelling of each term and write the definition in the space provided. Check definitions by looking the term up in the glossary.

Term	Pronunciation	Definition
abortion	☐ ah-**BOR**-shun	_____
abruptio placenta	☐ ah-**BRUP**-she-oh plah-**SEN**-tah	_____
alpha-fetoprotein	☐ **AL**-fah fee-toh-**PRO**-teen	_____
amenorrhea	☐ **ah**-men-oh-**REE**-ah	_____
amnion	☐ **AM**-nee-on	_____
amniotic fluid	☐ **am**-nee-**OT**-ik **FLOO**-id	_____
areola	☐ ah-**REE**-oh-lah	_____
ballottement	☐ bah-**LOT**-ment	_____
cerclage	☐ sair-**KLOGH**	_____
cervix	☐ **SER**-viks	_____
chloasma	☐ kloh-**AZ**-mah	_____
chorion	☐ **KOH**-ree-on	_____
coitus	☐ **KOH**-ih-tus	_____
colostrum	☐ koh-**LOSS**-trum	_____
conception	☐ con-**SEP**-shun	_____
copulation	☐ **kop**-yoo-**LAY**-shun	_____
corpus luteum	☐ **COR**-pus **LOO**-tee-um	_____
culdocentesis	☐ **kull**-doh-sen-**TEE**-sis	_____
dilation	☐ dye-**LAY**-shun	_____
eclampsia	☐ eh-**KLAMP**-see-ah	_____
ectopic pregnancy	☐ eck-**TOP**-ick **PREG**-nan-see	_____
edema	☐ eh-**DEE**-mah	_____
effacement	☐ eh-**FACE**-ment	_____
ejaculation	☐ eh-**jak**-yoo-**LAY**-shun	_____
embryo	☐ **EM**-bree-oh	_____
endometrium	☐ **en**-doh-**MEE**-tree-um	_____

Term	Pronunciation	Definition
episiotomy	☐ eh-**piz**-ee-**OT**-oh-mee	_____
estrogen	☐ **ESS**-troh-jen	_____
fallopian tubes	☐ fah-**LOH**-pee-**an** tubes	_____
fertilization	☐ **fer**-til-ih-**ZAY**-shun	_____
fetoscope	☐ **FEET**-oh-skohp	_____
fetus	☐ **FEE**-tus	_____
fimbriae	☐ **FIM**-bree-ay	_____
gamete	☐ **GAM**-eet	_____
gastroesophageal reflux	☐ **gas**-troh-eh-**soff**-ah-**JEE**-al **REE**-flucks	_____
gestation	☐ jess-**TAY**-shun	_____
gestational diabetes	☐ jess-**TA**Y-shun-al **dye**-ah-**BEE**-teez	_____
gestational hypertension	☐ jess-**TAY**-shun-al high-per-**TEN**-shun	_____
glycogen	☐ **GLYE**-koh-jen	_____
graafian follicles	☐ **GRAF**-ee-an-**FOL**-ik-kulz	_____
Hegar's sign	☐ **HAY**-garz sign	_____
hydatidiform mole	☐ **high**-dah-**TID**-ih-form mohl	_____
hyperemesis gravidarum	☐ **high**-per-**EM**-eh-sis **grav**-ih-**DAR**-um	_____
hyperpigmentation	☐ **high**-per-**pig**-men-**TAY**-shun	_____
hypertension	☐ **high**-per-**TEN**-shun	_____
hypotension	☐ **high**-poh-**TEN**-shun	_____
hypovolemic shock	☐ **high**-poh-voh-**LEE**-mik shock	_____
incompetent cervix	☐ in-**COMP**-eh-tent **SER**-viks	_____
labor	☐ **LAY**-bor	_____
lactation	☐ lak-**TAY**-shun	_____
lactiferous ducts	☐ lak-**TIF**-er-us ducts	_____
laparoscopy	☐ **lap**-ar-**OSS**-koh-pee	_____
leukorrhea	☐ **loo**-koh-**REE**-ah	_____
linea nigra	☐ **LIN**-ee-ah **NIG**-rah	_____
lordosis	☐ lor-**DOH**-sis	_____
multigravida	☐ **mull**-tih-**GRAV**-ih-dah	_____

Term	Pronunciation	Definition
multipara	☐ mull-**TIP**-ah-rah	_____
Nagele's rule	☐ **NAY**-geh-leez rule	_____
neonatology	☐ **nee**-oh-nay-**TOL**-oh-jee	_____
nullipara	☐ nuh-**LIP**-ah-rah	_____
obstetrician	☐ ob-steh-**TRISH**-an	_____
obstetrics	☐ ob-**STET**-riks	_____
ovary	☐ **OH**-vah-ree	_____
ovulation	☐ **ov**-you-**LAY**-shun	_____
ovum	☐ **OH**-vum	_____
parturition	☐ par-too-**RISH**-un	_____
pelvic ultrasound	☐ **PELL**-vik **ULL**-tra-sound	_____
pelvimetry	☐ pell-**VIM**-eh-tree	_____
perineum	☐ **pair**-ih-**NEE**-um	_____
placenta	☐ plah-**SEN**-tah	_____
placenta previa	☐ plah-**SEN**-tah **PRE**-vee-ah	_____
preeclampsia	☐ **pre**-eh-**KLAMP**-see-ah	_____
prenatal	☐ pre-**NAY**-tal	_____
primigravida	☐ **prye**-mih-**GRAV**-ih-dah	_____
primipara	☐ prye-**MIP**-ah-rah	_____
progesterone	☐ proh-**JES**-ter-ohn	_____
proteinuria	☐ **proh**-teen-**YOO**-ree-ah	_____
puberty	☐ **PEW**-ber-tee	_____
pyrosis	☐ pye-**ROH**-sis	_____
quickening	☐ **KWIK**-en-ing	_____
salpingectomy	☐ **sal**-pin-**JEK**-toh-mee	_____
striae gravidarum	☐ **STRIGH**-ay grav-ih-**DAR**-um	_____
symptoms	☐ **SIM**-toms	_____
tachycardia	☐ **tak**-eh-**CAR**-dee-ah	_____
testes	☐ **TESS**-teez	_____
transvaginal ultrasonography	☐ trans-**VAJ**-in-al ull-trah-son-**OG**-rah-fee	_____
trimester	☐ **TRY**-mes-ter	_____
ultrasonography	☐ **ull**-tra-son- **OG**-rah-fee	_____
umbilical cord	☐ um-**BILL**-ih-kal cord	_____

Term	Pronunciation	Definition
uterus	☐ **YOO**-ter-us	_____
vagina	☐ vah-**JIGH**-nah	_____
waddling gait	☐ **WOD**-ling **GATE**	_____

Review Checkpoint

Apply what you have learned in this chapter by completing the **Putting It All Together** exercise in your workbook.

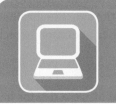

Online Resources

For additional study tools, such as PowerPoint® slides, go to the Student Companion Website.

Chapter Review Exercises

The following exercises provide a more in-depth review of the chapter material. Your goal in these exercises is to complete each section at a minimum 80% level of accuracy. If you score below 80% in any area, return to the appropriate section in the chapter and read the material again. A place has been provided for your score at the end of each section.

A. Spelling

Circle the correctly spelled term in each pairing of words. Each correct answer is worth 10 points. Record your score in the space provided at the end of the exercise.

1.	areola	ariola	6.	preclampsia	preeclampsia
2.	faloppian tubes	fallopian tubes	7.	cesarean	ceserean
3.	fimbrii	fimbria	8.	chloasthma	chloasma
4.	graafian follicles	graffian follicles	9.	effacement	efacement
5.	partuition	parturition	10.	obstetrics	obstetrix

Number correct _____ × ***10 points/correct answer: Your score*** _____ ***%***

B. Is She or Isn't She?

The following exercise will review some of the presumptive and probable signs of pregnancy. Read each statement carefully, decide if the symptom is a presumptive or probable sign of pregnancy, and check your choice in the space provided. Each correct response is worth 20 points. Record your score in the space provided at the end of the exercise.

1. April Jones is a 21-year-old junior in college. She and her fiancé are sexually active and use condoms as a means of birth control. She is usually regular with her menstrual periods but is two weeks late this month. At first she thought it might be because she is preparing for end-of-semester exams, but now she is not sure.

   ☐ Presumptive sign   ☐ Probable sign

2. Maria Quintana is a 35-year-old mother of three children, ages 2, 4, and 7. Lately she has experienced frequent fatigue and an increase in urination (urinary disturbances). Although Maria is using an IUD as a means of birth control, she is still concerned about the possibility of pregnancy, particularly in that she has had these symptoms with a previous pregnancy.

   ☐ Presumptive sign   ☐ Probable sign

3. Chin Soo-Young is a 26-year-old female who has come to the office today to find out if she is pregnant. She has done a pregnancy test at home and it was positive, but she continues to have her menstrual periods even though they are irregular. Her last "normal" period was four months ago. She has had no nausea or vomiting. For the last week, however, she has felt a slight flutter in her abdomen, which concerns her.

   ☐ Presumptive sign   ☐ Probable sign

4. Nicole Macormick is a 39-year-old mother of three children. She has come into the office today for her presurgery exam before having her tubal ligation next week. When the doctor performs the bimanual part of the pelvic examination, he notices that the lower segment of her uterus is soft and easy to palpate. He asks Nicole if she has missed a menstrual period. She confirms this, but states that it is not unusual for her to miss an occasional period.

   ☐ Presumptive sign   ☐ Probable sign

5. Theresa Bustos is a 24-year-old female who has been coming to the office for the past year for infertility studies. Today she is being seen for her third artificial insemination treatment (using her husband's sperm). When the doctor performs the pelvic examination prior to the procedure, he notices that Theresa's vagina has a bluish-violet color.

   ☐ Presumptive sign   ☐ Probable sign

Number correct _____ *× 20 points/correct answer: Your score* _____ %

C. Matching

Match the terms on the left with the applicable definitions on the right. Each correct answer is worth 10 points. Record your score in the space provided at the end of the exercise.

_____ 1. Chadwick's sign

_____ 2. Goodell's sign

_____ 3. embryo

_____ 4. fetus

_____ 5. chloasma

_____ 6. linea nigra

a. a technique that causes the fetus to bounce within the amniotic fluid, with the examiner feeling it rebound quickly

b. movement of the fetus felt by the mother

c. the name given to the product of conception from the second through the eighth week of pregnancy

d. a bluish-violet hue to the cervix and vagina

_____ 7. striae gravidarum

_____ 8. quickening

_____ 9. Braxton Hicks

_____ 10. ballottement

    e. absence of menstruation

    f. softening of the cervix, felt by the examiner

    g. "mask of pregnancy"

    h. the name given to the product of conception from the ninth week through the duration of the gestational period

    i. stretch marks on the abdomen, thighs, and breasts during pregnancy

    j. a dark line of pigmentation that may extend from the fundus to the symphysis pubis during pregnancy

    k. irregular contractions of the uterus that occur throughout pregnancy

_Number correct _____ × 10 points/correct answer: Your score _____%_

D. Word Element Review

The following words relate to the field of obstetrics. The prefixes and suffixes have been provided. Read the definition carefully and complete the word by filling in the blank, using the word elements provided in this chapter. If you have forgotten your word building rules, refer to Chapter 1. Each correct answer is worth 10 points. Record your score in the space provided at the end of this exercise.

1. Surgical puncture of the amniotic sac for the purpose of withdrawing amniotic fluid:
   _____ / centesis

2. Pertaining to before birth:
   pre / _____ / al

3. Surgical removal of a fallopian tube:
   _____ / ectomy

4. Pertaining to across the vagina:
   trans / _____ / al

5. A woman who is pregnant for the first time:
   primi / _____ / a

6. A woman who has borne no children:
   nulli / _____

7. Excessive vomiting:
   hyper / _____

8. Pertaining to the perineum:
   _____ / al

9. An instrument used to hear the fetal heartbeat through the mother's abdomen:
   _____ / _____ / scope

10. Difficult labor:
    dys / _____

_Number correct _____ × 10 points/correct answer: Your score _____%_

E. Completion

The following sentences provide a discussion of complications of pregnancy. Complete each sentence with the most appropriate word. Each correct answer is worth 10 points. Record your score in the space provided at the end of the exercise.

1. The premature separation of a normally implanted placenta from the uterine wall after the pregnancy has passed 20 weeks' gestation, or during labor, is known as:

    _____

2. The abnormal implantation of a fertilized ovum outside of the uterine cavity is known as:

    _____

3. Diabetes that develops during pregnancy is known as:

    _____

4. An abnormal condition of pregnancy characterized by severe vomiting that results in maternal dehydration and weight loss is known as:

    _____

5. A condition of pregnancy in which the placenta is implanted in the lower part of the uterus, and precedes the fetus during the birthing process, is known as:

    _____

6. A condition in which the cervical os dilates before the fetus reaches term, without uterine contractions, and results in a spontaneous abortion of the fetus is known as:

    _____

7. Hypertension that develops during pregnancy, after 20 weeks' gestation, with the presence of proteinuria or edema is known as:

    _____

8. The most severe form of hypertension during pregnancy that results in seizures is known as:

    _____

9. A miscarriage that occurs on its own as a result of abnormalities of the maternal environment or abnormalities of the embryo or fetus is known as:

    _____

10. An incompatibility between an Rh negative mother's blood with her Rh positive baby's blood, causing the mother's body to develop antibodies that will destroy the Rh positive blood, is known as:

    _____

Number correct _____ × *10 points/correct answer: Your score* _____%

F. Matching Abbreviations

Match the abbreviations on the left with the applicable definitions on the right. Each correct answer is worth 10 points. Enter your score in the space provided at the end of the exercise.

_____ 1. AFP

_____ 2. EDC

_____ 3. FHT

_____ 4. HCG

_____ 5. LMP

_____ 6. OB

_____ 7. CS

_____ 8. EDD

_____ 9. FHR

_____ 10. Multip

a. multipara

b. fetal heart tone

c. expected date of delivery

d. alpha-fetoprotein

e. cesarean section

f. fetal heart rate

g. last menstrual period

h. expected date of confinement

i. human chorionic gonadotropin

j. obstetrics

k. fetal heart reaction

l. electronic fetal monitoring

Number correct _____ × *10 points/correct answer: Your score* _____%

G. Multiple Choice

Read each statement carefully and select the correct answer from the choices provided. Each correct answer is worth 10 points. Record your score in the space provided at the end of the exercise.

1. The absence of menstruation is known as:
   a. amenorrhea
   b. oligomenorrhea
   c. metrorrhagia
   d. dysmenorrhea

2. The darker, pigmented, circular area surrounding the nipple of each breast is called the:
   a. chorion
   b. amnion
   c. areola
   d. alveoli

3. Patches of tan or brown pigmentation associated with pregnancy (occurring mostly on the forehead, cheeks, and nose and called the mask of pregnancy) is known as:
   a. corpus luteum
   b. cerclage
   c. effacement
   d. chloasma

4. Another name for sexual intercourse, other than coitus, is:
   a. copulation
   b. ballottement
   c. conception
   d. cerclage

(continued)

5. The most severe form of hypertension during pregnancy, evidenced by seizures (convulsions), is known as:

   a. Goodell's sign

   b. Chadwick's sign

   c. eclampsia

   d. Hegar's sign

6. A probable sign of pregnancy is softening of the lower segment of the uterus, which is called:

   a. Goodell's sign

   b. Chadwick's sign

   c. eclampsia

   d. Hegar's sign

7. The bluish-violet hue of the cervix and vagina after approximately the sixth week of pregnancy is known as:

   a. Goodell's sign

   b. Chadwick's sign

   c. eclampsia

   d. Hegar's sign

8. The fringelike end of the fallopian tube is called:

   a. fimbriae

   b. gamete

   c. fundus

   d. striae

9. The first feeling of movement of the fetus felt by the expectant mother, usually occurring between 18 and 20 weeks' gestation, is termed:

   a. lightening

   b. Hegar's sign

   c. Chadwick's sign

   d. quickening

10. The settling of the fetal head into the pelvis, occurring a few weeks prior to the onset of labor, is known as:

    a. lightening

    b. Hegar's sign

    c. Chadwick's sign

    d. quickening

Number correct _____ × *10 points/correct answer: Your score* _____%

H. True, False, or Nearing?

Read the following signs and symptoms, and determine if they are signs and symptoms of false labor, true labor, or nearing labor. Enter your choice with a check mark (✔) in the applicable column. Each correct answer is worth 10 points. Record your score in the space provided at the end of the exercise.

Signs/Symptoms	False	True	Nearing
1. Irregular contractions, not too intense	☐	☐	☐
2. Regular contractions (intense, longer duration)	☐	☐	☐
3. Lightening: the settling of the fetal head into the pelvis	☐	☐	☐
4. Cervix does not change	☐	☐	☐
5. Walking may relieve or decrease contractions	☐	☐	☐
6. A sudden burst of energy, feels like doing major house cleaning duties	☐	☐	☐
7. Discomfort felt in abdomen and groin area	☐	☐	☐
8. Discomfort felt in lower back, radiates to abdomen; cramping	☐	☐	☐
9. Walking strengthens contractions	☐	☐	☐
10. Cervix progressively enlarges and thins	☐	☐	☐

Number correct _____ *× 10 points/correct answer: Your score* _____%

I. Crossword Puzzle

Read the clues carefully and complete the puzzle. Each crossword answer is worth 10 points. When you have completed the crossword puzzle, total your points and enter your score in the space provided at the end of the puzzle.

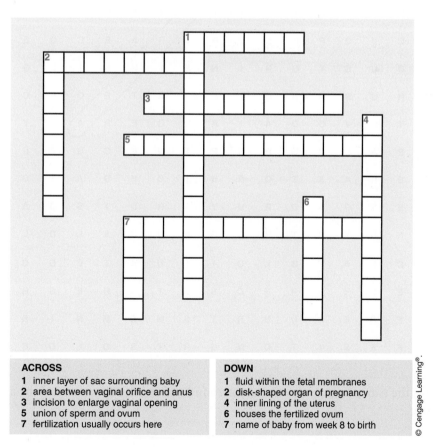

ACROSS
1 inner layer of sac surrounding baby
2 area between vaginal orifice and anus
3 incision to enlarge vaginal opening
5 union of sperm and ovum
7 fertilization usually occurs here

DOWN
1 fluid within the fetal membranes
2 disk-shaped organ of pregnancy
4 inner lining of the uterus
6 houses the fertilized ovum
7 name of baby from week 8 to birth

Number correct _____ *× 10 points/correct answer: Your score* _____%

J. Word Search

Read each definition carefully and identify the applicable word from the list that follows. Enter the word in the space provided and then find it in the puzzle and circle it. The words may be read up, down, diagonally, across, or backward. Each correct answer is worth 10 points. Record your score in the space provided at the end of the exercise.

amenorrhea	amnion	eclampsia
fetoscope	lightening	areola
estrogen	colostrum	cerclage
embryo	Braxton Hicks	

Example: Absence of menstruation.
<u>*amenorrhea*</u>

F	L	O	A	M	N	I	O	N	O	L	E	M	I	C
A	C	Y	N	M	E	S	M	S	I	D	A	S	T	T
M	I	O	T	T	E	C	L	A	M	P	S	I	A	R
C	A	O	N	M	E	N	O	S	D	I	C	C	B	O
I	L	C	B	D	E	P	O	C	S	O	T	E	F	S
N	U	R	E	I	Y	T	T	R	T	E	L	N	L	T
C	Y	O	P	H	L	L	B	I	R	A	E	C	O	E
O	U	S	T	G	N	I	N	E	T	H	G	I	L	O
N	U	R	R	P	O	I	P	I	A	T	E	O	E	C
T	U	V	O	D	A	I	A	L	O	E	R	A	M	Y
E	A	L	C	G	R	S	P	I	N	E	C	S	E	E
B	R	A	X	T	O	N	H	I	C	K	S	A	I	G
E	S	P	A	D	R	U	Y	A	R	D	I	S	G	A
N	U	E	S	T	R	O	G	E	N	U	A	L	D	L
C	R	A	T	B	L	O	I	I	U	A	T	C	O	C
E	E	N	E	R	H	C	S	U	T	U	R	E	S	R
F	R	E	R	U	U	R	I	S	M	E	M	N	I	E
P	E	R	I	T	O	M	U	R	T	S	O	L	O	C

1. The inner of the two membrane layers that surround and contain the fetus and the amniotic fluid during pregnancy.

   _____

2. The darker pigmented, circular area surrounding the nipple of each breast.

   _____

3. Irregular, ineffective contractions of the uterus that occur throughout pregnancy.

_____

4. Suturing the cervix to keep it from dilating prematurely during the pregnancy; sometimes referred to as the "purse string procedure."

_____

5. The thin, yellowish fluid secreted by the breasts during pregnancy and the first few days after birth, before lactation begins.

_____

6. The most severe form of hypertension during pregnancy, evidenced by seizures (convulsions).

_____

7. The name given to the product of conception from the second through the eighth week of pregnancy (through the second month).

_____

8. A female hormone that promotes the development of the female secondary sex characteristics.

_____

9. A special stethoscope for hearing the fetal heartbeat through the mother's abdomen.

_____

10. The settling of the fetal head into the pelvis, occurring a few weeks prior to the onset of labor.

_____

Number correct _____ × 10 points/correct answer: Your score _____%

K. Medical Scenario

The following scenario presents information on one of the complications of pregnancy discussed in this chapter. Read the scenario carefully and select the most appropriate answer for each question that follows. Each correct answer is worth 20 points. Record your score in the space provided at the end of the exercise.

Brooke Gray, a 29-year-old obstetric patient, has a scheduled prenatal visit with her obstetrician today. She is a primigravida and is at 12 weeks' gestation. Her obstetrician informed her on her last visit that she would discuss Brooke's specific blood type of B negative during today's visit. The health care professional prepared for this visit by refreshing her knowledge about pregnancy and clients with Rh negative blood type.

1. The health care professional found that the alarm about the mother having Rh negative blood is only a concern during and after pregnancy if the baby has:
    a. Rh negative blood type
    b. Rh positive blood type
    c. type AB blood
    d. type O blood

2. The health care professional identifies that the problem of Rh incompatibility is demonstrated with problems:
    a. during the first pregnancy only if the baby has Rh positive blood
    b. every baby delivered with Rh negative blood
    c. during the second pregnancy if both the first and second babies have Rh positive blood
    d. the third baby if he/she has Rh negative blood

(_continued_)

3. The health care professional learns that Brooke will likely be prescribed an injection of Rh immune globulin during the:

   a. visit today

   b. 20th week of pregnancy

   c. 28th week of pregnancy

   d. 30th week of pregnancy

4. The health care professional gained knowledge that if Brooke gives birth to an Rh positive baby, she will be administered:

   a. no further RhoGAM

   b. an injection of RhoGAM within 72 hours after the birth

   c. a blood transfusion of whole blood just after delivery

   d. a unit of fresh frozen plasma within 48 hours of delivery

5. The health care professional should remember the importance of instructing all of her patients with Rh negative blood that if the pregnancy ends in an abortion, the treatment regime is the same. This is important to prevent the formation of:

   a. antibodies that will affect her during future pregnancies

   b. an infection in the uterus and fallopian tubes

   c. an abruptio placenta in future pregnancies

   d. gestational diabetes toward the end of her next pregnancy

Number correct _____ × *20 points/correct answer: Your score* _____%

Child Health

CHAPTER CONTENT

OBJECTIVES

Upon completing this chapter and the review exercises at the end of the chapter, the learner should be able to:

1. Identify and define at least 20 pathological conditions common to children.

2. List and define 10 communicable diseases seen in children.

3. Correctly spell and pronounce terms listed on the Written and Audio Terminology Review, using the phonetic pronunciations provided.

4. Define at least 20 abbreviations common to the discussion of diseases and disorders of children.

5. State the recommended immunization schedule for infants and children.

6. Distinguish the differences between active and passive immunity.

Overview

Pediatrics is the field of medicine concerned with the **development** and care of children, specializing in the treatment and prevention of the diseases and disorders peculiar to children. In this chapter, the term *child health* is synonymous with **pediatrics**. The physician who specializes in **pediatrics** is known as a **pediatrician**. Some pediatric offices employ a **pediatric nurse practitioner (PNP)**, who is a registered nurse practitioner with advanced study and clinical practice in pediatric nursing. The pediatric specialty concerned with the diseases and abnormalities of the newborn **infant** is known as **neonatology**. The physician who specializes in **neonatology** is known as a **neonatologist**.

There are many subspecialties that deal with the care of children, such as pediatric oncology, pediatric cardiology, and child psychology. No matter what the specialty, the health professional who cares for children must possess a broad base of knowledge in the **growth** and development of children as well as a clear understanding of the illnesses and diseases peculiar to children. This knowledge will be applied when assisting in the care of both the healthy and the sick child.

An instrumental part of the prevention of disease and early detection of deviations from the norm in children is the **well-child** visit. During this visit, health professionals will assess the current health status of the child, the progression of growth and development, and the need for immunizations. The well-child visit also provides the opportunity for teaching the parents what to expect in the various stages of their child's growth and development. The physical examination, the immunizations, and the health teachings are all designed to promote optimal health for the child.

The field of **pediatrics** encompasses a wide range of terms that will be used by the health professional. This chapter covers terms and concepts that deal with the normal growth and development of the child, the well-child visit, immunizations, and diseases and disorders common to children.

Growth and Development

Normal growth and development proceeds in a predictable and orderly sequence. However, the rate of growth and development in individuals will vary.

Growth is defined as the physical increase in the whole or any of its parts. Growth is the result of biological change and an increase in the size and number of cells. The parameters of a child's growth can be measured easily with accuracy through acquiring the child's weight, **head circumference**, length or height, and **dentition**.

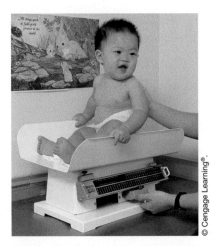

Figure 19-1 Measuring weight in the infant

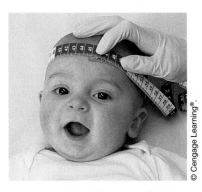

Figure 19-2 Measuring head circumference

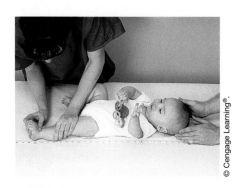

Figure 19-3 Recumbent length in infant

Weight is an important indicator of the child's nutritional status and general growth. It is also used to calculate medication dosages for children. Weight should be measured at every well-visit for general indications about growth and at every sick-visit to determine the effects of illness on weight. See *Figure 19-1*.

Recording the weight of the infant or child is important to measure the child's progress. Weights should be plotted on a **growth chart** so that the growth pattern can be visualized.

Head circumference is an important measurement because it is related to intracranial volume. Normal brain growth causes an increase in head circumference at an expected rate. Abnormal lags or surges in the increase of head circumference may indicate serious problems. Head circumference is measured during each well-child visit from birth to two to three years of age. See *Figure 19-2*.

An infant or child's head circumference is the measurement of the greatest circumference of the head. Head circumference is also plotted on a **nomogram** and is compared with weight and length for the particular age. Any inconsistencies in growth patterns will require further evaluation.

The **length** or **height** measurement is compared with the head circumference and weight measurement for an overall indicator of physical growth. Length or height is usually measured at every well-visit. The infant is measured from the crown of the head to the heel, with the child in a **recumbent** position. See *Figure 19-3*.

Standing height measurements are usually performed for children age three years or older. The child stands very still and straight, with his or her back against the measuring surface. Length or height is measured to the nearest 1/8 inch. This measurement is plotted on a growth chart for comparison with other measurements.

Dentition refers to the eruption of teeth and follows a sequential pattern. Twenty **primary teeth** erupt between 6 months and 30 months. At about the age of six years, the primary teeth are lost and permanent teeth begin to erupt. There are normally 32 permanent teeth. (See *Figure 19-5* later in the chapter.)

Development refers to an increase in function and complexity that results through learning, maturation, and growth. Development is much more complicated to measure than growth. Observation of problem-solving skills, interaction patterns, the performance of daily activities (playing, dressing, eating, etc.), and the communication patterns used all provide useful data to evaluate the child's development. The child communicates through his or her universal language, "play."

Developmental screening can be achieved through standardized assessment tools. Examples are as follows:

- **Brazelton Neonatal Behavior Assessment (BNBA) Scale for newborns**—a scale developed for evaluating and assessing an infant's alertness, motor maturity, irritability, consolability, and interaction with people. Used as a tool for the evaluation of the neurological condition and the behavior of a newborn, the BNBA scale consists of a series of 27 reaction tests, including response to inanimate objects, pin prick, light, and the sound of a bell or rattle.

- **Dubowitz for newborns**—a system for estimating the gestational age of a newborn according to such factors as posture, ankle dorsiflexion, and arm and leg recoil.

- **Ages & Stages Questionnaires (ASQ)**—a parent-completed method of at-home screening of infants and young children for developmental delays during the first five years of life. The questionnaires are written in simple words and are appropriate for parents from diverse backgrounds. The questionnaires consist of 30 items, divided into five categories that are designed to assess the children in their natural environments. The developmental areas being evaluated are communication, gross motor development, fine motor development, problem-solving skills, and personal/social skills. The parent observes the child and answers the questions. The responses are categorized as "yes," "sometimes," and "not yet." Once the questionnaire is completed, the professional converts the responses to a color-coded scoring sheet that makes it possible to determine the child's progress in each developmental area listed on the questionnaire.

When working with children, it is simple to refer to the child according to his or her age or stage of development. Following are stages of childhood growth and development.

- Newborn—birth to 1 month

- Infancy—1 month to 1 year

- Toddlerhood—1 to 3 years

- Preschool age—3 to 6 years

- School age—6 to 12 years

- Adolescents—12 to 18 years or 21 years

Growth and Development Principles

The patterns of growth and development are directional and predictable, including the following growth patterns.

cephalocaudal (**seff**-ah-loh-**KAW**-dal) cephal/o = head caud/o = tail -al = pertaining to	Growth and development proceeds from head to toe (cephalocaudal). See *Figure 19-4*. In the infant, muscular control follows the spine downward. For example, infants will hold up their head before they sit.

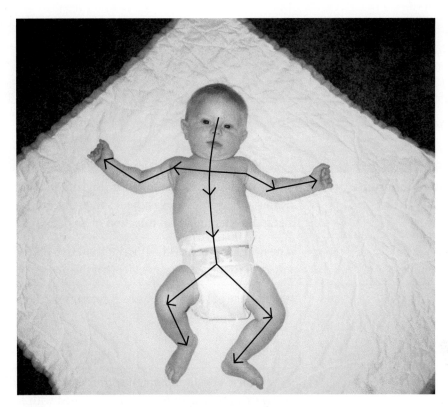

Figure 19-4 Cephalocaudal and proximodistal development
(*Courtesy of Vickie Rikard*)

proximodistal **proxim/o** = near **dist/o** = away from **-al** = pertaining to	Growth and development proceeds from the center outward or from the midline to the periphery (proximodistal). See *Figure 19-4*. For example, the large muscles of the arms and legs are subject to voluntary control sooner than the fine muscles of the hands and feet.
general to specific	Activities move from being generalized toward being more focused (general to specific). For example, the child will use the whole hand before picking up a small object between the thumb and forefinger.
simple to complex	Language, for example, develops from simple to complex.
growth spurts	Occur throughout childhood, alternating with periods of slow growth.

Children grow, learn, and mature with the assistance of many factors. The factors can be an inspiration or stimulus, or they can impede the process. Some of the factors that consistently have an influence on a child's growth and development include, but are not necessarily limited to, genetics, environment and culture, nutrition and health status, play, family and parental attitudes, and child rearing philosophies.

Review Checkpoint

Check your understanding of this section by completing the **Growth and Development** exercises in your workbook.

VOCABULARY

The following vocabulary words are frequently used when discussing child health.

Word	Definition
active acquired immunity (**AK**-tiv ah-**KWIRD** ih-**MEW**-nih-tee)	A form of long-term acquired **immunity** that protects the body against a new infection as the result of antibodies that develop naturally after an initial infection or artificially after a vaccination.
apical pulse (**AY**-pih-kal puhls)	The heart rate as heard with a stethoscope placed on the chest wall adjacent to the cardiac apex (top of the heart).
apnea (ap-**NEE**-ah) a- = without, not -pnea = breathing	An absence of spontaneous respiration.
autism (**AW**-tizm) aut/o = self -ism = condition	A pervasive developmental disorder characterized by the individual being extremely withdrawn and absorbed with fantasy. The individual suffers from impaired communication/social interaction skills, and activities and interest are very limited. **Autism** was first classified as a type of schizophrenia.
axillary temperature (**AK**-sih-lair-ee **TEMP**-per-ah-toor) axill/o = armpit -ary = pertaining to	The body temperature as recorded by a thermometer placed in the armpit. The reading is generally 0.5 to 1.0 degree less than the **oral temperature**.
congenital	Present at birth.
crackles (**CRACK**-ulz)	A common abnormal respiratory sound heard on auscultation of the chest during inspiration, characterized by discontinuous bubbling noises.
cyanosis (sigh-ah-**NOH**-sis) cyan/o = blue -osis = condition	Bluish discoloration of the skin and mucous membranes caused by an excess of deoxygenated hemoglobin in the blood or a structural defect in the hemoglobin molecule.
deciduous teeth (dee-**SID**-yoo-us **TEETH**)	Baby teeth; the first set of teeth, also known as primary teeth.
dentition (den-**TIH**-shun)	The eruption of teeth. This occurs in a sequential pattern, with 20 primary teeth erupting between the ages of 6 to 30 months. See *Figure 19-5*.
development	An increase in function and complexity that results through learning, maturation, and growth.
febrile (**FEE**-brill)	Pertaining to or characterized by an elevated body temperature, such as a **febrile** reaction to an infectious agent.

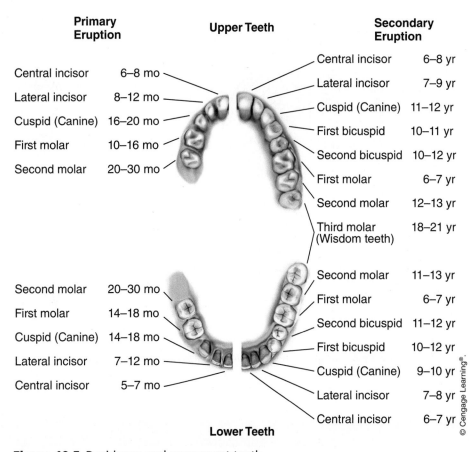

Primary Eruption	Upper Teeth		Secondary Eruption	
Central incisor	6–8 mo		Central incisor	6–8 yr
Lateral incisor	8–12 mo		Lateral incisor	7–9 yr
Cuspid (Canine)	16–20 mo		Cuspid (Canine)	11–12 yr
First molar	10–16 mo		First bicuspid	10–11 yr
Second molar	20–30 mo		Second bicuspid	10–12 yr
			First molar	6–7 yr
			Second molar	12–13 yr
			Third molar (Wisdom teeth)	18–21 yr
Second molar	20–30 mo		Second molar	11–13 yr
First molar	14–18 mo		First molar	6–7 yr
Cuspid (Canine)	14–18 mo		Second bicuspid	11–12 yr
Lateral incisor	7–12 mo		First bicuspid	10–12 yr
Central incisor	5–7 mo		Cuspid (Canine)	9–10 yr
			Lateral incisor	7–8 yr
			Central incisor	6–7 yr

Lower Teeth

© Cengage Learning®

Figure 19-5 Deciduous and permanent teeth

Word	Definition
friction rub (**FRICK**-shun rub)	A dry, grating sound heard with a stethoscope during auscultation.
growth	An increase in the whole or any of its parts physically.
grunting (**GRUNT**-ing)	Abnormal, short, audible, deep, hoarse sounds in exhalation that often accompany severe chest pain.
head circumference (HEAD sir-**KUM**-fer-ens)	The measurement around the greatest circumference of the head of an infant. This measurement is plotted according to normal growth and development patterns for the infant's head. Increased lags or surges in the increase of the head circumference may indicate serious problems.
hydrocephalus (high-droh-**SEFF**-ah-lus) hydr/o = water cephal/o = head -us = noun ending	A pathological condition characterized by an abnormal accumulation of cerebrospinal fluid, usually under increased pressure, within the cranial vault and subsequent dilation of the ventricles; also called hydrocephaly. See *Figure 19-6*.
immunity (ih-**MEW**-nih-tee)	The quality of being insusceptible to or unaffected by a particular disease or condition.
immunization (**im**-mew-nih-**ZAY**-shun)	A process by which resistance to an infectious disease is induced or augmented.

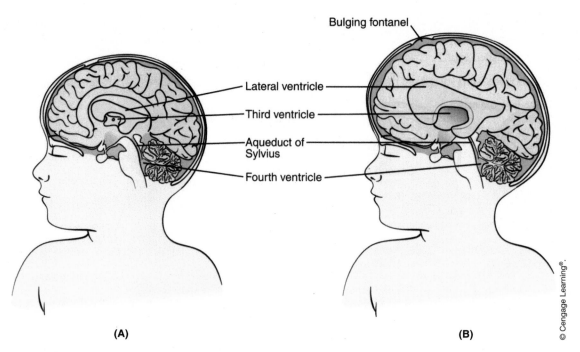

Figure 19-6 Comparison of (A) Normal size ventricles and (B) Enlarged ventricles associated with hydrocephalus

© Cengage Learning®.

Word	Definition
infant (**IN**-fant)	A child who is in the earliest stage of extrauterine life, a time extending from the first month after birth to approximately 12 months of age, when the baby is able to assume an erect posture. Some extend the period to 24 months of age.
length (recumbent) (**LENGTH** [ree-**KUM**-bent])	The measurement of the distance from the crown of the infant's head to the infant's heel while the infant is lying on the back with legs extended.
lumbar puncture (**LUM**-bar **PUNK**-choor)	The introduction of a hollow needle and stylet into the subarachnoid space of the lumbar portion of the spinal canal to obtain specimens of cerebrospinal fluid.
microcephalus (**my**-kroh-**SEFF**-ah-lus) micr/o = small cephal/o = head -us = noun ending	A **congenital** anomaly characterized by abnormal smallness of the head in relation to the rest of the body and by underdevelopment of the brain, resulting in some degree of mental retardation.
natural immunity (natural ih-**MEW**-nih-tee)	A usually innate and permanent form of **immunity** to a specific disease.
neonatologist (nee-oh-nay-**TOL**-oh-jist) neo- = new nat/o = birth -logist = one who specializes in the study of	A medical doctor who specializes in **neonatology**.

Word	Definition
neonatology (**nee**-oh-nay-**TOL**-oh-jee) neo- = new nat/o = birth -logy = the study of	The medical specialty concerned with the diseases and abnormalities of the newborn infant.
nomogram nom/o = of or relating to usage -gram = a record	A graphic representation, by any of various systems, of a numeric relationship.
omphalitis (om-fal-**EYE**-tis) omphal/o = navel -itis = inflammation of	An inflammation of the umbilical stump, marked by redness, swelling, and purulent exudate in severe cases.
omphalocele (om-**FAL**-oh-seel) omphal/o = navel -cele = swelling or herniation	Congenital herniation of intra-abdominal viscera through a defect in the abdominal wall around the umbilicus.
omphalorrhea (**om**-fal-oh-**REE**-ah) omphal/o = navel -rrhea = discharge; flow	Drainage from the umbilicus (navel).
oral temperature or/o = mouth -al = pertaining to	The mean body temperature of a normal person as recorded by a clinical thermometer placed in the mouth.
passive acquired immunity (passive ih-**MEW**-nih-tee)	A form of acquired immunity resulting from antibodies that are transmitted naturally through the placenta to a fetus, through the colostrum to an infant, or artificially by injection of antiserum for treatment or as a prophylaxis (protection against disease).
pediatrician (pee-dee-ah-**TRISH**-an) pedi/a = child -iatrician = one who treats; a physician	A physician who specializes in **pediatrics**.
pediatric nurse practitioner (pee-dee-**AT**-rik **NURSE** prac-**TIH**-shin-er) pedi/a = child -iatric = medicine, the medical profession, or physician	A registered nurse with advanced study and clinical practice in pediatric nursing.
pediatrics (pee-dee-**AT**-riks) pedi/a = child -iatrics = medicine, the medical profession, or physician	Pertaining to preventive and primary health care and treatment of children and the study of childhood diseases.

Word	Definition
primary teeth (**PRYE**-mair-ee **TEETH**)	Baby teeth; the first set of teeth, also known as **deciduous teeth**.
prodromal (pro-**DROH**-mal)	Pertaining to early signs or symptoms that mark the onset of a disease.
pyrexia (pie-**REK**-see-ah) pyr/o = fire, heat	Fever.
rectal temperature rect/o = rectum -al = pertaining to	Temperature as measured in the rectum.
recumbent (ree-**KUM**-bent)	Lying down.
retractions (rih-**TRAK**-shunz)	The displacement of tissues to expose a part or structure of the body; **retractions** may be seen around the ribs in a child or infant with respiratory distress.
stature (**STAT**-yoor)	Natural height of a person in an upright position.
stridor (**STRYE**-dor)	An abnormal, high-pitched, musical sound caused by an obstruction in the trachea or larynx.
toxoid (**TOKS**-oyd) tox/o = poisons -oid = resembling	A toxin that has been treated with chemicals or with heat to decrease its toxic effect but that retains its ability to cause the production of antibodies.
tympanic temperature (tim-**PAN**-ik **TEM**-per-ah-chur) tympan/o = eardrum -ic = pertaining to	The body temperature as measured electronically at the tympanic membrane.
vaccine (**VAK**-seen; vak-**SEEN**)	A suspension of attenuated or killed microorganisms administered intradermally, intramuscularly, orally, or subcutaneously to induce **active immunity** to infectious disease.
vertex (**VER**-teks)	The top of the head; crown.
well-child visit	Routine health visit in which health professionals assess the current health status of the child, the progression of growth and development, and the need for immunizations.
wheezing (**HWEEZ**-ing)	A breath sound, characterized by a high-pitched musical quality heard on both inspiration and expiration. Wheezes may be associated with **asthma** and chronic bronchitis as well as with other illnesses.

Review Checkpoint

Check your understanding of this section by completing the **Vocabulary** exercises in your workbook.

WORD ELEMENTS

The following word elements pertain to the specialty of child health. As you review the list, pronounce each word element aloud twice and check the box after you "say it." Write the definition for the example term given for each word element. Use your medical dictionary to find the definitions of the example terms.

Word Element	Pronunciation	"Say It"	Meaning
blast/o erythro**blast**osis fetalis	**BLASS**-toh eh-rith-roh-blass-**TOH**-sis fee-**TAL**-is	☐	embryonic stage of development
cephal/o hydro**cephal**us	**SEFF**-ah-loh high-droh-**SEFF**-ah-lus	☐	head
crypt/o **crypt**orchidism	**KRIPT**-toh kript-**OR**-kid-izm	☐	hidden
epi- **epi**spadias	**EP**-ih ep-ih-**SPAY**-dee-ass	☐	upon, over
esophag/o **esophag**eal atresia	ee-**SOFF**-ah-goh ee-**soff**-ah-**JEE**-al ah-**TREE**-zee-ah	☐	esophagus
hydro- **hydro**cele	**HIGH**-droh **HIGH**-droh-seel	☐	water
hypo- **hypo**spadias	**HIGH**-poh **high**-poh-**SPAY**-dee-ass	☐	under, below, beneath, less than normal
-iatric ped**iatric**ian	ee-**AH**-trik pee-dee-ah-**TRISH**-an	☐	relating to medicine, physicians, or medical treatment
micr/o **micr**ocephalus	**MY**-kroh my-kroh-**SEFF**-ah-lus	☐	small
nat/o neo**nat**al	**NAY**-toh nee-oh-**NAY**-tal	☐	birth

Word Element	Pronunciation	"Say It"	Meaning
neo- **neo**natologist	**NEE**-oh **nee**-oh-nay-**TOL**-oh-jist	☐	new
omphal/o **omphal**orrhea	om-**FAL**-oh om-fal-oh-**REE**-ah	☐	navel
pedi/a **pedi**atrics	**PEE**-dee-ah pee-dee-**AT**-riks	☐	child
pyr/o **pyr**exia	**PIE**-roh pie-**REK**-see-ah	☐	fire, heat
rose/o **rose**ola infantum	**ROH**-zee-oh roh-zee-**OH**-lah in-**FAN**-tum	☐	rose colored
tetr/a **tetr**alogy of Fallot	**TEH**-trah teh-**TRALL**-oh-jee of fal-**OH**	☐	four
tympan/o **tympan**ic temperature	tim-**PAN**-oh tim-**PAN**-ik **TEM**-per-ah-chur	☐	eardrum

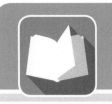

Review Checkpoint

Check your understanding of this section by completing the **Word Elements** exercises in your workbook.

Immunizations

An important part of the normal growth, development, and health of a child is the prevention of disease. This is achieved partly through the administration of immunizations. **Immunization** is the process of creating **immunity** to a specific disease in an individual. Not only does **immunization** refer to a process, but also the word *immunization* is used to describe the medication that is administered to the child. The actual medication administered in the immunizing process is called a **vaccine**, a suspension of infectious agents, or some part of them, that is given for the purpose of establishing resistance to an infectious disease. The state of being immune to or protected from a disease, especially an infectious disease, is known as **immunity**.

The health professional will be involved in the administration of immunizations as well as the education of parents concerning the need for and importance of immunizations. The parents need to understand the risks involved in the administration of immunizations and the common side effects. They also need to know what to do to promote the comfort of their child after administration of the **vaccine**. (Side effects are usually mild.) In addition, parents should be taught to recognize severe side effects of immunizations and should be instructed in emergency follow-up should serious reactions occur.

Immunizations are administered to the well child according to a specific schedule recommended by the American Academy of Pediatrics. Doctors responsible for the continuing health care of infants and children recommend a regular schedule of visits for both general physical checkups and immunizations throughout the childhood years. This general program of preventive care for infants is often referred to as "well-baby checkups." A typical schedule for well-baby care would include visits at the following ages: 2 weeks, 1 month, 2 months, 4 months, 6 months, 9 months, 12 months, 15 months, 18 months, 2 years, 3 years, 4 years, 5 years, and every two years until age 11. After the age of 11, the child is usually seen annually until the age of 18.

The recommended vaccination schedule for infants and children is based on the fact that repeated doses of **vaccine** are necessary to ensure proper development of antibodies. The goal of the administration of immunizations is to ensure complete vaccination of the child by the age of 15 to 18 months if no contraindications are present when immunizations are begun. *Table 19-1* illustrates the recommended **immunization** schedule for infants and children. *Table 19-2* illustrates the recommended catch-up immunization schedule for individuals aged 4 months through 18 years. These schedules are approved by the Centers for Disease Control and Prevention (CDC) Advisory Committee on Immunization Practices (ACIP), the American Academy of Pediatrics (AAP), and the American Academy of Family Physicians (AAFP).

Communicable Diseases

This section concentrates on communicable diseases common to the child. The child will often have generalized symptoms of a virus before the defining symptoms appear. These early symptoms that mark the onset of a disease are known as **prodromal** symptoms.

| **chickenpox (varicella)**

(**CHICK**-en-pox)

(**vair**-ah-**SELL**-ah)

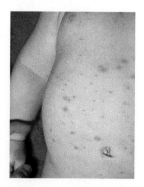 | A viral disease of sudden onset with slight fever, successive eruptions of macules, papules, and vesicles on the skin followed by crusting over of the lesions with a granular scab. Itching may be severe. (Macules are discolorations at normal skin level; papules are raised, pimplelike skin blemishes; and vesicles are blisterlike.) See *Figure 19-7*.

The infectious agent is the varicella-zoster virus, a member of the *Herpesvirus* group. **Chickenpox** is spread through direct contact, by droplet spread, or by contaminated objects. The incubation period is from 10 to 21 days. It is communicable from up to five days before skin eruptions occur until lesions are dry. The **immunization** for chickenpox is called the varicella **vaccine**.

Figure 19-7 Varicella (chickenpox)
(Courtesy of Robert A. Silverman, MD, Pediatric Dermatology, Georgetown University) |

Table 19-1 Recommended Immunization Schedule for Individuals Aged 0 through 18 years – 2014.

Figure 1. Recommended immunization schedule for persons aged 0 through 18 years – **United States, 2014.**

(FOR THOSE WHO FALL BEHIND OR START LATE, SEE THE CATCH-UP SCHEDULE [FIGURE 2]).

These recommendations must be read with the footnotes that follow. For those who fall behind or start late, provide catch-up vaccination at the earliest opportunity as indicated by the green bars in Figure 1. To determine minimum intervals between doses, see the catch-up schedule (Figure 2). School entry and adolescent vaccine age groups are in bold.

Vaccine	Birth	1 mo	2 mos	4 mos	6 mos	9 mos	12 mos	15 mos	18 mos	19–23 mos	2-3 yrs	4-6 yrs	7-10 yrs	11-12 yrs	13-15 yrs	16–18 yrs
Hepatitis B[1] (HepB)	1st dose	←2nd dose→			←————— 3rd dose —————→											
Rotavirus[2] (RV) RV1 (2-dose series); RV5 (3-dose series)			1st dose	2nd dose	See footnote 2											
Diphtheria, tetanus, & acellular pertussis[3] (DTaP: <7 yrs)			1st dose	2nd dose	3rd dose		←—— 4th dose ——→					5th dose				
Tetanus, diphtheria, & acellular pertussis[4] (Tdap: ≥7 yrs)														(Tdap)		
Haemophilus influenzae type b[5] (Hib)			1st dose	2nd dose	See footnote 5		3rd or 4th dose, See footnote 5									
Pneumococcal conjugate[6] (PCV13)			1st dose	2nd dose	3rd dose		←— 4th dose —→									
Pneumococcal polysaccharide[6] (PPSV23)																
Inactivated poliovirus[7] (IPV) (<18 yrs)			1st dose	2nd dose	←————— 3rd dose —————→							4th dose				
Influenza[8] (IIV; LAIV) 2 doses for some: See footnote 8						Annual vaccination (IIV only)							Annual vaccination (IIV or LAIV)			
Measles, mumps, rubella[9] (MMR)							←— 1st dose —→					2nd dose				
Varicella[10] (VAR)							←— 1st dose —→					2nd dose				
Hepatitis A[11] (HepA)							2-dose series, See footnote 11									
Human papillomavirus[12] (HPV2: females only; HPV4: males and females)														(3-dose series)		
Meningococcal[13] (Hib-Men-CY ≥ 6 weeks; MenACWY-D ≥9 mos; MenACWY-CRM ≥ 2 mos)			See footnote 13											1st dose		Booster

| Range of recommended ages for all children | | Range of recommended ages for catch-up immunization | | Range of recommended ages for certain high-risk groups | | Range of recommended ages during which catch-up is encouraged and for certain high-risk groups | | Not routinely recommended |

This schedule includes recommendations in effect as of January 1, 2014. Any dose not administered at the recommended age should be administered at a subsequent visit, when indicated and feasible. The use of a combination vaccine generally is preferred over separate injections of its equivalent component vaccines. Vaccination providers should consult the relevant Advisory Committee on Immunization Practices (ACIP) statement for detailed recommendations, available online at http://www.cdc.gov/vaccines/hcp/acip-recs/index.html. Clinically significant adverse events that follow vaccination should be reported to the Vaccine Adverse Event Reporting System (VAERS) online (http://www.vaers.hhs.gov) or by telephone (800-822-7967).Suspected cases of vaccine-preventable diseases should be reported to the state or local health department. Additional information, including precautions and contraindications for vaccination, is available from CDC online (http://www.cdc.gov/vaccines/recs/vac-admin/contraindications.htm) or by telephone (800-CDC-INFO [800-232-4636]).

This schedule is approved by the Advisory Committee on Immunization Practices (http://www.cdc.gov/vaccines/acip), the American Academy of Pediatrics (http://www.aap.org), the American Academy of Family Physicians (http://www.aafp.org), and the American College of Obstetricians and Gynecologists (http://www.acog.org).

NOTE: The above recommendations must be read along with the footnotes of this schedule.

Footnotes — Recommended immunization schedule for persons aged 0 through 18 years—United States, 2014

For further guidance on the use of the vaccines mentioned below, see: http://www.cdc.gov/vaccines/hcp/acip-recs/index.html.
For vaccine recommendations for persons 19 years of age and older, see the adult immunization schedule.

Additional information

- For contraindications and precautions to use of a vaccine and for additional information regarding that vaccine, vaccination providers should consult the relevant ACIP statement available online at http://www.cdc.gov/vaccines/hcp/acip-recs/index.html.
- For purposes of calculating intervals between doses, 4 weeks = 28 days. Intervals of 4 months or greater are determined by calendar months.
- Vaccine doses administered 4 days or less before the minimum interval are considered valid. Doses of any vaccine administered ≥5 days earlier than the minimum interval or minimum age should not be counted as valid doses and should be repeated as age-appropriate. The repeat dose should be spaced after the invalid dose by the recommended minimum interval. For further details, see MMWR, General Recommendations on Immunization and Reports / Vol. 60 / No. 2; Table 1. Recommended and minimum ages and intervals between vaccine doses available online at http://www.cdc.gov/mmwr/pdf/rr/rr6002.pdf.
- Information on travel vaccine requirements and recommendations is available at http://wwwnc.cdc.gov/travel/destinations/list.
- For vaccination of persons with primary and secondary immunodeficiencies, see Table 13, "Vaccination of persons with primary and secondary immunodeficiencies," in General Recommendations on Immunization (ACIP), available at http://www.cdc.gov/mmwr/pdf/rr/rr6002.pdf; and American Academy of Pediatrics. Immunization in Special Clinical Circumstances, in Pickering LK, Baker CJ, Kimberlin DW, Long SS eds. Red Book: 2012 report of the Committee on Infectious Diseases. 29th ed. Elk Grove Village, IL: American Academy of Pediatrics.

1. **Hepatitis B (HepB) vaccine. (Minimum age: birth)**
   Routine vaccination:
   At birth:
   - Administer monovalent HepB vaccine to all newborns before hospital discharge.
   - For infants born to hepatitis B surface antigen (HBsAg)-positive mothers, administer HepB vaccine and 0.5 mL of hepatitis B immune globulin (HBIG) within 12 hours of birth. These infants should be tested for HBsAg and antibody to HBsAg (anti-HBs) 1 to 2 months after completion of the HepB series, at age 9 through 18 months (preferably at the next well-child visit).
   - If mother's HBsAg status is unknown, within 12 hours of birth administer HepB vaccine regardless of birth weight. For infants weighing less than 2,000 grams, administer HBIG in addition to HepB vaccine within 12 hours of birth. Determine mother's HBsAg status as soon as possible and, if mother is HBsAg-positive, also administer HBIG for infants weighing 2,000 grams or more as soon as possible, but no later than age 7 days.

   Doses following the birth dose:
   - The second dose should be administered at age 1 or 2 months. Monovalent HepB vaccine should be used for doses administered before age 6 weeks.
   - Infants who did not receive a birth dose should receive 3 doses of a HepB-containing vaccine on a schedule of 0, 1 to 2 months, and 6 months starting as soon as feasible. See Figure 2.
   - Administer the second dose 1 to 2 months after the first dose (minimum interval of 4 weeks), administer the third dose at least 8 weeks after the second dose AND at least 16 weeks after the first dose. The final (third or fourth) dose in the HepB vaccine series should be administered no earlier than age 24 weeks.
   - Administration of a total of 4 doses of HepB vaccine is permitted when a combination vaccine containing HepB is administered after the birth dose.

   Catch-up vaccination:
   - Unvaccinated persons should complete a 3-dose series.
   - A 2-dose series (doses separated by at least 4 months) of adult formulation Recombivax HB is licensed for use in children aged 11 through 15 years.
   - For other catch-up guidance, see Figure 2.

2. **Rotavirus (RV) vaccines. (Minimum age: 6 weeks for both RV1 [Rotarix] and RV5 [RotaTeq])**
   Routine vaccination:
   Administer a series of RV vaccine to all infants as follows:
   1. If Rotarix is used, administer a 2-dose series at 2 and 4 months of age.
   2. If RotaTeq is used, administer a 3-dose series at ages 2, 4, and 6 months.
   3. If any dose in the series was RotaTeq or vaccine product is unknown for any dose in the series, a total of 3 doses of RV vaccine should be administered.

   Catch-up vaccination:
   - The maximum age for the first dose in the series is 14 weeks, 6 days; vaccination should not be initiated for infants aged 15 weeks, 0 days or older.
   - The maximum age for the final dose in the series is 8 months, 0 days.
   - For other catch-up guidance, see Figure 2.

3. **Diphtheria and tetanus toxoids and acellular pertussis (DTaP) vaccine. (Minimum age: 6 weeks. Exception: DTaP-IPV [Kinrix]: 4 years)**
   Routine vaccination:
   - Administer a 5-dose series of DTaP vaccine at ages 2, 4, 6, 15 through 18 months, and 4 through 6 years. The fourth dose may be administered as early as age 12 months, provided at least 6 months have elapsed since the third dose.

   Catch-up vaccination:
   - The fifth dose of DTaP vaccine is not necessary if the fourth dose was administered at age 4 years or older.
   - For other catch-up guidance, see Figure 2.

4. **Tetanus and diphtheria toxoids and acellular pertussis (Tdap) vaccine. (Minimum age: 10 years for Boostrix, 11 years for Adacel)**
   Routine vaccination:
   - Administer 1 dose of Tdap vaccine to all adolescents aged 11 through 12 years.
   - Tdap may be administered regardless of the interval since the last tetanus and diphtheria toxoid-containing vaccine.
   - Administer 1 dose of Tdap vaccine to pregnant adolescents during each pregnancy (preferred during 27 through 36 weeks gestation) regardless of time since prior Td or Tdap vaccination.

   Catch-up vaccination:
   - Persons aged 7 years and older who are not fully immunized with DTaP vaccine should receive Tdap vaccine as 1 (preferably the first) dose in the catch-up series; if additional doses are needed, use Td vaccine. For children 7 through 10 years who receive a dose of Tdap as part of the catch-up series, an adolescent Tdap vaccine dose at age 11 through 12 years should NOT be administered. Td should be administered instead 10 years after the Tdap dose.
   - Persons aged 11 through 18 years who have not received Tdap vaccine should receive a dose followed by tetanus and diphtheria toxoids (Td) booster doses every 10 years thereafter.
   - Inadvertent doses of DTaP vaccine:
     - If administered inadvertently to a child aged 7 through 10 years may count as part of the catch-up series. This dose may count as the adolescent Tdap dose, or the child can later receive a Tdap booster dose at age 11 through 12 years.
     - If administered inadvertently to an adolescent aged 11 through 18 years, the dose should be counted as the adolescent Tdap booster.
   - For other catch-up guidance, see Figure 2.

5. **Haemophilus influenzae type b (Hib) conjugate vaccine. (Minimum age: 6 weeks for PRP-T [ACTHIB, DTaP-IPV/Hib (Pentacel) and Hib-MenCY (MenHibrix)], PRP-OMP [PedvaxHIB or COMVAX], 12 months for PRP-T [Hiberix])**
   Routine vaccination:
   - Administer a 2- or 3-dose Hib vaccine primary series and a booster dose (dose 3 or 4 depending on vaccine used in primary series) at age 12 through 15 months to complete a full Hib vaccine series.
   - The primary series with ActHIB, MenHibrix, or Pentacel consists of 3 doses and should be administered at 2, 4, and 6 months of age. The primary series with PedvaxHIB or COMVAX consists of 2 doses and should be administered at 2 and 4 months of age; a dose at age 6 months is not indicated.
   - One booster dose (dose 3 or 4 depending on vaccine used in primary series) of any Hib vaccine should be administered at age 12 through 15 months. An exception is Hiberix vaccine. Hiberix should only be used for the booster (final) dose in children aged 12 months through 4 years who have received at least 1 prior dose of Hib-containing vaccine.

(continued)

For further guidance on the use of the vaccines mentioned below, see: http://www.cdc.gov/vaccines/hcp/acip-recs/index.html.

5. *Haemophilus influenzae type b (Hib) conjugate vaccine (cont'd)*
- For recommendations on the use of MenHibrix in patients at increased risk for meningococcal disease, please refer to the meningococcal vaccine footnotes and also to *MMWR* March 22, 2013; 62(RR02);1-22, available at http://www.cdc.gov/mmwr/pdf/rr/rr6202.pdf.

Catch-up vaccination:
- If dose 1 was administered at ages 12 through 14 months, administer a second (final) dose at least 8 weeks after dose 1, regardless of Hib vaccine used in the primary series.
- If the first 2 doses were PRP-OMP (PedvaxHIB or COMVAX), and were administered at age 11 months or younger, the third (and final) dose should be administered at age 12 through 15 months and at least 8 weeks after the second dose.
- If the first dose was administered at age 7 through 11 months, administer the second dose at least 4 weeks later and a third (and final) dose at age 12 through 15 months or 8 weeks after second dose, whichever is later, regardless of Hib vaccine used for first dose.
- If first dose is administered at younger than 12 months of age and second dose is given between 12 through 14 months of age, a third (and final) dose should be given 8 weeks later.
- For unvaccinated children aged 15 months or older, administer only 1 dose.
- For other catch-up guidance, see Figure 2. For catch-up guidance related to MenHibrix, please see the meningococcal vaccine footnotes and also *MMWR* March 22, 2013; 62(RR02);1-22, available at http://www.cdc.gov/mmwr/pdf/rr/rr6202.pdf.

Vaccination of persons with high-risk conditions:
- Children aged 12 through 59 months who are at increased risk for Hib disease, including chemotherapy recipients and those with anatomic or functional asplenia (including sickle cell disease), human immunodeficiency virus (HIV) infection, immunoglobulin deficiency, or early component complement deficiency, who have received either no doses or only 1 dose of Hib vaccine before 12 months of age, should receive 2 additional doses of Hib vaccine 8 weeks apart; children who received 2 or more doses of Hib vaccine before 12 months of age should receive 1 additional dose.
- For patients younger than 5 years of age undergoing chemotherapy or radiation treatment who received a Hib vaccine dose(s) within 14 days of starting therapy or during therapy, repeat the dose(s) at least 3 months following therapy completion.
- Recipients of hematopoietic stem cell transplant (HSCT) should be revaccinated with a 3-dose regimen of Hib vaccine starting 6 to 12 months after successful transplant, regardless of vaccination history; 3 doses should be administered at least 4 weeks apart.
- A single dose of any Hib-containing vaccine should be administered to unimmunized* children and adolescents 15 months of age and older undergoing an elective splenectomy; if possible, vaccine should be administered at least 14 days before procedure.
- Hib vaccine is not routinely recommended for patients 5 years or older. However, 1 dose of Hib vaccine should be administered to unimmunized* persons aged 5 years or older who have anatomic or functional asplenia (including sickle cell disease) and unvaccinated persons 5 through 18 years of age with human immunodeficiency virus (HIV) infection.

* Patients who have not received a primary series and booster dose or at least 1 dose of Hib vaccine after 14 months of age are considered unimmunized.

6. **Pneumococcal vaccines. (Minimum age: 6 weeks for PCV13, 2 years for PPSV23)**

Routine vaccination with PCV13:
- Administer a 4-dose series of PCV13 vaccine at ages 2, 4, and 6 months and at age 12 through 15 months.
- For children aged 14 through 59 months who have received an age-appropriate series of 7-valent PCV (PCV7), administer a single supplemental dose of 13-valent PCV (PCV13).

Catch-up vaccination with PCV13:
- Administer 1 dose of PCV13 to all healthy children aged 24 through 59 months who are not completely vaccinated for their age.
- For other catch-up guidance, see Figure 2.

Vaccination of persons with high-risk conditions with PCV13 and PPSV23:
- All recommended PCV13 doses should be administered prior to PPSV23 vaccination if possible.
- For children 2 through 5 years of age with any of the following conditions: chronic heart disease (particularly cyanotic congenital heart disease and cardiac failure); chronic lung disease (including asthma if treated with high-dose oral corticosteroid therapy); diabetes mellitus; cerebrospinal fluid leak; cochlear implant; sickle cell disease and other hemoglobinopathies; anatomic or functional asplenia; HIV infection; chronic renal failure; nephrotic syndrome; diseases associated with treatment with immunosuppressive drugs or radiation therapy, including malignant neoplasms, leukemias, lymphomas, and Hodgkin disease; solid organ transplantation; or congenital immunodeficiency:
  1. Administer 1 dose of PCV13 if 3 doses of PCV (PCV7 and/or PCV13) were received previously.
  2. Administer 2 doses of PCV13 at least 8 weeks apart if fewer than 3 doses of PCV (PCV7 and/or PCV13) were received previously.

6. **Pneumococcal vaccines (cont'd)**
  3. Administer 1 supplemental dose of PCV13 if 4 doses of PCV7 or other age-appropriate complete PCV7 series was received previously.
  4. The minimum interval between doses of PCV (PCV7 or PCV13) is 8 weeks.
  5. For children with no history of PPSV23 vaccination, administer PPSV23 at least 8 weeks after the most recent dose of PCV13.
- For children aged 6 through 18 years who have cerebrospinal fluid leak; cochlear implant; sickle cell disease and other hemoglobinopathies; anatomic or functional asplenia; congenital or acquired immunodeficiencies; HIV infection; chronic renal failure; nephrotic syndrome; diseases associated with treatment with immunosuppressive drugs or radiation therapy, including malignant neoplasms, leukemias, lymphomas, and Hodgkin disease; generalized malignancy; solid organ transplantation; or multiple myeloma:
  1. If neither PCV13 nor PPSV23 has been received previously, administer 1 dose of PCV13 now and 1 dose of PPSV23 at least 8 weeks later.
  2. If PCV13 has been received previously but PPSV23 has not, administer 1 dose of PPSV23 at least 8 weeks after the most recent dose of PCV13.
  3. If PPSV23 has been received but PCV13 has not, administer 1 dose of PCV13 at least 8 weeks after the most recent dose of PPSV23.
- For children aged 6 through 18 years with chronic heart disease (particularly cyanotic congenital heart disease and cardiac failure), diabetes mellitus, alcoholism, or chronic liver disease, who have not received PPSV23, administer 1 dose of PPSV23. If PCV13 has been received previously, then PPSV23 should be administered at least 8 weeks after any prior PCV13 dose.
- A single revaccination with PPSV23 should be administered 5 years after the first dose to children with sickle cell disease or other hemoglobinopathies; anatomic or functional asplenia; congenital or acquired immunodeficiencies; HIV infection; chronic renal failure; nephrotic syndrome; diseases associated with treatment with immunosuppressive drugs or radiation therapy, including malignant neoplasms, leukemias, lymphomas, and Hodgkin disease; generalized malignancy; solid organ transplantation; or multiple myeloma.

7. **Inactivated poliovirus vaccine (IPV). (Minimum age: 6 weeks)**

Routine vaccination:
- Administer a 4-dose series of IPV at ages 2, 4, 6 through 18 months, and 4 through 6 years. The final dose in the series should be administered on or after the fourth birthday and at least 6 months after the previous dose.

Catch-up vaccination:
- In the first 6 months of life, minimum age and minimum intervals are only recommended if the person is at risk for imminent exposure to circulating poliovirus (i.e., travel to a polio-endemic region or during an outbreak).
- If 4 or more doses are administered before age 4 years, an additional dose should be administered at age 4 through 6 years and at least 6 months after the previous dose.
- A fourth dose is not necessary if the third dose was administered at age 4 years or older and at least 6 months after the previous dose.
- If both OPV and IPV were administered as part of a series, a total of 4 doses should be administered, regardless of the child's current age. IPV is not routinely recommended for U.S. residents aged 18 years or older.
- For other catch-up guidance, see Figure 2.

8. **Influenza vaccines. (Minimum age: 6 months for inactivated influenza vaccine [IIV], 2 years for live, attenuated influenza vaccine [LAIV]**

Routine vaccination:
- Administer influenza vaccine annually to all children beginning at age 6 months. For most healthy, nonpregnant persons aged 2 through 49 years, either LAIV or IIV may be used. However, LAIV should NOT be administered to some persons, including 1) those with asthma, 2) children 2 through 4 years who had wheezing in the past 12 months, or 3) those who have any other underlying medical conditions that predispose them to influenza complications. For all other contraindications to use of LAIV, see *MMWR* 2013; 62 (No. RR-7):1-43, available at http://www.cdc.gov/mmwr/pdf/rr/rr6207.pdf.

For children aged 6 months through 8 years:
- For the 2013–14 season, administer 2 doses (separated by at least 4 weeks) to children who are receiving influenza vaccine for the first time. Some children in this age group who have been vaccinated previously will also need 2 doses. For additional guidance, follow dosing guidelines in the 2013-14 ACIP influenza vaccine recommendations, *MMWR* 2013; 62 (No. RR-7):1-43, available at http://www.cdc.gov/mmwr/pdf/rr/rr6207.pdf.
- For the 2014–15 season, follow dosing guidelines in the 2014 ACIP influenza vaccine recommendations.

For persons aged 9 years and older:
- Administer 1 dose.

For further guidance on the use of the vaccines mentioned below, see: http://www.cdc.gov/vaccines/hcp/acip-recs/index.html.

9. **Measles, mumps, and rubella (MMR) vaccine. (Minimum age: 12 months for routine vaccination)**

Routine vaccination:

- Administer a 2-dose series of MMR vaccine at ages 12 through 15 months and 4 through 6 years. The second dose may be administered before age 4 years, provided at least 4 weeks have elapsed since the first dose.
- Administer 1 dose of MMR vaccine to infants aged 6 through 11 months before departure from the United States for international travel. These children should be revaccinated with 2 doses of MMR vaccine, the first at age 12 through 15 months (12 months if the child remains in an area where disease risk is high), and the second dose at least 4 weeks later.
- Administer 2 doses of MMR vaccine to children aged 12 months and older before departure from the United States for international travel. The first dose should be administered on or after age 12 months and the second dose at least 4 weeks later.

Catch-up vaccination:

- Ensure that all school-aged children and adolescents have had 2 doses of MMR vaccine; the minimum interval between the 2 doses is 4 weeks.

10. **Varicella (VAR) vaccine. (Minimum age: 12 months)**

Routine vaccination:

- Administer a 2-dose series of VAR vaccine at ages 12 through 15 months and 4 through 6 years. The second dose may be administered before age 4 years, provided at least 3 months have elapsed since the first dose. If the second dose was administered at least 4 weeks after the first dose, it can be accepted as valid.

Catch-up vaccination:

- Ensure that all persons aged 7 through 18 years without evidence of immunity (see MMWR 2007; 56 [No. RR-4], available at http://www.cdc.gov/mmwr/pdf/rr/rr5604.pdf) have 2 doses of varicella vaccine. For children aged 7 through 12 years, the recommended minimum interval between doses is 3 months (if the second dose was administered at least 4 weeks after the first dose, it can be accepted as valid); for persons aged 13 years and older, the minimum interval between doses is 4 weeks.

11. **Hepatitis A (HepA) vaccine. (Minimum age: 12 months)**

Routine vaccination:

- Initiate the 2-dose HepA vaccine series at 12 through 23 months; separate the 2 doses by 6 to 18 months.
- Children who have received 1 dose of HepA vaccine before age 24 months should receive a second dose 6 to 18 months after the first dose.
- For any person aged 2 years and older who has not already received the HepA vaccine series, 2 doses of HepA vaccine separated by 6 to 18 months may be administered if immunity against hepatitis A virus infection is desired.

Catch-up vaccination:

- The minimum interval between the two doses is 6 months.

Special populations:

- Administer 2 doses of HepA vaccine at least 6 months apart to previously unvaccinated persons who live in areas where vaccination programs target older children, or who are at increased risk for infection. This includes persons traveling to or working in countries that have high or intermediate endemicity of infection; men having sex with men; users of injection and non-injection illicit drugs; persons who work with HAV-infected primates or with HAV in a research laboratory; persons with clotting-factor disorders; persons with chronic liver disease; and persons who anticipate close, personal contact (e.g., household or regular babysitting) with an international adoptee during the first 60 days after arrival in the United States from a country with high or intermediate endemicity. The first dose should be administered as soon as the adoption is planned, ideally 2 or more weeks before the arrival of the adoptee.

12. **Human papillomavirus (HPV) vaccines. (Minimum age: 9 years for HPV2 [Cervarix] and HPV4 [Gardisil])**

Routine vaccination:

- Administer a 3-dose series of HPV vaccine on a schedule of 0, 1-2, and 6 months to all adolescents aged 11 through 12 years. Either HPV4 or HPV2 may be used for females, and only HPV4 may be used for males.
- The vaccine series may be started at age 9 years.
- Administer the second dose 1 to 2 months after the first dose (minimum interval of 4 weeks), administer the third dose 24 weeks after the first dose and 16 weeks after the second dose (minimum interval of 12 weeks).

Catch-up vaccination:

- Administer the vaccine series to females (either HPV2 or HPV4) and males (HPV4) at age 13 through 18 years if not previously vaccinated.
- Use recommended routine dosing intervals (see above) for vaccine series catch-up.

13. **Meningococcal conjugate vaccines. (Minimum age: 6 weeks for Hib-MenCY [MenHibrix], 9 months for MenACWY-D [Menactra], 2 months for MenACWY-CRM [Menveo])**

Routine vaccination:

- Administer a single dose of Menactra or Menveo vaccine at age 11 through 12 years, with a booster dose at age 16 years.
- Adolescents aged 11 through 18 years with human immunodeficiency virus (HIV) infection should receive a 2-dose primary series of Menactra or Menveo with at least 8 weeks between doses.
- For children aged 2 months through 18 years with high-risk conditions, see below.

Catch-up vaccination:

- Administer Menactra or Menveo vaccine at age 13 through 18 years if not previously vaccinated.
- If the first dose is administered at age 13 through 15 years, a booster dose should be administered at age 16 through 18 years with a minimum interval of at least 8 weeks between doses.
- If the first dose is administered at age 16 years or older, a booster dose is not needed.
- For other catch-up guidance, see Figure 2.

Vaccination of persons with high-risk conditions and other persons at increased risk of disease:

Children with anatomic or functional asplenia (including sickle cell disease):

1. For children younger than 19 months of age, administer a 4-dose infant series of MenHibrix or Menveo at 2, 4, 6, and 12 through 15 months of age.
2. For children aged 19 through 23 months who have not completed a series of MenHibrix or Menveo, administer 2 primary doses of Menveo at least 3 months apart.
3. For children aged 24 months and older who have not received a complete series of MenHibrix or Menveo or Menactra, administer 2 primary doses of either Menactra or Menveo at least 2 months apart. If Menactra is administered to a child with asplenia (including sickle cell disease), do not administer Menactra until 2 years of age and at least 4 weeks after the completion of all PCV13 doses.

Children with persistent complement component deficiency:

1. For children younger than 19 months of age, administer a 4-dose infant series of either MenHibrix or Menveo at 2, 4, 6, and 12 through 15 months of age.
2. For children 7 through 23 months who have not initiated vaccination, two options exist depending on age and vaccine brand:
   a. For children who initiate vaccination with Menveo at 7 months through 23 months of age, a 2-dose series should be administered with the second dose after 12 months of age and at least 3 months after the first dose.
   b. For children who initiate vaccination with Menactra at 9 months through 23 months of age, a 2-dose series of Menactra should be administered at least 3 months apart.
   c. For children aged 24 months and older who have not received a complete series of MenHibrix, Menveo, or Menactra, administer 2 primary doses of either Menactra or Menveo at least 2 months apart.

- For children who travel to or reside in countries in which meningococcal disease is hyperendemic or epidemic, including countries in the African meningitis belt or the Hajj, administer an age-appropriate formulation and series of Menactra or Menveo for protection against serogroups A and W meningococcal disease. Prior receipt of MenHibrix is not sufficient for children traveling to the meningitis belt or the Hajj because it does not contain serogroups A or W.
- For children at risk during a community outbreak attributable to a vaccine serogroup, administer or complete an age- and formulation-appropriate series of MenHibrix, Menactra, or Menveo.
- For booster doses among persons with high-risk conditions, refer to MMWR 2013; 62(RR02);1-22, available at http://www.cdc.gov/mmwr/preview/mmwrhtml/rr6202a1.htm.

Catch-up recommendations for persons with high-risk conditions:

1. If MenHibrix is administered to achieve protection against meningococcal disease, a complete age-appropriate series of MenHibrix should be administered.
2. If the first dose of MenHibrix is given at or after 12 months of age, a total of 2 doses should be given at least 8 weeks apart to ensure protection against serogroups C and Y meningococcal disease.
3. For children who initiate vaccination with Menveo at 7 months of age, a 2-dose series should be administered with the second dose after 12 months of age and at least 3 months after the first dose.
4. For other catch-up recommendations for these persons, refer to MMWR 2013; 62(RR02);1-22, available at http://www.cdc.gov/mmwr/preview/mmwrhtml/rr6202a1.htm.

For complete information on use of meningococcal vaccines, including guidance related to vaccination of persons at increased risk of infection, see MMWR March 22, 2013; 62(RR02);1-22, available at http://www.cdc.gov/mmwr/pdf/rr/rr6202.pdf.

Source: Centers for Disease Control and Prevention

Table 19-2 Catch-up Immunization Schedule for Individuals Aged 4 Months through 18 years Who Start Late or Who Are More Than 1 Month behind–United States–2014.

FIGURE 2. Catch-up immunization schedule for persons aged 4 months through 18 years who start late or who are more than 1 month behind —United States, 2014.

The figure below provides catch-up schedules and minimum intervals between doses for children whose vaccinations have been delayed. A vaccine series does not need to be restarted, regardless of the time that has elapsed between doses. Use the section appropriate for the child's age. Always use this table in conjunction with Figure 1 and the footnotes that follow.

Vaccine	Minimum Age for Dose 1	Minimum Interval Between Doses			
		Dose 1 to dose 2	Dose 2 to dose 3	Dose 3 to dose 4	Dose 4 to dose 5
Persons aged 4 months through 6 years					
Hepatitis B[1]	Birth	4 weeks	8 weeks and at least 16 weeks after first dose; minimum age for the final dose is 24 weeks		
Rotavirus[2]	6 weeks	4 weeks	4 weeks[2]		
Diphtheria, tetanus, & acellular pertussis[3]	6 weeks	4 weeks	4 weeks	6 months	6 months[3]
Haemophilus influenzae type b[5]	6 weeks	4 weeks if first dose administered at younger than age 12 months / 8 weeks (as final dose) if first dose administered at age 12 through 14 months / No further doses needed if first dose administered at age 15 months or older	4 weeks[5] if current age is younger than 12 months and first dose administered at < 7 months old / 8 weeks (as final dose)[5] if current age is younger than 12 months through 59 months (as final dose); if current age is 12 months and age 12 months through 59 months and first dose administered between 7 through 11 months (regardless of Hib vaccine [PRP-T or PRP-OMP] used for first dose); OR if current age is 12 through 59 months and first dose administered at younger than age 12 months; OR first 2 doses were PRP-OMP and administered at younger than 12 months. / No further doses needed if previous dose administered at age 15 months or older	8 weeks (as final dose) This dose only necessary for children aged 12 through 59 months who received 3 (PRP-T) doses before age 12 months and started the primary series before age 7 months	
Pneumococcal[6]	6 weeks	4 weeks if first dose administered at younger than age 12 months / 8 weeks (as final dose for healthy children) if first dose administered at age 12 months or older / No further doses needed for healthy children if first dose administered at age 24 months or older	4 weeks if current age is younger than 12 months / 8 weeks (as final dose for healthy children) if current age is 12 months or older / No further doses needed for healthy children if previous dose administered at age 24 months or older	8 weeks (as final dose) This dose only necessary for children aged 12 through 59 months who received 3 doses before age 12 months or for children at high risk who received 3 doses at any age	
Inactivated poliovirus[7]	6 weeks	4 weeks[7]	4 weeks[7]	6 months[7] minimum age 4 years for final dose	
Meningococcal[13]	6 weeks	8 weeks[13]	See footnote 13	See footnote 13	
Measles, mumps, rubella[9]	12 months	4 weeks			
Varicella[10]	12 months	3 months			
Hepatitis A[11]	12 months	6 months			
Persons aged 7 through 18 years					
Tetanus, diphtheria; tetanus, diphtheria, & acellular pertussis[4]	7 years[4]	4 weeks	4 weeks if first dose of DTaP/DT administered at younger than age 12 months / 6 months if first dose of DTaP/DT administered at age 12 months or older and then no further doses needed for catch-up	6 months if first dose of DTaP/DT administered at younger than age 12 months	
Human papillomavirus[12]	9 years	Routine dosing intervals are recommended[12]			
Hepatitis A[11]	12 months	6 months			
Hepatitis B[1]	Birth	4 weeks	8 weeks (and at least 16 weeks after first dose)		
Inactivated poliovirus[7]	6 weeks	4 weeks	4 weeks[7]	6 months[7]	
Meningococcal[13]	6 weeks	8 weeks[13]	See footnote 13		
Measles, mumps, rubella[9]	12 months	4 weeks			
Varicella[10]	12 months	3 months if person is younger than age 13 years / 4 weeks if person is aged 13 years or older			

NOTE: The above recommendations must be read along with the footnotes of this schedule.

Footnotes — Recommended immunization schedule for persons aged 0 through 18 years—United States, 2014

For further guidance on the use of the vaccines mentioned below, see: http://www.cdc.gov/vaccines/hcp/acip-recs/index.html.
For vaccine recommendations for persons 19 years of age and older, see the adult immunization schedule.

Additional information

- For contraindications and precautions to use of a vaccine and for additional information regarding that vaccine, vaccination providers should consult the relevant ACIP statement available online at http://www.cdc.gov/vaccines/hcp/acip-recs/index.html.
- For purposes of calculating intervals between doses, 4 weeks = 28 days. Intervals of 4 months or greater are determined by calendar months.
- Vaccine doses administered 4 days or less before the minimum interval or minimum age should not be counted as valid doses and should be repeated as age-appropriate. The repeat dose should be spaced after the invalid dose by the recommended minimum interval. For further details, see *MMWR, General Recommendations on Immunization and Reports / Vol. 60 / No. 2; Table 1. Recommended and minimum ages and intervals between vaccine doses* available online at http://www.cdc.gov/mmwr/pdf/rr/rr6002.pdf.
- Information on travel vaccine requirements and recommendations is available at http://wwwnc.cdc.gov/travel/destinations/list.
- For vaccination of persons with primary and secondary immunodeficiencies, see Table 13, *"Vaccination of persons with primary and secondary immunodeficiencies,"* in General Recommendations on Immunization (ACIP), available at http://www.cdc.gov/mmwr/pdf/rr/rr6002.pdf; and American Academy of Pediatrics. Immunization in Special Clinical Circumstances, in Pickering LK, Baker CJ, Kimberlin DW, Long SS eds. *Red Book: 2012 report of the Committee on Infectious Diseases. 29th ed.* Elk Grove Village, IL: American Academy of Pediatrics.

1. **Hepatitis B (HepB) vaccine. (Minimum age: birth)**
   Routine vaccination:
   At birth:
   - Administer monovalent HepB vaccine to all newborns before hospital discharge.
   - For infants born to hepatitis B surface antigen (HBsAg)-positive mothers, administer HepB vaccine and 0.5 mL of hepatitis B immune globulin (HBIG) within 12 hours of birth. These infants should be tested for HBsAg and antibody to HBsAg (anti-HBs) 1 to 2 months after completion of the HepB series, at age 9 through 18 months (preferably at the next well-child visit).
   - If mother's HBsAg status is unknown, within 12 hours of birth administer HepB vaccine regardless of birth weight. For infants weighing less than 2,000 grams, administer HBIG in addition to HepB vaccine within 12 hours of birth. Determine mother's HBsAg status as soon as possible and, if mother is HBsAg-positive, also administer HBIG for infants weighing 2,000 grams or more as soon as possible, but no later than age 7 days.

   Doses following the birth dose:
   - The second dose should be administered at age 1 or 2 months. Monovalent HepB vaccine should be used for doses administered before age 6 weeks.
   - Infants who did not receive a birth dose should receive 3 doses of a HepB-containing vaccine on a schedule of 0, 1 to 2 months, and 6 months starting as soon as feasible. See Figure 2.
   - Administer the second dose 1 to 2 months after the first dose (minimum interval of 4 weeks), administer the third dose at least 8 weeks after the second dose AND at least 16 weeks after the first dose. The final (third or fourth) dose in the HepB vaccine series should be administered no earlier than age 24 weeks.
   - Administration of a total of 4 doses of HepB vaccine is permitted when a combination vaccine containing HepB is administered after the birth dose.

   Catch-up vaccination:
   - Unvaccinated persons should complete a 3-dose series.
   - A 2-dose series (doses separated by at least 4 months) of adult formulation Recombivax HB is licensed for use in children aged 11 through 15 years.
   - For other catch-up guidance, see Figure 2.

2. **Rotavirus (RV) vaccines. (Minimum age: 6 weeks for both RV1 [Rotarix] and RV5 [RotaTeq])**
   Routine vaccination:
   Administer a series of RV vaccine to all infants as follows:
   1. If Rotarix is used, administer a 2-dose series at 2 and 4 months of age.
   2. If RotaTeq is used, administer a 3-dose series at ages 2, 4, and 6 months.
   3. If any dose in the series was RotaTeq or vaccine product is unknown for any dose in the series, a total of 3 doses of RV vaccine should be administered.

   Catch-up vaccination:
   - The maximum age for the first dose in the series is 14 weeks, 6 days; vaccination should not be initiated for infants aged 15 weeks, 0 days or older.
   - The maximum age for the final dose in the series is 8 months, 0 days.
   - For other catch-up guidance, see Figure 2.

3. **Diphtheria and tetanus toxoids and acellular pertussis (DTaP) vaccine. (Minimum age: 6 weeks. Exception: DTaP-IPV [Kinrix]: 4 years)**
   Routine vaccination:
   - Administer a 5-dose series of DTaP vaccine at ages 2, 4, 6, 15 through 18 months, and 4 through 6 years. The fourth dose may be administered as early as age 12 months, provided at least 6 months have elapsed since the third dose.
   Catch-up vaccination:
   - The fifth dose of DTaP vaccine is not necessary if the fourth dose was administered at age 4 years or older.
   - For other catch-up guidance, see Figure 2.

4. **Tetanus and diphtheria toxoids and acellular pertussis (Tdap) vaccine. (Minimum age: 10 years for Boostrix, 11 years for Adacel)**
   Routine vaccination:
   - Administer 1 dose of Tdap vaccine to all adolescents aged 11 through 12 years.
   - Tdap may be administered regardless of the interval since the last tetanus and diphtheria toxoid-containing vaccine.
   - Administer 1 dose of Tdap vaccine to pregnant adolescents during each pregnancy (preferred during 27 through 36 weeks gestation) regardless of time since prior Td or Tdap vaccination.
   Catch-up vaccination:
   - Persons aged 7 years and older who are not fully immunized with DTaP vaccine should receive Tdap vaccine as 1 (preferably the first) dose in the catch-up series; if additional doses are needed, use Td vaccine. For children 7 through 10 years who receive a dose of Tdap as part of the catch-up series, an adolescent Tdap vaccine dose at age 11 through 12 years should NOT be administered. Td should be administered instead 10 years after the Tdap dose.
   - Persons aged 11 through 18 years who have not received Tdap vaccine should receive a dose followed by tetanus and diphtheria toxoids (Td) booster doses every 10 years thereafter.
   - Inadvertent doses of DTaP vaccine:
     - If administered inadvertently to a child aged 7 through 10 years may count as part of the catch-up series. This dose may count as the adolescent Tdap dose, or the child can later receive a Tdap booster dose at age 11 through 12 years.
     - If administered inadvertently to an adolescent aged 11 through 18 years, the dose should be counted as the adolescent Tdap booster.
   - For other catch-up guidance, see Figure 2.

5. **Haemophilus influenzae type b (Hib) conjugate vaccine. (Minimum age: 6 weeks for PRP-T [ACTHIB, DTaP-IPV/Hib (Pentacel) and Hib-MenCY (MenHibrix)], PRP-OMP [PedvaxHIB or COMVAX], 12 months for PRP-T [Hiberix])**
   Routine vaccination:
   - Administer a 2- or 3-dose Hib vaccine primary series and a booster dose (dose 3 or 4 depending on vaccine used in primary series) at age 12 through 15 months to complete a full Hib vaccine series.
   - The primary series with ActHIB, MenHibrix, or Pentacel consists of 3 doses and should be administered at 2, 4, and 6 months of age. The primary series with PedvaxHIB or COMVAX consists of 2 doses and should be administered at 2 and 4 months of age; a dose at age 6 months is not indicated.
   - One booster dose (dose 3 or 4 depending on vaccine used in primary series) of any Hib vaccine should be administered at age 12 through 15 months. An exception is Hiberix vaccine. Hiberix should only be used for the booster (final) dose in children aged 12 months through 4 years who have received at least 1 prior dose of Hib-containing vaccine.

(continued)

For further guidance on the use of the vaccines mentioned below, see: http://www.cdc.gov/vaccines/hcp/acip-recs/index.html.

5. *Haemophilus influenzae* type b (Hib) conjugate vaccine (cont'd)
- For recommendations on the use of MenHibrix in patients at increased risk for meningococcal disease, please refer to the meningococcal vaccine footnotes and also to *MMWR* March 22, 2013; 62(RR02);1-22, available at http://www.cdc.gov/mmwr/pdf/rr/rr6202.pdf.

Catch-up vaccination:
- If dose 1 was administered at ages 12 through 14 months, administer a second (final) dose at least 8 weeks after dose 1, regardless of Hib vaccine used in the primary series.
- If the first 2 doses were PRP-OMP (PedvaxHIB or COMVAX), and were administered at age 11 months or younger, the third (and final) dose should be administered at age 12 through 15 months and at least 8 weeks after the second dose.
- If the first dose was administered at age 7 through 11 months, administer the second dose at least 4 weeks later and a third (and final) dose at age 12 through 15 months or 8 weeks after second dose, whichever is later, regardless of Hib vaccine used for first dose.
- If first dose is administered at younger than 12 months of age and second dose is given between 12 through 14 months of age, a third (and final) dose should be given 8 weeks later.
- For unvaccinated children aged 15 months or older, administer only 1 dose.
- For other catch-up guidance, see Figure 2. For catch-up guidance related to MenHibrix, please see the meningococcal vaccine footnotes and also *MMWR* March 22, 2013; 62(RR02);1-22, available at http://www.cdc.gov/mmwr/pdf/rr/rr6202.pdf.

Vaccination of persons with high-risk conditions:
- Children aged 12 through 59 months who are at increased risk for Hib disease, including chemotherapy recipients and those with anatomic or functional asplenia (including sickle cell disease), human immunodeficiency virus (HIV) infection, immunoglobulin deficiency, or early component complement deficiency, who have received either no doses or only 1 dose of Hib vaccine before 12 months of age, should receive 2 additional doses of Hib vaccine 8 weeks apart; children who received 2 or more doses of Hib vaccine before 12 months of age should receive 1 additional dose.
- For patients younger than 5 years of age undergoing chemotherapy or radiation treatment who received a Hib vaccine dose(s) within 14 days of starting therapy or during therapy, repeat the dose(s) at least 3 months following therapy completion.
- Recipients of hematopoietic stem cell transplant (HSCT) should be revaccinated with a 3-dose regimen of Hib vaccine starting 6 to 12 months after successful transplant, regardless of vaccination history; doses should be administered at least 4 weeks apart.
- A single dose of any Hib-containing vaccine should be administered to unimmunized* children and adolescents 15 months of age and older undergoing an elective splenectomy; if possible, vaccine should be administered at least 14 days before procedure.
- Hib vaccine is not routinely recommended for patients 5 years or older. However, 1 dose of Hib vaccine should be administered to unimmunized* persons aged 5 years or older who have anatomic or functional asplenia (including sickle cell disease) and unvaccinated persons 5 through 18 years of age with human immunodeficiency virus (HIV) infection.
  *Patients who have not received a primary series and booster dose or at least 1 dose of Hib vaccine after 14 months of age are considered unimmunized.

6. Pneumococcal vaccines. (Minimum age: 6 weeks for PCV13, 2 years for PPSV23)

Routine vaccination with PCV13:
- Administer a 4-dose series of PCV13 vaccine at ages 2, 4, and 6 months and at age 12 through 15 months.
- For children aged 14 through 59 months who have received an age-appropriate series of 7-valent PCV (PCV7), administer a single supplemental dose of 13-valent PCV (PCV13).

Catch-up vaccination with PCV13:
- Administer 1 dose of PCV13 to all healthy children aged 24 through 59 months who are not completely vaccinated for their age.
- For other catch-up guidance, see Figure 2.

Vaccination of persons with high-risk conditions with PCV13 and PPSV23:
- All recommended PCV13 doses should be administered prior to PPSV23 vaccination if possible.
- For children 2 through 5 years of age with any of the following conditions: chronic heart disease (particularly cyanotic congenital heart disease and cardiac failure); chronic lung disease (including asthma if treated with high-dose oral corticosteroid therapy); diabetes mellitus; cerebrospinal fluid leak; cochlear implant; sickle cell disease and other hemoglobinopathies; anatomic or functional asplenia; HIV infection; chronic renal failure; nephrotic syndrome; diseases associated with treatment with immunosuppressive drugs or radiation therapy, including malignant neoplasms, leukemias, lymphomas, and Hodgkin disease; solid organ transplantation; or congenital immunodeficiency:
  1. Administer 1 dose of PCV13 if 3 doses of PCV (PCV7 and/or PCV13) were received previously.
  2. Administer 2 doses of PCV13 at least 8 weeks apart if fewer than 3 doses of PCV (PCV7 and/or PCV13) were received previously.

6. Pneumococcal vaccines (cont'd)
  3. Administer 1 supplemental dose of PCV13 if 4 doses of PCV7 or other age-appropriate complete PCV7 series was received previously.
  4. The minimum interval between doses of PCV (PCV7 or PCV13) is 8 weeks.
  5. For children with no history of PPSV23 vaccination, administer PPSV23 at least 8 weeks after the most recent dose of PCV13.
- For children aged 6 through 18 years who have cerebrospinal fluid leak; cochlear implant; sickle cell disease and other hemoglobinopathies; anatomic or functional asplenia; congenital or acquired immunodeficiencies; HIV infection; chronic renal failure; nephrotic syndrome; diseases associated with immunosuppressive drugs or radiation therapy, including malignant neoplasms, leukemias, lymphomas, and Hodgkin disease; generalized malignancy; solid organ transplantation; or multiple myeloma:
  1. If neither PCV13 nor PPSV23 has been received previously, administer 1 dose of PCV13 now and 1 dose of PPSV23 at least 8 weeks later.
  2. If PCV13 has been received previously but PPSV23 has not, administer 1 dose of PPSV23 at least 8 weeks after the most recent dose of PCV13.
  3. If PPSV23 has been received but PCV13 has not, administer 1 dose of PCV13 at least 8 weeks after the most recent dose of PPSV23.
- For children aged 6 through 18 years with chronic heart disease (particularly cyanotic congenital heart disease and cardiac failure), diabetes mellitus, alcoholism, or chronic liver disease, who have not received previously, then PPSV23 should be administered at least 8 weeks after any prior PCV13 dose.
- A single revaccination with PPSV23 should be administered 5 years after the first dose to children with sickle cell disease or other hemoglobinopathies; anatomic or functional asplenia; congenital or acquired immunodeficiencies; HIV infection; chronic renal failure; nephrotic syndrome; diseases associated with treatment with immunosuppressive drugs or radiation therapy, including malignant neoplasms, leukemias, lymphomas, and Hodgkin disease; generalized malignancy; solid organ transplantation; or multiple myeloma.

7. Inactivated poliovirus vaccine (IPV). (Minimum age: 6 weeks)

Routine vaccination:
- Administer a 4-dose series of IPV at ages 2, 4, 6 through 18 months, and 4 through 6 years. The final dose in the series should be administered on or after the fourth birthday and at least 6 months after the previous dose.

Catch-up vaccination:
- In the first 6 months of life, minimum age and minimum intervals are only recommended if the person is at risk for imminent exposure to circulating poliovirus (i.e, travel to a polio-endemic region or during an outbreak).
- If 4 or more doses are administered before age 4 years, an additional dose should be administered at age 4 through 6 years and at least 6 months after the previous dose.
- A fourth dose is not necessary if the third dose was administered at age 4 years or older and at least 6 months after the previous dose.
- If both OPV and IPV were administered as part of a series, a total of 4 doses should be administered, regardless of the child's current age. IPV is not routinely recommended for U.S. residents aged 18 years or older.
- For other catch-up guidance, see Figure 2.

8. Influenza vaccines. (Minimum age: 6 months for inactivated influenza vaccine [IIV], 2 years for live, attenuated influenza vaccine [LAIV])

Routine vaccination:
- Administer influenza vaccine annually to all children beginning at age 6 months. For most healthy, nonpregnant persons aged 2 through 49 years, either LAIV or IIV may be used. However, LAIV should NOT be administered to some persons, including 1) those with asthma, 2) children 2 through 4 years who had wheezing in the past 12 months, or 3) those who have any other underlying medical conditions that predispose them to influenza complications. For all other contraindications to use of LAIV, see *MMWR* 2013; 62 (No. RR-7):1-43, available at http://www.cdc.gov/mmwr/pdf/rr/rr6207.pdf.

For children aged 6 months through 8 years:
- For the 2013–14 season, administer 2 doses (separated by at least 4 weeks) to children who are receiving influenza vaccine for the first time. Some children in this age group who have been vaccinated previously will also need 2 doses. For additional guidance, follow dosing guidelines in the 2013-14 ACIP influenza vaccine recommendations, *MMWR* 2013; 62 (No. RR-7):1-43, available at http://www.cdc.gov/mmwr/pdf/rr/rr6207.pdf.
- For the 2014–15 season, follow dosing guidelines in the 2014 ACIP influenza vaccine recommendations.

For persons aged 9 years and older:
- Administer 1 dose.

For further guidance on the use of the vaccines mentioned below, see: http://www.cdc.gov/vaccines/hcp/acip-recs/index.html.

9. **Measles, mumps, and rubella (MMR) vaccine. (Minimum age: 12 months for routine vaccination)**

   Routine vaccination:
   - Administer a 2-dose series of MMR vaccine at ages12 through 15 months and 4 through 6 years. The second dose may be administered before age 4 years, provided at least 4 weeks have elapsed since the first dose.
   - Administer 1 dose of MMR vaccine to infants aged 6 through 11 months before departure from the United States for international travel. These children should be revaccinated with 2 doses of MMR vaccine, the first at age 12 through 15 months (12 months if the child remains in an area where disease risk is high), and the second dose at least 4 weeks later.
   - Administer 2 doses of MMR vaccine to children aged 12 months and older before departure from the United States for international travel. The first dose should be administered on or after age 12 months and the second dose at least 4 weeks later.

   Catch-up vaccination:
   - Ensure that all school-aged children and adolescents have had 2 doses of MMR vaccine; the minimum interval between the 2 doses is 4 weeks.

10. **Varicella (VAR) vaccine. (Minimum age: 12 months)**

    Routine vaccination:
    - Administer a 2-dose series of VAR vaccine at ages 12 through 15 months and 4 through 6 years. The second dose may be administered before age 4 years, provided at least 3 months have elapsed since the first dose. If the second dose was administered at least 4 weeks after the first dose, it can be accepted as valid.

    Catch-up vaccination:
    - Ensure that all persons aged 7 through 18 years without evidence of immunity (see *MMWR* 2007; 56 [No. RR-4], available at http://www.cdc.gov/mmwr/pdf/rr/rr5604.pdf) have 2 doses of varicella vaccine. For children aged 7 through 12 years, the recommended minimum interval between doses is 3 months (if the second dose was administered at least 4 weeks after the first dose, it can be accepted as valid); for persons aged 13 years and older, the minimum interval between doses is 4 weeks.

11. **Hepatitis A (HepA) vaccine. (Minimum age: 12 months)**

    Routine vaccination:
    - Initiate the 2-dose HepA vaccine series at 12 through 23 months; separate the 2 doses by 6 to 18 months.
    - Children who have received 1 dose of HepA vaccine before age 24 months should receive a second dose 6 to 18 months after the first dose.
    - For any person aged 2 years and older who has not already received the HepA vaccine series, 2 doses of HepA vaccine separated by 6 to 18 months may be administered if immunity against hepatitis A virus infection is desired.

    Catch-up vaccination:
    - The minimum interval between the two doses is 6 months.

    Special populations:
    - Administer 2 doses of HepA vaccine at least 6 months apart to previously unvaccinated persons who live in areas where vaccination programs target older children, or who are at increased risk for infection. This includes persons traveling to or working in countries that have high or intermediate endemicity of infection; men having sex with men; users of injection and non-injection illicit drugs; persons who work with HAV-infected primates or with HAV in a research laboratory; persons with clotting-factor disorders; persons with chronic liver disease; and persons who anticipate close, personal contact (e.g., household or regular babysitting) with an international adoptee during the first 60 days after arrival in the United States from a country with high or intermediate endemicity. The first dose should be administered as soon as the adoption is planned, ideally 2 or more weeks before the arrival of the adoptee.

12. **Human papillomavirus (HPV) vaccines. (Minimum age: 9 years for HPV2 [Cervarix] and HPV4 [Gardisil])**

    Routine vaccination:
    - Administer a 3-dose series of HPV vaccine on a schedule of 0, 1-2, and 6 months to all adolescents aged 11 through 12 years. Either HPV4 or HPV2 may be used for females, and only HPV4 may be used for males.
    - The vaccine series may be started at age 9 years.
    - Administer the second dose 1 to 2 months after the first dose (minimum interval of 4 weeks), administer the third dose 24 weeks after the first dose and 16 weeks after the second dose (minimum interval of 12 weeks).

    Catch-up vaccination:
    - Administer the vaccine series to females (either HPV2 or HPV4) and males (HPV4) at age 13 through 18 years if not previously vaccinated.
    - Use recommended routine dosing intervals (see above) for vaccine series catch-up.

13. **Meningococcal conjugate vaccines. (Minimum age: 6 weeks for Hib-MenCY [MenHibrix], 9 months for MenACWY-D [Menactra], 2 months for MenACWY-CRM [Menveo])**

    Routine vaccination:
    - Administer a single dose of Menactra or Menveo vaccine at age 11 through 12 years, with a booster dose at age 16 years.
    - Adolescents aged 11 through 18 years with human immunodeficiency virus (HIV) infection should receive a 2-dose primary series of Menactra or Menveo with at least 8 weeks between doses.
    - For children aged 2 months through 18 years with high-risk conditions, see below.

    Catch-up vaccination:
    - Administer Menactra or Menveo vaccine at age 13 through 18 years if not previously vaccinated.
    - If the first dose is administered at age 13 through 15 years, a booster dose should be administered at age 16 through 18 years with a minimum interval of at least 8 weeks between doses.
    - If the first dose is administered at age 16 years or older, a booster dose is not needed.
    - For other catch-up guidance, see Figure 2.

    Vaccination of persons with high-risk conditions and other persons at increased risk of disease:
    - Children with anatomic or functional asplenia (including sickle cell disease):
      1. For children younger than 19 months of age, administer a 4-dose infant series of MenHibrix or Menveo at 2, 4, 6, and 12 through 15 months of age.
      2. For children aged 19 through 23 months who have not completed a series of MenHibrix or Menveo, administer 2 primary doses of Menveo at least 3 months apart.
      3. For children aged 24 months and older who have not received a complete series of MenHibrix or Menveo or Menactra, administer 2 primary doses of either Menactra or Menveo at least 2 months apart. If Menactra is administered to a child with asplenia (including sickle cell disease), do not administer Menactra until 2 years of age and at least 4 weeks after the completion of all PCV13 doses.

    - Children with persistent complement component deficiency:
      1. For children younger than 19 months of age, administer a 4-dose infant series of either MenHibrix or Menveo at 2, 4, 6, and 12 through 15 months of age.
      2. For children 7 through 23 months who have not initiated vaccination, two options exist depending on age and vaccine brand:
         a. For children who initiate vaccination with Menveo at 7 months through 23 months of age, a 2-dose series should be administered with the second dose after 12 months of age and at least 3 months after the first dose.
         b. For children who initiate vaccination with Menactra at 9 months through 23 months of age, a 2-dose series of Menactra should be administered at least 3 months apart.
         c. For children aged 24 months and older who have not received a complete series of MenHibrix, Menveo, or Menactra, administer 2 primary doses of either Menactra or Menveo at least 2 months apart.

    - For children who travel to or reside in countries in which meningococcal disease is hyperendemic or epidemic, including countries in the African meningitis belt or the Hajj, administer an age-appropriate formulation and series of Menactra or Menveo for protection against serogroups A and W meningococcal disease. Prior receipt of MenHibrix is not sufficient for children traveling to the meningitis belt or the Hajj because it does not contain serogroups A or W.
    - For children at risk during a community outbreak attributable to a vaccine serogroup, administer or complete an age- and formulation-appropriate series of MenHibrix, Menactra, or Menveo.
    - For booster doses among persons with high-risk conditions, refer to *MMWR* 2013; 62(RR02):1-22, available at http://www.cdc.gov/mmwr/preview/mmwrhtml/rr6202a1.htm.

    Catch-up recommendations for persons with high-risk conditions:
    1. If MenHibrix is administered to achieve protection against meningococcal disease, a complete age-appropriate series of MenHibrix should be administered.
    2. If the first dose of MenHibrix is given at or after 12 months of age, a total of 2 doses should be given at least 8 weeks apart to ensure protection against serogroups C and Y meningococcal disease.
    3. For children who initiate vaccination with Menveo at 7 months through 9 months of age, a 2-dose series should be administered with the second dose after 12 months of age and at least 3 months after the first dose.
    4. For other catch-up recommendations for these persons, refer to *MMWR* 2013; 62(RR02);1-22, available at http://www.cdc.gov/mmwr/preview/mmwrhtml/rr6202a1.htm.

    For complete information on use of meningococcal vaccines, including guidance related to vaccination of persons at increased risk of infection, see *MMWR* March 22, 2013; 62(RR02);1-22, available at http://www.cdc.gov/mmwr/pdf/rr/rr6202.pdf.

Source: Centers for Disease Control and Prevention

diphtheria (diff-**THEE**-ree-ah)	Serious infectious disease affecting the nose, pharynx, or larynx, usually resulting in sore throat, dysphonia (difficult speaking or hoarseness), and fever. The disease is caused by the bacterium *Corynebacterium diphtheriae*, which forms a white coating over the affected airways as it multiplies.

The bacterium releases a toxin into the bloodstream that can quickly damage the heart and nerves, resulting in heart failure, paralysis, and death.

Diphtheria is uncommon in countries such as the United States, where a **vaccine** against the disease is routinely given to children. The **immunization** for **diphtheria** is one of the components of the DPT **immunization**.

erythema infectiosum **(fifth disease)** (**air**-ih-**THEE**-mah in-**fek**-she-**OH**-sum)	A viral disease characterized by a face that appears as "slapped cheeks," a fiery red rash on the cheeks. See *Figure 19-8*.

In approximately one to four days after the appearance of the facial rash, a maculopapular rash appears on the trunk and extremities. There are usually only mild systemic responses during the course of this disease. This disease may last from 2 to 5 days, but rash may recur for several weeks under certain conditions (stress, exposure to heat or cold).

The infectious agent is the human parvovirus. The transmission of **erythema infectiosum** is through respiratory droplets, airborne particles, blood, and blood products. The incubation period is from 4 to 14 days. Its communicability is unknown but believed to be up to 7 days before the initial rash on the face appears. Therefore, isolation is not required.

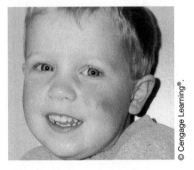

Figure 19-8 Erythema infectiosum

impetigo (im-peh-**TYE**-goh)	Contagious, superficial skin infection characterized by serous vesicles and pustules filled with millions of staphylococcus or streptococcus bacteria, usually forming on the face. See *Figure 19-9*.

Impetigo progresses to pruritic erosions and crusts with a honey-colored appearance. The discharge from the lesions allows the infection to be highly contagious.

Treatment for **impetigo** includes the use of oral and topical antibiotics. It is important to instruct the individual to complete the entire regime of systemic antibiotics to prevent the possibility of complications due to secondary infections such as acute glomerulonephritis (kidney infection, primarily in the glomeruli) and/or rheumatic fever.

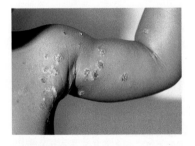

Figure 19-9 Impetigo

(Courtesy of Robert A. Silverman, MD, Clinical Associate Professor, Pediatric Dermatology, Georgetown University)

mumps **(infectious parotitis)** (in-**FEK**-shus pah-roh-**TYE**-tis)	Acute viral disease characterized by fever, swelling, and tenderness of one or more salivary glands, usually the parotid glands (below and in front of the ears). See *Figure 19-10*.

The infectious agent is the **mumps** virus. It is transmitted by droplet spread or by direct contact with the saliva of an infected person.

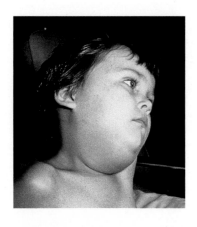

The incubation period is from 14 to 21 days. The period of maximum communicability is from immediately before to immediately after swelling begins. The **immunization** for **mumps (infectious parotitis)** is a part of the MMR **vaccine**.

Figure 19-10 Mumps (parotitis)
(Courtesy of the Centers for Disease Control and Prevention [CDC])

pertussis **(whooping cough)** (per-**TUSS**-is)	An acute, upper respiratory infectious disease caused by the *Bordetella pertussis* bacterium.

Pertussis (whooping cough) occurs mainly in children and infants. Early stages of **pertussis** are suggestive of the common cold, with slight elevation of fever, sneezing, rhinitis, dry cough, irritability, and loss of appetite.

As the disease progresses (approximately two weeks later), the cough is more violent and consists of a series of several short coughs followed by a long, drawn inspiration during which the typical whoop is heard. The coughing episode may be severe enough to cause vomiting. If diagnosed early, **pertussis** can be treated with oral antibiotics. Otherwise, antibiotics are ineffective and treatment (when needed) consists of supportive care, such as the administration of sedatives to reduce coughing and oxygen to facilitate respiration. **Pertussis** may be prevented by **immunization** of infants beginning at two months of age. The **immunization** for **pertussis** is one of the components of the DPT **immunization**.

roseola infantum (roh-zee-**OH**-lah in-**FAN**-tum) **rose/o** = rose colored	A viral disease with a sudden onset of a high fever for three to four days, during which time the child may experience mild cold-like symptoms and slight irritability. **Febrile** seizures may occur.

When the fever falls rapidly on the third or fourth day, a macular or maculopapular rash appears on the trunk, expanding to the rest of the body, only to fade in 24 hours.

The infectious agent is the herpesvirus 6. The transmission of **roseola infantum** is unknown, as is the incubation period and the period of communicability.

rubella (German measles; **3-day measles)** (roo-**BELL**-lah)	A mild **febrile** (fever-causing) infectious disease resembling both **scarlet fever** and measles but differing from these in its short course; characterized by a rash of both macules and papules that fades and disappears in three days. See *Figure 19-11*.

Koplik's spots and photophobia are not present with **rubella**. The infectious agent is the **rubella** virus, transmitted by direct contact or spread by infected persons (nasopharyngeal secretions) or by droplet spread.

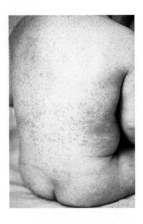

The incubation period for **rubella** is 14 to 21 days, and the period of communicability is from 7 days before to about 5 days after rash appears. The **immunization** for **rubella** is a part of the MMR **vaccine**.

Figure 19-11 Rubella
(Courtesy of the Centers for Disease Control and Prevention [CDC])

rubeola ("red measles," 7-day measles) (roo-bee-**OH**-lah) 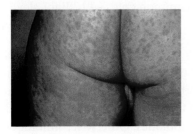	Acute, highly communicable viral disease that begins as an upper respiratory disorder with fever, sore throat, cough, runny nose, sensitivity to light, and possible conjunctivitis. Typical red, blotchy rash appears 4 to 5 days after onset of symptoms, beginning behind the ears, on the forehead, or cheeks and progressing to extremities and trunk and lasting about 5 days. See *Figure 19-12*.

Figure 19-12 Rubeola
(Courtesy of the Centers for Disease Control and Prevention [CDC])

Diagnosis is based on the presence of **Koplik's spots** in the mouth (spots with grayish centers and red, irregular outer rings). The measles virus is the infectious agent and is transmitted by droplet spread or by direct contact with secretions from an infected person.

The incubation period is from 10 to 20 days. **Rubeola** is communicable from 4 days before to 5 days after the rash appears. This **immunization** for measles is a part of the MMR **vaccine**.

scarlet fever (scarlatina) (**SCAR**-let **FEE**-ver) (scar-lah-**TEE**-nah) 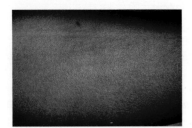	An acute, contagious disease characterized by sore throat, abrupt high fever, increased pulse, strawberry tongue (red and swollen), and punctiform (pointlike) bright red rash on the body. See *Figure 19-13*.

The infectious agent of **scarlet fever** (scarlatina) is group A, betahemolytic streptococci, transmitted by direct contact with an infected person or by droplet spread. Incubation period is 2 to 4 days, and the period of communicability is from onset until approximately 10 days after onset.

Figure 19-13 Scarlet fever
(Courtesy of the Centers for Disease Control and Prevention [CDC])

Review Checkpoint

Check your understanding of this section by completing the **Communicable Diseases** exercises in your workbook.

Pathological Conditions

The **basic definition** is in a green shaded box followed by a more detailed description in regular print. The phonetic pronunciation is directly beneath each term, as well as a breakdown of the component parts of the term where applicable.

asthma	Paroxysmal dyspnea (severe attack of difficult breathing) accompanied by **wheezing** caused by a spasm of the bronchial tubes or by swelling of the mucous membrane.
(**AZ**-mah)	

No age is exempt, but **asthma** occurs most frequently in childhood or early adulthood. **Asthma** differs from other obstructive lung diseases in that it is a reversible process. The attack may last from 30 minutes to several hours. In some circumstances the attack subsides spontaneously.

The asthmatic attack starts suddenly with coughing and a sensation of tightness in the chest; then slow, laborious, wheezy breathing begins. Expiration is much more strenuous and prolonged than inspiration, and the patient may assume a "hunched forward" position in an attempt to get more air.

Recurrence and severity of attacks are greatly influenced by secondary factors, by mental or physical fatigue, by exposure to fumes or secondhand cigarette smoke, by endocrine changes at various periods in life, and by emotional situations. Acute attacks of **asthma** may be relieved by a number of drugs (such as epinephrine). Status asthmaticus, a severe, prolonged **asthma** attack that is unresponsive to conventional therapy, is a medical emergency.

autism	**Autism** is a pervasive developmental disorder characterized by the individual being extremely withdrawn and absorbed with fantasy. The individual suffers from impaired communication/social interaction skills, and activities and interests are very limited.
(**AW**-tizm)	
aut/o = self	
-ism = condition	

Autism is usually first observed before the age of 3 and is first noticed by the mother or caretaker when the infant fails to be interested in others or fails to be socially responsive to others through eye contact and facial expressions. Autism occurs more frequently in boys than in girls. The etiology of autism is unknown.

Symptoms include but are not limited to language delay or total absence of language, **echolalia** (the repetition of sounds made by another person, such as the last word or words heard), withdrawal, bizarre body movements (rocking, waving, or flipping the hands back and forth), rigid adherence to routines and rituals, severe reactions to minor changes in routines, and repetitive actions. The play or behaviors of an autistic child will typically involve solitary activities.

Treatment is aimed at improving the overall functional status of the child by teaching communication, social, adaptive, and academic skills; decreasing unacceptable behavior patterns; helping the family manage stress associated with rearing a child with autism; and involving the caregivers in the therapy at home. It is extremely important to provide a highly structured environment with as much one-on-one instruction as possible. There is growing evidence that intense, early-intervention services for children with autism before the age of 5 years may lead to better outcomes.

cleft lip and palate
(**CLEFT LIP** and **PAL**-at)

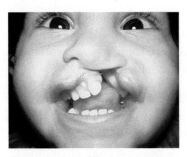

(A)

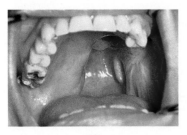

(B)

Cleft lip is a congenital defect in which there is an open space between the nasal cavity and the lip due to failure of the soft tissue and bones in this area to fuse properly during embryologic development. See *Figure 19-14A*. With **cleft palate**, the hard palate fails to fuse, resulting in a fissure (cracklike sore) in the middle of the palate. See *Figure 19-14B*.

As a result of these abnormalities, the newborn infant has difficulty with feeding and breathing. **Dentition** and speech can become problems as the child grows and develops.

The medical management of the child with a **cleft lip** and/or **palate** is based on the severity of the defect but is focused on feeding techniques that allow the newborn to have adequate intake and growth. The surgical management may begin for the **cleft lip** as early as two to four days but may wait until the child is 10 weeks old, weighs 10 pounds, and has a hemoglobin level of at least 10 g/dL. Cosmetic modifications may be done around the age of 4 to 5 years. For the child with a **cleft palate**, the repair will begin between six months and 2 years.

Figure 19-14 (A) Cleft lip; (B) Cleft palate
(Photos courtesy of Dr. Joseph Konzelman, School of Dentistry, Medical College of Georgia)

clubfoot
(talipes equinovarus)

(**TAL**-ih-peez **eh**-kwin-oh-**VAIR**-us)

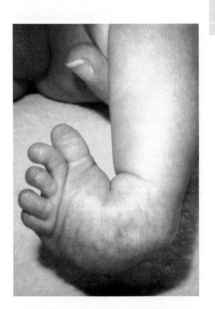

The medical term for clubfoot is *talipes equinovarus*. In this condition, the infant's foot is fixed in plantar flexion (turned downward) and deviates medially (turned inward), and the heel is in an elevated position. Therefore, the infant's foot cannot remain in normal position with the sole of the foot firmly on the floor. See *Figure 19-15*.

The diagnosis of **clubfoot** is made by physical examination soon after birth. Initial treatment is nonoperative, consisting of manipulation to improve the alignment of the foot, followed by application of a long-leg cast to maintain the alignment. Multiple casts are required to correct the clubfoot.

Most children who are born with clubfoot will walk at the appropriate age and will have normal use of their feet and ankles by school age because treatment is begun immediately after diagnosis. In rare cases, surgery is required to correct the deformity. If this is necessary, surgery is usually performed between 6 and 12 months of age.

Figure 19-15 Clubfoot (talipes equinovarus)
(Courtesy of the Centers for Disease Control and Prevention [CDC]/James W. Hanson, M.D.)

coarctation of the aorta (**koh**-ark-**TAY**-shun of the ay-**OR**-tah)	A congenital heart defect characterized by a localized narrowing of the aorta, which results in increased blood pressure in the upper extremities (area proximal to the defect) and decreased blood pressure in the lower extremities (area distal to the defect). Refer to the cardiovascular system for a visual reference. The classic sign of **coarctation of the aorta** is a contrast in pulsations and blood pressures in the arms and legs. The femoral, popliteal, and pedal pulses are weak or delayed in comparison with the strong, bounding pulses found in the arms and carotid arteries. Surgical correction of the defect is curative if the disease is diagnosed early.
croup (**CROOP**)	A childhood illness characterized by a barking cough, **stridor** (high-pitched musical sound when breathing in), and laryngeal spasm. The symptoms of **croup** can be dramatic and anxiety producing to the parent and the child. It is important to approach the child and parents in a calm manner to reduce fears and anxiety. Treatment includes providing a high-humidity atmosphere with cool moisture (cool mist vaporizer) and rest to relieve the symptoms. **Croup** may result from an acute obstruction of the larynx caused by an allergen, foreign body, viral infection, or new growth.
cryptorchidism (kript-**OR**-kid-izm) **crypt/o** = hidden **orchid/o** = testicle **-ism** = condition	Condition of undescended testicle(s); the absence of one or both testicles from the scrotum. The testicle may be located in the abdominal cavity or in the inguinal canal. If the testicle does not descend on its own, surgery will be necessary to correct the position, usually before age 3. The surgery for **cryptorchidism** (known as an **orchiopexy**) involves making an incision into the inguinal canal, locating the testicle, and bringing it back down into the scrotal sac. This surgery is usually done on an outpatient basis, with normal physical activity being restored within a few weeks to a month.
Down syndrome (**DOWN SIN**-drohm) 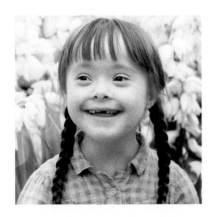	A congenital condition characterized by multiple defects and varying degrees of mental retardation. See *Figure 19-16.* The cause of **Down syndrome** (DS) is unknown. However, maternal age over 35 years has consistently been noted as a risk factor. It is also called **trisomy 21**, indicating that there are three 21st chromosomes present instead of the normal two. In addition to the mental retardation, specific clinical manifestations evident at birth include low-set ears; a short, broad appearance to the head (brachycephaly); protruding tongue; short, thick neck; simian line (transverse crease on palm); broad, short feet and hands; poor or diminished muscle tone; and hyperflexible joints. The diagnosis of DS can be made prenatally by testing the amniotic fluid. **Figure 19-16** Down syndrome *Denis Kuvaev/Shutterstock.com*

dwarfism (**DWARF**-ism) 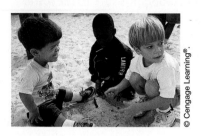 **Figure 19-17** Dwarfism	Generalized growth retardation of the body due to the deficiency of the human growth hormone; also known as congenital hypopituitarism or hypopituitarism. See *Figure 19-17*. The abnormal underdevelopment leaves the child extremely short, with a small body. There is an absence of secondary sex characteristics. The condition may have a connection with other defects or varying degrees of mental retardation. Treatment may include administration of human growth hormone or somatotropin until a height of 5 feet is reached. These children may need replacement of other hormones, especially just before and during puberty.
epispadias (**ep**-ih-**SPAY**-dee-as) epi- = upon, over	A congenital defect (birth defect) in which the urethra opens on the upper side of the penis at some point near the glans. See Chapter 16 for a visual reference. Treatment for **epispadias** is surgical correction, with redirection of the opening of the urethra to its normal position at the end of the penis.
erythroblastosis fetalis (eh-**rith**-roh-blass-**TOH**-sis fee-**TAL**-iss) erythr/o = red blast/o = embryonic stage of development -osis = condition	A form of hemolytic anemia that occurs in neonates due to a maternal–fetal blood group incompatibility involving the ABO grouping or the Rh factors. This is also known as hemolytic disease of the newborn (HDN). **Erythroblastosis fetalis** is caused by an antigen–antibody reaction. The incompatible antigens of fetal blood stimulate the mother to make antibodies against them. The hemolytic reaction typically occurs in subsequent pregnancies. This reaction can be prevented by giving the mother an injection of a high-titer anti-Rh gamma globulin after the delivery of an Rh positive fetus.
esophageal atresia (ee-**soff**-ah-**JEE**-al ah-**TREE**-zee-ah) esophag/o = esophagus -eal = pertaining to	A congenital abnormality of the esophagus due to its ending before it reaches the stomach either as a blind pouch or as a fistula connected to the trachea. Either type of **esophageal atresia** (EA) is a **neonatal** (newborn) surgical emergency. Death may result from aspiration pneumonia if prompt treatment is not instituted. The birth weight of infants with EA is significantly lower than average, and there is an unusually high incidence of prematurity in infants with this condition.
gigantism (**JYE**-gan-tizm)	A proportional overgrowth of the body's tissue due to the hypersecretion of the human growth hormone before puberty. The child experiences accelerated abnormal growth chiefly in the long bones. The cause of oversecretion of the human growth hormone is most often due to an adenoma of the anterior pituitary. The treatment is aimed at reducing the size of the pituitary gland through surgery or radiation.

hyaline membrane disease (**HIGH**-ah-lighn **MEM**-brayn dih-**ZEEZ**)	Also known as respiratory distress syndrome of the premature infant (RDS), **hyaline membrane disease** is severe impairment of the function of respiration in the premature newborn. This condition is rarely present in a newborn of greater than 37 weeks' gestation or in one weighing at least 5 pounds.

Shortly after birth, the premature infant will have a low Apgar score and will develop signs of acute respiratory distress due to collapse of lung tissue: tachypnea (rapid breathing), tachycardia (rapid heartbeat), retraction of the rib cage during inspiration, **cyanosis**, and **grunting** during expiration will be present.

hydrocele (**HIGH**-droh-seel) hydro- = water -cele = swelling or herniation	An accumulation of fluid in any saclike cavity or duct, particularly the scrotal sac or along the spermatic cord.

This condition is caused by inflammation of the epididymis or testis or by obstruction of lymphatic or venous flow within the spermatic cord. Treatment for a **hydrocele** is surgery to remove the fluid pouch.

hydrocephalus (high-droh-**SEFF**-ah-lus) hydro- = water cephal/o = head -us = noun ending	An abnormal increase of cerebrospinal fluid (CSF) in the brain that causes the ventricles of the brain to dilate, resulting in an increased head circumference in the infant with open fontanel(s); congenital disorder. See *Figure 19-18*.

The increase in CSF may be due to an increased production of CSF, a decreased absorption of CSF, or a blockage in the normal flow of CSF. The infant may also show frontal bossing (forehead protrudes out), which may cause the "setting sun" sign in which the upper scleras of the eyes show with the eyes directed downward. The infant will demonstrate other signs of increased pressure, such as a high-pitched cry, a bulging fontanel, extreme irritability, and inability to sleep for long periods of time.

Hydrocephalus in the young infant may be detected by increased head circumferences resulting in an abnormal graphing curve. This may be detected when checking the head circumference of the infant on well-baby checkups in the physician's office. Along with checking head circumference, the infant should be assessed for any signs and symptoms of increased intracranial pressure (IICP).

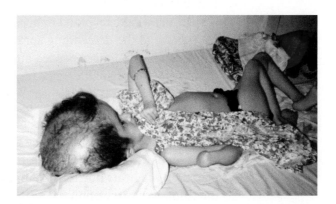

Figure 19-18 Untreated hydrocephalus
(Courtesy of Russell Cox, M.D., Gastonia, N.C.)

When the diagnosis of **hydrocephalus** is made, treatment to relieve or remove the obstruction is initiated. If there is no obstruction, a **shunt** is generally required to relieve the intracranial pressure by shunting the excess CSF into another body space, thus preventing permanent damage to the brain tissue. As the child grows, the shunt will have to be replaced with a longer one.

Hydrocephalus is often a complication of another disease or disorder. The infant with spina bifida cystica may develop **hydrocephalus**. It can also occur as a result of an intrauterine infection such as **rubella** or syphilis.

hypospadias (**high**-poh-**SPAY**-dee-as) hypo- = under, below, beneath, less than normal	A congenital defect in which the urethra opens on the underside of the penis instead of at the end. Refer to Chapter 16 for a visual reference. Treatment for **hypospadias** involves surgery to redirect the opening of the urethra to its normal location at the end of the penis.
intussusception (**in**-tuh-suh-**SEP**-shun)	Telescoping of a portion of proximal intestine into distal intestine (usually in the ileocecal region), causing an obstruction. Refer to Chapter 12 for a visual reference. **Intussusception** typically occurs in infants and young children. Clinical manifestations include intermittent, severe abdominal pain, vomiting, and a "currant jelly stool" (which indicates the presence of bloody mucus). **Intussusception** is diagnosed and medically treated with a barium enema. During examination, the telescoping is often reduced by the pressure created with a barium enema. When the obstruction is not reduced with the barium enema, immediate surgical intervention is necessary.
patent ductus arteriosus (**PAY**-tent **DUK**-tus ar-**tee**-ree-**OH**-suss)	An abnormal opening between the pulmonary artery and the aorta caused by failure of the fetal ductus arteriosus to close after birth. This defect is seen primarily in premature infants. Refer to Chapter 10 for a visual reference. During the prenatal period, the ductus arteriosus serves as a normal pathway in the fetal circulatory system. It is a large channel between the pulmonary artery and the aorta that is open, allowing fetal blood to bypass the lungs, passing from the pulmonary artery to the descending aorta, and ultimately to the placenta. This passageway is no longer needed after birth and usually closes during the first 24 to 72 hours of life, once the normal circulatory pattern of the cardiovascular system is established. If the ductus arteriosus remains open after birth, blood under pressure from the aorta is shunted into the pulmonary artery, resulting in oxygenated blood *recirculating* through the pulmonary circulation. A strain is placed on the heart due to the pumping of blood a second time through the pulmonary circulation. Treatment for **patent ductus arteriosus** is surgery to close the open channel. In some cases, medication can be used.

phimosis	A tightness of the foreskin (prepuce) of the penis of the male infant that prevents it from being pulled back. The opening of the foreskin narrows due to the tightness and may cause some difficulty with urination.
(fih-**MOH**-sis)	

The parents of the uncircumcised male infant may notice difficulty pulling the prepuce back for cleaning the area of the glans penis the prepuce covers. If this occurs, it should be reported to the physician immediately. However, the foreskin is not fully retractable until puberty and should never be forcibly retracted. Treatment for **phimosis** is **circumcision** (surgery to remove the foreskin).

Reye's syndrome	A syndrome marked by severe edema of the brain and increased intracranial pressure, hypoglycemia, and fatty infiltration and dysfunction of the liver. Symptoms may follow an acute viral infection, occurring in children younger than age 18, often with fatal results. There are confirmed studies linking the onset of **Reye's syndrome** to aspirin administration during a viral illness.
syn- = together, joined	
-drome = that which runs together	

The symptoms of Reye's syndrome typically follow a pattern through stages:

1. Vomiting, contusion, and lethargy (sluggish and apathetic)

2. Irritability, hyperactive reflexes, delirium, and hyperventilation

3. Changes in level of consciousness progressing to coma, and sluggish pupillary response

4. Fixed, dilated pupils; continued loss of cerebral function; and periods of absent breathing

5. Seizures, loss of deep tendon reflexes, and respiratory arrest

The prognosis is directly related to the stage of Reye's syndrome at the time of diagnosis and treatment. Treatment includes decreasing intracranial pressure to prevent seizures, controlling cerebral edema, and closely monitoring the child for changes in level of consciousness. In some cases, respiratory support and/or dialysis is necessary.

shaken baby syndrome (SBS)	**Shaken baby syndrome** is a serious form of child abuse that describes a group of unique symptoms resulting from repetitive, violent shaking. The violent shaking (forward and backward shaking) produces acceleration–deceleration forces within the head of the child that can cause brain injury. This whiplash-type injury is not caused by playful bouncing of the child and is not an accidental injury.

Shaken baby syndrome most often involves children under the age of 1. Crying usually triggers the episode of violent shaking. The individual responsible for the violent shaking usually grabs the infant by the shoulders or under the arms and repeatedly shakes the baby forcefully, causing the head to move back and forth rapidly.

This form of child abuse is sometimes difficult to detect because the damage is not always obvious. The symptoms produced by this type of injury may range from irritability and vomiting to more severe symptoms of seizures, retinal hemorrhages, respiratory distress, and signs of swelling of the brain. These infants may also have bruises on their backs and may suffer from rib fractures due to the violent shaking of the head and body. In extreme cases, the infant may suffer brain hemorrhage and die.

When the explanation of how the injury occurred does not match the infant's degree of injury, the health professional should be suspicious of abuse. Diagnostic imaging may be used to detect internal symptoms and confirm the diagnosis.

spina bifida occulta (**SPY**-nah **BIH**-fih-dah oh-**KULL**-tah)	A congenital defect of the central nervous system in which the back portion of one or more vertebrae is not closed. A dimpling over the area may occur.

Other symptoms include hair growing out of this area, a port wine nevus (pigmented blemish) over the area, and/or a subcutaneous lipoma (fatty tumor) in this area. **Spina bifida occulta** can occur anywhere along the vertebral column but usually occurs at the level of the fifth lumbar or first sacral vertebrae. There are usually very few neurological symptoms present. Without symptoms, no treatment is recommended.

sudden infant death syndrome (SIDS)	The completely unexpected and unexplained death of an apparently well, or virtually well, infant. SIDS is also known as "crib death."

SIDS is a worldwide syndrome that occurs more frequently in the second to fourth months of life, in premature infants, in males, and in infants living in poverty. The deaths usually occur during sleep and are more likely to happen in winter than in summer.

Infants at risk are monitored during their sleep and are sometimes placed on **apnea** monitors designed to sound an alarm when the infant ceases to breathe. Since the introduction of the "Back to Sleep" campaign, the rates of SIDS have declined by more than 50%. The "Back to Sleep" campaign is so named for its recommendation to place healthy babies on their backs to sleep. The American Academy of Pediatrics (AAP) indicates that back sleeping is the preferred sleep position for babies at nighttime and naptime.

Tay-Sachs disease (TAY-**SACKS** dih-**ZEEZ**)	A congenital disorder caused by altered lipid metabolism due to an enzyme deficiency.

An accumulation of a specific type of lipid occurs in the brain, leading to progressive neurological deterioration with both physical and mental retardation. The symptoms of neurological deterioration begin about the age of six months. Deafness, blindness with a cherry-red spot on each retina, convulsions, and paralysis all occur in the child with **Tay-Sachs disease** (until death occurs about the age of 2 to 4 years). There is no specific therapy for this condition. Therefore, supportive and symptomatic care are indicated.

Tay-Sachs disease occurs most frequently in families of Eastern European Jewish origin, specifically, the Ashkenazic Jews. This disease can be diagnosed in utero through amniocentesis.

tetralogy of Fallot

(teh-**TRALL**-oh-jee of fal-**OH**)

   tetr/a = four

   -logy = the study of

A congenital heart anomaly that consists of four defects: pulmonary stenosis, interventricular septal defect, dextroposition (shifting to the right) of the aorta so that it receives blood from both ventricles, and hypertrophy of the right ventricle; named for the French physician, Etienne Fallot, who first described the condition.

Refer to Chapter 10 for a visual reference. Further description of **tetralogy of Fallot** identifies the four defects in more detail.

1. The pulmonary stenosis restricts the flow of blood from the heart to the lungs.

2. The interventricular septal defect creates a right-to-left shunt between the ventricles, allowing deoxygenated blood from the right ventricle to communicate with the oxygenated blood in the left ventricle (which then exits the heart via the aorta).

3. The shifting of the aorta to the right causes it to override the right ventricle and thus communicate with the interventricular septal defect, allowing the oxygen-poor blood to pass more easily into the aorta.

4. The hypertrophy of the right ventricle occurs because of the increased work required to pump blood through the obstructed pulmonary artery.

Most infants born with **tetralogy of Fallot** display varying degrees of **cyanosis**, which may typically occur during activities that increase the need for oxygen (such as crying, feeding, or straining with a bowel movement). The **cyanosis** develops as a result of the decreased flow of blood to the lungs for oxygenation and as a result of the mixing of oxygenated and deoxygenated blood released into the systemic circulation. These babies are termed "blue babies." Treatment for **tetralogy of Fallot** involves surgery to correct the multiple defects.

transposition of the great vessels

(trans-poh-**SIH**-shun)

A condition in which the two major arteries of the heart are reversed in position, resulting in two noncommunicating circulatory systems.

The aorta arises from the right ventricle (instead of the left) and delivers unoxygenated blood to the systemic circulation. This blood is returned from the body tissues back to the right atrium and right ventricle without being oxygenated, because it does not pass through the lungs.

The pulmonary artery arises from the left ventricle (instead of the right) and delivers blood to the lungs for oxygenation. The oxygenated blood returns from the lungs, to the left atrium and the left ventricle, and back to the lungs without sending the oxygenated blood throughout the systemic circulation.

This congenital **anomaly** creates an oxygen deficiency to the body tissues and an excessive workload on the right and left ventricles. The infant is usually severely cyanotic at birth.

Treatment involves surgical correction of the defect and repositioning of the vessels to reestablish a normal pattern of blood flow through the circulatory system. Surgical correction of the defect is an arterial switch that must be done as early as possible, usually within the first two weeks of life. When surgery must be delayed until the infant can tolerate the procedure better, an immediate **palliative** surgery (aimed at achieving adequate mixing of oxygenated and unoxygenated blood) enables the child to survive until the corrective surgery can be performed.

umbilical hernia (um-**BILL**-ih-kahl **HER**-nee-ah)	An outward protrusion of the intestine through a weakness in the abdominal wall around the umbilicus (navel, or "belly button").

An **umbilical hernia** usually closes spontaneously within the first two years of life. If it remains beyond that point, surgical closure of the weakened abdominal wall may be necessary. This defect is more likely to be seen in girls than in boys, and in premature infants. See *Figure 19-19.*

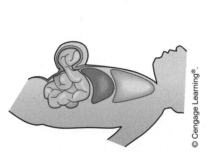
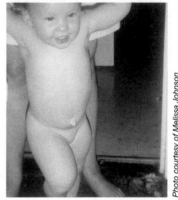

© Cengage Learning®.

Photo courtesy of Melissa Johnson

Figure 19-19 Umbilical hernia

Review Checkpoint

Check your understanding of this section by completing the **Pathological Conditions** exercises in your workbook.

Diagnostic Techniques, Treatments, and Procedures

circumcision (sir-kum-**SIH**-zhun)	A surgical procedure in which the foreskin (prepuce) of the penis is removed.

Circumcision is widely performed on newborn boys for religious or sociocultural reasons. It may also be performed on adult males who suffer from **phimosis** (tightness of the foreskin). It is usually performed on the infant during the first or second day of life.

With the infant lying flat on his back and restrained, the penis is exposed and the area is cleansed and draped. A clamp designed especially for circumcision is placed over the end of the penis, stretching the foreskin tightly. Some physicians apply a local anesthetic to numb the area before excising the foreskin.

After circumcision is performed, the glans penis is fully exposed. See *Figure 19-20*.

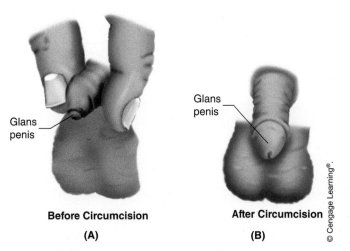

Before Circumcision

(A)

After Circumcision

(B)

© Cengage Learning®.

Figure 19-20 Circumcision (A) before and (B) after the procedure

| **heel puncture** | **Heel puncture** is a method of obtaining a blood sample from a newborn or premature infant by making a shallow puncture of the lateral or medial area of the plantar (sole of the foot) surface of the heel; also called a "heel stick." See *Figure 19-21*. |

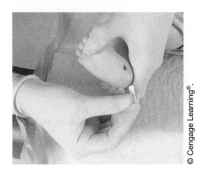

© Cengage Learning®.

Figure 19-21 Capillary heel puncture

| **pediatric urine collection**
(pee-dee-**AT**-rik) | A urine specimen may be requested as part of an infant's physical examination to determine the presence of a pathologic condition. |

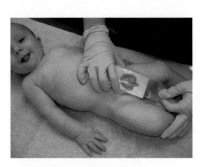

Figure 19-22 Application of a pediatric urine collector on a male
(Courtesy of Brandi Hall)

When a child is unable to produce a urine specimen upon request, a pediatric collection bag is used. Urine is collected as required for various diagnostic procedures. See *Figure 19-22*.

The disposable urine collection bag is applied to the perineal area of the infant so that urine can collect in the bag for a specimen. The skin must be completely dry for the bag to adhere to it. If the specimen is not needed immediately, the parent can attach the bag at home, place the diaper over the bag, and bring the infant to the office at a time when a specimen is available. The bag should be removed gently to avoid pulling or chafing the infant's skin. If urine is being collected for culture to rule out infection, a catheterized specimen should be obtained.

The following should be recorded in the patient's chart: the date, time of collection, and purpose of the specimen, and the results of any tests performed on the specimen. If the specimen is sent to a laboratory for testing, this should be noted on the chart.

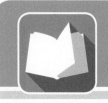

Review Checkpoint

Check your understanding of this section by completing the **Diagnostic Techniques, Treatments, and Procedures** exercises in your workbook.

COMMON ABBREVIATIONS

Abbreviation	Meaning	Abbreviation	Meaning
AAP	American Academy of Pediatrics	HMD	**hyaline membrane disease**
ASQ	Ages & Stages Questionnaire	MMR	measles-mumps-rubella [vaccine]
BCG	bacille Calmette-Guérin [vaccine]	PKU	phenylketonuria
		PNP	pediatric nurse practitioner
DPT	diphtheria, pertussis, and tetanus [vaccine]	RDS	respiratory distress syndrome
DS	**Down syndrome**	SBS	shaken baby syndrome
EA	**esophageal atresia**	SIDS	**sudden infant death syndrome**
HDN	hemolytic disease of the newborn (**erythroblastosis fetalis**)	Tb	tuberculosis
		Td	tetanus and diphtheria toxoid [vaccine]
HIB	*Haemophilus influenzae* type B [vaccine]		

Review Checkpoint

Check your understanding of this section by completing the **Common Abbreviations** exercises in your workbook.

WRITTEN AND AUDIO TERMINOLOGY REVIEW

Review each of the following terms from this chapter. Study the spelling of each term and write the definition in the space provided. Check definitions by looking the term up in the glossary.

Term	Pronunciation	Definition
active acquired immunity	☐ **AK**-tiv ah-**KWIRD** ih-**MEW**-nih-tee	_____
apical pulse	☐ **AY**-pih-kal pulhs	_____
apnea	☐ ap-**NEE**-ah	_____
asthma	☐ **AZ**-mah	_____
autism	☐ **AW**-tizm	_____
axillary temperature	☐ **AK**-sih-lair-ee **TEM**-per-ah-chur	_____
cephalocaudal	☐ **seff**-ah-loh-**KAW**-dal	_____
cleft lip	☐ **CLEFT LIP**	_____
cleft palate	☐ **CLEFT PAL**-at	_____
coarctation of the aorta	☐ **koh**-ark-**TAY**-shun of the ay-**OR**-tah	_____
crackles	☐ **CRACK**-ulz	_____
croup	☐ **CROOP**	_____
cryptorchidism	☐ kript-**OR**-kid-izm	_____
cyanosis	☐ **sigh**-ah-**NOH**-sis	_____
dentition	☐ den-**TIH**-shun	_____
diphtheria	☐ diff-**THEE**-ree-ah	_____
Down syndrome	☐ **DOWN SIN**-drom	_____
epispadias	☐ **ep**-ih-**SPAY**-dee-as	_____
erythema infectiosum	☐ **air**-ih-**THEE**-mah in-**fek**-she-**OH**-sum	_____
erythroblastosis fetalis	☐ eh-**rith**-roh-blass-**TOH**-sis fee-**TAL**-iss	_____
esophageal atresia	☐ ee-**soff**-ah-**JEE**-al ah-**TREE**-zee-ah	_____
febrile	☐ **FEE**-brill _or_ fee-**BRILL**	_____
friction rub	☐ **FRICK**-shun rub	_____
heel puncture	☐ heel **PUNK**-cher	_____
hyaline membrane disease	☐ **HIGH**-ah-lighn **MEM**-brayn dih-**ZEEZ**	_____

Term	Pronunciation	Definition
hydrocele	☐ **HIGH**-droh-seel	_____
hydrocephalus	☐ **high**-droh-**SEFF**-ah-lus	_____
hypospadias	☐ **high**-poh-**SPAY**-dee-as	_____
immunity	☐ ih-**MEW**-nih-tee	_____
immunization	☐ **ih**-mew-nih-**ZAY**-shun	_____
impetigo	☐ **im**-peh-**TYE**-goh	_____
infectious parotitis	☐ in-**FEK**-shus pair-oh-**TYE**-tis	_____
intussusception	☐ **in**-tus-suh-**SEP**-shun	_____
microcephalus	☐ **my**-kroh-**SEFF**-ah-lus	_____
mumps	☐ **MUMPS**	_____
neonatal	☐ **nee**-oh-**NAY**-tal	_____
neonatologist	☐ **nee**-oh-nay-**TOL**-oh-jist	_____
neonatology	☐ **nee**-oh-nay-**TOL**-oh-jee	_____
omphalocele	☐ om-**FAL**-oh-seel	_____
omphalorrhea	☐ om-**fal**-oh-**REE**-ah	_____
patent ductus arteriosus	☐ **PAY**-tent **DUK**-tus ar-**tee**-ree-**OH**-suss	_____
pediatrician	☐ **pee**-dee-ah-**TRISH**-an	_____
pediatrics	☐ **pee**-dee-**AT**-rikz	_____
pertussis	☐ per-**TUSS**-is	_____
phimosis	☐ fih-**MOH**-sis	_____
pyrexia	☐ pie-**REK**-see-ah	_____
retractions	☐ rih-**TRAK**-shuns	_____
roseola infantum	☐ **roh**-zee-**OH**-lah in-**FAN**-tum	_____
rubella	☐ roo-**BELL**-lah	_____
rubeola	☐ roo-bee-**OH**-la	_____
scarlatina, scarlet fever	☐ **scar**-lah-**TEE**-nah, **SCAR**-let **FEE**-ver	_____
spina bifida occulta	☐ **SPY**-nah **BIH**-fih-dah oh-**KULL**-tah	_____
stature	☐ **STAT**-yoor	_____
stridor	☐ **STRYE**-dor	_____
Tay-Sachs disease	☐ **TAY**-sack dih-**ZEEZ**	_____
tetralogy of Fallot	☐ teh-**TRALL**-oh-jee of fal-**OH**	_____
tympanic temperature	☐ tim-**PAN**-ik **TEM**-per-ah-chur	_____
vaccine	☐ vak-**SEEN** *or* **VAK**-seen	_____
vertex	☐ **VER**-teks	_____
wheezing	☐ **HWEEZ**-ing	_____

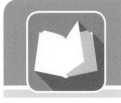

Review Checkpoint

Apply what you have learned in this chapter by completing the **Putting It All Together** exercise in your workbook.

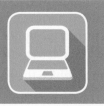

Online Resources

For additional study tools, such as PowerPoint® slides, go to the Student Companion Website.

Chapter Review Exercises

The following exercises provide a more in-depth review of the chapter material. Your goal in these exercises is to complete each section at a minimum 80% level of accuracy. If you score below 80% in any area, return to the applicable section in the chapter and read the material again. A space has been provided for your score at the end of each section.

A. Term to Definition

Define each diagnosis or procedure listed by writing the definition in the space provided. Check the box provided if you are able to complete this exercise correctly the first time (without referring to the answers). Each correct answer is worth 10 points. Record your score in the space provided at the end of the exercise.

☐ 1. transposition of the great vessels _____

☐ 2. scarlet fever _____

☐ 3. cleft lip _____

☐ 4. intussusception _____

☐ 5. cleft palate _____

☐ 6. hyaline membrane disease _____

☐ 7. phimosis _____

☐ 8. erythema infectiosum _____

☐ 9. impetigo _____

☐ 10. sudden infant death syndrome _____

Number correct _____ × *10 points/correct answer: Your score* _____%

B. Matching Conditions

Match the descriptions of the pathological condition on the right with the applicable pathological condition on the left. Each correct answer is worth 10 points. When you have completed the exercise, record your score in the space provided at the end of the exercise.

_____ 1. spina bifida occulta

_____ 2. Tay-Sachs disease

_____ 3. roseola infantum disease

_____ 4. rubella

_____ 5. rubeola

_____ 6. Down syndrome

_____ 7. esophageal atresia

_____ 8. tetralogy of Fallot

_____ 9. erythroblastosis fetalis

_____ 10. coarctation of the aorta

a. a congenital heart anomaly that consists of four defects: pulmonary stenosis, interventricular septal defect, dextroposition (shifting to the right) of the aorta so that it receives blood from both ventricles, and hypertrophy of the right ventricle

b. a congenital heart defect characterized by a localized narrowing of the aorta, which results in increased blood pressure in the upper extremities and decreased blood pressure in the lower extremities

c. a congenital defect of the central nervous system in which the back portion of one or more vertebrae is not closed

d. a form of hemolytic anemia, which occurs in neonates due to a maternal–fetal blood group incompatibility

e. a viral disease with sudden onset of a high fever for three to four days, during which time the child may experience mild coldlike symptoms and slight irritability

f. a mild febrile infectious disease characterized by a rash of both macules and papules that fade and disappear in three days

g. an acute, highly communicable viral disease with a red, blotchy rash that begins as an upper respiratory disorder with fever, sore throat, cough, runny nose, and sensitivity to light

h. a congenital condition characterized by multiple defects and varying degrees of mental retardation

i. a congenital abnormality of the esophagus due to its ending before it reaches the stomach either as a blind pouch or as a fistula connected to the trachea

j. a congenital disorder caused by altered lipid metabolism due to an enzyme deficiency

_Number correct _____ × 10 points/correct answer: Your score _____%_

C. Crossword Puzzle

Each crossword answer is worth 10 points. When you have completed the crossword puzzle, total your points and enter your score in the space provided.

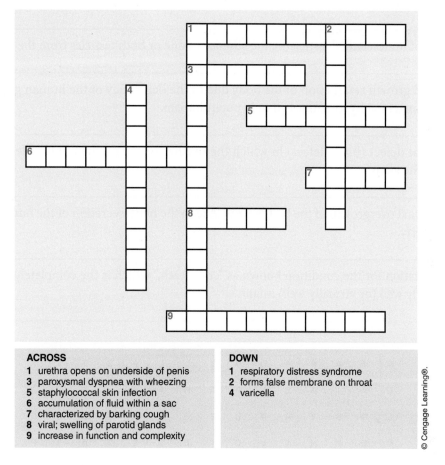

ACROSS
1 urethra opens on underside of penis
3 paroxysmal dyspnea with wheezing
5 staphylococcal skin infection
6 accumulation of fluid within a sac
7 characterized by barking cough
8 viral; swelling of parotid glands
9 increase in function and complexity

DOWN
1 respiratory distress syndrome
2 forms false membrane on throat
4 varicella

© Cengage Learning®.

Number correct _____ × 10 points/correct answer: Your score _____%

D. Word Search

Read each definition carefully and identify the applicable word from the list that follows. Enter the word in the space provided and then find it in the puzzle and circle it. The words may be read up, down, diagonally, across, or backward. Each correct answer is worth 10 points. Record your score in the space provided at the end of the exercise.

rubella	dwarfism	hydrocephalus
epispadias	growth	hypospadias
SIDS	pertussis	cryptorchidism
croup	gigantism	

Example: Also known as "German measles."

rubella _____

1. An increase in the whole or any of its parts physically.

_____

(continued)

2. A congenital defect in which the urethra opens on the underside of the penis instead of at the end.

_____

3. A childhood illness characterized by a barking cough, suffocative and difficult breathing, stridor, and laryngeal spasm.

_____

4. Condition of undescended testicle(s); the absence of one or both testicles from the scrotum.

_____

5. Generalized growth retardation of the body due to the deficiency of the human growth hormone; also known as congenital hypopituitarism or hypopituitarism.

_____

6. A congenital defect (birth defect) in which the urethra opens on the upper side of the penis at some point near the glans.

_____

7. A proportional overgrowth of the body's tissue due to the hypersecretion of the human growth hormone before puberty.

_____

8. The abbreviation for the condition known as "crib death," which is the completely unexpected death of an apparently well (or virtually well) infant.

_____

M	E	A	P	R	U	B	E	L	L	A	S	T	I	K
U	A	I	G	E	L	P	A	R	A	P	I	A	P	S
L	D	B	Y	A	C	U	T	E	I	M	G	E	N	E
C	E	P	H	A	L	G	I	A	S	S	E	A	S	P
R	R	H	R	S	I	F	L	E	X	I	I	N	O	T
Y	O	O	N	I	T	A	N	O	R	T	Z	D	C	L
P	S	S	U	T	H	I	M	B	R	N	N	H	S	K
T	E	L	A	P	M	S	I	F	R	A	W	D	Y	S
O	A	X	I	I	I	N	O	I	T	G	P	I	R	I
R	T	T	C	D	D	N	E	X	T	I	N	M	I	S
C	I	N	E	R	A	A	A	R	L	G	A	E	I	S
H	Y	D	R	O	C	E	P	H	A	L	U	S	C	U
I	N	S	H	D	R	R	P	S	I	P	R	S	N	T
D	S	I	A	I	E	S	U	M	O	O	S	U	P	R
I	O	O	L	S	S	A	I	D	A	P	S	I	P	E
S	U	N	U	S	E	N	E	U	R	O	Y	O	G	P
M	R	O	S	D	S	R	S	I	F	L	E	H	X	N
P	L	A	N	M	I	G	R	O	W	T	H	O	Y	O

9. Also called "whooping cough."

_____

10. An abnormal increase of cerebrospinal fluid (CSF) in the brain, which causes the ventricles of the brain to dilate, resulting in an increased head circumference in the infant with open fontanel(s).

_____

Number correct _____ **× 10 points/correct answer: Your score** _____**%**

E. Matching Abbreviations

Match the abbreviation on the left with the applicable definition on the right. Each correct response is worth 10 points. When you have completed the exercise, total your points and record your score in the space provided at the end of the exercise.

_____ 1. PKU a. sudden infant death syndrome

_____ 2. MMR b. tuberculosis

_____ 3. DPT c. Denver Placement Test

_____ 4. Td d. bacille Calmette-Guérin [vaccine]

_____ 5. HMD e. measles, mumps, rubella [vaccine]

_____ 6. ASQ f. phenylketonuria

_____ 7. HIB g. diphtheria, pertussis, tetanus [vaccine]

_____ 8. BCG h. tetanus and diphtheria toxoid [vaccine]

_____ 9. SIDS i. Standard Intelligence Developmental Screening

_____ 10. Tb j. hyaline membrane disease

                                      k. Ages & Stages Questionnaire.

                                      l. *Haemophilus influenzae* type B [vaccine]

                                      m. head circumference × months = dentition

Number correct _____ **× 10 points/correct answer: Your score** _____**%**

F. Spelling

Circle the correctly spelled term in each pairing of words. Each correct answer is worth 10 points. Record your score in the space provided at the end of the exercise.

1. dentition   dentishun   6. vacine   vaccine

2. immunization   immanization   7. pirexia   pyrexia

3. pediatrishun   pediatrician   8. impetigo   infantigo

4. omfalorrhea   omphalorrhea   9. rubeyola   rubeola

5. stridor   strider   10. hypospadias   hypospadius

Number correct _____ **× 10 points/correct answer: Your score** _____**%**

G. Completion

The following sentences relate to the chapter on child health. Complete each sentence with the most appropriate word. Each correct answer is worth 10 points. Record your score in the space provided at the end of the exercise.

1. A communicable disease in children (caused by the varicella-zoster virus) that is characterized by eruptions of macules, papules, and vesicles on the skin followed by crusting over of the lesions with a granular scab is known as _____.

2. A viral disease characterized by a face that appears as "slapped cheeks," with a fiery red rash on the cheeks, is called _____.

3. Another name for infectious parotitis is _____.

4. The medical term for whooping cough is _____.

5. The medical term for the three-day measles (or German measles) is _____.

6. The medical term for the seven-day measles (or "red measles") is _____.

7. A childhood illness characterized by a barking cough, suffocative and difficult breathing, stridor, and laryngeal spasms is called _____.

8. An accumulation of fluid in any saclike cavity or duct, particularly the scrotal sac or along the spermatic cord, is known as _____.

9. A congenital defect in which the urethra opens on the upper side of the penis at some point near the tip of the penis is known as _____.

10. A tightness of the foreskin (prepuce) of the penis of the male infant that prevents it from being pulled back and causes difficulty with urination is known as _____.

Number correct_____ × 10 points/correct answer: Your score_____%

H. Word Element Review

The following words relate to the chapter on child health. The word elements have been labeled (WR = word root, P = prefix, S = suffix, and V = combining vowel). Read the definition carefully, and complete the word by filling in the blank, using the word elements provided in this chapter. If you still have trouble with word building rules, see Chapter 1. Each correct word is worth 10 points. Record your score in the space provided at the end of this exercise.

1. A congenital anomaly characterized by abnormal smallness of the head in relation to the rest of the body and by underdevelopment of the brain:

   _____ / _____ / _____ / _____
       WR   V   WR   S

2. The medical specialty concerned with the diseases and abnormalities of the newborn infant:

   _____ / _____ / _____ / _____
       P   WR   V   S

3. A pathological condition characterized by an abnormal accumulation of cerebrospinal fluid, usually under increased pressure, within the cranium:

   _____ / _____ / _____
       P   WR   S

4. Congenital herniation of intra-abdominal viscera through a defect in the abdominal wall around the umbilicus (umbilical hernia):

_____ / _____ / _____
     WR   V   S

5. A condition of undescended testicle(s); the absence of one or both testicles from the scrotum:

_____ / _____ / _____
     WR   WR   S

6. A condition of blueness; bluish discoloration of the skin and mucous membranes caused by an excess of deoxygenated hemoglobin in the blood or a structural defect in the hemoglobin molecule:

_____ / _____
     WR   S

7. Pertaining to fever (other than pyrexia):

_____ / _____
     WR   S

8. Pertaining to the head and the tail, as in growth and development proceeding from the head to the toe:

_____ / _____ / _____ / _____
     WR   V   WR   S

9. Pertaining to near and away from, as in growth and development proceeding from the center outward or from the midline to the periphery:

_____ / _____ / _____ / _____
     WR   V   WR   S

10. Without breathing; an absence of spontaneous respiration:

_____ / _____
     P   S

Number correct _____ × 10 points/correct answer: Your score _____%

I. Definition to Term

Using the following definitions, identify and provide the word for the pathological condition to match the definition. Each correct answer is worth 10 points. Record your score in the space provided at the end of the exercise.

1. The heart rate as heard with a stethoscope placed on the chest wall adjacent to the cardiac apex (top of the heart):

_____

2. Abnormal, short, audible, gruntlike breaks in exhalation that often accompany severe chest pain:

_____

3. The eruption of teeth. This occurs in a sequential pattern, with 20 primary teeth erupting between the ages of 6 months to 36 months:

_____

4. A process by which resistance to an infectious disease is induced or augmented:

_____

(continued)

5. A medical doctor who specializes in neonatology:

_____

6. Drainage from the umbilicus (navel):

_____

7. A physician who specializes in pediatrics:

_____

8. Another name for fever other than febrile:

_____

9. The body temperature as measured electronically at the eardrum:

_____ temperature

10. A breath sound characterized by a high-pitched musical quality heard on both inspiration and expiration; associated with asthma and chronic bronchitis:

_____

Number correct _____ × *10 points/correct answer: Your score* _____%

J. Multiple Choice

Read each statement carefully and select the correct answer from the choices provided. Each correct answer is worth 10 points. Record your score in the space provided at the end of the exercise.

1. A process by which resistance to an infectious disease is induced or increased is called:
   a. immunization
   b. vaccine
   c. toxoid
   d. dentition

2. A graphic representation, by any of various systems, of a numeric relationship is called (a):
   a. stature
   b. nomogram
   c. head circumference
   d. growth spurt

3. A condition present at birth ("born with") is termed:
   a. grunting
   b. nomogram
   c. vertex
   d. congenital

4. The natural height of a person in an upright position is termed:
   a. stature
   b. nomogram
   c. vertex
   d. recumbent length

5. An acute, contagious disease characterized by sore throat, abrupt high fever, increased pulse, "strawberry" tongue, and a pointlike, bright red rash on the body is:

   a. rubella (German measles)

   b. rubeola (red measles)

   c. scarlet fever (scarlatina)

   d. roseola infantum

6. A congenital defect, in which there is an open space between the nasal cavity and the lip due to failure of the soft tissue and bones in this area to fuse properly during embryological development, is known as:

   a. coarctation of the aorta

   b. cleft lip

   c. croup

   d. tetralogy of Fallot

7. This condition is also known as respiratory distress syndrome of the premature infant:

   a. hyaline membrane disease

   b. esophageal atresia

   c. erythroblastosis fetalis

   d. epispadias

8. A congenital condition known as trisomy 21 (characterized by multiple defects and varying degrees of mental retardation) is called:

   a. dwarfism

   b. hyaline membrane disease

   c. Down syndrome

   d. patent ductus arteriosus

9. The telescoping of a portion of proximal intestine into distal intestine usually into the ileocecal region, causing an obstruction, is known as:

   a. phimosis

   b. intussusception

   c. Reye's syndrome

   d. Tay-Sachs disease

10. The completely unexpected and unexplained death of an apparently well, or virtually well, infant is known as SIDS or:

    a. crib death

    b. tetralogy of Fallot

    c. Reye's syndrome

    d. hyaline membrane disease

***Number correct* _____ × *10 points/correct answer: Your score* _____%**

K. Medical Scenario

The following medical scenario presents information on one of the pathological conditions discussed in this chapter. Read the scenario carefully and select the most appropriate answer for each question that follows. Each correct answer is worth 20 points. Record your score in the space provided at the end of the exercise.

(*continued*)

Hope Ivey, a five-month-old infant, is a patient of the pediatrician, Dr. Cane. Hope visited the pediatrician today because of a concern her mother had about her crying and having excessive vomiting. The pediatrician has scheduled a diagnostic test to determine whether Hope has intussusception. Hope's mother asks the health care professional several questions about this possible diagnosis.

1. The health care professional will base her responses to Mrs. Ivey's questions about intussusception on which of the following facts? An intussusception is:
   a. an abnormal opening between the pulmonary artery and the aorta caused by failure of the fetal ductus arteriosus to close after birth
   b. an outward protrusion of the intestine through a weakness in the abdominal wall around the umbilicus
   c. a congenital abnormality of the esophagus in which it ends (before reaching the stomach) as a blind pouch or as a fistula connected to the trachea
   d. telescoping of a portion of proximal intestine into distal intestine, usually in the ileocecal region, causing an intestinal obstruction

2. The health care professional reads on Hope's chart that she has had the classic symptom of intussusception, which is:
   a. currant-jelly stool
   b. projectile vomiting
   c. frequent choking and coughing spells with difficulty breathing
   d. increased blood pressure in upper extremities and decreased blood pressure in lower extremities

3. The health care professional explains to Mrs. Ivey that the diagnostic test used to diagnose the intussusception is a(n):
   a. echocardiogram
   b. barium swallow
   c. barium enema
   d. cardiac catheterization

4. The health care professional also explains to Mrs. Ivey that although the procedure is a diagnostic procedure, it often reduces the telescoping due to the:
   a. pressure created with a barium enema
   b. lack of pressure created
   c. introduction of the catheter into the heart
   d. passage of the barium into the esophagus

5. Mrs. Ivey questions the health care professional about the treatment for intussusception. Which of the following responses by the health care professional would be correct? If the intussusception is not corrected with the diagnostic procedure:
   a. an emergency shunt will be placed in the ventricle to relieve the excess pressure
   b. immediate surgical intervention will need to be done to resolve the intestinal obstruction
   c. surgery will be required to provide closure of the open channel
   d. administration of human growth hormone and somatotropin will be started

Number correct _____ × 20 points/correct answer: Your score _____%

Radiology and Diagnostic Imaging

CHAPTER CONTENT

OBJECTIVES

Upon completing this chapter and the review exercises at the end of the chapter, the learner should be able to:

1. Identify at least 20 diagnostic techniques/procedures relating to the specialty of radiology and diagnostic imaging.

2. Correctly spell and pronounce terms listed on the Written and Audio Terminology Review, using the phonetic pronunciations provided.

3. Identify at least 10 radiological positions and/or movements based on their descriptions.

4. Demonstrate the ability to create at least 10 medical terms related to the specialty of radiology and diagnostic imaging by completing the "Definition to Term" exercise at the end of the chapter.

5. Identify at least 20 abbreviations common to the specialty of radiology and diagnostic imaging.

Overview

The specialty of **radiology** and diagnostic imaging evolved from an accidental discovery that occurred over 100 years ago. In 1895, Wilhelm Conrad Roentgen (a German physicist) was experimenting with electrical discharges in an evacuated glass tube called a Crookes' tube (cathode-ray tube). He accidentally discovered a new form of electromagnetic energy rays that could penetrate a person's hand and cause the outline of bones to be seen on a chemically coated fluorescent screen behind the hand. Not knowing what the rays were, Roentgen coined the term *X-ray* (*X* represented the unknown). Roentgen developed a photographic film to replace the fluorescent screen to make lasting pictures of the image. The X-ray is also known as the roentgen ray, so named after its discoverer. Roentgen received the first Nobel prize for physics in 1901 for his discovery of the X-ray. From this simple beginning, an entirely new world was opened to medicine.

X-rays are high-energy electromagnetic waves that travel in straight lines and have a shorter wavelength than visible light, enabling them to penetrate solid materials of varying densities. These invisible waves of radiant energy are capable of exposing a photographic plate (X-ray film) in much the same way light rays expose the film in a camera. **X-rays** are used to visualize internal organs and structures of the body and provide a valuable means of verifying the presence of illness or disease. **Radiology** is the study of the diagnostic and therapeutic uses of **X-rays**. This branch of medicine is concerned with the use of **X-rays**, high-strength magnetic fields, high-frequency sound waves, and various radioactive compounds to diagnose and treat diseases. A **radiologist** is a medical doctor who specializes in **radiology**. A **radiologic technologist**, also known as a **radiographer**, is an allied health professional trained to use X-ray machines and other imaging equipment to produce images of the internal structures of the body. Most radiologic technologists are employed in hospital X-ray departments and work under the direction of a **radiologist** or other physicians.

Radiology and Diagnostic Imaging Procedures and Techniques

When the physician is confirming a diagnosis, he or she will sometimes find it necessary to view the internal structures of the body or observe them in action. Examples of procedures that aid in diagnosing include (but are not limited to) X-ray images of the body with or without a contrast medium, **ultrasound** images, body scans, and fluoroscopic procedures that allow the physician to observe the particular organ as it functions. This section provides a basic discussion of the most common radiologic and diagnostic imaging procedures and techniques used in medicine. The procedures and techniques are listed in alphabetical order.

angiocardiography (cardiac catheterization)

(an-jee-oh-kar-dee-**OG**-rah-fee

CAR-dee-ak **kath**-eh-ter-ih-**ZAY**-shun)

angi/o = vessel

cardi/o = heart

-graphy = process of recording

A specialized diagnostic procedure in which a catheter (a hollow, flexible tube) is introduced into a large vein or artery, usually of an arm or a leg, and then threaded through the circulatory system to the heart.

Cardiac catheterization is used to obtain detailed information about the structure and function of the heart chambers, valves, and great vessels. Pressures within the chambers of the heart can be measured, as can oxygen concentration, saturation, and tension. In the case of coronary artery disease, the patient may undergo a cardiac catheterization to determine the amount of occlusion of his or her coronary arteries for the physician to determine the most appropriate treatment. Treatment may consist of coronary artery bypass surgery or percutaneous transluminal coronary angioplasty.

Immediately after the injection of the contrast medium, a series of X-ray films allowing visualization of the heart is taken. This sequence of films taken during a cardiac catheterization allows the **radiologist** to follow the circulation of blood through the great vessels, heart, and lungs.

The three major approaches used for the **angiocardiography** procedure for indicating the exact location of the contrast injection are right-sided **angiocardiography**, left-sided **angiocardiography**, and selective coronary artery **angiocardiography**. This procedure is typically done in the special controlled environment of a cardiac catheterization lab under **fluoroscopy** and in the presence of a **radiologist** or a cardiologist. The person undergoing a cardiac catheterization is required to sign a consent form and is to have nothing by mouth (NPO) for six to eight hours before the procedure. This procedure may be contraindicated for persons with allergies to shellfish, iodine, or other contrast media due to the possibility of experiencing an anaphylactic reaction.

angiography

(an-jee-**OG**-rah-fee)

angi/o = vessel

-graphy = process of recording

A series of X-ray films allowing visualization of internal structures after the introduction of a **radiopaque** substance. See *Figure 20-1.*

This recording is made possible by contrast medium, which promotes the imaging (makes them visible) of those structures that are otherwise difficult to see on X-ray film. This substance is injected into an artery or vein.

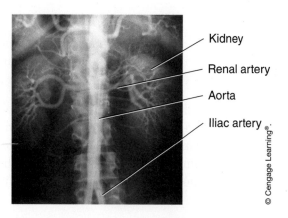

Kidney

Renal artery

Aorta

Iliac artery

© Cengage Learning®.

Figure 20-1 Angiogram of abdomen

Hypersensitivity tests are often performed before the radiographic material is used because the iodine in the contrast material has been known to cause severe allergic reactions in some persons. Various types of **angiography** are used to diagnose conditions such as myocardial infarction, occlusion of blood vessels, calcified atherosclerotic plaques, stroke (cerebrovascular accident), hypertension of the vessels leading to the liver (portal hypertension), and narrowing of the renal artery. The following are descriptions of some of the specific types of **angiography**.

cerebral angiography
 	
(**SER**-eh-bral or seh-**REE**-bral
an-jee-**OG**-rah-fee)
  cerebr/o = cerebrum
  -al = pertaining to
  angi/o = vessel
  -graphy = process of recording
	The injection of a **radiopaque** contrast medium into an arterial blood vessel (carotid, femoral, or brachial) to make visualization of the cerebral vascular system via X-ray possible.
	
	The arterial, capillary, and venous structures are outlined as the contrast medium flows through the brain. Through the **cerebral angiography**, cerebral circulation abnormalities such as occlusions or aneurysms are visualized. Vascular and nonvascular tumors can be noted as well as hematomas and abscesses.

renal angiography
 	
(**REE**-nal **an**-jee-**OG**-rah-fee)
  ren/o = kidney
  -al = pertaining to
  angi/o = vessel
  -graphy = process of recording
	X-ray visualization of the internal anatomy of the renal blood vessels after injection of a contrast medium.
	
	A **radiopaque** catheter is inserted into the femoral artery. Using **fluoroscopy**, the catheter is guided up the aorta to the level of the renal arteries. A contrast dye is then injected, and a series of **X-rays** is taken to visualize the renal vessels. **Renal angiography** is used to detect narrowing of the renal vessels, vascular damage, renal vein thrombosis (clots), cysts, and tumors.

arteriography
 	
(**ar**-tee-ree-**OG**-rah-fee)
  arteri/o = artery
  -graphy = process of recording
	Arteriography is X-ray visualization of arteries following the introduction of a **radiopaque** contrast medium into the bloodstream through a specific vessel by way of a catheter.

arthrography
 	
(ar-**THROG**-rah-fee)
  arthr/o = joint
  -graphy = process of recording
	Arthrography is the process of taking **X-rays** of the inside of a joint after a contrast medium (substance that makes the inside of the joint visible) has been injected into the joint.

barium enema (BE) **(lower GI series)** (**BAH**-ree-um **EN**-eh-mah)	Infusion of a **radiopaque** contrast medium, barium sulfate, into the rectum. The contrast medium is retained in the lower intestinal tract while X-ray films are obtained of the lower GI tract.

For the most definitive results, the colon should be empty of fecal material. Along with the use of a laxative and/or a cleansing enema, the person having a **barium enema (BE)** would be without food or drink from the midnight before the procedure. Abnormal findings include malignant tumors, colonic stenosis, colonic fistula, perforated colon, diverticula, and polyps. The barium will cause the stool (feces) to have a chalky appearance. Patients are encouraged to drink plenty of fluids to help eliminate the barium.

barium swallow (upper GI series) (BAH-ree-um SWALL-oh)	Oral administration of a **radiopaque** contrast medium, barium sulfate, which flows into the esophagus as the person swallows. See *Figure 20-2*.

During a **barium swallow**, X-ray films are obtained of the esophagus and borders of the heart in which esophageal varices (twisted veins) can be identified and esophageal strictures, tumors or obstructions, achalasia, or abnormal motility of the esophagus can be identifiable. As the barium sulfate continues to flow into the upper GI tract (lower esophagus, stomach, and duodenum), X-ray films are taken to reveal ulcerations, tumors, hiatal hernias, or obstructions.

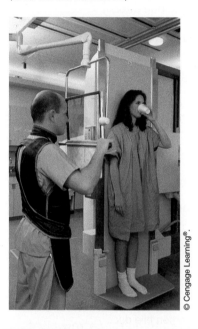

Figure 20-2 Barium swallow (upper GI series)

bronchography (brong-KOG-rah-fee) bronch/o = bronchus -graphy = process of recording	**Bronchography** is an X-ray examination of the interior passageways of the lower respiratory tract (larynx, trachea, and bronchi) following the coating of these structures with a **radiopaque** substance.

As the catheter or bronchoscope is inserted through the nose or mouth and advanced down the throat into the trachea and bronchi, the radiopaque substance is released, forming a coating on the lining of the interior walls of these structures. Abnormalities such as tumors, cavities, cysts, and obstructions may be revealed. Bronchography is less frequently used due to the improved technology of computerized tomography (CT scan) and bronchoscopy.

cholangiography (intravenous) (IVC) (koh-lan-jee-OG-rah-fee) (in-trah-VEE-nus) chol/e = bile angi/o = vessel -graphy = process of recording	Visualizing and outlining of the major bile ducts following an intravenous injection of a contrast medium.

The bile duct structure can be observed for obstruction, strictures, anatomic variations, malignant tumors, and congenital cysts during an intravenous **cholangiography**.

The IVC is less frequently used today and has been largely replaced by other diagnostic procedures, such as ERCP (endoscopic retrograde cholangiopancreatography), endoscopic ultrasound, and, increasingly, by MRI cholangiography.

cholangiography (percutaneous transhepatic) (PTC, PTHC)

(koh-**lan**-jee-**OG**-rah-fee)

(**per**-kyoo-**TAY**-nee-us **trans**-heh-**PAT**-ik)

chol/e = bile
angi/o = vessel
-graphy = process of recording
per- = through
cutane/o = skin
-ous = pertaining to
trans- = across
hepat/o = liver
-ic = pertaining to

An examination of the bile duct structure, using a needle to pass directly into an intrahepatic bile duct to inject a contrast medium. See *Figure 20-3.*

In bile duct structure, bile can be observed for obstruction, strictures, anatomic variations, malignant tumors, recording, and congenital cysts. If the cause is found to be extrahepatic in jaundiced persons, a catheter may be used for external drainage by leaving it in the bile duct.

Special procedures and care are required before, during, and after this procedure. It is an invasive procedure with significant morbidity due to potential complications. Abnormal findings include:

- Tumors, gallstones, or strictures of the common bile or hepatic duct
- Biliary sclerosis
- Cysts of the common bile duct
- Tumors, inflammation, or pseudocysts of the pancreatic duct
- Anatomic biliary or pancreatic duct abnormalities

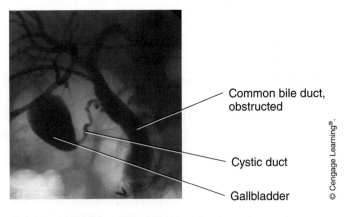

Common bile duct, obstructed

Cystic duct

Gallbladder

© Cengage Learning®.

Figure 20-3 PTHC with common bile duct obstruction

cholangiopancreatography (endoscopic retrograde) (ERCP)

(koh-**lan**-jee-oh-**pan**-kree-ah-**TOG**-rah-fee)

(en-doh-**SKOP**-ic **RET**-roh-grayd)

chol/e = bile
angi/o = vessel
pancreat/o = pancreas
-graphy = process of recording
endo- = within
scop/o = to view
-ic = pertaining to
retro- = backward, behind

A procedure that examines the size and filling of the pancreatic and biliary ducts through direct radiographic visualization with a fiberoptic endoscope. See *Figure 20-4.*

During the ERCP procedure, a fiberoptic scope (flexible tube with a lens and a light source) passes through the patient's esophagus and stomach into the duodenum. A small camera, which is attached to the end of the endoscope, transmits the image to a computer. Passage of the tube is observed on a fluoroscopic screen that makes it possible to view the procedure in action. The doctor locates the ampulla of Vater, a common passageway that connects the common bile duct and the pancreatic duct to the duodenum. Digestive enzymes can be removed from this area for analysis before a contrast medium is injected into the area for visualization upon X-ray.

This procedure requires the person to lie very still during the process. The patient is kept NPO (nothing by mouth) before the procedure and

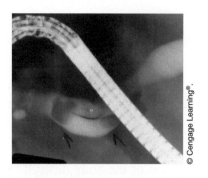

is mildly sedated during the procedure. Abnormal findings include strictures (narrowing) of the common bile duct, tumors, gallstones, cysts, and anatomic variations of the biliary or pancreatic ducts.

Figure 20-4 ERCP with stones

cholecystography (oral) (koh-lee-sis-**TOG**-rah-fee) chol/e = bile cyst/o = bladder, sac, or cyst -graphy = process of recording	Visualization of the gallbladder through X-ray following the oral ingestion of pills containing a **radiopaque** iodinated dye. The oral **cholecystography** is not as accurate as the gallbladder **ultrasound**. Abnormal findings would include gallstones, gallbladder polyps, gallbladder cancer, or cystic duct obstruction.
cineradiography (sin-eh-**ray**-dee-**OG**-rah-fee) cine- = pertaining to movement radi/o = radiation; also refers to radius -graphy = process of recording	**Cineradiography** is a diagnostic technique combining the techniques of **fluoroscopy**, radiography, and cinematography by filming the images that develop on a fluorescent screen with a movie camera.
computed axial tomography (CT, CAT) (kom-**PEW**-ted **AK**-see-al toh-**MOG**-rah-fee) tom/o = to cut -graphy = process of recording	A painless, noninvasive diagnostic X-ray procedure using ionizing radiation that produces a cross-sectional image of the body; also called **computed tomography**. The image created by the computer represents a detailed cross section of the tissue structure being examined. See *Figure 20-5*. **Computed axial tomography** (also called **CAT** or CT scan) is the analysis of a two-dimensional view of the tissue being evaluated as obtained from X-ray beams passing through successive horizontal layers of tissue. The computer detects the radiation absorption and the variation in tissue

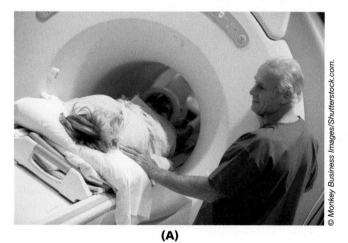
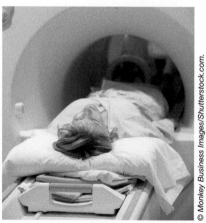

(A)   **(B)**

Figure 20-5 (A) Computed tomography (CT) scanning. Instruct patient to lie still (B) Instruct patient to breathe deeply and relax during procedure. Reassure patient that whirring and clicking sounds are normal

density in each layer. From this detection of radiation absorption and tissue density, a series of anatomic pictures is produced in varying shades of gray.

When contrast is indicated for the CT scan, IV iodinated dye is injected via a peripheral IV site. If the procedure is ordered with contrast, the person needs to be NPO for four hours prior to the study because the contrast dye can cause nausea and vomiting.

This diagnostic procedure is used for various areas and systems of the body. **CAT** scans are helpful in evaluating areas of the body difficult to assess using standard X-ray procedures. The CT scan provides information about the exact location, the extent of involvement, and the direction needed for treatment. The following are descriptions of specific CT scans.

1. **CT of the abdomen**: The CT scan of the abdomen aids in the diagnosis of tumors, abscesses, cysts, inflammation, obstructions, perforation, bleeding, and aneurysms.

2. **CT of the brain**: The analysis of a three-dimensional view of brain tissue obtained as X-ray beams pass through successive horizontal layers of the brain. The images provided are as though you were looking down through the top of the head.

   CT scans of the brain are helpful in identifying intracranial tumors, areas of hemorrhage within the brain, cerebral aneurysm, multiple sclerosis, hydrocephalus, and brain abscess.

3. **CT of lymphoid tissue**: Diagnosis of abnormalities in lymphoid organs are made in areas such as the spleen, thymus gland, and lymph nodes with the collection of X-ray images taken from various angles following injection of a contrast medium.

voiding cystourethrography (**VOYD**-ing **sis**-toh-yoo-ree-**THROG**-rah-fee) cyst/o = bladder, sac, or cyst urethr/o = urethra -graphy = process of recording	X-ray visualization of the bladder and urethra during the voiding process, after the bladder has been filled with a contrast material. The record produced is known as a **cystourethrogram.** A **radiopaque** dye is instilled into the bladder via a urethral catheter. The catheter is then removed and the patient is asked to void. X-ray pictures are taken as the patient is expelling the urine. The **voiding cystourethrography** is helpful in diagnosing urethral lesions, bladder and urethral obstructions, and vesicoureteral reflux (abnormal backflow of urine from the bladder to the ureter).
digital subtraction angiography (DSA) (**DIJ**-ih-tal sub-**TRAK**-shun **an**-jee-**OG**-rah-fee) angi/o = vessel -graphy = process of recording	X-ray images of blood vessels only, appearing without any background due to the use of a computerized digital video subtraction process. Through a central venous line, a smaller than normal amount of contrast medium is injected. The raw data, in digital form, are stored and can be recovered at any time. The best images of the vessels are selected for electronic manipulation. The image is manipulated to provide specific detail. A reaction to the contrast medium is the only potential complication of this procedure. The person undergoing a **digital subtraction angiography (DSA)** will need to be well hydrated and consume no solid food for

two hours prior to the procedure. Persons with the following may be candidates for a DSA:

- Transient ischemic attacks (TIAs)

- Intracranial tumors

- Serial follow-up for individuals with known stenoses in the carotid artery

- Postoperative aneurysm

DSA is being used less and less routinely in imaging departments as it is being replaced by computed tomography angiography (CTA), which can produce 3-D images, is faster, is noninvasive and has fewer complications. DSA is, however, still considered the gold standard for arterial imaging.

echocardiography

(**ek**-oh-**kar**-dee-**OG**-rah-fee)
  echo- = sound
  cardi/o = heart
  -graphy = process of recording

Echocardiography is a diagnostic procedure for studying the structure and motion of the heart. It is useful in evaluating structural and functional changes in a variety of heart disorders. This noninvasive procedure has no known risks or side effects. See *Figure 20-6*.

Ultrasound waves pass through the heart via a **transducer**, bounce off tissues of varying densities, and are reflected backward (or echoed) to the **transducer**, creating an image on the graph.

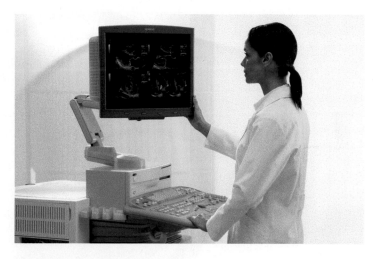

Figure 20-6 Echocardiography
(*Courtesy of Siemens Medical Solutions USA Inc.*)

fluoroscopy

(**floo**-**ROSS**-koh-pee)
  fluor/o = luminous
  -scopy = process of viewing

A radiological technique used to examine the function of an organ or a body part by using a fluoroscope.

Fluoroscopy provides immediate serial images essential in many clinical procedures. While this noninvasive exam visualizes the particular organ in motion, still images can also be captured and stored digitally on a computer.

hysterosalpingography

(**hiss**-ter-oh-**sal**-pin- **GOG**-rah-fee)
  hyster/o = uterus
  salping/o = fallopian tube
  -graphy = process of recording

Hysterosalpingography is an X-ray of the uterus and the fallopian tubes by injecting a contrast material into these structures.

The contrast medium is injected through a cannula inserted into the cervix. As the material is slowly injected, the filling of the uterus and fallopian tubes is observed with a fluoroscope. This procedure is performed to evaluate abnormalities in structure, to detect the presence of possible tumors, and to test for tubal obstructions. The patient may feel occasional menstrual-type cramping during the procedure and will have vaginal drainage for a couple of days after the procedure (from the drainage of the contrast material).

lymphangiography
 	
(lim-**fan**-jee-**OG**-rah-fee)
  lymph/o = lymph
  angi/o = vessel
  -graphy = process of recording
	An X-ray assessment of the lymphatic system following injection of a contrast medium into the lymph vessels in the hand or foot.
	
	The path of lymph flow is noted moving into the chest region. The assistance of a **lymphangiography** is helpful in diagnosing and staging lymphomas.

magnetic resonance imaging (MRI) (mag-**NET**-ik **REZ**-oh-nans **IM**-ij-ing)	A noninvasive **scanning** procedure that provides visualization of fluid, soft tissue, and bony structures by using electromagnetic energy. See *Figure 20-7*.

The person is placed inside a large electromagnetic, tubelike machine where specific radio frequency signals change the alignment of hydrogen atoms in the body. The absorbed radio frequency energy is analyzed by a computer, and an image is projected on the screen.

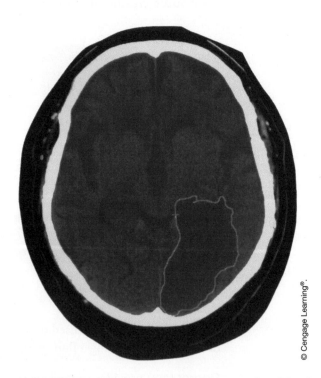

© Cengage Learning®.

Figure 20-7 MRI of a brain with the area of a "bleed" visible in the lower right

A strong magnetic field is used and radio frequency waves produce the imaging valuable in providing images of the heart, large blood vessels, brain, and soft tissue. **Magnetic resonance imaging (MRI)** is also used to examine the aorta to detect masses or possible tumors and pericardial disease. It can show the flow of blood and the beating of the heart. The **MRI** provides far more precision and accuracy than most diagnostic tools.

Those persons with implanted metal devices cannot undergo an **MRI** due to the strong magnetic field and the possibility of dislodging a chip or rod. Thus persons with pacemakers, any recently implanted wires or clips, or prosthetic valves are not eligible for **MRI**. Persons should be informed that **MRI** is a very confining procedure, because they are placed within a tube-like structure, and they should be asked if they are claustrophobic (fear enclosed spaces). Open **MRI** machines are available so that the magnet does not completely surround the patient; however, these machines may not be available in all medical centers.

mammography

(mam-**OG**-rah-fee)

mamm/o = breasts
-graphy = process of recording

The process of taking **X-rays** of the soft tissue of the breast to detect various benign and/or malignant growths before they can be felt.

The American College of Radiology recognizes the use of X-ray **mammography** as the approved method of screening for breast cancer. This procedure takes approximately 15 to 30 minutes to complete and can be performed in an X-ray department of a hospital or in a private **radiology** facility. Each facility should have equipment designed and used exclusively for mammograms.

During the examination, the breast tissue is compressed between two clear disks for each X-ray view. The first view requires compressing the breast from top to bottom to take a top-to-bottom (craniocaudal) view. The second view requires compressing the breast from side to side to take a side-to-side (mediolateral) view.

Figures 20-8A and *B* illustrate the Cleopatra view for a mammogram. This view provides local compression of the lateral aspect of the breast close to the pectoral muscle.

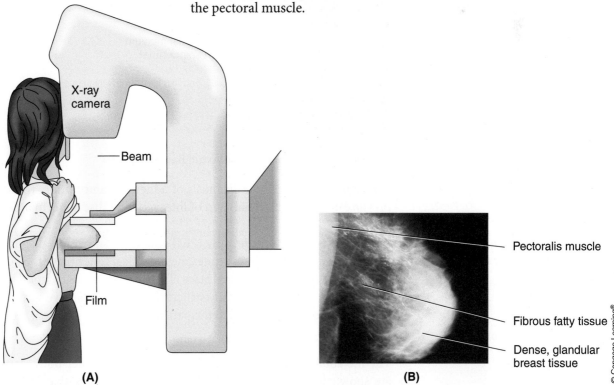

(A)

(B)

Pectoralis muscle

Fibrous fatty tissue

Dense, glandular breast tissue

© Cengage Learning®.

Figure 20-8 Mammography (A) positioning for Cleopatra view; (B) Cleopatra view radiograph

The patient having a mammogram may experience fleeting discomfort as the breast tissue is compressed between the plates. However, this is necessary to facilitate maximum visualization of the breast tissue.

The American Cancer Society recommends that women have their first mammogram (a baseline mammogram) at age 40 and should continue annually as long as the woman is in good health.

myelography

(my-eh-**LOG**-rah-fee)

   myel/o = spinal cord or bone marrow

   -graphy = process of recording

Introduction of contrast medium into the lumbar subarachnoid space through a lumbar puncture to visualize the spinal cord and vertebral canal through X-ray examination. See *Figure 20-9*.

If needed, a small amount of CSF (cerebrospinal fluid) may be withdrawn for lab studies. A **radiopaque** substance (contrast material) is slowly injected into the lumbar subarachnoid space. **Myelography** is accomplished on a tilt table in the **radiology** department. The X-ray table is tilted slowly, allowing the contrast material to reach different levels in the spinal canal.

The exam focuses on the areas of complaint by the patient, such as the lower back, the mid-back, or the neck.

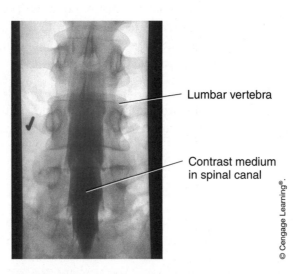

Lumbar vertebra

Contrast medium in spinal canal

© Cengage Learning®.

Figure 20-9 Posteroanterior (PA) lumbar myelogram

Myelography aids in the diagnosis of adhesions and tumors (producing pressure on the spinal canal) and of intervertebral disc abnormalities.

positron emission tomography (PET)

(**POZ**-ih-tron ee-**MISH**-un toh-**MOG**-rah-fee)

   tom/o = to cut

   -graphy = process of recording

Positron emission tomography (PET) scan is a noninvasive diagnostic imaging method that demonstrates the biological function of the body before anatomical changes take place. The scan produces computerized radiographic images of the body structures when radioactive substances (positrons) are administered to the patient (inhaled or injected). See *Figure 20-10*.

The metabolic activity of the brain and numerous other body structures are shown through computerized, color-coded images that indicate the degree and intensity of the metabolic process. The **positron emission**

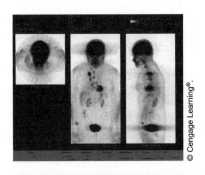

tomography **(PET)** scan exposes persons to very little radiation because the radioactive substances used are short-lived.

The PET scan is widely used for detecting cancer and cancer recurrences (metastasis) and for determining the presence and severity of cardiovascular disease and neurological conditions. One major disadvantage of the use of **positron emission tomography** is that it is very expensive.

Figure 20-10 PET body scan demonstrates tumor in the right lung

pyelography (intravenous) (IVP) (pye-eh-**LOG**-rah-fee) (**in**-trah-**VEE**-nus) pyel/o = renal pelvis -graphy = process of intra- = within ven/o = vein -ous = pertaining to	Also known as **intravenous pyelogram** or excretory urogram, this radiographic procedure provides visualization of the entire urinary tract; that is, the kidneys, ureters, bladder, and urethra. See *Figure 20-11*. A contrast dye is injected intravenously and multiple X-ray films are taken as the medium is cleared from the blood by the glomerular filtration of the kidney. The intravenous **pyelography** (IVP) is useful in diagnosing renal tumors, cysts, or stones, structural or functional abnormalities of the bladder, and ureteral obstruction.

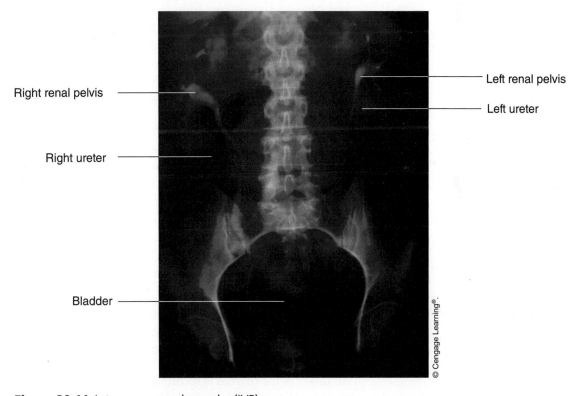

Right renal pelvis

Right ureter

Bladder

Left renal pelvis

Left ureter

Figure 20-11 Intravenous pyelography (IVP)

radiation therapy (ray-dee-**AY**-shun **THAIR**-ah-pee)	The delivery of ionizing radiation to accomplish one or more of the following: 1. Destruction of tumor cells 2. Reduction of tumor size 3. Decrease in pain 4. Relief of obstruction 5. To slow or stop the spread of cancer cells

The ionizing radiation of gamma and **X-rays** has proven **lethal** to the cell's DNA, especially rapidly dividing cells in faster-growing tissues and tumors. **Radiation therapy** (also called radiotherapy) will destroy the rapidly multiplying cells whether or not they are cancerous. The cells of the skin and mucous membranes normally divide rapidly and may be affected by **radiation therapy**.

The goal of therapy with radiation is to reach maximum tumor control with no, or minimum, normal tissue damage. **Radiation therapy** may be delivered by **teletherapy** (external radiation) or **brachytherapy** (internal radiation) or by a combination of both. A treatment method used to decrease the damage to normal tissue is fractionation, which involves giving radiation in repeated small doses at intervals.

The individual receiving external radiation (**teletherapy**) must lie still so that the radiation is delivered to the exact area it is directed (to prevent damage to other tissues). Side effects of external radiation include skin changes such as redness, blanching, scaling, sloughing, hyperpigmentation, pain or hemorrhage, ulcerations in the mucous membranes, and decreased secretions from the mucous membranes (thus posing the frequent ulcerations to become infected). Other common side effects are hair loss (hair cells multiply rapidly), tiredness, increased susceptibility to infection (bone marrow suppression), and GI symptoms (including nausea, vomiting, anorexia, diarrhea, and bleeding). **Radiation therapy** affects the lungs through the development of an interstitial exudate that may lead to radiation pneumonia.

Internal radiation allows the radioactive material to be placed directly into the tumor site to dispense a high dose to the tumor itself. (Thus the normal tissues receive a lower dose.) The ingested or implanted radiation can be hazardous to those taking care of, living with, or treating the individual. Precautions are necessary for caregivers to protect themselves by using specific safety measures for handling secretions, maintaining a distance, and limiting the time of exposure. The side effects of internal radiation are the same as those of the external radiation.

radioactive iodine uptake (RAIU) (**ray**-dee-oh-**AK**-tiv **EYE**-oh-dine **UP**-tayk)	**Radioactive iodine uptake** is an examination that determines the position, size, shape, and physiological function of the thyroid gland through the use of radionuclear **scanning**.

An image of the thyroid is recorded and visualized after a radioactive substance is given. Nodules are readily noted with this scan and are classified as hot (functioning) or cold (nonfunctioning). The thyroid scan is helpful in the diagnosis of the following cases:

1. Neck or substernal masses

2. Thyroid nodules (thyroid cancers are typically cold)

3. Cause of hyperthyroidism

4. Evaluating metastatic tumors with an unknown primary site

scanning (bone, brain, liver, lungs)

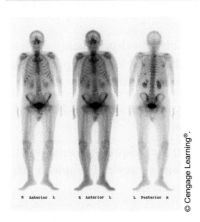

Figure 20-12 Complete bone scan

© Cengage Learning®.

Scanning is the process of recording the emission of radioactive waves using a **gamma camera** (scanner) after an intravenous injection of a **radionuclide** material (tracer) into the particular part of the body being studied. The tracer doesn't remain active for long, with radioactivity being completely eliminated by two days.

The image of the area being studied is displayed by recording the concentration or collection of a radioactive substance specifically drawn to that area. A variety of scans is used in diagnostic evaluations. The following are more distinct descriptions of some of the frequently used scans.

1. **Bone scan: A bone scan involves the intravenous injection of a radionuclide material absorbed by bone tissue. See *Figure 20-12*.**

   The degree of **uptake** of the **radionuclide** is directly related to the metabolism of the bone. After approximately three hours, the skeleton is scanned with a gamma camera (scanner), moving from one end of the body to the other. The scanner detects the areas of radioactive concentration (areas where the bone absorbs the isotope) and produces an image on a screen, where the concentrations show up as pinpoint dots cast in the image of a skeleton. Areas of greater concentration of the **radioisotope** appear darker than other areas of distribution and are called "hot spots," which represent new bone growth around areas of pathology. These areas of pathology can be detected months earlier with a bone scan as compared to an X-ray film.

   A bone scan is primarily used to detect the spread of cancer to the bones (metastasis), osteomyelitis, and other destructive changes in the bone. It can be used to detect bone fractures when pathological fractures are suspected and multiple **X-rays** are not in the best interest of the patient. The "hot spots" on the scan will pinpoint the areas needing X-ray.

2. **Brain nuclear medicine scan: Nuclear scanning of cranial content two hours after an intravenous injection of radioisotopes; also known as a brain PET scan.**

   Normally, blood does not cross the blood–brain barrier and come in contact with brain tissue. However, in localized pathological situations, this barrier is disrupted (allowing isotopes to gather). These isotopes concentrate in abnormal tissue of the brain, indicating a pathological process. The scanner can localize any abnormal tissue where the isotopes have accumulated, detecting energy given off by the radioactive substance and changing it into 3-D pictures. The images are displayed on a monitor for the health care provider to read.

   The brain scan can assist in diagnosing abnormal findings such as an acute cerebral infarction, cerebral neoplasm, cerebral hemorrhage, brain abscess, aneurysms, cerebral thrombosis, hematomas, hydrocephalus, cancer metastasis to the brain, and bleeds.

3. **Liver scan: A noninvasive scanning technique that enables the visualization of the shape, size, and consistency of the liver after the IV injection of a radioactive compound.**

This compound is readily taken up by the liver's Kupffer cells, and later the distribution is recorded by a radiation detector. This scan can detect cysts, abscesses, tumors, granulomas, or diffuse infiltrative processes affecting the liver.

4. **Lung scan: The visual imaging of the distribution of ventilation or blood flow in the lungs by scanning the lungs after the patient has been injected with or has inhaled radioactive material.**

The scanning device records the pattern of pulmonary radioactivity after the patient has received the medication.

5. **Spleen scan: A noninvasive scanning technique that enables the visualization of the shape, size, and consistency of the spleen after the IV injection of radioactive red blood cells.**

This scan can detect damage, tumors, or other problems.

single-photon emission computed tomography (SPECT)	Single-photon emission computed tomography (SPECT) is a nuclear imaging procedure that shows how blood flows to tissues and organs.

(single-**FOH**-ton ee-**MISH**-un kom-**PEW**-ted toh-**MOG**-rah-fee)
  tom/o = to cut
  -graphy = process of recording

The SPECT scan uses computed tomography and a radioactive material that can be detected by a gamma camera. The tracking of the radioactive material allows the physician to see the perfusion of blood to tissues and organs.

The radiopharmaceutical substance is injected into the patient before the SPECT scan. The gamma camera rotates around the patient's body, and the image is transmitted from the camera to a computer screen for interpretation. The SPECT scan differs from the PET scan in that the chemical substance stays in the patient's bloodstream instead of being absorbed into the surrounding tissues. This restricts the images produced to the areas where blood flows.

The SPECT scan is used primarily to visualize blood flow through arteries and veins in the brain. It is also used for myocardial perfusion studies, presurgical evaluation of medically uncontrolled seizures, and diagnosing stress fractures in the spine.

small bowel follow-through	Oral administration of a radiopaque contrast medium, barium sulfate, which flows through the GI system. X-ray films are obtained at timed intervals to observe the progression of the barium through the small intestine. See *Figure 20-13*.

Notable delays in the time for transit may occur with both malignant and benign forms of obstruction or diminished intestinal motility. In hypermotility states, and in malabsorption, the flow of barium is much quicker.

Small bowel tumors, obstructions, inflammatory disease, malabsorption syndrome, congenital defects, or perforation may be identified with a **small bowel follow-through** study.

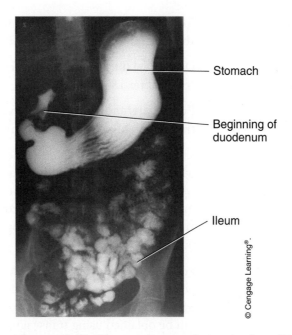

- Stomach
- Beginning of duodenum
- Ileum

© Cengage Learning®.

Figure 20-13 Fifteen-minute radiograph of small bowel study

tomography
 	
(toh-**MOG**-rah-fee)
 	
   tom/o = to cut; section
   -graphy = process of recording
	An X-ray technique used to construct a detailed cross section, at a predetermined depth, of a tissue structure.
	
	Tomography is a useful diagnostic tool for finding and identifying space-occupying lesions in the liver, brain, pancreas, and gallbladder.

ultrasonography
 	
(ull-trah-son-**OG**-rah-fee)
 	
   ultra- = beyond, excess
   son/o = sound
   -graphy = process of recording
	Also called **ultrasound**; **sonogram**. This is a procedure in which sound waves are transmitted into the body structures as a small **transducer** is passed over the patient's skin. See *Figure 20-14*.

The area to be examined is lubricated before applying the **transducer**. As the sound waves are reflected back into the **transducer**, they are interpreted by a computer (which in turn presents the composite in a picture form). Frequently used types of **ultrasonography** are as follows:

1. **Abdominal ultrasound: Through the use of reflected sound waves, abdominal ultrasound is able to provide reliable visualization of the liver, gallbladder, bile ducts, pancreas, and kidneys.**

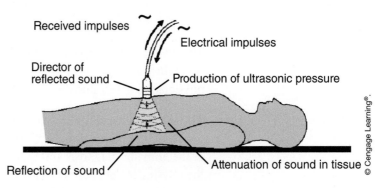

Received impulses

Electrical impulses

Director of reflected sound

Production of ultrasonic pressure

Reflection of sound

Attenuation of sound in tissue

© Cengage Learning®.

Figure 20-14 Ultrasonography

This noninvasive diagnostic procedure demonstrates normal or abnormal findings of the abdominal organs.

2. **Obstetrical ultrasound: For information on the obstetrical ultrasound, see Chapter 18.**

3. **Pelvic ultrasound: A noninvasive procedure that uses high-frequency sound waves to examine the structures within the pelvis.**

The sound waves pass through the abdominal wall from the **transducer**, which is moved back and forth across the abdomen. When the sound waves bounce from the internal organs in the abdominopelvic region, these waves are converted to electrical impulses eventually recorded on an oscilloscope screen. A photograph of the images is then taken for further study.

Pelvic **ultrasound** can be used to locate a pelvic mass, an ectopic pregnancy, or an intrauterine device and to inspect and assess the uterus, ovaries, and fallopian tubes. Clearer ultrasonic pictures of the pelvic organs can be obtained using transvaginal **ultrasonography**. This procedure produces the same type of picture as abdominal **ultrasound** but involves the use of a vaginal probe, which is inserted into the vagina while the patient is in lithotomy position. The probes are encased in a sterile sheath and placed in the **transducer** before it is inserted into the vagina. The sound waves function in the same way as those for the abdominopelvic **ultrasound**, but the transvaginal ultrasonic image is much clearer.

4. **Renal ultrasound: An ultrasound of the kidneys is useful in distinguishing between fluid-filled cysts and solid masses, detecting renal calculi, identifying obstructions, and evaluating transplanted kidneys.**

This noninvasive procedure requires no contrast medium.

5. **Thyroid echogram (ultrasound): An ultrasound examination important in distinguishing solid thyroid nodules from cystic nodules.**

The type of nodule will provide information for treatment. In addition to differentiating the type of nodule, the thyroid echogram is used to evaluate the reaction to the medical therapy for a thyroid mass.

venography
 	
(vee-**NOG**-rah-fee)
 	
  ven/o = vein
 	
  -graphy = process of recording
	Also called phlebography, **venography** is a technique used to prepare an X-ray image of veins that have been injected with a contrast medium that is **radiopaque**.
	
	The venography procedure involves injecting X-ray contrast material (dye) into a vein to show how blood flows through the veins, allowing the physician to determine the condition of the individual's veins.

X-rays	The use of high-energy electromagnetic waves, passing through the body onto a photographic film, to produce a picture of the internal structures of the body for diagnosis and therapy. A chest X-ray is a visualization of the interior of the chest, critical in the complete evaluation of the cardiac and pulmonary systems. See *Figure 20-15.*

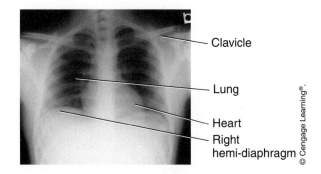

— Clavicle

— Lung

— Heart
— Right
hemi-diaphragm

© Cengage Learning®.

Figure 20-15 Anteroposterior (AP) view of the chest

Sites of abnormal density (such as collections of fluid or pus) can be seen. In addition, the chest X-ray provides diagnostic information about the following:

1. Tumors—primary or metastatic lung, chest wall, heart, and bony thorax

2. Inflammation—pneumonia, pleuritis, and pericarditis

3. Accumulation of fluid—pleural effusion, pericardial effusion, pulmonary edema

4. Accumulation of air—chronic obstructive pulmonary disease (COPD), pneumothorax

5. Bone fractures—thorax, vertebrae

6. Diaphragmatic hernia

7. Size of the heart

8. Calcification—old lung granulomas, large vessel deterioration

9. Placement of centrally located intravenous access devices

Most chest **X-rays** are taken with the person standing. The **supine** or sitting position can be used, but fluid levels cannot be visualized with chest **X-rays** taken in these positions. The chest X-ray can be viewed in the following ways:

1. **Anteroposterior (AP):** The X-rays pass through the front of the body (anterior) to the back of the body (posterior).

2. **Posteroanterior (PA):** The **X-rays** pass through the back of the body (posterior) to the front of the body (anterior). *See Figure 20-16.*

3. **Lateral:** The **X-rays** pass through the person's side.

4. **Oblique:** The **X-rays** are taken from different angles.

5. **Decubitus:** The **X-rays** are taken with the person in **recumbent** lateral position, which aids in localizing fluid. Decubitus position also refers to the patient being on his or her back or stomach.

A portable X-ray may be done at the bedside of a person who is in critical condition or who cannot be transported to an X-ray department. Persons having a chest X-ray must remove clothing above the waist (wear an X-ray

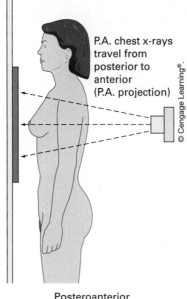

P.A. chest x-rays travel from posterior to anterior (P.A. projection)

© Cengage Learning®.

Posteroanterior
(P.A.) projection

Figure 20-16 Posteroanterior (PA) view of chest

gown) and be able to take a deep breath and hold it while the X-ray is being taken. Precautions must be taken to be sure that the person has no metal objects on his or her body and that protection is provided for the testicles and ovaries to prevent radiation-induced abnormalities.

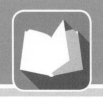

Review Checkpoint

Check your understanding of this section by completing the **Radiology and Diagnostic Imaging Procedures and Techniques** exercises in your workbook.

VOCABULARY

The following vocabulary words are frequently used when discussing radiology and diagnostic imaging.

Word	Definition
abduction (ab-**DUCK**-shun) ab- = from, away from	Movement of a limb away from the body.
adduction (add-**DUCK**-shun) ad- = toward, increase	Movement of a limb toward the axis of the body.

Word	Definition
anteroposterior (**an**-ter-oh-poss-**TEER**-ee-or) anter/o = front poster/o = back	From the front to the back of the body, commonly associated with the direction of the X-ray beam.
aortography (ay-or-**TOG**-rah-fee) aort/o = aorta -graphy = process of recording	A radiographic process in which the aorta and its branches are injected with any of various contrast media for visualization.
arthrography (ar-**THROG**-rah-fee) arthr/o = joint -graphy = process of recording	A method of radiographically visualizing the inside of a joint by injecting air or contrast medium.
axial (**AK**-see-al)	Pertaining to or situated on the axis of a structure or part of the body.
betatron (**BAY**-tah-tron)	A cyclic accelerator that produces high-energy electrons for radiotherapy treatments.
brachytherapy (**brak**-ee-**THAIR**-ah-pee)	The placement of radioactive sources in contact with or implanted into the tissues to be treated.
bronchography (brong-**KOG**-rah-fee) bronch/o = bronchus -graphy = process of recording	An X-ray examination of the interior passageways of the lower respiratory tract (larynx, trachea, and bronchi), following the coating of these structures with a **radiopaque** substance.
cineradiography (see-nee-ray-dee-**OG**-rah-fee) cine- = pertaining to movement radi/o = radiation; also refers to radius -graphy = process of recording	The filming with a movie camera of the images that appear on a fluorescent screen, especially those images of body structures that have been injected with a nontoxic **radiopaque** medium for diagnostic purposes; also called cinefluorography.
computed tomography (CT) (computed toh-**MOG**-rah-fee) tom/o = to cut; section -graphy = process of recording	An X-ray technique that produces a film representing a detailed cross section of tissue structure.
digital radiography (**DIJ**-ih-tal ray-dee-**OG**-rah-fee) radi/o = radiation; also refers to radius -graphy = process of recording	Any method of X-ray image formation that uses a computer to store and manipulate data.
Doppler effect (**DOP**-ler ee-fect)	The apparent change in frequency of sound or light waves emitted by a source as it moves away from or toward an observer.
eversion (ee-**VER**-zhun)	A turning outward or inside out, such as a turning of the foot outward at the ankle.

Word	Definition
extension (eks-**TEN**-shun)	A movement allowed by certain joints of the skeleton that increases the angle between two adjoining bones, such as extending the leg (which increases the angle between the femur and the tibia).
flexion (**FLEK**-shun)	A movement allowed by certain joints of the skeleton that decreases the angle between two adjoining bones, such as bending the elbow (which decreases the angle between the humerus and the ulna).
fluorescence (floo-**RES**-ens)	The emission of light of one wavelength (usually ultraviolet) when exposed to light of a different (usually shorter) wavelength; a property possessed by certain substances.
fluoroscopy (**floo-ROSS**-koh-pee) fluor/o = luminous -scopy = process of viewing	A technique in **radiology** for visually examining a part of the body or the function of an organ, using a fluoroscope.
gamma camera (**GAM**-ah **CAM**-er-ah)	A device that uses the emission of light from a crystal struck by **gamma rays** to produce an image of the distribution of radioactive material in a body organ.
gamma rays (**GAM**-ah)	An electromagnetic radiation of short wavelength emitted by the nucleus of an atom during a nuclear reaction. Also called gamma radiation.
half-life	The time required for a radioactive substance to lose 50% of its activity through decay.
interstitial therapy (in-ter-**STISH**-al therapy)	Radiotherapy in which needles or wires that contain radioactive material are implanted directly into tumor areas.
inversion (in-**VER**-zhun)	An abnormal condition in which an organ is turned inside out, such as a uterine **inversion**; also refers to turning inward, as in **inversion** of the ankle.
ionization (eye-oh-nye-**ZAY**-shun)	The process in which a neutral atom or molecule gains or loses electrons and thus acquires a negative or positive electric charge.
irradiation (ih-ray-dee-**AY**-shun)	Exposure to any form of radiant energy (such as heat, light, or X-ray).
lethal (**LEE**-thal)	Capable of causing death.
linear accelerator (**LIN**-ee-ar)	An apparatus for accelerating charged subatomic particles used in radiotherapy, physics research, and the production of radionuclides.
lymphangiography (lim-**fan**-jee-**OG**-rah-fee) lymph/o = lymph angi/o = vessel -graphy = process of recording	The X-ray examination of lymph glands and lymphatic vessels after an injection of contrast medium.

Word	Definition
magnetic resonance imaging (MRI) (mag-**NET**-ik **REZ**-oh-nans **IM**-ij-ing)	Medical imaging that uses radio frequency signals as its source of energy.
myelography (my-eh-**LOG**-rah-fee) myel/o = bone marrow or spinal cord -graphy = process of recording	A radiographic process by which the spinal cord and the spinal subarachnoid space are viewed and photographed after the introduction of a contrast medium.
nuclear medicine (**NOO**-klee-ar medicine)	A medical discipline that uses radioactive isotopes in the diagnosis and treatment of disease.
orthovoltage (**or**-thoh-**VOHL**-tij)	The voltage range of 100 KeV to 350 KeV supplied by some X-ray generators used for **radiation therapy**.
palliative (**PAL**-ee-ay-tiv)	To soothe or relieve.
piezoelectric (pie-**EE**-zoh-eh-**lek**-trik)	The generation of a voltage across a solid when a mechanical stress is applied.
positron emission tomography (PET) (**POZ**-ih-tron ee-**MISH**-un toh-**MOG**-rah-fee) tom/o = to cut; section -graphy = process of recording	A computerized radiographic technique that employs radioactive substances to examine the metabolic activity of various body structures.
posteroanterior (**poss**-ter-oh-an-**TEER**-ee-or) poster/o = back anter/o = front	The direction from back to front.
prone (**PROHN**)	Being in horizontal position when lying facedown.
pyelography (pie-eh-**LOG**-rah-fee) pyel/o = renal pelvis -graphy = process of recording	A technique in **radiology** for examining the structures and evaluating the function of the urinary system.
rad (**RAD**)	Abbreviation for *radiation absorbed dose*; the basic unit of absorbed dose of ionizing radiation.
radiation therapy (ray-dee-**AY**-shun **THAIR**-ah-pee)	The treatment of neoplastic disease by using **X-rays** or **gamma rays**, usually from a cobalt source, to deter the growth of malignant cells by decreasing the rate of cell division or impairing DNA synthesis. Also called radiotherapy.

Word	Definition
radioactivity (**ray**-dee-oh-**ak**-**TIV**-ih-tee)	The ability of a substance to emit rays or particles (alpha, beta, or gamma) from its nucleus.
radiographer (**ray**-dee-**OG**-rah-fer) radi/o = radiation; also refers to radius graph/o = to record -er = one who	An allied health professional trained to use X-ray machines and other imaging equipment to produce images of the internal structures of the body; also known as a radiologic technologist.
radioimmunoassay (**ray**-dee-oh-**im**-yoo-noh-**ASS**-ay) radi/o = radiation; also refers to radius immun/o = immune, protection -assay = to evaluate	A technique in **radiology** used to determine the concentration of an antigen, antibody, or other protein in the serum.
radioisotope (**ray**-dee-oh-**EYE**-soh-tohp)	A radioactive isotope (of an element) used for therapeutic and diagnostic purposes.
radiologist (ray-dee-**OL**-oh-jist) radi/o = radiation; also refers to radius -logist = one who specializes in the study of	A physician who specializes in **radiology**.
radiology (ray-dee-**ALL**-oh-jee) radi/o = radiation; also refers to radius -logy = the study of	The study of the diagnostic and therapeutic uses of X-rays; also known as **roentgenology**.
radiolucent (**ray**-dee-oh-**LOO**-sent)	Pertaining to materials that allow X-rays to penetrate with a minimum of absorption.
radionuclide (radioisotope) (ray-dee-oh-**NOO**-kleed) (**ray**-dee-oh-**EYE**-soh-tohp)	An isotope (or nuclide) that undergoes radioactive decay.
radiopaque (ray-dee-oh-**PAYK**)	Not permitting the passage of X-rays or other radiant energy.
radiopharmaceutical (ray-dee-oh-farm-ah-**SOO**-tih-kal) radi/o = radiation; also refers to radius pharmac/o = drugs, medicine	A drug that contains radioactive atoms.

Word	Definition
recumbent (ree-**KUM**-bent)	Lying down or leaning backward.
roentgenology (**rent**-jen-**OL**-oh-jee)	See **radiology**.
scanning	A technique for carefully studying an area, organ, or system of the body by recording and displaying an image of the area.
single-photon emission computed tomography (SPECT) (single-**FOH**-ton ee-**MISH**-un kom-**PEW**-ted toh-**MOG**-rah-fee)	A variation of computerized **tomography** (**CT**) **scanning** in which gamma camera detectors rotate around the patient's body, collecting data. The data are summarized into a three-dimensional representation.
supine (soo-**PIGHN**)	Lying horizontally on the back.

teletherapy
(tell-eh-**THAIR**-ah-pee)
  tel/e = distance
  -therapy = treatment
	Radiation therapy administered by a machine positioned at some distance from the patient.

tomography
(toh-**MOG**-rah-fee)
  tom/o = to cut; section
  -graphy = process of recording
	An X-ray technique that produces a film representing a detailed cross section of tissue structure at a predetermined depth.

transducer (trans-**DOO**-sir)	A handheld device that sends and receives a sound-wave signal.
ultrasound (**ULL**-trah-sound) ultra- = beyond	Sound waves at the very high frequency of more than 20,000 kHz (vibrations per second).
uptake (**UP**-tayk)	The drawing up or absorption of a substance.

Review Checkpoint

Check your understanding of this section by completing the **Vocabulary** exercises in your workbook.

WORD ELEMENTS

The following word elements appear in terms used to describe radiology and diagnostic imaging treatments and procedures. As you review the list, pronounce each word element aloud twice and check the applicable box after you "say it." Write the definition for the example term given for each word element. Use your medical dictionary to find the definitions of the example terms.

Word Element	Pronunciation	"Say It"	Meaning
angi/o **angi**ography	**AN**-jee-oh an-jee-**OG**-rah-fee	☐	vessel
anter/o **anter**oposterior	**AN**-ter-oh **an**-ter-oh-poss-**TEER**-ee-or	☐	front
aort/o **aort**ogram	ay-**OR**-toh ay-**OR**-toh-gram	☐	aorta
arthr/o **arthr**ography	**AR**-throh ar-**THROG**-rah-fee	☐	joint
arteri/o **arteri**ogram	ar-**TEE**-ree-oh ar-**TEE**-ree-oh-gram	☐	artery
bronch/o **bronch**ography	**BRONG**-koh brong-**KOG**-rah-fee	☐	bronchus
cardi/o **cardi**ocatheterization	**KAR**-dee-oh **kar**-dee-oh-**kath**-eh-ter-ih-**ZAY**-shun	☐	heart
chol/e **chol**ecystogram	**KOH**-lee **koh**-lee-**SIS**-toh-gram	☐	bile
cine- **cine**angiogram	**SIN**-ee sin-ee-**AN**-jee-oh-gram	☐	pertaining to movement
cyst/o **cyst**ourethrography	**SIS**-toh sis-toh-yoo-ree-**THROG**-rah-fee	☐	bladder, sac, or cyst
echo- **echo**cardiography	**ECK**-oh eck-oh-**kar**-dee-**OG**-rah-fee	☐	sound
fluor/o **fluor**oscopy	**FLOO**-roh floo-**ROSS**-koh-pee	☐	luminous
hyster/o **hyster**osalpingogram	**HIS**-ter-oh **hiss**-ter-oh-**sal**-**PING**-oh-gram	☐	uterus

Word Element	Pronunciation	"Say It"	Meaning
immun/o radio**immuno**assay	im-**YOO**-noh **ray**-dee-oh-im-yoo-noh-**ASS**-ay	☐	immune, protection
lymph/o **lymph**angiogram	**LIM**-foh lim-**FAN**-jee-oh-gram	☐	lymph
mamm/o **mamm**ography	**MAM**-oh mam-**OG**-rah-fee	☐	breast
myel/o **myel**ography	**MY**-el-oh my-el-**OG**-rah-fee	☐	bone marrow, spinal cord
pyel/o intravenous **pyel**ogram	**PIE**-eh-loh in-trah-**VEE**-nus **PIE**-eh-loh-gram	☐	renal pelvis
radi/o **radi**opaque	**RAY**-dee-oh ray-dee-oh-**PAYK**	☐	radiation; also refers to radius
ren/o **ren**al	**REE**-noh **REE**-nal	☐	kidney
son/o **son**ogram	**SOH**-noh **SOH**-noh-gram	☐	sound
tel/e **tel**etherapy	**TELL**-eh tel-eh-**THER**-ah-pee	☐	distance
tom/o **tom**ography	**TOH**-moh toh-**MOG**-rah-fee	☐	to cut
ultra- **ultra**sound	**ULL**-trah **ULL**-trah-sound	☐	beyond
ven/o **ven**ography	**VEE**-noh vee-**NOG**-rah-fee	☐	vein
xer/o **xer**oradiography	**ZEE**-roh zee-roh-ray-dee-**OG**-rah-fee	☐	dry

Review Checkpoint

Check your understanding of this section by completing the **Word Elements** exercises in your workbook.

COMMON ABBREVIATIONS

Abbreviation	Meaning	Abbreviation	Meaning
AP	anteroposterior	MRA	magnetic resonance angiography
Ba	barium	MRI	magnetic resonance imaging
BE	barium enema	NMR	nuclear magnetic resonance (imaging)
CAT	computed axial tomography		
C-spine	cervical spine (film)	NPO	nothing by mouth
CT	computed tomography	PA	posteroanterior
CXR	chest X-ray	PET	positron emission tomography
DSA	digital subtraction angiography	PTC, PTHC	percutaneous transhepatic cholangiography
DSR	dynamic spatial reconstructor	rad	radiation absorbed dose
ECHO	echocardiogram	RAI	radioactive iodine
ERCP	endoscopic retrograde cholangiopancreatography	RIA	radioimmunoassay
		RAIU	radioactive iodine uptake (scan)
Fx	fracture	SBS	small bowel series
IVC	intravenous cholangiography	SPECT	single-photon emission computed tomography
IVP	intravenous pyelogram		
IVU	intravenous urography	UGI	upper gastrointestinal (series)
KUB	kidneys, ureters, bladder	u/s	ultrasound
LGI	lower gastrointestinal (series)		

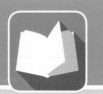

Review Checkpoint

Check your understanding of this section by completing the **Common Abbreviations** exercises in your workbook.

WRITTEN AND AUDIO TERMINOLOGY REVIEW

Review each of the following terms from this chapter. Study the spelling of each term and write the definition in the space provided. Check definitions by looking the term up in the glossary.

Term	Pronunciation	Definition
angiocardiography	☐ **an**-jee-oh-**kar**-dee-**OG**-rah-fee	_____
angiography	☐ **an**-jee-**OG**-rah-fee	_____
anteroposterior	☐ **an**-ter-oh-poss-**TEER**-ee-or	_____
aortogram	☐ ay-**OR**-toh-gram	_____
aortography	☐ **ay**-or-**TOG**-rah-fee	_____
arteriogram	☐ ar-**TEE**-ree-oh-gram	_____
arteriography	☐ **ar**-tee-ree-**OG**-rah-fee	_____
arthrography	☐ ar-**THROG**-rah-fee	_____
axial	☐ **AK**-see-al	_____
barium enema (BE)	☐ **BAIR**-ree-um **EN**-eh-mah (BE)	_____
barium swallow	☐ **BAIR**-ree-um **SWALL**-oh	_____
betatron	☐ **BAY**-tah-tron	_____
brachytherapy	☐ **brak**-ee-**THAIR**-ah-pee	_____
bronchography	☐ brong-**KOG**-rah-fee	_____
cardiocatheterization	☐ kar-dee-o-**kath**-eh-ter-ih-**ZAY**-shun	_____
cerebral angiography	☐ **SER**-eh-bral (seh-**REE**-bral) **an**-jee-**OG**-rah-fee	_____
cholangiography	☐ koh-**lan**-jee-**OG**-rah-fee	_____
cholecystogram	☐ **koh**-lee-**SIS**-toh-gram	_____
cholecystography	☐ **koh**-lee-sis-**TOG**-rah-fee	_____
cineangiogram	☐ **sin**-ee-**AN**-jee-oh-gram	_____
cineradiography	☐ **sin**-eh-**ray**-dee-**OG**-rah-fee	_____
computed axial tomography (CAT)	☐ kom-**PEW**-ted **AK**-see-al toh-**MOG**-rah-fee (CAT)	_____
cystourethrogram	☐ **sis**-toh-yoo-**REE**-**throw**-gram	_____

Term	Pronunciation	Definition
digital radiography	☐ **DIJ**-ih-tal ray-dee-**OG**-rah-fee	_____
digital subtraction angiography (DSA)	☐ **DIJ**-ih-tal sub-**TRAK**-shun **an**-jee-**OG**-rah-fee (DSA)	_____
echocardiography	☐ **eck**-oh-kar-dee-**OG**-rah-fee	_____
eversion	☐ ee-**VER**-shun	_____
extension	☐ ecks-**TEN**-shun	_____
flexion	☐ **FLEK**-shun	_____
fluorescence	☐ floo-**RES**-ens	_____
fluoroscopy	☐ floo-**ROSS**-koh-pee	_____
gamma rays	☐ **GAM**-ah rays	_____
hysterosalpingogram	☐ **hiss**-ter-oh-**sal**-**PING**-oh-gram	_____
hysterosalpingography	☐ **hiss**-ter-oh-**sal**-pin-**GOG**-rah-fee	_____
intravenous pyelogram	☐ **in**-trah-**VEE**-nus **PIE**-eh-loh-**gram**	_____
inversion	☐ in-**VER**-zhun	_____
ionization	☐ **eye**-oh-nye-**ZAY**-shun	_____
irradiation	☐ ih-**ray**-dee-**AY**-shun	_____
lethal	☐ **LEE**-thal	_____
linear accelerator	☐ **LIN**-ee-ar ak-**SELL**-er-**ay**-tor	_____
lymphangiogram	☐ lim-**FAN**-jee-oh-gram	_____
lymphangiography	☐ lim-**fan**-jee-**OG**-rah-fee	_____
magnetic resonance imaging (MRI)	☐ mag-**NET**-ik **REZ**-oh-nans **IM**-ij-ing (MRI)	_____
mammography	☐ mam-**OG**-rah-fee	_____
myelography	☐ **my**-eh-**LOG**-rah-fee	_____
nuclear medicine	☐ **NOO**-klee-ar medicine	_____
orthovoltage	☐ **or**-thoh-**VOHL**-tij	_____
palliative	☐ **PAL**-ee-ay-tiv	_____
piezoelectric	☐ pie-**EE**-zoh-eh-**lek**-trik	_____
positron emission tomography (PET)	☐ **POZ**-ih-tron ee-**MISH**-un toh-**MOG**-rah-fee (PET)	_____
posteroanterior	☐ **poss**-ter-oh-an-**TEER**-ee-or	_____
prone	☐ **PROHN**	_____
pyelography	☐ **pie**-eh-**LOG**-rah-fee	_____

Term	Pronunciation	Definition
rad	☐ **RAD**	_____
radiation therapy	☐ **ray**-dee-**AY**-shun **THAIR**-ah-pee	_____
radioactive iodine uptake	☐ **ray**-dee-oh-**AK**-tiv **EYE**-oh-dine **UP**-tayk	_____
radioactivity	☐ **ray**-dee-oh-ak-**TIV**-ih-tee	_____
radiographer	☐ **ray**-dee-**OG**-rah-fer	_____
radioimmunoassay	☐ **ray**-dee-oh-im-yoo-noh-**ASS**-ay	_____
radioisotope	☐ **ray**-dee-oh-**EYE**-soh-tohp	_____
radiologist	☐ **ray**-dee-**OL**-oh-jist	_____
radiology	☐ **ray**-dee-**OL**-oh-jee	_____
radiolucent	☐ **ray**-dee-oh-**LOO**-sent	_____
radionuclide	☐ **ray**-dee-oh-**NOO**-klyde	_____
radiopaque	☐ **ray**-dee-oh-**PAYK**	_____
radiopharmaceutical	☐ **ray**-dee-oh-farm-ah-**SOO**-tih-kal	_____
recumbent	☐ ree-**KUM**-bent	_____
renal angiography	☐ **REE**-nal an-jee-**OG**-rah-fee	_____
roentgenology	☐ **rent**-jen-**OL**-oh-jee	_____
scanning	☐ **SCAN**-ing	_____
single-photon emission computed tomography (SPECT)	☐ single **FOH**-ton ee-**MISH**-un kom-**PEW**-ted toh-**MOG**-rah-fee (SPECT)	_____
sonogram	☐ **SOH**-noh-gram	_____
supine	☐ soo-**PIGHN**	_____
teletherapy	☐ **tell**-eh-**THAIR**-ah-pee	_____
tomography	☐ toh-**MOG**-rah-fee	_____
transducer	☐ trans-**DOO**-sir	_____
ultrasonography	☐ **ull**-trah-son-**OG**-rah-fee	_____
ultrasound	☐ **ULL**-trah-sound	_____
uptake	☐ **UP**-tayk	_____
venography	☐ vee-**NOG**-rah-fee	_____
voiding cystourethrography	☐ **VOYD**-ing sis-toh-**yoo**-ree-**THROG**-rah-fee	_____
X-rays	☐ **ECKS**-rays	_____

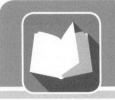

Review Checkpoint

Apply what you have learned in this chapter by completing the **Putting It All Together** exercise in your workbook.

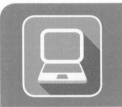

Online Resources

For additional study tools, such as PowerPoint® slides, go to the Student Companion Website.

Chapter Review Exercises

The following exercises provide a more in-depth review of the chapter material. Your goal in these exercises is to complete each section at a minimum 80% level of accuracy. If you score below 80% in any area, return to the applicable section in the chapter and read the material again. A place has been provided for your score at the end of each section.

A. Term to Definition

Define each term by writing the definition in the space provided. Check the box if you are able to complete this exercise correctly the first time (without referring to the answers). Each correct answer is worth 10 points. Record your score in the space provided at the end of the exercise.

☐ 1. mammography _____

☐ 2. intravenous pyelogram _____

☐ 3. hysterosalpingogram _____

☐ 4. posteroanterior _____

☐ 5. cystourethrogram _____

☐ 6. fluoroscopy _____

☐ 7. radiology _____

☐ 8. radiation therapy _____

☐ 9. lymphangiogram _____

☐ 10. lethal _____

Number correct _____ × 10 points/correct answer: Your score _____%

B. Matching Abbreviations

Match the abbreviations on the left with the correct definition on the right. Each correct response is worth 10 points. When you have completed the exercise, record your score in the space provided at the end of the exercise.

_____ 1. AP

_____ 2. BE

_____ 3. CXR

_____ 4. IVP

_____ 5. KUB

_____ 6. MRI

_____ 7. PET

_____ 8. RIA

_____ 9. CAT

_____ 10. SPECT

a. computed axial tomography

b. radioimmunoassay

c. computed tomography

d. retrograde pyelogram

e. intravenous pyelogram

f. anteroposterior

g. chest X-ray

h. barium enema

i. kidneys, ureters, bladder

j. magnetic resonance imaging

k. positron emission tomography

l. posteroanterior

m. single-photon emission computed tomography

Number correct _____ × 10 points/correct answer: Your score _____%

C. Crossword Puzzle

Read the clues carefully and complete the puzzle. Each crossword puzzle answer is worth 10 points. When you have completed the puzzle, total your points and enter your score in the space provided at the end of the exercise.

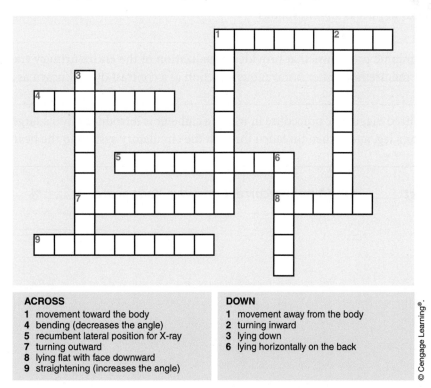

ACROSS
1 movement toward the body
4 bending (decreases the angle)
5 recumbent lateral position for X-ray
7 turning outward
8 lying flat with face downward
9 straightening (increases the angle)

DOWN
1 movement away from the body
2 turning inward
3 lying down
6 lying horizontally on the back

© Cengage Learning®.

Number correct _____ × 10 points/correct answer: Your score _____%

D. Completion

Complete each sentence with the most appropriate answer. Each correct answer is worth 10 points. Record your score in the space provided at the end of the exercise.

1. X-ray of the uterus and the fallopian tubes by injecting a contrast material into these structures is known as:

    _____

2. The introduction of contrast medium into the lumbar subarachnoid space through a lumbar puncture to visualize the spinal cord and vertebral canal through X-ray examination is known as:

    _____

3. The process of taking X-rays of the soft tissue of the breast to detect various benign and/or malignant growths before they can be felt is known as:

    _____

4. A procedure in which sound waves are transmitted into the body structures as a small transducer is passed over the patient's skin is called:

    _____

5. A diagnostic procedure for studying the structure and motion of the heart is known as:

    _____

6. A bronchial examination via X-ray following the coating of the bronchi with a radiopaque substance is termed:

    _____

7. The visualization of the gallbladder through X-ray following the oral ingestion of pills containing a radiopaque iodinated dye is known as an oral:

    _____

8. The visualization of the outline of the major bile ducts following an intravenous injection of a contrast medium is known as an intravenous:

    _____

9. A radiographic procedure that provides visualization of the entire urinary tract—the kidneys, ureters, bladder, and urethra—after intravenous injection of a contrast dye is known as an intravenous:

    _____

10. A specialized diagnostic procedure in which a catheter is introduced into a large vein or artery, usually of an arm or a leg, and is then threaded through the circulatory system to the heart is an:

    _____

Number correct _____ × *10 points/correct answer: Your score* _____%

E. Matching Procedures

Match the diagnostic procedures on the left with the applicable definition on the right. Each correct answer is worth 10 points. When you have completed the exercise, record your score in the space provided at the end of the exercise.

_____ 1. ERCP

_____ 2. voiding cystourethrography

_____ 3. lung scan

_____ 4. MRI

_____ 5. cerebral angiography

_____ 6. arthrography

_____ 7. X-rays

_____ 8. small bowel follow-through

_____ 9. pelvic ultrasound

_____ 10. renal ultrasound

a. the visual imaging of the distribution of ventilation or blood flow in the lungs by scanning the lungs after the patient has been injected with, or has inhaled, radioactive material

b. oral administration of a radiopaque contrast medium (barium sulfate), which flows through the GI system while X-ray films are obtained at timed intervals to observe the progression of the barium through the small intestines

c. the process of taking X-rays of the inside of a joint after a contrast medium has been injected into the joint

d. a type of cholangiopancreatography that examines the filling of the pancreatic and biliary ducts through direct radiographic visualization with a fiberoptic endoscope

e. visualization of the cerebrovascular system via X-ray made possible by the injection of a radiopaque contrast medium into an arterial blood vessel (carotid, femoral, or brachial)

f. the use of high-energy electromagnetic waves (passing through the body onto a photographic film) to produce a picture of the internal structures of the body for diagnosis and therapy

g. a noninvasive procedure that uses high-frequency sound waves to examine the pelvis

h. an ultrasound of the kidneys useful in distinguishing between fluid-filled cysts and solid masses, detecting renal calculi, identifying obstructions, and evaluating transplanted kidneys

i. a noninvasive scanning procedure that provides visualization of fluid, soft tissue, and bony structures without the use of radiation

j. X-ray visualization of the bladder and urethra during the voiding process after the bladder has been filled with a contrast material

Number correct _____ _× 10 points/correct answer: Your score_ _____%

F. Definition to Term

Using the following definitions, identify and provide the medical term(s) to match the definition. Each correct answer is worth 10 points. Record your score in the space provided at the end.

1. A series of X-ray films allowing visualization of internal structures after the IV introduction of a radio-paque substance.

   _____

   (one word)

2. Infusion of a radiopaque contrast medium into the rectum and held in the lower intestinal tract while X-rays are made of the lower GI tract.

   _____

   (two words)

3. A painless, noninvasive diagnostic X-ray using ionizing radiation and producing a cross-section image of the tissue structure being examined.

   _____

   (two or three words)

4. Images of blood vessels only, appearing without any background.

   _____

   (three words)

5. Visualization of the metabolic activity of body structures shown through computerized color-coded images, which indicate the degree and intensity of the metabolic process.

   _____

   (three words)

6. Radiographic visualization of the entire urinary tract.

   _____

   (one word)

7. Delivery of ionizing radiation to accomplish the destruction of rapidly multiplying tumor cells.

   _____

   (two words)

8. Detection of the degree of uptake of a previous IV injection of a radionuclide material that has been absorbed by bone tissue.

   _____

   (two words)

9. A noninvasive scanning technique that enables the visualization of the shape, size, and consistency of the spleen after the IV injection of radioactive red blood cells.

   _____

   (two words)

10. An ultrasound examination important in distinguishing solid thyroid nodules from cystic nodules.

    _____

    (two words)

Number correct _____ *× 10 points/correct answer: Your score* _____%

G. Word Search

Read each definition carefully and identify the applicable word from the list that follows. Enter the word in the space provided and then find it in the puzzle and circle it. The words may be read up, down, diagonally, across, or backward. Each correct answer is worth 10 points. Record your score in the space provided at the end of the exercise.

flexion	transducer	radiographer
radiopaque	irradiation	radiologist
MRI	arthrography	palliative
radiolucent	anteroposterior	

Example: Bending (decreases the angle)

flexion _____

1. A medical doctor who specializes in roentgenology is known as a:

   _____

2. A health professional who takes X-rays is known as a:

   _____

F	L	E	X	I	O	N	O	A	T	T	S	I	S	L
R	O	I	R	E	T	S	O	P	O	R	E	T	N	A
L	A	B	Y	A	T	U	T	E	A	A	G	R	Y	C
M	A	D	S	A	I	H	S	D	I	N	E	E	R	I
R	S	D	I	R	G	I	I	L	E	S	I	H	A	T
I	I	S	Y	O	M	O	A	N	O	D	R	P	D	U
L	T	E	D	E	L	H	I	M	M	U	I	A	I	E
E	I	E	E	U	T	O	E	X	I	C	N	R	O	C
D	V	X	C	V	I	N	G	N	T	E	P	G	P	A
C	N	E	C	I	I	N	E	I	T	R	N	O	A	M
L	N	U	U	R	M	T	A	R	S	I	A	I	Q	R
T	C	H	O	L	Y	M	A	J	W	T	V	D	U	A
R	N	O	I	S	O	R	T	I	E	P	R	A	E	H
O	U	I	A	I	A	S	U	M	L	O	S	R	P	P
S	J	O	L	S	Y	R	S	H	C	L	S	Y	A	O
I	N	N	U	N	O	I	T	A	I	D	A	R	R	I
S	O	O	S	D	S	R	S	L	F	L	E	P	X	D
P	C	A	N	M	I	G	A	I	U	E	H	P	Y	A
A	R	T	H	R	O	G	R	A	P	H	Y	L	T	R

(continued)

3. Abbreviation for a noninvasive scanning procedure that provides visualization of fluid, soft tissue, and bony structure, using electromagnetic energy:

_____

4. Something that does not permit passage of X-rays is said to be:

_____

5. Something that allows X-rays to penetrate is said to be:

_____

6. The part of the sonograph that sends and receives sound-wave signals is known as the:

_____

7. A treatment or medication that soothes or relieves is said to be:

_____

8. Exposure to radiant energy is called:

_____

9. Direction of X-ray beam from front to back is termed:

_____

10. The process of taking X-rays of the inside of a joint after contrast medium has been injected into the joint is known as:

_____

Number correct _____ × 10 points/correct answer: Your score _____%

H. Spelling

Circle the correctly spelled term in each pairing of words. Each correct answer is worth 10 points. Record your score in the space provided at the end of the exercise.

1. flouroscopy   fluoroscopy
2. angography   angiography
3. cinoradiography   cineradiography
4. myelography   mylography
5. brachitherapy   brachytherapy

6. arterography   arteriography
7. rentgenology   roentgenology
8. cystourethrogram   cystourethergram
9. phlebography   phelbography
10. echogram   eckogram

Number correct _____ × 10 points/correct answer: Your score _____%

I. Word Element Review

Read the following definitions carefully and write the correct word element in the space provided. (*Note:* Each word element should be written as it appears in your textbook, using the combining vowel.) Each correct answer is worth 10 points. Record your score in the space provided at the end of the exercise.

Example: The word element for vessel is *angi/o* _____

1. The word element for *joint* is _____
2. The word element for *bronchus* is _____
3. The word element for *bile* is _____
4. The prefix that means "pertaining to movement" is _____

5. The word element that means "luminous" is _____

6. The word element that means "breast" is _____

7. The word element that means "renal pelvis" is _____

8. The word element that means "to cut or section" is _____

9. The word element that means "dry" is _____

10. The prefix that means "beyond" is _____

Number correct _____ × 10 points/correct answer: Your score _____%

J. True or False

Read each statement carefully and circle the correct answer as true or false. HINT: Pay close attention to the word elements written in **bold** as you make your decision. If the statement is false, identify the meaning of that word element. Each correct answer is worth 10 points. Record your score in the space provided at the end of the exercise.

1. An angio**cardio**graphy is used to obtain detailed information about the structure and function of the heart chambers, valves, and the great vessels.

   True   False

   If your answer is False, what does *cardi/o* mean? _____

2. An **arterio**graphy is the X-ray visualization of arteries following the introduction of a radiopaque contrast medium into the bloodstream through a specific vessel by way of a catheter.

   True   False

   If your answer is False, what does *arteri/o* mean? _____

3. A **ren**al angiography is the X-ray visualization of the heart.

   True   False

   If your answer is False, what does *ren/o* mean? _____

4. An **arthro**graphy is the process of taking X-rays inside of a joint after a contrast medium has been injected into the joint.

   True   False

   If your answer is False, what does *arthr/o* mean? _____

5. A **broncho**graphy is the X-ray examination of the stomach after coating it with a contrast medium.

   True   False

   If your answer is False, what does *bronch/o* mean? _____

6. An intravenous **chol**angiography is the process of visualizing and outlining the major bile ducts following an intravenous injection of a contrast medium.

   True   False

   If your answer is False, what does *chol/e* mean? _____

7. A voiding **cysto**urethrography is the X-ray visualization of the bladder and urethra during the voiding process after the bladder has been filled with a contrast material.

   True   False

   If your answer is False, what does *cyst/o* mean? _____

(*continued*)

8. A **lymph**angiography is an X-ray assessment of the urinary system.

   True   False

   If your answer is False, what does *lymph/o* mean? _____

9. A hystero**salpingo**graphy is an X-ray of the uterus and the fallopian tubes by injecting a contrast material into these structures.

   True   False

   If your answer is False, what does *salping/o* mean? _____

10. **Mammo**graphy is the process of taking X-rays of the soft tissue of the thigh.

    True   False

    If your answer is False, what does *mamm/o* mean? _____

Number correct _____ × *10 points/correct answer: Your score* _____%

Oncology (Cancer Medicine)

CHAPTER CONTENT

OBJECTIVES

Upon completing this chapter and the review exercises at the end of the chapter, the learner should be able to:

1. Identify and define 15 pathological conditions and five treatment methods associated with oncology.

2. Identify at least 10 diagnostic techniques used in diagnosis and treatment of oncological disorders.

3. Correctly spell and pronounce terms listed on the Written and Audio Terminology Review, using the phonetic pronunciations provided.

4. Identify at least 10 abbreviations common to oncology.

5. List and define six surgical procedures used in the diagnosis or cure of malignant tumors.

6. List and define three tumor responses to radiation therapy.

Overview

When we hear that **cancer** causes more deaths in children between the ages of 3 and 15 than any other disease, it is a jolting reminder that **cancer** can strike at any age. It is estimated that one of every three Americans alive today will develop **cancer** during his or her lifetime. **Cancer** is now the second leading cause of death in the United States.

The term *cancer* does not refer to only one disease. It actually refers to a group of diseases, consisting of more than 200 types. Although **cancer** can originate in almost any body organ, the most common site for **cancer** in women is the breast and the most common site for **cancer** in men is the prostate gland. The prognosis, or outlook, for a patient diagnosed with **cancer** will depend on many factors, which include (but are not limited to) the type of **cancer**, the stage of the disease, the patient's age and general state of health, and the response to treatment.

The medical specialty concerned with the study of malignancy is known as **oncology**. The physician who specializes in the study and treatment of neoplastic diseases, particularly cancer, is known as an **oncologist**.

This chapter concentrates on a discussion of many of the terms associated with the study of **cancer**, the characteristics of **benign** and **malignant** tumors, predisposing factors that influence one's susceptibility to developing **cancer**, some of the more common types of **cancer**, and the diagnostic techniques and procedures associated with the treatment of **cancer**. It is not designed to provide an in-depth study of **cancer**.

Many pathological conditions in this chapter have already been discussed in previous body system chapters. This should reinforce the concept that **cancer** can affect almost any body system.

Cancer Terms

Any discussion of **cancer** should begin with a review of some terms that provide a foundation for understanding this complex disease. The term *neoplasia* is used to define the development of an abnormal growth of new cells that is unresponsive to normal growth control mechanisms. This development may be **benign** or **malignant**. The term *neoplasm* refers to the growth itself, that is, any abnormal growth of new tissue that serves no useful purpose. It, too, may be **benign** or **malignant**. The term *neoplasm* is used synonymously with **tumor**. When the term *neoplasm* is used in the discussion of **cancer**, the word *malignant* must precede it (as in **malignant neoplasm** equals **malignant** tumor).

During the developmental stages, cells are under the control of **deoxyribonucleic acid (DNA)**—the carrier of genetic information. They undergo changes in their structural and functional properties as they form the different tissues of the body. In other words, the immature cell changes many times in its process of becoming a mature cell with clearly defined functions. This process of cells becoming specialized and differentiated both physically and functionally is known as **differentiation**. Cells that look and act like the parent cell (tissue of origin) are said to be well differentiated.

Neoplasms that consist of cells that do not resemble the tissue of origin are said to be poorly differentiated or undifferentiated. The loss of cellular **differentiation** and reversion to a more primitive form is called **anaplasia**. Anaplastic cell division is not under the control of DNA. **Anaplasia** may occur as a response to overpowering destructive conditions in surrounding tissue or within the cell. **Anaplasia** is not reversible and is considered a classic characteristic of **malignant** tumors.

Abnormal cells multiply to form nests of **malignant** tumors (**malignant** neoplasms). **Malignant** tumors contain cells that can detach from the tumor mass, overrun surrounding tissues, and spread to distant sites in the body via the lymph or blood. Cancers are inclined to grow rapidly and to invade, crowd, and destroy normal tissues. They tend to recur when removed.

Malignant neoplasms that spread to the tissue of origin are called primary **malignant** tumors. Tumors that grow in tissues remote from the tissue of origin are called secondary (metastatic) neoplasms. **Malignant** neoplasms that are untreated are usually fatal.

If the established growth is **benign**, it is noncancerous and the cells are well differentiated. If the established growth is **malignant**, it is cancerous and the cells are poorly differentiated. *Metastasis* is the term used to describe the process by which **malignant** cells spread to other parts of the body.

VOCABULARY

The following vocabulary words are frequently used when discussing the study of cancer (oncology).

Word	Definition
adjuvant (**AD**-joo-vant)	A substance, especially a drug, added to a prescription to assist in the action of the main ingredient.
adjuvant therapy	Treatment of a disease with a substance, especially a drug, that enhances the main ingredient. For example, **chemotherapy** may be used as **adjuvant therapy** to **radiation**.
anaplasia (**an**-ah-**PLAY**-zee-ah) ana- = not, without -plasia = formation, growth	A change in the structure and orientation of cells characterized by a loss of specialization and reversion to a more primitive form.

Word	Definition
antimetabolite (**an**-tih-meh-**TAB**-oh-light)	A class of **antineoplastic** drugs used to treat **cancer**. These drugs are most effective against rapidly growing tumors.
antineoplastic (**an**-tih-**nee**-oh-**PLASS**-tik) anti- = against neo- = new plas/o = formation, development -tic = pertaining to	Of or pertaining to a substance, procedure, or measure that prevents the proliferation of **malignant** cells.
benign (bee-**NINE**)	Noncancerous and therefore not an immediate threat, even though treatment eventually may be required for health or cosmetic reasons; not life threatening.
cancer (**CAN**-sir)	A **neoplasm** characterized by the uncontrolled growth of anaplastic cells that tend to invade surrounding tissue and to metastasize to distant body sites.
carcinogen (kar-**SIN**-oh-jen) carcin/o = cancer -gen = that which generates	A substance or agent that causes the development or increases the incidence of **cancer**.
carcinoma (**kar**-sih-**NOH**-mah) carcin/o = cancer -oma = tumor	A **malignant neoplasm**.
carcinoma in situ (CIS) (kar-sih-**NOH**-mah in-**SIT**-oo) carcin/o = cancer -oma = tumor	A premalignant **neoplasm** that has not invaded the basement membrane but shows cytologic characteristics of **cancer**.
chemotherapy (**kee**-moh-**THAIR**-ah-pee) chem/o = pertaining to a chemical, drug -therapy = treatment	The use of chemical agents to destroy **cancer** cells on a selective basis.
cytotoxic (**sigh**-toh-**TOKS**-ik) cyt/o = cell tox/o = poisons -ic = pertaining to	Pertaining to being destructive to cells.
dedifferentiation (dee-diff-er-en-she-**AY**-shun)	See **anaplasia**.
deoxyribonucleic acid (DNA) (dee-ock-see-rye-boh-noo-**KLEE**-ic **ASS**-id)	A large nucleic acid molecule found principally in the chromosomes of the nucleus of a cell that is the carrier of genetic information.

Word	Definition
differentiation (diff-er-en-she-**AY**-shun)	A process in development in which unspecialized cells or tissues are systemically modified and altered to achieve specific and characteristic physical forms, physiologic functions, and chemical properties.
encapsulated (en-**CAP**-soo-**LAY**-ted)	Enclosed in fibrous or membranous sheaths.
fractionation (frak-shun-**AY**-shun)	In radiology, the division of the total dose of **radiation** into small doses administered at intervals in an effort to minimize tissue damage.
hyperplasia (high-per-**PLAY**-zee-ah) hyper- = excessive -plasia = formation, growth	An increase in the number of cells of a body part ("excessive formation").
infiltrative (in-fill-**TRAY**-tiv)	Possessing the ability to invade or penetrate adjacent tissue.
invasive (in-**VAY**-siv)	Characterized by a tendency to spread, infiltrate, and intrude.
ionizing radiation (**EYE**-oh-nigh-zing ray-dee-**AY**-shun)	High-energy X-rays that can kill cells or retard their growth.
linear accelerator (**LIN**-ee-ar ak-**SELL**-er-ay-tor)	An apparatus for accelerating charged subatomic particles used in **radiotherapy**, physics research, and the production of radionuclides.
lumpectomy (lum-**PEK**-toh mee)	Surgical removal of only the tumor and the immediate adjacent breast tissue; a method of treatment for **breast cancer** when detected in the early stage of the disease.
malignant (mah-**LIG**-nant)	Tending to become worse and cause death.
melanoma (**mell**-ah-**NOH**-mah) melan/o = black -oma = tumor	Darkly pigmented cancerous tumor.
metastasis (meh-**TASS**-tah-sis) meta- = beyond, after -stasis = stopping; controlling	The process by which tumor cells spread to distant parts of the body.
mitosis (my-**TOH**-sis)	A type of cell division that results in the formation of two genetically identical daughter cells.
mixed-tissue tumor (mixed-tissue **TOO**-mor)	A growth of more than one type of neoplastic tissue.
modality (moh-**DAL**-ih-tee)	A method of application (i.e., a treatment method).

Word	Definition
morbidity (mor-**BID**-ih-tee)	An illness or an abnormal condition or quality.
mutation (mew-**TAY**-shun)	A change or transformation in a gene.

neoplasm
(**NEE**-oh-plazm)
  neo- = new
  -plasm = living substance
	Any abnormal growth of new tissue, **benign** or **malignant**.

oncogene
(**ONG**-koh-jeen)
  onc/o = swelling, mass, or tumor
  -gene = that which generates
	A gene in a virus that can cause a cell to become **malignant**.

oncogenesis
(**ong**-koh-**JEN**-eh-sis)
  onc/o = swelling, mass, or tumor
  -genesis = production of,
      formation of
	The formation of a tumor.

oncologist
(ong-**KOL**-oh-jist)
  onc/o = swelling, mass, tumor
  -logist = one who specializes in
      the study of
	The physician who specializes in the study and treatment of neoplastic diseases, particularly cancer.

oncology
(ong-**KOL**-oh-jee)
  onc/o = swelling, mass, tumor
  -logy = the study of
	The medical specialty concerned with the study of malignancy.

papillary (**PAP**-ih-lar-ee)	Of or pertaining to a papilla (nipplelike projection).

papilloma
(pap-ih-**LOH**-mah)
  papill/o = resembling a nipple
  -oma = tumor
	A **benign** epithelial **neoplasm** characterized by a branching or lobular tumor.

pedunculated (peh-**DUN**-kyoo-**LAY**-ted)	Pertaining to a structure with a stalk.
protocol (**PROH**-toh-kol)	A written plan or description of the steps to be taken in a particular situation, such as conducting research.
radiation (ray-dee-**AY**-shun)	The emission of energy, rays, or waves.

Word	Definition
radiocurable tumor (**ray**-dee-oh-**KYOOR**-ah-bal **TOO**-mor)	Pertaining to the susceptibility of tumor cells to destruction by **ionizing radiation**.
radioresistant tumor (**ray**-dee-oh-ree-**SIS**-tant **TOO**-mor)	A tumor that resists the effects of **radiation**.
radioresponsive tumor (**ray**-dee-oh-ree-**SPON**-siv **TOO**-mor)	A tumor that reacts favorably to **radiation**.
radiosensitive tumor (**ray**-dee-oh-**SEN**-sih-tiv **TOO**-mor)	A tumor capable of being changed by or reacting to radioactive emissions such as X-rays, alpha particles, or gamma rays.
radiotherapy (ray-dee-oh-**THAIR**-ah-pee)	The treatment of disease by using X-rays or gamma rays.
relapse (ree-**LAPS**)	To exhibit again the symptoms of a disease from which a patient appears to have recovered.
remission (rih-**MISH**-un)	The partial or complete disappearance of the symptoms of a chronic or **malignant** disease.
ribonucleic acid (RNA) (**rye**-boh-**new**-**KLEE**-ik **ASS**-id)	A nucleic acid found in both the nucleus and cytoplasm of cells that transmits genetic instructions from the nucleus to the cytoplasm.
sarcoma (sar-**KOM**-ah) sarc/o = flesh -oma = tumor	A **malignant neoplasm** of the connective and supportive tissues of the body, usually first presenting as a painless swelling.
scirrhous (**SKIR**-us) scirrh/o = hard -ous = pertaining to	Pertaining to a **carcinoma** with a hard structure.
sessile (**SESS**-il)	Attached by a base rather than by a stalk or a peduncle.
staging (**STAY**-jing)	The determination of distinct phases or periods in the course of a disease.
stem cell (**STEM SELL**)	A formative cell; a cell whose daughter cells may give rise to other cell types.
tumor (**TOO**-mor)	A new growth of tissue characterized by progressive, uncontrolled proliferation (growth) of cells. The tumor may be localized or **invasive**, **benign** or **malignant**.
verrucous (ver-**ROO**-kus)	Rough; warty.

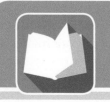

Review Checkpoint

Check your understanding of this section by completing the **Vocabulary** exercises in your workbook.

WORD ELEMENTS

The following word elements pertain to the medical specialty of oncology. As you review the list, pronounce each word element aloud twice and check the box after you "say it." Write the definition for the example term given for each word element. Use your medical dictionary to find the definitions of the example terms.

Word Element	Pronunciation	"Say It"	Meaning
ana- **ana**plasia	**AN**-ah an-ah-**PLAY**-zee-ah	☐	not, without
-blast melano**blast**	**BLAST** **MELL**-an-oh-**blast**	☐	embryonic stage of development
carcin/o **carcin**oma	kar-**SIH**-noh **kar**-sih-**NOH**-mah	☐	**cancer**
chem/o **chem**otherapy	**KEE**-moh kee-moh-**THAIR**-ah-pee	☐	pertaining to a chemical, drug
cry/o **cry**osurgery	**KRIGH**-oh krigh-oh-**SIR**-jer-ee	☐	cold
cyst/o **cyst**ic carcinoma	**SIS**-toh **SIS**-tik kar-sih-**NOH**-mah	☐	bladder, sac, or cyst
epi- **epi**dermoid carcinoma	**EP**-ih ep-ih-**DER**-moyd kar-sih-**NOH**-mah	☐	upon, over
fibr/o **fibr**osarcoma	**FY**-broh fy-broh-sar-**KOH**-mah	☐	pertaining to fiber
melan/o **melan**oma	**mell**-ah-**NOH** **mell**-ah-**NOH**-mah	☐	black
meta- **meta**stasis	**MEH**-tah meh-**TASS**-tah-sis	☐	beyond, after
-oma melan**oma**	**OH**-mah mell-ah-**NOH**-mah	☐	tumor

Word Element	Pronunciation	"Say It"	Meaning
onc/o **onc**ogenic	**ONG**-koh ong-koh-**JEN**-ik	☐	swelling, mass, or tumor
papill/o **papill**ocarcinoma	pap-**ILL**-oh **pap**-ill-oh-kar-sih-**NOH**-mah	☐	resembling a nipple
-plasia hyper**plasia**	**PLAY**-zee-ah **high**-per-**PLAY**-zee-ah	☐	formation or growth
-plasm neo**plasm**	**PLAZM** **NEE**-oh-plazm	☐	living substance
radi/o **radi**ocurable	**RAY**-dee-oh **ray**-dee-oh-**KYOOR**-ah-bal	☐	**radiation**; also refers to radius
sarc/o **sarc**oma	**SAR**-koh sar-**KOH**-mah	☐	flesh
scirrh/o **scirrh**ous carcinoma	**SKIR**-oh **SKIR**-us kar-sih-**NOH**-mah	☐	hard

Review Checkpoint

Check your understanding of this section by completing the **Word Elements** exercises in your workbook.

Benign versus Malignant Tumors

A **benign** tumor is a **neoplasm** that does not invade other tissues or metastasize to other sites. Characteristics of a **benign** tumor include the following:

- Usually **encapsulated** (tumor cells usually remain within a connective tissue capsule)
- Cells similar in structure to cells from which they originate (well differentiated)
- Well-defined borders
- Slow growing and limited to one area
- Possible growth displacement (but not invasion) to adjacent tissue

A **malignant** tumor is a **neoplasm** that can invade surrounding tissue and can metastasize to distant sites. Characteristics of a **malignant** tumor include the following:

- Not **encapsulated**; not cohesive, and irregular in shape and in pattern of growth
- No resemblance to cell of origin
- No well-defined borders; distinct separation from surrounding tissue difficult

- Growth into adjacent cells rather than displacing or pushing them aside

- Able to metastasize (spread) to distant sites through the blood or lymph systems

- Rapid growth through rapid cell division and multiplication

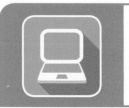

Media Link

To increase your understanding of this content, go to the Student Companion Website and view the **Cancer Metastasizing** animation.

Classification of Neoplasms

There is a system for naming, or classifying, neoplasms that uses a root word to indicate the type of body tissue that gives rise to the **neoplasm** and a suffix to indicate whether the tumor is **benign** or **malignant**. If the tumor is **benign**, the root word is usually followed by the suffix -*oma*. If the tumor is **malignant**, the root word will be followed by the suffix *carcinoma* or *sarcoma*. For example, a **benign** tumor of the epithelium is termed a *papilloma*, whereas a **malignant** tumor of the epithelium is termed a *carcinoma*. A **benign** tumor of the adipose tissue is called a *lipoma*, whereas a **malignant** tumor of the adipose tissue is called a *liposarcoma*. Exceptions to this rule include neoplastic disorders that have distinct names of their own, such as leukemia, Hodgkin's disease, **Wilms' tumor**, and lymphomas. **Cancers** are usually named according to the site of the primary tumor or to the type of tissue involved. Two main categories of neoplasms are carcinomas and sarcomas:

1. Carcinomas make up the largest group of neoplasms. They are solid tumors that originate from epithelial tissue (which covers the external and internal body surfaces, the lining of vessels, body cavities, glands, and organs). An example of a name of a carcinoma of the stomach follows:

   gastric adenocarcinoma

   gastr/o = stomach

   aden/o = gland

   carcin/o = **cancer**

   -oma = tumor

2. Sarcomas are less common than carcinomas. These tumors originate from supportive and connective tissue such as bone, fat, muscle, and cartilage. An example of a name of a **sarcoma** arising from bone tissue follows:

   osteosarcoma

   oste/o = bone

   sarc/o = connective tissue

   -oma = tumor

Additional categories include:

3. Lymphomas arise in infection-fighting organs such as lymphatic tissue.

4. Leukemias occur in blood-forming organs such as the spleen and bone marrow.

Grading of Neoplasms

Grading measures the extent to which tumor cells differ from their parent tissue. Well-differentiated cells function most like the parent tissue and are thus graded as the least **malignant**, or grade 1. Those cells that are the least differentiated (not like the parent tissue) and most rapidly increasing in number are grade 4. There may be some variation in the grading criteria with tumors of different type locations.

Staging of Neoplasms

Staging refers to the extent of disease and relative size of the tumor at the time of diagnosis. All of the following terms are used in the **staging** of neoplasms.

- The "TNM **staging** classification system" is an internationally recognized system used for **staging** neoplasms. Every metastatic disease will have specific criteria that will differ regarding the following categories:

  T: (0–4) = tumor size (primary)

  N: (0–3) = degree of regional lymph node involvement

  M: (0–3) = presence or absence of distant metastases

  In all of the previous, zero equals no evidence and the scale moves toward increased involvement as each number increases. Once the T, N, and M **staging** is complete, the tumor is then classified as a stage I, II, III, or IV (with I being the early stage and IV being the advanced stage).

- Cytologic examination of biopsied tissues, tumors, body fluids, and/or body secretions further evaluates the extent of the disease.

- Tumor markers are biochemical indicators that a malignancy is present in the body when these molecules (tumor markers) are detectable in any body fluids, particularly blood. If high levels are detected, a diagnostic follow-up is necessary.

- Oncologic imaging includes CT scans, MRIs, X-ray imaging, radioisotope scans, ultrasonography, use of tagged antibodies, angiography, and use of direct visualization (endoscopy, sigmoidoscopy, etc.).

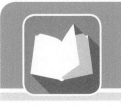

Review Checkpoint

Check your understanding of this section by completing the **Classification of Neoplasms** exercises in your workbook.

Risk Factors

Many factors have been identified by **cancer** researchers as those that predispose an individual (make one susceptible) to the development of **cancer**. Research indicates that a large majority of cancers are related to lifestyle and environmental factors such as tobacco, alcohol, diet, sunlight, **radiation**, industrial agents and chemicals, and hormones. These factors can be controlled to some degree. An uncontrollable factor that contributes to one's susceptibility to developing **cancer** is heredity.

Who is at risk of developing **cancer**? Anyone. **Cancer** researchers define two risk categories for developing **cancer**.

1. Lifetime risk refers to the probability that an individual, over the course of his or her lifetime, will develop **cancer** or will die from **cancer**. Men have a 1 in 2 lifetime risk of developing **cancer**; women have a 1 in 3 lifetime risk of developing **cancer**.

2. Relative risk measures the strength of the relationship between risk factors and particular types of **cancer**. For example, male smokers have a 23 times greater chance of developing **cancer** than do nonsmokers; and women who have a mother, sister, or daughter with a history of breast cancer are twice as likely to develop breast cancer as women who do not have a family history of breast cancer.

Some of the preventive measures recommended by the American Cancer Society in relation to risks of developing **cancer** include the following:

■ Avoid use of tobacco and heavy intake of alcohol. All cancers caused by cigarette, cigar and pipe smoking, smokeless tobacco forms (chewing tobacco and snuff), and heavy use of alcohol could be prevented completely.

■ Avoid excessive exposure to the sun's rays.

■ Participate in health screening examinations on a regular basis. Screening examinations conducted regularly by a health care professional are important in early detection of cancers, with treatment being more likely to be successful.

■ Know how to and perform self-examinations. For possible **cancer** of the breast, testicle, and skin, these may result in early detection (with more successful treatment results).

Warning Signs of Cancer

It is essential that all individuals know the warning signals of possible **cancer** to promote early detection because any delay in the diagnosis and treatment of **cancer** can influence the prognosis significantly. The American Cancer Society lists several warning signs of **cancer** that would indicate the need for immediate medical follow-up. These warning signs are listed in a particular order to make them easier to remember. By using the first letter of each statement and putting them together, one forms the acronym **CAUTION**. The individual is "cautioned" to report the following:

C = **C**hange in bowel or bladder habits

A = **A** sore that does not heal

U = **U**nusual bleeding or discharge

T = **T**hickening or lump in breast or elsewhere

I = **I**ndigestion or difficulty in swallowing

O = **O**bvious change in a wart or mole

N = **N**agging cough or hoarseness

When suspicious symptoms are present, further testing is indicated to rule out or confirm the possibility of **cancer**. A Pap test or a biopsy may be performed to establish a diagnosis. These procedures are discussed later in this chapter.

Specific Types of Cancers

For a general grouping of the leading sites of new **cancer** cases and deaths as estimated by a 2013 American Cancer Society Surveillance Research report, see *Figure 21-1*. The following is a discussion of some of the more common types of cancers.

basal cell carcinoma

(**BAY**-sal **SELL kar**-sih-**NOH**-mah)

carcin/o = cancer

-oma = tumor

A **malignant** epithelial cell tumor that begins as a slightly elevated nodule with a depression or ulceration in the center that becomes more obvious as the tumor grows. As the depression enlarges, the tissue breaks down, crusts, and bleeds. See *Figure 21-2*.

Basal cell carcinoma is the most common **malignant** tumor of the epithelial tissue, occurring most often on areas of the skin exposed to the sun (usually between the hairline and the upper lip).

If not treated, the basal cell carcinoma will invade surrounding tissue, which can lead to destruction of body parts (such as a nose). Treatment includes surgical excision, curettage and electrodesiccation, **cryosurgery**, or **radiation therapy**. Basal cell carcinomas rarely metastasize, but they tend to recur.

Leading New Cancer Cases and Deaths – 2013 Estimates

Estimated New Cases*		Estimated Deaths	
Male	**Female**	**Male**	**Female**
Prostate	Breast	Lung & bronchus	Lung & bronchus
238,590 (28%)	232,340 (29%)	87,260 (28%)	72,220 (26%)
Lung & bronchus	Lung & bronchus	Prostate	Breast
118,080 (14%)	110,110 (14%)	29,720 (10%)	39,620 (14%)
Colon & rectum	Colon & rectum	Colon & rectum	Colon & rectum
73,680 (9%)	69,140 (9%)	26,300 (9%)	24,530 (9%)
Urinary bladder	Uterine corpus	Pancreas	Pancreas
54,610 (6%)	49,560 (6%)	19,480 (6%)	18,980 (7%)
Melanoma of the skin	Thyroid	Liver & intrahepatic bile duct	Ovary
45,060 (5%)	45,310 (6%)	14,890 (5%)	14,030 (5%)
Kidney & renal pelvis	Non-Hodgkin's lymphoma	Leukemia	Leukemia
40,430 (5%)	32,140 (4%)	13,660 (4%)	10,060 (4%)
Non-Hodgkin's lymphoma	Melanoma of the skin	Esophagus	Non-Hodgkin's lymphoma
37,600 (4%)	31,630 (4%)	12,220 (4%)	8,430 (3%)
Oral cavity & pharynx	Kidney & renal pelvis	Urinary bladder	Uterine corpus
29,620 (3%)	24,720 (3%)	10,820 (4%)	8,190 (3%)
Leukemia	Pancreas	Non-Hodgkin's lymphoma	Liver & intrahepatic bile duct
27,880 (3%)	22,480 (3%)	10,590 (3%)	6,780 (2%)
Pancreas	Ovary	Kidney & renal pelvis	Brain & other nervous system
22,740 (3%)	22,240 (3%)	8,780 (3%)	6,150 (2%)
All sites	All sites	All sites	All sites
854,790 (100%)	805,500 (100%)	306,920 (100%)	273,430 (100%)

*Excludes basal and squamous cell skin cancers and in situ carcinoma except urinary bladder.

Figure 21-1 Leading sites of new cancer cases and deaths—2013 Estimates

(Source: American Cancer Society, Inc., Surveillance Research)

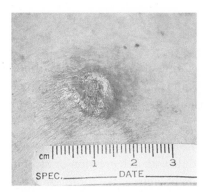

Figure 21-2 Basal cell carcinoma

(Courtesy of Robert A. Silverman, M.D., Pediatric Dermatology, Georgetown University)

breast cancer (carcinoma of the breast)	A **malignant** tumor of the breast tissue. The most common type, ductal **carcinoma**, originates in the mammary ducts.

(**kar**-sih-**NOH**-mah of the breast)

  carcin/o = cancer

  -oma = tumor

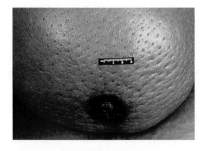

Figure 21-3 Peau d'orange

(Courtesy of Dr. S. Eva Singletary, University of Texas, Anderson Cancer Center)

Carcinoma of the breast can invade surrounding tissue if not detected early enough. Once the **cancer** cells penetrate the duct, they will metastasize (spread) through the surrounding breast tissue, eventually reaching the axillary lymph nodes. Through the lymph vessels, the **cancer** cells can spread to distant parts of the body.

In advanced cases, symptoms such as dimpling of the breast, peau d'orange appearance of the breast (breast skin will have the appearance of an orange peel), and retraction of the breast nipple may occur. See *Figure 21-3*.

The symptoms of breast cancer have a gradual onset. A painless, nontender lump, which may be movable, develops in the breast. This is usually noticed in the upper outer quadrant. Most breast lumps are discovered by either the woman or her sexual partner. Many women, however, fail to follow through with seeking medical attention when they discover a lump in their breast. Any lump, no matter how small, should be reported to a physician immediately! Nipple retraction or nipple discharge are other early symptoms. Some women have no noticeable symptoms or palpable lump but will have an abnormal mammogram.

Once a lump has been discovered in the female breast, and has been palpated (felt) by the physician, a mammogram is ordered to confirm the presence of a suspicious mass. This is usually followed with a biopsy of the lump to confirm the diagnosis.

Most women with early-stage breast cancer are successfully treated. Treatment involves surgical removal of the lump and any diseased tissue surrounding it. If the lump is detected in the early stage of the disease, a **lumpectomy** may be the only **surgery** necessary. This involves removal of only the tumor and the immediate adjacent breast tissue. Other treatment options include a simple mastectomy (in which only the breast is removed), a modified radical mastectomy (see *Figure 21-4*)—in which the breast is removed along with the lymph nodes in the axilla (armpit)— and a radical mastectomy (in which the breast, the chest muscles on the affected side, and the lymph nodes in the axilla are removed). **Surgery** is usually followed by a series of **radiation** treatments (**radiation** therapy), **chemotherapy**, or sometimes both.

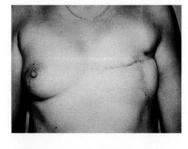

Figure 21-4 Modified radical mastectomy

(Courtesy of Dr. Steven Lynch)

Some women opt to have reconstructive breast **surgery** after having had a mastectomy. The type of material used to reconstruct the breast includes silicone implants and transplanting tissue from one part of the patient's body (such as the hips or thighs) to the breast. Patients considering breast reconstruction should discuss this thoroughly with the physician to ensure their understanding of this procedure.

Cancer of the breast ranks second among **cancer** deaths in women (American Cancer Society, *Cancer Facts & Figures,* 2013). It is estimated that one in eight women in the United States will develop breast cancer during her lifetime, based on a 100-year life expectancy. Factors that place some women in a higher risk category than others include a family history of breast cancer, nulliparity (having borne no children), early menarche, late menopause, hypertension, obesity, diabetes, chronic cystic breast disease, exposure to **radiation**, and possibly menopausal hormone therapy (MHT), formerly known as hormone replacement therapy (HRT).

Early detection and treatment is of the utmost importance when the diagnosis is **cancer**. Women should be encouraged to perform breast self-examinations monthly, have yearly physical examinations by their physicians, have a baseline mammogram done at age 40, and yearly thereafter. The procedure for breast self-examination is described in the section on diagnostic techniques.

bronchogenic carcinoma	A **malignant** lung tumor that originates in the bronchi; lung cancer.

(brong-koh-**JEN**-ik **kar**-sih-**NOH**-mah)
  bronch/o = bronchus
  -genic = producing
  carcin/o = cancer
  -oma = tumor

According to the American Cancer Society, lung cancer is the most common cancer-related death in both men and women.

Bronchogenic carcinoma is usually associated with a history of cigarette smoking. It is increasing at a greater rate in women than in men.

Since 1987, more women have died each year of lung cancer than of breast cancer—which, for over 40 years, was the major cause of **cancer** death in women (American Cancer Society, *Cancer Facts & Figures,* 2013).

Symptoms of bronchogenic (lung) **cancer** include (but may not be limited to) a persistent cough, blood-streaked sputum (hemoptysis), chest pain, and voice change. The five-year survival rate for lung cancer is low due to usually significant **metastasis** at the time of diagnosis. More than one-half of the tumors are advanced and inoperable when diagnosed.

cervical carcinoma	A **malignant** tumor of the cervix.

(**SER**-vih-kal **kar**-sih-**NOH**-mah)
  cervic/o = cervix
  -al = pertaining to
  carcin/o = cancer
  -oma = tumor

Cervical cancer is one of the most common malignancies of the female reproductive tract. Symptoms include an abnormal Pap smear and bleeding between menstrual periods, after sexual intercourse, or after menopause.

Cervical cancer appears to be most frequent in women from ages 30 to 50. Factors that increase the risk of developing cervical cancer at a later age are as follows:

■ First sexual intercourse before the age of 20

■ Having many sex partners

- Having certain sexually transmitted diseases

- History of smoking

- Presence of condylomata (genital warts)

In the earliest stage of cervical cancer, the **cancer** remains in place without spreading. This early stage is known as **carcinoma in situ (CIS)** (it just sits there). The progression into a more advanced stage that can metastasize to other parts of the body is usually slow. This particular quality of cervical cancer makes the prognosis excellent if the disease is detected in its earliest stage.

The Papanicolaou (Pap) smear is used to detect early changes in the cervical tissue that may indicate cervical **cancer**. The Pap test consists of obtaining scrapings from the cervix and examining them under a microscope to detect any abnormalities in cervical tissue. Approximately 90% of the early changes in the cervical tissue are detected by this test. The diagnosis of cervical cancer is confirmed with a tissue biopsy.

Treatment for cervical cancer includes **surgery** to remove the diseased tissue and a margin of healthy tissue. This may involve removing the cervix or may be more extensive, involving removal of the uterus, fallopian tubes, and ovaries as well. **Surgery** may be followed with **radiation therapy**.

As discussed earlier, studies now indicate that the human **papilloma** virus (HPV) has a strong correlation to risk for cervical cancer. The HPV is passed from one person to another through sexual contact. There are many types of HPVs. Some cause no harm, some cause genital warts, and others are associated with certain types of **cancer** (high-risk HPVs). When a woman becomes infected with certain high-risk types of HPV and the infection is not cleared by the body, abnormal cells can develop in the lining of the cervix. If this is not detected early and treated properly, the abnormal cells can lead to precancerous conditions and possibly to **cancer**. Most women are diagnosed with HPV as a result of an abnormal Pap smear.

The U.S. Food and Drug Administration (FDA) has approved a vaccine that is highly effective in preventing infections from two high-risk HPVs that cause approximately 70% of cervical cancers and two HPVs that cause approximately 90% of genital warts. This vaccine is given in three separate doses by injection over the course of six months. The vaccine, Gardasil, is recommended for 11- to 12-year-old girls (ideally before sexual activity begins) and can be given as early as 9 years of age through 26 years of age.

colorectal cancer	The presence of a **malignant neoplasm** in the large intestine.

(koh-loh-**REH**-tal **CAN**-sir)
  col/o = colon
  rect/o = rectum
  -al = pertaining to

Most neoplasms in the large intestine are adenocarcinomas and at least 50% originate in the rectum, causing bleeding and pain. **Colorectal cancer** is the third most common type of **cancer** in both men and women. The most common sign is a change in bowel habits.

A personal or family history of **colorectal cancer** or polyps and inflammatory bowel disease have been associated with increased **colorectal cancer** risk. Other possible risk factors include physical inactivity, obesity, long-term smoking, heavy alcohol consumption, a diet high in red or processed meats, and inadequate intake of fruits and vegetables

(American Cancer Society, *Cancer Facts & Figures,* 2013). The risk of colorectal cancer increases with age, with approximately 90% of the cases diagnosed being found in individuals over 50 years of age. Diagnostic procedures include a rectal examination, barium enema, sigmoidoscopy and/or colonoscopy, and examination of a stool specimen for occult blood. Beginning at age 50, it is recommended that both men and women who are at average risk for developing **colorectal cancer** begin screening for early detection by having a colonoscopy. Surgery is the most common treatment for **colorectal cancer**.

endometrial carcinoma
 	
(**en**-doh-**MEE**-tree-al
kar-sih-**NOH**-mah)
  endo- = within
  metri/o = uterus
  -al = pertaining to
  carcin/o = cancer
  -oma = tumor
	Malignant tumor of the inner lining of the uterus; also known as adenocarcinoma of the uterus; and/or cancer of the uterine corpus (body of the uterus).

This is the most common **cancer** of the female reproductive tract, occurring in women during or after menopause (peak incidence between the ages 50 and 60). The classic symptom of **endometrial carcinoma** is abnormal uterine bleeding. This includes any postmenopausal bleeding or recurrent metrorrhagia in the premenopausal patient. An abnormal discharge (mucoid or watery discharge) may precede the bleeding by weeks or months.

Diagnosis is usually confirmed with an endometrial biopsy or dilation and curettage, with microscopic examination of the tissue sample. Dilation involves enlarging the cervical opening, and curettage involves scraping tissue cells from the uterine lining for sampling. Treatment usually involves a total abdominal hysterectomy (removal of the uterus, fallopian tubes, and ovaries) followed by **radiation**, hormone, and/or chemotherapy.

lymphoma
 	
(**LIM**-foh-mah)
  lymph/o = lymph
  -oma = tumor
	Lymphoma is a lymphoid tissue **neoplasm** that is typically **malignant**, beginning with a painless enlarged lymph node(s) and progressing to anemia, weakness, fever, and weight loss. For information on Burkitt's **lymphoma**, Hodgkin's disease, and non-Hodgkin's **lymphoma**, see Chapter 9.

Kaposi's sarcoma
 	
(**KAP**-oh-seez sar-**KOH**-mah)
  sarc/o = flesh
  -oma = tumor
	Rare **malignant** lesions that begin as soft, purple-brown nodules or plaques on the feet and gradually spread throughout the skin. See *Figure 21-5.*

This is a systemic disease also involving the GI tract and lungs. **Kaposi's sarcoma** occurs most often in men, and there is an increased incidence in individuals infected with AIDS. It is also associated with diabetes and **malignant lymphoma** (tumor of lymphatic tissue).

Radiotherapy and **chemotherapy** are usually recommended as methods of treatment. Kaposi's sarcoma may also be treated with **cryosurgery** or laser **surgery**.

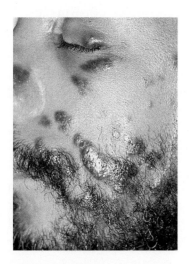

Figure 21-5 Kaposi's sarcoma

(Courtesy of Robert A. Silverman, MD, Pediatric Dermatology, Georgetown University)

malignant melanoma

(mah-**LIG**-nant **mell**-ah-**NOH**-mah)

melan/o = black, dark

-oma = tumor

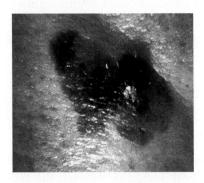

Figure 21-6 Malignant melanoma
(Courtesy of the Centers for Disease Control and Prevention [CDC]/Carl Washington, M.D., Emory University School of Medicine; Mona Saraiya, M.D., MPH.)

Malignant skin tumor originating from melanocytes in preexisting nevi (moles), freckles, or skin with pigment; darkly pigmented cancerous tumor. See *Figure 21-6*.

These tumors have irregular surfaces and borders and variable colors and are generally located on the trunk in men and on the legs in women.

Around the primary lesion, small satellite lesions are often noted.

Persons at risk for malignant melanomas include those with a family history of **melanoma** and those with fair complexions. There is also an increased risk with excessive sun exposure to develop particular forms of malignant melanomas. Generally, most melanomas are extremely **invasive** and spread first to the lymphatic system and then metastasize throughout the body to any organ (with fatal results).

All nevi and skin should be inspected and self-examined regularly, remembering the ABCD rule for **malignant melanoma:**

Asymmetry—Any pigmented lesion that has both flat and elevated parts should be considered potentially **malignant**.

Borders—Any leakage across the borders of brown pigment or irregular shaped margins are suspicious.

Color—Variations (including black, dark brown, or tan) are suspicious.

Diameter—Any lesions with the previous characteristics measuring more than 6 mm in diameter should be removed.

Treatment is surgical removal as well as **chemotherapy** and **radiation** therapy for distant metastases. The depth of surgical dissection and the prognosis depend on the **staging** classification of the tumor. The five-year survival rate is approximately 60% for all forms of malignant melanomas.

neuroblastoma

(**noo**-roh-blass-**TOH**-mah)

neur/o = nerve

blast/o = embryonic stage of
           development

-oma = tumor

A highly **malignant** tumor of the sympathetic nervous system.

Neuroblastoma most commonly occurs in the adrenal medulla, with early **metastasis** spreading widely to the liver, lungs, lymph nodes, and bone.

oral leukoplakia

(**OR**-al **loo**-koh-**PLAY**-kee-ah)

or/o = mouth

-al = pertaining to

leuk/o = white

Oral leukoplakia is a precancerous lesion occurring anywhere in the mouth.

These elevated, gray-white or yellow-white, leathery-surfaced lesions have clearly defined borders. Causative factors include chronic oral mucosal irritation, which occurs with the use of tobacco and alcohol. For a visual reference, see Chapter 12.

ovarian carcinoma

(oh-**VAIR**-ree-an **kar**-sih-**NOH**-mah)

ovari/o = ovary

-an = characteristic of

carcin/o = cancer

-oma = tumor

A **malignant** tumor of the ovaries, most commonly occurring in women in their 50s.

It is rarely detected in the early stage and is usually far advanced when diagnosed. **Ovarian carcinoma** accounts for approximately 5% of cancer deaths among women and causes more deaths than any other **cancer** of the female reproductive system (American Cancer Society, *Cancer Facts & Figures*, 2013).

Symptoms usually do not appear with ovarian cancer until the disease is well advanced. The earliest symptoms of ovarian cancer are swelling, bloating, or discomfort in the lower abdomen and mild digestive complaints (loss of appetite, feeling of fullness, indigestion, nausea, and weight loss). As the tumor increases in size, it may create pressure on adjacent organs, such as the urinary bladder or the rectum, causing frequent urination and dysuria or constipation. Later developments in the course of the disease include an accumulation of fluid within the abdominal cavity (ascites), resulting in swelling and discomfort.

Diagnosis is confirmed with examination of a sample of the tumor tissue under a microscope. This is achieved through surgical removal of the affected ovary. If the ovary is diseased with **cancer**, the surgeon will then remove the other ovary, the uterus, and the fallopian tubes. A process called **staging** is important to determine the amount of **metastasis**, if any. This process involves taking samples (biopsy) of nearby lymph nodes, and the diaphragm, and sampling the fluid from the abdomen.

Treatment involves the use of **surgery**, **chemotherapy**, or **radiation therapy**. It may involve one or a combination of the treatment choices, depending on the extent of the disease.

pancreatic cancer
 	
(**pan**-kree-**AT** -ik **CAN**-sir)
 	
  pancreat/o = pancreas
  -ic = pertaining to
	A life-threatening primary **malignant neoplasm** typically found in the head of the pancreas.

For all stages of diagnosed **pancreatic cancer**, the one-year relative survival rate is 24% and the five-year survival rate is about 5% (American Cancer Society, *Cancer Facts and Figures*, 2013). The occurrence of **pancreatic cancer** for smokers is twice that for nonsmokers. Other related risk factors include a diet high in fat, pancreatitis, exposure to chemicals and toxins, and diabetes mellitus.

With a slow onset, **pancreatic cancer** causes very nonspecific symptoms such as nausea, anorexia, dull epigastric pain, weight loss, and flatulence. As the tumor grows, the pain worsens. If there is an early diagnosis, surgical removal of the tumor may be possible.

prostatic cancer (carcinoma of the prostate)
 	
(**kar**-sih-**NOH**-mah of the **PROSS**-tayt)
 	
  carcin/o = cancer
  -oma = tumor
  prostat/o = prostate gland
  -e = noun ending
	Malignant growth within the prostate gland, creating pressure on the upper part of the urethra. It is the most frequently diagnosed **cancer** in men.

Cancer of the prostate is the second-leading cause of cancer deaths in men (American Cancer Society, *Cancer Facts & Figures*, 2013). Unfortunately, symptoms are not usually present in the early stages of **cancer** of the prostate. By the time symptoms are evident, the **cancer** may have already metastasized (spread) to other areas of the body. When symptoms of prostate **cancer** do occur, they may include any of the following:

1. A need to urinate frequently (i.e., urinary frequency), especially at night

2. Difficulty starting or stopping urine flow

3. Inability to urinate

4. Weak or interrupted flow of urine when urinating (patient may complain of "dribbling" instead of having a steady stream of urine)

5. Pain or burning when urinating

6. Pain or stiffness in the lower back, hips, or thighs

7. Painful ejaculation

Because the presence of symptoms usually means that the disease is more advanced, early detection of **cancer** of the prostate is essential to successful treatment. Beginning at age 50, men should have a yearly physical examination that includes a digital rectal examination of the prostate gland. The rectal examination can reveal a cancerous growth before symptoms appear. A **PSA blood test** may be performed during the examination to detect increased growth of the prostate (the growth could be **benign** or **malignant**). The PSA test measures a substance called prostate-specific antigen. The level of PSA in the blood may rise in men who have prostate **cancer** or **benign** prostatic hypertrophy. If the level is elevated, the physician will order additional tests to confirm a diagnosis of **cancer** of the prostate.

The most common procedure used to treat or relieve the urinary obstruction resulting from **cancer** of the prostate is **surgery** to remove the prostate tissue that is pressing against the upper part of the urethra. This procedure is also used to treat **benign** prostatic hypertrophy. This **surgery**, called transurethral resection of the prostate (TUR or TURP), is discussed in the diagnostic procedures section of Chapter 16.

Other methods of treatment include a radical prostatectomy (removal of the prostate gland), **radiation therapy**, hormone therapy, or **chemotherapy**. The treatment of choice depends on the patient's age and medical history, risks and benefits of treatment, and the stage of the disease.

renal cell carcinoma	A **malignant** tumor of the kidney, occurring in adulthood; cancer of the kidney.
(**REE**-nal **SELL** kar-sih-**NOH**-mah)	
ren/o = kidney	The patient is asymptomatic (symptom free) until the latter stages of the disease. The most common symptom of **renal cell carcinoma** is painless hematuria with later development of flank pain and intermittent fever. Once the diagnosis is confirmed, the treatment of choice is **surgery** to remove the tumor before it can metastasize. **Chemotherapy** and **radiation** treatment may also follow **surgery**.
-al = pertaining to	
carcin/o = cancer	
-oma = tumor	
squamous cell carcinoma	A malignancy of the squamous cells of epithelial tissue, which is a much faster growing **cancer** than basal cell carcinoma and has a greater potential for **metastasis** if not treated. See *Figure 21-7*.
(**SKWAY**-mus **SELL** kar-sih-**NOH**-mah)	
carcin/o = cancer	Squamous cell lesions are seen most frequently on sun-exposed areas such as the following:
-oma = tumor	

1. Top of the nose

2. Forehead

3. Margin of the external ear

4. Back of the hands

5. Lower lip

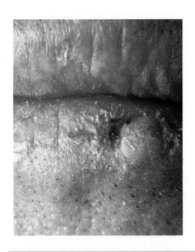

The squamous cell lesion begins as a flesh-colored or red, firm papule, sometimes with a crusted appearance. As the lesion grows it may bleed or ulcerate and become painful. When **squamous cell carcinoma** recurs, it can be highly **invasive** and present an increased risk of **metastasis**.

Treatment is surgical excision with the goal to remove the tumor completely, along with a margin of healthy surrounding tissue. **Cryosurgery** for low-risk squamous cell carcinomas is also common.

Figure 21-7 Squamous cell carcinoma
(Courtesy of Dr. Joseph Konzelman. School of Dentistry, Medical College of Georgia)

testicular cancer (carcinoma of the testes)	A **malignant** tumor of the testicle that appears as a painless lump in the testicle.
(**kar**-sih-**NOH**-mah of the **TESS**-teez) carcin/o = tumor -oma = tumor	This type of tumor is rare and usually occurs in men under the age of 40. The cause is basically unknown. The diagnosis of **testicular cancer** is usually confirmed by biopsy after the physician has palpated the lump in the testicle. Treatment of choice is **surgery** to remove the diseased testicle, followed by **radiation therapy** and **chemotherapy**. The healthy testicle is not removed, and thus fertility and potency should not be altered in the male. Chances for complete recovery are excellent if the malignancy is detected in the early stages. Testicular cancer can spread throughout the body via the lymphatic system if not treated in the early stages. Early treatment is essential to complete recovery. Therefore, it is recommended that all men perform monthly testicular self-examinations. If a lump is discovered, it should be reported immediately to a physician.
thyroid cancer (cancer of the thyroid gland)	**Malignant** tumor of the thyroid gland that leads to dysfunction of the gland and thus inadequate or excessive secretion of the thyroid hormone.
(**CAN**-sir of the **THIGH**-royd gland)	The presence of a palpable nodule or lump, in the neck, may be the first indication of **thyroid cancer**. A needle aspiration biopsy is used to confirm the diagnosis. A **malignant** tumor of the thyroid is classified and staged according to the site of origin, size of tumor, amount of lymph node involvement, and the presence of **metastasis**. Treatment typically consists of partial or complete removal of the thyroid gland. Lifelong thyroid hormone replacement is then required.
tumors, intracranial	**Intracranial tumors** occur in any structural region of the brain and may be **malignant** or **benign**. They are classified as primary or secondary and are named according to the tissue from which they originate.
(**TOO**-mors, in-trah-**KRAY**-nee-al) intra- = within crani/o = cranium, skull -al = pertaining to	An intracranial tumor causes the normal brain tissue to be displaced and compressed, leading to progressive neurological dysfunctions. The symptoms of **intracranial tumors** include headaches, dizziness, vomiting, problems with coordination and muscle strength, personality changes, altered mental function, seizures, paralysis, and sensory disturbances.

Surgical removal is the desired treatment when possible. **Radiation** and/or **chemotherapy** are used according to location, classification, and type of tumor.

tumors, metastatic intracranial (**TOO**-mors, **met**-ah-**STAT**-ik in-trah-**KRAY**-nee-al) 　intra- = within 　crani/o = cranium, skull 　-al = pertaining to 　meta- = beyond, after 　-static = stopping or controlling	Tumors occurring as a result of **metastasis** from a primary site such as the lung or breast.

A metastatic intracranial tumor is a common occurrence, comprising approximately 20% to 40% of **intracranial tumors**. The tissue in the brain reacts intensely to the presence of a metastatic tumor and usually progresses rapidly. Surgical removal of a single **metastasis** to the brain can be achieved if the tumor is located in an operable region. The removal may provide the individual with several months or years of life.

tumors, primary intracranial (**TOO**-mors, primary in-trah-**KRAY**-nee-al) 　intra- = within 　crani/o = cranium, skull 　-al = pertaining to	Tumors that arise from gliomas (**malignant** glial cells that are a support for nerve tissue) or from the meninges are known as **primary intracranial tumors**.

Gliomas are classified according to the principal cell type, shape, and size. The following are classified as gliomas.

1. *Glioblastoma multiforme* comprises approximately 20% of all **intracranial tumors**. They arise in the cerebral hemisphere and are the most rapidly growing of the gliomas.

2. *Astrocytoma* comprises approximately 10% of all **intracranial tumors** and is a slow-growing primary tumor of astrocytes. Astrocytomas tend to invade surrounding structures and over time become more anaplastic. A highly **malignant** glioblastoma may develop within the tumor mass.

3. *Ependymomas* comprise approximately 6% of all **intracranial tumors**. They commonly arise from the ependymomal cells that line the fourth ventricle wall and often extend into the spinal cord. An ependymoma occurs more commonly in children and adolescents and is usually **encapsulated** and **benign**.

4. *Oligodendrogliomas* comprise approximately 5% of all **intracranial tumors** and are usually slow growing. At times, the oligodendrogliomas imitate the glioblastomas with rapid growth. Oligodendrogliomas occur most often in the frontal lobe.

5. *Medulloblastoma* comprises approximately 4% of all **intracranial tumors**. Medulloblastoma occurs most frequently in children between five and nine years of age. It affects more boys than girls and typically arises in the cerebellum growing rapidly. The prognosis is poor.

6. *Meningiomas* comprise approximately 15% of all **intracranial tumors**. They originate from the meninges, grow slowly, and are largely vascular. Meningiomas largely occur in adults.

Wilms' tumor (**VILMZ TOO**-mor)	A **malignant** tumor of the kidney occurring predominantly in childhood.

The most frequent finding is a palpable mass in the abdomen. The child may also be experiencing abdominal pain, fever, anorexia, nausea, vomiting, and hematuria. Secondary hypertension may also occur.

Once diagnosis is confirmed, the treatment of choice is **surgery** to remove the tumor followed by **chemotherapy** and **radiation**. With treatment and no evidence of **metastasis**, the cure rate is high for patients with Wilms' tumors.

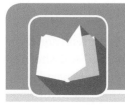

Review Checkpoint

Check your understanding of this section by completing the **Specific Types of Cancer** exercises in your workbook.

Treatment Techniques and Procedures

The treatment of **cancer** may be used in conjunction with some other course of treatment, may only provide symptomatic relief (palliative treatment), or may cure the **cancer**. Techniques used to treat **cancer** may be used alone or in combination. Following are three major treatment procedures used and one treatment procedure occasionally used against **cancer**.

chemotherapy (**kee**-moh-**THAIR**-ah-pee) chem/o = pertaining to a chemical, drug -therapy = treatment	The use of **cytotoxic** drugs and chemicals to achieve a cure, decrease **tumor** size, provide relief of pain, or slow **metastasis**.

Chemotherapy is often used in conjunction with **surgery**, **radiation** therapy, or **immunotherapy**. **Chemotherapy** destroys cells by disrupting the cell cycle in various phases of metabolism and reproduction. **Chemotherapy** also interferes with the **malignant** cell's ability to synthesize needed chemicals and enzymes. **Chemotherapy** drugs are phase specific (only work during a specific phase of the cell cycle) or non-phase specific (works throughout the cell cycle). The following describes some of the classes or categories of chemotherapeutic drugs.

Alkylating agents are non-phase specific and work by altering DNA synthesis and the cell's ability to replicate. The toxic effects include delayed, prolonged, or permanent bone marrow failure; a treatment-resistant form of acute myelogenous leukemia; irreversible infertility; hemorrhagic cystitis; and nephrotoxicity.

Antimetabolites are a group of **chemotherapy** drugs that are phase specific and alter the cell's ability to replicate or copy the DNA, consequently preventing cell replication. The toxic effects relate to cells that rapidly proliferate (GI, hair, skin, and WBCs) and include nausea and vomiting, stomatitis, decreased WBC count, diarrhea, and alopecia (baldness).

Cytotoxic antibiotics are non-phase specific and act in several ways to damage the cell membrane and kill cells. The main toxic effect occurs as damage to the cardiac muscle, which restricts the duration and amount of treatment.

Plant alkaloids include two groups: vinca alkaloids and etoposide. The vinca alkaloids are phase specific. The toxicity is seen as bone marrow depression, motor weakness, pain and altered sensation, paralytic ileus, and cranial nerve disruptions. Etoposide affects all phases of the cell cycle. The most common toxic effect is hypotension, which results from the IV administration being too rapid. Other toxic effects are nausea, vomiting, and bone marrow suppression.

Hormones and hormone antagonists, corticosteroids and prednisone, the main hormones used in **cancer** therapy are phase specific and alter cell function and growth. Side effects include hyperglycemia, hypertension, impaired healing, osteoporosis, fluid retention, and hirsutism. Hormone antagonists are used with hormone-binding tumors (prostate, breast, and endometrium) to deprive them of their hormones. The goal of these drugs is to cause regression of the tumor, not to cure it. Toxic effects include change in the secondary sex characteristics.

Side effects associated with **chemotherapy** can be very distressing and somewhat debilitating to the patient. Serious side effects—such as alopecia (hair loss), nausea and vomiting, open sores on the mucous membrane, and skin changes—can occur as a result of aggressive **chemotherapy**. Other side effects include (but may not be limited to) anxiety, sleep disturbance, and decreased mobility.

immunotherapy (**im**-yoo-noh-**THAIR**-ah-pee) immun/o = immune, protection -therapy = treatment	Agents that are capable of changing the relationship between a tumor and the host are known as biologic response modifiers (BRMs). These agents are used to strengthen the individual's immune responses.

Because the role of various immune cells against different malignancies is not clear, **immunotherapy** is used only to halt disease that is advanced and/or metastasizing.

Mohs surgery	**Mohs surgery** is an advanced treatment procedure for skin cancer. The cancerous tumor is removed in stages, the tissue is examined for evidence of **cancer**, and additional tissue is removed until negative boundaries are confirmed. This process allows the surgeon to excise the tumor, remove layers of tissue, and examine the fresh tissue immediately. Only tissue containing **cancer** is removed and the healthy tissue is kept intact.

Once the cancerous tumor is removed, the tissue specimens are marked with colored dye to mark a reference point. The tissue sample is then flattened and frozen. Horizontal sections are cut from the undersurface of the tissue sample and are examined microscopically for evidence of **cancer**. The advantage of the horizontal cuts is that this allows for complete examination of the peripheral tumor margins as opposed to making vertical cuts. Any positive tumor margins will be noted on a map drawn to the scale and shape of the original specimen.

Additional tissue from the tumor-positive area is removed and examined microscopically. This process is repeated until negative boundaries are confirmed. The **Mohs surgery** is most often used to treat basal cell carcinoma and squamous cell carcinoma.

radiation therapy (ray-dee-**AY**-shun **THAIR**-ah-pee)	The use of **ionizing radiation** to interrupt cellular growth. The goal of **radiation therapy** is to reach maximum tumor control with minimum normal tissue damage.

The delivery of **ionizing radiation** is used to accomplish one or more of the following:

1. Destruction of tumor cells

2. Reduction of tumor size

3. Decrease in pain

4. Relief of obstruction

5. To slow or stop **metastasis**

Low-energy beams called electron beams are used for the treatment of surface and skin tumors. High-energy X-ray beams are delivered by a large electronic device called a **linear accelerator** and are required for the treatment of deep-seated tumors.

Radiation therapy may be delivered by teletherapy (external radiation) or brachytherapy (internal radiation) or by a combination of both. A treatment method used to decrease damage to normal tissue is **fractionation**. With **fractionation**, the **radiation** is given in repeated small doses at intervals.

Radiocurable tumors are very sensitive to **radiation** and can be totally eradicated by **radiation therapy** (Hodgkin's disease and lymphomas). Drugs that increase the sensitivity of tumors to **radiation** are called radiosensitizers.

In a **radiosensitive tumor**, irradiation is able to cause cell death without seriously damaging normal surrounding tissue. Hematopoietic and lymphatic-origin tumors are radiosensitive.

Radioresistant tumors require large doses of **radiation** to produce death of the tumor cells. Connective tissue tumors are highly radioresistant.

surgery (**SIR**-jer-ee)	In more than 90% of all cancers, **surgery** is used for diagnosing and **staging**. In more than 60% of all cancers, **surgery** is the primary treatment. When feasible, the primary tumor is excised in its entirety.

Tumor removal may necessitate the reconstruction of tissues or organs affected by the **surgery**. An example is the creation of a colostomy when a portion of the colon is removed. Common surgical procedures used for diagnosis or cure of **malignant** tumors are as follows:

1. **Incisional biopsies** are used to remove a piece of a tumor for examination and diagnosing.

2. **Excisional biopsies** are used to remove the tumor and a portion of normal tissue, which provide a specimen for examination and diagnosis. Sometimes this excisional biopsy results in a cure when the **neoplasm** is small.

3. An **en bloc** resection includes the removal of a tumor and a large area of surrounding tissue that contains lymph nodes. An example is a modified radical mastectomy.

4. **Fulguration** is the destruction of tissue with electric sparks, and **electrocauterization** is destruction of tissue by burning.

5. **Cryosurgery** is often used to treat bladder or brain tumors by freezing the **malignant** tissue, which results in its destruction.

6. **Exenteration** is a wide resection that removes the organ of origin and surrounding tissue.

Review Checkpoint

Check your understanding of this section by completing the **Treatment Techniques and Procedures** exercises in your workbook.

COMMON ABBREVIATIONS

Abbreviation	Meaning	Abbreviation	Meaning
ACS	American Cancer Society	Pap smear	a simple smear method of examining stained exfoliative cells; the Papanicolaou test
Bx, bx	biopsy		
Ca	cancer	PSA	prostate-specific antigen
CEA	carcinoembryonic antigen	RNA	ribonucleic acid
DES	diethylstilbestrol	RTx	radiation therapy
DNA	deoxyribonucleic acid	TNM	tumor, nodes, and **metastasis** (a system for **staging** **malignant** neoplastic disease)
mets	metastasis		
NHL	non-Hodgkin's **lymphoma**		

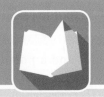

Review Checkpoint

Check your understanding of this section by completing the **Common Abbreviations** exercises in your workbook.

WRITTEN AND AUDIO TERMINOLOGY REVIEW

Review each of the following terms from this chapter. Study the spelling of each term and write the definition in the space provided. Check definitions by looking the term up in the glossary.

Term	Pronunciation	Definition
adjuvant	☐ **AD**-joo-vant	_____
anaplasia	☐ **an**-ah-**PLAY**-zee-ah	_____
antimetabolite	☐ **an**-tih-meh-**TAB**-oh-lite	_____
antineoplastic	☐ **an**-tih-**nee**-oh-**PLASS**-tik	_____
benign	☐ beh-**NINE**	_____
bronchogenic carcinoma	☐ **brong**-koh-**JEN**-ik **kar**-sih-**NOH**-mah	_____
cancer	☐ **CAN**-sir	_____
carcinogen	☐ kar-**SIN**-oh-jen	_____
carcinoma	☐ **kar**-sih-**NOH**-mah	_____
carcinoma in situ (CIS)	☐ **kar**-sih-**NOH**-mah in **SIT**-oo (CIS)	_____
chemotherapy	☐ **kee**-moh-**THAIR**-ah-pee	_____
colorectal cancer	☐ koh-loh-**REK**-tal **CAN**-sir	_____
cryosurgery	☐ **krigh**-oh-**SIR**-jer-ee	_____
cytotoxic	☐ **sigh**-toh-**TOKS**-ik	_____
dedifferentiation	☐ **dee**-diff-er-en-she-**AY**-shun	_____
deoxyribonucleic acid (DNA)	☐ **dee**-ock-see-**rye**-boh-noo-**KLEE**-ic **ASS**-id (DNA)	_____
differentiation	☐ **diff**-er-en-she-**AY**-shun	_____
encapsulated	☐ en-**CAP**-soo-lay-ted	_____
endometrial carcinoma	☐ **en**-doh-**MEE**-tree-al **kar**-sih-**NOH**-mah	_____
epidermoid carcinoma	☐ **ep**-ih-**DER**-moyd **kar**-sih-**NOH**-mah	_____
fibrosarcoma	☐ **fye**-broh-sar-**KOH**-mah	_____
fractionation	☐ **frak**-shun-**AY**-shun	_____
hyperplasia	☐ **high**-per-**PLAY**-zee-ah	_____
immunotherapy	☐ **im**-yoo-noh-**THAIR**-ah-pee	_____

Term	Pronunciation	Definition
infiltrative	☐ **in**-fill-**TRAY**-tiv	_____
intracranial tumors	☐ **in**-trah-**KRAY**-nee-al **TOO**-mors	_____
invasive	☐ in-**VAY**-siv	_____
ionizing radiation	☐ **EYE**-oh-nigh-zing ray-dee-**AY**-shun	_____
linear accelerator	☐ **LIN**-ee-ar ak-**SELL**-er-ay-tor	_____
lymphoma	☐ **LIM**-foh-mah	_____
malignant	☐ mah-**LIG**-nant	_____
melanoblast	☐ **MELL**-an-oh-blast	_____
melanoma	☐ mell-ah-**NOH**-mah	_____
metastasis	☐ meh-**TASS**-tah-sis	_____
metastatic intracranial tumors	☐ **met**-ah-**STAT**-ik in-trah-**KRAY**-nee-al **TOO**-mors	_____
mitosis	☐ my-**TOH**-sis	_____
mixed-tissue tumor	☐ mixed-tissue **TOO**-mor	_____
modality	☐ moh-**DAL**-ih-tee	_____
morbidity	☐ mor-**BID**-ih-tee	_____
mutation	☐ mew-**TAY**-shun	_____
neoplasm	☐ **NEE**-oh-plazm	_____
neuroblastoma	☐ **noo**-roh-blass-**TOH**-mah	_____
oncogene	☐ **ONG**-koh-jeen	_____
oncogenesis	☐ **ong**-koh-**JEN**-eh-sis	_____
oncogenic	☐ **ong**-koh-**JEN**-ik	_____
oncologist	☐ ong-**kOL**-oh-jist	_____
oral leukoplakia	☐ **OR**-al **loo**-koh-**PLAY**-kee-ah	_____
ovarian carcinoma	☐ oh-**VAIR**-ree-an **kar**-sih-**NOH**-mah	_____
pancreatic cancer	☐ **pan**-kree-**AT**-ik **CAN**-sir	_____
papillary	☐ **PAP**-ih-lar-ee	_____
papillocarcinoma	☐ **pap**-ill-oh-**kar**-sih-**NOH**-mah	_____
papilloma	☐ **pap**-ih-**LOH**-mah	_____
pedunculated	☐ peh-**DUN**-kyoo-lay-ted	_____
primary intracranial tumors	☐ primary in-trah-**KRAY**-nee-al **TOO**-mors	_____

Term	Pronunciation	Definition
protocol	☐ **PROH**-toh-kall	_____
radiation	☐ **ray**-dee-**AY**-shun	_____
radiation therapy	☐ **ray**-dee-**AY**-shun **THAIR**-ah-pee	_____
radiocurable tumor	☐ **ray**-dee-oh-**KYOOR**-ah-bul **TOO**-mor	_____
radioresistant tumor	☐ **ray**-dee-oh-ree-**SIS**-tant **TOO**-mor	_____
radioresponsive tumor	☐ **ray**-dee-oh-ree-**SPON**-siv **TOO**-mor	_____
radiotherapy	☐ **ray**-dee-oh-**THAIR**-ah-pee	_____
relapse	☐ ree-**LAPS**	_____
remission	☐ rih-**MISH**-un	_____
renal cell carcinoma	☐ **REE**-nal **SELL** **kar**-sih-**NOH**-mah	_____
ribonucleic acid (RNA)	☐ **rye**-boh-new-**KLEE**-ik **ASS**-id (RNA)	_____
sarcoma	☐ sar-**KOH**-mah	_____
scirrhous	☐ **SKIR**-us	_____
sessile	☐ **SESS**-il	_____
staging	☐ **STAY**-jing	_____
stem cell	☐ **STEM SELL**	_____
surgery	☐ **SIR**-jer-ee	_____
verrucous	☐ veh-**ROO**-kus	_____
Wilms' tumor	☐ **VILMZ TOO**-mor	_____

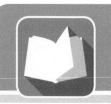

Review Checkpoint

Apply what you have learned in this chapter by completing the **Putting It All Together** exercise in your workbook.

Online Resources

For additional study tools, including PowerPoint® slides and animations, go to the Student Companion Website.

Chapter Review Exercises

The following exercises provide a more in-depth review of the chapter material. Your goal in these exercises is to complete each section at a minimum 80% level of accuracy. If you score below 80% in any area, return to the applicable section in the chapter and read the material again. A space has been provided for your score at the end of each section.

A. Term to Definition

Define each diagnosis or procedure by writing the definition in the space provided. Check the box if you are able to complete this exercise correctly the first time (without referring to the answers). Each correct answer is worth 10 points. Record your score in the space provided at the end.

☐   1. simple mastectomy _____

☐   2. modified radical mastectomy _____

☐   3. radical mastectomy _____

☐   4. Papanicolaou smear _____

☐   5. endometrial carcinoma _____

☐   6. Kaposi's sarcoma _____

☐   7. transurethral resection _____

☐   8. intracranial tumors _____

☐   9. Wilms' tumor _____

☐   10. oral leukoplakia _____

Number correct _____ × 10 points/correct answer: Your score _____ %

B. Matching

Match the descriptions of the tumor on the right with the applicable tumor name on the left. Each correct answer is worth 10 points. When you have completed the exercise, record your score in the space provided at the end of the exercise.

_____ 1. astrocytoma

_____ 2. glioblastoma

_____ 3. meningioma

_____ 4. medulloblastoma

_____ 5. ependymoma

_____ 6. oligodendroglioma

a. a malignant tumor of the cervix

b. the presence of a malignant multiform neoplasm in the large intestine

c. malignant skin tumor originating from melanocytes in preexisting nevi, freckles, or skin with pigment

d. arises in the cerebral hemisphere and is the most rapidly growing of the gliomas

_____ 7. bronchogenic carcinoma

_____ 8. cervical cancer

_____ 9. colorectal cancer

_____ 10. malignant melanoma

e. typically arises in the cerebellum and grows rapidly; occurs most frequently in children between five and nine years of age

f. originates from the meninges, grows slowly, and is largely vascular

g. comprises approximately 10% of all intracranial tumors; is a slow-growing primary tumor of star-shaped cells

h. commonly arises from the ependymomal cells that line the fourth ventricle wall and often extends into the spinal cord

i. occurs most often in the frontal lobe of the brain, usually grows slowly, and comprises approximately 5% of all intracranial tumors

j. a malignant lung tumor that originates in the bronchi; lung cancer usually associated with a history of cigarette smoking

Number correct _____ **× 10 points/correct answer: Your score** _____ **%**

C. Crossword Puzzle

Read the clues carefully and complete the puzzle. Each crossword answer is worth 10 points. When you have completed the crossword puzzle, total your points and enter your score in the space provided.

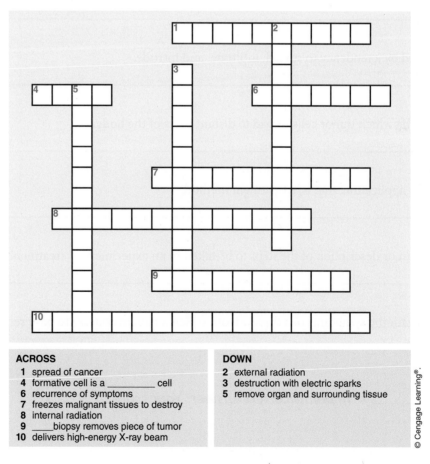

ACROSS

1 spread of cancer
4 formative cell is a _____ cell
6 recurrence of symptoms
7 freezes malignant tissues to destroy
8 internal radiation
9 ____biopsy removes piece of tumor
10 delivers high-energy X-ray beam

DOWN

2 external radiation
3 destruction with electric sparks
5 remove organ and surrounding tissue

Number correct _____ **× 10 points/correct answer: Your score** _____ **%**

D. Definition to Term

Using the following definitions, identify and provide the medical term(s) to match the definition. Each correct answer is worth 10 points. Record your score in the space provided at the end of the exercise.

1. A substance, especially a drug, added to a prescription to assist in the action of the main ingredient.

    _____

    (one word)

2. Noncancerous and therefore not an immediate threat.

    _____

    (one word)

3. A substance or agent that causes the development or increases the incidence of cancer.

    _____

    (one word)

4. A premalignant neoplasm that has not invaded the basement membrane but shows cytologic characteristics of cancer.

    _____

    (three words)

5. In radiology, the division of the total dose of radiation into small doses, administered at intervals, in an effort to minimize tissue damage.

    _____

    (one word)

6. Characterized by a tendency to spread, infiltrate, and intrude.

    _____

    (one word)

7. The process by which tumor cells spread to distant parts of the body.

    _____

    (one word)

8. A method of application, that is, a treatment method.

    _____

    (one word)

9. A written plan or description of the steps to be taken in an experiment or treatment plan.

    _____

    (one word)

10. To exhibit again the symptoms of a disease from which a patient appears to have recovered.

    _____

    (one word)

Number correct _____ × *10 points/correct answer: Your score* _____ %

E. Word Search

Read each definition carefully and identify the applicable word from the list that follows. Enter the word in the space provided and then find it in the puzzle and circle it. The words may be read up, down, diagonally, across, or backward. Each correct answer is worth 10 points. Record your score in the space provided at the end of the exercise.

benign	chemotherapy	radiocurable
melanoma	leukoplakia	metastasis
Wilms'	neuroblastoma	carcinoma
ovarian	basal	

Example: Noncancerous; not life threatening.

benign _____

1. A malignant skin tumor originating from melanocytes in preexisting moles, freckles, or skin with pigment.

   _____

2. A precancerous lesion occurring anywhere in the mouth, characterized by gray-white, leathery-surfaced lesions is known as oral

   _____ .

3. The use of cytotoxic drugs and chemicals to achieve a cure, decrease tumor size, provide relief of pain, or slow metastasis.

   _____

4. A malignant tumor of the kidney occurring predominantly in childhood is known as a

   _____ tumor.

5. A highly malignant tumor of the sympathetic nervous system.

   _____

6. The type of tumor very sensitive to radiation and can be totally eradicated by radiation.

   _____

7. The process by which tumor cells spread to distant parts of the body.

   _____

8. A malignant neoplasm; cancerous tumor.

   _____

9. _____ cell carcinoma is the most common malignant tumor of the epithelial tissue and occurs most often on areas of the skin exposed to the sun.

10. This carcinoma most commonly occurs in women in their 50s and is rarely detected in the early stage.

    _____

Number correct _____ × *10 points/correct answer: Your score* _____ *%*

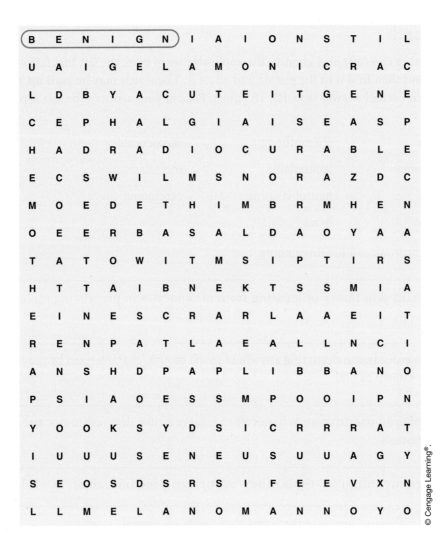

B E N I G N I A I O N S T I L

U A I G E L A M O N I C R A C

L D B Y A C U T E I T G E N E

C E P H A L G I A I S E A S P

H A D R A D I O C U R A B L E

E C S W I L M S N O R A Z D C

M O E D E T H I M B R M H E N

O E E R B A S A L D A O Y A A

T A T O W I T M S I P T I R S

H T T A I B N E K T S S M I A

E I N E S C R A R L A A E I T

R E N P A T L A E A L L N C I

A N S H D P A P L I B B A N O

P S I A O E S S M P O O I P N

Y O O K S Y D S I C R R R A T

I U U U S E N E U S U U A G Y

S E O S D S R S I F E E V X N

L L M E L A N O M A N N O Y O

© Cengage Learning®.

F. Matching Abbreviations

Match the abbreviations on the left with the correct definition on the right. Each correct answer is worth 10 points. When you have completed the exercise, record your score in the space provided at the end of the exercise.

_____ 1. bx

_____ 2. Ca

_____ 3. mets

_____ 4. NHL

_____ 5. PSA

_____ 6. RNA

_____ 7. TNM

_____ 8. DES

_____ 9. DNA

_____ 10. Pap smear

a. metastasis

b. deoxyribonucleic acid

c. a system for staging malignant neoplastic disease

d. a simple smear method of examining stained exfoliative cells

e. cancer

f. biopsy

g. carcinoembryonic antigen

h. ribonucleic acid

i. non-Hodgkin's lymphoma

j. prostate-specific antigen

k. diethylstilbestrol

Number correct _____ × *10 points/correct answer: Your score* _____ %

G. Spelling

Circle the correctly spelled term in each pairing of words. Each correct answer is worth 10 points. Record your score in the space provided at the end of the exercise.

1.	melanoma	melenoma	6.	incapsulated	encapsulated
2.	scirrous	scirrhous	7.	mytosis	mitosis
3.	neaplasm	neoplasm	8.	benign	bening
4.	metastasis	metastisis	9.	adjuvant	ajudvant
5.	papillary	papilarry	10.	antimetabolyte	antimetabolite

Number correct** _____ **× 10 points/correct answer: Your score** _____ **%

H. True or False

Read each statement carefully and circle the correct answer as true or false. HINT: Pay close attention to the word elements written in **bold** as you make your decision. If the statement is false, identify the meaning of the word element written in bold. Each correct answer is worth 10 points. Record your score in the space provided at the end of the exercise.

1. A **carcin**oma is a benign tumor.

   True   False

   If your answer is False, what does *carcin/o* mean? _____

2. **Meta**stasis is the process by which tumor cells spread beyond or to distant parts of the body.

   True   False

   If your answer is False, what does *meta-* mean? _____

3. The term ***scirrhous*** pertains to a carcinoma with a hard structure.

   True   False

   If your answer is False, what does *scirrh/o* mean? _____

4. The medical term ***ana*plasia** means complete formation.

   True   False

   If your answer is False, what does *ana-* mean? _____

5. **Cryo**surgery is the use of heat to treat tissues.

   True   False

   If your answer is False, what does *cry/o* mean? _____

6. The term *hyper**plasia*** refers to excessive formation or development.

   True   False

   If your answer is False, what does *-plasia* mean? _____

7. A melan**oma** is a dark spot on the nailbed.

   True   False

   If your answer is False, what does *-oma* mean? _____

8. **Chemo**therapy is treatment with a drug or chemical.

   True   False

   If your answer is False, what does *chem/o* mean? _____

(continued)

9. The term **antineoplastic** means "of or pertaining to a substance, procedure, or measure that prevents (works against) the proliferation (increase) of malignant cells."

   True   False

   If your answer is False, what does *anti-* mean? _____

10. The medical term *oncogenesis* means "destruction of a tumor."

    True   False

    If your answer is False, what does *-genesis* mean? _____

Number correct _____ × *10 points/correct answer: Your score* _____ %

I. Multiple Choice

Read each statement carefully and select the correct answer from the choices provided. Each correct answer is worth 10 points. Record your score in the space provided at the end of the exercise.

1. The medical term for rough or warty is:
   a. verrucous
   b. papillary
   c. neoplasm
   d. pedunculated

2. A substance, especially a drug, added to a prescription to assist in the action of the main ingredient is a(n):
   a. antimetabolite
   b. carcinogen
   c. adjuvant
   d. protocol

3. High-energy X-rays that can kill cells or retard their growth are known as:
   a. ionizing radiation
   b. linear accelerator
   c. fractionation
   d. protocol

4. A tumor or growth that is enclosed in a fibrous or membranous sheath is:
   a. infiltrative
   b. anaplastic
   c. sessile
   d. encapsulated

5. A tumor that can invade or penetrate adjacent tissue is:
   a. infiltrative
   b. anaplastic
   c. sessile
   d. encapsulated

6. The medical term that means "pertaining to a structure with a stalk" is:

   a. sessile

   b. pedunculated

   c. verrucous

   d. papillary

7. The medical term that means "pertaining to nipplelike projections" is:

   a. sessile

   b. pedunculated

   c. verrucous

   d. papillary

8. A written plan or description of the steps to be taken in an experiment is known as:

   a. protocol

   b. staging

   c. grading

   d. differentiation

9. The medical term that means to exhibit again the symptoms of a disease from which a patient appears to have recovered is:

   a. remission

   b. mutation

   c. relapse

   d. protocol

10. The medical term that means the partial or complete disappearance of the symptoms of a chronic or malignant disease is:

    a. remission

    b. mutation

    c. relapse

    d. protocol

Number correct _____ **× 10 points/correct answer: Your score** _____ **%**

J. Completion

Please complete the following statements with the most appropriate response. Each correct answer is worth 10 points. Record your score in the space provided at the end of the exercise.

1. High-energy X-rays that can kill cells or retard their growth are known as _____ radiation.

2. A gene in a virus that can cause a cell to become malignant is known as an _____.

3. To exhibit again the symptoms of a disease from which a patient appears to have recovered is known as _____.

4. The partial or complete disappearance of the symptoms of a chronic or malignant disease is known as _____.

(*continued*)

5. The probability that an individual, over the course of his or her lifetime, will develop cancer or will die from cancer is known as _____ risk.

6. The measure of the strength of the relationship between risk factors and particular types of cancer is known as _____ risk.

7. The most common malignant tumor of the epithelial tissue that occurs most often on areas of the skin exposed to the sun is _____ _____ carcinoma.

8. The classic symptom of endometrial cancer is inappropriate _____ bleeding.

9. A malignant skin tumor originating from melanocytes in the preexisting nevi, freckles, or skin with pigment is known as malignant _____.

10. A precancerous lesion occurring anywhere in the mouth and that has elevated gray-white or yellow-white, leathery surfaces with clearly defined borders is known as oral _____.

Number correct _____ **× 10 points/correct answer: Your score** _____ **%**

K. Medical Scenario

The following medical scenario presents information on one of the specific types of cancers discussed in this chapter. Read the scenario carefully and select the most appropriate answer for each question that follows. Each correct answer is worth 20 points. Record your score in the space provided at the end of the exercise.

Faith Hord, 53 years old, is a patient of the oncologist, Dr. Goodwin. She has been diagnosed with ovarian carcinoma. The health care professional reviews information about ovarian carcinoma to be prepared for Mrs. Hord's next visit.

1. The health care professional will base her responses to Mrs. Hord's questions about ovarian carcinoma on which of the following facts about ovarian carcinoma? Select all that apply.

   1. It is a malignant tumor of the ovaries, most commonly occurring in women in their 50s.
   2. It is frequently detected in the early stages and, therefore, in many cases, it is curable.
   3. Later developments in the course of the disease include an accumulation of fluid within the abdominal cavity (ascites), resulting in swelling and discomfort.
   4. If the ovary is found to be diseased with cancer, the surgeon will then remove the other ovary, the uterus, and the fallopian tubes.
      a. 1, 3, 4
      b. 2, 3, 4
      c. 1, 2, 4
      d. 1 only

2. The health care professional is reminded from review of the information that the earliest symptoms of ovarian carcinoma are:
   a. painless hematuria and flank pain
   b. seizures and projectile vomiting
   c. swelling, bloating, and/or discomfort in the lower abdomen
   d. increased blood pressure and pulse and respirations

3. The health care professional discovers that diagnosis is confirmed with examination of a sample of the tumor tissue under a microscope. This is achieved through:

   a. urinary catheterization

   b. punch biopsy

   c. surgical intervention

   d. radiation and needle biopsy

4. The health care professional finds that a process of staging is used to determine the amount of metastasis, if any, when a client has ovarian carcinoma. This process involves taking samples of:

   a. nearby lymph nodes and sampling the fluid from the abdomen

   b. the fallopian tubes, uterus, and the other ovary

   c. the cervix and ovaries

   d. the endometrium and cervix

5. Mrs. Hord questions the health care professional about the treatment for ovarian carcinoma. Which of the following responses by the health care professional would be most accurate? The ovarian cancer is treated according to the extent of the disease and may involve:

   a. surgery only

   b. radiation therapy only

   c. chemotherapy only

   d. surgery, radiation therapy, and/or chemotherapy

Number correct _____ × *20 points/correct answer: Your score* _____ *%*

CHAPTER 22

Pharmacology

CHAPTER CONTENT

OBJECTIVES

Upon completing this chapter and the review exercises at the end of the chapter, the learner should be able to:

1. Identify the laws and governing agencies that enforce the safe manufacture, distribution, and use of foods, drugs, and cosmetics.

996

2. List five drug schedules used for categorizing controlled substances as identified in this chapter.

3. List four drug references identified in this chapter.

4. Identify four sources of drugs, giving examples for each source, as identified in this chapter.

5. Identify five names given to drugs to identify their chemical formula, their manufacturer's original name, or the name under which they are sold.

6. Identify at least 10 drug actions/interactions that occur within the body.

7. Identify 10 forms of administration of medications.

8. Identify at least 14 classifications of drugs identified in this chapter.

9. Correctly spell and pronounce terms listed on the Written and Audio Terminology Review, using the phonetic pronunciations provided.

10. Identify at least 30 abbreviations related to pharmacology.

Overview

Health care professionals must know the basics of **pharmacology** and understand the interactions of drugs within the body. A knowledge of the sources, forms, routes of administration, classifications, indications, range of dosages, desired effects, and side effects of drugs is essential. In addition, health care professionals must know the laws regulating the distribution and use of medications. A concentrated study of **pharmacology** will provide the background necessary for understanding the need for safe administration of medications as prescribed by the physician and for acquiring a strong sense of responsibility concerning administering medications.

Pharmacology is the field of medicine that specializes in the study of drugs, including their sources, appearance, chemistry, actions, and uses. A **drug** is any substance that when taken into the body may modify one or more of its functions. **Pharmacodynamics** is the study of how drugs interact in the human body. A **pharmacist** is one who is licensed to prepare and dispense drugs. A **pharmacy** is a place where drugs are dispensed. **Chemotherapy** is the treatment with drugs that have a specific and deadly effect on disease-causing microorganisms (originally used in the treatment of infectious diseases). **Chemotherapy** now includes the treatment of mental illness and cancer with drugs. **Toxicology** is the study of poisons, their detection, and their effects and establishing antidotes (substances that oppose the action of poisons) and methods of treatment for conditions they produce.

There are many terms related to **pharmacology**. Health care professionals may use these terms on a day-to-day basis when involved in administering medications, instructing patients in the use of medications, charting the administration of medications, or transcribing information regarding medications in the patient's chart. This chapter is devoted to the study of terms that relate to the field of **pharmacology**. Where appropriate throughout the chapter, word elements are identified and defined.

Drug Laws

To ensure the safe manufacture, distribution, and use of medications, drugs are subject to numerous state and federal laws. The **Food, Drug, and Cosmetic Act (FDCA)** was passed in 1938. This law regulates the quality, purity, **potency**, effectiveness, safety, labeling, and packaging of food, drug, and cosmetic products. The government agency responsible for administering and enforcing the FDCA within the United States is the **Food and Drug Administration (FDA)**. The federal law concerned with the manufacture, distribution, and dispensing of **controlled substances** is the **Controlled Substances Act**. These drugs have the potential of being abused and of causing physical or psychological dependence. The government agency responsible for administering and enforcing the Controlled Substances Act is the **Drug Enforcement Administration (DEA)**. Physicians who administer controlled substances must enter their DEA number on the prescription. Drugs that fall under the Controlled Substances Act are known as controlled substances or **schedule drugs**. These drugs are identified by a classification system that categorizes them by their potential for abuse. The schedule is divided into five categories: Schedules I to V. The five schedules for controlled substances are listed in *Table 22-1*, with examples of specific medicines appearing in each schedule.

Table 22-1 Schedule of Controlled Substances

Drug Schedule	Description	Example Drugs
I	Schedule I drugs are not considered to be legitimate for medical use in the United States. They are used for research only and they cannot be prescribed, having a high risk for abuse.	LSD, heroin, marijuana*
II	Schedule II drugs have accepted medical use but have a high potential for abuse or addiction. These drugs must be ordered by written prescription and cannot be refilled without a new, written prescription.	Morphine, cocaine, oxycodone, Demerol, Dilaudid
III	Schedule III drugs have moderate potential for abuse or addiction and low potential for physical dependence. These drugs may be ordered by written prescription or by telephone order. Prescriptions expire in 6 months. They may not be refilled more than five times in a 6-month period.	Tylenol with codeine, Vicodin, Hycodan
IV	Schedule IV drugs have less potential for abuse or addiction than those of Schedule III, with limited physical dependence. These drugs may be ordered by written prescription or by telephone order. They may be refilled up to five times over a 6-month period. Prescription expires in 6 months.	Xanax, Valium, Darvon, Ambien, Soma
V	Schedule V drugs have a small potential for abuse or addiction. These drugs may be ordered by written prescription or by telephone order, and there is no limit on prescription refills. Some of these drugs may not need a prescription.	Robitussin A-C, Lyrica, Lomotil

Limited special permission has been obtained in some states for MDs to prescribe marijuana for treatment of side effects, such as nausea and vomiting, in patients receiving chemotherapy.

Drug Standards

The law requires that all preparations called by the same drug name must be of a uniform strength, quality, and purity. This ensures that the patient will obtain the same quality, purity, and strength of medication from the **pharmacy** each time it is prescribed and anywhere in the United States that it is prescribed. These rules (**standards**) have been established to control the strength, quality, and purity of medications prepared by various manufacturers. The *United States Pharmacopeia–National Formulary* (***USP–NF***) is an authorized publication of the United States Pharmacopeial Convention, Inc. It contains formulas and information that provide the standard for preparation and dispensation of drugs. The *USP–NF* is recognized by the U.S. government as the official listing of approved drugs in the United States. The FDCA specifies that a drug is official when it is listed in the *USP–NF*. This publication is updated every five years.

Drug References

Several reference books are available to physicians, nurses, and other health care professionals who are responsible for the safe administration of medications. These references normally provide the following information about drugs listed within them: composition, action, indications for use, contraindications for use, precautions, side effects, adverse reactions, **route of administration**, dosage range, and what forms are available.

The *Hospital Formulary* is a reference listing of all the drugs commonly stocked in the hospital **pharmacy**. This reference provides information about the characteristics of drugs and their clinical usage. This information is continuously revised to provide the most up-to-date information available.

The *Physicians' Desk Reference* (***PDR***) is published yearly by Thomson Reuters in cooperation with participating manufacturers. See *Figure 22-1*.

Manufacturers pay to list information about their products in the PDR. The information provided by the manufacturers is the same basic information found in **package inserts** that accompany each container of medication. The FDA requires that the drug's **generic name**, indications, contraindications, adverse effects, dosage, and route of administration be described in package inserts. Four additional references are listed as follows:

1. *Physicians' Desk Reference for Nonprescription Drugs*
2. *Physicians' Desk Reference for Ophthalmology*
3. *Drug Interactions and Side Effects Index*
4. *Indications Index*

The *Drug Facts and Comparisons* is a reference for health care professionals. It is issued yearly and is updated monthly. This loose-leaf binder reference provides information on drugs according to their therapeutic classifications. It contains the same basic facts as the other drug references listed and is particularly helpful in comparing the various drugs within each category to other products in reference to effectiveness, content, and cost.

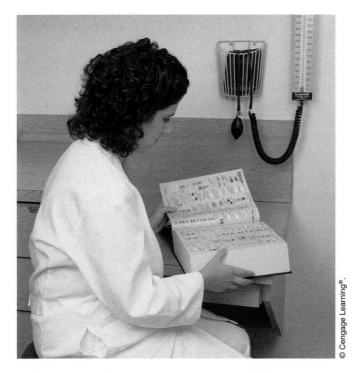

Figure 22-1 *Physicians' Desk Reference (PDR)*

© Cengage Learning®.

VOCABULARY

The following vocabulary words are frequently used when discussing pharmacology.

Word	Definition
adverse reaction	The body's reaction to a drug in an unexpected way that may endanger a patient's health and safety.
anaphylactic shock (**an**-ah-fih-**LAK**-tic **SHOCK**)	A life-threatening, hypersensitive reaction to food or drugs. The patient experiences acute respiratory distress; **hypotension**; edema; **tachycardia**; cool, pale skin; **cyanosis**; and possibly convulsions shortly after administration of the medication.
bacteriostatic bacteri/o = bacteria static = stopping or controlling	Stopping or controlling the growth of bacteria.
brand name	The name under which the drug is sold by a specific manufacturer. This name is owned by the manufacturer, and no other company may use that name. Each **brand name** carries a registered trademark symbol. Also known as **trade name**.

Word	Definition
buccal medication (**BUCK**-al med-ih-**KAY**-shun) bucc/o = cheek -al = pertaining to	Medication placed in the mouth next to the cheek, where it is absorbed into the mucous membrane lining of the mouth.
chemical name	The **chemical name** for a drug is the description of the chemical structure of the drug. It is listed in the *Hospital Formulary* along with the chemical formula diagram.
chemotherapy (**kee**-moh-**THAIR**-ah-pee) chem/o = pertaining to a chemical, drug -therapy = treatment	The treatment of diseases by using drugs that have a specific deadly effect on disease-causing microorganisms. These drugs are used in the treatment of certain infections and cancer.
contraindication (**kon**-trah-**in**-dih-**KAY**-shun)	Any special symptom or circumstance that indicates that the use of a particular drug or procedure is dangerous, not advised, or has not been proven safe for administration.
controlled substances	Drugs that have a potential for abuse. These drugs are placed into five categories, ranging from Schedule I drugs (which are the most dangerous and most likely to be abused) to Schedule V drugs, which are the least dangerous and least likely to be abused; also known as schedule drugs.
Controlled Substances Act	The federal law concerned with the manufacture, distribution, and dispensing of controlled substances. These drugs have the potential of being abused and of causing physical or psychological dependence.
cumulation (**KYOO**-mew-**lay**-shun)	**Cumulation** means that a drug level begins to accumulate in the body with repeated doses because the drug is not completely excreted from the body before another dose is administered.
desired effect	The effect that was intended; that is, if the drug lowered the blood pressure as was intended, the **desired effect** was achieved.
drug	Any substance that when taken into the body may modify one or more of its functions.
drug action	**Drug action** describes how a drug produces changes within the body.
drug effect	**Drug effect** describes the change that takes place in the body as a result of the drug action.
Drug Enforcement Administration	The government agency responsible for administering and enforcing the Controlled Substances Act.
Drug Facts and Comparisons	A reference book for health care professionals that provides information on drugs according to their therapeutic classifications. This reference compares the various drugs within each category with other products.

Word	Definition
first dose	Initial dose.
first-dose effect	An undesired effect of a medication that occurs within 30 to 90 minutes after administration of the first dose.
Food and Drug Administration	The government agency responsible for administering and enforcing the Food, Drug, and Cosmetic Act within the United States.
Food, Drug, and Cosmetic Act	A law that regulates the quality, purity, **potency**, effectiveness, safety, labeling, and packaging of food, drug, and cosmetic products.
generic name (jeh-**NAIR**-ik)	The name established when the drug is first manufactured. This name is protected for use by only the original manufacturer for a period of 17 years. After that time, the name of the drug becomes public property and can be used by any manufacturer.
Hospital Formulary (**FORM**-yoo-lair-ee)	A reference book that lists all of the drugs commonly stocked in the hospital **pharmacy**. This book provides information about the characteristics of drugs and their clinical usage.
hypotension (**high**-poh-**TEN**-shun) hypo- = under, below, beneath, less than normal tens/o = strain -ion = action; process	Low blood pressure; less than normal blood pressure.
idiosyncrasy (id-ee-oh-**SIN**-krah-see)	An unusual, inappropriate response to a drug or to the usual effective dose of a drug. This reaction can be life threatening.
inhalation medication (**in**-hah-**LAY**-shun)	Medication is sprayed or breathed into the nose, throat, and lungs. It is absorbed into the mucous membrane lining of the nose and throat and by the alveoli of the lungs.
initial dose	The first dose of a medication.
intradermal medication (**in**-trah-**DER**-mal) intra- = within derm/o = skin -al = pertaining to	Medication inserted just beneath the epidermis, using a syringe and needle.
intramuscular medication (in-trah-**MUSS**-kyoo-lar) intra- = within muscul/o = muscle -ar = pertaining to	Medication injected directly into the muscle.

Word	Definition
intravenous medication (in-trah-**VEE**-nus) intra- = within ven/o = vein -ous = pertaining to	Medication injected directly into the vein, entering the bloodstream immediately.
local effect	A response (to a medication) confined to a specific part of the body.
maintenance dose	The dose of a medication that will keep the concentration of the medication in the bloodstream at the desired level.
official name	Generic name.
over the counter (OTC)	Medication available without a prescription.
package insert	An information leaflet placed inside the container or package of prescription drugs. The FDA requires that the drug generic name, indications, contraindications, adverse effects, dosage, and route of administration be described in the leaflet.
parenteral medication (pah-**REN**-ter-al)	Any route of administration not involving the gastrointestinal tract, for example, **topical**, **inhalation**, or injection.
pharmacist (**FAR**-mah-sist) pharmac/o = drugs, medicine -ist = practitioner	One who is licensed to prepare and dispense drugs.
pharmacodynamics (far-mah-koh-dye-**NAM**-iks)	The study of how drugs interact in the human body.
pharmacology (far-mah-**KOL**-oh-jee) pharmac/o = drugs, medicine -logy = the study of	The field of medicine that specializes in the study of drugs, including their sources, appearance, chemistry, actions, and uses.
pharmacy (**FAR**-mah-see)	A place for preparing or dispensing drugs.
Physicians' Desk Reference (PDR)	A reference book that provides the same information found in package inserts that accompany each container of medication: description of the drug, actions, indications and usage (why medication is prescribed), contraindications, warnings, precautions, adverse reactions, overdosage, and dosage and administration.
potency (**POH**-ten-see)	Strength.
potentiation (poh-**ten**-she-**AY**-shun)	The effect that occurs when two drugs administered together produce a more powerful response than the sum of their individual effects.

Word	Definition
rectal medication (**REK**-tal) rect/o = rectum -al = pertaining to	Medication inserted into the rectum and slowly absorbed into the mucous membrane lining of the rectum. It is in the form of a suppository, which melts as the body temperature warms it, or a retention enema.
route of administration	The method of introducing a medication into the body.
side effect	An additional effect on the body by a drug that was not part of the goal for that medication. Nausea is a common **side effect** of many drugs.
standards	Rules that have been established to control the strength, quality, and purity of medications prepared by various manufacturers.
subcutaneous medication (**sub**-kyoo-**TAY**-nee-us) sub- = under, below cutane/o = skin -ous = pertaining to	Medication injected into the **subcutaneous** layer, or fatty tissue, of the skin.
sublingual medication (sub-**LING**-gwal) sub- = under, below lingu/o = tongue -al = pertaining to	Medication placed under the tongue, where it dissolves in the patient's saliva and is quickly absorbed through the mucous membrane lining of the mouth.
systemic effect (sis-**TEM**-ik effect)	A generalized response to a drug by the body. The drug has a widespread influence on the body because it is absorbed into the bloodstream.
tachycardia (tak-ee-**KAR**-dee-ah) tachy- = rapid cardi/o = heart -ia = noun ending	Rapid heartbeat, over 100 beats per minute.
therapeutic dose (thair-ah-**PEW**-tik)	The dose of a medication that achieves the desired effect.
tolerance (**TALL**-er-ans)	The body's decreased response to the effect of a drug after repeated dosages.
topical medication (**TOP**-ih-kal)	Medication applied directly to the skin or mucous membrane for a **local effect** to the area.
toxicology (tocks-ih-**KOL**-oh-jee) toxic/o = poisons -logy = the study of	The study of poisons, their detection, and their effects and establishing antidotes and methods of treatment for conditions they produce and prevention of poisoning.
trade name	Brand name copyrighted by a pharmaceutical company.

Word	Definition
United States Pharmacopeia–National Formulary (USP–NF) (**far**-mah-koh-**PEE**-ah)	An authorized publication of the United States Pharmacopeial Convention that contains formulas and information that provide a standard for preparation and dispensation of drugs. Recognized by the U.S. government as the official listing of standardized drugs.

vaginal medication (**VAJ**-in-al)
    vagin/o = vagina
    -al = pertaining to
	Medication inserted into the vagina; may be in the form of a suppository, cream, foam, or tablet.

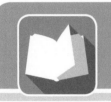

Review Checkpoint

Check your understanding of this section by completing the **Vocabulary** exercises in your workbook.

WORD ELEMENTS

The following word elements pertain to **pharmacology**. As you review the list, pronounce each word element aloud twice and check the box after you "say it." Write the definition for the example term given for each word element. Use your medical dictionary to find the definitions of the example terms.

Word Element	Pronunciation	"Say It"	Meaning
alges/o an**alges**ic	al-**JEE**-soh **an**-al-**JEE**-sik	☐	sensitivity to pain
anti- **anti**depressant	**AN**-tih **an**-tih-dee-**PRESS**-ant	☐	against
arrhythm/o anti**arrhythm**ic	ah-**RITH**-moh **an**-tee-ah-**RITH**-mik	☐	rhythm
bi/o anti**bi**otic	**BYE**-oh **an**-tih-bye-**OT**-ik	☐	life
bronch/o **bronch**odilator	**BRONG**-koh **brong**-koh-**DYE**-lay-tor	☐	bronchus
bucc/o **bucc**al medication	**BUCK**-oh **BUCK**-al	☐	cheek
chem/o **chem**otherapy	**KEE**-moh kee-moh-**THAIR**-ah-pee	☐	pertaining to a chemical, drug

Word Element	Pronunciation	"Say It"	Meaning
coagul/o anti**coagul**ant	koh-**AG**-yoo-loh an-tih-koh-**AG**-yoo-lant	☐	clotting
cutane/o sub**cutane**ous	kyoo-**TAY**-nee-oh sub-kyoo-**TAY**-nee-us	☐	skin
cyan/o **cyan**osis	sigh-**AN**-oh sigh-ah-**NOH**-sis	☐	blue
esthesi/o an**esthesi**a	ess-**THEEZ**-ee-oh an-ess-**THEEZ**-ee-ah	☐	feeling, sensation
fung/o anti**fung**al	**FUNG**-oh **an**-tih-**FUNG**-al	☐	fungus
gloss/o hypo**gloss**al	**GLOSS**-oh high-poh-**GLOSS**-al	☐	tongue
hyper- anti**hyper**tensive	**HIGH**-per an-tih-high-per-**TEN**-siv	☐	excessive
hypno- **hypno**tic	**HIP**-noh hip-**NOT**-ik	☐	sleep
-ia analges**ia**	**EE**-ah an-al-**JEE**-see-ah	☐	condition; noun ending
immun/o **immun**osuppressant	**IM**-yoo-noh **im**-yoo-noh-suh-**PRESS**-ant	☐	immune, protection
intra- **intra**dermal	**IN**-trah **in**-trah-**DER**-mal	☐	within
-ist pharmac**ist**	**IST** **FAR**-mah-sist	☐	practitioner
lingu/o sub**lingu**al	**LING**-yoo-oh sub-**LING**-gwal	☐	tongue
lip/o **lip**id	**LIP**-oh **LIP**-id	☐	fat
-logy pharmaco**logy**	**LOH**-jee **far**-mah-**KOL**-oh-jee	☐	the study of
muscul/o intra**muscul**ar medication	**MUSS**-kyoo-loh **in**-trah-**MUSS**-kyoo-lar	☐	muscle
neo- anti**neo**plastic	**NEE**-oh **an**-tih-**nee**-oh-**PLASS**-tic	☐	new
or/o **or**al medication	**OR**-oh **OR**-al	☐	mouth

Word Element	Pronunciation	"Say It"	Meaning
pharmac/o **pharma**cy	**FAR**-mah-koh **FAR**-mah-see	☐	drugs, medicine
pyr/o **pyr**etic	**PYE**-roh pye-**RET**-ick	☐	fire, heat
rect/o **rect**al medication	**REK**-toh **REK**-tal	☐	rectum
skelet/o **skelet**al muscle relaxant	**SKELL**-eh-toh **SKELL**-eh-tal muscle rih-**LAK**-sant	☐	skeleton
sub- **sub**ungual	**SUB** sub-**UNG**-gwal	☐	under, below
toxic/o **toxic**ology	**TOCKS**-ih-koh **tocks**-ih-**KOL**-oh-jee	☐	poison
vagin/o **vagin**al medication	**VAJ**-in-oh **VAJ**-in-al	☐	vagina
ven/o intra**ven**ous	**VEE**-noh in-trah-**VEE**-nus	☐	vein

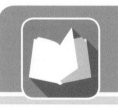

Review Checkpoint

Check your understanding of this section by completing the **Word Elements** exercises in your workbook.

Drug Sources

The origin of many of the drugs used today can be traced to ancient civilizations. Many drugs were prepared from plants, leaves, herbs, roots, and barks, with plants being a primary source of medicinal substances. Examples of plant sources of medications are the purple foxglove, which is a source for digitalis (a medication used to treat heart arrhythmias and congestive heart failure) and the poppy plant, which is a source of opium and is used in **antidiarrheal** medications and analgesics. Leaves and herbs were sources of medicinal-type teas in the earlier generations.

As time evolved, animals and minerals became additional sources of drugs. An example of an animal source for drugs commonly used today is insulin, which is extracted from the pancreas of animals (hogs and cows). An example of a mineral source of drugs is sulfa, which is used in many **bacteriostatic** medications.

A more recent source of drugs has been pharmaceutical laboratories that produce synthetic drugs. Medications such as Demerol (a narcotic **analgesic**) and Lomotil (an **antidiarrheal**) are examples of synthetic forms of medications. Insulin and sulfa drugs are also produced synthetically in pharmaceutical laboratories. See *Figure 22-2*.

Sources of Drugs	Example	Trade Name	Classification
Plants	Cinchona Bark	Quinidine	Antiarrhythmic
	Purple Foxglove Plant	Digitalis	Cardiotonic
	Poppy Plant (Opium)	Morphine, Codeine	Analgesic Analgesic, Antitussive
Minerals	Magnesium	Milk of Magnesia	Antacid, Laxative
	Zinc	Zinc Oxide Ointment	Sunscreen, Skin Protectant
	Gold	Auranofin	Anti-inflammatory; Used in the treatment of Rheumatoid Arthritis
Animals	Pancreas of Cow, Hog	Insulin: regular, NPH, PZI	Antidiabetic Hormone
	Stomach of Cow, Hog	Pepsin	Digestive Hormone
	Thyroid Gland of Animals	Thyroid, USP	Hormone
Synthetic	Meperidine	Demerol	Analgesic
	Diphenoxylate	Lomotil	Antidiarrheal
	Co-trimoxazole	Bactrim, Septra	Anti-infective Sulfonamide; Used in the treatment of urinary tract infections (UTI) and some other infections
DNA 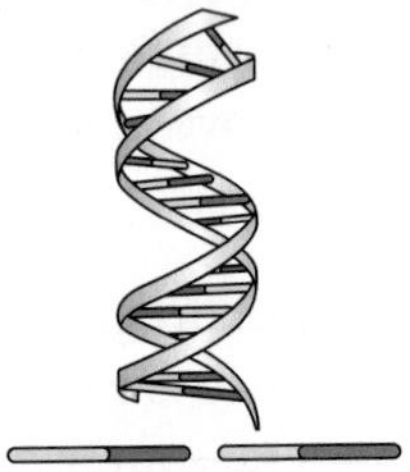 **Genetic Engineered**	Hepatitis B vaccine	Recombivax HB	Vaccine
	Insulin	Humulin, Novolin	Antidiabetic
	Growth hormone	Nutropin	Hormone

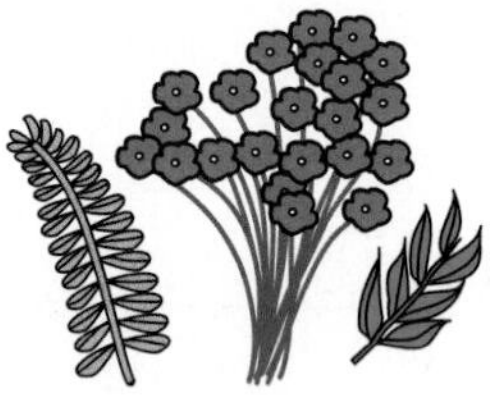

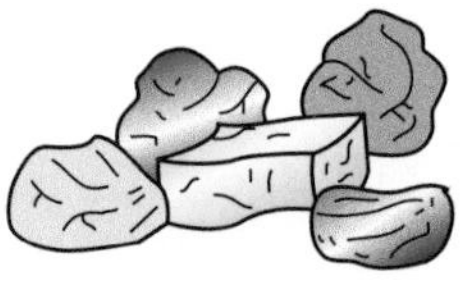

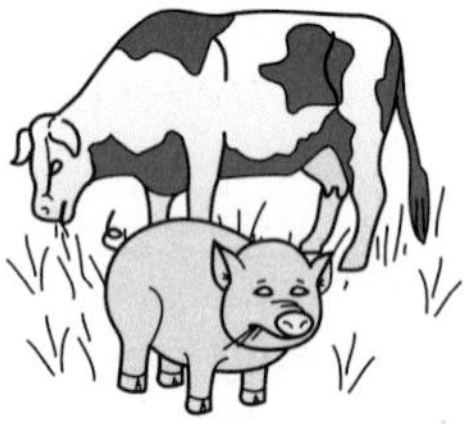

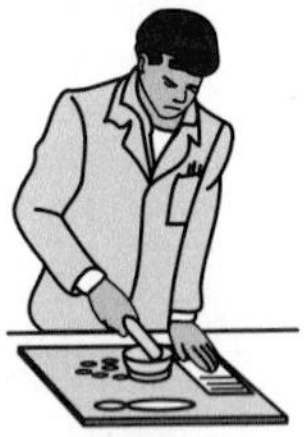

Figure 22-2 Drug sources

Drug Names

The **chemical name** of a drug describes the chemical structure of the drug. It is the formula that indicates the composition of the drug.

The generic name or **official name** of a drug is the name established when the drug is first manufactured. The spelling of the generic name is written in lowercase letters. The original manufacturer of the drug is the only company that can use the generic name for the drug for the first 17 years of its use. Then the name of the drug becomes public property and can be used by any manufacturer. Each drug has only one generic name. The official (generic) name for each drug is listed in the *USP–NF*.

The brand name or trade name of a drug is the name under which the drug is sold by a specific manufacturer. The name is owned by the drug company, and no other company may use that name. Each brand name drug carries a registered trademark symbol (®) after its name, showing that it is restricted to the particular manufacturer. A drug may be known by several brand names. The spelling of the brand name or trade name always begins with a capital letter.

Drug Actions/Interactions

When drugs are ingested or administered into the body, they are absorbed into the bloodstream or into the body tissues. The drugs then combine with or alter the molecules in the body cells, changing the way the cells work. How the drugs produce these changes within the body is known as drug action. The changes that take place in the body as a result of the drug action are known as the drug effect. Some drugs act in the body by either slowing down or speeding up the ordinary processes cells carry out. Other drugs destroy certain cells or parts of cells, such as drugs that destroy disease-producing microorganisms and cancer cells. Yet other drugs act by replacing substances the body lacks or fails to produce, such as vitamins.

The effect of the drug in the body may be a desired effect, achieving the response by the body that is intended; that is, the desired effect was to lower the blood sugar, and the patient's blood sugar level did drop. A drug is usually prescribed for its desired effect. A side effect is an additional effect on the body by the drug that was not part of the goal for that medication. Nausea is a common side effect of many drugs. Even though side effects are bothersome, they are not usually severe enough to warrant discontinuing the medication. An **adverse reaction** is one in which the body reacts to a drug in an unexpected way that may endanger a patient's health and safety. A **contraindication** is any special symptom or circumstance that indicates that the use of a particular drug or procedure is dangerous, not advised, or has not been proven safe for administration.

Drugs may affect only a specific part of the body (having a local effect) or they may affect the body as a whole, having a **systemic effect**. A local effect of a drug is one confined to a specific part of the body. For example, the dentist may administer a medication to numb only one tooth. (The medication has a local effect on that particular area of the body.)

A **systemic effect** of a drug is one that has a widespread influence on the body because it is absorbed into the bloodstream. The remaining terms in this section describe the action and interaction of drugs in the body after they have been absorbed into the bloodstream, that is, those having a **systemic effect** on the body.

cumulation (kyoo-mew-**LAY**-shun)	**Cumulation** occurs when a drug is not completely excreted from the body before another dose is given.

When repeated doses of the drug are given, the drug starts to accumulate in the body tissues and **toxic** effects may occur.

idiosyncrasy (**id**-ee-oh-**SIN**-krah-see)	An **idiosyncrasy** is an unusual, inappropriate response to a drug or to the usual effective dose of a drug.

This reaction may be life threatening. An example of a severe idiosyncratic reaction to a drug or its dosage is **anaphylactic shock**, in which the patient experiences acute respiratory distress; **hypotension**; edema; tachycardia; cool, pale skin; **cyanosis**; and possibly convulsions shortly after administration of the medication. Penicillin is a medicine known to cause anaphylactic reactions in some individuals.

potentiation (poh-**ten-she-AY**-shun)	**Potentiation** occurs when two drugs administered together produce a more powerful response than the sum of their individual effects.

Patients who are taking blood thinners are advised to avoid taking aspirin, which will potentiate the thinning effect on the blood.

tolerance (**TOL**-er-ans)	**Tolerance** is decreased response to the effect of a drug after repeated dosages.

The individual develops a decreased sensitivity to subsequent doses of the drug and requires increasing doses to get the full effect of the drug. **Tolerance** is also a characteristic of drug addiction.

When a drug is given for the first time by whatever method, it is called the initial dose. The initial dose is also known as the **first dose**. Sometimes patients will have an undesired effect after the initial or first dose of a medication, particularly with some medications given for treatment of hypertension—that is, a sharp drop in blood pressure and fainting within 30 to 90 minutes after the first dose of the medication. This response to the initial dose of a medication is known as **first-dose effect**.

The dose of a medication that achieves the desired effect is known as the **therapeutic dose**. Some medications have to be given in increasing doses until the desired level of concentration in the bloodstream is achieved. A **maintenance dose** will keep the concentration of the medication in the bloodstream at the desired level. Medications given to slow and strengthen the heartbeat are often given in increments until the maintenance dose level is achieved.

Routes of Administration for Medications

Medications can be introduced into the body by several methods, referred to as the route of administration. The route of administration determines how rapidly a drug is absorbed into the bloodstream, how well the **drug** is absorbed, and how long the drug acts within the body. The route of administration is usually based on the type of medication given, the dosage form, and the desired effect. The following is a list of the major routes of administration for medications. The list is not alphabetized but is presented in the order in which routes of administration of medications are usually discussed in **pharmacology** textbooks.

---

oral

(**OR**-al)

  or/o = mouth

  -al = pertaining to

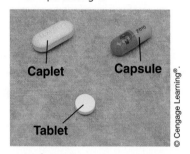

An **oral** medication is one that is given by mouth and swallowed. Oral medications may be given in a dry, solid, or powder form, or they may be given in the liquid form.

This drug is then slowly absorbed into the bloodstream through the lining of the stomach and intestines. See *Figure 22-3*.

> **Advantage:** easiest and safest method; most economical method.

> **Disadvantage:** slow method of absorption; possibility of being destroyed by the gastric juices.

Figure 22-3 Oral medications

---

sublingual

(sub-**LING**-gwal)

  sub- = under, below

  lingu/o = tongue

  -al = pertaining to

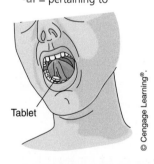

Tablet

A **sublingual medication** is one that is placed under the tongue. See *Figure 22-4*

It dissolves in the patient's saliva and is quickly absorbed through the mucous membrane lining of the mouth; also known as **hypoglossal**.

> **Advantage:** more rapid absorption rate than oral; higher concentration of medication reaches the bloodstream by not passing through the stomach.

> **Disadvantage:** not a convenient route of administration for bad-tasting medications or those that might irritate the mucous membrane.

Figure 22-4 Placement for sublingual medication

---

buccal

(**BUCK**-al)

  bucc/o = cheek

  -al = pertaining to

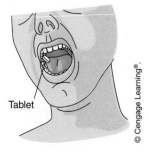

Tablet

A **buccal medication** is one that is placed in the mouth next to the cheek. It is in tablet form. See *Figure 22-5*.

The medication is absorbed into the mucous membrane lining of the mouth.

> **Advantage:** more rapid absorption rate than oral; higher concentration of medication reaches the bloodstream by not passing through the stomach; effects of the medication stop if the tablet is removed.

> **Disadvantage:** possibility of swallowing the pill.

Figure 22-5 Placement for buccal medication

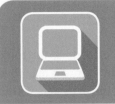

Media Link

Learn more about oral, sublingual, and buccal medication administration by viewing the **Oral Administration** video on the Student Companion Website.

inhalation (**in**-hah-**LAY**-shun)	Medications administered by inhalation are those that are sprayed or inhaled into the nose, throat, and lungs. See *Figure 22-6*.

The medication is absorbed into the mucous membrane lining of the nose and throat and by the alveoli of the lungs. These drugs are in the form of inhalers, sprays, mists, and sometimes steam vapor.

> **Advantage:** good absorption due to large surface contact area; provides rapid treatment.

> **Disadvantage:** sometimes difficult to regulate the dosage; not suitable for medications that might irritate the mucous membrane lining; sometimes considered an awkward method of administering medication.

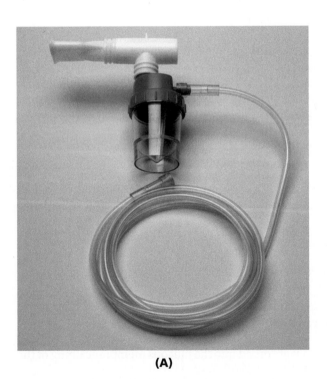

(A)

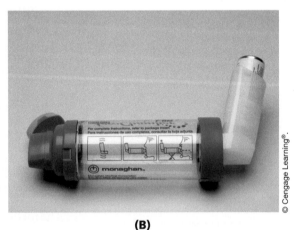

(B)

© Cengage Learning®.

Figure 22-6 (A) Small-volume aerosol nebulizer; (B) Metered-dose inhaler (MDI) with spacer

rectal (**REK**-tal) rect/o = rectum -al = pertaining to	Rectal medications are those inserted into the rectum and slowly absorbed into the mucous membrane lining of the rectum.

This medication is in the form of a suppository, which dissolves as the body temperature warms and melts it, or in liquid form administered by retention enema. See *Figure 22-7A*.

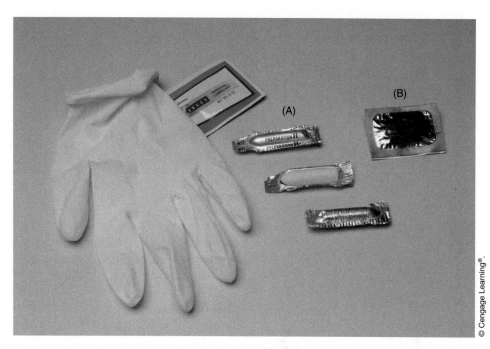

Figure 22-7 (A) Rectal medications; (B) Vaginal medications

Advantage: one method of choice when the patient is nauseated or cannot take medications orally.

Disadvantage: absorption is slow and irregular.

vaginal	Vaginal medications are those inserted into the vagina.
(**VAJ**-in-al) vagin/o = vagina -al = pertaining to	This medication may be in the form of a suppository, cream, foam, or tablet. The medication dissolves as the body temperature warms and melts it. See *Figure 22-7B*. Vaginal medications are usually given for their local effect on the mucous membrane lining the vagina.

Advantage: easiest method for treating the specific area.

Disadvantage: no particular disadvantage, other than the fact that medications sometimes stain underwear.

topical	A **topical medication** is one applied directly to the skin or mucous membrane for a local effect to the area.
(**TOP**-ih-kal)	

These medications are in the form of creams, ointments, sprays, lotions, liniments, liquids, and powders.

Advantage: easy method, convenient.

Disadvantage: slow absorption through the skin.

transdermal	A method of applying a drug to unbroken skin using an adhesive patch. See *Figure 22-8*. The drug is absorbed continuously and produces a **systemic effect**.
(tranz-**DER**-mal) trans- = across derm/o = skin -al = pertaining to	Medications administered by the **transdermal** infusion system are packaged in an adhesive-backed disk. The disk contains a premeasured amount of medication. When the disk is applied, the medication is released through the skin into the bloodstream at a controlled rate, producing

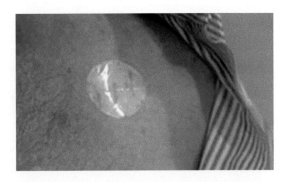

Figure 22-8 Transdermal delivery system
(Courtesy of Novartis)

a **systemic effect**. Examples of transdermal medications include vasodilators such as nitroglycerin, hormones such as estrogen, and medications used to help someone stop smoking.

> **Advantage:** good method for administering medications that need to be released slowly into the bloodstream over a period of time.

> **Disadvantage:** units can be dangerous if they come in contact with the skin of children or pets. A very limited number of drugs are available at this time that can be administered by the transdermal patch. Removal of the patch does not guarantee immediate stoppage of absorption of the medication should an **adverse reaction** occur.

parenteral	Any route of administration not involving the gastrointestinal tract, for example, topical, inhalation, or injection.
(pah-**REN**-ter-al)	
par- = apart from	
enter/o = intestine	
-al = pertaining to	

Parenteral medication for injection must be in a liquid form and administered by one of the following four methods: **intradermal**, **intramuscular**, **intravenous**, or subcutaneous. For a visual reference illustrating injection angles for various parental medications, see *Figure 22-9*.

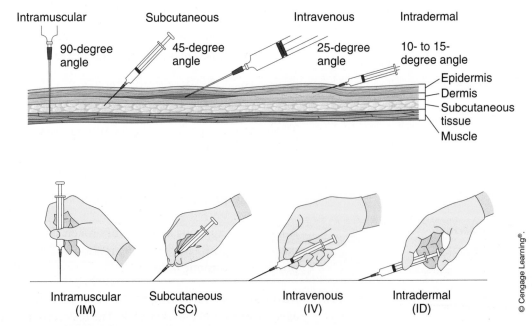

Figure 22-9 Parenteral medications

intradermal	A small amount of medication is injected just beneath the epidermis.
(**in**-trah-**DER**-mal) 　intra- = within 　derm/o = skin 　-al = pertaining to	Intradermal injections are used for allergy testing, tuberculin skin testing, and some vaccinations.
intramuscular	The medication is injected directly into large muscles.
(in-trah-**MUSS**-kyoo-lar) 　intra- = within 　muscul/o = muscle 　-ar = pertaining to	Intramuscular injections are used for administering antibiotics, medications that might be irritating to the layers of the skin, and medications that require dosages larger than the amount allowed for a subcutaneous injection.
intravenous	The medication is injected directly into the vein, entering the bloodstream immediately.
(in-trah-**VEE**-nus) 　intra- = within 　ven/o = vein 　-ous = pertaining to	Intravenous injections are used when medication is needed quickly and for administering medication over a period of time, by adding the medication to a bag of intravenous fluids (a process known as infusion).
subcutaneous	The medication is injected into the subcutaneous layer, or fatty tissue, of the skin.
(**sub**-kyoo-**TAY**-nee-us) 　sub- = under, below 　cutane/o = skin 　-ous = pertaining to	Subcutaneous injections are used for administering insulin, hormones, and local anesthetics.

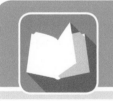

Review Checkpoint

Check your understanding of this section by completing the **Routes of Administration for Medication** exercises in your workbook.

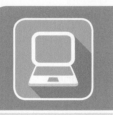

Media Link

Learn more about intradermal, intramuscular, and subcutaneous medications by viewing the **Intramuscular Injection** and **Subcutaneous Injection** videos on the Student Companion Website.

Drug Classification

Drugs are classified, or categorized, according to their primary or main effect(s) in the body. *Table 22-2* lists most of the major classifications of drugs along with a basic description of each category and a common example of a medicine from each classification. The generic name is written in lowercase letters, and the brand name begins with a capital letter.

Table 22-2 Major Drug Classifications

Drug Classification	General-Purpose Definition	Common Example
analgesic (**an**-al-**JEE**-sik) an- = without alges/o = pain -ic = pertaining to	Relieves pain	acetylsalicylic acid (aspirin, Bayer Children's Aspirin) acetaminophen (Tylenol)
anesthetic (**an**-ess-**THET**-ik) an- = without esthet/o = feeling, nervous sensation or sense of perception -ic = pertaining to	Partially or completely numbs or eliminates sensitivity with or without loss of consciousness	lidocaine (Xylocaine)
antiarrhythmic (**an**-tih-ah-**RITH**-mik) anti- = against arrhythm/o = rhythm -ic = pertaining to	Corrects cardiac arrhythmias (irregular beats)	digoxin (Lanoxin) propranolol hydrochloride (Inderal)
antibiotic (anti-infective) (**an**-tih-bye-**OT**-ik) anti- = against bi/o = life -tic = pertaining to	Stops or controls the growth of infection-causing microorganisms	phenoxymethyl-penicillin sodium (Pen-Vee-K, Penicillin VK, Veetids, V-Cillin K) trimethoprim and sulfamethoxazole (Bactrim, Bactrim DS)
anticoagulant (**an**-tih-koh-**AG**-yoo-lant) anti- = against coagul/o = clotting	Prevents clot continuation and formation	enoxaparin sodium (Lovenox) warfarin sodium (Coumadin)
anticonvulsant (**an**-tih-kon-**VULL**-sant)	Prevents or relieves convulsions (seizures)	clonazepam (Klonopin) phenobarbital (Luminal) diazepam (Valium)
antidepressant (**an**-tih-dee-**PRESS**-ant)	Prevents, cures, or alleviates mental depression	fluoxetine (Prozac) imipramine hydrochloride (Tofranil)
antidiabetic (**an**-tih-**dye**-ah-**BET**-ik)	Helps control the blood sugar level	chlorpropamide (Diabinese) metformin (Glucophage) insulin
antidiarrheal (**an**-tih-**dye**-ah-**REE**-ul)	Prevents or treats diarrhea	diphenoxylate-atropine sulfate (Lomotil) loperamide hydrochloride (Imodium)
antidiuretic (**an**-tih-dye-yoo-**REH**-tik)	Suppresses the formation of urine	vasopressin (Pitressin)

(continued)

Drug Classification	General-Purpose Definition	Common Example
antiemetic (**an**-tih-ee-**MET**-ik)	Prevents or relieves nausea and vomiting	chlorpromazine (Thorazine) meclizine hydrochloride (Bonine, Dramamine II, Antivert)

antifungal
(**an**-tih-**FUNG**-gal)
  anti- = against
  fung/o = fungus
  -al = pertaining to
	Destroys or inhibits the growth of fungi	miconazole (Monistat)
		fluconazole (Diflucan)
		clotrimazole (Gyne-Lotrimin)

antihistamine (**an**-tih-**HISS**-tah-meen)	Opposes the action of histamine, which is released in allergic reactions	diphenhydramine hydrochloride (Benadryl) cetirizine (Zyrtec)

antihypertensive
(**an**-tih-**high**-per-**TEN**-siv)
  anti- = against
  hyper- = excessive
	Prevents or controls high blood pressure	nadolol (Corgard)
		prazosin (Minipress)
		diltiazem hydrochloride
		(Cardizem, Cardizem CD)

anti-infective (antibiotic) (**an**-tih-in-**FEK**-tiv)	Stops or controls the growth of infection-causing microorganisms	amoxicillin (Amoxil, Polymox) doxycycline hyclate (Vibramycin)
anti-inflammatory (**an**-tih-in-**FLAM**-ah-toh-ree)	Counteracts inflammation in the body	nabumetone (Relafen) naproxen sodium (Anaprox, Aleve)

antineoplastic
(**an**-tih-**nee**-oh-**PLASS**-tik)
  anti- = against
  neo- = new
  plas/o = formation
  -tic = pertaining to
	Prevents the development, growth, or reproduction of cancerous cells	fluorouracil (Adrucil)
		methotrexate (Rheumatrex
		Dose Pack)

antipyretic
(**an**-tih-pye-**RET**-ick)
  anti = against
  pyr/o = fire, heat
  -tic = pertaining to
	Reduces fever	ibuprofen
		naproxen
		aspirin
		acetaminophen (Tylenol)

antitussive (**an**-tih-**TUSS**-iv)	Relieves cough due to various causes	dextromethorphan hydrobromide (Benylin DM, Robitussin Pediatric, Vick's Formula 44, Vick's Formula 44 Pediatric Formula) pseudoephedrine hydrochloride and guaifenesin (Novahistex Expectorant with Decongestant, Robitussin PE, Sudafed Expectorant)
antiulcer agent (**an**-tih-**ULL**-ser)	Treats and prevents peptic ulcer and gastric hypersecretion	ranitidine hydrochloride (Zantac) nizatidine (Axid)
antiviral agent (**an**-tih-**VYE**-ral)	Treats various viral conditions such as serious herpes virus infection, chickenpox, and influenza A	acyclovir (Zovirax) vidarabine (Vira-A)

(*continued*)

Drug Classification	General-Purpose Definition	Common Example
beta blocker (**BAY**-tah **BLOCK**-er)	Treats hypertension, angina, and various abnormal heart rhythms	metoprolol tartrate (Lopressor) carteolol hydrochloride (Ocupress, Cartrol)
bronchodilator (**brong**-koh-**DYE**-lay-tor) bronch/o = bronchus; airway	Expands the bronchial tubes by relaxing the bronchial muscles	theophylline (Bronkodyl, Quibron-T/SR, Theobid Duracaps) aminophylline (Aminophylline, Truphylline)
calcium channel blocker (**KAL**-see-um **CHAN**-ell **BLOCK**-er)	Treats hypertension, angina, and various abnormal heart rhythms	amlodipine (Norvasc) bepridil hydrochloride (Vascor)
diuretic (**dye**-yoor-**RET**-ik)	Increases urine secretion	furosemide (Lasix) hydrochlorothiazide (Hydro-Diuril)
hormone (**HOR**-mohn)	Treats deficiency states where specific hormone level is abnormally low	estrogen, conjugated (Premarin) glucagon (Glucagon)
hypnotic (hip-**NOT**-ik) hypno- = sleep -tic = pertaining to	Induces sleep or dulls the senses	pentobarbital (Nembutal) secobarbital sodium (Seconal Sodium)
immunosuppressant (**im**-yoo-noh-suh-**PRESS**-ant) immun/o = immunity	Suppresses the body's natural immune response to an antigen, as in treatment for transplant patients	cyclosporine (Sandimmune) azathioprine (Imuran)
laxative (**LACK**-sah-tiv)	Prevents constipation or promotes the emptying of the bowel contents with ease	docusate calcium (Surfak) bisacodyl (Dulcolax) psyllium hydrophilic mucilloid (Metamucil)
lipid-lowering agent (**LIP**-id) lip/o = fat	Reduces blood lipid (fat) levels	atorvastatin (Lipitor) lovastatin (Mevacor)
sedative (**SED**-ah-tiv)	Exerts a soothing or tranquilizing effect on the body	phenobarbital (Nembutal) diazepam (Valium) flurazepam hydrochloride (Dalmane)
skeletal muscle relaxant (**SKELL**-eh-tal muscle rih-**LAK**-sant) skelet/o = skeleton -al = pertaining to muscul/o = muscle -e = noun ending	Relieves muscle tension	dantrolene sodium (Dantrium) carisoprodol (Soma) cyclobenzaprine-hydrochloride (Flexeril)
vitamin (**VIGH**-tah-min)	Prevents and treats **vitamin** deficiencies and used as dietary supplement	vitamins A, D, E, etc. ascorbic acid (vitamin C) cyanocobalamin (vitamin B_{12})

Review Checkpoint

Check your understanding of this section by completing the **Drug Classification** exercises in your workbook.

COMMON CHARTING ABBREVIATIONS

Medical abbreviations serve as a universal language for medical professionals to provide specific information and orders in a shortened format. Individuals involved in all aspects of health care may use these abbreviations on a daily basis. It is essential that health care professionals commit these abbreviations to memory to transmit and receive clear and concise meanings.

It is also important that health care professionals remember that ambiguous medical notations are one of the most common and preventable causes of medication errors. Clarity in writing abbreviations is of the utmost importance. If an abbreviation is not written clearly, to minimize confusion, misinterpretation of the meaning may lead to mistakes that result in patient harm.

As you continue to study medical terminology and the various abbreviations for drug names, dosage units, and directions, you will learn that some abbreviations are error prone and should be spelled out completely or abbreviated very clearly to avoid confusion of the meaning. The Institute for Safe Medication Practices (ISMP) and the Food and Drug Administration (FDA) recommend that the ISMP's list of error-prone abbreviations be considered whenever medical information is communicated.

Some of the more commonly used abbreviations that relate to pharmacology and are used for charting follow this discussion. The list has been updated to eliminate the error-prone abbreviations.

Abbreviation	Meaning	Abbreviation	Meaning
a.c.	before meals	fl	fluid
ad lib	as desired	FDA	Food and Drug Administration
AM	morning	FDCA	Food, Drug, and Cosmetic Act
b.i.d.	twice a day	g	gram
C	Celsius (centigrade)	gr, Gr	grain
c̄	with	gt., gtt	drop, drops
caps	capsule, capsules	h, hr	hour
cm	centimeter	H_2O	water
DEA	Drug Enforcement Administration	ID	intradermal
		IM	intramuscular
elix	Elixir	ISMP	Institute for Safe Medication Practices
F	Fahrenheit		

Abbreviation	Meaning	Abbreviation	Meaning
IV	intravenous	q.h. or qh	every hour
kg	kilogram	q.2 h., q.3 h., ...	every 2 hours, every 3 hours ....
L	liter	q.i.d. or qid	four times a day
lb	pound	q.s. or qs	quantity sufficient
mcg	microgram	R$_x$	take; treatment; prescription
mg	milligram	s̄	without
mEq	milliequivalent	sig	write on label (let it be labeled)
mL	milliliter	SL	sublingual
NKA	no known allergies	sos	if necessary
NKDA	no known drug allergies	stat	immediately
n.p.o., NPO	nothing by mouth	subq	subcutaneous
O$_2$	oxygen	supp	suppository
OTC	**over the counter** (drugs that require no prescription)	tab	tablet
		t.i.d. or tid	three times a day
oz	ounce	tinc	tincture
p̄	after	ung, oint.	ointment
p.c. or pc	after meals	USP–NF	*United States Pharmacopeia–National Formulary*
PDR	*Physicians' Desk Reference*		
PM	afternoon	vag	vaginal
p.o., po, or PO	by mouth (per os)	VO	verbal order
p.r.n. or prn	as needed	x	times, multiplied by
q	every		
q.a.m.	every morning		

Review Checkpoint

Check your understanding of this section by completing the **Common Charting Abbreviations** exercises in your workbook.

Examples of Error-Prone Abbreviations

The Institute for Safe Medication Practices (ISMP) has compiled a list of Error-Prone Abbreviations, Symbols, and Dose Designations. The following are samples of some of the abbreviations that have been designated as error prone. The abbreviation and its intended meaning have been identified along with the proper way of charting to avoid misunderstanding. The abbreviations **OD**, **OS**, and **OU** are intended to mean (respectively) right eye, left eye, and each eye. These abbreviations should be written as "right eye," "left eye," and "each eye" to avoid confusing them with AD, AS, and AU (which refer to the ear).

The abbreviation **hs** is intended to mean bedtime "hour of sleep." This abbreviation should be written as "bedtime" to avoid confusing it with HS, which refers to half-strength. The abbreviation **U** is intended to mean "unit." This abbreviation should be written as "unit" to avoid confusing it with the number zero if poorly written. For a complete listing of error-prone abbreviations, visit the ISMP website at http://www.ismp.org.

WRITTEN AND AUDIO TERMINOLOGY REVIEW

Review each of the following terms from this chapter. Study the spelling of each term and write the definition in the space provided. Check definitions by looking the term up in the glossary.

Term	Pronunciation	Definition
adverse reaction	☐ **AD**-vers reaction	_____
analgesic	☐ an-al-**JEE**-sik	_____
anaphylactic shock	☐ an-ah-fih-**LAK**-tic **SHOCK**	_____
anesthesia	☐ an-ess-**THEEZ**-ee-ah	_____
anesthetic	☐ an-ess-**THET**-ik	_____
antiarrhythmic	☐ an-tee-ah-**RITH**-mik	_____
antibiotic	☐ an-tih-bye-**OT**-ik	_____
anticoagulant	☐ an-tih-koh-**AG**-yoo-lant	_____
anticonvulsant	☐ an-tih-kon-**VULL**-sant	_____
antidepressant	☐ an-tih-dee-**PRESS**-ant	_____
antidiabetic	☐ an-tih-**dye**-ah-**BET**-ik	_____
antidiarrheal	☐ an-tih-**dye**-ah-**REE**-al	_____
antiemetic	☐ an-tih-ee-**MET**-ik	_____
antifungal	☐ an-tih-**FUNG**-gal	_____

Term	Pronunciation	Definition
antihistamine	☐ **an**-tih-**HISS**-tah-meen	_____
antihypertensive	☐ **an**-tih-**high**-per-**TEN**-siv	_____
anti-infective	☐ **an**-tih-in-**FEK**-tiv	_____
anti-inflammatory	☐ **an**-tih-in-**FLAM**-ah-toh-ree	_____
antineoplastic	☐ **an**-tih-nee-oh-**PLASS**-tik	_____
antitussive	☐ **an**-tih-**TUSS**-iv	_____
antiulcer	☐ **an**-tih-**ULL**-ser	_____
antiviral	☐ **an**-tih-**VYE**-ral	_____
beta blocker	☐ **BAY**-tah blocker	_____
bronchodilator	☐ **brong**-koh-**DYE**-lay-tor	_____
buccal	☐ **BUCK**-al	_____
calcium channel blocker	☐ **KAL**-see-um **CHAN**-ell **BLOCK**-er	_____
chemical name	☐ **KEM**-ih-cal name	_____
chemotherapy	☐ **kee**-moh-**THAIR**-ah-pee	_____
contraindication	☐ **kon**-trah-**in**-dih-**KAY**-shun	_____
cumulation	☐ **kyoo**-mew-**LAY**-shun	_____
cyanosis	☐ **sigh**-ah-**NOH**-sis	_____
hormone	☐ **HOR**-mohn	_____
Hospital Formulary	☐ hospital **FORM**-yoo-**lair**-ee	_____
hypnotic	☐ hip-**NOT**-ik	_____
hypoglossal	☐ **high**-poh-**GLOSS**-al	_____
hypotension	☐ **high**-poh-**TEN**-shun	_____
idiosyncrasy	☐ **id**-ee-oh-**SIN**-krah-see	_____
immunosuppressant	☐ **im**-yoo-noh-suh-**PRESS**-ant	_____
intradermal	☐ **in**-trah-**DER**-mal	_____
intramuscular	☐ in-trah-**MUSS**-kyoo-lar	_____
intravenous	☐ in-trah-**VEE**-nus	_____
laxative	☐ **LACK**-sah-tiv	_____
lipid-lowering agent	☐ **LIP**-id lowering agent	_____
parenteral	☐ pah-**REN**-ter-al	_____
pharmacist	☐ **FAR**-mah-sist	_____
pharmacodynamics	☐ **far**-mah-koh-dye-**NAM**-iks	_____

Term	Pronunciation	Definition
pharmacology	☐ **far**-mah-**KOL**-oh-jee	_____
pharmacy	☐ **FAR**-mah-see	_____
potency	☐ **POH**-ten-see	_____
potentiation	☐ poh-**ten**-she-**AY**-shun	_____
sedative	☐ **SED**-ah-tiv	_____
skeletal muscle relaxant	☐ **SKELL**-eh-tal muscle rih-**LAK**-sant	_____
subcutaneous	☐ **sub**-kyoo-**TAY**-nee-us	_____
systemic effect	☐ sis-**TEM**-ik effect	_____
tolerance	☐ **TOL**-er-ans	_____
toxicology	☐ **tocks**-ih-**KOL**-oh-jee	_____
transdermal	☐ tranz-**DER**-mal	_____
vitamin	☐ **VIGH**-tah-min	_____

Review Checkpoint

Apply what you have learned in this chapter by completing the **Putting It All Together** exercise in your workbook.

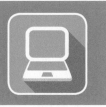

Online Resources

For additional study tools, including PowerPoint® slides and animations, go to the Student Companion Website.

Chapter Review Exercises

The following exercises provide a more in-depth review of the chapter material. Your goal in these exercises is to complete each section at a minimum 80% level of accuracy. If you score below 80% in any area, return to the applicable section in the chapter and read the material again. A space has been provided for your score at the end of each section.

A. Matching

Match the terms on the left with the most appropriate definition on the right. Each correct answer is worth 10 points. Record your score in the space provided at the end of the exercise.

_____ 1. pharmacology

_____ 2. drug

_____ 3. pharmacodynamics

_____ 4. pharmacist

_____ 5. pharmacy

_____ 6. chemotherapy

_____ 7. toxicology

_____ 8. standards

_____ 9. package insert

_____ 10. druggist

a. pharmacist

b. rules that have been established to control the strength, quality, and purity of medications

c. the field of medicine that specializes in the study of drugs

d. an information leaflet placed inside the container of a package of prescription drugs

e. any substance that when taken into the body may modify one or more of its functions

f. treatment using drugs that have a specific and deadly effect on disease-causing microorganisms

g. one who is licensed to prepare and dispense drugs

h. the study of poisons, their detection, their effects, and establishing antidotes and methods of treatment

i. place where drugs are dispensed

j. the study of how drugs interact in the human body

Number correct _____ × *10 points/correct answer: Your score* _____ %

B. Multiple Choice

Read each question carefully and circle the most appropriate response for each statement. Each correct answer is worth 10 points. When you have completed this exercise, record your score in the space provided at the end of the exercise.

1. The Food, Drug, and Cosmetic Act is a law that regulates:

   a. the quality, purity, potency, effectiveness, safety, labeling, and packaging of food, drugs, and cosmetics

   b. the quality, purity, potency, effectiveness, safety, labeling, and packaging of drugs only

   c. the quality, purity, potency, effectiveness, safety, labeling, and packaging of prescription cosmetics

   d. the quality, purity, labeling, and packaging of food only

2. The government agency responsible for administering and enforcing the Food, Drug, and Cosmetic Act within the United States is the:

    a. FDA

    b. FNA

    c. DEA

    d. CSA

3. The federal law concerned with the manufacture, distribution, and dispensing of drugs that have the potential of being abused and of causing physical or psychological dependence is the:

    a. Food, Drug, and Cosmetic Act

    b. Controlled Substance Act

    c. Drug Enforcement Act

    d. Schedule Drug Control Act

4. The government agency responsible for administering and enforcing the Controlled Substance Act within the United States is the:

    a. FDA

    b. FNA

    c. DEA

    d. CSA

5. The drug schedule that includes drugs that are not acceptable for medical use and are used for research only is the:

    a. Schedule I

    b. Schedule II

    c. Schedule III

    d. Schedule IV

6. The drug schedule that includes drugs that are considered to have a strong potential for abuse or addiction and cannot be refilled without a new, written prescription is:

    a. Schedule I

    b. Schedule II

    c. Schedule III

    d. Schedule IV

7. The drug schedule that includes drugs that have a small potential for abuse or addiction is:

    a. Schedule I

    b. Schedule II

    c. Schedule IV

    d. Schedule V

8. The official publication that contains formulas and information that provide a standard for preparation and dispensation of drugs is the:

    a. *Physicians' Desk Reference*

    b. *United States Pharmacopeia–National Formulary*

    c. *Drug Facts and Comparisons*

    d. *Compendium of New Drugs/New Standards*

(continued)

9. The drug reference published annually by Thomson Reuters in cooperation with participating manufacturers is:

   a. *Physicians' Desk Reference*

   b. *United States Pharmacopeia–National Formulary*

   c. *Drug Facts and Comparisons*

   d. *Compendium of New Drugs/New Standards*

10. The drug reference that lists all of the drugs commonly stocked by the hospital pharmacy is:

    a. *Physician's Hospital Reference*

    b. *Hospital Drug Facts and Comparisons*

    c. *Compendium of New Drugs/New Standards*

    d. *Hospital Formulary*

Number correct _____ **× 10 points/correct answer: Your score** _____ **%**

C. Completion

Complete each sentence with the most appropriate answer. Each correct answer is worth 10 points. Record your score in the space provided at the end of the exercise.

1. The name that describes the chemical structure of a drug is the _____ name.

2. The name of a drug established when the drug is first manufactured is known as the _____ name.

3. The name by which a drug is sold by a specific manufacturer is known as the _____ name.

4. The name that is the same as the official name of a drug is the _____ name.

5. The name that is the same as the trade name of a drug is the _____ name.

6. How the drug produces changes within the body is known as drug _____.

7. The change that takes place in the body as a result of the drug action is known as drug _____.

8. An additional effect on the body by a drug that was not part of the goal for that medication is known as a _____.

9. When the body reacts to a drug in an unexpected way that may endanger a patient's health and safety, the patient is said to have had the following type of reaction to the medication: _____.

10. Any special symptom or circumstance that indicates that the use of a particular drug or procedure is dangerous, not advised, or has not been proven safe for administration is known as a _____.

Number correct _____ **× 10 points/correct answer: Your score** _____ **%**

D. Crossword Puzzle

Identify the various routes of administration of medications based on the clues provided. Each correct answer is worth 10 points. When you have completed this exercise, record your score in the space provided at the end of the exercise.

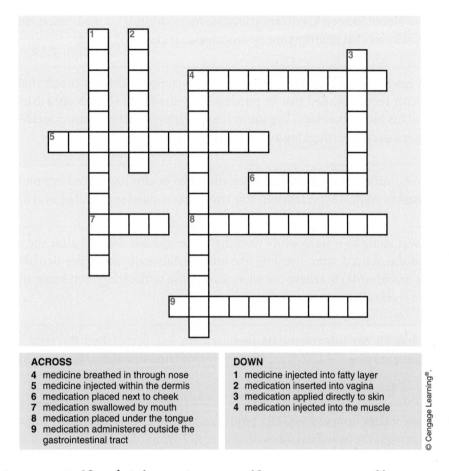

ACROSS
4 medicine breathed in through nose
5 medicine injected within the dermis
6 medication placed next to cheek
7 medication swallowed by mouth
8 medication placed under the tongue
9 medication administered outside the gastrointestinal tract

DOWN
1 medicine injected into fatty layer
2 medication inserted into vagina
3 medication applied directly to skin
4 medication injected into the muscle

© Cengage Learning®.

Number correct _____ × *10 points/correct answer: Your score* _____ %

E. Drug Classification Selection

Using the following drug classifications, enter the most appropriate response in the space provided. Each correct answer is worth 10 points. When you have completed the exercise, record your score in the space provided. If you can answer all of the questions without assistance from your text or notes, give yourself 10 extra bonus points!

antiulcer agent	antitussive	anticonvulsant
diuretic	antihistamine	anesthetic
antihypertensive	antiemetic	anticoagulant
antidepressant	antibiotic	antidiabetic
analgesic	bronchodilator	antifungal

(continued)

1. Juan Miguel is complaining of a headache. His doctor told him to take Tylenol (acetaminophen) to relieve the pain. You know that acetaminophen is classified as a(n):

   _____

2. Recently Judy Silverstein's mother died shortly after Judy lost her job. For the past two months, Judy has been having difficulty coping with her situation. She has been extremely depressed and cries excessively. The doctor has placed Judy on Elavil (amitriptyline hydrochloride), a medication used to alleviate mental depression. You know that amitriptyline hydrochloride is classified as a(n):

   _____

3. Aiden Allran has had a cold for three days. He has developed a scratchy cough that keeps him awake at night. His doctor recommended that he purchase Robitussin PE (pseudoephedrine hydrochloride and guaifenesin) at his local pharmacy. You know that pseudoephedrine hydrochloride and guaifenesin is a medication given to relieve coughing and is classified as a(n):

   _____

4. Pearl Henderson suffers from high blood pressure. The doctor has placed her on Corgard (nadolol), a medication used to control hypertension. You know that nadolol is classified as a(n):

   _____

5. Bette Daves was stung by a wasp while working in her garden. Shortly after the sting, her finger was throbbing and she noticed some swelling. She immediately took one of her Benadryl capsules (diphenhydramine hydrochloride) to relieve the allergic response to the sting. You know that diphenhydramine hydrochloride is classified as a(n):

   _____

6. Mark Jones has an ear infection. His pediatrician has prescribed Bactrim (trimethoprim and sulfamethoxazole) to stop the infection. You know that trimethoprim and sulfamethoxazole is classified as a(n):

   _____

7. Alicia Montoya suffers from asthma. Her physician has prescribed Bronkodyl (theophylline), a medication given to expand the bronchial tubes, to relieve her symptoms. You know that theophylline is classified as a(n):

   _____

8. Helen Bell has experienced a good bit of swelling in her legs lately. Her physician has prescribed Lasix (furosemide), a medication used to increase urine secretion, in hopes of relieving the edema in her legs. You know that furosemide is classified as a(n):

   _____

9. Jennifer Allran is preparing for her final exams in nursing school. She has not felt well for the past two days and is experiencing stomach cramps and nausea. Her physician states that she has a virus. He has prescribed medication for the stomach cramps and Bonine (meclizine hydrochloride) to relieve the nausea. You know that meclizine hydrochloride is classified as a(n):

   _____

10. Matt King went to the dentist today to have a filling replaced. His dentist used Xylocaine (lidocaine) to completely numb the tooth before replacing the filling. You know that lidocaine is classified as a(n):

    _____

Number correct _____ × *10 points/correct answer: Your score* _____ %

Bonus points for answering all questions without assistance: _____

Your score + bonus points: Grand total _____ %

F. Definition to Term

Using the word definitions in each statement, identify and provide the appropriate medical term to match the definition. Each correct response is worth 10 points. When you complete the exercise, record your score in the space provided at the end of the exercise.

1. Without sensitivity to pain (adjective):

   _____

2. Treatment with drugs:

   _____

3. Within the skin (adjective):

   _____

4. Without sensation or feeling:

   _____

5. Pertaining to the rectum (adjective):

   _____

6. The study of drugs:

   _____

7. Under the tongue (adjective):

   _____

8. The study of poisons:

   _____

9. Within the vein (adjective):

   _____

10. One who is licensed to dispense drugs:

   _____

Number correct _____ **× 10 points/correct answer: Your score** _____ **%**

G. Matching

Match the abbreviations on the left with the appropriate definition on the right. Each correct answer is worth 5 points. Record your score in the space provided at the end of the exercise.

_____	1. a.c.	a. ounce
_____	2. b.i.d.	b. rectal
_____	3. c̄	c. three times a day
_____	4. gm, g	d. as desired
_____	5. gr	e. quantity sufficient
_____	6. gtt	f. after meals
_____	7. ID	g. ointment
_____	8. IM	h. milliequivalent
_____	9. ml	i. intradermal
_____	10. mEq	j. drop

(*continued*)

_____ 11. NPO   k. gram

_____ 12. ung   l. twice a day

_____ 13. p̄   m. before meals

_____ 14. p.c.   n. with

_____ 15. p.r.n.   o. grain

_____ 16. q.s.   p. intramuscular

_____ 17. R$_x$ q. milliliter

_____ 18. ad. lib.   r. nothing by mouth

_____ 19. stat.   s. after

_____ 20. t.i.d.   t. as needed

                                      u. take

                                      v. immediately

                                      w. tablet

                                      x. every night

Number correct _____ × *5 points/correct answer: Your score* _____ %

H. Word Search

Read each definition carefully and identify the applicable word from the list that follows. Enter the word in the space provided and then find it in the puzzle and circle it. The words may be read up, down, diagonally, across, or backward. Each correct answer is worth 10 points. Record your score in the space provided at the end of the exercise.

local	action	adverse
systemic	side	cumulation
idiosyncrasy	tolerance	contraindication
potentiation	desired	

Example: A drug effect confined to a specific part of the body is known as a _____*local*_____ effect.

1. Drug _____ is defined as how the drugs produce changes within the body.

2. The _____ effect is when a drug achieves the response in the body that is intended.

3. A _____ effect is when a medication has a widespread influence on the body because it is absorbed into the bloodstream.

4. An _____ reaction is one in which the body reacts to a drug in an unexpected way that may endanger a patient's health and safety.

5. A _____ is a special symptom or circumstance that indicates that the use of a particular drug is dangerous.

6. A _____ effect is an additional effect on the body by the drug that was not part of the goal for that medication.

7. _____ occurs when a drug is not completely excreted from the body before another dose is given and the drug starts to accumulate within the body tissues with each successive dose.

8. _____ is an unusual, inappropriate response to a drug or to the usual effective dose of a drug.

9. _____ occurs when two drugs administered together produce a more powerful response than the sum of their individual effects.

10. _____ is the resistance to the effect of a drug. (The individual requires increasing doses to achieve the full effect of the drug.)

```
B  R  P  O  N  C  H  S  Y  S  T  E  M  I  C  B  R  E  A  T  H  I
A  N  A  O  G  E  S  I  C  A  N  E  S  T  H  E  T  I  C  R  A  D
M  I  C  K  T  M  N  M  E  T (L  O  C  A  L) N  O  T  O  M  E  I
C  A  R  V  E  E  O  O  S  D  I  A  C  B  A  C  R  F  E  S  R  O
I  L  E  T  Y  T  N  L  I  E  O  Y  N  T  I  C  H  A  I  Y  I  S
M  U  C  O  I  O  T  T  O  T  E  B  R  L  N  E  E  R  R  O  N  Y
L  R  O  T  H  L  O  E  I  U  A  S  C  O  A  S  E  I  D  R  T  N
P  U  D  L  M  E  I  D  N  A  U  L  I  R  R  D  I  B  I  C  R  C
L  E  U  V  D  R  N  I  A  C  T  Y  U  E  N  O  M  L  U  P  H  R
S  A  C  U  D  A  D  S  O  D  E  I  V  M  A  C  T  I  O  N  B  A
L  A  C  I  G  N  L  E  R  U  E  D  O  R  U  Q  W  E  A  R  Y  S
N  O  I  T  A  C  I  D  N  I  A  R  T  N  O  C  V  E  N  O  U  Y
B  U  T  T  E  E  R  U  M  A  I  D  I  S  G  O  O  D  Y  E  S  E
```

© Cengage Learning®.

Number correct _____ × *10 points/correct answer: Your score* _____%

I. Terms to Definition

Define the following drug classification terms. Where possible, break the word down into its word elements in the space provided. Each correct definition is worth 10 points and each correct "breakdown" of the word is worth 10 points. When you have completed the exercise, record your score in the space provided at the end of the exercise.

Term: analgesic

1. Definition: _____

2. Breakdown: _____ / _____ / _____
     (prefix)   (word root)   (suffix)

Term: antiarrhythmic

3. Definition: _____

4. Breakdown: _____ / _____ / _____
     (prefix)   (word root)   (suffix)

Term: anticonvulsant

5. Definition _____

Term: antidepressant

6. Definition: _____

Term: antifungal

7. Definition: _____

8. Breakdown: _____ / _____ / _____
     (prefix)   (word root)   (suffix)

(continued)

Term: antineoplastic

9. Definition: _____

10. Breakdown:_____ /_____ /_____ /_____

                    (prefix)   (prefix)   (word root)   (suffix)

Number correct _____ *× 10 points/correct answer: Your score* _____ *%*

J. Interpret the Doctor's Orders

The following is an example of some written orders that may be seen on a prescription or may have to be called in to the hospital for the physician. Read each order carefully in its abbreviated form and then write the definition for each abbreviation in the space provided. Each correct response is worth 10 points. Record your score in the space provided when you have completed the exercise.

1. Physician's order: Give Tylenol, gr. X for T. above 101 degrees F.

    a. gr. X _____

    b. T _____

    c. F _____

2. Physician's order: Seconal 100 mg at bedtime. for sleep, prn.

    a. 100 mg _____

    b. prn _____

3. Physician's order: Normal saline solution 0.5% IV × 8 hr.

    a. IV _____

    b. × _____

    c. hr _____

4. Physician's order: Glucophage, one tablet p.o., b.i.d.

    a. p.o. _____

    b. b.i.d _____

Number correct _____ *× 10 points/correct answer: Your score* _____ *%*

K. Medical Scenario

The following medical scenario presents information on one of the routes of administration for medications discussed in this chapter. Read the scenario carefully and select the most appropriate answer for each question that follows. Each correct answer is worth 20 points. Record your score in the space provided at the end of the exercise.

Sandra Lovelace, 63 years old, is a patient of the cardiologist Dr. Baldwin. She has been diagnosed with coronary artery disease. Dr. Baldwin has prescribed *Nitroderm* patches for her to use daily. The health care professional will teach Mr. and Mrs. Lovelace the correct usage of these transdermal patches.

1. The health care professional will describe to Mrs. Lovelace that transdermal administration of medications is the administration of:

    a. a small amount of medication injected just beneath the epidermis

    b. a parenteral medication placed inside the cheek or under the tongue

    c. a medication injected directly into the subcutaneous layer, or fatty tissue, of the skin and producing a local effect

    d. a medication applied to unbroken skin, using an adhesive-backed disk whereby the drug is absorbed continuously and produces a systemic effect

2. The health care professional will explain to Mrs. Lovelace that the transdermal medication will be:

   a. premeasured on the disk she receives from the pharmacy

   b. measured in a syringe that the health care professional will provide her with today

   c. measured by the amount of chest pain she has had the day before

   d. premeasured in a syringe she receives from the pharmacy

3. Mrs. Lovelace explains that her husband will administer the transdermal medication each day. The health care professional will instruct Mr. Lovelace to always:

   a. hold the syringe at a 10-degree angle prior to injecting the bubble

   b. place the medication under her tongue and remind her not to swallow until it is dissolved

   c. place a glove on the hand used to remove the old patch and apply the new patch

   d. put on gloves prior to removing the medication from the syringe and applying it to the skin

4. The health care professional talks to the Lovelaces about their young grandchildren and their dog Oscar. She will explain that if the children or the dog come in contact with the transdermal patch:

   a. it will not be a problem because it cannot be transferred to another living being

   b. it should be discarded and another one applied so that she will not miss any medication

   c. it is dangerous because the medication from the patch can be absorbed into the skin of children or animals from the skin of the client

   d. the child or dog would have to have the medication actually injected into them for the medication to harm them

5. The health care professional also explained to Mrs. Lovelace that one of the advantages of using the transdermal patch delivery system for medication is that it is:

   a. a good method of administering medications that need to be released slowly into the bloodstream over a period of time

   b. a good method of administering medications into the bloodstream immediately

   c. not a problem if the patch comes in contact with the skin when it is removed

   d. guaranteed that immediate stoppage of absorption of the medication will occur with removal of the patch in the case of an adverse reaction

Number correct _____ × *20 points/correct answer: Your score* _____ **%**

CHAPTER 23

Mental Health

CHAPTER CONTENT

OBJECTIVES

Upon completing this chapter and the review exercises at the end of the chapter, the learner should be able to:

1. Correctly spell and pronounce terms listed on the Written and Audio Terminology Review, using the phonetic pronunciations provided.

2. List and define 10 defense mechanisms studied in this chapter.

3. List and define at least five phobias studied in this chapter.

4. List and define at least 20 mental disorders discussed in this chapter.

5. Identify at least 10 abbreviations common to mental health.

6. Identify 10 treatments, therapies, and tests used in the practice of mental health.

Overview

Physical symptoms have been first and foremost in the previous chapters of this textbook as we have discussed the various pathological conditions of each body system. We now turn from the physical to the study of psychological symptoms that often affect the physical condition of the patient. A general discussion of defense mechanisms, phobias, **mental** disorders, and therapeutic treatments is included in this chapter. The topics of discussion are alphabetized under each category heading.

Mental health is a relative state of mind in which the person who is healthy is able to cope with and adjust to the recurrent stresses of everyday living in an acceptable way. **Mental** disorders are disturbances of emotional stability as manifested in maladaptive behavior and impaired functioning. This may be caused by genetic, physical, chemical, biological, psychological, or social and cultural factors. A **mental** disorder may be referred to as **mental** illness, emotional illness, or psychiatric disorder.

Many of us use **defense mechanisms** on a normal day-to-day basis when dealing with areas of conflict in our lives. It is when the defense mechanisms become a way of dealing with life that they may be indicative of the need for psychological or psychiatric help.

Psychology is the study of behavior and the processes of the mind, especially as they relate to the individual's social and physical environment. A **psychologist** is a professional who specializes in the study of the structure and function of the brain and related **mental** processes. A **psychologist** is not a physician but one who earns either a master's or doctoral degree in some area of **psychology**. A **clinical psychologist** provides testing and counseling services to patients with **mental** and emotional disorders. **Psychiatry** is the branch of medicine that deals with the causes, treatment, and prevention of **mental**, emotional, and behavioral disorders. A **psychiatrist** is a medical doctor who specializes in diagnosing, preventing, and treating **mental** disorders—an educational process that involves several additional years beyond medical school. Psychiatrists may specialize in various areas of practice in the field of **psychiatry**. If a **psychiatrist** chooses to specialize in **psychoanalysis**, he or she would be known as a **psychoanalyst** and would complete additional special training in psychotherapeutic techniques. **Psychoanalysis** involves the use of **free association**, dream interpretation, and the analysis of defense mechanisms. The **psychoanalyst** applies the techniques of psychoanalytic theory to help the patient become aware of repressed emotional conflicts and seeks ways to help the individual to bring the conflicts to a conscious level so that they can be resolved.

Defense Mechanisms

The body's unconscious reaction used to protect itself from conflicts or anxieties is known as a **defense mechanism**. There is, however, one conscious **defense mechanism** (**sublimation**), included in this section. Some defense mechanisms are designed to lessen or deal with **anxiety** or conflict, allowing normal function to continue. Others are designed to conceal the **anxiety** or conflict.

The following is an alphabetical listing and a general discussion of some of the more commonly used defense mechanisms, with an example of each. Keep in mind that each of these defense mechanisms operates on an unconscious level.

compensation (kom-pen-**SAY**-shun)	**Compensation** is an effort to overcome, or make up for, real or imagined inadequacies. An individual may compensate for a deficiency in physical size by excelling in academics.
denial (dee-**NYE**-al)	**Denial** is a refusal to admit or acknowledge the reality of something, thus avoiding emotional conflict or **anxiety**. A child may deny that he or she is being abused by a parent.
displacement (dis-**PLACE**-ment)	**Displacement** is the process of transferring a feeling or emotion from the original idea or object to a substitute idea or object. An individual is angry at the "boss" and cannot express that anger. The feelings are displaced by criticizing everyone else.
introjection (in-troh-**JEK**-shun)	An ego **defense mechanism** whereby an individual unconsciously identifies with another person or with some object. The individual assumes the supposed feelings and/or characteristics of the other personality or object. A child develops his or her conscience by internalizing what the parents believe is right and wrong. The child may say to a friend while playing, "Don't hit people. Nice people don't do that."
projection (proh-**JEK**-shun)	**Projection** is the act of transferring one's own unacceptable thoughts or feelings to someone else. A worker who dislikes his or her boss accuses the boss of disliking him or her.
rationalization (rash-un-al-ih-**ZAY**-shun)	**Rationalization** is attempting to make excuses or invent logical reasons to justify unacceptable feelings or behaviors. A student may rationalize that he or she failed a test because the questions were too confusing.
regression (rih-**GRESH**-un)	**Regression** is a response to stress in which the individual reverts to an earlier level of development and the comfort measures associated with that level of functioning. A child may regress to an earlier stage of development, such as bedwetting, when confronted with a stress in his or her life (such as a new baby in the family).
repression (rih-**PRESH**-un)	**Repression** is an involuntary blocking of unpleasant feelings and experiences from one's conscious mind. An individual involved in a tragic automobile accident may have no memory of the sequence of events.

sublimation (sub-lih-**MAY**-shun)	Rechanneling or redirecting one's unacceptable impulses and drives into constructive activities.
	Sublimation is a conscious **defense mechanism**. The positive aspect of **sublimation** is that the individual participates in constructive activities. Parents of children who were victimized by violence may redirect their expected anger and outrage into working with other victims of violent crimes.
suppression (suh-**PRESH**-un)	**Suppression** is the voluntary blocking of unpleasant feelings and experiences from one's mind.
	An individual faced with a frustrating or painful situation may consciously choose not to confront the situation.

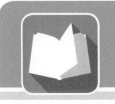

Review Checkpoint

Apply what you have learned in this chapter by completing the **Defense Mechanisms** exercise in your workbook.

VOCABULARY

The following vocabulary words are frequently used when discussing mental health.

Word	Definition
affect (**AFF**-fekt)	Observable evidence of a person's feelings or emotions.
amnesia (am-**NEE**-zee-ah)	Loss of memory caused by severe emotional trauma, brain injury, substance abuse, or reaction to medications or toxins.
amphetamines (am-**FET**-ah-meenz)	A group of nervous system stimulants that produce alertness and a feeling of well-being (**euphoria**).

anorexia
(an-oh-**REK**-see-ah)
  an- = without
  -orexia = appetite
	Lack of or loss of appetite, resulting in the inability to eat.

anorexia nervosa (an-oh-**REK**-see-ah ner-**VOH**-suh)	A disorder (seen primarily in adolescent girls) characterized by an emotional disturbance concerning body image; prolonged refusal to eat followed by extreme weight loss; amenorrhea; and a lingering, abnormal fear of becoming obese.

Word	Definition
anxiety (**ang-ZYE**-eh-tee)	A state of mind in which the individual feels increased tension, apprehension, a painfully increased sense of helplessness, a feeling of uncertainty, fear, jitteriness, and worry. Observable signs of **anxiety** include (but are not limited to) restlessness, poor eye contact, glancing about, facial tension, dilated pupils, increased perspiration, and a constant focus on self.
anxiety disorders	Disorders characterized by chronic worry.
apathy (**AP**-ah-thee)	Absence or **suppression** of observable emotion, feeling, concern, or passion.
autism (**AW**-tizm) aut/o = self -ism = condition	A pervasive developmental disorder characterized by the individual being extremely withdrawn and absorbed with fantasy. The individual suffers from impaired communication/social interaction skills, and activities and interests are very limited. Autism was first classified as a type of schizophrenia. (Autism is discussed in Chapter 19.)
behavior therapy	A form of **psychotherapy** that seeks to modify observable maladjusted patterns of behavior by substituting new responses to given stimuli.
bulimia nervosa (boo-**LIM**-ee-ah)	An uncontrolled craving for food, often resulting in eating binges, followed by vomiting to eliminate the food from the stomach. The individual may then feel depressed and go through a period of self-deprivation followed by another eating binge, and the cycle continues.
cannabis (**CAN**-ah-bis)	A mind-altering drug derived from the flowering top of hemp plants; also called **marijuana**. This drug is classified as a controlled substance, Schedule I drug.
cataplexy (**CAT**-ah-pleks-ee)	A sudden loss of muscle tone in which the individual's head may drop, the jaw may sag, the knees become weakened, and the individual may collapse or fall to the ground; may accompany a **narcolepsy** attack (sudden, uncontrollable attack of sleep).
compensation (kom-pen-**SAY**-shun)	An effort to overcome, or make up for, real or imagined inadequacies.
compulsions (kom-**PUHL**-shuns)	Irresistible, repetitive, irrational impulses to perform an act. These behavior patterns are intended to reduce **anxiety**, not provide pleasure or gratification.
conversion disorder (kon-**VER**-zhun)	A disorder in which the individual represses **anxiety** experienced by emotional conflicts by converting the anxious feelings into physical symptoms that have no organic basis but are perceived to be real by the individual. The individual may experience symptoms such as paralysis, pain, loss of sensation, or some other form of dysfunction of the nervous system; also called conversion hysteria.
cyclothymic disorder (sigh-cloh-**THIGH**-mic)	A chronic (of long duration) mood disorder characterized by numerous periods of mood swings from **depression** to happiness. The period of mood disturbance is at least two years.

Word	Definition
defense mechanism	An unconscious, intrapsychic (within one's mind) reaction that offers protection to the self from a stressful situation.
delirium (dee-**LEER**-ee-um)	A state of frenzied excitement or wild enthusiasm.
delirium tremens (DTs) (dee-**LEER**-ee-um **TREE**-menz)	An acute and sometimes fatal psychotic reaction caused by cessation of excessive intake of alcoholic beverages over a long period of time.
delusion (dee-**LOO**-zhun)	A persistent, abnormal belief or perception held firmly by a person despite evidence to the contrary. Two forms of delusions are delusions of persecution (in which the person thinks others are following him, spying on him, or trying to torment him) and delusions of grandeur, in which the person has a false sense of possessing wealth or power.
dementia (dee-**MEN**-shee-ah)	A progressive, **organic mental disorder** characterized by chronic personality disintegration, confusion, disorientation, stupor, deterioration of intellectual capacity and function, and impairment of control of memory, judgment, and impulses.
denial	A refusal to admit or acknowledge the reality of something, thus avoiding emotional conflict or **anxiety**.
depression	A mood disturbance characterized by exaggerated feelings of sadness, discouragement, and hopelessness that are inappropriate and out of proportion with reality; may be relative to some personal loss or tragedy.
displacement (dis-**PLACE**-ment)	The process of transferring a feeling or emotion from the original idea or object to a substitute idea or object.
dissociation (dis-**soh**-shee-**AY**-shun)	An unconscious **defense mechanism** by which an idea, thought, emotion, or other **mental** process is separated from the consciousness and thereby loses emotional significance.
drug therapy	The use of **psychotropic** drugs to treat **mental** disorders.
dysphoria (dis-**FOH**-ree-ah) dys- = bad, difficult, painful, disordered -phoria = emotional state	A disorder of **affect** (mood) characterized by **depression** and anguish.
electroconvulsive therapy (ECT)	The process of passing an electrical current through the brain to create a brief seizure in the brain.
euphoria (yoo-**FOR**-ee-ah) eu- = well, easily, good, normal -phoria = emotional state	A sense of well-being or elation.
exhibitionism	A sexual disorder involving the exposure of one's genitals to a stranger.

Word	Definition
factitious disorders	Disorders that are characterized by physical or psychological symptoms that are intentionally produced or feigned to assume the sick role.
family therapy	A form of **psychotherapy** that focuses the treatment on the process between family members that supports and sustains symptoms.
free association	The spontaneous, consciously unrestricted association of ideas, feelings, or **mental** images.
frotteurism	A sexual disorder in which the person gains sexual stimulation or excitement by rubbing against a nonconsenting person.
group therapy	The application of psychotherapeutic techniques within a small group of people who experience similar difficulties.
hallucination (hah-**loo**-sih-**NAY**-shun)	A subjective (existing in the mind) perception of something that does not exist in the external environment. Hallucinations may be visual, olfactory (smell), gustatory, (taste), tactile (touch), or auditory (hearing).
hallucinogens (hah-**LOO**-sih-noh-**jenz**)	Substances that cause excitation of the central nervous system, characterized by symptoms such as hallucinations, mood changes, **anxiety**, increased pulse and blood pressure, and dilation of the pupils.
hypnosis	A passive, trancelike state of existence that resembles normal sleep, during which perception and memory are altered, resulting in increased responsiveness to suggestion.
hypochondriasis (**high**-poh-kon-**DRY**-ah-sis)	A chronic, abnormal concern about the health of the body, characterized by extreme **anxiety**, **depression**, and an unrealistic interpretation of real or imagined physical symptoms as indications of a serious illness or disease despite rational medical evidence that no disorder is present. A person affected by **hypochondriasis** is referred to as a hypochondriac.
hypomania (**high**-poh-**MAY**-nee-ah) hypo- = under, below, beneath, less than normal -mania = madness	A mild degree of **mania** characterized by optimism, excitability, energetic and productive behavior, marked hyperactivity and talkativeness, heightened sexual interest, quickness to anger, irritability, and a decreased need for sleep.
intoxication (in-**toks**-ih-**KAY**-shun)	A state of being characterized by impaired judgment, slurred speech, loss of coordination, irritability, and mood changes; may be due to drugs, including alcohol.
introjection	An ego **defense mechanism** whereby an individual unconsciously identifies with another person or with some object, assuming the supposed feelings and/or characteristics of the other personality or object.
lithium (**LITH**-ee-um)	A drug that is particularly useful in treating the manic phase of **bipolar disorders** (manic-depressive disorders).

Word	Definition
major depressive disorder	A disorder characterized by one or more episodes of depressed mood that lasts at least two weeks and is accompanied by at least four additional symptoms of **depression**.
malingering (mah-**LING**-er-ing)	A willful and deliberate faking of symptoms of a disease or injury to gain some consciously desired end.
mania (**MAY**-nee-ah)	"Madness"; an unstable emotional state characterized by symptoms such as extreme excitement, hyperactivity, overtalkativeness, agitation, flight of ideas, fleeting attention, and sometimes violent, destructive, and self-destructive behavior.
marijuana	See **cannabis**.
mood disorders	An affective state characterized by any of a variety of periods of **depression** or **depression** elation.
mutism (**mew**-tizm)	The inability to speak because of a physical defect or emotional problem.

neurosis (noo-**ROH**-sis)
  neur/o = nerve
  -osis = condition
	A psychological or behavioral disorder in which **anxiety** is the primary characteristic; thought to be related to unresolved conflicts.

obsession (ob-**SESS**-shun)	A persistent thought or idea with which the mind is continually and involuntarily preoccupied.
panic attack	An episode of acute **anxiety** during which the individual may experience intense feelings of uneasiness or fright accompanied by dyspnea, dizziness, sweating, trembling, and palpitations of the heart. Panic attacks, which occur unexpectedly, may last a few minutes and may return.
panic disorder	A disorder characterized by recurrent panic attacks that come on unexpectedly.
paranoia (pair-ah-**NOY**-ah)	A **mental** disorder characterized by an elaborate, overly suspicious system of thinking, with delusions of persecution and grandeur usually centered on one major theme (such as a financial matter, a job situation, an unfaithful spouse, or other problem).

paraphilia (**pair**-ah-**FILL**-ee-ah)
  para- = near, beside, beyond, two like parts
  -philia = attraction to
	Sexual perversion or deviation; a condition in which the sexual instinct is expressed in ways that are socially prohibited, unacceptable, or biologically undesirable.

pedophilia (**ped**-oh-**FILL**-ee-ah)
  ped/o = child
  -philia = attraction to
	A sexual disorder in which the individual is sexually aroused and engages in sexual activity with children (generally age 13 or younger).

Word	Definition
personality disorders	Any of a large group of **mental** disorders characterized by rigid, inflexible, and maladaptive behavior patterns that impair a person's ability to function in society by severely limiting adaptive potential.
phobia (**FOH**-bee-ah)	An **anxiety** disorder characterized by an obsessive, irrational, and intense fear of a specific object, of an activity, or of a physical situation. Phobias are usually characterized by symptoms such as faintness, fatigue, palpitations, perspiration, nausea, tremor, and panic.
pica (**PYE**-kah)	**Pica** is an eating disorder characterized by a craving to eat nonfood substances such as chalk, charcoal, clay, dirt, glue, hair, ice, paint, paper, soap, or starch over a period of at least one month. This disorder may occur with pregnancy or as a result of some nutritional deficiency (for example, iron deficiency). **Pica** can usually be distinguished from the other eating disorders by the consumption of nonnutritive, nonfood substances.
play therapy	A form of **psychotherapy** in which a child plays in a protected and structured environment with games and toys provided by a therapist.
projection (proh-**JEK**-shun)	The act of transferring one's own unacceptable thoughts or feelings to someone else.
psychiatrist (sigh-**KIGH**-ah-trist) psych/o = mind, soul -iatrist = one who treats; a physician	A physician who specializes in the diagnosis, prevention, and treatment of **mental** disorders.
psychiatry (sigh-**KIGH**-ah-tree) psych/o = mind, soul -iatry = medical treatment, medical profession	The branch of medicine that deals with the causes, treatment, and prevention of **mental**, emotional, and behavioral disorders.
psychoanalysis (**sigh**-koh-an-**NAL**-ih-sis)	A form of **psychotherapy** that uses **free association**, dream interpretation, and analysis of defense mechanisms to help the patient become aware of repressed emotional conflicts.
psychoanalyst (**sigh**-koh-**AN**-ah-list)	A psychotherapist, usually a **psychiatrist**, who has had special training in **psychoanalysis** and who applies the techniques of psychoanalytic theory.
psychodrama (sigh-koh-**DRAH**-mah)	A form of group **psychotherapy** in which people act out their emotional problems through unrehearsed dramatizations; also called role-playing therapy.
psychologist (sigh-**KOL**-oh-jist) psych/o = mind, soul -logist = one who specializes in the study of	A person who specializes in the study of the structure and function of the brain and related **mental** processes of animals and humans. A clinical **psychologist** has a graduate degree with specialized training in providing testing and counseling to patients with **mental** and emotional disorders.

Word	Definition

psychology
(sigh-**KOL**-oh-jee)
  psych/o = mind, soul
  -logy = the study of
	The study of behavior and the processes of the mind, especially as it relates to the individual's social and physical environment.

psychosis
(sigh-**KOH**-sis)
  psych/o = mind, soul
  -osis = condition
	Any major **mental** disorder of organic or emotional origin characterized by a loss of contact with reality.

psychosomatic
(**sigh**-koh-soh-**MAT**-ik)
  psych/o = mind, soul
  somat/o = body
  -ic = pertaining to
	Pertaining to the expression of an emotional conflict through physical symptoms.

psychotherapy
(sigh-koh-**THAIR**-ah-pee)
  psych/o = mind, soul
  -therapy = treatment
	Any of a large number of related methods of treating **mental** and emotional disorders by using psychological techniques instead of physical means of treatment.

psychotropic (sigh-koh-**TROH**-pik)	Any substance capable of affecting the mind, emotions, and behavior; drugs used in the treatment of **mental** illness.
purging (**PERJ**-ing)	The means of ridding the body of what has been consumed; that is, the individual may induce vomiting or use laxatives to rid the body of food that has just been eaten.
rationalization (**rash**-un-al-ih-**ZAY**-shun)	Attempting to make excuses or invent logical reasons to justify unacceptable feelings or behaviors; most commonly used **defense mechanism**.
regression (rih-**GRESH**-un)	A response to stress in which the individual reverts to an earlier level of development and the comfort measures associated with that level of functioning.
repression (rih-**PRESH**-un)	An involuntary blocking of unpleasant feelings and experiences from one's conscious mind.

schizophrenia
(skiz-oh-**FREN**-ee-ah)
  schiz/o = split
  phren/o = mind; also refers to
         the diaphragm
  -ia = condition
	Any of a large group of psychotic disorders characterized by gross distortion of reality, disturbances of language and communication, withdrawal from social interaction, and the disorganization and fragmentation of thought, perception, and emotional reaction.

sedative	An agent that decreases functional activity and has a calming effect on the body.

Word	Definition
senile dementia (**SEE**-nile dee-**MEN**-shee-ah)	An **organic mental disorder** of the aged, resulting from the generalized atrophy (wasting) of the brain with no evidence of cerebrovascular disease. This condition is characterized by loss of memory, impaired judgment, decreased moral and ethical values, inability to think abstractly, and periods of confusion and irritability. These symptoms may range from mild to severe.
sexual sadism/sexual masochism	A sexual disorder that involves the act (real, not simulated) of being humiliated, beaten, bound, or otherwise made to suffer; or the act of inflicting psychological or physical suffering on the victim.
somatic disorders (soh-**MAT**-oh-form)	Any group of neurotic disorders characterized by symptoms suggesting physical illness or disease for which there are no demonstrable organic causes or physiologic dysfunctions.
sublimation (sub-lih-**MAY**-shun)	Rechanneling or redirecting one's unacceptable impulses and drives into constructive activities.
suppression (suh-**PRESH**-un)	The voluntary blocking of unpleasant feelings and experiences from one's mind.
tolerance (**TAHL**-er-ans)	The ability to endure unusually large doses of a drug without apparent adverse effects and, with continued use of the drug, to require increased dosages to produce the same effect.

Review Checkpoint

Check your understanding of this section by completing the **Vocabulary** exercises in your workbook.

WORD ELEMENTS

The following word elements pertain to the specialty of mental health. As you review the list, pronounce each word element aloud twice and check the box after you "say it." Write the definition for the example term given for each word element. Use your medical dictionary to find the definitions of the example terms.

Word Element	Pronunciation	"Say It"	Meaning
aut/o **aut**ism	**AW**-toh **AW**-tizm	☐	self
cata- **cata**tonia	**KAT**-ah kat-ah-**TOH**-nee-ah	☐	down, under, against, lower

Word Element	Pronunciation	"Say It"	Meaning
hypn/o **hypn**otize	**HIP**-noh **HIP**-noh-tize	☐	sleep
-iatrist, iatr/o psych**iatrist**	**EYE**-ah-trist, **EYE**-ah-troh sigh-**KIGH**-ah-trist	☐	one who treats; a physician
-mania klepto**mania**	**MAY**-nee-ah **klep**-toh-**MAY**-nee-ah	☐	a **mental** disorder; a "madness"
ment/o **ment**al	**MEN**-toh **MEN**-tal	☐	mind
neur/o psycho**neur**osis	**NOO**-roh **sigh**-koh-noo-**ROH**-sis	☐	nerves
-philia necro**philia**	**FILL**-ee-ah nek-roh-**FILL**-ee-ah	☐	attraction to
-phobia claustro**phobia**	**FOH**-bee-ah **klaws**-troh-**FOH**-bee-ah	☐	abnormal fear
-phoria eu**phoria**	**FOR**-ee-ah yoo-**FOR**-ee-ah	☐	emotional state
phren/o schizo**phren**ia	**FREN**-oh **skiz**-oh-**FREN**-ee-ah	☐	mind
psych/o **psych**osis	**SIGH**-koh sigh-**KOH**-sis	☐	mind
schiz/o **schiz**oid	**SKIZ**-oh **SKIZ**-oyd	☐	split
somat/o psycho**somat**ic disorder	soh-**MAT**-oh **sigh**-koh-soh-**MAT**-ik dis-**OR**-der	☐	body
-thymia cyclo**thymia**	**THIGH**-mee-ah **sigh**-kloh-**THIGH**-mee-ah	☐	condition of the mind or will

Review Checkpoint

Check your understanding of this section by completing the **Word Elements** exercises in your workbook.

Mental Disorders

The *Diagnostic and Statistical Manual of Mental Disorders* is the principal guide for mental health professionals today and serves as a universal authority for the diagnosis of psychiatric disorders. While the *DSM-5* was officially released in May 2013, it is not expected to be fully implemented until October 1, 2015. Effective on that date, the United States will begin using the *ICD-10* diagnostic coding system as a common nomenclature in all health care transactions. The *ICD-10* codes have been incorporated into the *DSM-5* and will thus make the simultaneous transition to both of these systems much easier for clinicians.

The *DSM-5* contains several major changes from the previous edition (*DSM-IV-TR*), including the removal of the multiaxial system, an expansion of the assessment of disability and functioning, and changes to disorders to include removals, additions, and revisions of diagnostic criteria. The scope of these changes are too broad to cover in this chapter but may be reviewed at http://www.DSM-5.org or through the American Psychiatric Association's website at http://www.psychiatry.org.

The disorders presented in this chapter in no way reflect the depth of the material covered in the *DSM-5*. The discussion of **mental** disorders will be limited to the following topics:

- Cognitive disorders
- Substance-related disorders
- **Schizophrenia**
- Bipolar and related disorders
- Depressive disorders
- Anxiety disorders
- Somatic symptom, sleep, and **factitious disorders**
- Sleep-wake disorders
- Dissociative identity disorders
- Paraphilic disorders
- Eating disorders
- **Personality disorders**
- Neurodevelopmental disorders

Cognitive Disorders

Cognitive disorders are those that affect the individual's ability to perceive, think, reason, and remember. The following cognitive disorders deal with a deficiency in memory. They may also be termed *organic* **mental** disorders. The incidence of these disorders, which may be related to the aging of the brain or to the body's reaction to the ingestion of a substance, is increasing and is expected to continue increasing in this century.

amnesia disorders (am-**NEE**-zee-ah)	**Amnesia disorders**, or amnestic disorders, are characterized by short-term and long-term memory deficits.

These individuals have normal attention but are unable to learn new information (short-term memory) and are unable to recall previously learned information (long-term memory). Individuals with **amnesia** are able to remember things from the distant past easier than things from the recent past. These individuals have no personality change, no impairment in judgment, and no impairment in abstract thinking.

Causes of amnestic disorders include, but are not limited to, medical conditions such as head injury, cerebrovascular disease, poorly controlled insulin-dependent diabetes mellitus, substance abuse, reaction to medications, and exposure to toxins. Treatment is directed at the underlying cause.

delirium (dee-**LEER**-ee-um)	A **delirium** is a state of frenzied excitement. It occurs rapidly and is characterized by difficulty maintaining and shifting attention.

The individual is easily distracted and must be constantly reminded to focus attention. Thinking is disorganized and speech is irrelevant, rambling, and sometimes incoherent. The individual is disoriented to time and place and has lost the ability to reason.

Causes of **delirium** include (but are not limited to) medical conditions such as systemic infections, severe hypoglycemia, injury to the head, substance abuse, and withdrawal from certain substances. One particular type of **delirium** is **delirium tremens (DTs)**, an acute and sometimes fatal psychotic reaction caused by cessation of excessive intake of alcoholic beverages over a long period of time. The duration of **delirium** is usually short term and subsides completely after treating the underlying cause.

dementia (dee-**MEN**-shee-ah)	**Dementia** is a progressive, **organic mental disorder** characterized by chronic personality disintegration, confusion, disorientation, stupor, deterioration of intellectual capacity and function, and impairment of control of memory, judgment, and impulses.

Dementia of the Alzheimer's type is the most common form of **dementia**. The onset of symptoms is slow and not easily detected at first, with the course of the disorder becoming progressive and deteriorating. If the onset is early, the symptoms will appear before the age of 65. If the onset is late, the symptoms will appear after the age of 65. A definitive diagnosis of Alzheimer's disease is not possible until death because biopsy or autopsy examination of the brain tissue is required for a diagnosis.

However, the symptoms of **dementia** of the Alzheimer's type may begin as forgetfulness, followed by the individual becoming suspicious of others as his or her memory deteriorates. The individual may become apathetic and socially withdrawn or more untidy in appearance. Irritability, moodiness, and sudden outbursts over trivial issues may become apparent. These individuals may wander away from home, forgetting where they are and where they live. As the condition progresses, the ability to work or care for personal needs independently is no longer possible and the individual requires supervised care.

Substance-Related Disorders

Substance-related disorders are divided into two groups: substance-use disorders and substance-induced disorders (*DSM-5*, 2013, p. 481). This section concentrates on substance-use disorders. Characteristics include psychological dependence on the substance, daily use, frequent **intoxication** by the ingestion of the substance and an inability to control use of the substance. Physical dependence on the substance involves serious withdrawal problems if use of the substance is stopped. The following drugs are involved in most of the substance-related disorders.

- Central nervous system depressants: substances that slow the activity of the central nervous system, causing impaired motor activity, judgment, and concentration. Examples of central nervous system depressants are alcohol, barbiturates, and opium derivatives.

- Central nervous system stimulants: substances that increase the activity of the central nervous system, causing an increase in heart rate and blood pressure, heightened behavioral activity, and increased alertness. Examples of central nervous system stimulants are cocaine and amphetamines.

- **Hallucinogens**: substances that create perceptual distortions of the mind. Examples of **hallucinogens** are LSD and **cannabis** (**marijuana**).

The misuse of drugs may lead to a state of **intoxication**, characterized by impaired judgment, slurred speech, loss of coordination, irritability, and mood changes. Continued use of drugs will lead to a pattern of maladaptive behavior and dependence on the drug. The individual develops a pattern of substance abuse in which the drug is used excessively on a regular basis, allowing it to become a major part of his or her life. The drug is used for a nontherapeutic effect. Drug abuse may begin to affect the individual's relationships with family members, friends, and employers.

The continued abuse of the drug will create a physical dependence in which serious withdrawal symptoms would occur if the use of the drug were stopped. Withdrawal symptoms include a physical craving for the drug characterized by muscle aches, cramps, **anxiety**, sweating, and nausea. In addition to the physical dependence, the individual develops a **tolerance** to the drug and requires increasing strengths of the drug with each use to achieve the desired effect. Physical dependence and **tolerance** are classic symptoms of drug addiction.

Individuals who become physically dependent on drugs or alcohol may need to enroll in a detoxification program. This medically supervised treatment program is designed to counteract or destroy toxic properties within the patient. Withdrawal may take several days and may require a week or more of treatment in a medical center. After detoxification, the patient should attend **drug therapy** sessions to learn the steps necessary to remain free of drugs or alcohol.

Schizophrenia

A **psychosis** is described as a condition characterized by loss of contact with reality. The individual's ability to comprehend and react to environmental stimuli becomes impaired and distorted. The impairment can become so severe that the individual may be reduced to limited functioning and may withdraw into a private world. Most commonly, **psychosis** appears in the form of **schizophrenia**.

schizophrenia

(**skiz**-oh-**FREN**-ee-ah)

   schiz/o = split

   phren/o = mind; also refers to
           the diaphragm

   -ia = condition

Any of a large group of psychotic disorders characterized by gross distortion of reality, disturbances of language and communication, withdrawal from social interaction, and the disorganization and fragmentation of thought, perception, and emotional reaction. See *Figure 23-1.*

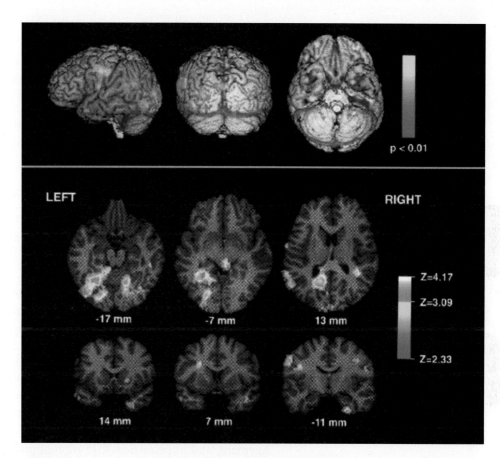

Figure 23-1 Surface and slice images of the brain of a patient with schizophrenia *(Courtesy of D. Silbersweig, M.D., and E. Stern, M.D., Functional Neuroimaging Laboratory, The New York Hospital–Cornell Medical Center. [1995]. In D. Silbersweig, E. Stern, et al., Functional Neuroanatomy of Hallucinations in Schizophrenia. Nature 378 [176–179])*

This complex disorder is diagnosed most frequently in the early 20s for men and the late 20s for women. The diagnosis of **schizophrenia** requires not only the presence of distinct symptoms but the persistence of those symptoms over a period of time; that is, the symptoms must be present for at least six months (with two or more of the characteristic symptoms being present for at least a one-month period during that time frame).

Characteristic symptoms of **schizophrenia** include the following:

1. Hallucinations—in which the person perceives something that does not exist in the external environment. The **hallucination** may be visual, olfactory (smell), gustatory (taste), tactile (touch), or auditory (hearing). The most common form of **hallucination** in **schizophrenia** is hearing voices that are distinct from the person's own thoughts. The voices may be friendly or hostile.

2. Delusions—in which the person firmly holds to a persistent abnormal belief or perception despite evidence to the contrary. Two forms of delusions are delusions of persecution (in which the person believes others are following him, spying on him, or trying to torment him) and delusions of grandeur, in which the person believes that newspaper articles or radio-television stories are about him or her.

3. Disorganized speech—in which the person may move rapidly from one topic to another, making little sense.

4. Disorganized or catatonic (unresponsive) behavior—in which the person may alternate between agitation and nonpurposeful or random body movements to little or no behavioral response to the environment.

5. Flattened **affect**—in which the individual shows little or no emotional response to the environment, that is, diminished emotional expression.

Bipolar and Related Disorders

Bipolar disorders are characterized by disturbances in physical, emotional, and behavioral response patterns. These patterns range from extreme elation and agitation to extreme **depression** with suicidal potential.

bipolar disorders **(manic-depressive)** (by-**POHL**-ar)	A psychological disorder characterized by episodes of **mania** and **depression**, alternations between the two, or a mixture of the two moods simultaneously.
	The **mania** is characterized by extreme excitement, hyperactivity, agitation, overly talkative, flight of ideas, fleeting attention, and sometimes violent, destructive, and self-destructive behavior. The individual may have a decreased need for sleep and seemingly limitless energy. The **depression** is characterized by exaggerated feelings of sadness, discouragement, and hopelessness that are inappropriate and out of proportion with reality.
cyclothymic disorder (sigh-cloh-**THIGH**-mic)	A chronic mood disorder characterized by numerous periods of mood swings from **depression** to happiness. The period of mood disturbance is at least two years in duration.
	The symptoms of the **cyclothymic disorder** are similar to, but less severe than, those of **major depressive disorder**.

Depressive Disorders

The common feature of all of the depressive disorders is the presence of sad, empty, or irritable mood, accompanied by somatic and cognitive changes that significantly affect the individual's capacity to function (*DSM-5*, 2013, p. 156). This section will concentrate on major depressive disorder.

major depressive disorder	A disorder characterized by one or more episodes of depressed mood that last at least two weeks and are accompanied by at least five additional symptoms of **depression**.

These symptoms of **depression** must exist for most of the day and must exist for at least two consecutive weeks to be categorized as a major depressive episode. **Major depressive disorder** is characterized by exaggerated feelings of sadness, discouragement, hopelessness, worthlessness, or guilt that are inappropriate and out of proportion with reality. The individual may experience changes in appetite, weight, or sleep; have decreased energy; have difficulty concentrating or making decisions; and have recurrent thoughts of death or suicide. The depressive episode may be relative to some personal loss or tragedy. However, it is different from the normal sadness and grief that follow a personal loss or tragedy.

Symptoms of a major depressive episode usually develop over a period of time. If a full major depressive episode is left untreated, the **depression** may last six months or more.

Anxiety Disorders

Anxiety is state of mind in which the individual feels increased tension, apprehension, a painfully increased sense of helplessness, a feeling of uncertainty, fear, jitteriness, and worry. Observable signs of **anxiety** include (but are not limited to) restlessness, poor eye contact, glancing about, facial tension, dilated pupils, increased perspiration, and a constant focus on self. **Anxiety** is usually considered a normal reaction to a realistic danger or threat to the body or self-concept. Normal **anxiety** disappears when the danger or threat is no longer present. The discussion that follows deals with disorders that precipitate unrealistic feelings of **anxiety** in individuals.

generalized anxiety disorder	A disorder characterized by chronic, unrealistic, and excessive **anxiety** and worry. The symptoms have usually existed for at least six months or more and have no relation to any specific causes.

Symptoms of **generalized anxiety disorder** include excessive worry about numerous events, restlessness, feeling keyed up and being easily fatigued. Generalized **anxiety** tends to be chronic with recurrence being associated with stress-related situations.

panic disorder	**Panic disorder** is characterized by recurrent panic attacks that come on unexpectedly, followed by at least one month of persistent concern about having another **panic attack**.

The individual experiences intense apprehension, fear, or terror, often associated with feelings of impending doom. The person may experience dyspnea, dizziness, sweating, trembling, and chest pain or palpitations of the heart. The attack may last a few seconds, to several minutes, to an hour or longer and may repeat itself in certain situations.

phobia (**FOH**-bee-ah)	A phobia is an **anxiety** disorder characterized by an obsessive, irrational, and intense fear of a specific object, of an activity, or of a physical situation.

Phobias are usually characterized by symptoms such as faintness, fatigue, palpitations, perspiration, nausea, tremor, and panic. The individual recognizes that the fear is excessive or unreasonable in proportion to the actual danger of the object, activity, or situation even though the feelings are still present.

Phobias are normal, common experiences in childhood with fear of animals, darkness, strangers, and so on. However, phobias in adulthood can become a debilitating experience. A list of several specific phobias follows:

1. Acrophobia: fear of high places that results in extreme **anxiety**

2. Aerophobia: morbid fear of fresh air or drafts

3. Agoraphobia: fear of being in an open, crowded, or public place (such as a field, congested street, or busy department store) where escape may be difficult

4. Arachnophobia: fear of spiders

5. **Claustrophobia** : fear of being in or becoming trapped in enclosed or narrow places; fear of closed spaces

6. Nyctophobia: an obsessive, irrational fear of darkness

7. Zoophobia: a persistent, irrational fear of animals, particularly of dogs, snakes, insects, or mice

obsessive-compulsive disorder (ob-**SESS**-iv kom-**PUHL**-siv)	A disorder characterized by recurrent obsessions or **compulsions** that are severe enough to be time consuming (they take more than one hour a day) or to cause obvious distress or a notable handicap.

Obsessions are repeated, persistent thoughts or impulses that are irrational and with which the mind is continually and involuntarily preoccupied. Examples of obsessions are repetitive doubts that something is not right, that a tragic event may occur, thoughts of contamination, or thoughts of violence. **Compulsions** are irresistible, repetitive, irrational impulses to perform an act. These behavior patterns are intended to reduce **anxiety**, not to provide pleasure or gratification. Examples of **compulsions** are touching repeatedly, often combined with counting, washing the hands repeatedly when they have come in contact with contaminants, or checking repeatedly to make sure that no disaster has occurred.

The individual affected with **obsessive-compulsive disorder** recognizes that his or her behavior is excessive or unreasonable. The disorder also causes obvious distress, is time consuming, and interferes with the individual's normal daily routine.

post-traumatic stress disorder (PTSD) (post-trah-**MAT**-ik)	A disorder in which the individual experiences characteristic symptoms following exposure to an extremely traumatic event. The individual reacts with horror, extreme fright, or helplessness to the event.

Experiences that may produce this type of response include (but are not limited to) military combat, being kidnapped, being raped, being tortured, or enduring natural or manmade disasters or automobile accidents. Symptoms may include reexperiencing the traumatic event, flashbacks, feeling emotionally detached, startling easily, having trouble sleeping, and having difficulty concentrating when awake.

Post-traumatic stress disorder may last from a few months to several years, depending on the severity of the trauma. It is often more severe or long lasting when the trauma was due to an act of human violence such as rape. Complete recovery can occur within a few months in approximately half of individuals. Relapse can also occur.

Somatic Symptom, Sleep, and Factitious Disorders

Somatic symptom disorders are described as any group of neurotic disorders characterized by symptoms suggesting physical illness or disease for which there are no demonstrable organic causes or physiologic dysfunctions. Sleep disorders are a problem for many individuals, be they temporary or long standing. The causes of sleep disorders may be related to stress, **anxiety**, or physiological problems. Factitious disorders are characterized by physical or psychological symptoms that are intentionally produced or feigned to assume the sick role.

Malingering is a term used to describe a willful and deliberate faking of symptoms of a disease or injury to gain some consciously desired end. It differs from **somatic symptom disorders** in that it is of the conscious mind instead of being unconsciously motivated, and it usually results in secondary gain as opposed to the **somatic symptom disorders** resulting in reduction of **anxiety**.

conversion disorder	A disorder in which the individual represses **anxiety** experienced by emotional conflicts by converting the anxious feelings into physical symptoms that have no organic basis but are perceived to be real by the individual.

The individual may experience symptoms such as paralysis, pain, loss of sensation, or some other form of dysfunction of the nervous system, also called conversion hysteria.

The symptoms that occur with **conversion disorder** usually occur after a situation that produces extreme psychological stress. The conversion symptoms, which usually appear suddenly, prevent the individual from experiencing the internal conflict and pain associated with the incident. The individual's lack of concern with the problem, however, is not in keeping with the severity of the symptoms. This relative lack of concern for the severity of the symptoms displayed is often a clue to the physician that the problem may be psychological rather than physiological.

hypochondriasis (**high**-poh-kon-**DRY**-ah-sis)	A chronic, abnormal concern about the health of the body, characterized by extreme **anxiety, depression**, and an unrealistic interpretation of real or imagined physical symptoms as indications of a serious illness or disease despite rational medical evidence that no disorder is present.

The individual is preoccupied with fear of having a serious illness. This fear becomes disabling despite reassurance that no organic disease exists.

Individuals with **hypochondriasis** complain of minor physical problems, worry unrealistically about having or developing a serious illness, constantly seek professional care, and consume multiple over-the-counter remedies. They are so consumed with their fears of illness that it impairs their social and/or occupational functioning.

These individuals are so convinced that their symptoms are related to organic disease that they firmly reject any implication that their problems may be due to stress or psychosocial problems instead of true medical conditions. Their fear of serious illness may persist for a period of six months or more despite medical reassurance. They may become irritated with their physician's suggestion of something other than medical problems. Individuals with **hypochondriasis** often have a long history of "doctor shopping" and are convinced that they are not receiving the proper care.

Munchausen syndrome (by proxy) (mun-**CHOW**-zen **SIN**-drom)	A somewhat rare form of child abuse in which a parent of a child falsifies an illness in a child by fabricating or creating the symptoms and then seeks frequent medical attention for the child; the *DSM-5* refers to this condition as a factitious disorder imposed on another.

The children usually range in age from infancy to about six years. The parent will take the child to the doctor for repeated treatment and possible hospitalization for acute illnesses. Frequently, the mother is the one who actually triggers the symptoms in the child by giving insulin to induce hypoglycemia, laxatives to induce diarrhea, or syrup of ipecac to induce vomiting. When the child is admitted to the hospital for testing and treatment, the mother rarely leaves the child's bedside and appears genuinely concerned about her child's illness.

The most common symptoms the child will present with are bleeding, vomiting, diarrhea, fever, seizures, and apnea. **Munchausen syndrome by proxy** may be suspected when the following criteria become evident.

1. The child is presented for recurrent illnesses for which a cause cannot be identified.

2. The symptoms described by the parent are unusual, and they do not make sense or come together as a particular illness/condition.

3. The symptoms are observed only by the parent.

4. The child's history and the physical findings by the physician do not match.

5. The child has frequent hospital visits (particularly emergency room visits), resulting in normal physical findings.

6. The child has had numerous hospital admissions at several hospitals (if this can be determined).

Munchausen syndrome in adults is characterized by the adult making habitual pleas for treatment and hospitalization for a symptomatic but imaginary illness. The affected person may logically and convincingly present the symptoms and history of a real illness or disease. Often, the individual has enough health-related background to make the information appear believable. The symptoms may disappear after treatment, but the individual may seek further treatment for another imaginary illness or condition.

Adults with **Munchausen syndrome** are mentally ill and need treatment. When they do not get the necessary help, they frequently turn their "perceived illnesses and symptoms" toward their child in the form of **Munchausen syndrome by proxy**.

narcolepsy
 	
(**NAR**-koh-**lep**-see)
  narc/o = sleep
  -lepsy = seizure, attack
	A sleep disorder characterized by a repeated, uncontrollable desire to sleep—often several times a day. The sleep attacks must occur daily over a period of at least three months to establish the diagnosis of **narcolepsy**.

The individual cannot prevent falling asleep. He or she may be in the middle of a task or a conversation when the attack occurs. **Cataplexy** may accompany the sleep attack. This is characterized by a sudden loss of muscle tone in which the individual's head may drop, the jaw may sag, the knees may become weakened, and the individual may collapse and fall to the ground. The individual will regain full muscle strength after the sleep episode.

The attacks of sleep usually last 10 to 20 minutes, but can last for as long as an hour. They can occur at any time, are unpredictable, and therefore can be dangerous if the individual is driving or operating heavy equipment or machinery. The condition is treated effectively with amphetamines and other stimulant drugs.

Dissociative Identity Disorders

Dissociative identity disorders are those in which the individual has emotional conflicts that are so repressed into the subconscious mind that a separation or split in personality occurs. This results in an altered state of consciousness or a confusion in identity. Examples of dissociative disorder include **amnesia**, fugue, and multiple personality. These disorders are discussed individually.

dissociative amnesia (formerly: psychogenic amnesia) (diss-**SOH**-see-ah-tiv am-**NEE**-zee-ah)	**Dissociative amnesia** is a disorder in which the individual is unable to recall important personal information, usually of a traumatic or stressful nature. The loss of memory is more than simple forgetting.

This disorder, although rare, is more common in adolescents and young adult women.

dissociative identity disorder (formerly: multiple personality disorder)	A disorder in which there is the presence of two or more distinct personalities within one individual. At some point in time, each personality takes complete control of the person's behavior.

Paraphilic Disorders

Paraphilias are characterized by recurrent, intense sexual urges, fantasies, or behaviors that involve unusual objects, activities, or situations. These sexual perversions or deviations are expressed in ways that are socially prohibited or unacceptable or are biologically undesirable.

exhibitionism (egs-hih-**BIH**-shun-izm)	**Exhibitionism** is a sexual disorder involving the exposure of one's genitals to a stranger.
	The episode may or may not be accompanied by masturbation. In some cases, the individual is aware of a desire to surprise or shock the observer. In other cases, the individual has the sexually arousing fantasy that the observer will become sexually aroused.
frotteurism (**FROH**-chur-izm)	**Frotteurism** is a sexual disorder in which the person gains sexual stimulation or excitement by rubbing against a nonconsenting person. The sexual arousal is achieved through the act of rubbing and/or touching, which includes fondling.
	The incident usually occurs in crowded places such as buses and subway transportation and involves the rubbing of the individual's genitalia against the victim's thighs or buttocks (or fondling the victim). During this brief encounter, the individual fantasizes a relationship with the victim. Escape is usually easy after the episode due to the victim's initial shock and disbelief that something of this nature could occur in such a public place.
pedophilia (**ped**-oh-**FILL**-ee-ah) **ped/o** = child; foot **-philia** = attraction to	**Pedophilia** is a sexual disorder in which the individual is sexually aroused and engages in sexual activity with children (generally age 13 or younger). This individual is known as a pedophile.
	The child usually knows the pedophile, who may be a family member, neighbor, or older friend. The pedophile is at least 16 years of age and is at least 5 years older than the child. In addition to rape, the molestation by pedophiles may involve exposing genitalia to the child, genital touching and fondling of the child, masturbating in the presence of a child, or undressing and looking at the child.
sexual sadism/sexual masochism	A sexual disorder that involves the act (real, not simulated) of being humiliated, beaten, bound, or otherwise made to suffer or the act of inflicting psychological or physical suffering on the victim.
	Examples of **sexual sadism** or **sexual masochism** include (but are not limited to) restraining by holding down or tying down, slapping, spanking, blindfolding, beating, burning, rape, cutting, and torturing. If the sadistic urges are intense enough, there is danger of serious harm or even death to the victim.

Eating Disorders

The eating disorders discussed in this section are characterized by severe disturbances in eating behavior. The individuals have a morbid fear of gaining weight. **Anorexia nervosa** is characterized by a refusal to maintain a minimally normal body weight. **Bulimia nervosa** is characterized by repeated episodes of binge eating followed by inappropriate behaviors such as self-induced vomiting, excessive exercise, misuse of laxatives, or fasting. A disturbance in perception of body shape and weight is an essential feature of both **anorexia nervosa** and **bulimia nervosa**. A discussion of each disorder follows.

anorexia nervosa	A disorder seen primarily in adolescent girls, characterized by an emotional disturbance concerning body image, prolonged refusal to eat followed by extreme weight loss, amenorrhea, and a lingering abnormal fear of becoming obese. See *Figure 23-2*.
(an-oh-**REK**-see-ah ner-**VOH**-suh)	

This potentially life-threatening disorder is most common in young women, beginning sometimes as early as the age of 12. Weight loss is usually achieved by reduction in food intake (may be as little as 300 calories per day) and considerable exercise. The individual may also abuse laxatives and diuretics and induce vomiting after meals to ensure the weight loss.

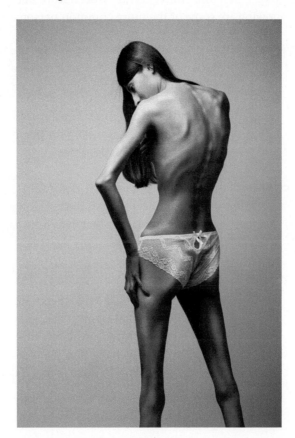

Figure 23-2 Physical manifestations of wasting with anorexia nervosa *(PutilichD/Shutterstock.com)*

bulimia nervosa	An uncontrolled craving for food, often resulting in eating binges followed by vomiting to eliminate the food from the stomach. The individual may then feel depressed and go through a period of self-deprivation followed by another eating binge, and the cycle continues.
(boo-**LIM**-ee-ah ner-**VOH**-suh)	

The individual may consume as many as 5,000 or more calories in one eating binge episode, with several episodes occurring within one day. Immediately after the episode, the individual feels depressed, guilty, and ashamed of the binge episode. This may be followed by **purging**, a means of ridding the body of what has been consumed; that is, the individual may induce vomiting or use laxatives or diuretics to rid the body of the food. Vomiting is the most common method used for **purging** following an eating binge. Individuals with bulimia often avoid social eating events, disappear after meals, and are overly concerned about their body weight. They may experience some weight fluctuations due to the alternating food binges and food fasting, although the weight of the bulimic individual usually stays close to the normal ranges.

Personality Disorders

Personality disorders are rigid, inflexible, and maladaptive patterns of behavior that impair a person's ability to function well in society due to a limited ability to adapt. Following are some of the more common personality disorders.

antisocial personality disorder (**an**-tih-**SOH**-shal)	**Antisocial personality disorder** is characterized by repetitive behavioral patterns that lack moral and ethical standards, keeping the individual in continuous conflict with society.

The individual demonstrates socially irresponsible, guiltless behavior. He or she manipulates others for personal gain, deceives others, and fails to establish stable relationships.

borderline personality disorder	**Borderline personality disorder** is characterized by an extensive pattern of instability of interpersonal relationships, self-image, and marked impulsivity that begins by early adulthood and is present in a variety of contexts.

Characteristics of this disorder include the following:

1. Frantic efforts to avoid real or imagined abandonment. These individuals experience intense abandonment fears and inappropriate anger even when faced with a realistic, time-limited separation or when there are unavoidable changes in plans (for example, panic or fury when someone important to them arrives late or cancels an appointment).

2. A pattern of unstable and intense interpersonal relationships characterized by alternating between extremes of idealization and devaluation.

3. An unstable self-image or sense of self. There may be sudden changes in opinions and plans about career, sexual identity, values, and types of friends.

4. Impulsivity in at least two areas that are potentially self-damaging (for example, they may gamble, spend money irresponsibly, binge eat, abuse substances, engage in unsafe sex, or drive recklessly).

5. May express inappropriate, intense anger or have difficulty controlling anger as evidenced by frequent displays of temper, constant anger, or verbal outbursts.

Because of the similarity of characteristics, **borderline personality disorder** must be distinguished from personality changes due to a general medical condition. It should also be distinguished from symptoms that may develop in association with chronic substance abuse.

narcissistic personality disorder (nar-sis-**SIST**-ik)	**Narcissistic personality disorder** is characterized by an abnormal interest in oneself, especially in one's own body and sexual characteristics.

This individual has an exaggerated sense of self-worth, lacks empathy, appears to lack humility, and tends to exploit others to fulfill his or her own needs and desires. The narcissistic individual is usually jealous of others and feels that others are jealous of him or her. Due to his or her fragile self-esteem, the narcissistic individual is hypersensitive to the evaluation of others and may quickly shift from an optimistic, cheerful mood to a mood of shame, humiliation, or rage. Following this feeling of disapproval, the narcissistic individual may withdraw from others and fantasize or rationalize about his or her continued superiority over others.

paranoid personality disorder (**PAIR**-ah-noyd)	**Paranoid personality disorder** is characterized by a generalized distrust and suspiciousness of others, so much so that the individual blames them for his or her own mistakes and failures.

These individuals are constantly "on guard" for any real or imagined threat, they appear tense and irritable, and they feel that others are trying to take advantage of them. The paranoid personality trusts no one and anticipates humiliation and betrayal by others. As a result of this distrust and suspicion, the paranoid individual is quick to react angrily or to counterattack when perceiving that someone has attacked his or her character or reputation.

Neurodevelopmental Disorders

The neurodevelopmental disorders usually become evident early in development, often before the child enters grade school. These individuals almost always choose solitary activities, are quiet and rarely speak to coworkers or neighbors, and have no close friends.

Disorders in this category include, but may not be limited to, intellectual developmental disorder (mental retardation); learning disorders of math, reading, and written expression; communication disorders; attention-deficit disorders; and tic disorders. The discussion in this section is limited to attention-deficit hyperactivity disorder (ADHD).

attention-deficit hyperactivity disorder (ADHD) (ah-ten-shun-**DEF**-ih-sit **HIGH**-per-ak-tiv-ih-tee diss-**OR**-der)	**ADHD** is a condition of persistent inattention and hyperactivity, impulsivity, or both; formerly known as attention-deficit disorder (ADD).

It is a condition that becomes obvious in some children in the preschool and early school years. It is difficult for these children to control their behavior or pay attention. Boys are more likely to be diagnosed with **ADHD** than are girls.

The inattention or attention deficit may not become apparent until the child enters elementary school and faces the day-to-day challenges in school. These children may have difficulty paying attention to detail and are easily distracted. This often leads to a situation in which the child finds it impossible to complete school assignments. Disorganization and mistake making are common. Many times, the textbook assignments are completely forgotten.

The hyperactivity is usually obvious before the age of seven. Symptoms of hyperactivity include fidgeting, getting up frequently out of one's seat to walk or run around, difficulty playing quietly, and sometimes talking excessively.

The exact cause of **ADHD** is unknown. There is suggestion of hereditary causes as well as of nongenetic factors.

Diagnosis of **ADHD** should be made by a professional with training in **ADHD** or in the diagnosis of **mental** disorders. The specialist will gather information on the child's continuing behavior to compare these behaviors to the symptoms and diagnostic criteria listed in the *DSM-5*. Making a correct diagnosis usually involves talking with the child and observing the child in various settings, particularly those that may elicit the symptoms.

ADHD may go undetected in childhood and is sometimes not diagnosed until adulthood. Treatment for **ADHD** varies from pharmacological treatment stimulants for the child to behavioral training for the parent and the teacher.

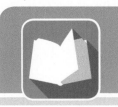

Review Checkpoint

Check your understanding of this section by completing the **Mental Disorders** exercises in your workbook.

Treatments and Therapies

Psychotherapy is defined as any of a large number of related methods of treating **mental** and emotional disorders, using psychological techniques instead of physical means of treatment. It may involve talking, interpreting, listening, rewarding, and role play. Many people seek therapy at some point in their lives. We often think of therapy for the obvious needs such as receiving help in overcoming the trauma of physical or emotional abuse or seeking help in overcoming fears and depressions.

Therapy can also be used to improve the quality of one's life. In any case, the therapies are designed to help the individual learn ways of dealing with emotional conflict and helping them to find positive ways to heal and move forward with their lives. These treatment methods may be conducted by a **psychiatrist** or by a clinical **psychologist**. Following are some of the more commonly practiced treatments and therapies in the field of **psychiatry** or **psychology**, with a brief definition of each.

| **behavior therapy** | A form of **psychotherapy** that seeks to modify observable, maladjusted patterns of behavior by substituting new responses to given stimuli; also called behavior modification. |

Behavior therapy is used to treat conditions such as anxieties, phobias, panic disorders, and stuttering. The therapist strives to change the individual's feelings of fear and panic to a belief that he or she is able to master the situation.

drug therapy	The use of psychotropic drugs to treat **mental** disorders. Psychotropic drugs are those prescribed for their effects in relieving symptoms of **anxiety**, **depression**, or other **mental** disorders (such as **schizophrenia**).

This section is devoted to the discussion of three main types of psychotherapeutic drugs: antianxiety agents, antidepressants, and antipsychotic agents.

1. **Antianxiety agents**, commonly known as minor tranquilizers, are used for *short-term* treatment to calm anxious or agitated people without decreasing their consciousness. Popular antianxiety drugs used are Xanax, Valium, and Ativan; also known as anxiolytics.

2. **Antidepressants** regulate mood and reduce the symptoms of **depression**. Some common agents used to relieve or reduce the symptoms of **depression** are Elavil, Prozac, and Nardil.

3. **Antipsychotic agents** are major tranquilizers that work to block the receptors in the brain responsible for psychotic behavior, including hallucinations, delusions, and **paranoia**. These agents lessen agitated behavior, reduce tension, decrease hallucinations and delusions, improve the individual's social behavior, and produce better sleep patterns of the disturbed individual. Some of the most effective drugs used to treat **schizophrenia** are Clozaril, Zyprexa, Haldol, and Risperdal.

electroconvulsive therapy (ECT) (ee-**lek**-troh-kon-**VULL**-siv)	The process of passing an electrical current through the brain to create a brief seizure in the brain, much like a spontaneous seizure from some forms of epilepsy; also called shock therapy.

Electroconvulsive therapy is used mainly to treat severe **depression** that has not responded to drug treatment. The patient is given anesthesia and muscle relaxants before the current is applied, and usually sleeps through the procedure. A small electric current lasting no longer than a second passes through two electrodes that have been placed on the individual's head. The current excites the nerve tissue and stimulates a brain seizure that lasts from 60 to 90 seconds. Upon awakening after the procedure, the individual usually has no conscious memory of the treatment. Positive results are usually seen after several treatments, as evidenced by the reduction of **depression**.

family therapy	A form of **psychotherapy** that focuses the treatment on the process between family members that supports and sustains symptoms. It is a **group therapy** with family members composing the group.

The therapist may focus on validating the importance of each member in the family, concentrating on the fact that the problem is a "family" problem—not an individual's problem—and leading the family members toward focusing on ways to solve the central conflict within the family.

group therapy	The application of psychotherapeutic techniques within a small group of people who experience similar difficulties; also known as encounter groups.
	Although **group therapy** is not as popular today as 20 years ago, the sessions are designed to promote self-understanding through candid group interactions. These encounter groups are not necessarily positive experiences nor helpful to all participants. **Group therapy** has been found to be effective in treating various addictions.
hypnosis (hip-**NOH**-sis)	A passive, trancelike state of existence that resembles normal sleep during which perception and memory are altered, resulting in increased responsiveness to suggestion.
	Hypnosis is used in **psychotherapy**, medicine, and in some criminal investigations. While the individual is in the trancelike state of existence, the hypnotist may direct the individual to stop certain behaviors (such as smoking or overeating), may question the individual about forgotten events (as in a criminal investigation), or may suggest the absence of pain upon awakening (as in use with dentistry or medicine).
play therapy	A form of **psychotherapy** in which a child plays in a protected and structured environment with games and toys provided by a therapist who observes the behavior, affect, and conversation of the child to gain insight into thoughts, feelings, and fantasies.
	The therapist will help the child work through any conflicts that are discovered during the sessions.
psychoanalysis (**sigh**-koh-ah-**NAL**-ih-sis)	A form of **psychotherapy** that analyzes the individual's unconscious thought, using **free association**, questioning, probing, and analyzing.
	The therapist uses a technique known as **free association**, which allows the individual to say aloud anything that comes to mind no matter how minor or embarrassing. The therapist interprets the statements to understand what is truly causing the individual's conflict. This form of **psychotherapy** is designed to bring the unconscious thoughts, often repressed since childhood, to a conscious level so that the individual can deal with the emotional conflict.
psychoeducation	**Psychoeducation** refers to education offered to individuals who live with a psychological disturbance. It involves teaching people about their illness, how to treat it, and how to recognize signs of relapse so they can seek treatment before the condition worsens or returns.
	Training frequently involves patients with **schizophrenia**, **bipolar disorder**, attention-deficit hyperactivity disorder (ADHD), **anxiety** disorders, eating disorders, and personality disorders. A goal of the training sessions is to help the patient understand and be better able to deal with the presented illness, thus equipping the patient to live with the condition.
	Family psychoeducation involves educating the family concerning symptoms and the process of certain psychological disturbances. This will help them deal more effectively with their ill relative. Psychoeducation training for family reduces distress, confusion, and anxieties within the family.

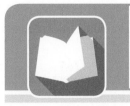

Review Checkpoint

Check your understanding of this section by completing the **Treatments and Therapies** exercises in your workbook.

Personality and Intelligence Tests

Psychologists use a variety of scientifically developed tests and methods to evaluate personality and intelligence. The reasons for evaluating personality are varied. For example, a clinical or school **psychologist** may assess personality to gain a better understanding of an individual's psychological problems, an industrial **psychologist** may evaluate personality to help an individual trying to select a career, and a research **psychologist** may assess personality to investigate theories of personality. **Intelligence testing** may be performed to determine the individual's ability to comprehend and perform at certain levels. It has become one of the primary tools for identifying children with **mental** retardation and learning disabilities. The following list is a sample of some of the more commonly used personality and intelligence tests today in the field of **psychiatry** or **psychology**.

| **Draw-a-Person (DAP) test** | A personality test that is based on the interpretation of drawings of human figures of both sexes. See *Figure 23-3*. |

The individual is asked to draw human figures and talk about them. Evaluations of the drawings are based on the quality and shape of the drawings, the location of the drawing on the paper, how solid the pencil stroke lines appear, the features of the figures drawn, and whether the

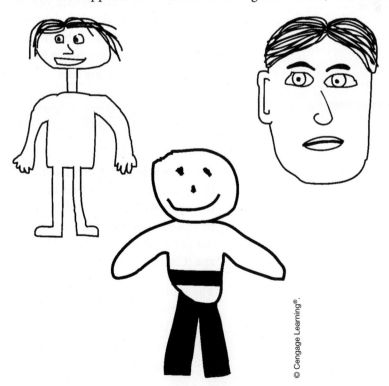

© Cengage Learning®.

Figure 23-3 Draw-a-Person (DAP) test

individual used any background in the drawing. It is believed that the individual's interpretations of the drawings will reveal valuable information about his or her personality.

Minnesota Multiphasic Personality Inventory (MMPI) (mull-tih-**FAYZ**-ic)	A self-report personality inventory test that consists of 550 statements that can be answered "true," "false," or "cannot say." The statements vary widely in content and are sometimes repeated in various ways throughout the test.
	The individual's answers are grouped according to clinical categories that detect various disorders such as **depression, schizophrenia**, and social introversion.
Rorschach inkblot test (**ROR**-shak)	**Rorschach inkblot test** is a personality test that involves the use of 10 inkblot cards, half black-and-white and half in color. The cards are shown to the individual one at a time. The person is shown a card and asked to describe what he or she sees in the card.
	The examiner records the responses and notes the individual's mannerisms, gestures, and attitude during the responses. After the 10 cards have been shown and described, the examiner presents each inkblot again and this time asks the individual questions about the previous responses that were made, that is, "how" and "what" questions to determine characteristics about the individual's true personality.
thematic apperception test (TAT) (thee-**MAT**-ik **ap**-er-**SEP**-shun)	**Thematic apperception test** is designed to elicit stories that reveal something about an individual's personality. This test consists of a series of 30 black-and-white pictures, each on an individual card.
	When the cards are shown, the individual being tested is asked to tell a story about each picture, providing all of the background information and all of the details of the story. The assumption in this test is that the individual will project his or her own unconscious feelings and thoughts into the story he or she tells.
intelligence testing	Intelligence testing was designed to measure an individual's ability to adapt and constructively solve problems in the environment.
	The first successful test of intelligence was developed by Alfred Binet, a French **psychologist**. He tested children in French public schools to identify those at risk of falling behind their peers in academic achievement. The test items were graded in difficulty according to age. The scoring of the test produced a number called the child's **mental age (MA)**: the age level at which one functions intellectually. This was compared to the child's **chronological age (CA)**: the age of the individual expressed as time beyond birth.
	The numeric expression of an individual's intellectual level is known as that person's **intelligence quotient (IQ)**. The intellectual level is measured against the statistical average of the individual's age group. The IQ is determined by dividing the **mental** age (MA) by the chronological age (CA) and multiplying the result by 100:

$$IQ = MA/CA \times 100$$

If the **mental** age and the chronological age are the same, the IQ would be 100 (considered average). If the **mental** age is above the chronological age, the IQ is above 100. Conversely, if the **mental** age is lower than the chronological age, the IQ is below 100.

Numerous tests have been developed over the years to measure IQ. They include (but may not be limited to) the following.

- **Stanford-Binet Intelligence Scale** has been revised several times. The fifth edition (SB5) is in use today. This is the American translation of the original Binet-Simon intelligence test developed by Alfred Binet. SB5 is appropriate for a wider age range, with norms for children of 24 months up to adults age 90.

- **WAIS-III: Wechsler Adult Intelligence Scale-III**, which measures verbal IQ, performance IQ, and overall IQ. This test is used for persons 16 and older.

- **WISC-III: Wechsler Intelligence Scale for Children-III** is used for children between the ages of 6 and 16.

- **WPPSI-III: Wechsler Preschool and Primary Scale of Intelligence-R, third edition**, is used for children between the ages of two and six.

COMMON ABBREVIATIONS

Abbreviation	Meaning	Abbreviation	Meaning
ADD	attention-deficit disorder	MMPI	**Minnesota Multiphasic Personality Inventory**
ADHD	attention-deficit hyperactivity disorder	OCD	obsessive-compulsive disease
CA	chronological age	PCP	phencyclidine (a psychoactive drug)
CNS	central nervous system		
DAP	Draw-a-Person personality test	PTSD	post-traumatic stress disorder
DSM	*Diagnostic and Statistical Manual of Mental Disorders*	TAT	**thematic apperception test** (personality test)
DTs	**delirium tremens**	WAIS	Wechsler Adult Intelligence Scale
ECT	**electroconvulsive therapy**	WISC	Wechsler Intelligence Scale for Children
IQ	intelligence quotient		
LSD	lysergic acid diethylamide (a hallucinogenic drug)	WPPSI	Wechsler Preschool and Primary Scale of Intelligence
MA	**mental age**		

Review Checkpoint

Check your understanding of this section by completing the **Common Abbreviations** exercises in your workbook.

WRITTEN AND AUDIO TERMINOLOGY REVIEW

Review each of the following terms from this chapter. Study the spelling of each term and write the definition in the space provided. Check definitions by looking the term up in the glossary.

Term	Pronunciation	Definition
affect	☐ **AFF**-fekt	_____
amnesia	☐ am-**NEE**-zee-ah	_____
amphetamine	☐ am-**FET**-ah-meen	_____
anorexia nervosa	☐ **an**-oh-**REK**-see-ah ner-**VOH**-suh	_____
antisocial personality disorder	☐ **an**-tih-**SOH**-shal per-son-**AL**-ih-tee dis-**OR**-der	_____
anxiety	☐ **ang**-**ZY**-eh-tee	_____
apathy	☐ **AP**-ah-thee	_____
autism	☐ **AW**-tizm	_____
behavior therapy	☐ bee-**HAYV**-yer **THAIR**-ah-pee	_____
bipolar disorder	☐ by-**POHL**-ar dis-**OR**-der	_____
borderline personality disorder	☐ **BOR**-der-line per-son-**AL**-ih-tee dis-**OR**-der	_____
bulimia nervosa	☐ boo-**LIM**-ee-ah ner-**VOH**-suh	_____
cannabis	☐ **CAN**-ah-bis	_____
cataplexy	☐ **CAT**-ah-pleks-ee	_____
catatonia	☐ **kat**-ah-**TOH**-nee-ah	_____
claustrophobia	☐ **kloss**-troh-**FOH**-bee-ah	_____
compensation	☐ **kom**-pen-**SAY**-shun	_____
compulsions	☐ kom-**PUHL**-shuns	_____
conversion disorder	☐ kon-**VER**-zhun dis-**OR**-der	_____
cyclothymia	☐ **sigh**-kloh-**THIGH**-mee-ah	_____

Term	Pronunciation	Definition
cyclothymic disorder	☐ **sigh**-cloh-**THIGH**-mic dis-**OR**-der	_____
defense mechanism	☐ dee-**FENCE MEH**-kan-izm	_____
delirium	☐ dee-**LEER**-ee-um	_____
delirium tremens (DTs)	☐ dee-**LEER**-ee-um **TREE**-menz (DTs)	_____
delusion	☐ dee-**LOO**-zhun	_____
dementia	☐ dee-**MEN**-she-ah	_____
denial	☐ dee-**NYE**-al	_____
depression	☐ dee-**PRESH**-un	_____
displacement	☐ dis-**PLACE**-ment	_____
dissociation	☐ **dis**-soh-shee-**AY**-shun	_____
dissociative amnesia	☐ diss-**OH**-see-ah-tiv am-**NEE**-zee-ah	_____
dysphoria	☐ dis-**FOH**-ree-ah	_____
electroconvulsive therapy (ECT)	☐ ee-**lek**-troh-kon-**VULL**-siv **THAIR**-ah-pee (ECT)	_____
euphoria	☐ yoo-**FOR**-ee-ah	_____
exhibitionism	☐ **egs**-hih-**BIH**-shun-izm	_____
free association	☐ free ah-**soh**-shee-**AY**-shun	_____
frotteurism	☐ **FROH**-chur-izm	_____
generalized anxiety disorder	☐ generalized ang-**ZYE**-eh-tee dis-**OR**-der	_____
group therapy	☐ groop **THAIR**-ah-pee	_____
hallucination	☐ hah-**loo**-sih-**NAY**-shun	_____
hallucinogens	☐ hah-**LOO**-sih-noh-jens	_____
hypnosis	☐ hip-**NOH**-sis	_____
hypnotize	☐ **HIP**-noh-tize	_____
hypochondriasis	☐ **high**-poh-kon-**DRY**-ah-sis	_____
hypomania	☐ **high**-poh-**MAY**-nee-ah	_____
intoxication	☐ in-**toks**-ih-**KAY**-shun	_____
kleptomania	☐ **klep**-toh-**MAY**-nee-ah	_____
lithium	☐ **LITH**-ee-um	_____
major depressive disorder	☐ **MAY**-jer dee-**PRESS**-iv dis-**OR**-der	_____
malingering	☐ mah-**LING**-er-ing	_____
mania	☐ **MAY**-nee-ah	_____

Term	Pronunciation	Definition
marijuana	☐ mar-ih-**WAH**-nah	_____
mental	☐ **MEN**-tal	_____
Minnesota Multiphasic Personality Inventory (MMPI)	☐ min-eh-**SOH**-tah mull-tih-**FAYZ**-ic per-son-**AL**-ih-tee **IN**-ven-toh-ree (MMPI)	_____
Munchausen syndrome (by proxy)	☐ mun-**CHOW**-zen **SIN**-drom by **PROCKS**-ee	_____
mutism	☐ **MEW**-tism	_____
narcissistic personality disorder	☐ **na**r-sis-**SIST**-ik per-son-**AL**-ih-tee dis-**OR**-der	_____
narcolepsy	☐ **NAR**-coh-**lep**-see	_____
necrophilia	☐ **nek**-roh-**FILL**-ee-ah	_____
neurosis	☐ noo-**ROH**-sis	_____
obsession	☐ ob-**SESS**-shun	_____
obsessive-compulsive disorder	☐ ob-**SESS**-siv kom-**PUHL**-siv dis-**OR**-der	_____
panic disorder	☐ **PAN**-ik dis-**OR**-der	_____
paranoia	☐ pair-ah-**NOY**-ah	_____
paranoid personality disorder	☐ **PAIR**-ah-noyd per-son-**AL**-ih-tee dis-**OR**-der	_____
paraphilia	☐ **pair**-ah-**FILL**-ee-ah	_____
pedophilia	☐ **pee**-doh-**FILL**-ee-ah	_____
phobia	☐ **FOH**-bee-ah	_____
post-traumatic stress disorder	☐ **post**-trah-**MAT**-ik stress dis-**OR**-der	_____
projection	☐ proh-**JEK**-shun	_____
psychiatrist	☐ sigh-**KIGH**-ah-trist	_____
psychiatry	☐ sigh-**KIGH**-ah-tree	_____
psychoanalysis	☐ **sigh**-koh-ah-**NAL**-ih-sis	_____
psychoanalyst	☐ **sigh**-koh-**AN**-ah-list	_____
psychodrama	☐ **sigh**-koh-**DRAH**-mah	_____
psychologist	☐ sigh-**KOL**-oh-jist	_____
psychology	☐ sigh-**KOL**-oh-jee	_____
psychoneurosis	☐ **sigh**-koh-noo-**ROH**-sis	_____
psychosis	☐ sigh-**KOH**-sis	_____

Term	Pronunciation	Definition
psychosomatic	☐ **sigh**-koh-soh-**MAT**-ik	_____
psychotherapy	☐ **sigh**-koh-**THAIR**-ah-pee	_____
purging	☐ **PERJ**-ing	_____
rationalization	☐ **rash**-un-al-ih-**ZAY**-shun	_____
regression	☐ rih-**GRESH**-un	_____
repression	☐ rih-**PRESH**-un	_____
Rorschach inkblot test	☐ **ROR**-shak **INK**-blot test	_____
schizophrenia	☐ **skiz**-oh-**FREN**-ee-ah	_____
sedative	☐ **SED**-ah-tiv	_____
senile dementia	☐ **SEE**-nile dee-**MEN**-she-ah	_____
sexual masochism	☐ **SEKS**-yoo-al **MASS**-oh-kism	_____
sexual sadism	☐ **SEKS**-yoo-al **SAY**-dizm	_____
somatic symptom disorders	☐ soh-**MAT**-ik **SIM**-tohm dis-**OR**-ders	_____
sublimation	☐ sub-lih-**MAY**-shun	_____
suppression	☐ suh-**PRESH**-un	_____
thematic apperception test	☐ thee-**MAT**-ik ap-er-**SEP**-shun test	_____
tolerance	☐ **TAHL**-er-ans	_____

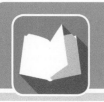

Review Checkpoint

Apply what you have learned in this chapter by completing the **Putting It All Together** exercise in your workbook.

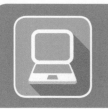

Online Resources

For additional study tools, such as PowerPoint® slides, go to the Student Companion Website.

Chapter Review Exercises

The following exercises provide a more in-depth review of the chapter material. Your goal in these exercises is to complete each section at a minimum 80% level of accuracy. If you score below 80% in any area, return to the applicable section in the chapter and read the material again. A place has been provided for your score at the end of each section.

A. Spelling

Circle the correctly spelled term in each pairing of words. Each correct answer is worth 10 points. Record your score in the space provided at the end of the exercise.

1. bulemia   bulimia
2. hypochondriasis   hypocondriasis
3. schizophrenia   skitzophrenia
4. bipoler   bipolar
5. claustrophobia   claustraphobia

6. malingering   melingering
7. Munchousen   Munchausen
8. frotteurism   frotturism
9. narcalepsy   narcolepsy
10. hallucination   halucination

Number correct _____ **× 10 points/correct answer: Your score** _____ **%**

B. Crossword Puzzle

Read the clues carefully and complete the puzzle. Each crossword answer is worth 10 points. When you have completed the crossword puzzle, total your points and enter your score in the space provided.

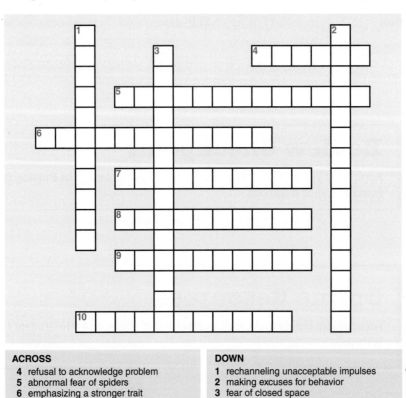

ACROSS
4 refusal to acknowledge problem
5 abnormal fear of spiders
6 emphasizing a stronger trait
7 abnormal fear of heights
8 blocking unpleasant thoughts
9 to assign one's feelings to another
10 abnormal fear of open spaces

DOWN
1 rechanneling unacceptable impulses
2 making excuses for behavior
3 fear of closed space

© Cengage Learning®.

Number correct _____ **× 10 points/correct answer: Your score** _____ **%**

C. Term to Definition

Define each term listed by writing the definition in the space provided. Check the box if you are able to complete this exercise correctly the first time (without referring to the answers). Each correct answer is worth 10 points. Record your score in the space provided at the end of the exercise.

☐ 1. affect _____

☐ 2. amnesia _____

☐ 3. apathy _____

☐ 4. delirium _____

☐ 5. euphoria _____

☐ 6. malingering _____

☐ 7. phobia _____

☐ 8. tolerance _____

☐ 9. sedative _____

☐ 10. compulsion _____

Number correct _____ × *10 points/correct answer: Your score* _____%

D. Matching Mental Disorders

Match the mental disorders on the left with the appropriate description on the right. Each correct answer is worth 10 points. Record your score in the space provided at the end of the exercise.

_____ 1. anorexia nervosa

_____ 2. bipolar disorder

_____ 3. paranoid personality disorder

_____ 4. cyclothymic disorder

_____ 5. obsessive-compulsive disorder

_____ 6. conversion disorder

_____ 7. Munchausen syndrome (by proxy)

_____ 8. narcolepsy

_____ 9. exhibitionism

_____ 10. pedophilia

a. characterized by recurrent obsessions or compulsions severe enough to be time consuming

b. the individual converts anxious feelings into physical symptoms that have no organic basis

c. a parent makes up an illness in a child by creating the symptoms and then seeks medical care for the child

d. a sleep disorder characterized by an uncontrollable desire to sleep

e. a sexual disorder in which an individual repeatedly exposes himself to unsuspecting women or girls

f. a sexual disorder in which the person becomes sexually aroused by inanimate objects

g. a sexual disorder in which the individual engages in sexual activity with children

h. a disorder characterized by a prolonged refusal to eat

i. a chronic mood disorder characterized by mood swings; lasts approximately two years

j. a psychological disorder alternating between mania and depression

k. a condition characterized by a general distrust and suspiciousness of others, so much so that the individual blames them for his or her own mistakes and failures.

Number correct _____ × *10 points/correct answer: Your score* _____%

E. Matching Abbreviations

Match the abbreviations on the left with the correct definition on the right. Each correct answer is worth 10 points. Record your score in the space provided at the end of the exercise.

_____	1. MA	a. Minnesota Math Placement Test
_____	2. TAT	b. intelligence quotient
_____	3. DSM	c. obsessive-compulsive disorder
_____	4. ECT	d. mental age
_____	5. IQ	e. Wechsler Adult Intelligence Scale
_____	6. MMPI	f. seasonal affective disorder
_____	7. WAIS	g. Thematic Apperception Test
_____	8. OCD	h. *Diagnostic and Statistical Manual of Mental Disorders*
_____	9. DTs	i. Minnesota Multiphasic Personality Inventory
_____	10. ADHD	j. electroconvulsive therapy
		k. delirium tremens
		l. attention-deficit hyperactivity disorder

Number correct _____ × 10 points/correct answer: Your score _____%

F. Word Search

Read each definition carefully and identify the appropriate word from the list that follows. Enter the word in the space provided and then find it in the puzzle and circle it. The words may be read up, down, diagonally, across, or backward. Each correct answer is worth 10 points. Record your score in the space provided at the end of the exercise.

exhibitionism	narcolepsy	anorexia
hypochondriasis	Munchausen	sadism
malingering	frotteurism	bulimia
narcissistic	pedophilia	

Example: A sexual disorder involving the exposure of one's genitals to strangers. In some cases, the individual is aware of a desire to shock the observer.
   *exhibitionism*_____

1. A sexual disorder in which the individual is sexually aroused and engages in sexual activity with children (generally age 13 or younger).

   _____

2. A personality disorder characterized by an abnormal interest in oneself, especially in one's own body and sexual characteristics, is known as a _____ personality disorder.

3. An uncontrollable craving for food, often resulting in eating binges, followed by vomiting to eliminate the food from the stomach.

   _____

4. A disorder characterized by an emotional disturbance concerning body image, prolonged refusal to eat followed by extreme weight loss, amenorrhea, and a lingering abnormal fear of becoming obese is known as _____ nervosa.

5. A sexual disorder in which the individual derives sexual excitement or gratification from inflicting pain and suffering on another person, either a consenting or nonconsenting partner.

_____

6. A sexual disorder in which the person gains sexual stimulation or excitement by rubbing against a non-consenting person.

_____

7. A willful and deliberate faking of symptoms of a disease or injury to gain some consciously desired outcome.

_____

8. A sleep disorder characterized by a repeated, uncontrollable desire to sleep, often several times a day.

_____

9. A somewhat rare form of child abuse in which a parent of a child falsifies an illness in a child by fabricating or creating the symptoms, and then seeks medical care for the child, is known as _____ syndrome by proxy.

10. A chronic, abnormal concern about the health of the body, characterized by extreme anxiety, depression, and unrealistic worry over the possibility of having a serious illness or disease despite rational medical evidence that no disorder is present.

_____

B	R	H	O	N	C	H	S	Y	S	T	N	M	I	M
A	N	Y	O	G	E	S	M	S	I	D	A	S	T	A
M	I	P	K	T	M	N	M	E	T	T	R	N	V	L
C	A	O	V	E	E	O	O	S	D	I	C	C	B	I
I	L	C	T	Y	T	N	L	I	E	O	O	N	T	N
M	U	H	O	I	O	T	T	O	T	E	L	R	L	G
L	R	O	T	H	L	O	B	I	U	A	E	C	O	E
P	U	N	L	M	E	I	U	N	A	R	P	I	R	R
P	E	D	O	P	H	I	L	I	A	T	S	U	E	I
S	A	R	U	D	A	D	I	N	D	E	Y	V	M	N
L	A	I	I	G	R	L	M	R	U	E	D	O	R	G
N	I	A	N	A	R	C	I	S	S	I	S	T	I	C
B	S	S	N	E	R	U	A	A	I	D	I	S	G	O
P	U	I	A	I	X	E	R	O	N	A	L	I	R	R
L	R	S	T	H	L	O	E	I	U	A	S	C	O	A
N	E	S	U	A	H	C	N	U	M	I	A	C	B	A
F	R	O	T	T	E	U	R	I	S	M	E	M	I	C
E	X	H	I	B	I	T	I	O	N	I	S	M	N	T

© Cengage Learning®.

Number correct _____ × *10 points/correct answer: Your score* _____ %

G. Completion

The following statements describe various treatments and therapies used in the field of psychiatry and psychology. Read each statement carefully and complete the sentences with the most appropriate answer. Each correct answer is worth 10 points. Record your score in the space provided at the end of the exercise.

1. A form of psychotherapy that analyzes the individual's unconscious thought (using free association, questioning, probing, and analyzing) is known as:

   _____

2. The application of psychotherapeutic techniques with a small number of people who experience similar difficulties is known as:

   _____

3. A form of psychotherapy that seeks to modify observable, maladjusted patterns of behavior by substituting new responses to given stimuli is known as:

   _____

4. A passive, trancelike state of existence that resembles normal sleep (during which perception and memory are altered, resulting in increased responsiveness to suggestion) is known as:

   _____

5. The process of passing an electrical current through the brain to create a brief seizure in the brain (much like a spontaneous seizure from some forms of epilepsy) is known as:

   _____

6. A form of psychotherapy in which a child plays in a protected and structured environment with games and toys provided by a therapist (who observes the behavior, affect, and conversation of the child to gain insight into thoughts, feelings, and fantasies) is known as:

   _____

7. A personality test in which 10 inkblot cards are shown to the individual, one at a time, and the person is asked to describe what he or she sees in the card is known as the:

   _____

8. A form of psychotherapy that focuses treatment on the process between family members that supports and sustains symptoms is known as:

   _____

9. A personality test based on the interpretation of drawings of human figures of both sexes is known as the:

   _____

10. A personality test in which the person is shown 30 black-and-white picture cards and is asked to tell an elaborate story about each picture, filling in all of the details, is known as:

   _____

Number correct _____ × *10 points/correct answer: Your score* _____%

H. Multiple Choice

Read the definition of each commonly used defense mechanism and select the correct answer from the choices provided. Each correct answer is worth 10 points. Record your score in the space provided at the end of the exercise.

1. An effort to overcome, or make up for, real or imagined inadequacies is known as:
   a. repression
   b. regression
   c. compensation
   d. projection

2. The voluntary blocking of unpleasant feelings and experiences from one's mind is known as:
   a. repression
   b. regression
   c. suppression
   d. sublimation

3. A refusal to admit or acknowledge the reality of something, thus avoiding emotional conflict or anxiety, is known as:
   a. displacement
   b. denial
   c. rationalization
   d. suppression

4. The process of transferring a feeling or emotion from the original idea or object to a substitute idea or object is known as:
   a. displacement
   b. introjection
   c. projection
   d. rationalization

5. Rechanneling or redirecting one's unacceptable impulses and drives into constructive activities is known as:
   a. projection
   b. sublimation
   c. compensation
   d. displacement

6. An involuntary blocking of unpleasant feelings and experiences from one's conscious mind is known as:
   a. denial
   b. regression
   c. repression
   d. suppression

(*continued*)

7. An ego defense mechanism whereby an individual unconsciously identifies with another person or with some object and assumes the supposed feelings and/or characteristics of the other personality or object is known as:

    a. introjection

    b. rationalization

    c. compensation

    d. sublimation

8. A response to stress in which the individual reverts to an earlier level of development and the comfort measures associated with that level of functioning is known as:

    a. repression

    b. regression

    c. rationalization

    d. projection

9. The act of transferring one's own unacceptable thoughts or feelings on to someone else is known as:

    a. compensation

    b. displacement

    c. projection

    d. sublimation

10. Attempting to make excuses or invent logical reasons to justify unacceptable feelings or behaviors is known as:

    a. rationalization

    b. projection

    c. denial

    d. introjection

Number correct _____ **× 10 points/correct answer: Your score** _____ **%**

I. Definition to Term

Using the following definitions, identify and provide the word for the pathological condition to match the definition. Each correct answer is worth 10 points. Record your score in the space provided at the end of the exercise.

1. Observable evidence of a person's feelings or emotions.

    _____

2. Loss of memory caused by severe emotional trauma, brain injury, substance abuse, or reaction to medications or toxins.

    _____

3. A mental disorder characterized by the individual being extremely withdrawn and absorbed with fantasy.

    _____

4. Absence or suppression of observable emotion, feeling, concern, or passion.

    _____

5. A state of frenzied excitement or wild enthusiasm.

    _____

6. A passive, trancelike state of existence that resembles normal sleep (during which perception and memory are altered, resulting in increased responsiveness to suggestion).

_____

7. A persistent thought or idea with which the mind is continually and involuntarily preoccupied.

_____

8. The inability to speak because of a physical defect or emotional problem.

_____

9. A willful and deliberate faking of symptoms of a disease or injury to gain some consciously desired end.

_____

10. Any major mental disorder of organic or emotional origin characterized by a loss of contact with reality.

_____

Number correct _____ **× 10 points/correct answer: Your score** _____ **%**

J. True or False

Read each statement carefully and circle the correct answer as true or false. HINT: Pay close attention to the word elements written in **bold** as you make your decision. If the statement is false, identify the meaning of the word element written in bold. Each correct answer is worth 10 points. Record your score in the space provided at the end of the exercise.

1. The term **hypn**osis means "condition of sleep" or "a passive, trancelike state of existence."

   True   False

   If your answer is False, what does *hypn/o* mean? _____

2. The term **psych**iatry refers to the branch of medicine that deals with physical therapy.

   True   False

   If your answer is False, what does *psych/o* mean? _____

3. **Dys**phoria is a disorder of affect (mood) characterized by difficult or bad feelings such as depression and anguish.

   True   False

   If your answer is False, what does *dys-* mean? _____

4. The term **eu**phoria is used to express a sense of well-being or elation.

   True   False

   If your answer is False, what does *eu-* mean? _____

5. Psycho**somat**ic means "pertaining to the expression of an emotional conflict by making excuses."

   True   False

   If your answer is False, what does *somat/o* mean? _____

6. **Schiz**ophrenia literally means "split mind."

   True   False

   If your answer is False, what does *schiz/o* mean? _____

7. A person suffering from klepto**mania** has a love for shopping.

   True   False

   If your answer is False, what does *-mania* mean? _____

(continued)

8. Someone with *claustro**phobia*** has an abnormal fear of enclosed spaces.

   True   False

   If your answer is False, which does *-phobia* mean? _____

9. Someone suffering from *necro**philia*** has an abnormal fear of dead bodies.

   True   False

   If your answer is False, what does *-philia* mean? _____

10. The term *psycho**neurosis*** literally means "a condition of the mind and nerves."

    True   False

    If your answer is False, what does *neur/o* mean? _____

Number correct _____ × 10 points/correct answer: Your score _____%

K. Medical Scenario

The following medical scenario presents information on one of the anxiety disorders discussed in this chapter. Read the scenario carefully and select the most appropriate answer for each question that follows. Each correct answer is worth 20 points. Record your score in the space provided at the end of the exercise.

Johnny Burrows, a 48-year-old, is a patient of the psychiatrist, Dr. Ryan. Mr. Burrows was diagnosed with a phobia nine months ago. Most recently, he has experienced an increase in the recurrence of the phobia. Mr. Burrow's wife has many questions for the health care professional about this disorder.

1. The health care professional will base her responses to Mrs. Burrows' questions about phobias on which of the following facts? A phobia is described as a(n):

   a. anxiety disorder characterized by recurrent obsessions or compulsions that are severe enough to be time consuming and/or cause obvious distress

   b. anxiety disorder characterized by an obsessive, irrational, and intense fear of a specific object, of an activity, or of a physical situation

   c. disorder characterized by gross distortion of reality, disturbances of language and communication, withdrawal from social interactions, and the disorganization and fragmentation of thought, perception, and emotional reaction

   d. a disorder in which the individual represses anxiety experienced by emotional conflicts by converting the anxious feelings into physical symptoms that have no organic basis

2. When Mrs. Burrows asks the health care professional about the symptoms normally seen in patients experiencing a phobia, the health care professional's best response would be one or more of the following:

   a. faintness, fatigue, palpitations, perspiration, nausea, tremor, and panic

   b. hallucinations, delusions, disorganized speed, flattened affect, and catatonic behavior

   c. exaggerated feeling of sadness, discouragement, hopelessness, worthlessness, and guilt

   d. paralysis, pain, loss of sensation, or some other form of dysfunction of the nervous system

3. Mrs. Burrows asks the health care professional what will possibly help Mr. Burrows get through this disorder. The health care professional explains to Mrs. Burrows that the typical treatment used to treat phobias is:

   a. behavior therapy

   b. electroconvulsive therapy

   c. administration of antipsychotic agents

   d. play therapy

4. Mrs. Burrows asks the health care professional to explain what the classification "nyctophobia" means. The health care professional would explain to her that nyctophobia is a(n):

   a. fear of being in an open, crowded, or public place (such as a field, congested street, or busy department store) where escape may be difficult

   b. persistent, irrational fear of animals, particularly of dogs, snakes, insects, and mice

   c. obsessive, irrational fear of darkness

   d. fear of high places that result in extreme anxiety

5. Mrs. Burrow's final question for the health care professional was, "What is it called when he is unreasonably afraid of our neighbor's dog?" The health care professional explained that this phobia is called:

   a. aerophobia

   b. arachnophobia

   c. claustrophobia

   d. zoophobia

***Number correct* _____ × *10 points/correct answer: Your score* _____ %**

CHAPTER 24

Gerontology

CHAPTER CONTENT

OBJECTIVES

Upon completing this chapter and the review exercises at the end of the chapter, the learner should be able to:

1. Identify and define 10 pathological conditions related to gerontology.

2. Identify at least five diagnostic techniques and procedures used in diagnosis and treatment of disorders of older adults.

3. Correctly spell at least 20 medical terms that relate to gerontology.

4. Identify at least 10 medical terms related to gerontology based on their descriptions.

5. Create at least 10 medical terms related to gerontology and identify the appropriate combining form(s) for each term.

6. Identify at least 10 abbreviations related to gerontology.

7. Identify and define 10 word elements related to gerontology.

Overview

"Come grow old with me, the best is yet to be." Is it? "Life begins at 40." Does it? The poetic statements regarding **aging** are sometimes quite different from reality. Abraham Lincoln once said, "And in the end, it's not the years in your life that count. It's the life in your years." People age in different ways and at different rates. For those who enjoy good health and a clear mind, the years beyond the age of 60 can be most productive and rewarding. For others who do not enjoy good health, the scenario is quite different. Longevity (living a long life) can be influenced by many factors such as heredity, improved medical treatments, and lifestyle. The term *young-old* is used to describe an individual between the ages of 65 and 74 years of age. The term *middle-old* is used to describe an individual between the ages of 75 and 84 years of age. The term *old-old* is used to describe an individual 85 years of age and older. In the United States, the fastest growing age group is individuals over the age of 85. The health care professional must have an understanding of the normal changes that occur with aging—versus changes or signs that indicate a disease process—to provide the best care possible for the patient.

Aging, or **senescence**, is the process of growing old. This process can be positive in that the individual possesses desirable traits such as increased wisdom and experience. On the other hand, the aging process can have negative traits—such as decreased capacity to remember things, poorer vision, and a less steady gait (way of walking). The study of all aspects of the aging process—including the clinical, psychological, economic, and sociological issues encountered by older persons and the consequences for both the individual and society—is known as **gerontology**. The branch of medicine that deals with the physiological characteristics of aging and the diagnosis and treatment of diseases affecting the aged is known as **geriatrics**. A **geriatrician** is a physician who has specialized postgraduate education and experience in the medical care of the older person. A **geriatric nurse practitioner** is a registered nurse with additional education obtained through a master's degree program that prepares the nurse to deliver primary health care to older adults. **Gerontic nursing** is the nursing care of older adults, a compromise between caring for older adults who are ill (geriatric nursing) and a more holistic view of the nursing care of older adults (gerontological nursing). A **gerontologist** is one who specializes in the study of **gerontology**.

This chapter is devoted to discussion of some of the changes and conditions that occur in the older adult. Many of the pathological conditions in this chapter have already been discussed in previous body system chapters. They are presented again in this chapter as they relate to older adults and are presented by body systems.

Assessing the Older Adult

When conducting a physical assessment on an older adult, some of the following observations may be noted. There will be a decrease in adipose tissue. The skin becomes drier and the individual experiences a decrease in skin **turgor**. The individual also may notice some flaking of the skin on the extremities due to the dryness. In addition, the skin in the older adult may be thin—almost transparent. There may be an increase in skin tags as well as age spots.

There will be evidence of graying of the hair (**hypopigmentation**) as well as a decrease in the amount of hair on the head. Male pattern baldness may be evident. Men may develop thicker eyebrow hair, coarse nasal hair, and hair in the ear canal. The nailbeds may become more brittle, and there is usually a thickening of the toenails. The toenails may also become malformed and yellowish.

Observation of the face will reveal wrinkles and sagging of the skin. The lips may wrinkle due to the degeneration of elastin. The individual may have a pursed-lip appearance. Further observation of the mouth may reveal receding gum lines, some exposure of the root of the tooth, and some yellowing of the teeth. The eyes may appear sunken and the lids may droop due to loss of fatty tissue in the area. Visual acuity for far vision (hyperopia) will increase with aging, and visual acuity for near vision (**myopia**) will decrease. The change that occurs in the near vision due to the aging process is known as **presbyopia** (poor vision due to the natural aging process).

The stature (height) of the older adult female may be several inches shorter than in earlier years as a result of estrogen depletion. The abdomen of both the male and female may have a rounder appearance due to the redistribution of subcutaneous (fatty) tissue. The female breasts become more elongated and appear flatter with advanced age.

Accurate observations by the health care professional will assist the physician in proper diagnosis of the patient's condition. Not all deviations from the norm, in the older adult patient, are due to pathological conditions. Some are simply the normal process of aging. Every body system undergoes change with aging.

As you read through the chapter section on pathological conditions, you will find observations concerning the normal changes that occur in the particular body system as it ages (at the beginning of each body system discussed), followed by a discussion of the various pathological conditions related to that particular body system.

VOCABULARY

The following vocabulary words are frequently used when discussing the diseases and disorders of older adults.

Word	Definition
acrochordon (ak-roh-**KOR**-don)	Skin tag; a benign growth that hangs from a short stalk, commonly occurring on the neck, eyelids, axilla, or groin.
aging	The process of growing old.
alopecia (al-oh-**PEE**-she-ah)	Partial or complete loss of hair. **Alopecia** may result from normal aging, a reaction to a medication such as anticancer medications, an endocrine disorder, or a skin disease.

Word	Definition
anastomosis (ah-nas-toh-**MOH**-sis)	A surgical joining of two ducts, blood vessels, or bowel segments to allow flow from one to the other. **Anastomosis** of blood vessels may be performed to bypass an occluded area and restore normal blood flow to the area.
anorexia nervosa (an-oh-**REK**-see-ah) an- = without -orexia = appetite	Lack or loss of appetite, resulting in the inability to eat. **Anorexia nervosa** is seen in individuals who are depressed, with the onset of fever and illness, with stomach disorders, or as a result of excessive intake of alcohol or drugs.
ascites (ah-**SIGH**-teez)	An abnormal intraperitoneal (within the peritoneal cavity) accumulation of a fluid containing large amounts of protein and electrolytes.
atherosclerosis (**ath**-er-**oh**-skleh-**ROH**-sis) ather/o = fatty scler/o = hard -osis = condition	A form of **arteriosclerosis** (hardening of the arteries) characterized by fatty deposit buildup within the inner layers of the walls of larger arteries.
atrophic (aye-**TROH**-fik) a- = without troph/o = development -ic = pertaining to	Characterized by a wasting of tissues, usually associated with general malnutrition or a specific disease state.
atrophy (**AT**-roh-fee) a- = without troph/o = development -y = noun ending	Wasting or decrease in size or physiological activity of a part of the body; literally, "without development."
biomicroscopy (**BYE**-oh-mye-**kros**-koh-pee) bi/o = life micr/o = small -scopy = process of viewing	Ophthalmic examination of the eye by use of a slit lamp and a magnifying lens; also known as a slit-lamp exam.
bruit (brew-**EE**) plural: bruits (brew-**EEZ**)	An abnormal sound or murmur heard when listening to a carotid artery, organ, or gland with a stethoscope (e.g., during auscultation).
bunionectomy (bun-yun-**ECK**-toh-mee) -ectomy = surgical removal	Surgical removal of a **bunion**; removing the bony overgrowth and the bursa.
claudication (klaw-dih-**KAY**-shun)	Cramplike pains in the calves of the legs caused by poor circulation to the muscles of the legs; commonly associated with **atherosclerosis**.
crepitation (crep-ih-**TAY**-shun)	Clicking or crackling sounds heard upon joint movement.

Word	Definition
cryosurgery (cry-oh-**SER**-jer-ee) cry/o = cold	A noninvasive treatment for nonmelanoma skin cancer by using liquid nitrogen, which freezes the tissue. It is also used to remove benign skin tumors and growths such as warts.
curettage (koo-reh-**TAZH**)	The process of scraping material from the wall of a cavity or other surface for the purpose of removing abnormal tissue or unwanted material.

dyskinesia (dis-kih-**NEE**-see-ah)
  dys- = bad, difficult, painful, disordered
  -kinesia = movement
	An impairment of the ability to execute voluntary movements.

ectropion (ek-**TROH**-pee-on)	Eversion (turning outward) of the edge of the eyelid.
edema (eh-**DEE**-ma)	The abnormal accumulation of fluid in interstitial spaces of tissues.
electrodesiccation (ee-**lek**-troh-**des**-ih-**KAY**-shun) electr/o = electrical; electricity	A technique using an electrical spark to burn and destroy tissue; used primarily for the removal of surface lesions.
entropion (en-**TROH**-pee-on)	Inversion (turning inward) of the edge of the eyelid.
geriatrician (**jer**-ee-ah-**TRIH**-shun)	A physician who has specialized postgraduate education and experience in the medical care of the older person.
geriatric nurse practitioner (jer-ee-**AT**-rik)	A registered nurse with additional education obtained through a master's degree program that prepares the nurse to deliver primary health care to older adults.
geriatrics (jer-ee-**AT**-riks)	The branch of medicine that deals with the physiological characteristics of aging and the diagnosis and treatment of diseases affecting the aged.

gerontics (jer-**ON**-tiks)
  geront/o = old age
  -ics = pertaining to
	Pertaining to old age.

gerontologist (jer-on-**TOL**-oh-jist)
  geront/o = old age
  -logist = one who specializes in the study of
	One who specializes in the study of **gerontology**.

gerontology (**jer**-on-**TOL**-oh-jee)
  geront/o = old age
  -logy = the study of
	The study of all aspects of the aging process, including the clinical, psychological, economic, and sociologic issues encountered by older persons and their consequences for both the individual and society.

Word	Definition
gerontophobia (jer-on-toh-**FOH**-bee-ah) geront/o = old age -phobia = abnormal fear	An abnormal fear of growing old; fear of aging and of old people.
geropsychiatry	The study and treatment of psychiatric aspects of aging and mental disorders of older adults.
glucagon (**GLOO**-kah-gon)	A hormone produced by the alpha cells of the pancreas that stimulates the liver to convert glycogen into glucose when the blood sugar level is dangerously low.
glycosuria (glye-kohs-**YOO**-ree-ah) glyc/o = sugar, sweet -uria = urine condition	The presence of sugar in the urine.
hyperglycemia (high-per-glye-**SEE**-mee-ah) hyper- = excessive glyc/o = sugar, sweet -emia = blood condition	Elevated blood sugar level.
hypopigmentation (**high**-poh-pig-min-**TAY**-shun) hypo- = under, below, beneath, less than normal	Unusual lack of skin color.
ischemia (iss-**KEY**-mee-ah) -emia = blood condition	Decreased supply of oxygenated blood to a body part or organ.
ketones (**KEE**-tohnz)	Substances that increase in the blood as a result of incomplete fat metabolism. Fats are broken down for energy when the body is unable to use carbohydrates for energy, and the result is a buildup of ketone bodies in the blood and the urine.
kyphosis (kye-**FOH**-sis)	An abnormal outward curvature of a portion of the spine, commonly known as humpback or hunchback.
lichenification (lye-**ken**-ih-fih-**KAY**-shun)	Thickening and hardening of the skin.
malabsorption (**mal**-ab-**SORP**-shun)	Impaired absorption of nutrients into the bloodstream from the gastrointestinal tract.
middle-old	A term used to describe an individual between the ages of 75 and 84 years.
myopia (my-**OH**-pee-ah) my/o = muscle -opia = visual condition	A refractive error in which the lens of the eye cannot focus on an image accurately, resulting in impaired distant vision that is blurred due to the light rays being focused in front of the retina because the eyeball is longer than normal; nearsightedness.

Word	Definition
nocturia (nok-**TOO**-ree-ah) noct/o = night -uria = urine condition	Urination at night.
old-old	A term used to describe an individual 85 years of age and older. The highest number of older adults is in the old-old age group.
pitting edema (pitting ee-**DEE**-mah)	Swelling, usually of the skin of the extremities, that when pressed firmly with a finger will maintain the dent produced by the finger.
presbycusis (**prez**-bee-**KOO**-sis) presby/o = old age	Loss of hearing due to the natural aging process.
presbyopia (**prez**-bee-**OH**-pee-ah) presby/o = old -opia = visual condition	Loss of accommodation for near vision; poor vision due to the natural aging process.
senescence (seh-**NESS**-ens)	The process of growing old.
senile lentigines (**SEE**-nyle lin-**TIH**-jeh-nez)	Age spots; brown macules found on areas of the skin that are frequently exposed to the sun such as the face, neck, or back of the hands of many older people. The singular form of the word is *lentigo*.
stent	A rod or threadlike device (mesh tube) for supporting tubular structures during surgical **anastomosis** or for holding arteries open during angioplasty.
turgor (**TURH**-gor)	A reflection of the skin's elasticity. **Turgor** can be checked by lightly pinching the skin of the forearm between the examiner's thumb and forefinger and releasing it. The time it takes for the skin to return to its normal position is the measure of skin **turgor**, with the normal return time being approximately three seconds.
urinary incontinence (**YOO**-rih-**nair**-ee in-**CON**-tin-ens) urin/o = urine -ary = pertaining to	Inability to control urination; the inability to retain urine in the bladder.
young-old	A term used to describe an individual between the ages of 65 and 74 years.

Review Checkpoint

Check your understanding of this section by completing the **Vocabulary** exercises in your workbook.

WORD ELEMENTS

The following word elements pertain to **gerontology** and diseases and disorders of older adults. As you review the list, pronounce each word element aloud twice and check the box after you "say it." Write the definition for the example term given for each word element. Use your medical dictionary to find the definitions of the example terms.

Word Element	Pronunciation	"Say It"	Meaning
ankyl/o **ankyl**osis	**ANG**-kih-loh ang-kih-**LOH**-sis	☐	stiff
arter/o, arteri/o **arteri**osclerosis	ar-**TEE**-roh, ar-**TEE**-ree-oh ar-tee-ree-oh-sklair-**ROH**-sis	☐	artery
arthr/o **arthr**itis	**AR**-throh ar-**THRYE**-tis	☐	joint
carcin/o **carcin**oma	kar-**SIN**-noh kar-sih-**NOH**-mah	☐	cancer
corne/o **corne**itis	**COR**-nee-oh cor-nee-**EYE**-tis	☐	cornea
coron/o **coron**ary arteries	cor-**OH**-no **KOR**-oh-nah-ree **AR**-ter-eez	☐	heart
cry/o **cry**osurgery	**KRY**-oh kry-oh-**SIR**-jeer-ee	☐	cold
geront/o **geront**ics	jer-**ON**-toh jer-**ON**-tiks	☐	old age
glauc/o **glau**coma	**GLAW**-koh glaw-**KOH**-mah	☐	gray, silver
glyc/o **glyc**ogen	**GLIGH**-koh **GLIGH**-koh-jen	☐	sugar, sweet
hyper- **hyper**glycemia	**HIGH**-per high-per-glye-**SEE**-mee-ah	☐	excessive
hypo- **hypo**glycemia	**HIGH**-poh high-poh-glye-**SEE**-mee-ah	☐	under, below, beneath, less than normal
-itis prosta**titis**	**EYE**-tiss pross-tah-**TYE**-tis	☐	inflammation

Word Element	Pronunciation	"Say It"	Meaning
kerat/o **kerat**osis	kair-**AH**-toh kair-ah-**TOH**-sis	☐	hard, horny; also refers to the cornea of the eye
-malacia osteo**malacia**	mah-**LAY**-she-ah **oss**-tee-oh-mah-**LAY**-she-**ah**	☐	softening
myx/o **myx**edema	**MIKS**-oh miks-eh-**DEE**-mah	☐	relating to mucus
neur/o **neur**opathy	**NOO**-roh noo-**ROP**-ah-thee	☐	nerve
-opia my**opia**	**OH**-pee-ah my-**OH**-pee-ah	☐	visual condition
-osis thromb**osis**	**OH**-sis throm-**BOH**-sis	☐	condition
oste/o **oste**oarthritis	**OSS**-tee-oh oss-tee-oh-ar-**THRYE**-tis	☐	bone
ovari/o **ovari**an carcinoma	oh-**VAIR**-ree-oh oh-**VAIR**-ree-an car-sin-**OH**-ma	☐	ovary
-porosis osteo**porosis**	por-**ROW**-sis **oss**-tee-oh-por-**ROW**-sis	☐	porous, lessening in density
presby/o **presby**opia	**PRES**-bee-oh **pres**-bee-**OH**-pee-ah	☐	old age
prostat/o **prostat**itis	pross-**TAH**-toh pross-tah-**TYE**-tis	☐	prostate gland
pulmon/o **pulmon**ary	pull-**MON**-oh **PULL**-mon-air-ee	☐	lung
retin/o **retin**itis	**RET**-in-oh ret-in-**EYE**-tis	☐	retina
scler/o **scler**osis	**SKLAIR**-oh sklair-**OH**-sis	☐	hard
spondyl/o **spondyl**osis	**SPON**-dih-loh spon-dih-**LOH**-sis	☐	spine
troph/o hyper**trophy**	**TROH**-foh high-**PER**-troh-fee	☐	development, growth

Word Element	Pronunciation	"Say It"	Meaning
urin/o **urin**ary incontinence	**YOO**-rih-noh **YOO**-rih-nair-ee in-**CON**-tin-ens	☐	urine
urethr/o **urethr**itis	yoo-**REE**-throh yoo-ree-**THRIGH**-tis	☐	urethra
-uria poly**uria**	**YOO**-ree-ah pall-ee-**YOO**-ree-ah	☐	urine condition

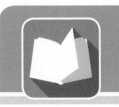

Review Checkpoint

Check your understanding of this section by completing the **Word Elements** exercises in your workbook.

Pathological Conditions and Changes in the Older Adult

The following is a discussion of some of the more commonly occurring pathological conditions and changes in the older adult than in other age groups. However, many of these conditions also occur at younger ages. These conditions and changes are presented by body systems.

Integumentary System

When observing the older adult and considering the integumentary system, the obvious changes due to the aging process are the graying of hair and the wrinkling of skin. Wrinkling of the skin is caused by the loss of subcutaneous fat and water in the epidermal layers of the skin and exposure to the sun over the course of a lifetime. The older adult will also have reduced skin **turgor**, possible dry scaly skin, and thinning epidermis (paper-thin skin). Sometimes the skin seems almost transparent over the underlying blood vessels. See *Figure 24-1*.

The nails of the older adult may become thick and prone to splitting. In addition, the older adult will develop brown, pigmented areas on the back of the hands, arms, and face. These spots are known as age spots. The older adult may also be prone to the development of precancerous and cancerous skin growths due to the lifetime exposure to the sun. The pathological conditions related to aging skin include (but are not limited to) the following.

acrochordon

(ak-roh-**KOR**-don)

A benign growth that hangs from a short stalk, commonly occurring on the neck, eyelids, axilla, or groin of an older person.

Acrochordon is also known as cutaneous papilloma or skin tag.

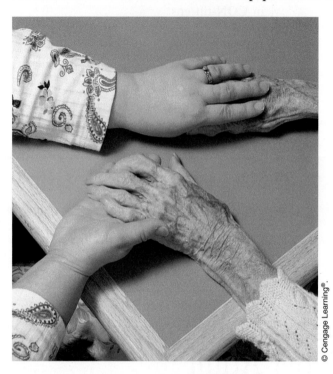

Figure 24-1 Transparent appearance of aging skin

actinic keratosis

(ak-**TIN**-ic kair-ah-**TOH**-sis)

  kerat/o = hard

  -osis = condition

Actinic keratosis is identified by raised areas that appear scaly and may bleed at the edges. An area of inflammation around the border of the lesion may be noted.

This premalignant warty lesion, occurring on the sun-exposed skin of the face or hands in aged, light-skinned persons, should be checked by a physician if any change in its status occurs.

carcinoma, basal cell

(**kar**-sih-**NOH**-mah, **BAY**-sal sell)

  carcin/o = cancer

  -oma = tumor

A malignant epithelial cell tumor that begins as a slightly elevated nodule with a depression or ulceration in the center that becomes more obvious as the tumor grows. As the depression enlarges, the tissue breaks down, crusts, and bleeds. See *Figure 24-2*.

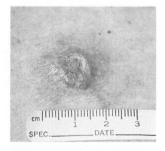

Figure 24-2 Basal cell carcinoma

(Courtesy of Robert A. Silverman, M.D., Pediatric Dermatology, Georgetown University)

Basal cell carcinoma is the most common malignant tumor of the epithelial tissue, occurring most often on areas of the skin exposed to the sun (usually between the hairline and the upper lip). Older adults exposed to the sun or other irritants for long intervals are susceptible to the development of skin cancer on the exposed surfaces of the skin.

If not treated, the basal cell carcinomas will invade surrounding tissue, which can lead to destruction of body parts (such as a nose). Treatment includes surgical excision, **curettage** and **electrodesiccation**, **cryosurgery**, or radiation therapy. (See the section on diagnostic tests and procedures for description.) Basal cell carcinomas rarely metastasize, but they tend to recur (especially those larger than 2 cm in diameter).

carcinoma, squamous cell

(**kar**-sih-**NOH**-mah, **SKWAY**-mus sell)

  carcin/o = cancer

  -oma = tumor

A malignancy of the squamous, or scalelike, cells of the epithelial tissue. Squamous cell carcinoma is a much faster growing cancer than basal cell carcinoma and has a greater potential for metastasis if not treated. See *Figure 24-3*.

These squamous cell lesions are seen most frequently on these sunexposed areas:

1. Top of the nose

2. Forehead

3. Margin of the external ear

4. Back of the hands

5. Lower lip

The squamous cell lesion begins as a firm, flesh-colored or red papule sometimes with a crusted appearance. As the lesion grows, it may bleed or ulcerate and become painful. When squamous cell carcinoma recurs, it can be highly invasive and present an increased risk of metastasis.

Treatment is surgical excision with the goal to remove the tumor completely along with a margin of healthy surrounding tissue. Cryosurgery for low-risk squamous cell carcinomas is also common.

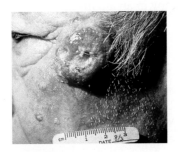

Figure 24-3 Squamous cell carcinoma
(*Courtesy of Robert A. Silverman, M.D., Pediatric Dermatology, Georgetown University*)

eczema

Eczema is an acute or chronic inflammatory skin condition characterized by erythema, papules, vesicles, pustules, scales, crusts, or scabs; accompanied by intense itching.

These lesions may occur alone or in any combination. They may be dry or may produce a watery discharge with resultant itching. Although **eczema** is not limited to the older adult, it is discussed in this section because it also affects the aging skin.

Long-term effects of **eczema** may result in thickening and hardening of the skin, known as **lichenification**, which is due to irritation caused from repeated scratching of the itchy area. Redness and scaling of the skin may also accompany the condition. Severe itching predisposes the areas to secondary infections and possible invasion by viruses.

An estimated 9% to 12% of the population is affected by **eczema**, occurring most commonly during infancy and childhood. The incidence decreases in adolescence and adulthood. The exact cause is not known. However, statistics support a convincing genetic component in that when both mother and father are affected, the child has an 80% chance of developing **eczema**. This inflammatory response is believed to be initiated by histamine release, with lesions usually occurring on the flexor surfaces of the arms and legs, hands, feet, and upper trunk of the body.

There is no specific treatment to cure **eczema**. However, local and systemic medications may be prescribed to prevent itching. It is important to stress daily skin care and avoidance of known irritants. Chronic **eczema** is often frustrating to control and may have to be dealt with throughout most of the individual's life because it is prone to recurrence.

psoriasis

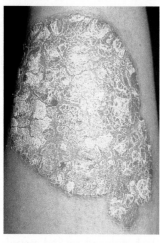

Psoriasis is a common, noninfectious, chronic disorder of the skin manifested by silvery white scales over round, raised, reddened plaques, producing pruritus.

The process of hyperkeratosis produces various-size lesions occurring largely on the scalp, ears, extensor surfaces of the extremities, bony prominences, and perianal and genital areas. See *Figure 24-4* for a visual reference.

Onset of psoriasis is usually between the ages of 10 and 40, but no age is exempt. Treatment includes topical application of various medications, phototherapy, and ultraviolet light therapy in an attempt to slow the hyperkeratosis.

Figure 24-4 Psoriasis
(*Courtesy of Robert A. Silverman, M.D., Pediatric Dermatology, Georgetown University*)

seborrheic keratosis

(seb-oh-**REE**-ik kair-ah-**TOH**-sis)

   kerat/o = hard

   -osis = condition

Seborrheic keratosis appears as a brown or waxy yellow wartlike lesion(s), 5 to 20 mm in diameter, loosely attached to the skin surface.

Seborrheic keratosis is also known as seborrheic warts.

Skeletal System

The normal age-related changes of the musculoskeletal system generally affect mobility. After about the age of 50, the process of bone formation and resorption becomes unstable, causing the musculoskeletal system to gradually lose bone mass. When discussing the skeletal system of the older adult, one must consider the decrease in total body mass, bone mass, and bone density. The older adult will also experience an increase in bone fragility and a decrease in bone strength. These factors influence the types of skeletal system diseases and disorders experienced by older adults. The pathological conditions related to the aging skeletal system include (but are not limited to) the following.

fracture of the hip

A break in the continuity of the bone involving the upper third of the femur.

A hip fracture is classified as either intracapsular (within the joint capsule) or extracapsular (outside the joint capsule). See *Figure 24-5*.

Hip fractures occur most often in older adults. This may be partly because the senses that help maintain equilibrium, coordination, and body position are diminished in the older adult, resulting in a general unsteadiness and a lack of coordination in movements.

Women who have **osteoporosis** are more susceptible to fractures of the hip. Most hip fractures, impactions (the adjacent fragmented ends of the fractured bone are wedged together), or dislocations (femoral head is out of the hip joint) are caused by falls.

Repair of hip fractures has rapidly become one of the most common surgeries among older adults. Many of the older adult patients who sustain

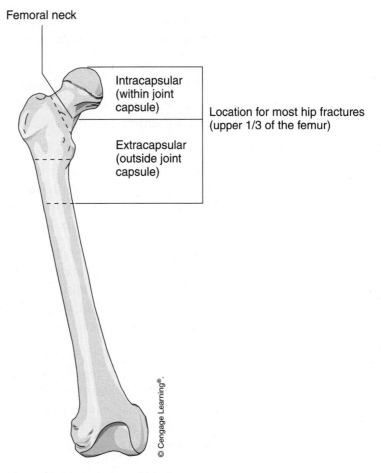

Femoral neck

Intracapsular
(within joint
capsule)

Extracapsular
(outside joint
capsule)

Location for most hip fractures
(upper 1/3 of the femur)

© Cengage Learning®.

Figure 24-5 Location of hip fractures

a hip fracture do not experience a rapid or full recovery. Some may die within a year of injury due to medical complications or immobility as a result of the fracture.

The treatment of choice for a fractured hip is surgery, which may involve open reduction and internal fixation. (*Figure 24-16* later in the chapter provides a visual reference for internal fixation of a fracture.)

osteomalacia

(**oss**-tee-oh-mah-**LAY**-shee-ah)

oste/o = bone

-malacia = softening

Osteomalacia is a disease in which the bones become abnormally soft due to a deficiency of calcium and phosphorus in the blood (which is necessary for bone mineralization). This disease results in fractures and noticeable deformities of the weight-bearing bones. This disease is the adult equivalent of rickets.

The deficiency of these minerals is due to a lack of vitamin D, which is necessary for the absorption of calcium and phosphorus by the body. The vitamin D deficiency may be caused by a diet lacking in vitamin D, a lack of exposure to sunlight, or by a metabolic disorder causing malabsorption.

Treatment includes daily administration of vitamin D in addition to a diet sufficient in calcium, phosphorus, and protein. Supplemental calcium may also be prescribed. The older adult should be encouraged to be as active as possible because active exercise and a nutritionally adequate diet are now thought to decrease the speed at which muscle mass and bone density decrease.

osteoporosis

(**oss**-tee-oh-poh-**ROW**-sis)

oste/o = bone

-porosis = porous, lessening in density

Osteoporosis literally means porous bones; that is, bones that were once strong become fragile due to loss of bone density.

Osteoporosis is a common manifestation of bone abnormality in older adults and occurs more frequently and at an earlier age in women than in men. The patient is more susceptible to fractures, especially in the wrist, hip, and vertebral column.

Osteoporosis occurs most frequently in postmenopausal women, in sedentary or immobilized individuals, and in patients on long-term steroid treatment. A major factor in **osteoporosis** is hormonal: postmenopausal women are at a high risk for **osteoporosis** because estrogen production and bone calcium storage decrease with menopause. Other risk factors tend to be hereditary.

Classic characteristics of **osteoporosis** are fractures that occur in response to normal activity or minimal trauma, a loss of standing height of greater than 2 inches, and the development of the typical **kyphosis** (dowager's hump). See *Figure 24-6*.

Treatment includes (but is not limited to) prescribing drug therapy such as estrogen replacement and calcium supplements, promoting calcium intake, and promoting active weight-bearing exercises. Studies indicate that women aged 65 years and older should consume dairy products to provide 1,500 mg calcium daily or take calcium fortified with vitamin D.

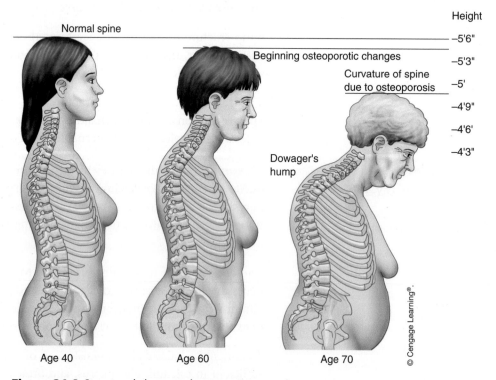

Figure 24-6 Structural changes due to osteoporosis

Paget's disease
 	
(**PAJ**-ets dih-**ZEEZ**)
osteitis deformans
(oss-tee-**EYE**-tis de-**FOR**-manz)
   oste/o = bone
   -itis = inflammation
	A nonmetabolic disease of the bone, characterized by excessive bone destruction (breakdown of bone tissue by the osteoclasts) and unorganized bone formation by the osteoblasts. The bone is weak and prone to fractures. After symptoms are present, the diseased bone takes on a characteristic mosaic pattern that can be detected with X-ray or bone scan; also known as osteitis deformans.

Paget's disease may occur in one bone or in several sites. The most common areas of occurrence are the vertebrae, femur, tibia, pelvis, and skull. Individuals with symptoms may develop pathological fractures, complain of bone pain, and may experience skeletal deformity such as bowing of the leg bones (tibia or femur) or **kyphosis**. The exact cause of this disease is unknown. Paget's disease more commonly affects the middle-aged and older adults, with a higher incidence in men than in women.

Muscles and Joints

Loss of muscle mass due to a decline in the number of muscle fibers is significant in the aging individual. This process occurs more slowly in men than in women because men have more muscle mass than women. Many older adults also experience a decline in muscle strength, depending on the muscle group. By the time a person is 80 years old, he or she may lose 30% or more skeletal muscle mass.

Cartilage in the joints eventually erodes in the older adult, increasing stress on the underlying bone. This leads to changes secondary to inflammation, which decreases flexibility. Joint mobility in the older adult is also hampered by the elastic synovial tissue being replaced with collagen fibers and the synovial fluid within the joint increasing in viscosity.

The ability to move around independently is one of the most important issues to older adults. Many of the diseases and disorders of the musculoskeletal system limit mobility. The pathological conditions related to the aging muscles and joints include, but are not limited to, the following.

ankylosing spondylitis
 	
(**ang**-kih-**LOH**-sing **spon**- dih-**LYE**-tis)
   ankyl/o = stiff
   spondyl/o = spine
   -itis = inflammation
	Ankylosing spondylitis is a type of **arthritis** that affects the vertebral column and causes deformities of the spine; also known as Marie-Strümpell disease and as rheumatoid spondylitis.

Patient symptoms include other joint involvement, arthralgia (pain in the joints), weight loss, and generalized malaise (weakness). As the disease progresses, the spine becomes increasingly stiff, with fusion of the spine into a position of **kyphosis** (humpback).

Treatment includes prescribing medications to reduce inflammation and relieve pain as well as physical therapy to keep the spine as straight as possible and to promote mobility.

bunion (hallux valgus) (**BUN**-yun) (**HAL**-uks **VAL**-gus)	An abnormal enlargement of the joint at the base of the great toe. See *Figure 24-7*.

The great toe deviates laterally, causing it either to override or undercut the second toe. As the condition worsens, the bony prominence enlarges at the base of the great toe, causing pain and swelling of the joint.

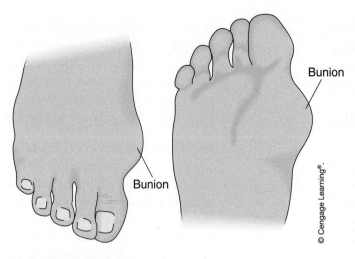

Figure 24-7 Bunion

A bunion often occurs as a result of **arthritis** or as a result of chronic irritation and pressure from wearing poorly fitting shoes, although it can be congenital. Treatment for a bunion may include application of padding between the toes or around the bunion to relieve pressure when wearing shoes, medications to relieve the pain and inflammation, or a **bunionectomy**, which involves removal of the bony overgrowth and the bursa.

gout

(GOWT)

Gout is a metabolic disease in which uric acid crystals are deposited in joints or other tissues. It is characterized by inflammation of the first metatarsal joint of the great toe. Although the great toe is the most common site for gout, it can occur in other parts of the foot and body. Men between the ages of 40 and 60 are more commonly affected by gout than women. Gout usually appears in women in the postmenopausal period.

Gout, also known as gouty **arthritis**, can be a hereditary disease in which the individual does not metabolize uric acid properly. It may also be a complication of another disease or secondary to the use of certain drugs or may arise from unknown causes. Large amounts of uric acid accumulate in the blood and in the synovial fluid of the joints. (The body produces uric acid from metabolism of ingested purines in the diet, especially from eating red meats.) The uric acid crystals are responsible for the inflammatory reaction that develops in the joint, causing intense pain. The pain reaches a peak after several hours and then gradually declines. The attack may be accompanied by a slight fever and chills. Symptoms are recurrent.

Treatment for gout may include bed rest, immobilizing the affected part, and application of a cold pack (if the area is not too painful to touch). Anti-inflammatory medications may be given to lessen the inflammation of the area, analgesics may be given to relieve the pain, and medications such as allopurinol may be prescribed to lower the uric acid level in the blood. The individual will be instructed to avoid eating foods high in purine (that is, decrease the red meats) and increase fluid intake.

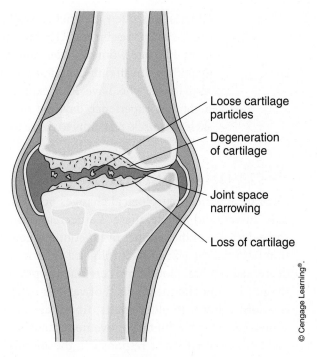

Loose cartilage
particles

Degeneration
of cartilage

Joint space
narrowing

Loss of cartilage

© Cengage Learning®.

Figure 24-8 Osteoarthritis (knee joint)

osteoarthritis	**Osteoarthritis** is also known as degenerative joint disease. It is the most common form of **arthritis**, having universal prevalence in those age 80 and over. It results from wear and tear on the joints, especially weight-bearing joints such as the hips and knees.

(**oss**-tee-oh-ar-**THRYE**-tis)

oste/o = bone

arthr/o = joint

-itis = inflammation

As this chronic disease progresses, the repeated stress to the joints results in degeneration of the joint cartilage. The joint space becomes narrower, taking on a flattened appearance. See *Figure 24-8.*

Symptoms include joint soreness and pain; stiffness, especially in the mornings; and aching, particularly with changes in the weather. Joint movement may elicit clicking or crackling sounds, known as **crepitation**. The individual may also experience a decrease in the range of motion of a joint and increased pain with use of the joint.

The objectives of treatment for **osteoarthritis** are to reduce inflammation, lessen the pain, and maintain the function of the affected joints. **Osteoarthritis** cannot be cured. Medications may be prescribed to reduce the inflammation and to relieve the pain. Physical therapy may be prescribed to promote the function of the joint. If the condition becomes severe, joint replacement surgery may become necessary.

restless legs syndrome (RLS)	A condition of the legs involving annoying sensations of uneasiness, tiredness, itching, or tingling of the leg muscles while resting. The individual feels an overwhelming desire to get up and move around due to the jerking sensation and painful twitching of the muscles.

Older adults often experience **restless legs syndrome**, although it is not limited to this age group. **RLS** tends to run in families and is most common in middle-age women, older adults, pregnancy, people who drink large quantities of caffeine-containing drinks, and people who smoke heavily. Individuals who have **RLS** experience repeated awakenings during the night and experience daytime sleepiness. Treatment involves the use of skeletal muscle relaxants to decrease the movements and awakenings.

Nervous System

The rate at which neurological changes occur in the older adult vary among individuals. In very old people, there is a decrease in the size and weight of the brain, with some decrease in the number of functioning neurons, although there is no real correlation between the size of the brain and functioning. Changes in the brain can include decreased cerebral blood flow, cerebral atrophy, ventricular dilation, and alterations in the production and metabolism of various neurotransmitters. Generally, nerve transmission is slower in older adults. About age 70, the individual may be noted to have somewhat slower voluntary movement, may be slower in decision-making processes, and have a slowed startle response. In the absence of pathology, intellect and the capacity for learning remain unchanged with aging.

Noticeable nervous system changes common in the older adult may include (but are not limited to) slower voluntary movement; stooped, forward-flexed posture; slowed gait (way of walking); dry eyes; impaired ability to hear high-pitched sounds; and decreased ability to maintain balance and correct imbalance. The pathological conditions related to the **aging** nervous system include (but are not limited to) the following.

Alzheimer's disease (AD)	A progressive, degenerative disease that affects the cortex of the brain and results in deterioration of a person's intellectual functioning. **Alzheimer's disease (AD)** is progressive and extremely debilitating. It begins with minor memory loss and progresses to complete loss of mental, emotional, and physical functioning, frequently occurring in persons over 65 years of age.
(**ALTS**-high-merz dih-**ZEEZ**)	

Approximately 10% of individuals over the age of 65 and almost 50% of those over the age of 85 will develop **Alzheimer's disease**, although it can strike in those aged 40 to 50. This process occurs through three identified stages over a number of years.

Stage 1 lasts for approximately one to three years and includes loss of short-term memory; decreased ability to pay attention or learn new information; gradual personality changes such as increased irritability, denial, and **depression**; and difficulties in depth perception. The person with Alzheimer's disease in stage 1 will often recognize and attempt to adjust or cover up mental errors.

Stage 2 lasts approximately 2 to 10 years, during which time the person loses the ability to write, to identify objects by touch, to accomplish purposeful movements, and to perform simple tasks such as getting dressed. During this progressive deterioration, safety is a major concern. Also during the second stage, the person with Alzheimer's disease loses the ability to communicate socially with others. He or she uses the wrong words in conversation, tends to repeat phrases, and may eventually develop total loss of language function (called aphasia).

Stage 3 lasts for 8 to 10 years, during which time the person with Alzheimer's disease has very little, if any, communication skills due to disorientation to time, place, and person. Bowel and bladder incontinence, posture flexion, and limb rigidity are noted during this stage as well. This increasing deterioration tends to render the person with Alzheimer's disease dependent on others to provide for basic needs. This individual may be cared for by family members or need placement in a long-term care facility. The person with Alzheimer's disease is prone to additional complications such as malnutrition, dehydration, and **pneumonia**.

There is no single clinical test to identify **Alzheimer's disease**. Before a diagnosis is made, other conditions that mimic the symptoms must be excluded. A clinical diagnosis of Alzheimer's disease is then based on tests such as physical, psychological, neurological, and psychiatric examinations plus various laboratory tests. With today's new diagnostic tools and criteria, it is possible for physicians to make a positive clinical diagnosis of Alzheimer's with approximately 90% accuracy. A confirmation of the diagnosis of **Alzheimer's disease** is not possible until death, because biopsy or autopsy examination of the brain tissue is required for diagnosis.

Treatment for **Alzheimer's disease** includes the use of medications such as donepezil (Aricept) or galantamine (Razadyne). An earlier drug, tacrine (Cognex) is rarely used today because of its significant liver toxicity. Antidepressants and tranquilizers are also frequently used to treat the symptoms of Alzheimer's disease. The persons and families experiencing Alzheimer's disease need a great deal of education and support to endure this difficult disease.

cerebrovascular accident (CVA)	Neurological deficit(s) resulting from a decrease in blood (**ischemia**) to a specific localized area in the brain; also called "stroke" or "brain attack."
(seh-**ree**-broh-**VASS**-kyoo-lar **AK**-sih-dent)	

The deficits will differ widely according to the degree of involvement, the amount of time the blood flow is decreased or stopped, and the region of the brain involved. If only a small area of the brain is involved for a short period of time, the deficit may be small or even go unnoticed. However, if there is significant loss of blood supply to a large area, the deficit may be a severe disability or death. Due to the crossing of the sensory-motor pathways at the junction of the medulla and spinal cord, neurological deficits from the **cerebrovascular accident (CVA)** on one side of the brain will show manifestations on the opposite side of the body.

Cellular death and altered level of consciousness occur if the ischemia is severe and prolonged. Vasospasm and increased blood viscosity may also occur with a CVA and cause decreased circulation to the specific area(s) of the brain, causing even more complex deficits. Other typical clinical manifestations of the person experiencing a **CVA** are motor deficits (frequently hemiplegia), language disorders, visual alterations, headache, dizziness, and various sensory deficits. Older adults have a higher mortality rate than younger individuals. However, those who do survive a stroke have an excellent chance of recovery with proper care.

The onset of a **CVA** may be gradual or rapid. A number of factors that cause the alteration in cerebral blood flow leading to neurological deficits include transient ischemic attacks, cerebral **thrombosis**, cerebral embolism, and cerebral hemorrhage. These are described as follows.

Transient ischemic attacks (TIAs) are very brief periods of ischemia in the brain, lasting from minutes to hours, which can cause a variety of symptoms. **TIAs** ("mini strokes") often precede a full-blown thrombolytic **CVA**. The neurological symptoms range according to the amount of ischemia and the location of the vessels involved. The person experiencing a **TIA** may complain of numbness or weakness in the extremities or corner of the mouth, difficulty communicating, or maybe a visual disturbance. Sometimes the symptoms are vague and difficult to describe. The person may simply complain of a "funny feeling."

Cerebral thrombosis (clot), also called thrombolytic **CVA**, makes up 50% of all **CVAs** and occurs largely in individuals older than 50—and often during rest or sleep. The cerebral clot is typically caused by **atherosclerosis**, which is a thickened fibrotic vessel wall causing the diameter of the vessel to be decreased or completely closed off from the buildup of plaque. The thrombolytic **CVA** is often preceded by one or many **TIAs**. The occurrence of the **CVA** caused by a cerebral **thrombosis** is rapid, but the progression is slow. It is often called a "stroke in evolution," sometimes taking three days to become a "completed stroke" when the maximum neurological deficit has been accomplished and the affected area of the brain is swollen and necrotic.

Cerebral embolism occurs when an embolus or fragments of a blood clot, fat, bacteria, or tumor lodge in a cerebral vessel and cause an occlusion. This occlusion renders the area supplied by this vessel ischemic. A heart problem may lead to the occurrence of a cerebral embolus such as endocarditis, atrial fibrillation, and valvular conditions. A piece of a **thrombosis** may break off in the carotid artery and move into the circulation, causing a cerebral embolism. A fat emboli can occur from the fracture of a long bone. The cerebral emboli will cause immediate neurological deficits. If the emboli breaks up and is consumed by the body, the deficits will disappear. If not, the deficits will remain. Even when the emboli breaks up, the vessel wall is often left weakened, thus increasing the possibility of a cerebral hemorrhage at this site.

Cerebral hemorrhage occurs when a cerebral vessel ruptures, allowing bleeding into the CSF, brain tissue, or the subarachnoid space. High blood pressure is the most common cause of a cerebral hemorrhage. The symptoms occur rapidly and generally include a severe headache along with other neurological deficits (related to the area involved).

Parkinson's disease

(**PARK**-in-sons dih-**ZEEZ**)

A degenerative, slowly progressive, deterioration of nerves in the brain stem's motor system, characterized by a gradual onset of symptoms (such as a stooped posture with the body flexed forward; a bowed head; a shuffling gait; pill-rolling gestures; an expressionless, masklike facial appearance; muffled speech; and swallowing difficulty).

The cause of **Parkinson's disease** is not known, although a neurotransmitter deficiency (dopamine) has been clinically noted in persons with **Parkinson's disease**. **Parkinson's disease** is seen more often in males, with the onset of symptoms beginning during the ages of 50 to 60 years. The clinical symptoms can be divided into three groups.

1. **Motor dysfunction** demonstrated by the nonintentional tremors (pill-rolling), slowed movements, inability to start voluntary movements, speech problems, muscle rigidity, and gait and posture disturbances.

2. **Autonomic system dysfunction** demonstrated by mottled skin, drooling, dysphagia, problems from seborrhea and excess sweating on the upper neck and face, absence of sweating on the lower body, abnormally low blood pressure when standing, heat intolerance, and **constipation**.

3. **Mental and emotional dysfunction** demonstrated by loss of memory, declining mental processes, lack of problem-solving skill, uneasiness, and depression.

Treatment for **Parkinson's disease**, in addition to drug therapy, consists of control of symptoms and supportive measures, with physical therapy playing a very important role in keeping the person's mobility maximized. A recent surgical technique used for the person with **Parkinson's disease** is a **pallidotomy**. This procedure involves the destruction of the involved tissue in the brain to reduce tremors and severe **dyskinesia**. The goal of this procedure, to restore a more normal ambulatory function to the individual, is not always successful.

shingles (herpes zoster)

(**HER**-peez **ZOS**-ter)

An acute viral infection seen mainly in adults, characterized by inflammation of the underlying spinal or cranial nerve pathway, producing painful vesicular eruptions on the skin following along these nerve pathways.

This acute eruption is caused by reactivation of latent varicella virus (the same virus that causes chickenpox). **Herpes zoster** affects 10% to 20% of the population, with the highest incidence in adults over 50.

Symptoms include severe pain before and during eruption, fever, itching, GI disturbances, headache, general tiredness, and increased sensitivity of the skin around the area. The lesions usually take three to five days to erupt and then progress to crusting and drying (with recovery in approximately three weeks). Treatment with antiviral medications, analgesics, and sometimes corticosteroids aids in decreasing the severity of symptoms.

Blood and Lymphatic Systems

The effect of the aging process on the blood results mainly from the reduced capacity to make new blood cells quickly when disease has occurred. After about the age of 70, the percentage of bone marrow space occupied by tissue that produces blood cells declines progressively. This decreased ability to produce new blood cells when disease has occurred can be a problem for older adults.

Age-related changes in the lymphatic system affect the immune responses. The aging process impairs specific antibody responses to foreign antigens. Due to the decreased immunity, the older adult may be more susceptible to infections and malignancy. Infections are a leading cause of morbidity and mortality among older adults. The pathological conditions related to the aging blood and lymphatic systems include, but are not limited to, the following.

purpura	Collection of blood beneath the skin in the form of pinpoint hemorrhages appearing as red-purple skin discolorations.
(**PER**-pew-rah)	

Purpura are small hemorrhages caused from a decreased number of circulating platelets (thrombocytopenia). The body may produce an antiplatelet factor that will damage its own platelets.

Idiopathic thrombocytopenic purpura is a disorder in which the individual produces antibodies that destroy his or her own platelets. The cause of the prolonged bleeding time is unknown. Corticosteroids are administered and, many times, the individuals require the removal of the spleen to stop platelet destruction. **Purpura** is also seen in persons with low platelet counts for other associated reasons such as drug reactions and leukemia.

Cardiovascular System

As one ages, the workload and efficiency of the heart may be compromised due to accumulation of excess fat surrounding the heart. This may be brought about by poor dietary and exercise habits. Studies have shown that cardiovascular disease is nearly twice as likely to develop in sedentary people than in those who continue to be active. Cardiovascular disease can be quite severe in older adults, with approximately 85% of all cardiovascular deaths occurring in those over the age of 65. The risk for cardiovascular disease increases significantly in women after menopause. After the age of 65, the incidence of coronary heart disease in women is about one in three. The pathological conditions related to the aging cardiovascular system include, but are not limited to, the following.

arteriosclerosis	An arterial condition in which there is thickening, hardening, and loss of elasticity of the walls of the arteries, resulting in decreased blood supply, especially to the lower extremities and cerebrum; also called hardening of the arteries.
(ar-**tee**-ree-oh-sklair-**ROH**-sis)	
arteri/o = artery	
scler/o = hard	
-osis = condition	

Symptoms include intermittent **claudication**, changes in skin temperature and color, altered peripheral pulses, **bruits** over the involved artery, headache, dizziness, and memory defects (depending on the organ system involved). Risk factors for **arteriosclerosis** include hypertension, increased blood **lipids** (particularly cholesterol and triglycerides), obesity, diabetes, cigarette smoking, inability to cope with stress, and family history of early-onset **atherosclerosis**. Treatment options may include a diet low in saturated fatty acids, medications to lower the blood lipid levels (in conjunction with the low-fat diet), proper rest and regular exercise, avoidance of stress, discontinuing cigarette smoking, and additional treatment specific to the condition for factors (such as hypertension, diabetes, and obesity).

congestive heart failure (CHF) (kon-**JESS**-tiv heart failure)	Condition characterized by weakness, breathlessness, and abdominal discomfort. **Edema** in the lower portions of the body results from the flow of the blood through the vessels being slowed (venous stasis) and the outflow of blood from the left side of the heart being reduced. The pumping ability of the heart is progressively impaired to the point that it no longer meets bodily needs; also known as cardiac failure. **Congestive heart failure** is the single most frequent cause of hospitalization for those individuals 65 years of age and older.

The principal feature in congestive heart failure is increased intravascular volume. Congestion of the tissues results from increased arterial and venous pressure due to decreased cardiac output in the failing heart.

Left-sided cardiac failure is more common in older adults. It occurs when the left ventricle is unable to pump the blood sufficiently that enters it from the lungs. This causes increased pressure in the pulmonary circulation, which results in the forcing of fluid into the pulmonary tissues, creating **pulmonary edema** ("congestion"). The patient experiences dyspnea, cough (mostly moist sounding), fatigue, tachycardia, restlessness, and anxiety.

Right-sided cardiac failure occurs when the right side of the heart is unable to empty its blood volume sufficiently and cannot accommodate all of the blood it receives from the venous circulation. This results in congestion of the viscera and the peripheral tissues. The patient experiences edema of the lower extremities (**pitting edema**), weight gain, enlargement of the liver (hepatomegaly), distended neck veins, **ascites**, anorexia, **nocturia**, and weakness.

Treatment involves promoting rest to reduce the workload on the heart, medications to increase the strength and efficiency of the heartbeat, and medications to eliminate the accumulation of fluids within the body. Dietary sodium may also be restricted. The older adult with moderate to severe symptoms may require hospital admission for proper treatment.

coronary artery disease (CAD) (**KOR**-ah-nair-ree **AR**-ter-ee dih-**ZEEZ**) coron/o = heart -ary = pertaining to arter/o = artery -y = noun ending	Narrowing of the coronary arteries to the extent that adequate blood supply to the myocardium is prevented.

Coronary artery disease is usually caused by **atherosclerosis**. It may progress to the point that the heart muscle is damaged due to lack of blood supply (ischemia) as the lumen of the coronary artery narrows. When the lumen of the artery is narrowed and the wall is rough, there is a great tendency for clots to form, creating the possibility for **thrombotic occlusion** of the vessel.

As a result of the ischemia of the myocardial muscle, the individual experiences a burning, squeezing, or tightness in the chest that may radiate to the neck, shoulder blade, and left arm. Nausea, vomiting, sweating, and anxiety may also accompany the pain.

Accepted treatments for occluded coronary arteries (that reduce or prevent sufficient flow of blood to the myocardium) include medications, which may be used alone or in conjunction with other types of therapy, and diagnostic and treatment procedures such as percutaneous transluminal coronary angioplasty (PTCA), **directional coronary atherectomy** (DCA), and coronary bypass graft (CABG). The PTCA, DCA, and CABG procedures are discussed later in the chapter.

Respiratory System

When considering the respiratory system of the older adult, it is important to remember some of the changes that occur in the aging lungs. Most notably, the older adult experiences decreased volume during inspiration and expiration. Aging also affects the mechanical aspects of ventilation. Pulmonary tissue in the older adult has an altered level of function because of loss of elasticity, which leads to some degree of hyperinflation of the lung. The cilia within the respiratory tract show decreased action as the lung ages, and the respiratory muscle strength and endurance also decrease. With these changes, there is a corresponding decrease in strength for breathing or coughing. The respiratory system generally is able to meet the needs of a normal older adult. However, when illness or stress triggers a need for increased respiratory function, the reserve capacity may be inadequate to meet the need. The pathological conditions related to the **aging** respiratory system include, but are not limited to, the following.

emphysema

(em-fih-**SEE**-mah)

A chronic pulmonary disease characterized by increase beyond the normal in the size of air spaces distal to the terminal bronchiole, either from dilation of the alveoli or from destruction of their walls. See *Figure 24-9*.

This nonuniform pattern of abnormal permanent distention of the air spaces appears to be the end stage of a process that has progressed slowly for many years. By the time the patient develops the symptoms of **emphysema**, pulmonary function is often so impaired that it is irreversible.

The major cause of emphysema is cigarette smoking. The person with emphysema has a chronic obstruction (increase in airway resistance) to the inflow and outflow of air from the lungs. The lungs lose their elasticity and are in a chronic state of hyperexpansion, making expiration of air more difficult. The act of expiration then becomes one of active muscular movement to force the air out. The patient takes on a "barrel chest" appearance due to the loss of elasticity of lung tissue, becoming increasingly short of breath.

Treatment for emphysema is directed at improving the quality of life for the patient and slowing the progression of the disease. This may involve measures to improve the patient's ventilation (with the use of bronchodilators and medicine to thin the mucous secretions), the administration of medications to treat any infection present, and the administration of oxygen to treat the hypoxia that may be present.

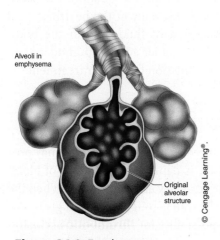

Alveoli in emphysema

Original alveolar structure

© Cengage Learning®.

Figure 24-9 Emphysema

influenza (in-floo-**IN**-zah)	A highly contagious viral infection of the respiratory tract transmitted by airborne droplet infection; also known as the flu. **Influenza** can occur in isolated cases or can be epidemic. The incubation period is usually one to three days after exposure. Older adults may be more prone to developing bacterial influenza, as are those individuals who have chronic pulmonary disease.

Symptoms of the flu include sore throat, cough, fever, muscular pains, and generalized weakness. The onset is usually sudden, with the individual experiencing fever, chills, respiratory symptoms, headache, muscle pain, and extreme tiredness.

Treatment for influenza is symptomatic and involves bed rest, plenty of fluids, and medications for pain. Recovery usually occurs within 3 to 10 days. Yearly vaccination with the current prevailing strain of influenza virus is recommended for older adults or debilitated individuals.

pneumonia	An acute inflammation of the lungs caused mainly by inhaled pneumococci of the *Streptococcus pneumoniae* species. It may also be caused by other bacteria as well as by viruses.

Pneumonia is a common infection in older adults and one of the leading causes of death. Aging tends to predispose the older adult to pneumonia as a result of the lowered immune status and less efficient ventilation. Some of the predisposing factors to older adults developing pneumonia are chronic obstructive pulmonary disease (COPD), nutritional deficiencies, or changes in mental status.

Treatment for pneumonia includes medication for the causative organism or virus, proper diet, increased fluid intake, analgesics for pain and/or nonsteroidal anti-inflammatory drugs (NSAIDs) for inflammation, plenty of rest, and proper clearing of mucus from the respiratory passages. Depending on the age of the individual and the general health status, the individual may be treated at home. The recovery period for the older adult varies. It may take weeks to feel normal again.

Prevention is important in the older adult patient. This can be achieved through administration of the pneumonia vaccine. The general rule of thumb is to administer the pneumonia vaccine once before the age of 80 and to repeat it every five to seven years thereafter.

pulmonary edema (**PULL**-mon-air-ree eh-**DEE**-mah) pulmon/o = lung -ary = pertaining to	Swelling of the lungs caused by an abnormal accumulation of fluid in the lungs, in either the alveoli or the interstitial spaces.

The most common cause of pulmonary edema is cardiac disease. The pulmonary congestion occurs when the pulmonary vessels receive more blood from the right ventricle of the heart than the left ventricle can accommodate and remove. This congestion (or backup of fluid) causes the fluid to leak through the capillary walls and permeate into the airways, creating a sudden onset of breathlessness and a sense of suffocation. The patient's nailbeds become cyanotic and the skin becomes gray. As the condition progresses, breathing is noisy and moist. The patient needs immediate medical attention.

pulmonary heart disease (cor pulmonale)	Hypertrophy of the right ventricle of the heart (with or without failure) resulting from disorders of the lungs, pulmonary vessels, or chest wall; heart failure resulting from disorders of the lungs; pulmonary disease.
(**PULL**-mon-air-ree heart dih-**ZEEZ**) (**COR**-pull-mon-**ALL**-ee) **pulmon/o** = lung **-ary** = pertaining to	

Pulmonary heart disease reduces proper ventilation to the lungs, resulting in increased resistance in the pulmonary circulation. This, in turn, raises the pulmonary blood pressure. **Cor pulmonale** develops because of the pulmonary hypertension, which causes the right side of the heart to work harder to pump the blood against the resistance of the pulmonary vascular circulation, thus creating hypertrophy of the right ventricle of the heart.

Chronic obstructive pulmonary disease (COPD), the most frequent cause of cor pulmonale, produces shortness of breath and cough. The patient develops edema of the feet and legs, distended neck veins, an enlarged liver, pleural effusion, ascites, and a heart murmur.

Treatment is related to treating the underlying cause of cor pulmonale and is often a long-term process. In the case of COPD, treatment involves improving the patient's ventilation (airways must be dilated to improve gas exchange within the lungs). The improved transport of oxygen to the blood and body tissues will reduce the strain on the pulmonary circulation, thus relieving the pulmonary hypertension that leads to cor pulmonale.

Digestive System

As the digestive system ages, many older adults experience significant changes in the gastrointestinal system that not only affect the nutritional status but also cause pain and discomfort. For the most part, however, gastrointestinal function remains intact even when some changes are present.

Some of the notable changes include loss of teeth related to dental or periodontal problems, decrease in the quality and quantity of saliva, some decrease in normal peristalsis in the esophagus, a weakness in the musculature of the large intestine that results in decreased forcefulness of contractions and a slowing of peristaltic activity, and a tendency toward formation of diverticula or herniations of the mucosa into the weakened intestinal musculature. The older adult may also experience some difficulty metabolizing some medications, making it necessary to adjust medication dosages to prevent cumulative effects and to ensure proper excretion of drugs. The pathological conditions related to the aging digestive system include, but are not limited to, the following.

achalasia (**ack**-al-**LAY**-zee-ah)	Decreased mobility of the lower two-thirds of the esophagus along with constriction of the lower esophageal sphincter (LES), making it difficult for food and liquids to move down the esophagus.

Due to the lack of nerve impulses and the absence of sympathetic receptors, the relaxation of the lower LES fails to happen with swallowing. Food and fluid accumulate in the lower esophagus due to the decreased mobility there and the constriction of the LES. **Achalasia** is a progressive disease and generally gets worse.

The individual may complain of difficulty in swallowing fluids and food, retrosternal chest pain or discomfort (a sensation of great fullness in the lower chest), and regurgitation of undigested food. Among the diagnostic tests used to diagnose achalasia are **barium swallow** and endoscopy studies. Medical intervention may be more suitable for the older adult, although achalasia can also be treated surgically.

colorectal cancer (**koh**-lo-**REK**-tal **CAN**-sir)	The presence of a malignant neoplasm in the large intestine.

Most neoplasms in the large intestine are adenocarcinomas and at least 50% originate in the rectum, causing bleeding and pain. Next to cancer of the lung, colon cancer is the third most commonly occurring cause of death. The incidence of **colorectal cancer** increases in individuals over 70 years of age, with a death rate of almost 50% of those affected.

Symptoms of colorectal cancer vary according to tumor location. Two-thirds of all colorectal cancers occur in the lower sigmoid colon and the rectum. The most common symptoms include rectal bleeding, followed by bowel changes, abdominal pain or cramping, unexplained weight loss, and anemia.

Although the cause of colorectal cancer is unknown, it has been suggested that a diet high in beef and refined carbohydrates and low in roughage leads to the formation of bacteria, boosting the amount of fatty acids and bile (which behave as carcinogens). Other factors that predispose one to colorectal cancer are history of Crohn's disease, ulcerative colitis, irritable bowel syndrome, or familial polyposis.

Along with the rectal exam, a **barium enema**, sigmoidoscopy and/or **colonoscopy**, and stool exam for occult blood will be used for diagnosis. Prognosis depends on the extent of the disease, and surgery is usually the treatment of choice.

constipation (**KON**-stih-**PAY**-shun)	A state in which the individual's pattern of bowel elimination is characterized by a decrease in the frequency of bowel movements and the passage of hard, dry stools. The individual experiences difficult defecation.

Constipation is a common complaint among older adult patients. Contributing factors include decreased peristalsis in the intestinal tract, decreased appetite, inadequate fluid intake, and lack of exercise. Repeated overuse or abuse of laxatives over the years worsens the problem.

Dietary concerns are important in preventing **constipation** in the older adult. The individual should be encouraged to eat small frequent meals, increase dietary fiber, and drink plenty of fluids daily.

diverticular disease (**dye**-ver-**TIK**-yoo-lar dih-**ZEEZ**)	An expression used to characterize both diverticulosis and diverticulitis. Diverticulosis describes the noninflamed outpouchings or herniations through the muscular layer of the intestine, typically the sigmoid colon. Inflammation of the outpouchings called diverticulum is referred to as diverticulitis.

Diverticular disease is an increasingly common occurrence in persons over 45 years of age. Persons eating diets low in fiber predispose themselves to the formation of diverticulum.

Symptoms of diverticulosis may include mild cramps, bloating, and **constipation**. The most common symptom of diverticulitis is abdominal pain. More severe symptoms include cramping, fever, increased flatus, and elevated WBC count (leukocytosis). The severity of symptoms depend on the extent of the infection and complications. Proctoscopy and barium enemas are used in the diagnostic process.

Endocrine System

When considering the aging endocrine system, there is a noted overall decline in hormone secretion and diminished tissue sensitivity to secreted hormones. The most notable decrease in hormones is that of estrogen and testosterone. The older adult also experiences a change in glucose tolerance, which results in a prolonged elevated blood sugar level in response to a meal. As a result of the physiological changes that occur in the endocrine system, endocrine diseases are most common in later years. The pathological conditions related to the aging endocrine system include, but are not limited to, the following.

diabetes mellitus (dye-ah-**BEE**-teez **MELL**-ih-tus)	A disorder of the pancreas in which the beta cells of the islets of Langerhans of the pancreas fail to produce an adequate amount of insulin, resulting in the body's inability to appropriately metabolize carbohydrates, fats, and proteins.

Diabetes mellitus affects approximately 10% of individuals over 65 years of age and approximately 20% of individuals over 80 years of age. The classic characteristic of the disease is **hyperglycemia**. First, the individual will experience abnormally elevated blood glucose levels (known as hyperglycemia) due to the body's inability to use glucose for energy. Insulin is necessary for the body cells to use glucose for energy. Second, when the body cannot use glucose for energy, the cells begin to break down fats and proteins for energy. This breakdown of fats and proteins releases waste products known as **ketones** into the bloodstream, which spill over into the urine due to abnormal accumulations.

The classic symptoms of **diabetes mellitus** are **glycosuria**, **polydipsia**, and **polyuria**. Other symptoms include increased eating (**polyphagia**) and weight loss, presence of **ketones** in the urine, itching (pruritus), muscle weakness, and fatigue.

Diabetes mellitus is classified as either type 1 diabetes (formerly known as insulin-dependent diabetes) or type 2 diabetes (formerly known as non-insulin-dependent diabetes). All people with diabetes are encouraged to wear emergency alert bracelets. This discussion is limited to type 2 diabetes, which usually occurs later in life.

Type 2 diabetes usually appears in adults after the age of 30, having a gradual onset. The majority of these individuals are obese. Individuals with type 2 diabetes usually have some pancreatic activity but experience insulin resistance (reduced ability of most cells to respond to insulin) or impaired insulin secretion. For these individuals, losing weight and gaining muscle helps the body use insulin more efficiently. Sometimes oral antidiabetic drugs are used in addition to control blood sugar levels. Approximately 90% of all people with diabetes have type 2 diabetes.

Some people with type 2 diabetes, however, become insulin dependent. Type 2 diabetes is a progressive disease that is often present for 3 to 12 years prior to diagnosis. Although these individuals are usually able to control their diabetes with diet and exercise in the beginning, they eventually have to convert to the administration of insulin injections for proper control when the body is unable to get enough glucose because of insulin resistance or decreased ability to produce insulin. Individuals with type 2 diabetes who do require insulin injections to control the disease experience all of the symptoms and problems that accompany type 1 diabetes. They are not as likely to develop diabetic ketoacidosis (DKA) early in the disease as are those with type 1 diabetes, due to the small amount of insulin they continue to secrete. However, later in the disease, if they have become completely dependent on insulin, they have just as great a likelihood.

An abnormally high blood glucose level is the main criterion for a diagnosis of **diabetes mellitus**. A random blood glucose level of more than 200 mg/dL of blood on more than one occasion, or a fasting blood glucose level of more than 126 mg/dL of blood, is diagnostic of diabetes.

Individuals with early type 2 diabetes usually control their diabetes with diet and exercise, eventually requiring the use of oral **hypoglycemia** agents to stimulate the production of insulin by the pancreas or supplemental insulin by injection or inhalation. Complications of long-term diabetes vary according to the individual and the type of diabetes. These complications include poor circulation in the extremities, especially the lower legs and feet; infections that heal poorly due to the decreased circulation; kidney disease and renal failure; **diabetic retinopathy**, which is a leading cause of blindness; and involvement of the nervous system (diabetic neuropathy), characterized by numbness (decreased sensitivity of the fingers to touch and grasp) and intermittent but severe episodes of pain in the extremities. People with diabetes who maintain near-normal blood glucose levels can reasonably expect to live for many years without major complications.

Special Senses (Eye and Ear)

Impairment of vision is one of the three most common medical problems among older adults. Of older adults over the age of 85, at least 25% have significant visual difficulties to cause trouble reading or difficulty conducting daily activities independently. The size of the pupil decreases with aging, which necessitates a brighter light for vision. Sensitivity to glare also increases with age because of changes in the opacity of the lens. Color discrimination decreases with aging, and depth perception is altered.

Hearing impairment is the second most common health problem affecting the older adult population. The ability to discriminate among high frequencies is often impaired by the age of 50 and shows a marked decline after the age of 65. The older adult who is described as "hard of hearing" may actually have more of a high-frequency loss than a generalized decline in hearing perception. It is, therefore, easier for an older adult to hear voices, telephones, doorbells, and horns that have lower tones and high intensity. The pathological conditions related to the aging eye and ear include, but are not limited to, the following.

cataract (**KAT**-ah-rakt)	The lens in the eye becomes progressively cloudy, losing its normal transparency and thus altering the perception of images due to the interference of light transmission to the retina.

The occurrence of cataracts can be classified as senile or secondary on the basis of etiology. See *Figure 24-10.*

Senile cataracts typically begin after the age of 50 years, at which time degenerative changes occur that result in the gradual clouding of the crystalline lens due to wear and tear and the change in fibers and protein as it ages. Senile cataracts are common and can be found in an estimated 95% of persons over 65 years.

Secondary cataracts result from trauma, radiation injury, inflammation, taking certain medications (such as corticosteroids), and metabolic diseases such as **diabetes mellitus**. Immature cataracts, those in which only a portion of the lens is affected, are diagnosed through **biomicroscopy** and the person's history. Mature cataracts, those in which the entire lens is clouded, can be visualized with the naked eye and appear as a gray-white area behind the pupil. A loss of the red reflex is noted as the **cataract** matures.

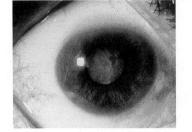

Figure 24-10 Cataract
(Courtesy of the National Eye Institute, NIH)

Treatment includes surgical intervention to remove the **cataract**. Surgery is indicated when the vision loss handicaps the person in the accomplishment of daily activities or when **glaucoma** or other secondary conditions occur. Surgical intervention for **cataract** removal is typically completed on an outpatient basis. No medical treatment is available for cataracts at present other than surgical removal.

deafness, sensorineural (sen-soh-ree-**NOO**-ral) **neur/o** = nerve **-al** = pertaining to	Hearing loss caused by the inability of nerve stimuli to be delivered to the brain from the inner ear due to damage to the auditory nerve or the cochlea.

The results vary from a mild hearing loss to a profound hearing loss. This sensorineural hearing loss can occur due to the aging process or damaged hair cells of the organ of Corti, which may occur in relation to loud machinery noise, loud music, or medication side effects. Other causes of sensorineural hearing loss include tumors, infections (such as bacterial meningitis), trauma altering the central auditory pathways, vascular disorders, and degenerative or demyelinating diseases. **Sensorineural deafness** makes speech discrimination difficult, primarily in noisy surroundings.

Diagnosis is based on the person's history and the results of the audiometry test. The best treatment is prevention when possible, accomplished by avoiding exposure to loud noises and being aware of medication with ototoxic effects (both of which may cause this damage). If the person cannot totally avoid the loud noises, wearing earplugs will be helpful to prevent or escape further damage. **Hearing aids** are helpful in some cases. However, the person with sensorineural hearing loss may require a cochlear implant to have sound perception restored.

diabetic retinopathy
 	
(dye-ah-**BET**-ik reh-tin-**OP**-ah-thee)
  retin/o = retina
  -pathy = disease
	Occurs as a consequence of an 8- to 10-year duration of **diabetes mellitus** in which the capillaries of the retina experience scarring due to the following:

1. Abnormal dilation and constriction of vessels

2. Hemorrhages

3. Microaneurysm

4. Abnormal formation of new vessels, causing leakage of blood into the vitreous humor

The scarring and leakage of blood causes a permanent decline in the sharpness of vision. The inability to get the oxygen and nutrients needed for good vision to the retina will eventually lead to permanent loss of vision. In the United States, **diabetic retinopathy** is the leading cause of blindness.

Diagnosis is made from the person's history and a thorough examination of the internal eye via biomicroscopy, during which the changes in the retinal vasculature can be seen. The person with **diabetes mellitus** should be followed regularly with dilated-eye exams to identify the changes taking place due to the available treatment with vitrectomy (removal of vitreous hemorrhages) and laser photocoagulation, which are normally useful in managing **diabetic retinopathy**.

ectropion (eck-**TROH**-pee-on)	"Turning out" or eversion of the eyelash margins (especially the lower eyelid) from the eyeball, leading to exposure of the eyelid and eyeball surface and lining. See *Figure 24-11.*

When an individual is affected by **ectropion**, tears are unable to flow into the tear ducts (which normally drain the tears) to keep the eyes moist and therefore flow down the face. This exposure and lack of moisture leads to dryness and irritation of the eye.

Ectropion frequently affects the older adult population as a result of aging. This occurs with the development of a weakened muscle in the lower eyelid, resulting in eversion of the eyelid (causing the outward turning of the eyelid). Facial nerve paralysis, eyelid tissue atrophy, and scarring of the cheek or eyelid (which pull down on the eyelid) are also causes of **ectropion**.

Ectropion is diagnosed through a visual exam. Treatment with a minor surgical process to correct **ectropion** is usually required because the condition rarely resolves on its own. The dryness and irritation remain a constant threat to the cornea and the development of permanent damage and corneal ulcers or severe dry eye.

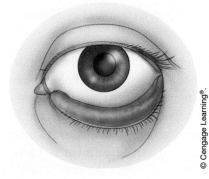

© Cengage Learning®.

Figure 24-11 Ectropion

entropion

(en-**TROH**-pee-on)

"Turning in" of the eyelash margins (especially the lower margins), resulting in the sensation similar to that of a foreign body in the eye (redness, tearing, burning, and itching). See *Figure 24-12*.

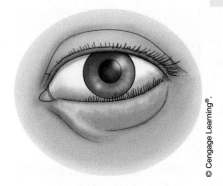

© Cengage Learning®.

Figure 24-12 Entropion

Entropion may result in damage to the cornea in the form of corneal scratches or corneal ulcers due to the constant irritation of the lashes rubbing on the surface.

Entropion frequently affects the older population as a result of aging. This occurs with the development of loose fibrous tissue in the lower eyelid, resulting in extreme tightening of the eyelid muscle (causing the inward turning of the eyelid). This is diagnosed through a visual exam. Treatment with a minor surgical process to correct **entropion** is required if the condition does not resolve and remains a constant irritant to the conjunctiva and cornea.

glaucoma

(glau-**KOH**-mah)

Ocular disorders identified as a group due to the increase in intraocular pressure. This increase in intraocular pressure may be primary or secondary, acute or chronic, and described as open or closed angle.

These disorders occur due to a barrier in the normal outflow of aqueous humor or an increased production of aqueous humor. Increased intraocular pressure leads to an inhibited blood supply of the optic neurons, which will lead to degeneration and atrophy of the optic nerve and finally total loss of vision. **Glaucoma** is the second leading cause of blindness in the United States. The incidence of **glaucoma** increases rapidly after 40 years of age. Chronic open-angle **glaucoma**, acute closed-angle **glaucoma**, and secondary **glaucoma** are discussed.

Chronic open-angle **glaucoma** occurs as a primary disorder, with a breakdown in the drainage system of the circulation of aqueous humor. A gradual elevation of internal pressure leads to a decreased blood supply to the optic nerve and the retina. The most common type of **glaucoma**, chronic open angle, is so gradual that the presence in most individuals is long-standing before any symptoms are recognized.

When chronic open-angle **glaucoma** is untreated, peripheral vision is gradually lost in advanced **glaucoma**. The central vision will eventually be lost as well, rendering the individual completely blind. Routine ophthalmic examinations, which include optic nerve evaluation and readings of intraocular pressure, are important for the detection and evaluation of chronic open-angle **glaucoma**.

Along with the person's history and the identified symptoms, the diagnosis of open-angle **glaucoma** can be confirmed through an ophthalmic exam with tonometry (measurement of intraocular pressure). Corneal thickness is an important factor in determining the final pressure measurement for intraocular pressure. The process of measuring corneal thickness is known as pachymetry. When diagnosis is made and early treatment is started with medication to open the drainage system or reduce the production of aqueous humor, the intraocular pressure is controlled to a certain extent. When medication does not adequately control the intraocular pressure, surgery may be required to bypass the faulty drainage system.

Acute angle-closure **glaucoma** is a rapid primary occurrence of increased intraocular pressure in a short period of time. It is due to the mouth of the drainage system being narrow and closing completely, allowing no flow of aqueous humor. This rapid occurrence is characterized by severe pain, blurred vision, photophobia, redness, and seeing "halos" around light. Within several days, the person with untreated acute angle-closure **glaucoma** can lose his or her sight.

Treatment is aimed at quickly reducing the pressure inside the eye to avoid vision loss. The creation of a small hole between the posterior and anterior chambers through a procedure called laser iridotomy has been effective in opening the filtering angle, allowing the aqueous humor to flow, and thus decreasing the intraocular pressure.

Secondary **glaucoma** occurs as a complication of another disorder, trauma, or surgery. Swelling of eye tissue from the trauma of surgery, injury, or inflammation causes the flow pattern or system to be affected. This leads to impeded drainage of aqueous humor and increased intraocular pressure.

macular degeneration (**MAK**-yoo-lar dee-**jin**-er-**RAY**-shun)	Progressive deterioration of the retinal cells in the macula due to aging. Known as senile or age-related **macular degeneration** (ARMD), this condition is a common and progressive cause of visual deficiency and permanent reading impairment in the adult over 65 years of age.

The macular area is the area of central vision. During the aging process, the macula may undergo a degenerative process that results in the loss of central vision. The peripheral or side vision remains intact. The older adult with age-related macular degeneration rarely experiences complete blindness. Because only the macula is affected, these individuals maintain their peripheral vision and can walk without assistance and carry out many activities by using side vision.

There are two types of macular degeneration. The dry form causes a slow, gradual deterioration of the function of the macula. Individuals affected by this form of macular degeneration may note distortion or blind spots in their vision. They experience slow, progressive, and painless decrease in vision.

The second type is the wet form, which is more serious and is responsible for the majority of the cases of severe visual loss due to macular degeneration. Individuals affected by the wet form of macular degeneration experience a leakage of fluid from abnormal vessels under the retina.

There is no known treatment for the dry type of ARMD. The wet type of macular degeneration is often treatable with laser therapy in the early stages. However, the laser is not used in the center of the macula if abnormal vessels already occupy it, because the laser destroys the area treated.

presbyopia	A refractive error occurring after the age of 40, when the lens of the eye(s) cannot focus on an image accurately due to its decreasing elasticity.
(**pres**-bee-**OH**-pee-ah)	
presby/o = old age	
-opia = visual condition	

This results in a decline in refraction and accommodation for close vision. There is diminished ability to focus clearly on close objects and fine print. **Presbyopia** usually results in hyperopia, or farsightedness.

In addition to blurred vision of close objects, the individual may also complain of headaches and frequent squinting. The diagnosis of **presbyopia** is verified through an ophthalmoscopic exam and is corrected through the use of contact lenses or eyeglasses.

The Urinary System

During the aging process, there are both structural and functional changes in the kidneys. The aging kidney is more susceptible to trauma or disease. The number of nephron units of the kidney decreases during the aging process, and there is a gradual degenerative change in the remaining number of nephrons. By the time the older adult reaches the age of 70 to 80 years, the glomerular filtration rate is approximately 50% of what it was when the individual was 30 years of age. With this decreased glomerular filtration, drugs may not be excreted as rapidly as possible and they may remain in the bloodstream, producing toxic levels.

The aging kidney is inefficient in its ability to regain normal fluid and electrolyte balance after a rapid loss of fluids, thus requiring a longer time to correct fluid and electrolyte imbalances. The ureters and bladder tend to lose muscle tone, and the bladder loses enough tone to result in incomplete emptying that leads to accumulation of residual urine, increasing the risk of retention and cystitis. The pathological conditions related to the aging urinary system include, but are not limited to, the following.

urinary incontinence	The inability to retain urine in the bladder; the loss of urine from the bladder due to loss of sphincter control. This involuntary loss of urine is severe enough to cause social or hygienic problems.
(**YOO**-rih-nair-ee in-**CON**-tin-ens)	
urin/o = urine	
-ary = pertaining to	

Urinary incontinence affects mostly older adults. However, it is not a normal consequence of aging. Bladder incontinence may be due to abnormalities of bladder contraction, abnormalities of urethral relaxation, or, in some older adults, **dementia**.

Many older women suffer from **stress incontinence**, which is the inability to hold urine when the bladder is stressed by sneezing, coughing, laughing, or lifting. A common method of treating stress incontinence is through the use of isometric exercises known as **Kegel exercises**. The woman executes a series of voluntary contractions or squeezing of the muscles required to stop the urinary stream while voiding (a tightening and relaxation of the pelvic muscles). Repetition of this tightening and relaxation exercise, 20 to 40 times several times a day, has proven successful in controlling some types of stress incontinence. The older adult may also suffer other types of **urinary incontinence**, such as the following.

1. *Functional incontinence*: The individual experiences an involuntary, unpredictable passage of urine. This is characterized by the urge to void, or bladder contractions that are strong enough to result in loss of urine before reaching an appropriate receptacle.

2. *Urge incontinence*: The urge to empty the bladder is sudden and uncontrollable, and the individual experiences involuntary passage of urine soon after the strong sense of urgency to void. The individual may not be able to reach a toilet in time when suffering from urge incontinence.

3. *Overflow incontinence*: The involuntary loss of urine is associated with overdistention of the bladder, when the bladder's capacity has reached its maximum. The individual may experience a constant dribbling of urine. This type of incontinence may be the result of complications of long-term diabetes (diabetic neuropathy) or the side effect of medication.

It is estimated that up to 30% of older adults over the age of 60, not living in nursing homes, are affected by **urinary incontinence** and that over 50% of those residing in nursing homes are affected by **urinary incontinence**. In many cases, once the underlying cause of the **urinary incontinence** is determined, it can be treated (and often cured).

The Male Reproductive System

As men age, they experience a decrease in testosterone level, sperm production, muscle tone of the scrotum, and the size and firmness of the testicles. The prostate gland enlarges considerably with age. Sexual activity is normal and possible in the older age group if there are no major health problems. The pathological conditions related to the aging male reproductive system include, but are not limited to, the following.

benign prostatic hypertrophy	A benign (noncancerous) enlargement of the prostate gland, creating pressure on the upper part of the urethra or neck of the bladder, causing obstruction of the flow of urine.

(bee-**NINE** pross-**TAT**-ik
high-**PER**-troh-fee)

   prostat/o = prostate gland
   -ic = pertaining to
   hyper- = excessive
   -trophy = development, growth

This is a common condition occurring in men over the age of 50. Approximately 25% of males older than 80 years will require prostatic surgery due to the obstructive symptoms caused by the enlarged prostate gland.

Men with **benign prostatic hypertrophy** (**BPH**) may complain of symptoms such as difficulty in starting urination, a weak stream of urine (not being able to maintain a constant stream), the inability to empty the bladder completely, or "dribbling" at the end of voiding.

Diagnosis is usually confirmed by thorough patient history and a rectal examination by the physician to confirm prostatic enlargement. The physician may order a urinalysis and culture of the urine to check for urinary tract infection or any abnormalities in the urine such as blood. Other diagnostic tests may be a cystourethroscopy to visualize the interior of the bladder and the urethra; a **KUB** (kidneys, ureters, bladder) X-ray to visualize the urinary tract; or a **residual urine test** to check for incomplete emptying of the bladder. If a malignancy (cancer) is suspected, a biopsy of the prostatic tissue may be ordered.

Treatment for BPH depends on the degree of urinary obstruction noted. For patients with mild cases of prostatic enlargement (which is normal as the male ages), the condition may simply be monitored. For patients with recurrent and obstructive problems due to hyperplasia of the prostate gland, surgery is usually indicated to remove the prostate gland. Two types of surgery used are **transurethral resection of the prostate (TURP)** and **suprapubic prostatectomy**, both of which are discussed in the diagnostic procedures section of this chapter.

carcinoma of the prostate	Malignant growth within the prostate gland, creating pressure on the upper part of the urethra.
(kar-sih-**NOH**-mah of the **PROSS**-tayt)	
carcin/o = cancer	
-oma = tumor	

Cancer of the prostate is the most common cancer among men and the most common cause of cancer death in men over the age of 55. Unfortunately, symptoms are not usually present in the early stages of cancer of the prostate. By the time symptoms are evident, the cancer may have already metastasized (spread) to other areas of the body. When symptoms of prostate cancer occur, they may include any of the following.

1. A need to urinate frequently (i.e., urinary frequency), especially at night

2. Difficulty starting or stopping urine flow

3. Inability to urinate

4. Weak or interrupted flow of urine when urinating (patient may complain of "dribbling" instead of having a steady stream of urine)

5. Pain or burning when urinating

6. Pain or stiffness in the lower back, hips, or thighs

7. Painful ejaculation

Because the presence of symptoms usually means that the disease is more advanced, early detection of cancer of the prostate is essential to successful treatment. All men over the age of 50 should have a yearly physical exam that includes a digital rectal examination of the prostate gland.

The rectal exam can reveal a cancerous growth before symptoms appear. A prostate-specific antigen (PSA) blood test may be performed during the exam to detect increased growth of the prostate. (The growth could be benign or malignant.) The level of PSA in the blood may rise in men who have prostate cancer or **benign prostatic hypertrophy**. If the level is elevated, the physician will order additional tests to confirm a diagnosis of cancer of the prostate.

The most common procedure used to treat or relieve the urinary obstruction resulting from cancer of the prostate is surgery (TURP) to remove the prostate tissue that is pressing against the upper part of the urethra. TURP is also used to treat **benign prostatic hypertrophy**.

Other methods of treatment include a radical prostatectomy (removal of the prostate gland), radiation therapy, hormone therapy, or chemotherapy. The treatment of choice depends on the patient's age, medical history, risks and benefits of treatment, and the stage of the disease.

The Female Reproductive System

Physical changes occur in women after menopause. The ovaries cease to produce ova (eggs) and have less estrogen hormone, which may cause physiological symptoms. As women age, they experience a general **atrophy** of the genitalia related to the hormonal changes. These changes in the genitalia include less fat, external hair loss, and flattening of the labia. The uterus of the older female is approximately one-half the size of the uterus of the young adult female. The vagina becomes drier and narrower. As a result of less vaginal lubrication, postmenopausal women may experience dyspareunia (pain during sexual intercourse).

After menopause and the decrease in estrogen levels, women experience changes in breast tissue that result in less glandular tissue, reduced elasticity, and more connective tissue and fat. These changes can cause sagging breasts, although the size of the breasts may not change. The pathological conditions related to the aging female reproductive system include, but are not limited to, the following.

atrophic vaginitis (aye-**TROH**-fik vaj-in-**EYE**-tis) a- = without troph/o = development -ic = pertaining to vagin/o = vagina -itis = inflammation	Degeneration of the vaginal mucous membrane after menopause. Also known as senile vaginitis, this condition is common in estrogen-deprived older women. The tissues of the vagina become drier and thinner. Symptoms of **atrophic vaginitis** include pruritus (itching), burning, dyspareunia (pain during sexual intercourse), and bleeding. Treatment includes estrogen replacement therapy, vaginal hormone creams, and lubricants.
ovarian carcinoma (oh-**VAY**-ree-an car-sin-**OH**-mah) ovari/o = ovary -an = characteristic of carcin/o = cancer -oma = tumor	A malignant tumor of the ovaries, most commonly occurring in women in their 50s. It is rarely detected in the early stage and is usually far advanced when diagnosed. Symptoms usually do not appear with **ovarian cancer** until disease is well advanced. The earliest symptoms of ovarian cancer are swelling, bloating, or discomfort in the lower abdomen and mild digestive complaints (loss of appetite, feeling of fullness, indigestion, nausea, and weight loss). As the tumor increases in size, it may create pressure on adjacent organs, such as the urinary bladder or the rectum, causing frequent urination and dysuria or **constipation**. Later developments in the course of the disease include an accumulation of fluid within the abdominal cavity (ascites), resulting in swelling and discomfort. Diagnosis is confirmed with examination of a sample of the tumor tissue under a microscope. This is achieved through surgical removal of the affected ovary. If the ovary is diseased with cancer, the surgeon will then remove the other ovary, the uterus, and the fallopian tubes. A process called staging is important to determine the amount of metastasis, if any. This process involves taking samples (biopsy) of nearby lymph nodes and the diaphragm and sampling the fluid from the abdomen. Treatment involves the use of surgery, chemotherapy, or radiation therapy. It may involve one or a combination of the treatment choices, depending on the extent of the disease.

Mental Health

Oliver Wendell Holmes (U.S. physician, poet, and humorist) once commented, "To be 70 years young is sometimes far more cheerful and hopeful than to be 40 years old." How true! Can you think of an older adult friend or relative who seems young, although this person is over 65? What is it that allows this individual to age successfully and enjoy a mentally healthy attitude about aging?

Many factors contribute to successful aging and a continued sense of self-worth. Factors such as maintaining positive social relationships, continuing to be independent, having adequate personal income, and maintaining the best possible level of health contribute to successful aging. It is important that aging adults become acquainted with the normal changes that occur with aging and understand that some adjustments may be required to meet these changes. Normal physiological changes do occur with aging but at an individualized pace and in a unique manner for each individual. Some approach these changes in a positive way; others find aging to be a negative event.

Although normal aging does not imply disease, the incidence of chronic diseases increases with age. This has been clearly depicted in the previous pages of this chapter. Mental health is defined as a relative state of mind in which a person is able to cope with and adjust to the repeated stresses of everyday living in an acceptable way. The majority of older adults have successfully coped with life crises and the aging process. A small percentage find difficulty in coping with life changes as they age. For those individuals, a common mental health problem is depression, which often goes undiagnosed. Furthermore, many older adults experience a co-occurrence of depression with heart disease. This segment of the chapter is devoted to the discussion of **dementia** and depression as related to older adults.

dementia	A progressive, organic mental disorder characterized by chronic personality disintegration, confusion, disorientation, stupor, deterioration of intellectual capacity and function, and impairment of control of memory, judgment, and impulses.
(dee-**MEN**-she-ah)	

Dementia of the Alzheimer's type is the most common form. The onset of symptoms is slow and not easily detected at first, with the course of the disorder becoming progressive and deteriorating. If the onset is early, the symptoms will appear before the age of 65. If the onset is late, the symptoms will appear after the age of 65. It has been projected that approximately 10% of individuals over the age of 65 and 50% of those over the age of 85 will develop **Alzheimer's disease**.

The symptoms of **dementia** of the Alzheimer's type may begin as forgetfulness, followed by the individual becoming suspicious of others as the memory deteriorates. The individual may become apathetic and socially withdrawn or untidier in appearance. Irritability, moodiness, and sudden outbursts over trivial issues may become apparent. These individuals may wander away from home, forgetting where they are and where they live. As the condition progresses, the ability to work or care for personal needs independently is no longer possible and the individual requires supervised care.

depression (dee-**PRESS**-shun)	A mood disturbance characterized by exaggerated feelings of sadness, discouragement, and hopelessness that are inappropriate and out of proportion to reality; may be relative to some personal loss or tragedy.

Depression is one of the most common, and most treatable, of all mental disorders in older adults—if it is recognized. Many factors in the lives of older adults place them at high risk for the development or recurrence of depression, such as biological, psychological, and social changes. The lack of treatment, however, for depression in the older adult may be attributed to the reluctance of the older adult to seek psychiatric care, the tendency of older adults to insist that physical illness rather than an emotional problem is at the root of their concern, and the failure of many health care professionals to recognize that depressive symptoms are not a natural part of growing old.

Depression can affect every aspect of an older adult's life. It may be characterized by some of the following behavioral signs: sadness, discouragement, crying, irritability, withdrawing from usual activities, being critical of self and others, becoming passive, decreased or increased appetite, fatigue, weight loss or sometimes weight gain, and thoughts of death. Some of these symptoms can be easily overlooked by the health care professional because physical illness can mask the symptoms of depression.

Several types of therapies have been found to be beneficial in treating depression in the older adult. The goals of treatment are designed to improve the quality of life and functional ability of these individuals as well as reducing morbidity and mortality.

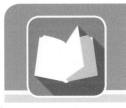

Review Checkpoint

Check your understanding of this section by completing the **Pathological Conditions** exercises in your workbook.

Diagnostic Techniques, Treatments, and Procedures

barium enema (lower GI series) (**BEAR**-ee-um **EN**-eh-mah)	Infusion of a radiopaque contrast medium, barium sulfate, into the rectum and held in place in the lower intestinal tract while X-ray films are obtained of the lower GI tract.

For the most definitive results, the colon should be empty of fecal material. Along with the use of a laxative and/or a cleansing enema, the person having a barium enema should be without food or drink from midnight before the procedure. Abnormal findings include malignant tumors, colonic stenosis, colonic fistula, perforated colon, diverticula, and polyps.

barium swallow (upper GI series) (**BEAR**-ee-um swallow)	Oral administration of a radiopaque contrast medium, barium sulfate, which flows into the esophagus as the person swallows. X-ray films are obtained of the esophagus and borders of the heart in which varices can be identified as well as strictures, tumors, obstructions, achalasia, or abnormal motility of the esophagus. As the barium sulfate continues to flow into the upper GI tract (lower esophagus, stomach, and duodenum), X-ray films are taken to reveal ulcerations, tumors, hiatal hernias, or obstruction.

colonoscopy
 	
(koh-lon-**OSS**-koh-pee)
  colon/o = colon
  -scopy = the process of viewing
	The direct visualization of the lining of the large intestine by using a fiberoptic colonoscope.
	
	A colonoscopy is indicated for individuals with a history of undiagnosed **constipation** and diarrhea, loss of appetite (anorexia), persistent rectal bleeding, or lower abdominal pain. The procedure is also used to check for colonic polyps or possible malignant tumors.

coronary artery bypass graft (CABG) surgery (**KOR**-ah-nair-ree **AR**-ter-ee **BYE**-pass graft **SIR**-jer-ree)	A surgical procedure (designed to increase the blood flow to the myocardial muscle) that involves bypass grafts to the coronary arteries that reroute the blood flow around the occluded area of the coronary artery. See *Figure 24-13*. Grafts are made from veins taken from other parts of the body (usually the saphenous vein from the leg) that are connected to the coronary artery above and below the occlusion. This anastomosis (plural: *anastomoses*) joins the two vessels, restoring the normal flow of oxygenated blood to the myocardium.

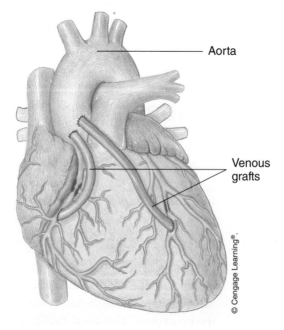

Aorta

Venous grafts

© Cengage Learning®.

Figure 24-13 Coronary artery bypass surgery

directional coronary atherectomy

(dih-**REK**-shun-al **KOR**-ah-nair-ree
ath-er-**REK**-toh-mee)

A procedure that uses a catheter (AtheroCath), which has a small mechanically driven cutter that shaves the plaque and stores it in a collection chamber. See *Figure 24-14.*

The plaque is then removed from the artery when the device is withdrawn. This procedure usually lasts from one to three hours and requires overnight hospitalization.

During the atherectomy procedure, the patient remains awake but is sedated. The catheter is inserted into the femoral artery and is advanced into position using X-ray visualization as a guide. Once in place, the catheter balloon is inflated, pressing the cutting device against the plaque on the opposite wall of the artery. This causes the plaque to protrude into the window of the cutting device. As this happens, the rotating blade of the cutting device then shaves off the plaque, storing it in the tip of the catheter until removal from the body. The process is repeated several times to widen the opening of the artery at the blockage site.

If the medications, angioplasty, and atherectomy are not successful methods of treatment (or if the **coronary artery disease** is severe), coronary bypass surgery will be the treatment of choice.

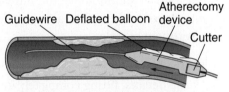

1. In coronary atherectomy procedures, a special cutting device with a deflated balloon on one side and an opening on the other is pushed over a wire down the coronary artery.

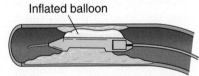

2. When the device is within a coronary artery narrowing, the balloon is inflated so that part of the atherosclerotic plaque is "squeezed" into the opening of the device.

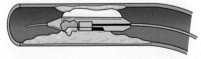

3. When the physician starts rotating the cutting blade, pieces of plaque are shaved off into the device.

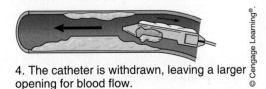

4. The catheter is withdrawn, leaving a larger opening for blood flow.

© Cengage Learning®.

Figure 24-14 Directional coronary atherectomy

dual-energy X-ray absorptiometry (DEXA)	This technique is also a noninvasive procedure that measures bone density. In the **dual-energy X-ray absorptiometry (DEXA)** procedure, an X-ray machine generates the energy photons that pass through the bones. A computer evaluates the amount of radiation absorbed by the bones, and the findings are interpreted by a physician.

This procedure is the most commonly used technique to measure bone density, taking less time and emitting less radiation. It is considered the "gold standard" for bone density measurement.

extracapsular cataract extraction (ECCE) (eks-trah-**KAP**-syoo-lar **KAT**-ah-rakt eks-**TRAK**-shun)	**Extracapsular cataract extraction** is the surgical removal of the anterior segment of the lens capsule and the lens, allowing for the insertion of an **intraocular lens implant**.

The insertion of a posterior chamber intraocular lens has proven to result in fewer complications.

hearing aids	Devices that amplify sound to provide more precise perception and interpretation of words communicated to the individual with a hearing deficit.

This improved interpretation and perception is made possible by the amplification of sound above the individual's hearing threshold because it is introduced to the ear's hearing apparatus. Hearing aids are accessible in an assortment of styles.

1. The "in-canal style" hearing aid is the newest and least conspicuous of the devices, fitting completely into the ear canal and allowing for exercise and talking on the telephone without being obtrusive. The disadvantages of using this style of hearing aid occur for those individuals who do not have good dexterity with their hands. Due to the size of the hearing aid, the handling, cleaning, and changing of batteries require good manual dexterity (which can be difficult for many older individuals). Cleaning is important because of the possible accumulation of earwax, which will plug the small portals and disrupt sound transmission.

2. The "in-ear style" hearing aid is worn in the external ear and is larger and more noticeable than the in-canal style. The care of the in-ear style also requires manual dexterity, which is often a concern for the older individual. Advantages of the in-ear style include a greater degree of amplification and toggle switches that allow for usage of the telephone. Cleaning is important because of the possible accumulation of earwax, which will plug the small portals and disrupt sound transmission. See *Figure 24-15A*.

3. The "behind-ear style" hearing aid allows for even greater amplification of sound than the in-ear style and is much easier to manipulate manually for care and control. If the user wears glasses, components are available that fit into the earpiece of the eyeglasses for convenience and comfort. See *Figure 24-15B*.

4. A "body hearing aid" is used by individuals who have a profound hearing loss. Sound is delivered to the ear canal by way of a microphone and amplifier clipped on the clothing in a pocket-sized container connected to a receiver, which is clipped onto the ear mold.

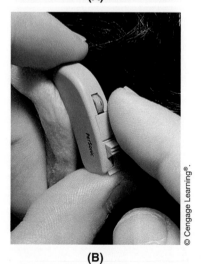

(A)

(B)

© Cengage Learning®.

Figure 24-15 Hearing aids: (A) In-ear style; (B) Behind-ear style

internal fixation devices

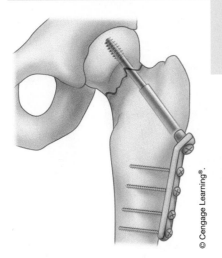

© Cengage Learning®.

The treatment of choice for a fractured hip is usually surgery. Devices such as screws, pins, wires, and nails may be used to internally maintain the bone alignment while healing takes place. These **internal fixation devices** are more commonly used with fractures of the femur and fractures of joints. See *Figure 24-16*.

Figure 24-16 Internal fixation device

intraocular lens implant

(in-trah-**OCK**-yoo-lar **LENZ IM**-plant)
  intra- = within
  ocul/o = eye
  -ar = pertaining to

An **intraocular lens implant** is the surgical process of **cataract** extraction and the insertion of an artificial lens into the patient's eye. This restores visual acuity and provides improved depth perception, light refraction, and binocular vision.

The lens can be implanted in the anterior chamber or posterior chamber.

percutaneous transluminal coronary angioplasty (PTCA)

(**per**-kyoo-**TAY**-nee-us
trans-**LOOM**-ih-nal
KOR-ah-nair-ree
AN-jee-oh-**plass**-tee)

A nonsurgical procedure in which a catheter, equipped with a small inflatable balloon on the end, is inserted into the femoral artery and is threaded up the aorta (under X-ray visualization) into the narrowed coronary artery.

When properly positioned, the balloon is carefully inflated, compressing the fatty deposits against the side of the walls of the artery and thus enlarging the opening of the artery to increase blood flow through the artery. Once the plaque is compressed against the walls of the artery, the balloon-tipped catheter is then removed or replaced with a **stent** (a mesh tube used to hold the artery open). Typically, the stent remains in place permanently unless reocclusion occurs. This procedure is also called a balloon catheter dilation or a balloon angioplasty. See *Figure 24-17*.

retinal photocoagulation

(**RET**-in-al
foh-toh-coh-**ag**-yoo-**LAY**-shun)
  retin/o = retina
  -al = pertaining to
  phot/o = light

Retinal photocoagulation is a surgical procedure that uses an argon laser to treat conditions such as **glaucoma**, retinal detachment, and **diabetic retinopathy**.

The following are different treatment methods.

1. In retinal detachment, the argon laser is used to create an area of inflammation, which will develop adhesions, causing a "welding" of the layers.

2. In **diabetic retinopathy**, the argon laser is used to seal microaneurysms and to reduce the risk of hemorrhage.

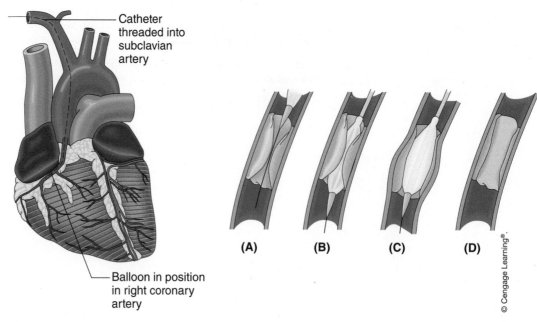

Figure 24-17 Balloon angioplasty

| **serum glucose tests** | Measures the amount of glucose in the blood at the time the sample was drawn. |
| | True serum glucose elevations are indicative of **diabetes mellitus**. However, the value must be evaluated according to the time of day and the last time the person has eaten. A glucose level can be collected in a tube or evaluated with a finger stick. |

suprapubic prostatectomy
(**soo**-prah-**PEW**-bik
pross-tah-**TEK**-toh-mee)
  supra- = above
  pub/o = pubis
  -ic = pertaining to
  prostat/o = prostate gland
  -ectomy = surgical removal of
	The surgical removal of the prostate gland by making an incision into the abdominal wall just above the pubis.

	A small incision is then made into the bladder, which has been distended with fluid. The prostate gland is removed through the bladder cavity.
	The removal of the prostate gland by the suprapubic approach is done when the surgeon believes the prostate gland is too enlarged to be removed through the urethra and is also used to remove the prostate gland when cancer is present.

| **transurethral resection of the prostate (TURP)**
(trans-you-**REE**-thral
REE-sek-shun of the **PROSS**-tayt)
  trans- = across
  urethr/o = urethra
  -al = pertaining to | The surgical removal of the prostate gland by inserting a resectoscope (an instrument used to remove tissue from the body) through the urethra and into the bladder to remove small pieces of tissue from the prostate gland. |

Review Checkpoint

Check your understanding of this section by completing the **Diagnostic Techniques, Treatments, and Procedures** exercises in your workbook.

COMMON ABBREVIATIONS

Abbreviation	Meaning	Abbreviation	Meaning
AAA	Area Agency on Aging	ECHO	echocardiogram
AD	Alzheimer's disease	GCNS	gerontological clinical nurse specialist
ADL	activities of daily living		
BPH	benign prostatic hypertrophy	GNP	gerontological nurse practitioner
CABG	coronary artery bypass graft	KUB	kidneys, ureters, bladder (an X-ray)
CAD	coronary artery disease	PTCA	percutaneous transluminal coronary angioplasty
Cath	catheterization		
CHF	congestive heart failure	RSVP	retired seniors volunteer program
CVA	cerebrovascular accident; stroke	SOB	shortness of breath
CVD	cardiovascular disease	TIA	transient ischemic attack
DEXA	dual-energy X-ray absorptiometry	TURP	transurethral resection of the prostate
ECG, EKG	electrocardiogram	URI	upper respiratory infection

Review Checkpoint

Check your understanding of this section by completing the **Common Abbreviations** exercises in your workbook.

WRITTEN AND AUDIO TERMINOLOGY REVIEW

Review each of the following terms from this chapter. Study the spelling of each term and write the definition in the space provided. Check definitions by looking the term up in the glossary.

Term	Pronunciation	Definition
acrochordon	☐ **ak**-roh-**KOR**-don	_____
actinic keratosis	☐ ak-**TIN**-ik kair-ah-**TOH**-sis	_____
alopecia	☐ **al**-oh-**PEE**-shee-ah	_____
Alzheimer's disease	☐ **ALTS**-high-merz dih-**ZEEZ**	_____
ankylosing spondylitis	☐ **ang**-kih-**LOH**-sing spon-dih-**LYE**-tis	_____
anorexia nervosa	☐ an-oh-**REK**-see-ah ner-**VOH**-suh	_____
arteriosclerosis	☐ ar-**tee**-ree-oh-skleh-**ROH**-sis	_____
arthritis	☐ ar-**THRYE**-tis	_____
atherosclerosis	☐ ath-er-**oh**-skleh-**ROH**-sis	_____
atrophic vaginitis	☐ aye-**TROH**-fik vaj-in-**EYE**-tis	_____
benign prostatic hypertrophy	☐ bee-**NINE** pross-**TAT**-ik high-**PER**-troh-fee	_____
bunionectomy	☐ **bun**-yun-**ECK**-toh-mee	_____
cataract	☐ **KAT**-ah-rakt	_____
cerebrovascular accident (CVA)	☐ seh-**ree**-broh-**VASS**-kyoo-lar **AK**-sih-dent	_____
claudication	☐ **klaw**-dih-**KAY**-shun	_____
colonoscopy	☐ **koh**-lon-**OSS**-koh-pee	_____
constipation	☐ **kon**-stih-**PAY**-shun	_____
coronary artery disease (CAD)	☐ **KOR**-ah-nair-ree **AR**-ter-ee dih-**ZEEZ**	_____
crepitation	☐ **crep**-ih-**TAY**-shun	_____
deafness, sensorineural	☐ **DEFF**-ness, **sen**-soh-ree-**NOO**-ral	_____
dementia	☐ dee-**MEN**-shee-ah	_____
diabetes mellitus	☐ **dye**-ah-**BEE**-teez **MELL**-ih-tus	_____
diabetic retinopathy	☐ **dye**-ah-**BET**-ik ret-in-**OP**-ah-thee	_____
ectropion	☐ eck-**TROH**-pee-on	_____

Term	Pronunciation	Definition
eczema	☐ **ECK**-zeh-mah	_____
entropion	☐ en-**TROH**-pee-on	_____
geriatrician	☐ **jer**-ee-ah-**TRIH**-shun	_____
geriatrics	☐ **jer**-ee-**AT**-riks	_____
gerontologist	☐ **jer**-on-**TOL**-oh-jist	_____
gerontology	☐ **jer**-on-**TOL**-oh-jee	_____
gerontophobia	☐ jer-**on**-toh-**FOH**-bee-ah	_____
glaucoma	☐ glah-**KOH**-mah	_____
herpes zoster	☐ **HER**-peez **ZOS**-ter	_____
intraocular lens implant	☐ **in**-trah-**OCK**-yoo-lar **LENZ IM**-plant	_____
ketones	☐ **KEY**-tonz	_____
kyphosis	☐ kye-**FOH**-sis	_____
lichenification	☐ lye-**ken**-ih-fih-**KAY**-shun	_____
nocturia	☐ nok-**TOO**-ree-ah	_____
osteoarthritis	☐ **oss**-tee-oh-ar-**THRYE**-tis	_____
osteoporosis	☐ **oss**-tee-oh-poh-**ROW**-sis	_____
Parkinson's disease	☐ **PARK**-in-sons dih-**ZEEZ**	_____
presbycusis	☐ **pres**-bee-**KOO**-sis	_____
presbyopia	☐ pres-bee-**OH**-pee-ah	_____
purpura	☐ **PER**-pew-rah	_____
retinal photocoagulation	☐ **RET**-in-al **foh**-toh-coh-**ag**-yoo-**LAY**-shun	_____
seborrheic keratosis	☐ **seb**-or-**REE**-ik kair-ah-**TOH**-sis	_____
senescence	☐ seh-**NESS**-ens	_____
senile lentigines	☐ **SEE**- nile lin-**TIH**-jeh-nez	_____
suprapubic prostatectomy	☐ **soo**-prah-**PEW**-bik **pross**-tah-**TEK**-toh-mee	_____
thrombosis	☐ throm-**BOH**-sis	_____
transurethral resection of the prostate (TURP)	☐ **trans**-yoo-**REE**-thral **REE**-sek-shun of the **PROSS**-tayt	_____
turgor	☐ **TURH**-gor	_____
urinary incontinence	☐ **YOO**-rih-nair-ee in-**CON**-tin-ens	_____

Review Checkpoint

Apply what you have learned in this chapter by completing the **Putting It All Together** exercise in your workbook.

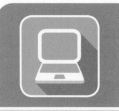

Online Resources

For additional study tools, such as PowerPoint® slides, go to the Student Companion Website.

Chapter Review Exercises

The following exercises provide a more in-depth review of the chapter material. Your goal in these exercises is to complete each section at a minimum 80% level of accuracy. A space has been provided for your score at the end of each section.

A. Define the Abbreviation

Define each abbreviation by writing the definition in the space provided. Confirm your answers with the text. Place a check in the space provided if you were able to complete this exercise correctly the first time (without referring to the text). Each correct answer is worth 10 points. Record your score in the space provided at the end of the exercise.

( ) 1. CVA _____

( ) 2. CAD _____

( ) 3. CABG _____

( ) 4. CHF _____

( ) 5. BPH _____

( ) 6. TURP _____

( ) 7. SOB _____

( ) 8. PTCA _____

( ) 9. ECG _____

( ) 10. KUB _____

Number correct _____ × 10 points/correct answer: Your score _____ %

B. Name the Pathological Condition

Read the descriptions of the pathological conditions on the right and match them with the applicable pathological condition on the left. Each correct answer is worth 10 points. When you have completed the exercise, record your score in the space provided at the end of the exercise.

_____ 1. eczema

_____ 2. seborrheic keratosis

_____ 3. psoriasis

_____ 4. achalasia

_____ 5. osteoporosis

_____ 6. osteomalacia

_____ 7. Paget's disease

_____ 8. osteoarthritis

_____ 9. gout

_____ 10. bunion

a. a common, noninfectious, chronic disorder of the skin manifested by silvery white scales over round, raised, reddened plaques producing pruritus

b. bones that were once strong become fragile due to loss of bone density

c. an abnormal enlargement of the joint at the base of the great toe

d. an acute or chronic inflammatory skin condition characterized by erythema, papules, vesicles, pustules, scales, crusts, or scabs; accompanied by intense itching

e. osteitis deformans

f. also known as degenerative joint disease, results from wear and tear on the joints—especially weight-bearing joints such as the hips and knees

g. abnormal softening of the bones due to a deficiency of calcium and phosphorus in the blood (which is necessary for bone mineralization)

h. brown or yellow wartlike lesions loosely attached to the skin surface; also known as senile warts

i. decreased mobility of the lower two-thirds of the esophagus along with constriction of the lower esophageal sphincter

j. a form of acute arthritis characterized by inflammation of the first metatarsal joint of the great toe

Number correct _____ × _10 points/correct answer: Your score_ _____ %

C. Word Element Review

The following words relate to this chapter. The word elements have been labeled (WR = word root, P = prefix, S = suffix, and V = combining vowel). Read the definition carefully and complete the word by filling in the blank, using the word elements provided in this chapter. If you have forgotten the word building rules, see Chapter 1. Each correct answer is worth 10 points. Record your score in the space provided at the end of this exercise.

1. A refractive error in which the lens of the eye cannot focus on an image accurately, resulting in impaired distant vision that is blurred due to the image being focused in front of the retina; nearsightedness.

   _____ / _____
   WR   S

2. A form of arteriosclerosis (hardening of the arteries) characterized by fatty deposits building up within the inner layers of the walls of larger arteries.

   _____ / _____ / _____ / _____
   WR   V   WR   S

(continued)

3. Urination at night.

_____ / _____

WR   S

4. Elevated blood sugar level.

_____ / _____ / _____

P   WR   S

5. Poor vision due to the natural aging process.

_____ / _____

WR   S

6. Pertaining to the heart.

_____ / _____

WR   S

7. An arterial condition in which there is thickening, hardening, and loss of elasticity of the walls of the arteries; hardening of the arteries.

_____ / _____ / _____ / _____

WR   V   WR   S

8. Any disease of the retina.

_____ / _____ / _____

WR   V   S

9. A cancerous tumor.

_____ / _____

WR   S

10. A condition of hardness.

_____ / _____

WR   S

Number correct _____ **× 10 points/correct answer: Your score** _____ **%**

D. Spelling

Circle the correctly spelled term in each pairing of words. Each correct answer is worth 10 points. Record your score in the space provided at the end of the exercise.

1. geriatrics	geriatricks	6. purpera	purpura
2. turger	turgor	7. Alzhimer's	Alzheimer's
3. ekzema	eczema	8. arteriosclerosis	arteriosclerosus
4. soriasis	psoriasis	9. emphyzema	emphysema
5. osteomalacia	osteomalasha	10. cateract	cataract

Number correct _____ **× 10 points/correct answer: Your score** _____ **%**

E. Word Search

Read each definition carefully and identify the applicable word from the list that follows. Enter the word in the space provided and then find it in the puzzle and circle it. The words may be read up, down, diagonally, across, or backward. Each correct answer is worth 10 points. Record your score in the space provided at the end of the exercise.

aging	gerontology	anorexia
turgor	bruit	alopecia
kyphosis	crepitation	edema
nocturia	myopia	

Example: The process of growing old.

aging _____

1. The study of all aspects of the aging process.

   _____

2. Partial or complete loss of hair.

   _____

3. A reflection of the skin's elasticity.

   _____

4. An abnormal sound or murmur heard when listening to a carotid artery, organ, or gland with a stethoscope.

   _____

5. Another name for nearsightedness.

   _____

6. Another name for humpback.

   _____

7. Clicking or crackling sounds heard upon joint movement.

   _____

8. Another name for swelling.

   _____

9. Lack or loss of appetite.

   _____

10. Urination at night.

   _____

(*continued*)

```
G  E  R  O  N  T  O  L  O  G  Y  N  M  I  A
P  L  E  U  R  U  I  D (A  G  I  N  G) M  L
E  I  O  K  T  R  N  M  E  T  T  R  N  V  O
X  A  O  N  E  G  L  O  S  D  I  C  C  B  P
I  L  C  T  D  O  P  A  R  A  G  M  D  N  E
M  U  H  O  B  R  U  I  T  E  L  R  O  T  C
C  R  O  T  H  L  Y  P  U  A  S  C  P  E  I
R  U  R  R  E  P  N  O  M  A  T  O  F  E  A
E  U  D  O  S  I  X  Y  T  U  I  P  E  E  E
P  D  R  C  D  A  D  M  R  D  E  Y  S  M  N
I  R  E  I  N  O  R  I  H  E  A  D  S  R  P
T  I  A  M  A  R  A  H  S  S  S  S  A  I  Y
A  S  S  N  A  T  U  Y  A  I  D  I  S  G  D
T  U  I  T  C  E  S  P  I  N  A  E  N  P  A
I  R  S  O  H  L  O  S  I  S  O  H  P  Y  K
O  A  N  O  R  E  X  I  A  T  U  R  E  S  B
N  R  O  T  T  E  U  R  I  S  M  E  M  I  C
E  X  H  I  B  I  T  D  I  O  M  A  S  E  S
```

Number correct _____ **×10 points/correct answer: Your score** _____ **%**

F. True or False

Read each statement carefully and circle the correct answer as true or false. HINT: Pay close attention to the word elements written in **bold** as you make your decision. If the statement is false, identify the meaning of that word element. Each correct answer is worth 10 points. Record your score in the space provided at the end of the exercise.

1. Urination at night is known as **noct**uria.

   True   False

   If your answer is False, what does *noct/o* mean? _____

2. **Hyper**glycemia means a low blood sugar level.

   True   False

   If your answer is False, what does *hyper* mean? _____

3. Diabetic **retin**opathy is a disease of the retina of the eye in which the capillaries of the retina experience scarring.

   True   False

   If your answer is False, what does *retin/o* mean? _____

4. Loss of vision due to the aging process is known as **presby**opia.

   True   False

   If your answer is False, what does *presby/o* mean? _____

5. Benign **prostat**ic hypertrophy is enlargement of the epididymis.

   True   False

   If your answer is False, what does *prostat/o* mean? _____

6. **Endo**metrial carcinoma refers to a malignant tumor of the outside of the uterus.

   True   False

   If your answer is False, what does *endo-* mean? _____

7. Osteo**porosis** refers to softening of the bones.

   True   False

   If your answer is False, what does *-porosis* mean? _____

8. Osteo**malacia** is a disease in which the bones become porous.

   True   False

   If your answer is False, what does *-malacia* mean? _____

9. **Kyph**osis is another name for humpback.

   True   False

   If your answer is False, what does *kyph/o* mean? _____

10. Osteo**arthr**itis is inflammation of the bones and the cartilage.

   True   False

   If your answer is False, what does *arthr/o* mean? _____

Number correct _____ *× 10 points/correct answer: Your score* _____ *%*

G. Completion

The following sentences relate to this chapter. Complete each sentence with the most appropriate word. Each correct answer is worth 10 points. Record your score in the space provided at the end of the exercise.

1. A condition of the legs involving annoying sensations of uneasiness, tiredness, itching, or tingling of the leg muscles while resting is known as _____.

2. An abnormal enlargement of the joint at the base of the great toe is known as a _____.

3. A form of acute arthritis characterized by inflammation of the first metatarsal joint of the great toe is known as _____.

4. A disease in which the bones become abnormally soft due to a deficiency of calcium and phosphorus in the blood, resulting in fractures and noticeable deformities of the weight-bearing bones, is known as

   _____.

5. A type of arthritis, also known as Marie-Strümpell disease, that affects the vertebral column and causes deformities of the spine is known as _____.

6. Cramplike pains in the calves of the legs caused by poor circulation to the muscles of the legs, and commonly associated with atherosclerosis, is known as _____.

7. A progressive and extremely debilitating disease that results in deterioration of a person's intellectual functioning is _____.

8. A degenerative, slowly progressive deterioration of nerves in the brain stem's motor system (characterized by stooped posture, bowed head, shuffling gait, pill-rolling gestures, and an expressionless, masklike facial appearance) is known as _____.

9. _____ is an acute viral infection seen mainly in adults, characterized by inflammation of the underlying spinal or cranial nerve pathway, producing painful, vesicular eruptions on the skin following along these nerve pathways.

10. Another name for a cerebrovascular accident is a _____.

Number correct _____ *× 10 points/correct answer: Your score* _____ *%*

H. Crossword Puzzle

Each crossword answer is worth 10 points. When you have completed the crossword puzzle, total your points and enter your score in the space provided.

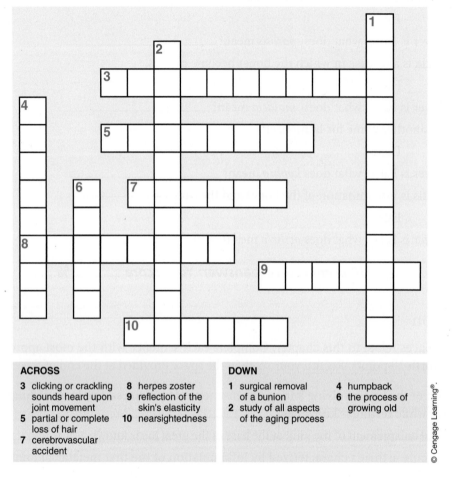

ACROSS

3 clicking or crackling sounds heard upon joint movement
5 partial or complete loss of hair
7 cerebrovascular accident
8 herpes zoster
9 reflection of the skin's elasticity
10 nearsightedness

DOWN

1 surgical removal of a bunion
2 study of all aspects of the aging process
4 humpback
6 the process of growing old

© Cengage Learning®.

Number correct _____ *× 10 points/correct answer: Your score* _____ *%*

I. Matching Abbreviations

Match the abbreviations on the left with the most appropriate definition on the right. Each correct response is worth 10 points. When you have completed the exercise, record your score in the space provided at the end of the exercise.

_____ 1. ECG
_____ 2. KUB
_____ 3. TURP
_____ 4. CVD
_____ 5. CVA
_____ 6. TIA
_____ 7. DEXA

a. benign prostatic hypertrophy
b. electroencephalogram
c. coronary artery bypass graft
d. electrocardiogram
e. coronary artery disease
f. kidneys, ureters, bladder
g. transient urinary retrograde pyelogram

_____ 8. CAD   h. cardiovascular disease

_____ 9. CABG   i. transient ischemic attack

_____ 10. BPH   j. dual-energy X-ray absorptiometry

                                 k. cerebrovascular accident; stroke

                                 l. transurethral resection of the prostate

Number correct _____ × *10 points/correct answer: Your score* _____ *%*

J. Term to Definition

Define each term by writing the definition in the space provided. Check the box if you are able to complete this exercise correctly the first time (without referring to the answers). Each correct answer is worth 10 points. Record your score in the space provided at the end of the exercise.

☐ 1. kyphosis _____

_____

☐ 2. crepitation _____

_____

☐ 3. edema _____

_____

☐ 4. ascites _____

_____

☐ 5. lichenification _____

_____

☐ 6. myopia _____

_____

☐ 7. alopecia _____

_____

☐ 8. acrochordon _____

_____

☐ 9. senile lentigines _____

_____

☐ 10. senescence _____

_____

Number correct _____ × *10 points/correct answer: Your score* _____ *%*

K. Medical Scenario

The following medical scenario presents information on one of the pathological conditions discussed in this chapter. Read the scenario carefully and select the most appropriate answer for each question that follows. Each correct answer is worth 20 points. Record your score in the space provided at the end of the exercise.

Sally Dodd is a 75-year-old patient visiting her internist. Mrs. Dodd has come to her physician, complaining of abdominal pain and fatigue. She is normally a very active 75-year-old who drives herself to exercise class,

(continued)

church, and garden club. She has not had the energy to participate in these activities for about two months now. Mrs. Dodd's blood evaluation showed that her hemoglobin was extremely low. Based on the history and physical, Mrs. Dodd's physician suspects that she may have colorectal cancer. The physician expressed to Mrs. Dodd that she would order some diagnostic tests to confirm or deny this diagnosis. Mrs. Dodd has some questions for the health care professional as she is about to leave the exam room.

1. The health care professional bases her response to her questions about colorectal cancer on which of the following facts about colorectal cancer?
    a. It is an inherited gastrointestinal disease characterized by a tumor or neoplasm in the small intestine due to the effects of the basal ganglia on the neurons.
    b. The pain and inflammation are caused by a degenerative inflammatory disease of the small intestines attacking the lining of the small and large bowels.
    c. It can probably be treated with bed rest, anti-inflammatory medication, and blood transfusions.
    d. The incidence increases in individuals over 70 years of age, with a death rate of almost 50% of those affected.

2. The health care professional explains to Mrs. Dodd that the cause of colorectal cancer is:
    a. unknown but suggested that a high-fat, low-fiber diet may increase occurrence
    b. most likely a hemorrhage of duodenal ulcer in the past, leading to this inflammation
    c. sometimes due to fat emboli in the cecum
    d. due to smoking and to drinking alcohol

3. Mrs. Dodd asks the health care professional why she is so tired all the time. She is concerned that this is due to something other than the colorectal cancer. The health care professional would explain to her that with colorectal cancer:
    a. there is bleeding from the tumor leading to anemia, which will cause the tiredness and fatigue
    b. her low hemoglobin targets the CNS, and this leads to a feeling of fatigue and tiredness
    c. along with her age, this symptom is possibly a result of atherosclerosis
    d. her blood pressure is high and thus she does not feel as energetic

4. Mrs. Dodd asked the health care professional what other symptoms are associated with colorectal cancer. She discussed with her that the most common symptoms of colorectal cancer are:
    a. constipation, excessive urination, increased thirst, and weight gain
    b. numbness in the extremities, nausea and vomiting, and hypertension
    c. difficulty swallowing, retrosternal chest pain, occult blood in the stool, and regurgitation of undigested food
    d. rectal bleeding, bowel changes, abdominal pain or cramping, anemia, and unexplained weight loss

5. Mrs. Dodd asks the health care professional if there are any factors that would predispose her to colorectal cancer. The health care professional explains that the factors that predispose one to colorectal cancer are:
    a. excessive fat stores, especially around the waist
    b. history of constipation and appendicitis
    c. history of Crohn's disease, ulcerative colitis, irritable bowel syndrome, or familial polyposis
    d. hypertension, increased blood lipids, obesity, diabetes, and inability to cope with stress

Number correct _____ *× 20 points/correct answer: Your score* _____ *%*

24-hour urine specimen (24-hour **YOO**-rin **SPEH**-sih-men) a collection of all of the urine excreted by the individual over a 24-hour period. The urine is collected in one large container. This urine specimen is also called composite urine specimen.

48-hour pH study a procedure used to measure and monitor the amount of gastric acid reflux into the esophagus during the specified period. The monitoring system will determine how often stomach contents reflux into the esophagus, how long the acid stays in the esophagus, and how much reflux occurs at nighttime. This test is used to determine if the patient has GERD (gastroesophageal reflux disease) and if so, the severity of the GERD; also known as 48-hour wireless esophageal pH monitoring.

A

Abdomen (**AB**-dah-men) the portion of the body between the thorax (chest) and the pelvis; the diaphragm separates the abdominal cavity from the thoracic cavity. The stomach is located in the upper left quadrant of the abdomen.

Abdominal cavity the cavity beneath the thoracic cavity that is separated from the thoracic cavity by the diaphragm; contains the liver, gallbladder, spleen, stomach, pancreas, intestines, and kidneys.

Abdominal ultrasound (ab-**DOM**-ih-nal **ULL**-trah-sound) the use of very-high-frequency sound waves to provide visualization of the internal organs of the abdomen (liver, gallbladder, bile ducts, pancreas, kidneys, bladder, and ureters); also known as an abdominal sonogram.

Abdominocentesis (paracentesis) (ab-**dom**-ih-noh-sen-**TEE**-sis, **pair**-ah-sen-**TEE**-sis) involves insertion of a needle or trocar into the abdominal cavity to remove excess fluid, with the person in a sitting position.

Abdominopelvic cavity describes the abdominal and pelvic cavity collectively; refers to the space between the diaphragm and the groin.

Abduction (ab-**DUCK**-shun) the movement of a bone away from the midline of the body.

Ablation (ab-**LAY**-shun) removal of a part, pathway, or function by one of the following methods: surgery, chemical destruction, electrocautery, or radiofrequency.

Abortion (ah-**BOR**-shun) termination of a pregnancy before the fetus has reached a viable age, that is, an age at which the fetus could live outside of the uterine environment.

Abrasion (ah-**BRAY**-zhun) a scraping or rubbing away of skin or mucous membrane as a result of friction to the area.

Abruptio placenta (ah-**BRUP**-she-oh pla-**SEN**-tah) the premature separation of a normally implanted placenta from the uterine wall after the pregnancy has passed 20 weeks' gestation or during labor (the birthing process).

Abscess (**AB**-sess) a localized collection of pus in any body part that results from invasion of pus-forming bacteria.

Absence seizure (**AB**-senz **SEE**-zyoor) a small seizure in which there is a sudden temporary loss of consciousness lasting only a few seconds.

Absorption (ab-**SORP**-shun) the passage of substances across and into tissues, such as the passage of digested food molecules into intestinal cells or the passage of liquids into kidney tubules.

Abstinence (**AB**-stih-nens) to abstain from having vaginal intercourse.

Acetabulum (ass-eh-**TAB**-you-lum) the hip socket.

Acetylcholine (ah-seh-till-**KOH**-leen) a chemical substance in the body tissues that facilitates the transmission of nerve impulses from one nerve to another. It has a stimulant (or excitatory) effect on some parts of the body (such as the skeletal muscles) and a depressant (or inhibitory) effect on other parts of the body (such as the heart muscle); also known as a neurotransmitter.

Achalasia (ak-al-**LAY**-zee-ah) decreased mobility of the lower two-thirds of the esophagus along with constriction of the lower esophageal sphincter (LES) making it difficult for food and liquids to move down the esophagus.

Acne vulgaris (**ACK**-nee vul-**GAY**-ris) a common inflammatory disorder seen on the face, chest, back, and neck; appears as papules, pustules, and comedos; commonly known as acne.

Acoustic (ah-**KOOS**-tik) pertaining to sound or hearing.

Acquired immunity (ah-**KWIRD** im-**YOO**-nih-tee) immunity that is a result of the body developing the ability to defend itself against a specific agent, as a result of having had the disease or from having received an immunization against a disease.

Acquired immunodeficiency syndrome (AIDS) (im-yoo-noh-dee-**FIH**-shen-see **SIN**-drom) involves clinical conditions that destroy the body's immune system in the last or final phase of a human immunodeficiency virus (HIV) infection, which primarily damages helper T-cell lymphocytes with CD4 receptors.

Acrochordon (ak-roh-**KOR**-don) a skin tag; a benign growth that hangs from a short stalk, commonly occurring on the neck, eyelids, axilla, or groin.

Acromegaly (ak-roh-**MEG**-ah-lee) a chronic metabolic condition characterized by the gradual noticeable enlargement and elongation of the bones of the face, jaw, and extremities due to hypersecretion of the human growth hormone after puberty.

Actinic keratosis (ak-**TIN**-ic kair-ah-**TOH**-sis) a premalignant, gray or red-to-brown, hardened lesion caused by excessive exposure to sunlight.

Active acquired immunity (**AK**-tiv ah-**KWIRD** im-**YOO**-nih-tee) a form of long-term acquired immunity that protects the body against a new infection as the result of antibodies that develop naturally after an initial infection or artificially after a vaccination.

Addison's disease (**AD**-ih-son's dih-**ZEEZ**) a life-threatening disease process due to failure of the adrenal cortex to secrete adequate mineralocorticoids and glucocorticoids resulting from an autoimmune process, a neoplasm, an infection, or a hemorrhage in the gland.

Adduction (ad-**DUCK**-shun) the movement of a bone toward the midline of the body.

Adenohypophysis (ad-eh-noh-high-**POFF**-ih-sis) the anterior pituitary gland.

Adenoids (**ADD**-eh-noydz) masses of lymphatic tissue located near the opening of the nasal cavity into the pharynx; also called the pharyngeal tonsils.

Adenoma (**ad**-eh-**NOH**-mah) a glandular tumor.

Adenopathy (**ad**-eh-**NOP**-ah-thee) any disease of a gland, characterized by enlargement.

Adhesive capsulitis (add-**HE**-sive cap-sool-**EYE**-tis) a shoulder condition characterized by stiffness of the shoulder, limited shoulder movement, and pain; also known as "frozen shoulder." The condition may be idiopathic (cause unknown) or due to an underlying cause such as trauma, osteoarthritis, or systemic diseases. Adhesive capsulitis is divided into three stages: the painful stage, the adhesive stage, and the recovery stage.

Adjuvant (**AD**-joo-vant) a substance, especially a drug, added to a prescription to assist in the action of the main ingredient.

Adjuvant therapy treatment of a disease with a substance, especially a drug, which enhances the main ingredient. For example, chemotherapy may be used as adjuvant therapy to radiation.

Adnexa (add-**NEK**-sah) tissues or structures in the body that are next to or near another. As in the uterus, the adnexa consists of the fallopian tubes, ovaries, and ligaments of the uterus.

Adrenalectomy (ad-ree-nal-**EK**-toh-mee) surgical removal of one or both of the adrenal glands.

Adrenalitis (ah-dree-nal-**EYE**-tis) inflammation of the adrenal glands.

Adrenocortical (ad-ree-noh-**KOR**-tih-kal) pertaining to the cortex of the adrenal gland(s).

Adverse reaction the body's reaction to a drug in an unexpected way that may endanger a patient's health and safety.

Aerophagia (ay-er-oh-**FAY**-jee-ah) the swallowing of air; excessive swallowing of air while eating or drinking, which may result in belching and gas.

Affect (**AFF**-fekt) observable evidence of a person's feelings or emotions.

Afferent nerves (**AFF**-er-ent nerves) transmitters of nerve impulses toward the CNS; also known as sensory nerves.

AFP screening (alpha-fetoprotein) a serum screening test that checks the level of AFP in a pregnant woman's blood. The amount of AFP in the pregnant woman's blood—along with her age and other factors—help the health care provider estimate the chance that the baby may have certain problems or birth defects such as spina bifida (defective closure of the vertebrae of the spinal column), trisomy 21 (Down syndrome), and trisomy 18 (severe mental retardation and severe birth defects).

Afterbirth the placenta, the amnion, the chorion, some amniotic fluid, blood, and blood clots expelled from the uterus after childbirth.

Agglutination (ah-gloo-tih-**NAY**-shun) the clumping of cells as a result of interaction with specific antibodies called agglutinins. Agglutinins are used in blood typing and in identifying or estimating the strength of immunoglobulins or immune serums.

Aging the process of growing old.

Agnosia (ag-**NOH**-zee-ah) loss of mental ability to understand sensory stimuli (such as sight, sound, or touch) even though the sensory organs themselves are functioning properly (e.g., the inability to recognize or interpret the images the eye is seeing is known as optic agnosia).

Agraphia (ah-**GRAFF**-ee-ah) the inability to convert one's thoughts into writing.

Alanine aminotransferase (ALT) (**AL**-ah-neen ah-mee-noh-**TRANS**-fer-ays) a hepatocellular enzyme released in elevated amounts due to liver dysfunction; also known as serum glutamic pyruvic transaminase (SGPT).

Albinism (**AL**-bin-izm) a condition characterized by absence of pigment in the skin, hair, and eyes.

Albumin (al-**BYOO**-min) a plasma protein. Various albumins are found in practically all animal tissues and in many plant tissues. In blood, albumin helps maintain blood volume and blood pressure.

Aldosterone (al-**DOSS**-ter-ohn) a hormone secreted by the adrenal cortex that regulates sodium and potassium balance in the blood.

Alexia (ah-**LEK**-see-ah) the inability to understand written words.

Alimentary canal (al-ih-**MEN**-tar-ee can-**NAL**) a musculomembranous tube, about 30 feet long, extending from the mouth to the anus and lined with mucous membrane. Also called the digestive tract or the gastrointestinal tract.

Alkaline phosphatase (ALP) (**AL**-kah-line **FOSS**-fah-tays) alkaline phosphatase enzyme is found in the highest concentrations in the liver, biliary tract, and bone.

Allergen (**AL**-er-jin) a substance that can produce a hypersensitive reaction in the body.

Allergy (**AL**-er-jee) a hypersensitive reaction to normally harmless antigens, most of which are environmental.

Allergy testing various procedures used to identify specific allergens in an individual by exposing the person to a very small quantity of the allergen.

Allogenic (**al**-oh-**JEN**-ick) pertaining to originating from a different origin, as in a transplant of tissue from a matching donor but not of the individual (recipient).

Alopecia (**al**-oh-**PEE**-she-ah) partial or complete loss of hair; baldness. Alopecia may result from normal aging, a reaction to a medication such as anticancer medications, an endocrine disorder, or a skin disease.

Alveoli (**al**-**VEE**-oh-lye) air cells of the lungs; known as the pulmonary parenchyma (functional units of the lungs).

Alzheimer's disease (**ALTS**-high-merz dih-**ZEEZ**) a progressive, degenerative disease that affects the cortex of the brain and results in deterioration of a person's intellectual functioning. It begins with minor memory loss and progresses to complete loss of mental, emotional, and physical functioning, frequently occurring in persons over 65 years of age.

Ambiopia (**am**-bee-**OH**-pee-ah) double vision caused by each eye focusing separately; also known as diplopia.

Amblyopia (**am**-blee-**OH**-pee-ah) reduced vision that is not correctable with lenses and with no obvious pathological or structural cause ("dullness or dimness of vision").

Amenorrhea (**ah**-men-oh-**REE**-ah) absence of menstrual flow.

Ametropia (**am**-eh-**TROH**-pee-ah) a condition in which there is an error of refraction, causing the eye not to focus parallel rays of light on the retina.

Amino acids (**ah**-**MEE**-noh acids) an organic chemical compound composed of one or more basic amino groups and one or more acidic carboxyl groups.

Amnesia (**am**-**NEE**-zee-ah) loss of memory caused by severe emotional trauma, brain injury, substance abuse, or reaction to medications or toxins.

Amnesia disorders (**am**-**NEE**-zee-ah) characterized by short-term and long-term memory deficits; also called amnestic disorders.

Amniocentesis (**am**-nee-oh-sen-**TEE**-sis) a surgical puncture of the amniotic sac for the purpose of removing amniotic fluid for examination.

Amnion (**AM**-nee-on) inner of the two membrane layers that surround and contain the fetus and the amniotic fluid during pregnancy.

Amniotic fluid (**am**-nee-**OT**-ik fluid) a liquid produced by and contained within the fetal membranes during pregnancy. This fluid protects the fetus from trauma and temperature variations, helps maintain fetal oxygen supply, and allows for freedom of movement by the fetus during pregnancy.

Amniotic sac (**am**-nee-**OT**-ik sack) the double-layered sac that contains the fetus and the amniotic fluid during pregnancy.

Amphetamines (**am**-**FET**-ah-meenz) a group of nervous system stimulants that produce alertness and a feeling of well-being (euphoria).

Amputation (**am**-pew-**TAY**-shun) the surgical removal of a part of the body or a limb or a part of a limb; performed to treat recurrent infections or gangrene of a limb.

Amylase (**AM**-ih-lays) an enzyme secreted normally from the pancreatic cells that travels to the duodenum by way of the pancreatic duct and aids in digestion.

Amyotrophic lateral sclerosis (ALS) (ah-**my**-oh-**TROH**-fick **LAT**-er-al skleh-**ROH**-sis) a severe weakening and wasting of the involved muscle groups, usually beginning with the hands and progressing to the shoulders, upper arms, and legs. It is caused by decreased nerve innervation to the muscle groups.

Anal fistula an abnormal passageway in the skin surface near the anus usually connecting with the rectum.

Analgesia (an-al-**JEE**-zee-ah) without sensitivity to pain.

Analgesic (**an**-al-**JEE**-sik) pertaining to relieving pain; a medication that relieves pain.

Anaphylactic shock (**an**-ah-fih-**LAK**-tic **SHOCK**) a life-threatening, hypersensitive reaction to food or drugs. The patient experiences acute respiratory distress; hypotension; edema; tachycardia; cool, pale skin; cyanosis; and possibly convulsions shortly after administration of the medication.

Anaphylaxis (**an**-ah-fih-**LAK**-sis) an exaggerated, life-threatening hypersensitivity reaction to a previously encountered antigen.

Anaplasia (**an**-ah-**PLAY**-zee-ah) a change in the structure and orientation of cells, characterized by a loss of differentiation and reversion to a more primitive form.

Anastomosis (ah-**nas**-toh-**MOH**-sis) a surgical joining of two ducts, blood vessels, or bowel segments to allow flow from one to the other. Anastomosis of blood vessels may be performed to bypass an occluded area and restore normal blood flow to the area.

Anatomical position the standard reference position for the body as a whole: the person is standing with arms at the sides and palms turned forward; the individual's head and feet are also pointing forward.

Androgen (**AN**-droh-jen) any steroid hormone (e.g., testosterone) that increases male characteristics.

Andropause (**AN**-droh-pawz) a change of life for men, occurring in their late forties or early fifties, in which there is a decrease in male hormone (androgen) levels.

Anemia (an-**NEE**-mee-ah) a condition in which there is a decrease in hemoglobin in the blood to levels below the normal range, resulting in a deficiency of oxygen being delivered to the cells.

Anemia, aplastic (an-**NEE**-mee-ah, ah-**PLAST**-ik) also called bone marrow depression anemia, aplastic anemia is characterized by pancytopenia—an inadequacy of the formed blood elements (RBCs, WBCs, and platelets).

Anemia, hemolytic (an-**NEE**-mee-ah, **hee**-moh-**LIT**-ik) hemolytic anemia is characterized by the extreme reduction in circulating RBCs due to their destruction.

Anemia, iron deficiency (an-**NEE**-mee-ah, **EYE**-urn **dee-FIH**-shen-see) iron deficiency anemia is characterized by deficiency of hemoglobin level due to a lack of iron in the body. There is a greater demand on the stored iron than can be supplied by the body.

Anemia, pernicious (an-**NEE**-mee-ah, per-**NISH**-us) results from a deficiency of mature RBCs and the formation and circulation of megaloblasts (large, nucleated, immature, poorly functioning RBCs) with marked poikilocytosis (RBC shape variation) and anisocytosis (RBC size variation).

Anemia, sickle cell (an-**NEE**-mee-ah, **SIK-ul SELL**) a chronic hereditary form of hemolytic anemia in which the RBCs become shaped like a crescent in the presence of low oxygen concentration.

Anencephaly (**an**-en-**SEFF**-ah-lee) an absence of the brain and spinal cord at birth, a congenital disorder.

Anesthesia (**an**-ess-**THEE**-zee-ah) without feeling or sensation.

Anesthetic (**an**-es-**THET**-ick) pertaining to partially or completely numbing or eliminating sensitivity with or without loss of consciousness.

Aneurysm (**AN**-yoo-rihzm) a localized dilation of an artery formed at a weak point in the vessel wall. This weakened area balloons out with each pulsation of the artery.

Aneurysmectomy (**AN**-yoo-riz-**MEK**-toh-mee) surgical removal of the sac of an aneurysm.

Angina pectoris (an-**JI**-nah or **AN**-jin-nah **PECK**-tor-is) severe pain and constriction about the heart, usually radiating to the left shoulder and down the left arm, creating a feeling of pressure in the anterior chest.

Angiocardiography (cardiac catheterization) (**an**-jee-oh-**kar**-dee-**OG**-rah-fee **CAR**-dee-ak **kath**-eh-ter-ih-**ZAY**-shun) a specialized diagnostic procedure in which a catheter (a hollow, flexible tube) is introduced into a large vein or artery, usually of an arm or a leg, and then threaded through the circulatory system to the heart.

Angiography (**an**-jee-**OG**-rah-fee) X-ray visualization of the internal anatomy of the heart and blood vessels after introducing a radiopaque substance (contrast medium) that promotes the imaging (makes them visible) of internal structures that are otherwise difficult to see on X-ray film. This substance is injected into an artery or a vein.

Anisocoria (an-ih-soh-**KOH**-ree-ah) inequality in the diameter of the pupils of the eyes.

Anisocytosis (an-**ih**-soh-sigh-**TOH**-sis) an abnormal condition of the blood characterized by red blood cells of variable and abnormal size.

Ankylosing spondylitis (**ang**-kih-**LOH**-sing spon-dih-**LYE**-tis) affects the vertebral column and causes deformities of the spine; also known as Marie-Strümpell disease and as rheumatoid spondylitis.

Anomaly (ah-**NOM**-ah-lee) deviation from normal; birth defect; for example, congenital anomaly.

Anorchism (an-**OR**-kizm) the absence of one or both testicles.

Anorexia (an-oh-**REK**-see-ah) lack or loss of appetite, resulting in the inability to eat. Anorexia is seen in individuals who are depressed, with the onset of fever and illness, with stomach disorders, or as a result of excessive intake of alcohol or drugs.

Anorexia nervosa (an-oh-**REK**-see-ah ner-**VOH**-suh) a disorder (seen primarily in adolescent girls) characterized by an emotional disturbance concerning body image; prolonged refusal to eat followed by extreme weight loss; amenorrhea; and a lingering, abnormal fear of becoming obese.

Anterior (an-**TEE**-ree-or) pertaining to the front of the body or toward the belly of the body.

Anteroposterior (**an**-ter-oh-poss-**TEER**-ee-or) from the front to the back of the body, commonly associated with the direction of the X-ray beam.

Anthracosis (an-thrah-**KOH**-sis) the accumulation of carbon deposits in the lungs due to breathing smoke or coal dust (black lung disease); also called coal worker's pneumoconiosis.

Antibodies (**AN**-tih-bod-eez) substances produced by the body in response to bacteria, viruses, or other foreign substances. Each class of antibody is named for its action.

Antidiuretic (an-tye-dye-yoo-**RET**-ik) pertaining to the suppression of urine production; an agent given to suppress the production of urine.

Antigen (**AN**-tih-jen) a substance, usually a protein, that causes the formation of an antibody and reacts specifically with that antibody.

Antimetabolite (**an**-tih-meh-**TAB**-oh-light) a class of antineoplastic drugs used to treat cancer. These drugs are most effective against rapidly growing tumors.

Antineoplastic (**an**-tih-**nee**-oh-**PLASS**-tik) of or pertaining to a substance, procedure, or measure that prevents the proliferation of malignant cells.

Antiseptic (**an**-tih-**SEP**-tik) a substance that tends to inhibit the growth and reproduction of microorganisms.

Antisocial personality disorder (**an**-tih-**SOH**-shal) characterized by repetitive behavioral patterns that lack moral and ethical standards, keeping the individual in continuous conflict with society.

Anus (**AY**-nus) the opening through which the solid wastes (feces) are eliminated from the body.

Anxiety (ang-**ZYE**-eh-tee) a state of mind in which the individual feels increased tension, apprehension, a painfully increased sense of helplessness, a feeling of uncertainty, fear, jitteriness, and worry. Observable signs of anxiety include (but are not limited to) restlessness, poor eye contact, glancing about, facial tension, dilated pupils, increased perspiration, and a constant focus on self.

Anxiety disorders disorders characterized by chronic worry.

Aortography (ay-or-**TOG**-rah-fee) a radiographic process in which the aorta and its branches are injected with any of various contrast media for visualization.

Apathy (**AP**-ah-thee) absence or suppression of observable emotion, feeling, concern, or passion.

Apex (**AY**-peks) (of the lung) the upper portion of the lung, rising about 2.5 to 5 cm above the collarbone.

Aphakia (ah-**FAY**-kee-ah) absence of the lens of the eye.

Aphasia (ah-**FAY**-zee-ah) inability to communicate through speech, writing, or signs because of an injury to or disease in certain areas of the brain.

Aphonia (ah-**FOH**-nee-ah) without sound.

Aphthous stomatitis (**AFF**-thus stoh-mah-**TYE**-tis) small, inflammatory, noninfectious, ulcerated lesions occurring on the lips, tongue, and inside the cheeks of the mouth; also called canker sores.

Apical pulse (**AY**-pih-kal puhls) the heart rate as heard with a stethoscope placed on the chest wall adjacent to the cardiac apex (top of the heart).

Aplasia (ah-**PLAY**-zee-ah) a developmental failure resulting in the absence of any organ or tissue.

Aplastic (ay-**PLAS**-tick) without development.

Apnea (ap-**NEE**-ah) an absence of spontaneous respiration.

Appendectomy (ap-en-**DEK**-toh-mee) the surgical removal of an inflamed appendix.

Appendicitis (ap-**pen**-dih-**SIGH**-tis) the inflammation of the vermiform appendix.

Apraxia (ah-**PRAK**-see-ah) inability to perform coordinated movements or use objects properly; not associated with sensory or motor impairment or paralysis.

Aqueous (**AY**-kwee-us) watery.

Arachnoid membrane (ah-**RAK**-noyd **MEM**-brayn) the weblike middle layer of the three membranous layers surrounding the brain and spinal cord.

Areola (ah-**REE**-oh-lah) the darker pigmented, circular area surrounding the nipple of each breast; also known as the areola mammae or the areola papillaris. Plural: *areolae* (ah-**REE**-oh-lee)

Argyll-Robertson pupil (ar-**GILL ROB**-ert-son pupil) a pupil that constricts upon accommodation but not in response to light. This can be due to miosis or advanced neurosyphilis.

Arteriography (**ar**-tee-ree-**OG**-rah-fee) X-ray visualization of arteries following the introduction of a radiopaque contrast medium into the bloodstream through a specific vessel by way of a catheter.

Arteriole (ar-**TEE**-ree-ohl) the smallest branch of an artery.

Arteriosclerosis (ar-**tee**-ree-oh-skleh-**ROH**-sis) an arterial condition in which there is thickening, hardening, and loss of elasticity of the walls of arteries, resulting in decreased blood supply, especially to the lower extremities and cerebrum. This is also called hardening of the arteries.

Arthralgia (ar-**THRAL**-jee-ah) joint pain.

Arthritis (ar-**THRYE**-tis) inflammation of joints.

Arthrocentesis (ar-throh-sen-**TEE**-sis) the surgical puncture of a joint with a needle for the purpose of withdrawing fluid for analysis.

Arthrodesis (**ar**-throh-**DEE**-sis) the surgical fusion of a joint.

Arthrogram (**AR**-throh-gram) an X-ray of a joint after injection of a contrast medium.

Arthrography (ar-**THROG**-rah-fee) the process of X-raying the inside of a joint after a contrast medium (a substance that makes the inside of the joint visible) has been injected into the joint.

Arthroplasty (**AR**-throh-**plas**-tee) the surgical reconstruction (repair) of a joint.

Articular cartilage (ar-**TIK**-yoo-lar **CAR**-tih-laj) thin layer of cartilage protecting and covering the connecting surfaces of the bones.

Articulation (ar-tik-yoo-**LAY**-shun) the point at which two bones come together; a joint.

Arthrography (ar-**THROG**-rah-fee) a method of radiographically visualizing the inside of a joint by injecting air or contrast medium.

Asbestosis (**as**-beh-**STOH**-sis) a lung disease resulting from inhalation of asbestos particles.

Ascites (ah-**SIGH**-teez) an abnormal collection of fluid within the peritoneal cavity (the peritoneum is the serous membrane that lines the entire abdominal cavity). This fluid contains large amounts of protein and electrolytes. General abdominal swelling occurs with ascites.

Ascitic fluid (ah-**SIT**-ik fluid) a watery fluid containing albumin, glucose, and electrolytes that accumulates in the peritoneal cavity in association with certain disease conditions (such as liver disease).

Aseptic technique (ay-**SEP**-tic tek-**NEEK**) any health care procedure in which precautions are taken to prevent contamination of a person, object, or area by microorganisms.

Aspiration biopsy (as-pih-**RAY**-shun **BYE**-op-see) an invasive procedure in which a needle is inserted into an area of the body, such as the breast, to withdraw a tissue or fluid sample for microscopic examination and diagnosis.

Asthma (**AZ**-mah) paroxysmal dyspnea (severe attack of difficult breathing) accompanied by wheezing caused by a spasm of the bronchial tubes or by swelling of the mucous membrane.

Astigmatism (ah-**STIG**-mah-tizm) a refractive error causing light rays entering the eye to be focused irregularly on the retina due to an abnormally shaped cornea or lens.

Astrocyte (**ASS**-troh-sight) a star-shaped neuroglial cell found in the CNS.

Astrocytoma (ass-troh-sigh-**TOH**-mah) a tumor of the brain or spinal cord composed of astrocytes.

Asymptomatic (ay-simp-toh-**MAT**-ik) without symptoms.

Asystole (ay-**SIS**-toh-lee) absence of contractions of the heart.

Ataxia (ah-**TAK**-see-ah) without muscular coordination.

Atelectasis (at-ee-**LEK**-tah-sis) incomplete expansion of part or all of a lung.

Atherosclerosis (ath-er-oh-skleh-**ROH**-sis) form of arteriosclerosis (hardening of the arteries) characterized by fatty deposit buildup within the inner layers of the walls of larger arteries.

Atrial flutter (**AY**-tree-al flutter) condition in which the contractions of the atria become extremely rapid, at the rate of between 250 and 350 beats per minute.

Atrophic (aye-**TROH**-fik) characterized by a wasting of tissues, usually associated with general malnutrition or a specific disease state.

Atrophic vaginitis (aye-**TROH**-fik vaj-in-**EYE**-tis) degeneration of the vaginal mucous membrane after menopause. Also known as senile vaginitis, this condition is common in estrogen-deprived older women. The tissues of the vagina become drier and thinner.

Atrophy (**AT**-roh-fee) wasting away; literally "without development."

Attention-deficit hyperactivity disorder (ADHD) (ah-ten-shun-**DEF**-ih-sit **HIGH**-per-ak-tiv-ih-tee diss-**OR**-der) ADHD is a condition of persistent inattention and hyperactivity, impulsivity, or both; formerly known as attention-deficit disorder (ADD).

Audiogram (**AW**-dee-oh-gram) a recording of the faintest sounds an individual is able to hear.

Audiometry (aw-dee-**OM**-eh-tree) the process of measuring how well an individual hears various frequencies of sound waves.

Auditory (**AW**-dih-tor-ee) pertaining to the sense of hearing.

Aura (**AW**-rah) the sensation an individual experiences prior to the onset of a migraine headache or an epileptic seizure. It may be a sensation of light or warmth and may precede the attack by hours or only a few seconds.

Aural (**AW**-ral) pertaining to the ear.

Auriculotemporal (aw-rik-yoo-loh-**TEM**-poh-ral) pertaining to the ear and the temporal area of the skull.

Auscultation (oss-kull-**TAY**-shun) process of listening for sounds within the body, usually to sounds of thoracic or abdominal viscera, to detect some abnormal condition or to detect fetal heart sounds.

Autism (**AW**-tizm) a pervasive developmental disorder characterized by the individual being extremely withdrawn and absorbed with fantasy. The individual suffers from impaired communication/social interaction skills, and activities and interest are very limited. Autism was first classified as a type of schizophrenia.

Autonomic nervous system (aw-toh-**NOM**-ik **NER**-vus **SIS**-tem) the part of the nervous system that regulates the involuntary vital functions of the body, such as the activities involving the heart muscle, smooth muscles, and the glands. The autonomic nervous system has two divisions: the SNS and the PNS (defined separately).

Axial (**AK**-see-al) pertaining to or situated on the axis of a structure or part of the body.

Axillary temperature (**AK**-sih-lair-ee **TEMP**-per-ah-toor) the body temperature as recorded by a thermometer placed in the armpit. The reading is generally 0.5 to 1.0 degree less than the oral temperature.

Axon (**AK**-son) the part of the nerve cell that transports nerve impulses away from the nerve cell body.

Azotemia (azz-oh-**TEE**-mee-ah) the presence of excessive amounts of waste products of metabolism (nitrogenous compounds) in the blood caused by failure of the kidneys to remove urea from the blood. Azotemia is characteristic of uremia.

B

Babinski's reflex (bah-**BIN**-skeez **REE**-fleks) can be tested by stroking the sole of the foot, beginning at midheel and moving upward and lateral to the toes. A positive Babinski's occurs when there is dorsiflexion of the great toe and fanning of the other toes.

Bacteriostatic stopping or controlling the growth of bacteria.

Balanitis (bal-ah-**NYE**-tis) inflammation of the glans penis and the mucous membrane beneath it.

Ball-and-socket joint allows movements in many directions around a central point. A ball-shaped head that fits into the concave depression of another bone allows the bone with the ball-shaped head to move in many directions. Examples of a ball-and-socket joint are the shoulder joint and the hip joint.

Ballottement (bah-**LOT**-ment) a technique of using the examiner's finger to tap against the uterus, through the vagina, to cause the fetus to "bounce" within the amniotic fluid and feeling it rebound quickly.

Barium enema (BE) (lower GI series) (**BAH**-ree-um **EN**-eh-mah) infusion of a radiopaque contrast medium, barium sulfate, into the rectum and held in the lower intestinal tract while X-ray films are obtained of the lower GI tract.

Barium swallow (UGI) (upper GI series) (**BAH**-ree-um swallow) involves oral administration of a radiopaque contrast medium, barium sulfate, which flows into the esophagus as the person swallows.

Barotitis media (bar-oh-**TYE**-tis **MEE**-dee-ah) inflammation or bleeding of the middle ear caused by sudden changes in atmospheric pressure, as in scuba diving or descent of an airplane (especially when one has a cold or an upper respiratory infection).

Barrier methods methods of birth control that place physical barriers between the cervix and the sperm so that the sperm cannot pass the cervix and enter the uterus, and, thus, the fallopian tubes.

Bartholin's glands (**BAR**-toh-linz glands) two small, mucus-secreting glands located on the posterior and lateral aspects of the entrance to the vagina.

Basal layer (**BAY**-sal layer) the deepest of the five layers of the epidermis.

Base (of the lung) the lowest part of the lung, resting on the diaphragm.

Basophil (**BAY**-soh-fill) a granulocytic white blood cell characterized by cytoplasmic granules that stain blue when exposed to a basic dye. Basophils represent 1% or less of the total white blood cell count.

Behavior therapy a form of psychotherapy that seeks to modify observable maladjusted patterns of behavior by substituting new responses to given stimuli; also called behavior modification.

Bell's palsy (**BELLZ PAWL**-zee) a temporary or permanent unilateral weakness or paralysis of the muscles in the face following trauma to the face, an unknown infection, or a tumor pressing on the facial nerve rendering it paralyzed.

Benign (bee-**NINE**) noncancerous and therefore not an immediate threat, even though treatment eventually may be required for health or cosmetic reasons; not life threatening.

Benign prostatic hypertrophy (bee-**NINE** pross-**TAT**-ik high-**PER**-troh-fee) a benign (noncancerous) enlargement of the prostate gland, creating pressure on the upper part of the urethra or neck of the bladder (causing obstruction of the flow of urine).

Betatron (**BAY**-tah-tron) a cyclic accelerator that produces high-energy electrons for radiotherapy treatments.

Bicuspid tooth (bye-**CUSS**-pid) one of the two teeth between the molars and canines of the upper and lower jaw, the bicuspid teeth have a flat surface with multiple projections (cusps) for crushing and grinding food; also known as premolar tooth.

Bile (**BYE**-al) a bitter, yellow-green secretion of the liver.

Bilirubin (bill-ih-**ROO**-bin) the orange-yellow pigment of bile formed principally by the breakdown of hemoglobin in red blood cells after termination of their normal life span.

Biomicroscopy (**BYE**-oh-mye-**kros**-koh-pee) ophthalmic examination of the eye by use of a slit lamp and a magnifying lens; also known as a slit-lamp exam.

Bipolar disorders (manic-depressive) (by-**POHL**-ar) a psychological disorder characterized by episodes of mania and depression, alternations between the two, or a mixture of the two moods simultaneously.

Birth control patch a thin, flexible square patch that continuously delivers hormones through the skin and into the bloodstream for a full seven days to prevent pregnancy. The birth control patch contains hormones similar to those in birth control pills but must be changed every seven days.

Blackhead an open comedo, caused by accumulation of keratin and sebum within the opening of a hair follicle.

Bleeding time measurement of the time required for bleeding to stop.

Blepharitis (blef-ah-**RYE**-tis) acute or chronic inflammation of the eyelid margins stemming from seborrheic, allergic, or bacterial origin.

Blepharochalasis (blef-ah-roh-**KAL**-ah-sis) relaxation of the skin of the eyelid (usually the upper eyelid). The skin may droop over the edge of the eyelid when the eyes are open; also known as dermatochalasis.

Blepharoptosis (ptosis) (blef-ah-roh-**TOH**-sis) occurs when the eyelid partially or entirely covers the eye as a result of a weakened muscle.

Blepharospasm (blef-ah-roh-**SPAZM**) a twitching of the eyelid muscles; may be due to eyestrain or nervous irritability.

Blindness loss of the sense of sight, or extreme visual limitations.

Blister a small, thin-walled skin lesion containing clear fluid; a vesicle.

Blood–brain barrier (**BLUD-BRAIN BAIR**-ree-er) a protective characteristic of the capillary walls of the brain that prevents the passage of harmful substances from the bloodstream into the brain tissue or CSF.

Blood transfusion (**BLUD** trans-**FEW**-zhun) an administration of blood or a blood component to an individual to replace blood lost through surgery, trauma, or disease.

Blood urea nitrogen (BUN) (**BLUD** yoo-**REE**-ah **NIGH**-troh-jen) a blood test performed to determine the amount of urea and nitrogen (waste products normally excreted by the kidney) present in the blood.

Bloody show a vaginal discharge that is a mixture of thick mucus and pink or dark brown blood. It may begin a few weeks prior to the onset of labor and occurs as a result of the softening, dilation, and effacement (thinning) of the cervix in preparation for childbirth. The bloody show will continue and will increase during labor as the cervix continues to dilate and efface.

Boil a localized pus-producing infection originating deep in a hair follicle; a furuncle.

Bolus (**BOH**-lus) a ball-like mass of chewed food (mixed with saliva) that is ready to be swallowed.

Bone depressions concave, indented areas or openings in bones.

Bone markings specific features of individual bones.

Bone marrow aspiration the process of removing a small sample of bone marrow from a selected site with a needle for the purpose of examining the specimen under a microscope.

Bone marrow biopsy (bone marrow **BY**-op-see) the microscopic exam of bone marrow tissue, which fully evaluates hematopoiesis by revealing the number, shape, and size of the RBCs and WBCs and platelet precursors.

Bone marrow transplant after receiving an intravenous infusion of aggressive chemotherapy or total-body irradiation to destroy all malignant cells and to inactivate the immune system, a donor's bone marrow cells are infused intravenously into the recipient.

Bone processes projections or outgrowths of bones.

Bone scan the intravenous injection of a radioisotope, which is absorbed by bone tissue. After approximately 3 hours, the skeleton is scanned with a gamma camera (scanner) moving from one end of the body to the other. The scanner detects the areas of radioactive concentration (areas where the bone absorbs the isotope) and converts the radioactive image to a screen on which the concentrations show up as pinpoint dots cast in the image of a skeleton.

Borderline personality disorder characterized by an extensive pattern of instability of interpersonal relationships, self-image, and marked impulsivity that begins by early adulthood and is present in a variety of contexts.

Bowel (**BOW**-el) the portion of the alimentary canal extending from the pyloric opening of the stomach to the anus.

Bowman's capsule (**BOW**-manz **CAP**-sool) the cup-shaped end of a renal tubule containing a glomerulus; also called glomerular capsule.

Brachytherapy (**brak**-ee-**THAIR**-ah-pee) the placement of radioactive sources in contact with or implanted into the tissues to be treated.

Bradycardia (**brad**-ee-**KAR**-dee-ah) a slow heart rate characterized by a pulse rate under 60 beats per minute.

Bradykinesia (**brad**-ee-kih-**NEE**-zee-ah) abnormally slow movement.

Brain abscess (**BRAIN AB**-sess) a localized accumulation of pus located anywhere in the brain tissue due to an infectious process—either a primary local infection or an infection secondary to another infectious process in the body (such as bacterial endocarditis, sinusitis, otitis, or dental abscess).

Brain scan a nuclear counter scanning of cranial content two hours after an intravenous injection of radioisotopes.

Brain stem the stemlike portion of the brain that connects the cerebral hemisphere with the spinal cord. The brain stem contains the midbrain, the pons, and the medulla oblongata.

Brand name the name under which the drug is sold by a specific manufacturer. This name is owned by the manufacturer, and no other company may use that name. Each brand name carries a registered trademark symbol. Also known as trade name.

Braxton Hicks contractions mild, irregular contractions that occur throughout pregnancy. As full term approaches, these contractions intensify and are sometimes mistaken for true labor.

Breast self-examination a procedure in which the woman examines her breasts and surrounding tissue for evidence of any changes that could indicate the possibility of malignancy.

Bronchi (**BRONG**-kigh) the two main branches leading from the trachea to the lungs, providing the passageway for air movement.

Bronchiectasis (brong-key-**EK**-tah-sis) chronic dilation of a bronchus or bronchi, with secondary infection that usually involves the lower portion of the lung.

Bronchiole (**BRONG**-key-ohl) one of the smaller subdivisions of the bronchial tubes.

Bronchitis (brong-**KIGH**-tis) inflammation of the mucous membrane of the bronchial tubes. Infection is often preceded by the common cold.

Bronchogenic carcinoma (**brong**-koh-**JEN**-ic kar-sih-**NOH**-mah) a malignant lung tumor that originates in the bronchi; lung cancer.

Bronchography (brong-**KOG**-rah-fee) an X-ray examination of the interior passageways of the lower respiratory tract (larynx, trachea, and bronchi) following the coating of these structures with a radiopaque substance. As the catheter or bronchoscope is inserted through the nose or mouth and advanced down the throat into the trachea and bronchi, the radiopaque substance is released, forming a coating on the lining of the interior walls of these structures. Abnormalities such as tumors, cavities, cysts, and obstructions may be revealed. Bronchography is less frequently used due to the improved technology of computerized tomography (CT scan) and bronchoscopy.

Bronchorrhea (**brong**-koh-**REE**-ah) discharge or drainage from the bronchial tubes.

Bronchoscopy (brong-**KOSS**-koh-pee) the examination of the interior of the bronchi using a lighted, flexible tube known as a bronchoscope (or endoscope).

Brudzinski's sign (broo-**JIN**-skeez **SIGN**) a positive sign of meningitis, in which there is an involuntary flexion of the arm, hip, and knee when the patient's neck is passively flexed.

Bruise a bluish-black discoloration of an area of the skin or mucous membrane caused by an escape of blood into the tissues as a result of an injury to the area. See also *ecchymosis*.

Bruit (brew-**EE**) an abnormal sound or murmur heard when listening to a carotid artery, organ, or gland with a stethoscope (e.g., during auscultation). Plural: *bruits* (brew-**EEZ**)

Buccal medication (**BUCK**-al med-ih-**KAY**-shun) medication placed in the mouth next to the cheek, where it is absorbed into the mucous membrane lining of the mouth. It is in tablet form.

Bulbourethral glands (buhl-boh-yoo-**REE**-thral glands) a pair of pea-sized glands that empty into the urethra just before it extends through the penis; also known as Cowper's glands.

Bulimia nervosa (boo-**LIM**-ee-ah ner-**VOH**-suh) an uncontrolled craving for food, often resulting in eating binges, followed by vomiting to eliminate the food from the stomach. The individual may then feel depressed and go through a period of self-deprivation followed by another eating binge, and the cycle continues.

Bulla (**BULL**-ah) a large blister.

Bunion (hallux valgus) (**BUN**-yun) (**HAL**-uks **VAL**-gus) a bunion, or hallux valgus, is an abnormal enlargement of the joint at the base of the great toe.

Bunionectomy (bun-yun-**ECK**-toh-mee) surgical removal of a bunion; removing the bony overgrowth and the bursa.

Burns tissue injury produced by flame, heat, chemicals, radiation, electricity, or gases. The extent of the damage to the underlying tissue is determined by the mode and duration of exposure, the thermal intensity or temperature, and the anatomic site of the burn. Burn degree is classified according to the depth of injury.

Burr hole a hole drilled into the skull using a form of drill.

Bursa (**BER**-sah) a small sac that contains synovial fluid for lubricating the area around the joint where friction is most likely to occur.

Byssinosis (bis-ih-**NOH**-sis) a lung disease resulting from inhalation of cotton, flax, and hemp; also known as brown lung disease.

C

Cachexia (kah-**KEKS**-eeh-ah) a condition of general ill health and malnutrition; physical wasting with loss of weight and muscle mass due to a disease.

Calculus (**KAL**-kew-lus) an abnormal stone formed in the body tissues by an accumulation of mineral salts; usually formed in the gallbladder and kidney. See also *renal calculus.*

Callus a common (usually painless) thickening of the epidermis at sites of external pressure or friction, such as the weight-bearing areas of the feet and on the palmar surface of the hands. This localized hyperplastic area of up to 1 inch in size is also known as a callosity.

Calyx (**KAY**-liks) the cup-shaped division of the renal pelvis through which urine passes from the renal tubules. Plural: *calyces* (**KAL**-ih-seez)

Cancellous bone (**CAN**-sell-us) spongy bone, not as dense as compact bone.

Cancer a neoplasm characterized by the uncontrolled growth of anaplastic cells that tend to invade surrounding tissue and to metastasize to distant body sites.

Cancer, thyroid gland malignant tumor of the thyroid gland, which leads to dysfunction of the gland and thus inadequate or excessive secretion of the thyroid hormone.

Candidiasis (kan-dih-**DYE**-ah-sis) a type of yeast infection (most often fom the fungi *Candida albicans*). Affected sites may be skin, oral mucosa, respiratory tract or vagina. The characteristic symptom with candidiasis is severe itching (pruritus) and a milky-white discharge.

Canine tooth (**KAY**-nine) any one of the four teeth, two in each jaw, situated immediately lateral to the incisor teeth in the human dental arches; also called cuspid tooth.

Cannabis (**CAN**-ah-bis) a mind-altering drug derived from the flowering top of hemp plants; also called marijuana. This drug is classified as a controlled substance, Schedule I drug.

Capillaries (**CAP**-ih-**lair**-eez) any of the minute (tiny) blood vessels. The capillaries connect the ends of the smallest arteries (arterioles) with the beginnings of the smallest veins (venules).

Capsule endoscopy (**CAP**-sool en-**DOSS**-koh-pee) the process of viewing the entire length of the small intestine by using an ingestible video camera with a light source, which is enclosed in a capsule (about the size of a large vitamin pill). This tiny video camera, known as the camera pill, produces digital images of the entire length of the small intestine and can visualize areas that other diagnostic techniques cannot. Use of the camera pill is not disruptive to the normal activities of the digestive tract; also known as wireless endoscopy.

Carbuncle (**CAR**-bung-kul) a circumscribed inflammation of the skin and deeper tissues that contains pus, which eventually discharges to the skin surface.

Carcinogen (kar-**SIN**-oh-jen) a substance or agent that causes the development or increases the incidence of cancer.

Carcinoma (**kar**-sih-**NOH**-mah) a malignant neoplasm.

Carcinoma, basal cell (kar-sih-**NOH**-mah, **BAY**-sal sell) a malignant epithelial cell tumor that begins as a slightly elevated nodule with a depression or ulceration in the center that becomes more obvious as the tumor grows. As the depression enlarges, the tissue breaks down, crusts, and bleeds.

Carcinoma of the breast (kar-sih-**NOH**-mah) a malignant (cancerous) tumor of the breast tissue. The most common type (ductal carcinoma) originates in the mammary ducts. This tumor has the ability to invade surrounding tissue if not detected early enough. Once the cancer cells penetrate the duct, they will metastasize (spread) through the surrounding breast tissue, eventually reaching the axillary lymph nodes. Through the lymph vessels, the cancer cells can spread to distant parts of the body.

Carcinoma in situ (CIS) a premalignant neoplasm that has not invaded the basement membrane but shows cytologic characteristics of cancer.

Carcinoma of the prostate (**kar**-sih-**NOH**-mah of the **PROSS**-tayt) malignant growth within the prostate gland, creating pressure on the upper part of the urethra.

Carcinoma, squamous cell (**kar**-sih-**NOH**-ma, **SKWAY**-mus sell) a malignancy of the squamous (or scalelike) cells of the epithelial tissue, which is a much faster growing cancer than basal cell carcinoma and which has a greater potential for metastasis if not treated.

Carcinoma of the testes (kar-sih-**NOH**-mah of the **TESS**-teez) a malignant tumor of the testicle that appears as a painless lump in the testicle; also called testicular cancer.

Cardiac catheterization (**CAR**-dee-ak **cath**-eh-ter-ih-**ZAY**-shun) a diagnostic procedure in which a catheter (a hollow, flexible tube) is introduced into a large vein or artery (usually of an arm or a leg) and then threaded through the circulatory system to the heart. Cardiac catheterization is used to obtain detailed information about the structure and function of the heart chambers, valves, and the great vessels.

Cardiac enzymes test (**CAR**-dee-ak **EN**-zyms test) performed on samples of blood obtained by venipuncture to determine the presence of damage to the myocardial muscle.

Cardiac muscle the muscle that makes up the muscular wall of the heart. Cardiac muscle is a type of involuntary muscle.

Cardiac sphincter (**CAR**-dee-ak **SFINGK**-ter) the muscular ring (sphincter) in the stomach that controls the passage of food from the esophagus into the stomach; also known as the lower esophageal sphincter.

Cardiac tamponade (**CAR**-dee-ak **TAM**-poh-nod) compression of the heart caused by the accumulation of blood or other fluid within the pericardial sac. (There is normally just enough fluid within this cavity to lubricate the area.) The accumulation of fluid in the pericardial cavity prevents the ventricles from adequately filling or pumping blood. Cardiac tamponade is a life-threatening emergency if untreated.

Cardiomyopathy (**CAR**-dee-oh-my-**OP**-ah-thee) disease of the heart muscle itself, primarily affecting the pumping ability of the heart. This noninflammatory disease of the heart results in enlargement of the heart (cardiomegaly) and dysfunction of the ventricles of the heart.

Carotid endarterectomy (kah-**ROT**-id **end**-ar-ter-**ECK**-toh-mee) a surgical procedure performed to remove plaque buildup in the carotid arteries and facilitate blood flow; performed to reduce the risk of stoke caused by disruption of the blood flow.

Carpal tunnel syndrome (**CAR**-pal **TUN**-el **SIN**-drom) a pinching or compression of the median nerve within the carpal tunnel due to inflammation and swelling of the tendons, causing intermittent or continuous pain that is greatest at night.

Cartilaginous joint (car-tih-**LAJ**-ih-nus) in a cartilaginous joint, the bones are connected by cartilage, as in the symphysis (joint between the pubic bones of the pelvis). This type of joint allows limited movement.

Castration (kass-**TRAY**-shun) the surgical removal of the testicles in the male (or the ovaries in the female); also known as an orchidectomy or orchiectomy in the male and as an oophorectomy in the female.

Cataplexy (**CAT**-ah-pleks-ee) a sudden loss of muscle tone in which the individual's head may drop, the jaw may sag, the knees become weakened, and the individual may collapse or fall to the ground; may accompany a narcolepsy attack (sudden, uncontrollable attack of sleep).

Cataract (**KAT**-ah-rakt) the lens in the eye becomes progressively cloudy, losing its normal transparency and thus altering the perception of images due to the interference of light transmission to the retina.

Catheter (**CATH**-eh-ter) a hollow, flexible tube that can be inserted into a body cavity or vessel for the purpose of instilling or withdrawing fluid.

Catheterization (kath-eh-ter-**EYE**-zay-shun) the introduction of a catheter (flexible, hollow tube) into a body cavity or organ to instill a substance or to remove a fluid.

Catheterized specimen (sterile specimen) (**CATH**-eh-ter-eyezd **SPEH**-sih-men) using aseptic techniques, a very small straight catheter is inserted into the bladder via the urethra to withdraw a urine specimen. The urine flows through the catheter into a sterile specimen container.

Cauda equina (**KAW**-dah ee-**KWY**-nah) the lower end of the spinal cord and the roots of the spinal nerves that occupy the spinal canal below the level of the first lumbar vertebra; so named because it resembles a horse's tail.

Caudal (**KAWD**-al) pertaining to the tail.

Causalgia (kaw-**ZAL**-jee-ah) a sensation of an acute burning pain along the path of a peripheral nerve, sometimes accompanied by erythema of the skin; due to injury to peripheral nerve fibers.

Cautery (**KAW**-ter-ree) heat or caustic substances that burn and scar the skin (coagulation of tissue).

Cecum (**SEE**-kum) a cul-de-sac containing the first part of the large intestine. It joins the ileum, the last segment of the small intestine.

Celiac disease (**SEE**-lee-ak dih-**ZEEZ**) nutrient malabsorption due to damaged small-bowel mucosa.

Cell the smallest and most numerous structural unit of living matter.

Cell body the part of the cell that contains the nucleus and the cytoplasm.

Cell membrane the semipermeable barrier that is the outer covering of a cell.

Cellulitis (sell-yoo-**LYE**-tis) a diffuse acute infection of the skin and subcutaneous tissue, characterized by localized heat, deep redness, pain, and swelling.

Central nervous system one of the two main divisions of the nervous system, consisting of the brain and the spinal cord.

Cephalalgia (seff-ah-**LAL**-jee-ah) pain in the head; headache.

Cephalocaudal (seff-ah-loh-**KAW**-dal) growth and development proceeds from head to toe (cephalocaudal). In the infant, muscular control follows the spine downward.

Cerclage (sair-**KLAZH**) suturing the cervix to keep it from dilating prematurely during the pregnancy. This procedure is sometimes referred to as a "purse string procedure." The sutures are removed near the end of the pregnancy.

Cerebellum (ser-eh-**BELL**-um) the part of the brain responsible for coordinating voluntary muscular movement; located behind the brain stem.

Cerebral angiography (seh-**REE**-bral an-jee-**OG**-rah-fee) visualization of the cerebral vascular system via X-ray after the injection of a radiopaque contrast medium into an arterial blood vessel (carotid, femoral, or brachial).

Cerebral concussion (seh-**REE**-bral con-**KUSH**-un) a brief interruption of brain function, usually with a loss of consciousness lasting for a few seconds.

Cerebral contusion (seh-**REE**-bral con-**TOO**-zhun) a small, scattered venous hemorrhage in the brain (or better described as a "bruise" of the brain tissue) occurring when the brain strikes the inner skull.

Cerebral cortex (seh-**REE**-bral **COR**-teks) the thin outer layer of nerve tissue, known as gray matter, that covers the surface of the cerebrum.

Cerebral palsy (CP) (seh-**REE**-bral **PAWL**-zee) is a collective term used to describe congenital (at birth) brain damage that is permanent but not progressive. It is characterized by the child's lack of control of voluntary muscles.

Cerebrospinal fluid (ser-eh-broh-**SPY**-nal **FLOO**-id) the fluid flowing through the brain and around the spinal cord that protects them from physical blow or impact.

Cerebrospinal fluid analysis (ser-eh-broh-**SPY**-nal **FLOO**-id an-**AL**-ah-sis) cerebrospinal fluid (CSF) obtained from a lumbar puncture is analyzed for the presence of bacteria, blood, or malignant cells as well as for the amount of protein and glucose present.

Cerebrovascular accident (CVA) (seh-**REE**-broh-**VASS**-kyoo-lar **AK**-sih-dent) Neurological deficit(s) resulting from a decrease in blood (ischemia) to a specific localized area in the brain; also called "stroke" or "brain attack."

Cerebrum (seh-**REE**-brum) the largest and uppermost part of the brain. It controls consciousness, memory, sensations, emotions, and voluntary movements.

Cerumen (seh-**ROO**-men) earwax.

Ceruminous gland (seh-**ROO**-mih-nus gland) a modified sweat gland that lubricates the skin of the ear canal with a yellowish-brown waxy substance called cerumen (or ear wax).

Cervical carcinoma (**SER**-vih-kal kar-sih-**NOH**-mah) a malignant tumor of the cervix. Cervical cancer is one of the most common malignancies of the female reproductive tract. Symptoms include an abnormal Pap smear and bleeding between menstrual periods, after sexual intercourse, or after menopause.

Cervical dysplasia (**SIR**-vih-kal dis-**PLAY**-see ah) the presence of abnormal tissue in the uterine cervix; this atypical tissue may be precancerous.

Cervical radiculopathy (**SIR**-vih-kal rah-**dick**-you-**LOP**-ah-thee) any disease of the spinal nerve roots in the neck; caused by pressure on the nerve roots.

Cervical vertebrae (**SER**-vic-al **VER**-teh-bray) the first seven segments of the spinal column; identified as C1 through C7.

Cervicitis (ser-vih-**SIGH**-tis) an acute or chronic inflammation of the uterine cervix.

Cervix (**SER**-viks) the part of the uterus that protrudes into the cavity of the vagina; the neck of the uterus.

Cesarean section (see-**SAYR**-ee-an section) a surgical procedure in which the abdomen and uterus are incised and a baby is delivered transabdominally. Also called cesarean birth or cesarean delivery.

Chadwick's sign the bluish-violet hue of the cervix and vagina after approximately the sixth week of pregnancy.

Chalazion (kah-**LAY**-zee-on) a cyst or nodule on the eyelid, resulting from an obstruction of a meibomian gland, which is responsible for lubricating the margin of the eyelid.

Chancre (**SHANG**-ker) a skin lesion, usually of primary syphilis, that begins at the site of infection as a small raised area and develops into a red painless ulcer with a scooped-out appearance; also known as a venereal sore.

Cheiloplasty (**KYE**-loh-plas-tee) surgically correcting a defect of the lip is known as cheiloplasty.

Chemical name the chemical name for a drug is the description of the chemical structure of the drug. It is listed in the *Hospital Formulary* along with the chemical formula diagram.

Chemotherapy (kee-moh-**THAIR**-ah-pee) the treatment of diseases by using drugs that have a specific deadly effect on disease-causing microorganisms. These drugs are used in the treatment of certain infections and cancer.

Chest pain a feeling of discomfort in the chest area.

Chest X-ray the use of high-energy electromagnetic waves passing through the body onto a photographic film to produce a picture of the internal structures of the body for diagnosis and therapy.

Cheyne-Stokes respirations (**CHAIN-STOHKS** res-pir-**AY**-shunz) an abnormal pattern of breathing characterized by periods of apnea followed by deep rapid breathing.

Chickenpox (varicella) (**CHICK**-en-pox) a viral disease of sudden onset with slight fever, successive eruptions of macules, papules, and vesicles on the skin followed by crusting over of the lesions with a granular scab. Itching may be severe. (Macules are discolorations at normal skin level; papules are raised pimplelike skin blemishes; and vesicles are blisterlike.)

Chlamydia (klah-**MID**-ee-ah) a sexually transmitted bacterial infection that causes inflammation of the cervix (cervicitis) in women and inflammation of the urethra (urethritis) and the epididymis (epididymitis) in men.

Chloasma (kloh-**AZ**-mah) patches of tan or brown pigmentation associated with pregnancy, occurring mostly on the forehead, cheeks, and nose; also called the "mask of pregnancy."

Cholangiogram (koh-**LAN**-jee-oh-**gram**) a record, or X-ray film, of the bile ducts following the injection of a radiopaque contrast medium.

Cholangiography (intravenous) (IVC) (koh-**lan**-jee-**OG**-rah-fee) (in-trah-**VEE**-nus) visualizing and outlining of the major bile ducts following an intravenous injection of a contrast medium.

Cholangiography (percutaneous transhepatic) (PTC, PTHC) (koh-**lan**-jee-**OG**-rah-fee) (**per**-kyoo-**TAY**-nee-us trans-heh-**PAT**-ik) examination of the bile duct structure, using a needle to pass directly into an intrahepatic bile duct to inject a contrast medium.

Cholecystectomy (koh-lee-sis-**TEK**-toh-mee) the surgical removal of the gallbladder.

Cholecystography (oral) (koh-lee-sis-**TOG**-rah-fee) visualization of the gallbladder through X-ray following the oral ingestion of pills containing a radiopaque iodinated dye.

Choledocholithiasis (koh-lee-**dock**-oh-lih-**THIGH**-ah-sis) the presence of a stone (calculus) in the common bile duct.

Cholelithiasis (koh-lee-lih-**THIGH**-ah-sis) abnormal presence of gallstones in the gallbladder.

Cholesteatoma (koh-lee-stee-ah-**TOH**-mah) a slow-growing cystic mass made up of epithelial cell debris in the middle ear.

Chordotomy (kor-**DOT**-oh-mee) a neurosurgical procedure for pain control accomplished through a laminectomy, in which there is surgical interference of pathways within the spinal cord that control pain.

Chorion (**KOH**-ree-on) the outer of the two membrane layers that surround and contain the fetus and the amniotic fluid during pregnancy.

Chorionic villus sampling (CVS) (koh-ree-**ON**-ik **VILL**-us sampling) a prenatal diagnostic test performed in the first trimester of pregnancy to detect chromosomal abnormalities (such as Down syndrome) in an unborn child.

Chromosomes (**KROH**-moh-sohm) the threadlike structures within the nucleus that control the functions of growth, repair, and reproduction for the body.

Chyme (KIGHM) the liquidlike material of partially digested food and digestive secretions found in the stomach just before it is released into the duodenum.

Cicatrix (SIK-ah-trix or sik-**AY**-trix) a scar; the pale, firm tissue that forms in the healing of a wound.

Cineradiography a diagnostic technique combining the techniques of fluoroscopy, radiography, and cinematography by filming the images that develop on a fluorescent screen with a movie camera.

Circumcision (sir-kum-**SIH**-zhun) a surgical procedure in which the foreskin (prepuce) of the penis is removed.

Circumduction (sir-kum-**DUCK**-shun) the movement of an extremity around in a circular motion. This motion can be performed with ball-and-socket joints, as in the shoulder and hip.

Circumscribed (SIR-kum-skrybd) confined to a limited space or well-defined area (as if a circle were drawn around it).

Cirrhosis (sih-**ROH**-sis) a disease of the liver that is chronic and degenerative, causing injury to the hepatocytes (functional cells of the liver).

Cisternal puncture (sis-**TER**-nal **PUNK**-chur) insertion of a short, beveled spinal needle into the cisterna magna (a shallow reservoir of CSF between the medulla and the cerebellum) to drain CSF or to obtain a CSF specimen.

Claudication (klaw-dih-**KAY**-shun) cramplike pains in the calves of the legs caused by poor circulation to the muscles of the legs; commonly associated with atherosclerosis.

Clean-catch specimen (midstream specimen) (CLEAN-CATCH SPEH-sih-men) this collection is used to avoid contamination of the urine specimen from the microorganisms normally present on the external genitalia.

Cleft lip and palate (CLEFT LIP and **PAL**-at) a congenital defect in which there is an open space between the nasal cavity and the lip due to failure of the soft tissue and bones in this area to fuse properly during embryologic development. With cleft palate, the hard palate fails to fuse, resulting in a fissure (cracklike sore) in the middle of the palate.

Climacteric (kly-**MAK**-ter-ik) the cessation of menstruation. See also *menopause*.

Clitoris (KLIT-oh-ris) the vaginal erectile tissue (structure) corresponding to the male penis.

Closed manipulation the manual forcing of a joint back into its original position without making an incision; also called closed reduction.

Closed reduction see *closed manipulation*.

Clubfoot (talipes equinovarus) (TAL-ih-peez **eh**-kwin-oh-**VAIR**-us) in this condition, the infant's foot is fixed in plantar flexion (turned downward) and deviates medially (turned inward) and the heel is in an elevated position. Therefore, the infant's foot cannot remain in normal position with the sole of the foot firmly on the floor.

Cluster headache (KLUSS-ter headache) occurs typically two to three hours after falling asleep; described as extreme pain around one eye that wakens the person from sleep.

Coagulation (koh-**ag**-yoo-**LAY**-shun) the process of transforming a liquid into a solid, especially of the blood.

Coarctation of the aorta (KOH-ark-**TAY**-shun) a congenital heart defect characterized by a localized narrowing of the aorta, which results in increased blood pressure in the upper extremities (area proximal to the defect) and decreased blood pressure in the lower extremities (area distal to the defect).

Coccyx (COCK-siks) the tailbone. Located at the end of the vertebral column, the coccyx results from the fusion of four individual coccygeal bones in the child.

Cochlear (KOK-lee-ar) pertaining to a snail-shaped structure within the middle ear.

Coitus (KOH-ih-tus) the sexual union of two people of the opposite sex in which the penis is introduced into the vagina; also known as sexual intercourse or copulation.

Collagen (KOL-ah-jen) the protein substance that forms the glistening inelastic fibers of connective tissue such as tendons, ligaments, and fascia.

Colon (COH-lon) the portion of the large intestine extending from the cecum to the rectum.

Colonoscopy (koh-lon-**OSS**-koh-pee) the direct visualization of the lining of the large intestine using a fiberoptic colonoscope.

Color blindness (monochromatism) (mon-oh-**KROH**-mah-tizm) an inability to perceive visual colors sharply.

Colorectal cancer (koh-loh-**REK**-tal **CAN**-sir) the presence of a malignant neoplasm in the large intestine.

Colostomy (koh-**LAHS**-toh-mee) the surgical creation of a new opening on the abdominal wall through which the feces will be expelled (an abdominal-wall anus) by bringing the incised colon out to the abdominal surface.

Colostrum (koh-**LOSS**-trum) the thin, yellowish fluid secreted by the breasts during pregnancy and the first few days after birth, before lactation begins.

Colposcopy (kol-**POSS**-koh-pee) visual examination of the vagina and cervix with a colposcope.

Coma (COH-mah) a deep sleep in which the individual cannot be aroused and does not respond to external stimuli.

Comatose (COH-mah-tohs) pertains to being in a coma.

Comedo (KOM-ee-doh) the typical lesion of acne vulgaris, caused by accumulation of keratin and sebum within the opening of a hair follicle (closed comedo = whitehead; open comedo = blackhead).

Common bile duct the duct formed by the joining of the cystic duct and hepatic duct.

Compact bone hard outer shell of the bone.

Compensation (kom-pen-**SAY**-shun) an effort to overcome, or make up for, real or imagined inadequacies.

Complete blood cell count (CBC) a series of tests performed on peripheral blood, which inexpensively screens for problems in the hematologic system as well as in several other organ systems.

Compulsions (kom-**PUHL**-shuns) irresistible, repetitive, irrational impulses to perform an act. These behavior patterns are intended to reduce anxiety, not provide pleasure or gratification.

Computed axial tomography (CAT) (computed **AK**-see-al toh-**MOG**-rah-fee) a diagnostic X-ray technique that uses ionizing radiation to produce a cross-sectional image of the body. It is often used to detect aneurysms of the aorta. X-ray signals are fed into a computer, which then turns them into a cross-sectional picture of the section of the body being scanned; called CAT scan; also known as a CT scan.

Conception (con-**SEP**-shun) the union of a male sperm and a female ovum; also termed fertilization.

Condyle (**CON**-dial) knucklelike projection at the end of a bone.

Cone biopsy (**KOHN BY**-op-see) surgical removal of a cone-shaped segment of the cervix for diagnosis or treatment; also known as a conization.

Congenital present at birth.

Congestive heart failure (kon-**JESS**-tiv heart failure) condition characterized by weakness, breathlessness, abdominal discomfort. Edema in the lower portions of the body resulting from the flow of the blood through the vessels being slowed (venous stasis) and the outflow of blood from the left side of the heart is reduced. The pumping ability of the heart is progressively impaired to the point that it no longer meets bodily needs; also known as cardiac failure. Congestive heart failure is the single most frequent cause of hospitalization for those individuals 65 years of age and older.

Conjunctivitis, acute (kon-junk-tih-**VYE**-tis) inflammation of the mucous membrane lining the eyelids and covering the front part of the eyeball; often called "pink eye." Three types of conjunctivitis are viral, bacterial, and allergic.

Conn's disease (primary aldosteronism) (al-**DOSS**-ter-ohn-izm) a condition characterized by excretion of excessive amounts of aldosterone, the most influential of the mineralo-corticoids, which causes the body to retain extra sodium and excrete extra potassium, leading to an increased volume of blood (hypervolemia) and hypertension.

Connective tissue tissue that supports and binds other body tissue and parts.

Constipation (**kon**-stih-**PAY**-shun) a state in which the individual's pattern of bowel elimination is characterized by a decrease in the frequency of bowel movements and the passage of hard, dry stools. The individual experiences difficult defecation.

Contraceptive ring a flexible ring (placed into the vagina) that slowly releases a low dose of hormones that prevent pregnancy.

Contract/contraction (con-**TRAK**-shun) a reduction in size, especially of muscle fibers.

Contraction stress test a stress test used to evaluate the ability of the fetus to tolerate the stress of labor and delivery (CST); also known as oxytocin challenge test.

Contracture (con-**TRAK**-cher) an abnormal (usually permanent) bending of a joint into a fixed position; usually caused by atrophy and shortening of muscle fibers.

Contraindication (**kon**-trah-**in**-dih-**KAY**-shun) any special symptom or circumstance that indicates that the use of a particular drug or procedure is dangerous, not advised, or has not been proven safe for administration.

Controlled substances drugs that have a potential for abuse. These drugs are placed into five categories, ranging from Schedule I drugs (which are the most dangerous and most likely to be abused) to Schedule V drugs, which are the least dangerous and least likely to be abused; also known as schedule drugs.

Controlled Substances Act the federal law concerned with the manufacture, distribution, and dispensing of controlled substances. These drugs have the potential of being abused and of causing physical or psychological dependence.

Contusion (kon-**TOO**-zhun) an injury to a part of the body without a break in the skin.

Conversion disorder (kon-**VER**-zhun) a disorder in which the individual represses anxiety experienced by emotional conflicts by converting the anxious feelings into physical symptoms that have no organic basis but are perceived to be real by the individual. The individual may experience symptoms such as paralysis, pain, loss of sensation, or some other form of dysfunction of the nervous system; also called conversion hysteria.

Convolution (kon-voh-**LOO**-shun) one of the many elevated folds of the surface of the cerebrum; also called a gyrus.

Copulation (kop-yoo-**LAY**-shun) sexual intercourse; coitus.

Corneal (**COR**-nee-al) pertaining to the cornea.

Corneal abrasion (**COR**-nee-al ah-**BRAY**-zhun) a disruption of the cornea's surface epithelium commonly caused by an eyelash, a small foreign body, contact lenses, or a scratch from a fingernail.

Corneal transplant (**COR**-nee-al) surgical transplantation of a donor cornea (cadaver's) into the eye of a recipient, often under general anesthesia.

Coronary artery bypass graft surgery (CABG) (**KOR**-ah-nair-ree **AR**-ter-ee **BYE**-pass graft **SIR**-jer-ree) a surgical procedure (designed to increase the blood flow to the myocardial muscle) that involves bypass grafts to the coronary arteries that reroute the blood flow around the occluded area of the coronary artery.

Coronary artery disease (**KOR**-ah-nair-ree **AR**-ter-ee dih-**ZEEZ**) the narrowing of the coronary arteries to the extent that adequate blood supply to the myocardium is prevented.

Corpus luteum (**KOR**-pus **LOO**-tee-um) a yellowish mass that forms within the ruptured ovarian follicle after ovulation, containing high levels of progesterone and some estrogen. It functions as a temporary endocrine gland for the purpose of secreting estrogen and large amounts of progesterone, which will sustain pregnancy (should it occur) until the placenta forms. If pregnancy does not occur, the corpus luteum will degenerate approximately three days prior to the beginning of menstruation.

Corpuscle (**KOR**-pus-ul) any cell of the body; a red or white blood cell.

Cortex (**COR**-tex) pertaining to the outer region of an organ or structure.

Cortisol (**COR**-tih-sal) a steroid hormone occurring naturally in the body; also called hydrocortisone.

Coryza (kor-**RYE**-zuh) inflammation of the respiratory mucous membranes, known as rhinitis or the common cold. The term *common cold* is usually used when referring to symptoms of an upper respiratory tract infection.

Cowper's glands (**KOW**-perz) see *bulbourethral glands.*

Crackles (**CRACK**-ulz) a common abnormal respiratory sound heard on auscultation of the chest during inspiration, characterized by discontinuous bubbling noises.

Cranial (**KRAY**-nee-al) pertaining to the skull or cranium.

Craniotomy (kray-nee-**OTT**-oh-mee) a surgical procedure that makes an opening into the skull.

Creatinine clearance test (kree-**AT**-in-in clearance test) a diagnostic test for kidney function that measures the filtration rate of creatinine, a waste product (of muscle metabolism) normally removed by the kidney.

Crepitation (crep-ih-**TAY**-shun) clicking or crackling sounds heard upon joint movement.

Crest distinct border or ridge, as in iliac crest.

Cretinism (**KREE**-tin-izm) a congenital condition (one that occurs at birth) caused by a lack of thyroid secretion. This condition is characterized by dwarfism, slowed mental development, puffy facial features, dry skin, and large tongue.

Crohn's disease (**KROHNZ** dih-**ZEEZ**) digestive tract inflammation of a chronic nature, causing fever, cramping, diarrhea, weight loss, and anorexia.

Croup (**KROOP**) a childhood disease characterized by a barking cough, hoarseness, tachypnea, inspiratory stridor, and laryngeal spasm.

Crown the part of the tooth that is visible above the gum line.

Cryosurgery (**krigh**-oh-**SER**-jer-ee) the destruction of tissue by rapid freezing with substances such as liquid nitrogen.

Cryptorchidism (kript-**OR**-kid-izm) condition of undescended testicle(s); the absence of one or both testicles from the scrotum.

CT of the abdomen (**CT** of the **AB**-doh-men) a painless, noninvasive X-ray procedure that produces an image created by the computer representing a detailed cross section of the tissue structure within the abdomen, for example, computerized tomography (CT) of the abdomen.

CT colonography (CT koh-lon-**OG**-rah-fee) uses CT scanning (or MRI) to obtain an interior view of the colon that is usually seen using an endoscope inserted into the rectum. This noninvasive, painless procedure provides two- and three-dimensional images that can show polyps and other lesions as clearly as when they are seen with direct visual colonoscopy. Use of the CT colonography allows these growths to be detected in their early stages; also called a virtual colonoscopy (virtual colonoscopy) (virtual koh-lon-OSS-koh-pee).

CT (CAT) scan a collection of X-ray images taken from various angles following injection of a contrast medium.

CT scan of the brain analysis of a three-dimensional view of brain tissue obtained as X-ray beams pass through successive horizontal layers of the brain; also called computerized axial tomography (CAT scan).

Cul-de-sac (kull-dih-**SAK**) a pouch located between the uterus and rectum within the peritoneal cavity. This pouch is formed by one of the ligaments that serves as support to the uterus. Because it is the lowest part of the abdominal cavity, blood, pus, and other drainage collect in the cul-de-sac.

Culdocentesis (kull-doh-sen-**TEE**-sis) the surgical puncture through the posterior wall of the vagina into the cul-de-sac to withdraw intraperitoneal fluid for examination.

Cumulation (**KYOO**-mew-**lay**-shun) a drug level begins to accumulate in the body with repeated doses because the drug is not completely excreted from the body before another dose is administered.

Curettage (kyoo-reh-**TAHZH**) process of scraping material from the wall of a cavity or other surface for the purpose of removing abnormal tissue or unwanted material.

Curettage and electrodesiccation (koo-reh-**TAHZ** and ee-**lek**-troh-**des**-ih-**KAY**-shun) a combination procedure of curettage that involves scraping away abnormal tissue and electrodesiccation, which involves destroying the tumor base with a low-voltage electrode.

Cushing's syndrome (**CUSH**-ings **SIN**-drom) a condition of the adrenal gland in which a cluster of symptoms occur as a result of an excessive amount of cortisol or ACTH circulating in the blood.

Cuspid tooth (**CUSS**-pid tooth) see *canine tooth.*

Cyanosis (**sigh**-ah-**NOH**-sis) slightly bluish, grayish, slatelike, or dark discoloration of the skin due to the presence of abnormal amounts of reduced hemoglobin in the blood.

Cycloplegia (sigh-kloh-**PLEE**-jee-ah) paralysis of the ciliary muscle of the eye.

Cyclothymic disorder (**sigh**-cloh-**THIGH**-mic) a chronic mood disorder characterized by numerous periods of mood swings from depression to happiness. The period of mood disturbance is at least two years.

Cyst (**SIST**) a closed sac or pouch in or within the skin that contains fluid, semifluid, or solid material.

Cystitis (siss-**TYE**-tis) inflammation of the urinary bladder.

Cystocele (**SIS**-toh-seel) herniation or downward protrusion of the urinary bladder through the wall of the vagina.

Cystometer (siss-**TOM**-eh-ter) an instrument that measures bladder capacity in relation to changing pressure.

Cystometrography (**siss**-toh-meh-**TROG**-rah-fee) an examination performed to evaluate bladder tone; measuring bladder pressure during filling and voiding.

Cystoscope (**SISS**-toh-skohp) an instrument used to view the interior of the bladder. It consists of an outer sheath with a lighting system, a scope for viewing, and a passage for catheters and devices used in surgical procedures; may also be referred to as a "cysto."

Cystoscopy (siss-**TOSS**-koh-pee) the process of viewing the interior of the bladder, using a cystoscope.

Cytology (sigh-**TOL**-oh-jee) the study of cells.

Cytomegalovirus (**sigh**-toh-**meg**-ah-loh-**VYE**-rus) a large species-specific herpes-type virus with a wide variety of disease effects. It causes serious illness in persons with AIDS, in newborns, and in individuals who are being treated with immunosuppressive drugs (as in individuals who have received an organ transplant). The virus usually results in retinal or gastrointestinal infection.

Cytoplasm (**SIGH**-toh-plazm) a gel-like substance that surrounds the nucleus of a cell. The cytoplasm contains cell organs, called organelles, which carry out the essential functions of the cell.

Cytotoxic (**sigh**-toh-**TOKS**-ik) pertaining to being destructive to cells.

D

Dacryoadenitis (dak-ree-oh-ad-en-**EYE**-tis) inflammation of the lacrimal (tear) gland.

Dacryorrhea (dak-ree-oh-**REE**-ah) excessive flow of tears.

Deafness, conductive (kon-**DUK**-tiv) hearing loss caused by the breakdown of the transmission of sound waves through the middle or external ear.

Deafness, sensorineural (sen-soh-ree-**NOO**-ral) hearing loss caused by the inability of nerve stimuli to be delivered to the brain from the inner ear due to damage to the auditory nerve or the cochlea or to lesions of the 8th cranial nerve (auditory).

Debridement (day-breed-**MENT**) removal of debris, foreign objects, and damaged or necrotic tissue from a wound to prevent infection and to promote healing.

Deciduous teeth (dee-**SID**-yoo-us) the first set or primary teeth; baby teeth.

Dedifferentiation (**dee**-diff-er-en-she-**AY**-shun) see *anaplasia*.

Deep away from the surface and toward the inside of the body.

Defecation (deff-eh-**KAY**-shun) the act of expelling feces from the rectum through the anus.

Defense mechanism an unconscious, intrapsychic (within one's mind) reaction that offers protection to the self from a stressful situation.

Deficit (**DEFF**-ih-sit) any deficiency or variation of the normal, as in a weakness deficit resulting from a cerebrovascular accident.

Degenerative disk (deh-**JEN**-er-ah-tiv **DISK**) the deterioration of the intervertebral disk, usually due to constant motion and wear on the disk.

Deglutition (**dee**-gloo-**TISH**-un) swallowing.

Delirium (dee-**LEER**-ee-um) a state of frenzied excitement or wild enthusiasm.

Delirium tremens (DTs) (dee-**LEER**-ee-um **TREE**-menz) an acute and sometimes fatal psychotic reaction caused by cessation of excessive intake of alcoholic beverages over a long period of time. It occurs rapidly and is characterized by difficulty maintaining and shifting attention.

Delusion (dee-**LOO**-zhun) a persistent, abnormal belief or perception held firmly by a person despite evidence to the contrary. Two forms of delusions are delusions of persecution (in which the person thinks others are following him, spying on him, or trying to torment him) and delusions of grandeur, in which the person has a false sense of possessing wealth or power.

Dementia (dee-**MEN**-shee-ah) a progressive, organic mental disorder characterized by chronic personality disintegration, confusion, disorientation, stupor, deterioration of intellectual capacity and function, and impairment of control of memory, judgment, and impulses.

Demyelination (dee-**MY**-eh-lye-**NAY**-shun) destruction or removal of the myelin sheath that covers a nerve or nerve fiber.

Dendrite (**DEN**-dright) a projection that extends from the nerve cell body. It receives impulses and conducts them on to the cell body.

Denial a refusal to admit or acknowledge the reality of something, thus avoiding emotional conflict or anxiety.

Dental caries (**DEN**-tal **KAIR**-eez) tooth decay caused by acid-forming microorganisms.

Dentin (**DEN**-tin) the chief material of teeth surrounding the pulp and situated inside of the enamel and cementum.

Dentition (den-**TIH**-shun) the eruption of teeth. This occurs in a sequential pattern, with 20 primary teeth erupting between the ages of 6 to 30 months.

Deoxyribonucleic acid (DNA) (**dee**-ock-see-**rye**-boh-noo-**KLEE**-ic **ASS**-id) A large nucleic acid molecule found principally in the chromosomes of the nucleus of a cell that is the carrier of genetic information.

Depo-Provera injection (**DEP**-oh proh-**VAIR**-ah) is a form of contraception administered intramuscularly, approximately once every 12 weeks.

Depression a mood disturbance characterized by exaggerated feelings of sadness, discouragement, and hopelessness that are inappropriate and out of proportion with reality; may be relative to some personal loss or tragedy.

Dermabrasion (der-mah-**BRAY**-zhun) removal of the epidermis and a portion of the dermis with sandpaper or brushes to eliminate superficial scars or unwanted tattoos.

Dermatitis (der-mah-**TYE**-tis) inflammation of the skin, seen in several forms. Dermatitis may be acute or chronic, contact or seborrheic.

Dermatoplasty (**DER**-mah-toh-**plas**-tee) skin transplantation to a body surface damaged by injury or disease.

Dermis (**DER**-mis) the layer of skin immediately beneath the epidermis; the corium.

Desired effect the effect that was intended; that is, if the drug lowered the blood pressure as was intended, the desired effect was achieved.

Development an increase in function and complexity that results through learning, maturation, and growth.

Diabetes, gestational (dye-ah-**BEE**-teez, jess-**TAY**-shun-al) a condition occurring in pregnancy characterized by the signs and symptoms of diabetes mellitus (such as impaired ability to metabolize carbohydrates due to insulin deficiency, and elevated blood sugar level). These symptoms usually disappear after delivery of the baby.

Diabetes insipidus (dye-ah-**BEE**-teez in-**SIP**-ih-dus) a condition caused by a deficiency in the secretion of antidiuretic hormone (ADH) by the posterior pituitary gland, characterized by large amounts of urine and sodium being excreted from the body.

Diabetes mellitus (dye-ah-**BEE**-teez **MELL**-ih-tus) a disorder of the pancreas in which the beta cells of the islets of Langerhans of the pancreas fail to produce an adequate amount of insulin, resulting in the body's inability to metabolize carbohydrates, fats, and proteins appropriately.

Diabetic ketoacidosis (dye-ah-**BEH**-tik kee-toh-ass-ih-**DOH**-sis) a dangerous condition that occurs as a result of severe lack of insulin, causing the body to break down body fats instead of glucose for energy. The stored fat is broken down into fatty acids and glycerol. The liver changes the fatty acids into ketone bodies (acids) which leads to an increase in acidity of the blood (acidosis) called diabetic ketoacidosis (DKA). Also known as diabetic coma.

Diabetic retinopathy (dye-ah-**BET**-ik ret-in-**OP**-ah-thee) a disorder of the blood vessels of the retina of the eye, in which the capillaries of the retina experience localized areas of bulging (microaneurysms) hemorrhages, leakage, and scarring.

Dialysate (dye-**AL**-ih-**SAYT**) solution that contains water and electrolytes that passes through the artificial kidney to remove excess fluids and wastes from the blood; also called "bath."

Dialysis (dye-**AL**-ih-sis) process of removing waste products from the blood when the kidneys are unable to do so. Hemodialysis involves passing the blood through an artificial kidney for filtering out impurities. Peritoneal dialysis involves introducing fluid into the abdomen through a catheter. Through the process of osmosis, this fluid draws waste products out of the capillaries into the abdominal cavity. It is then removed from the abdomen via a catheter.

Diaphoresis (dye-ah-foh-**REE**-sis) the secretion of sweat.

Diaphragm (**DYE**-ah-fram) the musculomembranous wall separating the abdomen from the thoracic cavity; also a term used in gynecology to represent a form of contraception.

Diaphysis (dye-**AFF**-ih-sis) main shaftlike portion of a bone.

Diencephalon (dye-en-**SEFF**-ah-lon) the part of the brain located between the cerebrum and the midbrain. Its main structures consist of the thalamus, hypothalamus, and pineal gland.

Dietitian (dye-ah-**TIH**-shun) an allied health professional trained to plan nutrition programs for sick as well as healthy people. This may involve planning meals for a hospital or large organization or individualized diet counseling with patients.

Differentiation (diff-er-en-she-**AY**-shun) a process in development in which unspecialized cells or tissues are systemically modified and altered to achieve specific and characteristic physical forms, physiologic functions, and chemical properties.

Digestion (dye-**JEST**-shun) the process of altering the chemical and physical composition of food so that it can be used by the body cells. This occurs in the digestive tract.

Digestive tract (dye-**JESS**-tiv **TRAKT**) see *alimentary canal.*

Digital radiography (**DIJ**-ih-tal ray-dee-**OG**-rah-fee) any method of X-ray image formation that uses a computer to store and manipulate data.

Digital subtraction angiography (DSA) (**DIJ**-ih-tal sub-**TRAK**-shun **an**-jee-**OG**-rah-fee) X-ray images of blood vessels only, appearing without any background due to the use of a computerized digital video subtraction process.

Dilation and curettage (dye-**LAY**-shun and koo-reh-**TAHZ**) dilation or widening of the cervical canal with a dilator, followed by scraping of the uterine lining with a curet; also termed D&C.

Dilation (of cervix) (dye-**LAY**-shun) the enlargement of the diameter of the cervix during labor. The calculation of the amount of dilation is measured in centimeters (cm). When the cervix has dilated to 10 cm, it is said to be completely dilated. Also known as dilatation.

Diphtheria (diff-**THEE**-ree-ah) serious infectious disease affecting the nose, pharynx, or larynx, usually resulting in sore throat, dysphonia (difficult speaking or hoarseness) and fever. The disease is caused by the bacterium *Corynebacterium diphtheriae*, which forms a white coating over the affected airways as it multiplies.

Diplopia (dip-**LOH**-pee-ah) double vision caused by each eye focusing separately. See also *ambiopia.*

Direct antiglobulin test (Coombs Test) (dih-**RECT** an-tih-**GLOB**-yoo-lin test) used to discover the presence of antierythrocyte antibodies present in the blood of an Rh-negative woman. The production of these antibodies is associated with an Rh incompatibility between a pregnant Rh negative woman and her Rh positive fetus.

Directional coronary atherectomy (dih-**REK**-shun-al **KOR**-ah-nair-ree ath-er-**REK**-toh-mee) procedure that uses a catheter (AtheroCath), which has a small mechanically driven cutter that shaves the plaque and stores it in a collection chamber.

Dislocation (diss-loh-**KAY**-shun) the displacement of a bone from its normal location within a joint, causing loss of function of the joint.

Displacement the process of transferring a feeling or emotion from the original idea or object to a substitute idea or object.

Dissociation (dis-**soh**-shee-**AY**-shun) an unconscious defense mechanism by which an idea, thought, emotion, or other mental process is separated from the consciousness and thereby loses emotional significance.

Dissociative amnesia (diss-**SOH**-see-ah-tiv am-**NEE**-zee-ah) (formerly: psychogenic amnesia) a disorder in which the individual is unable to recall important personal information, usually of a traumatic or stressful nature. The loss of memory is more than simple forgetting.

Dissociative identity disorder (formerly: multiple personality disorder) a disorder in which there is the presence of two or more distinct personalities within one individual. At some point in time, each personality takes complete control of the person's behavior.

Distal (**DISS**-tal) away from or farthest from the trunk of the body or farthest from the point of attachment of a body part.

Diverticular disease (**dye**-ver-**TIK**-yoo-lar dih-**ZEEZ**) an expression used to characterize both diverticulosis and diverticulitis. Diverticulosis describes the noninflamed out-pouchings or herniations of the muscular layer of the intestine, typically the sigmoid colon. Inflammation of these outpouchings (called diverticula) is referred to as diverticulitis.

Doppler (**DOP**-ler) a technique used in ultrasound imaging to monitor the behavior of a moving structure such as flowing blood or a beating heart. Fetal heart monitors operate on the Doppler sound wave principle to determine the fetal heart rate.

Doppler effect (**DOP**-ler ee-**FECT**) the apparent change in frequency of sound or light waves emitted by a source as it moves away from or toward an observer.

Dormant (**DOOR**-mant) inactive.

Dorsal pertaining to the back.

Dorsiflexion (dor-sih-**FLECK**-shun) dorsiflexion of the foot narrows the angle between the leg and the top of the foot (i.e., the foot is bent backward, or upward, at the ankle).

Dorsum the back or posterior surface of a part; in the foot, the top of the foot.

Down syndrome (**DOWN SIN**-drohm) a congenital condition characterized by multiple defects and varying degrees of mental retardation.

Draw-a-Person (DAP) test a personality test that is based on the interpretation of drawings of human figures of both sexes.

Drug any substance that when taken into the body may modify one or more of its functions.

Drug action describes how a drug produces changes within the body.

Drug effect describes the change that takes place in the body as a result of the drug action.

Drug Enforcement Administration the government agency responsible for administering and enforcing the Controlled Substances Act.

Drug Facts and Comparisons a reference book for health care professionals that provides information on drugs according to their therapeutic classifications. This reference compares the various drugs within each category with other products.

Drug therapy the use of psychotropic drugs to treat mental disorders. Psychotropic drugs are those prescribed for their effects in relieving symptoms of anxiety, depression, or other mental disorders (such as schizophrenia).

Dual energy X-ray absorptiometry (ab-sorp-she-**AHM**-eh-tree) **(DEXA)** a noninvasive procedure that measures bone density. In the DEXA procedure, an X-ray machine generates the energy photons that pass through the bones. A computer then evaluates the amount of radiation absorbed by the bones, and the findings are interpreted by a physician.

Duodenum (doo-oh-**DEE**-num *or* do-**OD**-eh-num) the first portion of the small intestine. The duodenum is the shortest, widest, and most fixed portion of the small intestine, taking an almost circular course from the pyloric valve of the stomach so that its termination is close to its starting point.

Dura mater (**DOO**-rah **MAH**-ter) the outermost of the three membranes (meninges) surrounding the brain and spinal cord.

Dwarfism (**DWARF**-ism) generalized growth retardation of the body due to the deficiency of the human growth hormone; also known as congenital hypopituitarism (or hypopituitarism).

Dwell time length of time the dialysis solution stays in the peritoneal cavity during peritoneal dialysis.

Dyscrasia (dis-**KRAY**-zee-ah) an abnormal condition of the blood or bone marrow, such as leukemia, aplastic anemia, or prenatal Rh incompatibility.

Dysentery (**DISS**-en-**ter**-ee) a term used to describe painful intestinal inflammation typically caused by ingesting water or food containing bacteria, protozoa, parasites, or chemical irritants.

Dyskinesia (dis-kih-**NEE**-see-ah) an impairment of the ability to execute voluntary movements.

Dyslexia (dis-**LEK**-see-ah) by an impairment of the ability to read. Letters and words are often reversed when reading.

Dysphasia (dis-**FAY**-zee-ah) difficult speech.

Dysphonia (diss-**FOH**-nee-ah) difficulty in speaking; hoarseness.

Dysphoria (dis-**FOH**-ree-ah) a disorder of affect (mood) characterized by depression and anguish.

Dysplasia (dis-**PLAY**-zee-ah) any abnormal development of cells, tissues, or organs.

Dyspnea (**DISP**-nee-ah) difficult breathing; air hunger resulting in labored or difficult breathing, sometimes accompanied by pain (normal when caused by vigorous work or athletic activity).

Dysuria (dis-**YOO**-ree-ah) painful urination.

E

Ecchymosis (ek-ih-**MOH**-sis) a bluish-black discoloration of an area of the skin or mucous membrane caused by an escape of blood into the tissues as a result of injury to the area; also known as a bruise or a black-and-blue mark.

Echocardiogram (ek-oh-**CAR**-dee-oh-**gram**) the graphic outline, or record of movements of structures of the heart produced by ultrasonography (ultrasound).

Echocardiography (eck-oh-car-dee-**OG**-rah-fee) a diagnostic procedure for studying the structure and motion of the heart. It is useful in evaluating structural and functional changes in a variety of heart disorders. This noninvasive procedure has no known risks or side effects.

Echoencephalography (eck-oh-en-**sef**-ah-**LOG**-rah-fee) ultrasound used to analyze the intracranial structures of the brain.

Eclampsia (eh-**KLAMP**-see-ah) the most severe form of hypertension during pregnancy, evidenced by seizures (convulsions).

Ectopic pregnancy (ek-**TOP**-ic **PREG**-nan-see) abnormal implantation of a fertilized ovum outside the uterine cavity; also called a tubal pregnancy.

Ectropion (eck-**TROH**-pee-on) "turning out" or eversion of the eyelash margins (especially the lower eyelid) from the eyeball, leading to exposure of the eyelid and eyeball surface and lining.

Eczema (**ECK**-zeh-mah) an acute or chronic inflammatory skin condition characterized by erythema, papules, vesicles, pustules, scales, crusts, or scabs and accompanied by intense itching.

Edema (eh-**DEE**-mah) a local or generalized condition in which the body tissues contain an excessive amount of tissue fluid; swelling. Generalized edema is sometimes called dropsy.

Effacement (eh-**FACE**-ment) thinning of the cervix, which allows it to enlarge the diameter of its opening in preparation for childbirth. This occurs during the normal processes of labor.

Efferent nerves (**EE**-fair-ent nerves) transmitters of nerve impulses away from the CNS; also known as motor nerves.

Ejaculation (ee-**jack**-yoo-**LAY**-shun) the process of ejecting, or expelling, the semen from the male urethra.

Electrocardiogram (ee-lek-troh-**CAR**-dee-oh-**gram**) a graphic record (visual representation) of the electrical action of the heart as reflected from various angles to the surface of the skin; known as an EKG or ECG.

Electroconvulsive therapy (ECT) the process of passing an electrical current through the brain to create a brief seizure in the brain, much like a spontaneous seizure from some forms of epilepsy; also called shock therapy.

Electrodesiccation (ee-lek-troh-**des**-ih-**KAY**-shun) a technique that uses an electrical spark to burn and destroy tissue; used primarily for the removal of surface lesions.

Electroencephalography (EEG) (ee-**leck**-troh-en-**sef**-ah-**LOG**-rah-fee) measurement of electrical activity produced by the brain and recorded through electrodes placed on the scalp.

Electromyography (EMG) (ee-lek-troh-my-**OG**-rah-fee) is the process of recording the electrical activity of muscle by inserting a small needle into the muscle and delivering a small current that stimulates the muscle.

Electronystagmography (ee-lek-troh-**niss**-tag-**MOG**-rah-fee) a group of tests used in evaluating the vestibulo-ocular reflex.

Electrophoresis (ee-**lek**-troh-for-**EE**-sis) the movement of charged suspended particles through a liquid medium in response to changes in an electric field. Charged particles of a given substance migrate in a predictable direction and at a characteristic speed.

Electroretinogram (ERG) (ee-lek-troh-**RET**-ih-noh-gram) a recording of the changes in the electrical potential of the retina after the stimulation of light.

Electrosurgery (ee-**lek**-troh-**SER**-jer-ee) the removal or destruction of tissue with an electrical current.

Embolism (**EM**-boh-lizm) an abnormal condition in which a blood clot (embolus) becomes lodged in a blood vessel, obstructing the flow of blood within the vessel.

Embryo (**EM**-bree-oh) the name given to the product of conception from the second through the eighth week of pregnancy (through the second month).

Emmetropia (em-eh-**TROH**-pee-ah) a state of normal vision. The eye is at rest and the image is focused directly on the retina.

Emphysema (em-fih-**SEE**-mah) a chronic pulmonary disease characterized by increase beyond the normal in the size of air spaces distal to the terminal bronchiole, either from dilation of the alveoli or from destruction of their walls.

Empyema (em-pye-**EE**-mah) pus in a body cavity, especially in the pleural cavity (pyothorax); usually the result of a primary infection in the lungs.

Emulsify (eh-**MULL**-sih-figh) to disperse a liquid into another liquid, making a colloidal suspension. Bile is released from the gallbladder into the small intestine in response to the presence of fatty content; its purpose in the digestive process is to emulsify, or break down, the fats into small droplets so the body can use them as nutrients.

Enamel (en-**AM**-el) a hard, white substance that covers the dentin of the crown of a tooth. Enamel is the hardest substance in the body.

Encapsulated (en-**CAP**-soo-**LAY**-ted) enclosed in fibrous or membranous sheaths.

Encephalitis (en-**seff**-ah-**LYE**-tis) the inflammation of the brain largely caused by a virus that enters the CNS when the person experiences a viral disease such as measles or mumps or through the bite of a mosquito or tick.

Endocarditis (**en**-doh-car-**DYE**-tis) inflammation of the membrane lining of the valves and chambers of the heart caused by direct invasion of bacteria or other organisms and leading to deformity of the valve cusps. Abnormal growths called vegetations are formed on or within the membrane.

Endocrine gland (**EN**-doh-krin) a ductless gland that produces a chemical substance called a hormone, which is secreted directly into the bloodstream instead of exiting the body through ducts.

Endocrinologist (**en**-doh-krin-**OL**-oh-jist) a physician who specializes in the medical practice of treating the diseases and disorders of the endocrine system.

Endocrinology (**en**-doh-krin-**OL**-oh-jee) the field of medicine that deals with the study of the endocrine system and of the treatment of the diseases and disorders of the endocrine system.

Endometrial biopsy (en-doh-**MEE**-tree-al **BYE**-op-see) is an invasive test for obtaining a sample of endometrial tissue (with a small curet) for examination.

Endometrial carcinoma (en-doh-**MEE**-tree-al kar-sih-**NOH**-mah) malignant tumor of the inner lining of the uterus; also known as adenocarcinoma of the uterus; and/or cancer of the uterine corpus (body of the uterus).

Endometriosis (en-doh-**mee**-tree-**OH**-sis) the presence and growth of endometrial tissue in areas outside the endometrium (lining of the uterus).

Endometrium (en-doh-**MEE**-tree-um) the inner lining of the uterus.

Endoscopic retrograde cholangiopancreatography (ERCP) (en-doh-**SKOP**-ic **RET**-roh-grayd koh-**lan**-jee-oh-**pan**-kree-ah-**TOG**-rah-fee) a procedure that examines the size of and the filling of the pancreatic and biliary ducts through direct radiographic visualization with a fiberoptic endoscope.

Entropion (en-**TROH**-pee-on) "turning in" of the eyelash margins (especially the lower margins) resulting in the sensation similar to that of a foreign body in the eye (redness, tearing, burning, and itching).

Enzyme (**EN**-zime) an organic substance that initiates and accelerates a chemical reaction.

Enzyme-linked immunosorbent assay (**EN**-zym **LINK'T** im-yoo-noh-**SOR**-bent **ASS**-say) a blood test used for screening for an antibody to the AIDS virus.

Eosinophil (**ee**-oh-**SIN**-oh-fill) a granulocytic, bilobed leukocyte somewhat larger than a neutrophil characterized by large numbers of coarse, refractile, cytoplasmic granules that stain with the acid dye eosin.

Epicardium (ep-ih-**CARD**-ee-um) the inner layer of the pericardium, which is the double-folded membrane that encloses the heart.

Epidermis (ep-ih-**DER**-mis) the outermost layer of the skin.

Epidermoid cyst (ep-ih-**DER**-moid) a cyst filled with a cheesy material composed of sebum and epithelial debris that has formed in the duct of a sebaceous gland; also known as a sebaceous cyst.

Epididymectomy (ep-ih-**did**-ih-**MEK**-toh-mee) surgical removal of the epididymis.

Epididymis (ep-ih-**DID**-ih-mis) a tightly coiled tubule that resembles a comma. Its purpose is that of housing the sperm until they mature, becoming fertile and motile. Mature sperm are stored in the lower portion of the epididymis.

Epididymitis (ep-ih-**did**-ih-**MY**-tis) acute or chronic inflammation of the epididymis. This condition can be the result of a urinary tract infection, prolonged use of indwelling catheters, or venereal disease in the male.

Epidural space (ep-ih-**DOO**-ral space) the space immediately outside the dura mater that contains a supporting cushion of fat and other connective tissues.

Epigastric region (ep-ih-**GAS**-trik **REE**-jun) the region of the abdomen located between the right and left hypochondriac regions in the upper section of the abdomen, beneath the cartilage of the ribs.

Epiglottis (ep-ih-**GLOT**-iss) a thin, leaf-shaped structure located immediately posterior to the root of the tongue; covers the entrance of the larynx when the individual swallows.

Epilepsy (**EP**-ih-**lep**-see) a syndrome of recurring episodes of excessive irregular electrical activity of the brain resulting in involuntary muscle movements called seizures.

Epinephrine (ep-ih-**NEF**-rin) a hormone produced by the adrenal medulla. This hormone plays an important role in the body's response to stress by increasing the heart rate, dilating the bronchioles, and releasing glucose into the bloodstream.

Epiphyseal line (ep-ih-**FIZZ**-ee-al) a layer of cartilage that separates the diaphysis from the epiphysis of a bone; also known as the epiphyseal plate.

Epiphysis (eh-**PIFF**-ih-sis) the end of a bone.

Episcleritis (ep-ih-skleh-**RYE**-tis) inflammation of the outermost layers of the sclera.

Episiotomy (eh-**pis**-ee-**OT**-oh-mee) a surgical procedure in which an incision is made into the woman's perineum to enlarge the vaginal opening for delivery of the baby. This incision is usually made shortly before the baby's birth (second stage of labor) to prevent tearing of the perineum.

Epispadias (ep-ih-**SPAY**-dee-as) a congenital defect (birth defect) in which the urethra opens on the upper side of the penis at some point near the glans.

Epistaxis (ep-ih-**STAKS**-is) hemorrhage from the nose; nosebleed.

Epithelial tissue (ep-ih-**THEE**-lee-al **TISH**-yoo) the tissue that covers the internal and external organs of the body; it also lines the vessels, body cavities, glands, and body organs.

Epithelium (ep-ih-**THEE**-lee-um) the tissue that covers the internal and external surfaces of the body.

Erythema (eh-rih-**THEE**-mah) redness of the skin due to capillary dilation. An example of erythema is nervous blushing or a mild sunburn.

Erythema infectiosum (air-ih-**THEE**-mah in-fek-she-**OH**-sum) a viral disease characterized by a face that appears as "slapped cheeks," a fiery red rash on the cheeks; fifth disease.

Erythremia (er-ih-**THREE**-mee-ah) an abnormal increase in the number of red blood cells; polycythemia vera.

Erythroblast (eh-**RITH**-roh-blast) an immature red blood cell.

Erythroblastosis fetalis (eh-**rith**-roh-blass-**TOH**-sis fee-**TAL**-iss) a form of hemolytic anemia that occurs in neonates due to a maternal–fetal blood group incompatibility involving the ABO grouping or the Rh factors. This is also known as hemolytic disease of the newborn (HDN).

Erythrocyte (eh-**RITH**-roh-sight) a mature red blood cell.

Erythrocyte sedimentation (eh-**RITH**-roh-sight sed-ih-men-**TAY**-shun **RATE**) a test performed on the blood, which measures the rate at which red blood cells settle out in a tube of unclotted blood. The ESR is determined by measuring the settling distance of RBCs in normal saline over one hour.

Erythroderma (eh-**rith**-roh-**DER**-mah) see *erythema*.

Erythropoiesis (eh-**rith**-roh-poy-**EE**-sis) the process of red blood cell production.

Erythropoietin (eh-**rith**-roh-**poy**-**EE**-tin) a hormone synthesized mainly in the kidneys and released into the bloodstream in response to anoxia (lack of oxygen). The hormone acts to stimulate and regulate the production of erythrocytes and is thus able to increase the oxygen-carrying capacity of the blood.

Escharotomy (es-kar-**OT**-oh-mee) an incision made into the necrotic tissue resulting from a severe burn.

Esophageal atresia (ee-**soff**-ah-**JEE**-al ah-**TREE**-zee-ah) a congenital abnormality of the esophagus due to its ending before it reaches the stomach either as a blind pouch or as a fistula connected to the trachea.

Esophagogastroduodenoscopy (EGD) (eh-**soff**-ah-goh-**gass**-troh-**doo**-oh-den-**OSS**-koh-pee) the process of direct visualization of the esophagus, stomach, and duodenum, using a lighted fiberoptic endoscope; also known as an upper endoscopy.

Esophagus (eh-**SOF**-ah-gus) a muscular canal about 9.4 inches long, extending from the pharynx to the stomach.

Esotropia (ess-oh-**TROH**-pee-ah) an obvious inward turning of one eye in relation to the other eye; also called crosseyes.

Estrogen (**ESS**-troh-jen) one of the female hormones that promotes the development of female secondary sex characteristics.

Euphoria (yoo-**FOR**-ee-ah) a sense of well-being or elation.

Euthyroid (yoo-**THIGH**-royd) pertaining to a normally functioning thyroid gland.

Event monitor similar to the Holter monitor in that it also records the electrical activity of the heart while the patient goes about usual daily activities. A cardiac event monitor can be used for a longer period of time than a Holter monitor (usually a month).

Eversion (ee-**VER**-zhun) a turning outward or inside out, such as a turning of the foot outward at the ankle.

Ewing's sarcoma (**YOO**-wings sar-**KOH**-mah) a malignant tumor of the bones common to young adults, particularly adolescent boys.

Exanthematous viral diseases (eks-an-**THEM**-ah-tus **VYE**-ral dih-**ZEEZ**-ez) a skin eruption or rash accompanied by inflammation, having specific diagnostic features of an infectious viral disease.

Excoriation (eks-koh-ree-**AY**-shun) an injury to the surface of the skin caused by trauma, such as scratching or abrasions.

Exercise stress testing a means of assessing cardiac function by subjecting the patient to carefully controlled amounts of physical stress (for example, using the treadmill).

Exfoliation (eks-foh-lee-**AY**-shun) peeling or sloughing off of tissue cells, as in peeling of the skin after a severe sunburn.

Exhibitionism a sexual disorder involving the exposure of one's genitals to a stranger.

Exocrine gland (**EKS**-oh-krin) a gland that opens onto the surface of the skin through ducts in the epithelium, such as an oil gland or a sweat gland.

Exophthalmia (**eck**-sof-**THAL**-mee-ah) an abnormal protrusion of the eyeball(s) typically due to an expanded volume of the orbital contents. The eye(s) appear to bulge forward.

Exophthalmos (**eck**-sof-**THAL**-mohs) see *exophthalmia*.

Exotropia (eks-oh-**TROH**-pee-ah) an obvious outward turning of one eye in relation to the other eye; also called walleye.

Extension (eks-**TEN**-shun) a straightening motion. It increases the angle between two bones.

Extracapsular cataract extract (eks-trah-**KAP**-syoo-lar) surgical removal of the anterior segment of the lens capsule along with the lens, allowing for the insertion of an intraocular lens implant.

Extracorporeal lithotripsy (ex-trah-cor-**POR**-ee-al **LITH**-oh-trip-see) also known as extracorporeal shock-wave lithotripsy. This is a noninvasive mechanical procedure for using sound waves to break up renal calculi so that they can pass through the ureters.

Extracorporeal shock wave lithotripsy (ESWL) (**eks**-trah-kor-**POR**-ee-al shockwave **LITH**-oh-**trip**-see) an alternative treatment for gallstones by using ultrasound to align the computerized lithotripter and source of shock waves with the stones to crush the gallstones and thus enable the contraction of the gallbladder to remove stone fragments.

Extraocular (eks-trah-**OCK**-yoo-lar) pertaining to outside the eye.

Exudate (**EKS**-yoo-dayt) fluid, pus, or serum slowly discharged from cells or blood vessels through small pores or breaks in cell membranes.

F

Factitious disorders characterized by physical or psychological symptoms that are intentionally produced or feigned to assume the sick role.

Fallopian tubes (fah-**LOH**-pee-an **TOOBS**) one of a pair of tubes opening at one end into the uterus and at the other end into the peritoneal cavity, over the ovary.

False ribs rib pairs 8 through 10, which connect to the vertebrae in the back but not to the sternum in the front because they join the seventh rib in the front.

Family therapy a form of psychotherapy that focuses the treatment on the process between family members that supports and sustains symptoms. It is a group therapy with family members composing the group.

Fascia (**FASH**-ee-ah) thin sheets of fibrous connective tissue that penetrate and cover the entire muscle, holding the fibers together.

Fasting blood sugar (FBS) blood glucose sample taken usually early in the morning after the person has been without food or drink since midnight.

Fatigue (**FAH**-teeg) a feeling of tiredness or weariness resulting from continued activity or as a side effect from some psychotropic drug.

Fatty acids any of several organic acids produced by the hydrolysis of neutral fats.

Febrile (**FEE**-brill) pertaining to or characterized by an elevated body temperature, such as a febrile reaction to an infectious agent, alternating with periods of slow growth.

Feces (**FEE**-seez) waste or excrement from the digestive tract that is formed in the intestine and expelled through the rectum.

Fertilization (fer-til-eye-**ZAY**-shun) the union of a male sperm and a female ovum.

Fetal monitoring (electronic) (**FEE**-tal **MON**-ih-tor-ing) the use of an electronic device to monitor the fetal heart rate and the maternal uterine contractions. This procedure can be done with external or internal devices.

Fetoscope (**FEET**-oh-skohp) a special stethoscope for hearing the fetal heartbeat through the mother's abdomen.

Fetus (**FEE**-tus) the name given to the developing baby from approximately the eighth week after conception until birth.

Fever (**FEE**-ver) elevation of temperature above the normal.

Fibrillation (atrial/ventricular) (fih-brill-**AY**-shun) atrial fibrillation is extremely rapid, incomplete contractions of the atria resulting in disorganized and uncoordinated twitching of the atria.

Fibrin (**FYE**-brin) a stringy, insoluble protein that is the substance of a blood clot.

Fibrinogen (fye -**BRIN**-oh-jen) a plasma protein converted into fibrin by thrombin in the presence of calcium ions.

Fibrocystic breast disease (figh-broh-**SIS**-tik) the presence of single or multiple fluid-filled cysts that are palpable in the breasts.

Fibroid tumor (**FIGH**-broyd tumor) a benign, fibrous tumor of the uterus.

Fibrous joint (**FYE**-bruss) in a fibrous joint, the surfaces of the bones fit closely together and are held together by fibrous connective tissue (as in a suture between the skull bones). This is an immovable joint.

Fimbriae (**FIM**-bree-ay) the fringelike end of the fallopian tube.

First dose initial dose.

First-dose effect an undesired effect of a medication that occurs within 30 to 90 minutes after administration of the first dose.

First trimester screening consists of a blood test (maternal serum sample) and an ultrasound to identify pregnancies at risk for birth defects such as Down syndrome and trisomy 18.

First-voided specimen (FIRST-VOYD-ed **SPEH**-sih-men) **(early-morning specimen)** the patient is instructed to collect the first-voided specimen of the morning and to refrigerate it until it can be taken to the medical office or laboratory.

Fissure (**FISH**-ur) a cracklike sore or groove in the skin or mucous membrane.

Fistula (**FISS**-tyoo-lah) an abnormal passageway between two tubular organs (e.g., rectum and vagina) or from an organ to the body surface.

Flaccid (**FLAK**-sid) weak; lacking normal muscle tone.

Flat bones bones that are broad and thin with flat or curved surfaces, such as the sternum.

Flexion (**FLEK**-shun) a bending motion. It decreases the angle between two bones.

Floating ribs rib pairs 11 and 12, which connect to the vertebrae in the back but are free of any attachment in the front.

Floaters one or more spots that appear to drift, or "float," across the visual field.

Fluorescein staining (floo-oh-**RESS**-ee-in) application of a fluorescein-stained sterile filter paper strip moistened with a few drops of sterile saline or sterile anesthetic solution to the lower cul-de-sac of the eye to visualize a corneal abrasion. A corneal abrasion is stained bright green when fluorescein stain is applied.

Fluorescence (floo-**RES**-ens) the emission of light of one wavelength (usually ultraviolet) when exposed to light of a different (usually shorter) wavelength; a property possessed by certain substances.

Fluoroscopy (**floo**-ROSS-koh-pee) a radiological technique used to examine the function of an organ or a body part by using a fluoroscope.

Fontanelle or fontanel (fon-tah-**NELL**) a space covered by tough membrane between the bones of an infant's cranium, called a "soft spot."

Food and Drug Administration the government agency responsible for administering and enforcing the Food, Drug, and Cosmetic Act within the United States.

Food, Drug, and Cosmetic Act a law that regulates the quality, purity, potency, effectiveness, safety, labeling, and packaging of food, drug, and cosmetic products.

Foramen (for-**AY**-men) hole in a bone through which blood vessels or nerves pass.

Foreskin (**FOR**-skin) a loose, retractable fold of skin covering the tip of the penis; also called the prepuce.

Fossa (**FOSS**-ah) hollow or concave depression in a bone.

Fourchette (foor-**SHET**) a tense band of mucous membranes at the posterior rim of the vaginal opening: the point at which the labia minora connect.

Fractionation (frak-shun-**AY**-shun) in radiology, the division of the total dose of radiation into small doses administered at intervals in an effort to minimize tissue damage.

Fracture a broken bone; a sudden breaking of a bone.

Fracture of the hip a break in the continuity of the bone involving the upper third of the femur.

Free association the spontaneous, consciously unrestricted association of ideas, feelings, or mental images.

Friction rub (**FRICK**-shun rub) a dry, grating sound heard with a stethoscope during auscultation.

Frontal plane any of the vertical planes passing through the body from the head to the feet, perpendicular to the sagittal planes and dividing the body into front and back portions.

Frotteurism a sexual disorder in which the person gains sexual stimulation or excitement by rubbing against a nonconsenting person. The sexual arousal is achieved through the act of rubbing or touching, which includes fondling.

FTA-ABS test a serological test for syphilis (performed on blood serum). The acronym stands for fluorescent treponemal antibody-absorption test.

Fulguration (ful-goo-**RAY**-shun) see *electrodesiccation.*

Fundoscopy (fund-**DOSS**-koh-pee) the examination of the fundus of the eye, the base or the deepest part of the eye, with an instrument called an ophthalmoscope through a procedure called ophthalmoscopy.

Fundus (**FUN**-dus) the dome-shaped central, upper portion of the uterus between the points of insertion of the fallopian tubes.

Furuncle (**FYOO**-rung-kul) a localized pus-producing infection originating deep in a hair follicle, characterized by pain, redness, and swelling; also known as a boil.

G

Gait (**GAYT**) the style of walking.

Gallbladder (**GALL**-blad-er) a pear-shaped excretory sac lodged in a fossa on the visceral surface of the right lobe of the liver.

Gallstones (cholelithiasis) (koh-lee-lih-**THIGH**-ah-sis) pigmented or hardened cholesterol stones formed as a result of bile crystallization.

Gamete (**GAM**-eet) a mature sperm or ovum.

Gamma camera (**GAM**-ah **CAM**-er-ah) a device that uses the emission of light from a crystal struck by gamma rays to produce an image of the distribution of radioactive material in a body organ.

Gamma rays (**GAM**-ah) an electromagnetic radiation of short wavelength emitted by the nucleus of an atom during a nuclear reaction. Also called gamma radiation.

Ganglion (**GANG**-lee-on) a knotlike mass of nerve tissue found outside the brain or spinal cord (plural: *ganglia*).

Ganglionectomy (gang-lee-on-**ECK**-toh-mee) surgical removal of a ganglion.

Gangrene (**GANG**-green) tissue death due to the loss of adequate blood supply, invasion of bacteria, and subsequent decay of enzymes (especially proteins) producing an offensive, foul odor.

Gastric analysis (**GAS**-trik analysis) study of the stomach content to determine the acid content and to detect the presence of blood, bacteria, bile, and abnormal cells.

Gastric lavage (**GAS**-trik lavage) the irrigation, or washing out, of the stomach with sterile water or a saline solution.

Gastroenterologist (gas-troh-en-ter-**OL**-oh-jist) a medical doctor who specializes in the study of the diseases and disorders affecting the gastrointestinal tract (including the stomach, intestines, gallbladder, and bile duct).

Gastroesophageal reflux (gas-troh-eh-soff-ah-**JEE**-al **REE**-flucks) a return, or reflux, of gastric juices into the esophagus, resulting in a burning sensation.

Gastrointestinal tract (gas-troh-in-**TESS**-tih-nal **TRAKT**) see *alimentary canal.*

Gavage (gah-**VAZH**) a procedure in which liquid or semiliquid food is introduced into the stomach through a tube.

General to specific activities move from being generalized toward being more focused (general to specific). For example, the child will use the whole hand before picking up a small object between the thumb and forefinger.

Generalized anxiety disorder a disorder characterized by chronic, unrealistic, and excessive anxiety and worry. The symptoms have usually existed for at least six months or more and have no relation to any specific causes.

Generic name (jeh-**NAIR**-ik) the name established when the drug is first manufactured. This name is protected for use by only the original manufacturer for a period of 17 years. After that time, the name of the drug becomes public property and can be used by any manufacturer.

Genes segments of chromosomes that transmit hereditary characteristics.

Genital herpes (**JEN**-ih-tal **HER**-peez) a highly contagious viral infection of the male and female genitalia; also known as venereal herpes. Caused by the herpes simplex virus (usually HSV-2), genital herpes is transmitted by direct contact with infected body secretions (usually through sexual intercourse). Genital herpes differs from other sexually transmitted diseases in that it can recur spontaneously once the virus has been acquired.

Genital warts (**JEN**-ih-tal warts) small, cauliflower-like, fleshy growths usually seen along the penis in the male and in or near the vagina in women. Genital warts are transmitted from person to person through sexual intercourse. They are caused by the human papillomavirus (HPV). The time span from initial contact with the virus to occurrence of symptoms can be from one to six months.

Geriatrician (jer-ee-ah-**TRIH**-shun) a physician who has specialized postgraduate education and experience in the medical care of the older person.

Geriatric nurse practitioner (jer-ee-**AT**-rik) a registered nurse with additional education obtained through a master's degree program that prepares the nurse to deliver primary health care to older adults.

Geriatrics (jer-ee-**AT**-riks) the branch of medicine that deals with the physiological characteristics of aging and the diagnosis and treatment of diseases affecting the aged.

Gerontics pertaining to old age.

Gerontologist one who specializes in the study of gerontology.

Gerontology (**jer**-on-**TOL**-oh-jee) the study of all aspects of the aging process, including the clinical, psychological, economic, and sociologic issues encountered by older persons and their consequences for both the individual and society.

Gerontophobia an abnormal fear of growing old; fear of aging and of old people.

Geropsychiatry the study and treatment of psychiatric aspects of aging and mental disorders of older adults.

Gestation (jess-**TAY**-shun) the term of pregnancy, which equals approximately 280 days from the onset of the last menstrual period. The period of intrauterine development of the fetus from conception through birth; also termed the gestational period.

Gestational hypertension (jess-**TAY**-shun-al **high**-per-**TEN**-shun) a complication of pregnancy in which the expectant mother develops high blood pressure after 20 weeks' gestation, with no signs of proteinuria or edema.

Gigantism (**JYE**-gan-tizm) a proportional overgrowth of the body's tissue due to the hypersecretion of the human growth hormone before puberty.

Gingiva (**JIN**-jih-vah *or* jin-**JYE**-vah) gum tissue (plural: *gingivae*).

Gingivitis (jin-jih-**VIGH**-tis) inflammation of the gums.

Glans penis (**GLANS PEE**-nis) the tip of the penis.

Glaucoma (glau-**KOH**-mah) ocular disorders identified as a group due to the increase in intraocular pressure, causing damage to the optic nerve. This increase in intraocular pressure may be primary or secondary, acute or chronic, and described as open or closed angle.

Globin (**GLOH**-bin) a group of four globulin protein molecules that become bound by the iron in heme molecules to form hemoglobin.

Globulin (**GLOB**-yoo-lin) a plasma protein made in the liver. Globulin helps in the synthesis of antibodies.

Glomerular filtrate (glom-**AIR**-yoo-lar **FILL**-trayt) substances that filter out of the blood through the thin walls of the glomeruli (e.g., water, sugar, salts, and nitrogenous waste products such as urea, creatinine, and uric acid).

Glomerulonephritis (acute) (gloh-**mair**-yoo-loh-neh-**FRYE**-tis) an inflammation of the glomerulus of the kidneys.

Glomerulus (glom-**AIR**-yoo-lus) a ball-shaped collection of very tiny coiled and intertwined capillaries, located in the cortex of the kidney.

Glottis (**GLOT**-iss) the sound-producing apparatus of the larynx consisting of the two vocal folds and the intervening space (the epiglottis protects this opening).

Glucagon (**GLOO**-kah-gon) a hormone produced by the alpha cells of the pancreas that stimulates the liver to convert glycogen into glucose when the blood sugar level is dangerously low.

Glucogenesis (gloo-koh-**JEN**-eh-sis) the formation of glycogen from fatty acids and proteins instead of from carbohydrates.

Glucose (**GLOO**-kohs) the simplest form of sugar in the body; a simple sugar found in certain foods, especially fruits; also a major source of energy for the human body.

Glucose tolerance test (GTT) (**GLOO**-kohs **TOL**-er-ans) a test that evaluates the person's ability to tolerate a concentrated oral glucose load by measuring the glucose levels.

Glycogen (**GLIGH**-koh-jen) the form of sugar stored in body cells, primarily the liver.

Glycogenesis (gligh-koh-**JEN**-eh-sis) the conversion of simple sugar (glucose) into a complex form of sugar (starch) for storage in the liver.

Glycogenolysis (gligh-koh-jen-**OL**-ih-sis) the breakdown of glycogen into glucose by the liver, releasing it back into the circulating blood in response to a very low blood sugar level.

Glycosuria (glye-kohs-**YOO**-ree-ah) the presence of sugar in the urine.

Goiter (**GOY**-ter) enlargement of the thyroid gland due to excessive growth (hyperplasia).

Gonads (**GOH**-nadz) a gamete-producing gland such as an ovary or a testis.

Gonioscopy (gah-nee-**OSS**-kah-pee) the process of viewing the anterior chamber angle of the eye for evaluation, management, and classification of normal and abnormal angle structures. The examination involves using a gonioprism (mirrored contact lens) and a slit-lamp biomicroscope to observe the anterior chamber of the eye (area between the cornea and the iris). This painless examination is used to determine whether the drainage angle of the eye (area where the fluid drains out of the eye) is open or closed.

Gonorrhea (**gon**-oh-**REE**-ah) a sexually transmitted bacterial infection of the mucous membrane of the genital tract in men and women. It is spread by sexual intercourse with an infected partner and can also be passed on from an infected mother to her infant during the birth process (as the baby passes through the vaginal canal). *Neisseria gonorrhoeae* is the causative organism.

Goodell's sign the softening of the uterine cervix, a probable sign of pregnancy.

Gout (**GOWT**) a metabolic disease in which uric acid crystals are deposited in joints or other tissues. It is most often characterized by inflammation of the first metatarsal joint of the great toe. It may also be found in the hands and in the spine.

Graafian follicles (**GRAF**-ee-an **FOL**-ih-kuls) a mature, fully developed ovarian cyst containing the ripe ovum.

Grand mal seizure (grand **MALL SEE**-zyoor) an epileptic seizure characterized by a sudden loss of consciousness and by generalized involuntary muscular contraction, vacillating between rigid body extension and an alternating contracting and relaxing of muscles.

Granulocyte (**GRAN**-yoo-loh-sight) a type of leukocyte characterized by the presence of cytoplasmic granules.

Granulocytosis (**gran**-yoo-loh-sigh-**TOH**-sis) an abnormally elevated number of granulocytes in the circulating blood as a reaction to any variety of inflammation or infection.

Graves' disease (hyperthyroidism) (high-per-**THIGH**-royd-izm) hypertrophy of the thyroid gland resulting in an excessive secretion of the thyroid hormone that causes an extremely high body metabolism, thus creating multisystem changes.

Gravida a woman who is pregnant. She may be identified as gravida I if this is her first pregnancy, gravida II for a second pregnancy, and so on.

Gray matter the part of the nervous system consisting of axons that are not covered with myelin sheath, giving a gray appearance.

Group therapy application of psychotherapeutic techniques within a small group of people who experience similar difficulties; also known as encounter groups.

Growth an increase in the whole or any of its parts physically.

Grunting (**GRUNT**-ing) abnormal, short, audible, deep, hoarse sounds in exhalation that often accompany severe chest pain.

Guillain-Barré syndrome (**GHEE**-yon bah-**RAY SIN**-drohm) acute polyneuritis ("inflammation of many nerves") of the PNS in which the myelin sheaths on the axons are destroyed, resulting in decreased nerve impulses, loss of reflex response, and sudden muscle weakness, which usually follows a viral gastrointestinal or respiratory infection.

Gynecologist (gigh-neh-**KOL**-oh-jist) a physician who specializes in the medical specialty that deals with diseases and disorders of the female reproductive system.

Gynecology (gigh-neh-**KOL**-oh-jee) the branch of medicine that deals with the study of diseases and disorders of the female reproductive system.

H

Hair follicle (**FOL**-ih-kul) the tiny tube within the dermis that contains the root of a hair shaft.

Hair root the portion of a strand of hair that is embedded in the hair follicle.

Hair shaft the visible part of the hair.

Half-life the time required for a radioactive substance to lose 50% of its activity through decay.

Hallucination (hah-**loo**-sih-**NAY**-shun) a subjective (existing in the mind) perception of something that does not exist in the external environment. Hallucinations may be visual, olfactory (smell), gustatory (taste), tactile (touch), or auditory (hearing).

Hallucinogens (hah-**LOO**-sih-noh-jens) substances that cause excitation of the central nervous system, characterized by symptoms such as hallucinations, mood changes, anxiety, increased pulse and blood pressure, and dilation of the pupils.

Haversian canals (ha-**VER**-shan) system of small canals within compact bone that contain blood vessels, lymphatic vessels, and nerves.

Headache (cephalalgia) (**seff**-ah-**LAL**-jee-ah) cephalalgia involves pain (varying in intensity from mild to severe) anywhere within the cranial cavity. It may be chronic or acute and may occur as a result of a disease process or be totally benign. The majority of headaches are transient and produce mild pain relieved by a mild analgesic.

Head circumference (**HEAD** sir-**KUM**-fer-ens) the measurement around the greatest circumference of the head of an infant. This measurement is plotted according to normal growth and development patterns for the infant's head. Increased lags or surges in the increase of the head circumference may indicate serious problems.

Hearing aids devices that amplify sound to provide more precise perception and interpretation of words communicated to the individual with a hearing deficit. They may be analog (makes continuous sound waves louder) or digital (amplifies the sound, but also filters out unwanted sounds like feedback and background noise).

Heart block (AV) an interference with the normal conduction of electric impulses that control activity of the heart muscle.

Heartburn, pregnancy related also known as pyrosis. This discomfort occurs mainly in the last few weeks of pregnancy due to the pressure exerted on the esophagus by the enlarged, pregnant uterus. This pressure may also cause a return, or reflux, of gastric juices into the esophagus, resulting in a burning sensation, a condition known as gastroesophageal reflux.

Heel puncture a method of obtaining a blood sample from a newborn or premature infant by making a shallow puncture of the lateral or medial area of the plantar (sole of the foot) surface of the heel; also called a "heel stick."

Hegar's sign (**HAY**-garz sign) softening of the lower segment of the uterus; a probable sign of pregnancy.

HELLP syndrome the acronym *HELLP* stands for **H** (hemolysis: breaking down of red blood cells), **EL** (elevated liver enzymes), and **LP** (low platelet count); a serious obstetrical complication that occurs in approximately 10% of pregnant women with preeclampsia or eclampsia.

Hemangioma (hee-**man**-jee-**OH**-mah) a benign (nonmalignant) tumor that consists of a mass of blood vessels and has a reddish-purple color.

Hematemesis (he-mah-**TEM**-eh-sis) vomiting of blood.

Hematocrit (hee-**MAT**-oh-krit) an assessment of RBC percentage in the total blood volume.

Hematologist (hee-mah-**TOL**-oh-jist) a medical specialist in the field of hematology.

Hematology (hee-mah-**TOL**-oh-jee) the scientific study of blood and blood-forming tissues.

Hematoma, epidural (hee-mah-**TOH**-mah) a collection of blood (hematoma) located above the dura mater and just below the skull.

Hematoma, subdural (hee-mah-**TOH**-mah, **SUB**-doo-ral) a collection of blood below the dura mater and above the arachnoid layer of the meninges.

Hematopoiesis (hem-ah-toh-poy-**EE**-sis) the normal formation and development of blood cells in the bone.

Heme (**HEEM**) the pigmented, iron-containing, nonprotein portion of the hemoglobin molecule. Heme binds and carries oxygen in the red blood cells, releasing it to tissues that give off excess amounts of carbon dioxide.

Hemianopsia (**hem**-ee-ah-**NOP**-see-ah) loss of vision, or blindness, in one-half of the visual field; also known as *hemianopia*.

Hemochromatosis (**hee**-moh-**kroh**-mah-**TOH**-sis) a rare iron metabolism disease characterized by iron deposits throughout the body, usually as a complication of one of the hemolytic anemias.

Hemoglobin (**hee**-moh-**GLOH**-bin) a complex protein–iron compound in the blood that carries oxygen to the cells from the lungs and carbon dioxide away from the cells to the lungs.

Hemoglobin A1c test (**HbA1c**) a blood test that shows the average level of glucose in an individual's blood during the past 3 months. A small sample of blood is collected from a vein (usually an arm vein) and is sent to the lab for analysis.

Hemoglobin test (**hee**-moh-**GLOH**-bin) concentration measurement of the hemoglobin in the peripheral blood. As a vehicle for transport of oxygen and carbon dioxide, hemoglobin levels provide information about the body's ability to supply tissues with oxygen.

Hemolysis (**hee**-**MOL**-ih-sis) the breakdown of red blood cells and the release of hemoglobin that occurs normally at the end of the life span of a red cell.

Hemophilia (**hee**-moh-**FILL**-ee-ah) involves different hereditary inadequacies of coagulation factors resulting in prolonged bleeding times.

Hemorrhage (**HEM**-eh-rij) a loss of a large amount of blood in a short period of time, either externally or internally. Hemorrhage may be arterial, venous, or capillary.

Hemorrhoids, pregnancy related swollen veins of the rectum and anus that develop as a result of the increasing pressure on the area due to the progressing pregnancy. They usually disappear after delivery but can cause discomfort in the pregnant female.

Hemostasis (**hee**-moh-**STAY**-sis) the termination of bleeding by mechanical or chemical means or by the complex coagulation process of the body, consisting of vasoconstriction, platelet aggregation, and thrombin and fibrin synthesis.

Heparin (**HEP**-er-in) a natural anticoagulant substance produced by the body tissues; heparin is also produced in laboratories for therapeutic use as heparin sodium.

Hepatitis (**hep**-ah-**TYE**-tis) acute or chronic inflammation of the liver due to a viral or bacterial infection, drugs, alcohol, toxins, or parasites.

Hepatocyte (**HEP**-ah-toh-sight) liver cell.

Hepatomegaly (**heh**-pat-oh-**MEG**-ah-lee) enlargement of the liver.

Hernia (**HER**-nee-ah) an irregular protrusion of tissue, organ, or a portion of an organ through an abnormal break in the surrounding cavity's muscular wall.

Herniated disk (**HER**-nee-ay-ted **DISK**) a rupture or herniation of the disk center (nucleus pulposus) through the disk wall and into the spinal canal, causing pressure on the spinal cord or nerve roots.

Herniorrhaphy (her-nee-**OR**-ah-fee) the surgical repair of a hernia by closing the defect, using sutures, mesh, or wire.

Herpes zoster (shingles) (**HER**-peez **ZOS**-ter) an acute viral infection characterized by painful vesicular eruptions on the skin following along the nerve pathways of underlying spinal or cranial nerves.

Herpetic stomatitis (her-**PEH**-tic stoh-mah-**TYE**-tis) inflammatory infectious lesions in or on the oral cavity occurring as a primary or a secondary viral infection caused by herpes simplex.

Hilum (**HIGH**-lum) the depression, or pit, of an organ where the vessels and nerves enter.

Hinge joint (**HINJ** joint) allows movement in one direction—a back-and-forth type of motion. An example of a hinge joint is the elbow.

Hirschsprung's disease (congenital megacolon) (**HIRSH**-sprungz dih-**ZEEZ**) (kon-**JEN**-ih-tal meg-ah-**KOH**-lon) absence at birth of the autonomic ganglia in a segment of the intestinal smooth muscle wall that normally stimulates peristalsis.

Hirsutism (**HER**-soot-izm) excessive body hair in an adult male distribution pattern, occurring in women.

Histamine (**HISS**-tah-min) or (**HISS**-tah-meen) a substance (found in all cells) that is released in allergic inflammatory reactions.

Histiocyte (**HISS**-tee-oh-sight) macrophage; a large phagocytic cell (cell that ingests microorganisms, other cells, and foreign particles) occurring in the walls of blood vessels and loose connective tissue.

Histologist (hiss-**TOL**-oh-jist) a medical scientist who specializes in the study of tissues.

Hives circumscribed, slightly elevated lesions of the skin that are paler in the center than its surrounding edges. See also *wheal*.

Holter monitoring a small, portable monitoring device that makes prolonged electrocardiograph recordings on a portable tape recorder. The continuous EKG (ambulatory EKG) is recorded on a magnetic tape recording while the patient conducts normal daily activities.

Homan's sign pain felt in the calf of the leg, or behind the knee, when the examiner is purposely dorsiflexing the foot of the patient (bending the toes upward toward the foot). If the patient feels pain, it is called a positive Homan's sign (indicating thrombophlebitis).

Hordeolum (stye) (hor-**DEE**-oh-lum) bacterial infection of an eyelash follicle or sebaceous gland originating with redness, swelling, and mild tenderness in the margin of the eyelash.

Hospital Formulary (**FORM**-yoo-lair-ee) a reference book that lists all of the drugs commonly stocked in the hospital pharmacy. This book provides information about the characteristics of drugs and their clinical usage.

Huntington's chorea (**HUNT**-ing-tonz koh-**REE**-ah) an inherited neurological disease characterized by rapid, jerky, involuntary movements and increasing dementia due to the effects of the basal ganglia on the neurons.

Hyaline membrane disease (**HIGH**-ah-lighn membrane dih-**ZEEZ**) also known as respiratory distress syndrome (RDS) of the premature infant, hyaline membrane disease is severe impairment of the function of respiration in the premature newborn. This condition is rarely present in a newborn of greater than 37 weeks' gestation or in one weighing at least 5 pounds.

Hydatidiform mole (high-dah-**TID**-ih-form **MOHL**) an abnormal condition that begins as a pregnancy and deviates from normal development very early. The diseased ovum deteriorates (not producing a fetus) and the chorionic villi of the placenta (small vessels protruding from the outer layer) change to a mass of cysts resembling a bunch of grapes.

Hydrocele (**HIGH**-droh-seel) a collection of fluid located in the area of the scrotal sac in the male.

Hydrocephalus (**high**-droh-**SEFF**-ah-lus) an abnormal increase of cerebrospinal fluid in the brain that causes the ventricles of the brain to dilate, resulting in an increased head circumference in the infant with open fontanel(s); a congenital disorder.

Hydrochloric acid (**high**-droh-**KLOH**-rik acid) a compound consisting of hydrogen and chlorine.

Hydronephrosis (high-droh-neh-**FROH**-sis) distension of the pelvis and calyces of the kidney caused by urine that cannot flow past an obstruction in a ureter.

Hydrostatic pressure pressure exerted by a liquid.

Hydroureter (**high**-droh-yoo-**REE**-ter) the distension of the ureter with urine due to blockage from an obstruction.

Hymen (**HIGH**-men) a thin layer of elastic, connective tissue membrane that forms a border around the outer opening of the vagina and may partially cover the vaginal opening.

Hyperalbuminemia (high-per-al-**byoo**-mih-**NEE**-mee-ah) an increased level of albumin in the blood.

Hyperbilirubinemia (high-per-**bill**-ih-roobin-**EE**-mee-ah) greater than normal amounts of the bile pigment, bilirubin, in the blood.

Hypercalcemia (high-per-kal-**SEE**-mee-ah) elevated blood calcium level.

Hyperemesis gravidarum (high-per-**EM**-eh-sis grav-ih-**DAR**-um) an abnormal condition of pregnancy characterized by severe vomiting that results in maternal dehydration and weight loss.

Hyperglycemia (high-per-glye-**SEE**-mee-ah) elevated blood sugar level.

Hypergonadism (high-per-**GOH**-nad-izm) excessive activity of the ovaries or testes.

Hyperinsulinism (high-per-**IN**-soo-lin-izm) an excessive amount of insulin in the body.

Hyperkalemia (high-per-kal-**EE**-mee-ah) an elevated blood potassium level.

Hyperkeratosis (**high**-per-**kair**-ah-**TOH**-sis) an overgrowth of the horny layer of the epidermis.

Hyperlipemia (**high**-per-lip-**EE**-mee-ah) an excessive level of blood fats, usually caused by a lipoprotein lipase deficiency or a defect in the conversion of low-density lipoproteins to high-density lipoproteins; also called hyperlipidemia.

Hyperlipidemia (**high**-per-lip-ih-**DEE**-mee-ah) an excessive level of fats in the blood.

Hypernatremia (high-per-nah-**TREE**-mee-ah) an elevated blood sodium level.

Hyperopia (high-per-**OH**-pee-ah) a refractive error in which the lens of the eye cannot focus on an image accurately, resulting in impaired close vision that is blurred due to the light rays being focused behind the retina because the eyeball is shorter than normal.

Hyperparathyroidism (hypercalcemia) (**high**-per-pair-ah-**THIGH**-royd-izm) (high-per-kal-**SEE**-mee-ah) overactivity of any one of the parathyroid glands, which leads to high levels of calcium in the blood and low levels of calcium in the bones.

Hyperpigmentation (**high**-per-**pig**-men-**TAY**-shun) an increase in the pigmentation of the skin.

Hyperpituitarism (high-per-pih-**TOO**-ih-tair-izm) overactivity of the anterior lobe of the pituitary gland.

Hyperplasia (**high**-per-**PLAY**-zee-ah) an increase in the number of cells of a body part.

Hypersensitivity (**high**-per-**sens**-sih-**TIV**-ih-tee) tissue damage resulting from exaggerated immune responses.

Hypersplenism (**high**-per-**SPLEN**-izm) a syndrome involving a deficiency of one or more types of blood cells and an enlarged spleen.

Hypertension (**high**-per-**TEN**-shun) elevated blood pressure persistently higher than 140/90 mmHg; high blood pressure; also known as arterial hypertension.

Hypertensive heart disease (high-per-**TEN**-siv heart dih-**ZEEZ**) a result of long-term hypertension. The heart is affected because it must work against increased resistance due to increased pressure in the arteries.

Hyperthyroidism (high-per-**THIGH**-roy-dizm) overactivity of the thyroid gland; also called Graves' disease.

Hyphema (hyphemia) (high-**FEE**-mah) a bleed into the anterior chamber of the eye, resulting from a postoperative complication or from a blunt eye injury.

Hypnosis a passive, trancelike state of existence that resembles normal sleep, during which perception and memory are altered, resulting in increased responsiveness to suggestion.

Hypocalcemia (high-poh-kal-**SEE**-mee-ah) less than normal blood calcium level.

Hypochondriac region (**high**-poh-**KON**-dree-ak **REE**-jun) the right and left regions of the upper abdomen, beneath the cartilage of the lower ribs; located on either side of the epigastric region.

Hypochondriasis (**high**-poh-kon-**DRY**-ah-sis) a chronic, abnormal concern about the health of the body, characterized by extreme anxiety, depression, and an unrealistic interpretation of real or imagined physical symptoms as indications of a serious illness or disease despite rational medical evidence that no disorder is present.

Hypogastric region (**high**-poh-**GAS**-trik **REE**-jun) the middle section of the lower abdomen, beneath the umbilical region.

Hypoglycemia (high-poh-glye-**SEE**-mee-ah) less than normal blood sugar level.

Hypokalemia (high-poh-kal-**EE**-mee-ah) less than normal blood potassium level.

Hypomania (high-poh-**MAY**-nee-ah) a mild degree of mania characterized by optimism, excitability, energetic and productive behavior, marked hyperactivity and talkativeness, heightened sexual interest, quickness to anger, irritability, and a decreased need for sleep.

Hyponatremia (high-poh-nah-**TREE**-mee-ah) less than normal blood sodium level.

Hypoparathyroidism (**high**-poh-pair-ah-**THIGH**-royd-izm) decreased production of parathyroid hormone, resulting in hypocalcemia, characterized by nerve and muscle weakness with muscle spasms or tetany (a state of continual contraction of the muscles).

Hypophysectomy (high-poff-ih-**SEK**-toh-mee) surgical removal of the pituitary gland.

Hypopigmentation (**high**-poh-pig-min-**TAY**-shun) unusual lack of skin color.

Hypopituitarism (**high**-poh-pih-**TOO**-ih-tah-rizm) a complex syndrome resulting from the absence or deficiency of the pituitary hormone(s).

Hypoplasia (**high**-poh-**PLAY**-zee-ah) incomplete or underdeveloped organ or tissue, usually the result of a decrease in the number of cells.

Hypospadias (high-poh-**SPAY**-dee-as) a congenital defect in which the urethra opens on the underside of the penis instead of at the end.

Hypotension (**high**-poh-**TEN**-shun) low blood pressure; less than normal blood pressure reading.

Hypothyroidism (high-poh-**THIGH**-royd-izm) a condition in which there is a shortage of thyroid hormone, causing an extremely low body metabolism due to a reduced usage of oxygen; also called myxedema in the most severe form.

Hypovolemic shock (**high**-poh-voh-**LEE**-mik) a state of extreme physical collapse and exhaustion due to massive blood loss; "less than normal" blood volume.

Hypoxemia (high-pox-**EE**-mee-ah) insufficient oxygenation of arterial blood.

Hysterosalpingography (**hiss**-ter-oh-**sal**-pin-**GOG**-rah-fee) X-ray of the uterus and the fallopian tubes by injecting a contrast material into these structures.

I

Ichthyosis (ik-thee-**OH**-sis) an inherited dermatological condition in which the skin is dry, hyperkeratotic (hardened) and fissured—resembling fish scales.

Idiosyncrasy (id-ee-oh-**SIN**-krah-see) an unusual, inappropriate response to a drug or to the usual effective dose of a drug. This reaction can be life threatening.

Ileum (**ILL**-ee-um) the distal portion of the small intestine extending from the jejunum to the cecum.

Ileus (**ILL**-ee-us) a term used to describe an obstruction of the intestine.

Immune reaction (immune response) (im-**YOON**) a defense function of the body that produces antibodies to destroy invading antigens and malignancies.

Immunity (im-**YOO**-nih-tee) the state of being resistant to or protected from a disease.

Immunization (im-yoo-nigh-**ZAY**-shun) the process of creating immunity to a specific disease.

Immunologist (**im**-yoo-**NOL**-oh-jist) the health specialist whose training and experience is concentrated in immunology.

Immunology (**im**-yoo-**NOL**-oh-jee) the study of the reaction of tissues of the immune system of the body to antigenic stimulation.

Immunotherapy (**im**-yoo-noh-**THAIR**-ah-pee) a special treatment of allergic responses that administers increasingly large doses of the offending allergens to gradually develop immunity.

Impacted cerumen (seh-**ROO**-men) an excessive accumulation of the waxlike secretions from the glands of the external ear canal.

Impetigo (im-peh-**TYE**-goh *or* im-peh-**TEE**-goh) contagious superficial skin infection characterized by serous vesicles and pustules filled with millions of staphylococcus or streptococcus bacteria, usually forming on the face.

Implantable cardioverter defibrillator (ICD) a small, lightweight, electronic device placed under the skin or muscle in either the chest or abdomen to monitor the heart's rhythm. If an abnormal rhythm occurs, the ICD helps return the heart to its normal rhythm.

Impotence (**IM**-poh-tens) the inability of a male to achieve or sustain an erection of the penis.

Incisor (in-**SIGH**-zor) one of the eight front teeth, four in each dental arch, that first appear as primary teeth during infancy are replaced by permanent incisors during childhood and last until old age.

Incompetent cervix (in-**COMP**-eh-tent **SER**-viks) a condition in which the cervical os (opening) dilates before the fetus reaches term, without labor or uterine contractions; usually occurring during the second trimester of pregnancy and resulting in a spontaneous abortion of the fetus.

Infant (**IN**-fant) a child who is in the earliest stage of extrauterine life, a time extending from the first month after birth to approximately 12 months of age, when the baby is able to assume an erect posture. Some extend the period to 24 months of age.

Infarction (in-**FARC**-shun) a localized area of necrosis (death) in tissue, a vessel, an organ, or a part resulting from lack of oxygen (anoxia) due to interrupted blood flow to the area.

Inferior below or downward toward the tail or feet.

Infiltrative (**in**-fill-**TRAY**-tiv) possessing the ability to invade or penetrate adjacent tissue.

Influenza (in-floo-**EN**-zah) a highly contagious viral infection of the respiratory tract transmitted by airborne droplet infection; also known as the flu. Influenza can occur in isolated cases or can be epidemic. The incubation period is usually one to three days after exposure. Older adults may be more prone to developing bacterial influenza, as are those individuals who have chronic pulmonary disease.

Inguinal hernia (**ING**-gwih-nal **HER**-nee-ah) a protrusion of a part of the intestine through a weakened spot in the muscles and membranes of the inguinal region of the abdomen. The intestine pushes into and sometimes fills the entire scrotal sac in the male.

Inguinal region (**ING**-gwih-nal **REE**-jun) the right and left regions of the lower section of the abdomen; also called the iliac region.

Inhalation medication (in-hah-**LAY**-shun) medication is sprayed or breathed into the nose, throat, and lungs. It is absorbed into the mucous membrane lining of the nose and throat and by the alveoli of the lungs.

Initial dose the first dose of a medication.

Insertion (in-**SIR**-shun) the point of attachment of a muscle to a bone it moves.

Inspection (in-**SPEK**-shun) visual examination of the external surface of the body as well as of its movements and posture.

Insulin (**IN**-soo-lin) a naturally occurring hormone secreted by the beta cells of the islets of Langerhans in the pancreas in response to increased levels of glucose in the blood.

Insulin shock (**IN**-soo-lin) a state of shock due to extremely low blood sugar level caused by an overdose of insulin, a decreased intake of food, or excessive exercise by a patient who is diabetic and insulin dependent. Severe hypoglycemia is a medical emergency.

Integument (in-**TEG**-yoo-ment) the skin. See also *cutaneous membrane.*

Integumentary system (in-**teg**-yoo-**MEN**-tah-ree **SIS**-tem) the body system consisting of the skin, hair, nails, sweat glands, and sebaceous glands.

Intercostal spaces (in-ter-**COS**-tal) spaces between the ribs.

Internal fixation devices the treatment of choice for a fractured hip is usually surgery. Devices such as screws, pins, wires, and nails may be used to internally maintain the bone alignment while healing takes place. These internal fixation devices are more commonly used with fractures of the femur and fractures of joints.

Interstitial therapy (in-ter-**STISH**-al therapy) radiotherapy in which needles or wires that contain radioactive material are implanted directly into tumor areas.

Intervertebral disc (in-ter-**VER**-teh-bral disk) a flat, circular, platelike structure of cartilage that serves as a cushion (or shock absorber) between the vertebrae.

Intestinal obstruction (in-**TESS**-tin-al ob-**STRUCK**-shun) complete or partial alteration in the forward flow of the content in the small or large intestines.

Intoxication (in-**toks**-ih-**KAY**-shun) a state of being characterized by impaired judgment, slurred speech, loss of coordination, irritability, and mood changes; may be due to drugs, including alcohol.

Intracranial tumors (in-trah-**KRAY**-nee-al **TOO**-morz) occur in any structural region of the brain. They may be malignant or benign, classified as primary or secondary, and are named according to the tissue from which they originate.

Intradermal medication (**in**-trah-**DER**-mal) medication inserted just beneath the epidermis, using a syringe and needle.

Intramuscular medication (in-trah-**MUSS**-kyoo-lar) medication injected directly into the muscle.

Intraocular lens implant an intraocular lens implant is the surgical process of cataract extraction and the insertion of an artificial lens in the patient's eye. This restores visual acuity and provides improved depth perception, light refraction, and binocular vision.

Intrauterine device (in-trah-**YOO**-ter-in) a small, plastic T-shaped object with strings attached to the leg of the T. It is inserted into the uterus, through the vagina, and remains in place in the uterus.

Intravenous medication (in-trah-**VEE**-nus) medication injected directly into the vein, entering the bloodstream immediately.

Intravenous pyelogram (IVP) (in-trah-**VEE**-nuss **PYE**-el-oh-gram) also known as intravenous pyelography or excretory urogram, this radiographic procedure provides visualization of the entire urinary tract (kidneys, ureters, bladder, and urethra). A contrast dye is injected intravenously, and multiple X-ray films are taken as the medium is cleared from the blood by the glomerular filtration of the kidney.

Introjection (in-troh-**JEK**-shun) an ego defense mechanism whereby an individual unconsciously identifies with another person or with some object. The individual assumes the supposed feelings and/or characteristics of the other personality or object.

Intussusception (in-tuh-suh-**SEP**-shun) telescoping of a portion of proximal intestine into distal intestine, usually in the ileocecal region (causing an obstruction).

Inversion (in-**VER**-zhun) an abnormal condition in which an organ is turned inside out, such as a uterine inversion; also refers to turning inward, as in inversion of the ankle.

Involuntary muscles muscles that act without conscious control. They are controlled by the autonomic nervous system and hormones.

Ion (**EYE**-on) an electrically charged particle.

Ionization (**eye**-oh-nye-**ZAY**-shun) process in which a neutral atom or molecule gains or loses electrons and thus acquires a negative or positive electric charge.

Iridectomy (ir-id-**EK**-toh-mee) extraction of a small segment of the iris to open an anterior chamber angle and permit the flow of aqueous humor between the anterior and posterior chambers, thus relieving the person's intraocular pressure.

Iridocyclitis (ir-id-oh-sigh-**KLEYE**-tis) inflammation of the iris and ciliary body of the eye.

Iritis (ih-**RYE**-tis) inflammation of the iris.

Irradiation (ih-**ray**-dee-**AY**-shun) exposure to any form of radiant energy (such as heat, light, or X-ray).

Irritable bowel syndrome (IBS) (**EAR**-it-ah-bul **BOW**-el **SIN**-drom) increased motility of the small or large intestinal wall, resulting in spastic colon, abdominal pain, flatulence, nausea, anorexia, and the trapping of gas throughout the intestines.

Ischemia (iss-**KEY**-mee-ah) decreased supply of oxygenated blood to a body part or organ.

J

Jejunum (jee-**JOO**-num) the intermediate or middle of the three portions of the small intestine, connecting proximally with the duodenum and distally with the ileum.

Joint cavity the space between two connecting bones.

K

Kaposi's sarcoma (**CAP**-oh-seez sar-**KOH**-mah) a locally destructive malignant neoplasm of the blood vessels associated with AIDS, typically forming lesions on the skin, visceral organs, or mucous membranes. These lesions appear initially as tiny red to purple macules and evolve into sizable nodules or plaques.

Keloid (**KEE**-loyd) an enlarged, irregularly shaped, and elevated scar that forms due to the presence of large amounts of collagen during the formation of the scar.

Keratin (**KAIR**-ah-tin) a hard fibrous protein found in the epidermis, hair, nails, enamel of the teeth, and horns of animals.

Keratitis (kair-ah-**TYE**-tis) corneal inflammation caused by a microorganism, trauma to the eye, a break in the sensory innervation of the cornea, a hypersensitivity reaction, or a tearing defect (may be due to dry eyes or ineffective eyelid closure).

Keratoconjunctivitis (kair-ah-toh-kon-junk-tih-**VYE**-tis) inflammation of the cornea and the conjunctiva of the eye.

Keratoconus (kair-ah-toh-**KOH**-nus) a cone-shaped protrusion (bulging) of the center of the cornea, not accompanied by

inflammation, usually associated with thinning of the cornea. The bulging results in distored vision.

Keratolytic (**KAIR**-ah-toh-**LIT**-ic) an agent used to break down or loosen the horny (hardened) layer of the skin.

Keratomycosis (kair-ah-toh-my-**KOH**-sis) a fungal growth present on the cornea.

Keratoplasty (**KAIR**-ah-toh-**plass**-tee) the transplantation of corneal tissue from one human eye to another to improve vision in the affected eye; also called corneal grafting.

Keratosis (kerr-ah-**TOH**-sis) skin condition in which there is a thickening and overgrowth of the cornified epithelium.

Ketones (**KEE**-tohnz) substances that increase in the blood as a result of incomplete fat metabolism. Fats are broken down for energy when the body is unable to use carbohydrates for energy, and the result is a buildup of ketone bodies in the blood and the urine.

Kidney transplantation (kidney tranz-plan-**TAY**-shun) involves the surgical implantation of a healthy human donor kidney into the body of a patient with irreversible renal failure. Kidney function is restored with a successful transplant, and the patient no longer depends on dialysis.

KUB (kidneys, ureters, bladder) an X-ray of the lower abdomen that defines the size, shape, and location of the kidneys, ureters, and bladder. A contrast medium is not used with this X-ray.

Kyphosis (kye-**FOH**-sis) humpback.

L

Labia majora (**LAY**-bee-ah mah-**JOR**-ah) two folds of skin containing fatty tissue and covered with hair that lie on either side of the vaginal opening, extending from the mons pubis to the perineum. The outer surface of the labia majora is covered by pubic hair; the inner surface is smooth and moist.

Labia minora (**LAY**-bee-ah mih-**NOR**-ah) two folds of hairless skin located within the folds of the labia majora. The labia minora extend from the clitoris downward toward the perineum.

Labor (**LAY**-bor) the time and the processes that occur during birth, from the beginning of cervical dilation to the delivery of the placenta.

Labyrinthitis (lab-ih-rin-**THIGH**-tis) infection or inflammation of the labyrinth or the inner ear—specifically, the three semicircular canals in the inner ear, which are fluid-filled chambers and control balance.

Laceration (lass-er-**AY**-shun) a tear in the skin; a torn, jagged wound.

Lacrimal (**LAK**-rim-al) pertaining to tears.

Lacrimation (lak-rih-**MAY**-shun) the secretion of tears from the lacrimal glands.

Lactation (lak-**TAY**-shun) the production and secretion of milk from the female breasts as nourishment for the infant.

Lactation can be referred to as a process or as a period of time during which the female is breastfeeding.

Lactiferous ducts (lak-**TIF**-er-us ducts) channels or narrow tubular structures that carry milk from the lobes of each breast to the nipple.

Laminectomy (**lam**-ih-**NEK**-toh-mee) the surgical removal of the bony arches from one or more vertebrae to relieve pressure on the spinal cord.

Lanugo (lan-**NOO**-go) soft, very fine hair that covers the body of the developing fetus; this hairy coating is almost completely gone by birth.

Laparoscope (**LAP**-ah-rah-scope) a thin-walled, flexible tube with a telescopic lens and light that is inserted through an incision in the abdominal wall to examine or perform minor surgery within the abdominal or pelvic cavities.

Laparoscopy (lap-ar-**OS**-koh-pee) the process of viewing the abdominal cavity with a laparoscope (a thin-walled flexible tube with a telescopic lens and light).

Laryngalgia (**lair**-ring-**GAL**-jee-ah) pain in the larynx.

Laryngitis (**lair**-in-**JYE**-tis) inflammation of the larynx, usually resulting in dysphonia (hoarseness) cough, and difficulty swallowing.

Laryngopharynx (lah-**ring**-go-**FAIR**-inks) lower portion of the pharynx that extends from the vestibule of the larynx (the portion just above the vocal cords) to the lowermost cartilage of the larynx.

Laryngoscopy (**lar**-in-**GOSS**-koh-pee) the examination of the interior of the larynx using a lighted, flexible tube known as a laryngoscope (or endoscope).

Larynx (**LAIR**-inks) the enlarged upper end of the trachea below the root of the tongue; the voice box.

Laser in situ keratomileusis (LASIK) the LASIK (laser in situ keratomileusis) procedure is a form of laser vision correction for nearsightedness (myopia).

Lateral toward the side of the body, away from the midline of the body.

Lavage (lah-**VAZH**) the process of irrigating (washing out) an organ—usually the bladder, bowel, paranasal sinuses, or stomach—for therapeutic purposes.

Leiomyoma (**ligh**-oh-my-**OH**-mah) a benign, smooth-muscle tumor of the uterus. Uterine leiomyomas are often mislabeled as fibroid tumors, when in fact they are not.

Length (recumbent) (ree-**KUM**-bent) the measurement of the distance from the crown of the infant's head to the infant's heel while the infant is lying on the back with legs extended.

Lesion (**LEE**-zhun) any visible damage to the tissues of the skin, such as a wound, sore, rash, or boil.

Lethal (**LEE**-thal) capable of causing death.

Leukemia (ALL, AML, CML) (loo-**KEE**-mee-ah) an excessive uncontrolled increase of immature WBCs in the blood eventually leading to infection, anemia, and thrombocytopenia (decreased number of platelets).

Leukocyte (**LOO**-koh-sight) a white blood cell, one of the formed elements of the circulating blood system.

Leukocytopenia (**loo**-koh-**sigh**-toh-**PEE**-nee-ah) an abnormal decrease in number of white blood cells to fewer than 5,000 cells per cubic millimeter.

Leukoplakia (loo-koh-**PLAY**-kee-ah) white, hard, thickened patches firmly attached to the mucous membrane in areas such as the mouth, vulva, or penis.

Leukorrhea (**loo**-koh-**REE**-ah) a white discharge from the vagina.

Lichenification (lye-**ken**-ih-fih-**KAY**-shun) thickening and hardening of the skin.

Ligaments (**LIG**-ah-ments) connective tissue bands that join bone to bone, offering support to the joint.

Lightening the settling of the fetal head into the pelvis, occurring a few weeks prior to the onset of labor.

Linea nigra (**LIN**-ee-ah **NIG**-rah) a darkened vertical midline appearing on the abdomen of a pregnant woman, extending from the fundus to the symphysis pubis.

Linear accelerator (**LIN**-ee-ar) an apparatus for accelerating charged subatomic particles used in radiotherapy, physics research, and the production of radionuclides.

Lipase (**LIH**-pays *or* **LIGH**-pays) an enzyme that aids in the digestion of fats.

Lipid (**LIP**-id) any of a group of fats or fatlike substances found in the blood. Examples of lipids are cholesterol, fatty acids, and triglycerides.

Lipid profile (**LIP**-id profile) a lipid profile measures the lipids in the blood.

Lipocyte (**LIP**-oh-sight) a fat cell.

Liposuction (**LIP**-oh-suck-shun) aspiration of fat through a suction cannula or curette to alter the body contours.

Liquid-based Pap (LBP) a process of collecting a tissue sample from the endocervix and the exocervix with a sampling device that is placed directly into a liquid fixative instead of being spread onto a glass slide. This process provides immediate fixation and improves specimen adequacy. The LBP has not completely replaced the traditional Pap smear but is an increasingly popular alternative to conventional cervical cytology smears.

Lithium (**LITH**-ee-um) a drug that is particularly useful in treating the manic phase of bipolar disorders (manic-depressive disorders).

Lithotomy position (lih-**THOT**-oh-mee position) a position in which the patient lies on her back, buttocks even with the end of the table, with her knees bent back toward her abdomen and the heel of each foot resting in an elevated foot rest at the end of the examination table.

Liver the largest gland of the body and one of its most complex organs.

Liver biopsy (**LIV**-er **BYE**-op-see) a piece of liver tissue is obtained for examination by inserting a specially designed needle into the liver through the abdominal wall.

Liver scan (**LIV**-er **SCAN**) a noninvasive scanning technique, which enables the visualization of the shape, size, and consistency of the liver after the IV injection of a radioactive compound.

Local effect a response (to a medication) confined to a specific part of the body.

Local reaction a reaction to treatment that occurs at the site it was administered.

Long axis the long axis of the body; the imaginary line created by directing a vertical line through the middle of the body from the top of the head to a space equidistant between the feet; essentially the midline of the body.

Long bones bones that are longer than they are wide and with distinctive shaped ends, such as the femur.

Loop electrosurgical excision procedure (LEEP) a procedure used to remove abnormal cells from the surface of the cervix using a thin wire loop that acts like a scalpel. A painless electrical current passes through the loop as it cuts away a thin layer of surface cells from the cervix.

Lordosis (lor-**DOH**-sis) a forward curvature of the spine, noticeable if the person is observed from the side.

Lower esophageal sphincter (LES) (lower eh-**soff**-ah-**JEE**-al **SFINGK**-ter) see *cardiac sphincter*.

Lower GI tract the lower portion of the gastrointestinal tract consisting of the small and large intestines.

Lumbar puncture (**LUM**-bar **PUNK**-chur) the insertion of a hollow needle and stylet into the subarachnoid space, generally between the third and fourth lumbar vertebrae below the level of the spinal cord under strict aseptic technique.

Lumbar region the right and left regions of the middle section of the abdomen.

Lumbar vertebrae the largest and strongest of the vertebrae of the spinal column, located in the lower back. The lumbar vertebrae consist of five large segments of the movable part of the spinal column; identified as L1 through L5.

Lumen (**LOO**-men) a cavity or the channel within any organ or structure of the body; the space within an artery, vein, intestine, or tube.

Lumpectomy (lum-**PEK**-toh-mee) surgical removal of only the tumor and the immediate adjacent breast tissue; a method of treatment for breast cancer when detected in the early stage of the disease.

Lunar month (**LOON**-ar) four weeks or 28 days; approximately the amount of time it takes the moon to revolve around the earth.

Lung abscess (lung **AB**-sess) a localized collection of pus formed by the destruction of lung tissue and microorganisms by white blood cells that have migrated to the area to fight infection.

Lung scan the visual imaging of the distribution of ventilation or blood flow in the lungs by scanning the lungs after the patient has been injected with or has inhaled radioactive material.

Lunula (**LOO**-noo-lah) the crescent-shaped pale area at the base of the fingernail or toenail.

Lyme disease (**LYME** dih-**ZEEZ**) an acute, recurrent, inflammatory infection transmitted through the bite of an infected deer tick.

Lymph (**LIMF**) interstitial fluid picked up by the lymphatic capillaries and eventually returned to the blood. Once the interstitial fluid enters the lymphatic vessels, it is known as lymph.

Lymphadenopathy (lim-**fad**-eh-**NOP**-ah-thee) any disorder of the lymph nodes or lymph vessels, characterized by localized or generalized enlargement.

Lymphangiogram (lim-**FAN**-jee-oh-gram) an X-ray assessment of the lymphatic system following injection of a contrast medium into the lymph vessels in the hand or foot.

Lymphangiography (lim-**fan**-jee-**OG**-rah-fee) an X-ray assessment of the lymphatic system following injection of a contrast medium into the lymph vessels in the hand or foot.

Lymphocyte (**LIM**-foh-sight) small, agranulocytic leukocytes originating from fetal stem cells and developing in the bone marrow.

Lymphoma (**LIM**-foh-mah) a lymphoid tissue neoplasm that is typically malignant, beginning with a painless enlarged lymph node(s) and progressing to anemia, weakness, fever, and weight loss.

Lysosomes (**LIGH**-soh-sohmz) cell organs (or organelles) that contain various types of enzymes that function in intracellular digestion. Lysosomes destroy bacteria by digesting them.

M

Macrophage (**MACK**-roh-fayj) any phagocytic cell involved in the defense against infection and in the disposal of the products of the breakdown of cells. Macrophages are found in the lymph nodes, liver, spleen, lungs, brain, and spinal cord.

Macular degeneration (**MACK**-yool-ar dee-jen-er-**RAY**-shun) progressive deterioration of the retinal cells in the macula due to aging. Known as senile or age-related macular degeneration (ARMD) this condition is a common and progressive cause of visual deficiency and permanent reading impairment in the adult over 65 years of age.

Macule (**MACK**-yool) a small, flat discoloration of the skin that is neither raised nor depressed. Some common examples of macules are bruises, freckles, and the rashes of measles and roseola.

Magnetic resonance imaging (MRI) (mag-**NEH**-tic **REHZ**-oh-nans imaging) involves the use of a strong magnetic field and radiofrequency waves to produce imaging that is valuable in providing images of the heart, large blood vessels, brain, and soft tissue.

Maintenance dose the dose of a medication that will keep the concentration of the medication in the bloodstream at the desired level.

Major depressive disorder a disorder characterized by one or more episodes of depressed mood that lasts at least two weeks and is accompanied by at least four additional symptoms of depression.

Malabsorption (**mal**-ab-**SORP**-shun) impaired absorption of nutrients into the bloodstream from the gastrointestinal tract.

Malaise (mah-**LAYZ**) a vague feeling of body weakness or discomfort, often indicating the onset of an illness or disease.

Malignant melanoma (mah-**LIG**-nant **mel**-ah-**NOH**-mah) malignant skin tumor originating from melanocytes in preexisting nevi, freckles, or skin with pigment; darkly pigmented cancerous tumor.

Malingering (mah-**LING**-er-ing) a willful and deliberate faking of symptoms of a disease or injury to gain some consciously desired end.

Malodorous (mal-**OH**-dor-us) foul smelling; having a bad odor.

Mammary glands (**MAM**-ah-ree glands) the female breasts.

Mammography (mam-**OG**-rah-fee) the process of examining with X-ray the soft tissue of the breast to detect various benign or malignant growths before they can be felt.

Mania (**MAY**-nee-ah) "Madness"; an unstable emotional state characterized by symptoms such as extreme excitement, hyperactivity, overtalkativeness, agitation, flight of ideas, fleeting attention, and sometimes violent, destructive, and self-destructive behavior.

Marijuana see *cannabis*.

Mask of pregnancy patches of tan or brown pigmentation associated with pregnancy, occurring mostly on the forehead, cheeks, and nose; also known as chloasma.

Mast cell a cell (found within the connective tissue) that contains heparin and histamine; these substances are released from the mast cell in response to injury and infection.

Mastectomy (mass-**TEK**-toh-mee) surgical removal of the breast as a treatment method for breast cancer; can be simple (breast only), modified radical (breast plus lymph nodes in axilla), or radical (breast, lymph nodes, and chest muscles on affected side).

Mastication (mass-tih-**KAY**-shun) chewing, tearing, or grinding food with the teeth while it becomes mixed with saliva.

Mastitis (mass-**TYE**-tis) inflammation of the breast.

Mastoiditis (mass-toyd-**EYE**-tis) inflammation of the mastoid process, which is usually an acute expansion of an infection in the middle ear (otitis media).

McBurney's point a point on the right side of the abdomen, about two-thirds of the distance between the umbilicus and the anterior bony prominence of the hip. When tenderness exists upon McBurney's point, a physician might suspect appendicitis.

Meatus (mee-**AY**-tus) an opening or tunnel through any part of the body, as in the urinary meatus, which is the external opening of the urethra.

Medial (**MEE**-dee-al) toward the midline of the body.

Mediastinum (**mee**-dee-as-**TYE**-num) the area between the lungs in the chest cavity that contains the heart, aorta, trachea, esophagus, and bronchi.

Mediolateral (**MEE**-dee-oh-**LAT**-er-al) pertaining to the middle and side of a structure.

Medulla (meh-**DULL**-lah) the internal part of a structure or organ.

Medullary cavity (**MED**-u-lair-ee) the center portion of the shaft of a long bone containing the yellow marrow.

Megakaryocyte (**meg**-ah-**KAIR**-ee-oh-sight) an extremely large bone marrow cell.

Melanin (**MEL**-an-in) a black or dark pigment (produced by melanocytes within the epidermis) that contributes color to the skin and helps filter ultraviolet light.

Melanocytes (**MEL**-an-oh-sights *or* mel-**AN**-oh-sights) cells responsible for producing melanin.

Melanoma (**mel**-ah-**NOH**-mah) darkly pigmented tumor.

Membrane a thin layer of tissue that covers a surface, lines a cavity, or divides a space, such as the abdominal membrane that lines the abdominal wall.

Menarche (meh-**NAR**-kee) onset of menstruation; the first menstrual period.

Ménière's disease (may-nee-**ARYZ**) chronic inner ear disease in which there is an overaccumulation of endolymph (fluid in the labyrinth) characterized by recurring episodes of vertigo (dizziness), hearing loss, feeling of pressure or fullness in the affected ear, and tinnitus; usually unilateral, but occurs bilaterally in about 10% to 20% of patients.

Meninges (men-**IN**-jeez) the three layers of protective membranes that surround the brain and spinal cord.

Meningitis (acute bacterial) (men-in-**JYE**-tis ah-**KYOOT** back-**TEE**-ree-al) a serious bacterial infection of the meninges—the covering of the brain and spinal cord—that can have residual debilitating effects or even a fatal outcome if not diagnosed and treated promptly with appropriate antibiotic therapy.

Meningocele (meh-**NING**-goh-**seel**) a cystlike sac covered with skin or a thin membrane protruding through the bony defect in the vertebrae containing meninges and CSF.

Meningomyelocele (men-**in**-goh-my-**ELL**-oh-seel) a cystlike sac covered with skin or a thin membrane protruding through the bony defect in the vertebrae that contains meninges, CSF, and spinal cord segments.

Menopause (**MEN**-oh-pawz) the permanent cessation (stopping) of the menstrual cycles.

Menorrhea (men-oh-**REE**-ah) menstrual flow; menstruation.

Menses (**MEN**-seez) another name for menstruation or menstrual flow.

Menstruation (men-stroo-**AY**-shun) the periodic shedding of the lining of the nonpregnant uterus through a bloody discharge that passes through the vagina to the outside of the body. It occurs at monthly intervals and lasts for 3 to 5 days.

Metabolism (meh-**TAB**-oh-lizm) the sum of all physical and chemical processes that take place within the body.

Metastatic intracranial tumors (secondary) (met-ah-**STAT**-ik in-trah-**KRAY**-nee-al **TOO**-morz) occur as a result of metastasis tumors (secondary) from a primary site such as the lung or breast. They occur more frequently than primary neoplasms.

Microcephalus (**my**-kroh-**SEFF**-ah-lus) a congenital anomaly characterized by abnormal smallness of the head in relation to the rest of the body and by underdevelopment of the brain, resulting in some degree of mental retardation.

Microglia (my-**KROG**-lee-ah) small neuroglial cells found in the interstitial tissue of the nervous system that engulf cellular debris, waste products, and pathogens within the nerve tissue.

Micro-insert system an alternative to tubal ligation that provides bilateral occlusion of the fallopian tubes by inserting a soft, flexible micro-insert into each fallopian tube.

Micturition the act of eliminating urine from the bladder; also called *voiding* or *urination*.

Midbrain the uppermost part of the brain stem.

Middle-old a term used to describe an individual between the ages of 75 and 84 years.

Midline of the body the imaginary "line" created when the body is divided into equal right and left halves.

Midsagittal plane (mid-**SADJ**-ih-tal) the plane that divides the body (or a structure) into right and left equal portions.

Migraine headache (**MY**-grain headache) a recurring, pulsating, vascular headache usually developing on one side of the head. It is characterized by a slow onset that may be preceded by an aura, during which a sensory disturbance occurs such as confusion or some visual interference (e.g., flashing lights).

Minnesota Multiphasic Personality Inventory (MMPI) (mull-tih-**FAYZ**-ic) a self-report personality inventory test that consists of 550 statements that can be answered "true," "false," or "cannot say." The statements vary widely in content and are sometimes repeated in various ways throughout the test.

Miosis (my-**OH**-sis) abnormal constriction of the pupil of the eye.

Miotic (my-**OT**-ik) an agent that causes the pupil of the eye to constrict.

Mitochondria (my-toh-**KON**-dree-ah) cell organs (or organelles) that provide the energy needed by the cell to carry on its essential functions.

Mitral valve prolapse (**MY**-tral valve proh-**LAPS**) drooping of one or both cusps of the mitral valve back into the left atrium during ventricular systole (when the and heart is pumping blood), resulting in incomplete closure of the valve mitral insufficiency. (Normally the mitral valve would completely close to prevent the backflow of blood into the left atrium during systole.) This is also known as click-murmur syndrome, Barlow's syndrome, and floppy mitral valve.

Modality (moh-**DAL**-ih-tee) a method of application (i.e., a treatment method).

Mohs surgery an advanced treatment procedure for skin cancer. The cancerous tumor is removed in stages, the tissue is examined for evidence of cancer, and additional tissue is removed until negative boundaries are confirmed. This process allows the surgeon to excise the tumor, remove layers of tissue, and examine the fresh tissue immediately. Only tissue containing cancer is removed and the healthy tissue is kept intact.

Molar tooth (**MOH**-lar) any of 12 molar teeth, 6 in each dental arch, located posterior to the premolar teeth. The molar teeth have a flat surface with multiple projections (cusps) for crushing and grinding food.

Monocyte (**MON**-oh-sight) a large mononuclear leukocyte.

Mononucleosis (mon-oh-**noo**-klee-**OH**-sis) usually caused by the Epstein–Barr virus (EBV), typically a benign, self-limiting acute infection of the B lymphocytes.

Motility (moh-**TILL**-ih-tee) the ability to move spontaneously.

Motor nerves (**MOH**-tor nerves) see *efferent nerves.*

Mucopurulent (mew-koh-**PEWR**-yoo-lent) characteristic of a combination of mucus and pus.

Multigravida (**mull**-tih-**GRAV**-ih-dah) a woman who has been pregnant more than once.

Multipara (mull-**TIP**-ah-rah) a woman who has given birth two or more times after 20 weeks' gestation.

Multiple myeloma (plasma cell myeloma) (**MULL**-tih-pul my-eh-**LOH**-mah) a malignant plasma cell neoplasm, multiple myeloma causes an increase in the number of both mature and immature plasma cells, which often entirely replace the bone marrow and destroy the skeletal structure.

Multiple sclerosis (MS) (**MULL**-tih-pal **SKLEH**-roh-sis) a degenerative inflammatory disease of the CNS attacking the myelin sheath in the spinal cord and brain, leaving it sclerosed (hardened) or scarred and interrupting the flow of nerve impulses.

Mumps (infectious parotitis) (in-**FEK**-shus pah-roh-**TYE**-tis) acute viral disease characterized by fever, swelling, and tenderness of one or more salivary glands, usually the parotid glands (below and in front of the ears).

Munchausen syndrome (by proxy) (mun-**CHOW**-zen **SIN**-drom) somewhat rare form of child abuse in which a parent of a child falsifies an illness in a child by fabricating or creating the symptoms and then seeks frequent medical attention for the child; the *DSM-5* refers to this condition as a factitious disorder imposed on another.

Murmur, a low-pitched humming or fluttering sound, as in a "heart murmur," heard on auscultation.

Muscle biopsy (muscle **BYE**-op-see) extraction of a specimen of muscle tissue, through either a biopsy needle or an incisional biopsy, for the purpose of examining it under a microscope.

Muscle fiber the name given to the individual muscle cell.

Muscle tissue the tissue capable of producing movement of the parts and organs of the body by contracting and relaxing its fibers.

Muscular dystrophy (**MUSS**-kew-lar **DIS**-troh-fee) muscular dystrophy is a group of genetically transmitted disorders characterized by progressive symmetrical wasting of skeletal muscles; there is no evidence of nerve involvement or degeneration of nerve tissue. The onset of muscular dystrophy is early in life.

Mutism (**mew**-tizm) the inability to speak because of a physical defect or emotional problem.

Myasthenia gravis (my-as-**THEE**-nee-ah **GRAV**-iss) a chronic progressive neuromuscular disorder causing severe skeletal muscle weakness (without atrophy) and fatigue, which occurs at different levels of severity.

Mydriasis (mid-**RYE**-ah-sis) abnormal dilation of the pupil of the eye.

Mydriatic (mid-ree-**AT**-ik) an agent that causes the pupil of the eye to dilate.

Myelin sheath (**MY**-eh-lin **SHEETH**) a protective sheath that covers the axons of many nerves in the body. It acts as an electrical insulator and helps speed the conduction of nerve impulses.

Myelography (my-eh-**LOG**-rah-fee) the introduction of contrast medium into the lumbar subarachnoid space through a lumbar puncture to visualize the spinal cord and vertebral canal through X-ray examination.

Myeloid (**MY**-eh-loyd) of or pertaining to the bone marrow or the spinal cord.

Myocardial infarction (my-oh-**CAR**-dee-al in-**FARC**-shun) heart attack: a condition caused by occlusion of one or more of the coronary arteries. This life-threatening condition results when myocardial tissue is destroyed in areas of the heart that are deprived of an adequate blood supply due to the occluded vessels.

Myocarditis (my-oh-car-**DYE**-tis) inflammation of the myocardium may be caused by viral or bacterial infections or may be a result of systemic diseases such as rheumatic fever. This may also be caused by fungal infections, serum sickness, or a chemical agent.

Myocardium (my-oh-**CAR**-dee-um) the middle muscular layer of the heart.

Myometrium (my-oh-**MEE**-tree-um) the muscular layer of the uterine wall.

Myopia (my-**OH**-pee-ah) a refractive error in which the lens of the eye cannot focus on an image accurately, resulting in impaired distance vision that is blurred due to the light rays being focused in front of the retina because the eyeball is longer than normal; nearsightedness.

Myringoplasty (mir-**IN**-goh-plass-tee) surgical repair of the eardrum with a tissue graft. This procedure is performed to correct hearing loss. It may also be called a tympanoplasty.

Myringotomy (mir-in-**GOT**-oh-mee) surgical incision into the eardrum. This procedure is performed to relieve pressure or release fluid from the middle ear. It is also called tympanotomy. A myringotomy is usually accompanied by the insertion of a pressure-equalizing tube (PET) into the tympanic membrane to promote drainage of fluid from the middle ear.

Myxedema (miks-eh-**DEE**-mah) the most severe form of hypothyroidism in the adult. This condition is characterized by puffiness of the hands and face; coarse, thickened edematous skin; an enlarged tongue; slow speech; loss of and dryness of the hair; sensitivity to cold; drowsiness; and mental apathy.

N

Nagele's rule (**NAY**-geh-leez) a formula that is used to calculate the date of birth: Subtract three months from the first day of the last normal menstrual period and add one year and seven days to that date to arrive at the estimated date of birth.

Nail body the visible part of the nail.

Narcissistic personality disorder (nar-sis-**SIST**-ik) characterized by an abnormal interest in oneself, especially in one's own body and sexual characteristics.

Narcolepsy (**NAR**-koh-**lep**-see) a rare syndrome of uncontrolled sudden attacks of sleep. The main features of narcolepsy are daytime sleepiness and cataplexy. The sleep attacks must occur daily over a period of at least three months to establish the diagnosis of narcolepsy.

Nares (**NAIRZ**) external nostrils.

Nasal endoscopy (**NAY**-sal en-**DOSS**-koh-pee) the process of viewing the inside of the nose and sinuses using a thin, usually flexible, fiberoptic tube with a telescopic lens.

Nasogastric intubation (nay-zoh-**GAS**-trik **in**-too-**BAY**-shun) tube placement through the nose into the stomach for the purpose of relieving gastric distension by removing gastric secretions, gas, or food.

Nasolacrimal (nay-zoh-**LAK**-rim-al) pertaining to the nose and the lacrimal (tear) ducts.

Nasopharynx (**nay**-zoh-**FAIR**-inks) part of the pharynx located above the soft palate (postnasal space).

Natural immunity (ih-**MEW**-nih-tee) immunity with which we are born; also called genetic immunity.

Nausea (**NAW**-zee-ah) unpleasant sensation usually preceding vomiting.

Navel (**NAY**-vel) the umbilicus; the belly button.

Needle aspiration (needle ass-per-**AY**-shun) the insertion of a needle into a cavity for the purpose of withdrawing fluid.

Neonatologist (**nee**-oh-nay-**TOL**-oh-jist) a medical doctor who specializes in neonatology.

Neonatology (**nee**-oh-nay-**TOL**-oh-jee) the branch of medicine that specializes in the treatment and care of the diseases and disorders of the newborn through the first four weeks of life.

Neoplasia (**nee**-oh-**PLAY**-zee-ah) the new and abnormal development of cells that may be benign or malignant.

Nephrolith (**NEF**-roh-lith) a kidney stone; also called a renal calculus.

Nephrolithiasis (**nef**-roh-lith-**EYE**-ah-sis) a condition of kidney stones; also known as renal calculi.

Nephrotic syndrome (neh-**FROT**-ic **SIN**-drohm) a group of clinical symptoms occurring when damage to the glomerulus of the kidney is present and large quantities of protein are lost through the glomerular membrane into the urine, resulting in severe proteinuria (presence of large amounts of protein in the urine); also called nephrosis.

Nerve a cordlike bundle of nerve fibers that transmit impulses to and from the brain and spinal cord to other parts of the body. A nerve is macroscopic (i.e., able to be seen without the aid of a microscope).

Nerve block the injection of a local anesthetic along the course of a nerve or nerves to eliminate sensation to the area supplied by the nerve(s); also called conduction anesthesia.

Nervous tissue tissue that transmits impulses throughout the body, thereby activating, coordinating, and controlling the many functions of the body.

Neuralgia (noo-**RAL**-jee-ah) severe, sharp, spasmlike pain that extends along the course of one or more nerves.

Neurectomy (noo-**REK**-toh-mee) a neurosurgical procedure to relieve pain in a localized or small area by incision of cranial or peripheral nerves.

Neuritis (noo-**RYE**-tis) inflammation of a nerve.

Neuroblastoma (**noo**-roh-blass-**TOH**-mah) highly malignant tumor of the sympathetic nervous system.

Neuroglia (noo-**ROG**-lee-ah) supporting tissue of the nervous system.

Neurologist (noo-**RAL**-oh-jist) physician who specializes in treating the diseases and disorders of the nervous system.

Neurology (noo-**RAL**-oh-jee) study of the nervous system and its disorders.

Neuron (**NOO**-ron) a nerve cell.

Neurosis (noo-**ROH**-sis) a psychological or behavioral disorder in which anxiety is the primary characteristic; thought to be related to unresolved conflicts.

Neurosurgeon (noo-roh-**SIR**-jun) a physician who specializes in surgery of the nervous system.

Neurosurgery (noo-roh-**SIR**-jer-ee) any surgery involving the nervous system (i.e., of the brain, spinal cord, or peripheral nerves).

Neurotransmitter (noo-roh-**TRANS**-mit-er) a chemical substance within the body that activates or inhibits the transmission of nerve impulses at synapses.

Neutrophil (**NOO**-troh-fill) a polymorphonuclear (multilobed nucleus) granular leukocyte that stains easily with neutral dyes.

Nevus (mole) (**NEE**-vus) a visual accumulation of melanocytes, creating a flat or raised rounded macule or papule with definite borders.

Nipple stimulation test noninvasive technique that produces basically the same results as the contraction stress test by having the pregnant woman stimulate the nipples of her breasts by rubbing them between her fingers.

Nocturia (nok-**TOO**-ree-ah) urination at night.

Nodule (**NOD**-yool) a small, circumscribed swelling protruding above the skin; a small node.

Norepinephrine (nor-ep-ih-**NEH**-frin) a hormone produced by the adrenal medulla. This hormone plays an important role in the body's response to stress by raising the blood pressure.

Nuchal rigidity (**NOO**-kal rih-**JID**-ih-tee) rigidity of the neck. The neck is resistant to flexion. This condition is seen in patients with meningitis.

Nuclear medicine (**NOO**-klee-ar medicine) a medical discipline that uses radioactive isotopes in the diagnosis and treatment of disease.

Nucleus (**NOO**-klee-us) the central controlling body within a living cell that is enclosed within the cell membrane.

Nullipara (nuh-**LIP**-ah-rah) woman who has never completed a pregnancy beyond 20 weeks' gestation.

Nutritionist (noo-**TRIH**-shun-ist) allied health professional who studies and applies the principles and science of nutrition.

Nystagmus (niss-**TAG**-mus) involuntary, rhythmic jerking movements of the eye. These "quivering" movements may be from side to side, up and down, or a combination of both.

O

Obsession (ob-**SESS**-shun) a persistent thought or idea with which the mind is continually and involuntarily preoccupied.

Obsessive-compulsive disorder (ob-**SESS**-iv kom-**PUHL**-siv) disorder characterized by recurrent obsessions or compulsions that are severe enough to be time consuming (they take more than one hour a day) or to cause obvious distress or a notable handicap.

Obstetrical ultrasound (ob-**STET**-rik-al **ULL**-trah-sound) (also called ultrasonography) a noninvasive procedure that uses high-frequency sound waves to examine internal structures of the body. In the field of obstetrics, ultrasonography is used to examine the internal structures and contents of the uterus. It can be used to detect very early pregnancy as well as the size and development of the fetus. It is also used to confirm complications of pregnancy such as placenta previa, breech presentation, and other abnormal positions of the fetus. Ultrasonography is also a valuable tool for diagnosis of multiple gestations.

Obstetrician (ob-steh-**TRISH**-an) physician who specializes in the care of women during pregnancy, the delivery of the baby, and the first six weeks following the delivery (known as the immediate postpartum period).

Obstetrics (ob-**STET**-riks) the field of medicine that deals with pregnancy, the delivery of the baby, and the first six weeks after delivery (the immediate postpartum period).

Occlusion (oh-**KLOO**-zhun) blockage.

Official name generic name.

Oil gland one of the many small glands located in the dermis; its secretions provide oil to the hair and surrounding skin. See also *sebaceous gland.*

Oligodendrocyte (ol-ih-goh-**DEN**-droh-sight) a type of neuroglial cell found in the interstitial tissue of the nervous system. Its dendrite projections coil around the axons of many neurons to form the myelin sheath.

Omphalitis (om-fal-**EYE**-tis) an inflammation of the umbilical stump, marked by redness, swelling, and purulent exudate in severe cases.

Oncologist (ong-**KOL**-oh-jist) the physician who specializes in the study and treatment of neoplastic diseases, particularly cancer.

Oncology (ong-**KOL**-oh-jee) the medical specialty concerned with the study of malignancy.

Onycholysis (**on**-ih-**KOL**-ih-sis) separation of a fingernail from its bed, beginning at the free margin. This condition is associated with dermatitis of the hand, psoriasis, and fungal infections.

Onychocryptosis (**on**-ih-koh-krip-**TOH**-sis) ingrown nail. The nail pierces the lateral fold of skin and grows into the dermis, causing swelling and pain.

Onychomycosis (**on**-ih-koh-my-**KOH**-sis) any fungal infection of the nails.

Onychophagia (**on**-ih-koh-**FAY**-jee-ah) the habit of biting the nails.

Ophthalmia neonatorum (off-**THAL**-mee-ah nee-oh-nay-**TOR**-um) purulent (contains pus) inflammation of the conjunctiva and/or cornea in the newborn.

Ophthalmologist (off-thal-**MOL**-oh-jist) a medical doctor (M.D.) who specializes in the comprehensive care of the eyes and visual system in the prevention and treatment of eye disease and injury. The ophthalmologist is the medically trained specialist who can deliver total eye care and diagnose general diseases of the body affecting the eye.

Ophthalmology (off-thal-**MOL**-oh-jee) the branch of medicine that specializes in the study of the diseases and disorders of the eye.

Ophthalmopathy (off-thal-**MOP**-ah-thee) any disease of the eye.

Ophthalmoscopy (off-thal-**MOSS**-koh-pee) examination of the external and internal structures of the eye with an instrument called an ophthalmoscope.

Opportunistic infection (op-or-**TOON**-is-tik in-**FEK**-shuns) an infection caused by normally non-disease-producing organisms that sets up in a host whose resistance has been decreased by surgery, illnesses, and disorders such as AIDS.

Optic (**OP**-tik) pertaining to the eyes or to sight.

Optician (op-**TISH**-an) health professional (not an M.D.) who specializes in filling prescriptions for corrective lenses for glasses or for contact lenses.

Optometrist (op-**TOM**-eh-trist) a doctor of optometry (O.D.) is responsible for examination of the eye, and associated structures—to determine vision problems. He or she can also prescribe lenses or optical aids.

Oral contraceptives (**ORAL** con-trah-**SEP**-tivz) birth control pills that contain synthetic forms of the estrogen and progesterone hormones and are taken by mouth.

Oral medication (**OR**-al) medication that is given by mouth and swallowed. Oral medications may be given in a dry, solid, or powder form, or they may be given in the liquid form.

Oral leukoplakia (**OR**-al **loo**-koh-**PLAY**-kee-ah) a precancerous lesion occurring anywhere in the mouth.

Orchidectomy (orchiectomy) (or-kid-**EK**-toh-mee) (or-kee-**EK**-toh-mee) the surgical removal of a testicle.

Orchidopexy (**or**-kid-oh-**PECK**-see) surgical fixation of an undescended testicle.

Orchiopexy (**or**-kee-oh-**PECK**-see) see *orchidopexy.*

Orchitis (or-**KIGH**-tis) inflammation of the testes due to a virus, bacterial infection, or injury. The condition may affect one or both testes. Orchitis typically results from the mumps virus.

Organ tissues arranged together to perform a special function.

Orifice (**OR**-ih-fis) entrance or outlet of any body cavity; as in the vaginal orifice.

Origin the point of attachment of a muscle to a bone that is less movable (i.e., the more fixed end of attachment).

Oropharynx (**or**-oh-**FAIR**-inks) central portion of the pharynx lying between the soft palate and upper portion of the epiglottis.

Orthopnea (or-**THOP**-nee-ah) an abnormal condition in which a person sits up straight or stands up to breathe comfortably.

Orthovoltage (or-thoh-**VOHL**-tij) voltage range of 100 to 350 KeV supplied by some X-ray generators used for radiation therapy.

Ossification (**oss**-sih-fih-**KAY**-shun) the conversion of cartilage and fibrous connective tissue to bone; the formation of bone.

Osteoarthritis (**oss**-tee-oh-ar-**THRYE**-tis) also known as degenerative joint disease. It is the most common form of arthritis, having universal prevalence in those age 80 and over. It results from wear and tear on the joints, especially weight-bearing joints such as the hips and knees.

Osteoblasts (**OSS**-tee-oh-blasts) immature bone cells that actively produce bony tissue.

Osteochondroma (**oss**-tee-oh-kon-**DROH**-mah) the most common benign bone tumor. The femur and the tibia are most frequently involved.

Osteoclasts (**OSS**-tee-oh-clasts) large cells that absorb or digest old bone tissue.

Osteocytes (**OSS**-tee-oh-sites) mature bone cells.

Osteogenic sarcoma (oss-tee-oh-**JEN**-ic sar-**KOH**-mah) a malignant tumor arising from bone. Also known as osteosarcoma, it is the most common malignant bone tumor, with common sites being the distal femur (just above the knee) the proximal tibia (just below the knee) and the proximal humerus (just below the shoulder joint).

Osteomalacia (oss-tee-oh-mah-**LAY**-she-ah) a disease in which the bones become abnormally soft due to a deficiency of calcium and phosphorus in the blood (which is necessary for bone mineralization). This disease results in fractures and noticeable deformities of the weight-bearing bones. When the disease occurs in children, it is called rickets.

Osteomyelitis (oss-tee-oh-mah-**LAY**-she-ah) a local or generalized infection of the bone and bone marrow, resulting from a bacterial infection that has spread to the bone tissue through the blood.

Osteoporosis (oss-tee-oh-poh-**ROW**-sis) literally means porous bones; that is, bones that were once strong become fragile due to loss of bone density.

Otalgia (oh-**TAL**-jee-ah) pain in the ear; earache. It is also called otodynia.

Otitis externa (OE) (swimmer's ear) (oh-**TYE**-tis eks-**TER**-nah) inflammation of the outer or external ear canal; also called "swimmer's ear." This inflammation is produced from the growth of bacteria or fungi in the external ear. In addition to the occurrence after swimming, otitis externa can develop due to conditions such as psoriasis or seborrhea, injury to the ear canal when trying to scratch or clean it with a foreign object, and frequent use of earphones or earplugs.

Otitis media (oh-**TYE**-tis **MEE**-dee-ah) inflammation of the middle ear.

Otitis media, acute (AOM) (oh-**TYE**-tis **MEE**-dee-ah) a middle ear infection, which predominantly affects infants, toddlers, and preschoolers.

Otodynia (oh-toh-**DIN**-ee-ah) see *otalgia*.

Otomycosis (oh-toh-my-**KOH**-sis) a fungal infection of the external auditory meatus of the ear.

Otoplasty (**OH**-toh-plass-tee) removal of a portion of ear cartilage to bring the pinna and auricle nearer the head.

Otorrhea (oh-toh-**REE**-ah) drainage from the ear; usually associated with inflammation of the ear.

Otosclerosis (oh-toh-sklair-**OH**-sis) condition in which the footplate of the stapes becomes immobile and secured to the oval window, resulting in a hearing loss.

Otoscopy (oh-**TOSS**-koh-pee) the use of an otoscope to view and examine the tympanic membrane and various parts of the outer ear.

Ovarian carcinoma (oh-**VAIR**-ree-an kar-sih-**NOH**-mah) a malignant tumor of the ovaries, most commonly occurring in women in their 50s. It is rarely detected in the early stage and is usually far advanced when diagnosed.

Ovarian cysts (oh-**VAIR**-ree-an **SISTS**) benign, globular sacs (cysts) that form on or near the ovaries. These cysts may be fluid filled or may contain semisolid material.

Ovary (**OH**-vah-ree) one of a pair of female gonads responsible for producing mature ova (eggs) and releasing them at monthly intervals (ovulation); also responsible for producing the female hormones, estrogen and progesterone.

Over the counter (OTC) medication available without a prescription.

Ovulation (ov-yoo-**LAY**-shun) the release of the mature ovum from the ovary, occurring approximately 14 days prior to the beginning of menses.

Ovum (**OH**-vum) the female reproductive cell; female sex cell or egg.

Oxytocin (ok-see-**TOH**-sin) hormone secreted by the posterior pituitary gland. This hormone stimulates the contractions of the uterus during childbirth and stimulates the release of milk from the breasts of lactating women (women who breastfeed) in response to the suckling reflex of the infant.

P

Pacemaker the SA node (sinoatrial) of the heart located in the right atrium. It is responsible for initiating the heartbeat, influencing the rate and rhythm of the heart beat. The cardiac pacemaker (artificial pacemaker) is an electric apparatus used for maintaining a normal heart rhythm by electrically stimulating the heart muscle to contract.

Pachyderma (pak-ee-**DER**-mah) abnormal thickening of the skin.

Pachymetry (pah-**KIM**-eh-tree) the measurement of the thickness of the cornea.

Package insert an information leaflet placed inside the container or package of prescription drugs. The FDA requires that the drug generic name, indications, contraindications, adverse effects, dosage, and route of administration be described in the leaflet.

Paget's disease (**PAJ**-ets dih-**ZEEZ**) a nonmetabolic disease of the bone, characterized by excessive bone destruction (breakdown of bone tissue by the osteoclasts) and unorganized bone formation by the osteoblasts. The bone is weak and prone to fractures. After symptoms are present, the diseased bone takes on a characteristic mosaic pattern that can be detected with X-ray or bone scan; also known as osteitis deformans.

Palate (**PAL**-at) structure that forms the roof of the mouth.

Palatine tonsils (**PAL**-ah-tyne **TON**-sills) lymphatic tissue located in the depression of the mucous membrane of fauces (the constricted opening leading from the mouth and the oral pharynx) and the pharynx.

Palliative (**PAL**-ee-ay-tiv) soothing.

Pallor (**PAL**-or) lack of color; paleness; an unnatural paleness or absence of color in the skin.

Palpable (**PAL**-pah-bul) detectable by touch.

Palpation (pal-**PAY**-shun) the process of examining by application of the hands or fingers to the external surface of the body to detect evidence of disease or abnormalities in the various organs.

Palpebral (**PAL**-peh-brahl) pertaining to the eyelid.

Palpitation (pal-pih-**TAY**-shun) a pounding or racing of the heart, associated with normal emotional responses or with heart disorders.

Pancreas (**PAN**-kree-as) an elongated organ approximately 6 to 9 inches long, located in the upper left quadrant of the abdomen that secretes various substances such as digestive enzymes, insulin, and glucagon.

Pancreatic cancer (**pan**-kree-**AT**-ik **CAN**-sir) a life-threatening primary malignant neoplasm typically found in the head of the pancreas.

Pancreatitis (pan-kree-ah-**TYE**-tis) an acute or chronic destructive inflammatory condition of the pancreas.

Pancytopenia a marked reduction in the number of the red blood cells, white blood cells, and platelets.

Panic attack episode of acute anxiety during which the individual may experience intense feelings of uneasiness or fright accompanied by dyspnea, dizziness, sweating, trembling, and palpitations of the heart. Panic attacks, which occur unexpectedly, may last a few minutes and may return.

Panic disorder disorder characterized by recurrent panic attacks that come on unexpectedly, followed by at least one month of persistent concern about having another panic attack.

Papanicolaou (Pap) smear (pap-ah-**NIK**-oh-low smear) a diagnostic test for cervical cancer, that is, a microscopic examination of cells scraped from within the cervix (endocervix) from around the cervix (ectocervix) and from the posterior part of the vagina (near the cervix) to test for cervical cancer; also called Pap test.

Papillae (pah-**PILL**-ay) a small, nipple-shaped projection (such as the conoid papillae of the tongue and the papillae of the corium) that extend from collagen fibers, the capillary blood vessels, and sometimes the nerves of the dermis.

Papillary (**PAP**-ih-lar-ee) of or pertaining to a papilla (nipplelike projection).

Papilledema (pap-ill-eh-**DEE**-mah) swelling of the optic disc, visible upon ophthalmoscopic examination of the interior of the eye.

Papilloma (pap-ih-**LOH**-mah) a benign epithelial neoplasm characterized by a branching or lobular tumor.

Papule (**PAP**-yool) a small, solid, circumscribed elevation on the skin.

Para woman who has produced an infant regardless of whether the infant was alive or stillborn. This term applies to any pregnancies carried to more than 20 weeks' gestation. The term may be written para II, para III, and so on, to indicate the number of pregnancies lasting more than 20 weeks' gestation, regardless of the number of off spring produced by the pregnancy. A woman who has had only one pregnancy resulting in multiple births is still a para I.

Paranasal sinuses (pair-ah-**NAYZ**-al **SIGH**-nuss-ez) hollow areas or cavities within the skull that communicate with the nasal cavity.

Paranoia (pair-ah-**NOY**-ah) mental disorder characterized by an elaborate, overly suspicious system of thinking, with delusions of persecution and grandeur usually centered on one major theme (such as a financial matter, a job situation, an unfaithful spouse, or other problem).

Paranoid personality disorder (**PAIR**-ah-noyd) characterized by a generalized distrust and suspiciousness of others, so much so that the individual blames them for his or her own mistakes and failures.

Paraphilia (pair-ah-**FILL**-ee-ah) sexual perversion or deviation; a condition in which the sexual instinct is expressed in ways that are socially prohibited, unacceptable, or biologically undesirable.

Paraplegia (par-ah-**PLEE**-jee-ah) paraplegia (paralysis of the lower extremities) is caused by severe injury to the spinal cord in the thoracic or lumbar region, resulting in loss of sensory and motor control below the level of injury.

Parasympathetic nerves (**pair**-ah-sim-pah-**THET**-ik) nerves of the ANS that regulate essential involuntary body functions such as slowing the heart rate, increasing peristalsis of the intestines, increasing glandular secretions, and relaxing sphincters.

Parasympathomimetic (**pair**-ah-**sim**-pah-thoh-mim-**ET**-ik) copying or producing the same effects as those of the parasympathetic nerves; "to mimic" the parasympathetic nerves.

Parenteral medication (par-**EN**-ter-al) any route of administration not involving the gastrointestinal tract, for example, topical, inhalation, or injection.

Paresthesia (pair-ess-**THEE**-zee-ah) a sensation of numbness or tingling.

Parietal pleura (pah-**RYE**-eh-tal **PLOO**-rah) portion of the pleura that is closest to the ribs.

Parkinson's disease (**PARK**-in-sons dih-**ZEEZ**) a degenerative, slowly progressive deterioration of nerves in the brain stem's motor system characterized by a gradual onset of symptoms such as a stooped posture with the body flexed forward; a bowed head; a shuffling gait; pill-rolling gestures; an expressionless, masklike facial appearance; muffled speech; and swallowing difficulty.

Paronychia (par-oh-**NIK**-ee-ah) inflammation of the fold of skin surrounding the fingernail; also called runaround.

Parotid gland (pah-**ROT**-id gland) one of the largest pairs of salivary glands that lie at the side of the face just below and in front of the external ear.

Partial thromboplastin (throm-boh-**PLAST**-tin) a blood test used to evaluate the common pathway and system of clot formation within the body.

Parturition (par-too-**RISH**-un) the act of giving birth.

Patent ductus arteriosus (**PAY**-tent **DUCK**-tus ar-**TEE**-ree-**OH**-sis) an abnormal opening between the pulmonary artery and the aorta caused by failure of the fetal ductus arteriosus to close after birth. This defect is seen primarily in premature infants.

Pathogens (**PATH**-oh-jenz) disease-producing microorganisms.

Pediatric urine collection (pee-dee-**AT**-rik) a urine specimen may be requested as part of an infant's physical examination to determine the presence of a pathologic condition.

Pediculosis (pee-**dik**-yoo-**LOH**-sis) a highly contagious parasitic infestation caused by blood-sucking lice.

Pedophilia (pee-doh-**FILL**-ee-ah) sexual disorder in which the individual is sexually aroused and engages in sexual activity with children (generally age 13 or younger). This individual is known as a pedophile.

Pedunculated (peh-**DUN**-kyoo-**LAY**-ted) pertaining to a structure with a stalk.

Pelvic cavity the lower front cavity of the body, located beneath the abdominal cavity; contains the urinary bladder and reproductive organs.

Pelvic girdle weakness (**PELL**-vik **GER**-dul **WEAK**-ness) weakness of the muscles of the pelvic girdle (the muscles that extend the hip and the knee). In muscular dystrophy, the pelvic girdle weakness causes the child to use one or both hands to assist in rising from a sitting position by "walking" the hands up the lower extremities until he or she is in an upright position.

Pelvic inflammatory disease (**PELL**-vik in-**FLAM**-mah-tor-ee) inflammation of the upper female genital tract (cervix, uterus, ovaries and fallopian tubes (also known as salpingitis); may be associated with sexually transmitted diseases.

Pelvic ultrasound (**PELL**-vik **ULL**-trah-sound) a noninvasive procedure that uses high-frequency sound waves to examine the abdomen and pelvis.

Pelvimetry (pell-**VIM**-eh-tree) the process of measuring the female pelvis, manually or by X-ray, to determine its adequacy for childbearing.

Pemphigus (**PEM**-fih-gus) a rare incurable disorder manifested by blisters in the mouth and on the skin which spread to involve large areas of the body, including the chest, face, umbilicus, back, and groin.

Peptic ulcers (gastric, duodenal, perforated) (PEP-tik **ULL**-sirz) (**GAS**-tric, doo-**OD**-en-al, **PER**-foh-ray-ted) a break in the continuity of the mucous membrane lining of the gastrointestinal tract as a result of hyperacidity or the bacterium *Helicobacter pylori*.

Percussion (per-**KUH**-shun) use of the fingertips to tap the body lightly but sharply to determine position, size, and consistency of an underlying structure and the presence of fluid or pus in a cavity.

Percutaneous transhepatic cholangiography (PTC) (**per**-kyoo-**TAY**-nee-us trans-heh-**PAT**-ik koh-**lan**-jee-**OG**-rah-fee) an examination of the bile duct structure by using a needle to pass directly into an intrahepatic bile duct to inject a contrast medium; also abbreviated as PTHC.

Percutaneous transluminal coronary angioplasty (PTCA) (**per**-kyoo-**TAY**-nee-us trans-**LOOM**-ih-nal **KOR**-ah-nair-ree **AN**-jee-oh-**plass**-tee) a nonsurgical procedure in which a catheter, equipped with a small inflatable balloon on the end, is inserted into the femoral artery and is threaded up the aorta (under X-ray visualization) into the narrowed coronary artery.

Perforation of the tympanic membrane (per-for-**AY**-shun of the tim-**PAN**-ik) rupture of the tympanic membrane or eardrum.

Pericardial pertaining to the pericardium.

Pericarditis (pair-ih-car-**DYE**-tis) inflammation of the pericardium (the saclike membrane that covers the heart muscle). It may be acute or chronic.

Pericardium (pehr-ih-**KAR**-dee-um) double membranous sac that encloses the heart and the origins of the great blood vessels.

Perineum (pair-ih-**NEE**-um) area between the scrotum and the anus in the male and between the vulva and anus in the female.

Periodontal disease (pair-ee-oh-**DON**-tal dih-**ZEEZ**) a term used to describe a group of inflammatory gum disorders, which may lead to degeneration of teeth, gums, and sometimes surrounding bones.

Periosteum (pair-ee-**AH**-stee-um) the thick, white, fibrous membrane that covers the surface of a long bone.

Peripheral arterial occlusive disease (per-**IF**-er-al ar-**TEE**-ree-al oh-**KLOO**-siv dih-**ZEEZ**) obstruction of the arteries in the extremities (predominantly the legs). The leading cause of this disease is atherosclerosis, which leads to narrowing of the lumen of the artery. The classic symptom of peripheral arterial occlusive disease is intermittent claudication, which is a cramplike pain in the muscles brought on by exercise and relieved by rest.

Peripheral neuritis (per-**IF**-er-al noo-**RYE**-tis) general term indicating inflammation of one or more peripheral nerves, the effects being dependent on the particular nerve involved.

Peripheral nervous system (per-**IF**-er-al nervous system) the part of the nervous system outside the CNS, consisting of 12 pairs of cranial nerves and 31 pairs of spinal nerves.

Peristalsis (pair-ih-**STALL**-sis) coordinated, rhythmic, serial contraction of smooth muscle that forces food through the digestive tract, bile through the bile duct, and urine through the ureters.

Peritoneal dialysis (**pair**-ih-toh-**NEE**-al dye-**AL**-ih-sis) mechanical filtering process used to cleanse the blood of waste products, draw off excess fluids, and regulate body chemistry when the kidneys fail to function properly. Instead of using the hemodialysis machine as a filter, the peritoneal membrane (also called the peritoneum) is used as the filter in peritoneal dialysis.

Peritoneum (pair-ih-toh-**NEE**-um) a specific serous membrane that covers the entire abdominal wall of the body and is reflected over the contained viscera.

Peritonitis (pair-ih-**ton**-**EYE**-tis) inflammation of the peritoneum (the membrane lining the abdominal cavity).

Permanent teeth the full set of teeth (32 teeth) that replace the deciduous or temporary teeth.

Personality disorders any of a large group of mental disorders characterized by rigid, inflexible, and maladaptive behavior patterns that impair a person's ability to function in society by severely limiting adaptive potential.

Perspiration the clear, watery fluid produced by the sweat glands. See also *sweat*.

Pertussis (per-**TUH**-sis) an acute upper respiratory infectious disease caused by the *Bordetella pertussis* bacterium; "whooping cough."

Petechiae (peh-**TEE**-kee-ee) small, purplish, hemorrhagic spots on the skin; may be due to abnormality in the blood-clotting mechanism of the body.

Petit mal seizure (pet-**EE MALL SEE**-zyoor) small seizure in which there is a sudden temporary loss of consciousness lasting only a few seconds; also known as an absence seizure.

Phacoemulsification (fak-oh-ee-**MULL**-sih-fih-**kay**-shun) phacoemulsification is a method of removing a lens by using ultrasound vibrations to split up the lens material into tiny particles that can be suctioned out of the eye.

Phagocytosis (fag-oh-sigh-**TOH**-sis) the process by which certain cells engulf and destroy microorganisms and cellular debris.

Pharmacist (**FAR**-mah-sist) one who is licensed to prepare and dispense drugs.

Pharmacodynamics (far-mah-koh-dye-**NAM**-iks) the study of how drugs interact in the human body.

Pharmacology (far-mah-**KOL**-oh-jee) the field of medicine that specializes in the study of drugs, including their sources, appearance, chemistry, actions, and uses.

Pharmacy (**FAR**-mah-see) a place for preparing or dispensing drugs.

Pharyngitis (**fair**-in-**JYE**-tis) inflammation of the pharynx, usually resulting in sore throat.

Pharynx (**FAIR**-inks) the throat; a tubular structure about 5.1 inches long that extends from the base of the skull to the esophagus and is situated just in front of the cervical vertebrae. The pharynx serves as a passageway for air from the nasal cavity to the larynx and for food from the mouth to the esophagus. It serves both the respiratory and digestive systems.

Pheochromocytoma (fee-oh-**kroh**-moh-sigh-**TOH**-mah) a vascular tumor of the adrenal medulla that produces extra epinephrine and norepinephrine, leading to persistent or intermittent hypertension and heart palpitations.

Phimosis (fih-**MOH**-sis) a tightness of the foreskin (prepuce) of the penis that prevents it from being pulled back. The opening of the foreskin narrows due to the tightness and may cause some difficulty with urination.

Phobia (**FOH**-bee-ah) anxiety disorder characterized by an obsessive, irrational, and intense fear of a specific object, of an activity, or of a physical situation. Phobias are usually characterized by symptoms such as faintness, fatigue, palpitations, perspiration, nausea, tremor, and panic.

Phobic disorder (**FOH**-bik) anxiety disorder characterized by an obsessive, irrational, and intense fear of a specific object, of an activity, or of a physical situation; also called phobia disorder.

Photophobia (foh-toh-**FOH**-bee-ah) abnormal sensitivity to light, especially by the eyes.

Photo-refractive keratectomy (foh-toh-ree-**FRAK**-tiv kair-ah-**TEK**-toh-mee) surgical procedure in which a few layers of corneal surface cells are shaved off by an excimer laser beam to flatten the cornea and reduce myopia (nearsightedness).

Photosensitivity (**foh**-toh-sen-sih-**TIH**-vih-tee) increased reaction of the skin to exposure to sunlight.

Phrenic nerve (**FREN**-ic nerve) the nerve known as the motor nerve to the diaphragm.

Physicians' Desk Reference a reference book that provides the same information found in package inserts that accompany each container of medication: description of the drug, actions, indications and usage (why medication is prescribed) contraindications, warnings, precautions, adverse reactions, overdosage, and dosage and administration.

Pia mater (**PEE**-ah **MAHT**-er) the innermost of the three membranes (meninges) surrounding the brain and spinal cord.

Pica (**PIE**-kah) an eating disorder characterized by a craving to eat nonfood substances such as chalk, charcoal, clay, dirt, glue, hair, ice, paint, paper, soap, or starch over a period of at least one month.

Piezoelectric (pie-**EE**-zoh-eh-**lek**-trik) generation of a voltage across a solid when a mechanical stress is applied.

Pilonidal cyst (**pye**-loh-**NYE**-dal) a closed sac located in the sacrococcygeal area of the back, sometimes noted at birth as a dimple.

Pimple a papule or pustule of the skin.

Pineal body (**PIN**-ee-al body) a small cone-shaped structure (located in the diencephalon of the brain) thought to be involved in regulating the body's biological clock and that produces melatonin; also called the pineal gland.

Pineal gland (**PIN**-ee-al gland) see *pineal body*.

Pitting edema (pitting ee-**DEE**-mah) swelling, usually of the skin of the extremities, that when pressed firmly with a finger will maintain the dent produced by the finger.

Placenta (plah-**SEN**-tah) highly vascular, disc-shaped organ that forms in the pregnant uterine wall for exchange of gases and nutrients between the mother and the fetus. The maternal side of the placenta attaches to the uterine wall, whereas the fetal side of the placenta gives rise to the umbilical cord (which connects directly to the baby). After the delivery of the baby, when the placenta is no longer needed, it separates from the uterine wall and passes to the outside of the body through the vagina (at which time it is called the afterbirth).

Placenta previa (plah-**SEN**-tah **PRE**-vee-ah) condition of pregnancy in which the placenta is implanted in the lower part of the uterus and precedes the fetus during the birthing process.

Plane imaginary slices (or cuts) made through the body as if a dividing sheet were passed through the body at a particular angle and in a particular direction, permitting a view from a different angle.

Plantar (**PLANT**-ar) pertaining to the sole or bottom of the foot.

Plantar flexion (**PLAN**-tar **FLEK**-shun) increases the angle between the leg and the top of the foot (i.e., the foot is bent downward at the ankle, with the toes pointing downward, as in ballet dancing).

Plasma (**PLAZ**-mah) the watery, straw-colored, fluid portion of the lymph and the blood in which the leukocytes, erythrocytes, and platelets are suspended.

Platelet (**PLAYT**-let) a clotting cell; a thrombocyte.

Platelet count (**PLAYT**-let count) the count of platelets per cubic millimeter of blood.

Play therapy form of psychotherapy in which a child plays in a protected and structured environment with games and toys provided by a therapist who observes the behavior, affect, and conversation of the child to gain insight into thoughts, feelings, and fantasies.

Pleura (**PLOO**-rah) the double-folded membrane that lines the thoracic cavity.

Pleural effusion (**PLOO**-ral eh-**FYOO**-zhun) accumulation of fluid in the pleural space, resulting in compression of the underlying portion of the lung, with resultant dyspnea.

Pleural space (**PLOO**-ral space) the space that separates the visceral and parietal pleurae, which contains a small amount of fluid that acts as a lubricant to the pleural surfaces during respiration.

Pleuritis (pleurisy) (ploor-**EYE**-tis) (**PLOOR**-ih-see) inflammation of both the visceral and parietal pleura.

Plexus (**PLEKS**-us) a network of interwoven nerves.

Pneumocystis carinii pneumonia (PCP) (**noo**-moh-**SIS**-tis kah-**rye**-nee-eye noo-**MOH**-nee-ah) caused by a common worldwide parasite, *Pneumocystis carinii*, for which most people have immunity if they are not severely immunocompromised.

Pneumoencephalography (noo-moh-en-**seff**-ah-**LOG**-rah-fee) used to visualize radiographically one of the ventricles or fluid-occupying spaces in the CNS.

Pneumonia (new-**MOH**-nee-ah) acute inflammation of the lungs caused mainly by inhaled pneumococci of the *Streptococcus pneumoniae* species. It may also be caused by other bacteria as well as by viruses.

Pneumothorax (new-moh-**THOH**-racks) collection of air or gas in the pleural cavity. The air enters as the result of a perforation through the chest wall or the pleura covering the lung (visceral pleura), causing the lung to collapse.

Poliomyelitis (poh-lee-oh-**my**-eh-**LYE**-tis) an infectious viral disease entering through the upper respiratory tract and affecting the ability of spinal cord and brain motor neurons to receive stimulation. Muscles affected become paralyzed without the motor nerve stimulation (i.e., respiratory paralysis requires ventilatory support).

Polycystic kidney disease (pol-ee-**SISS**-tik kidney disease) a hereditary disorder of the kidneys in which grapelike, fluid-filled sacs or cysts replace normal kidney tissue.

Polycythemia vera (pol-ee-sigh-**THEE**-mee-ah **VAIR**-ah) an abnormal increase in the number of RBCs, granulocytes, and thrombocytes, leading to an increase in blood volume and viscosity (thickness).

Polydipsia (pol-ee-**DIP**-see-ah) excessive thirst.

Polymyositis (pol-ee-my-oh-**SIGH**-tis) polymyositis is a chronic, progressive disease affecting the skeletal (striated) muscles. It is characterized by muscle weakness of hips and arms and degeneration (atrophy).

Polyp (**POL**-ip) a small, stalklike growth that protrudes upward or outward from a mucous membrane surface, resembling a mushroom stalk.

Polyphagia (pol-ee-**FAY**-jee-ah) excessive eating.

Polyps, colorectal (**POL**-ips koh-loh-**REK**-tal) colorectal polyps are small growths projecting from the mucous membrane of the colon or rectum.

Polysomnogram (polly-**SOHM**-no-gram) a polysomnogram (PSG) is a sleep study or sleep test that evaluates physical factors affecting sleep. Physical activity and level of sleep are monitored by a technician while the patient sleeps.

Polyuria (pol-ee-**YOO**-ree-ah) the excretion of excessively large amounts of urine.

Pons (**PONZ**) the part of the brain located between the medulla oblongata and the midbrain. It acts as a bridge to connect the medulla oblongata and the cerebellum to the upper portions of the brain.

Pores openings of the skin through which substances such as water, salts, and some fatty substances are excreted.

Positron emission tomography (PET) (**PAHZ**-ih-tron *or* **PAWZ**-ih-tron ee-**MISH**-un toh-**MOG**-rah-fee) a computerized X-ray technique that uses radioactive substances to examine the blood flow and the metabolic activity of various body structures such as the heart and blood vessels. The patient is given doses of strong radioactive tracers by injection or inhalation. The radiation emitted is measured by the PET camera.

Posterior (poss-**TEE**-ree-or) pertaining to the back of the body.

Posteroanterior (**poss**-ter-oh-an-**TEER**-ee-or) the direction from back to front.

Postpolio syndrome (**POST-POH**-lee-oh **SIN**-drom) progressive weakness occurring at least 30 years after the initial poliomyelitis attack.

Post-traumatic stress disorder a disorder in which the individual experiences characteristic symptoms following exposure to an extremely traumatic event. The individual reacts with horror, extreme fright, or helplessness to the event.

Potency (**POH**-ten-see) strength.

Potentiation (poh-**ten**-she-**AY**-shun) the effect that occurs when two drugs administered together produce a more powerful response than the sum of their individual effects.

Preeclampsia (**pre**-eh-**KLAMP**-see-ah) a state during pregnancy in which the expectant mother develops high blood pressure, accompanied by proteinuria or edema, or both, after 20 weeks' gestation.

Pregnancy (**PREG**-nan-see) the period of intrauterine development of the fetus from conception through birth. The average pregnancy lasts approximately 40 weeks; also known as the gestational period.

Pregnancy-induced hypertension development of hypertension (high blood pressure) during pregnancy in women who had normal blood pressure readings (normotensive) prior to pregnancy.

Pregnancy testing tests performed on maternal urine and blood to determine the presence of the hormone HCG (human chorionic gonadotropin). HCG is detected shortly after the first missed menstrual period.

Premature ejaculation (premature ee-**jack**-yoo-**LAY**-shun) the discharge of seminal fluid prior to complete erection of the penis or immediately after the penis has been introduced into the vaginal canal.

Premenstrual syndrome (pre-**MEN**-stroo-al **SIN**-drom) a group of symptoms that include irritability, fluid retention, tenderness of the breasts, and a general feeling of depression occurring shortly before the onset of menstruation; also called PMS.

Premolars see *bicuspid tooth.*

Prenatal (pre-**NAY**-tal) pertaining to the period of time during pregnancy, that is, before the birth of the baby.

Prepuce (**PRE**-pus) see *foreskin.*

Presbycusis (prez-bye-**KOO**-sis) loss of hearing due to the natural aging process.

Presbyopia (pres-bee-**OH**-pee-ah) a refractive error occurring after the age of 40, when the lens of the eye(s) cannot focus on an image accurately due to its decreasing loss of elasticity.

Pressure ulcer an inflammation, sore, or ulcer in the skin over a bony prominence of the body, resulting from loss of blood supply and oxygen to the area due to prolonged pressure on the body part; also known as a decubitus ulcer or pressure sore.

Primary intracranial tumors (**PRIGH**-mair-ree in-trah-**KRAY**-nee-al **TOO**-morz) arise from gliomas, malignant glial cells that are a support for nerve tissue, and from tumors that arise from the meninges.

Primigravida (prye-mih-**GRAV**-ih-dah) a woman who is pregnant for the first time.

Primipara (prye-**MIP**-ah-rah) a woman who has given birth for the first time, after a pregnancy of at least 20 weeks' gestation.

Prodromal (pro-**DROH**-mal) pertaining to early signs or symptoms that mark the onset of a disease.

Progesterone (proh-**JES**-ter-on) a female hormone secreted by the corpus luteum and the placenta. It is primarily responsible for the changes that occur in the endometrium in anticipation of a fertilized ovum and for development of the maternal placenta after implantation of a fertilized ovum. Also known as progestin.

Projection (proh-**JEK**-shun) the act of transferring one's own unacceptable thoughts or feelings to someone else.

Pronation (proh-**NAY**-shun) the act of turning the palm down or backward.

Prone (**PROHN**) lying facedown on the abdomen.

Prophylactic (proh-fih-**LAK**-tik) an agent that protects against disease.

Prostate gland (**PROSS**-tayt gland) a gland that surrounds the base of the urethra, which secretes a milky-colored secretion into the urethra during ejaculation. This secretion enhances the motility of the sperm and helps neutralize the secretions within the vagina.

Prostatectomy (pross-tah-**TEK**-toh-mee) removal of all or part of the prostate gland. A discussion of two approaches to removing the prostate gland is presented in the section on diagnostic techniques.

Prostatitis (pross-tah-**TYE**-tis) inflammation of the prostate gland.

Proteinuria (proh-teen-**YOO**-ree-ah) the presence of protein (albumin) in the urine; also called albuminuria. This can be a sign of pregnancy-induced hypertension (PIH).

Prothrombin (proh-**THROM**-bin) a plasma protein precursor of thrombin. It is synthesized in the liver if adequate vitamin K is present.

Prothrombin time (PT) (proh-**THROM**-bin) a blood test used to evaluate the common pathway and extrinsic system of clot formation.

Protocol (**PROH**-toh-kall) a written plan or description of the steps to be taken in a particular situation, such as conducting research.

Proximal (**PROCK**-sih-mal) toward or nearest to the trunk of the body or nearest to the point of attachment of a body part.

Proximodistal growth and development proceeds from the center outward or from the midline to the periphery.

Pruritus (proo-**RYE**-tus) itching.

Pseudohypertrophic muscular dystrophy (soo-doh-**high**-per-**TROH**-fic **MUSS**-kew-lar **DIS**-troh-fee) a form of muscular dystrophy that is characterized by progressive weakness and muscle fiber degeneration without evidence of nerve involvement or degeneration of nerve tissue; also known as Duchenne's muscular dystrophy.

Psoriasis (soh-**RYE**-ah-sis) a common, noninfectious, chronic disorder of the skin manifested by silvery-white scales covering round, raised, reddened plaques producing itching (pruritus).

Psychiatrist (sigh-**KIGH**-ah-trist) a physician who specializes in the diagnosis, prevention, and treatment of mental disorders.

Psychiatry (sigh-**KIGH**-ah-tree) the branch of medicine that deals with the causes, treatment, and prevention of mental, emotional, and behavioral disorders.

Psychoanalysis (**sigh**-koh-an-**NAL**-ih-sis) a form of psychotherapy that analyzes the individual's unconscious thought, using free association, questioning, probing, and analyzing.

Psychoanalyst (**sigh**-koh-**AN**-ah-list) a psychotherapist, usually a psychiatrist, who has had special training in psychoanalysis and who applies the techniques of psychoanalytic theory.

Psychodrama (sigh-koh-**DRAH**-mah) a form of group psychotherapy in which people act out their emotional problems through unrehearsed dramatizations; also called role-playing therapy.

Psychoeducation refers to education offered to individuals who live with a psychological disturbance. It involves teaching people about their illness, how to treat it, and how to recognize signs of relapse so they can seek treatment before the condition worsens or returns.

Psychologist (sigh-**KOL**-oh-jist) a person who specializes in the study of the structure and function of the brain and related mental processes of animals and humans. A clinical psychologist has a graduate degree with specialized training in providing testing and counseling to patients with mental and emotional disorders.

Psychology (sigh-**KOL**-oh-jee) the study of behavior and the processes of the mind, especially as it relates to the individual's social and physical environment.

Psychosis (sigh-**KOH**-sis) any major mental disorder of organic or emotional origin characterized by a loss of contact with reality.

Psychosomatic (**sigh**-koh-soh-**MAT**-ik) pertaining to the expression of an emotional conflict through physical symptoms.

Psychotherapy (sigh-koh-**THAIR**-ah-pee) any of a large number of related methods of treating mental and emotional disorders by using psychological techniques instead of physical means of treatment.

Psychotropic (sigh-koh-**TROH**-pik) any substance capable of affecting the mind, emotions, and behavior; drugs used in the treatment of mental illness.

Pterygium (ter-**IJ**-ee-um) an irregular growth of fibrovascular tissue from the conjunctiva onto the cornea, usually on the nasal side of the cornea, that can disrupt vision if it extends over the pupil.

Puberty (**PEW**-ber-tee) the period of life at which the ability to reproduce begins.

Pulmonary artery (**PULL**-moh-neh-ree **AR**-ter-ee) one of a pair of arteries that transports deoxygenated blood from the right ventricle of the heart to the lungs for oxygenation. The pulmonary arteries are the only arteries in the body to carry deoxygenated blood.

Pulmonary circulation (**PULL**-moh-neh-ree) the circulation of deoxygenated blood from the right ventricle of the heart to the lungs for oxygenation and back to the left atrium of the heart, that is, from the heart, to the lungs, back to the heart.

Pulmonary edema (**PULL**-mon-air-ree eh-**DEE**-mah) swelling of the lungs caused by an abnormal accumulation of fluid in the lungs, either in the alveoli or the interstitial spaces.

Pulmonary embolism (**PULL**-mon-air-ree **EM**-boh-lizm) the obstruction of one or more pulmonary arteries by a thrombus (clot) that dislodges from another location and is carried through the venous system to the vessels of the lung.

Pulmonary function tests physicians use this variety of tests to assess respiratory function.

Pulmonary heart disease (cor pulmonale) (**PULL**-mon-air-ree heart dih-**ZEEZ**) (cor pull-mon-**ALL**-ee) hypertrophy of the right ventricle of the heart (with or without failure) resulting from disorders of the lungs, pulmonary vessels, or chest wall; heart failure resulting from pulmonary disease.

Pulmonary parenchyma (**PULL**-mon-air-ee par-**EN**-kih-mah) the functional units of the lungs (for example, the alveoli) which have very thin walls that allow for the exchange of gases between the lungs and the blood.

Pulmonary vein (**PULL**-moh-neh-ree vein) one of four large veins (two from each lung) that returns oxygenated blood from the lungs back to the left atrium of the heart. The pulmonary veins are the only veins in the body to carry oxygenated blood.

Pulp any soft, spongy tissue such as that contained within the spleen, the pulp chamber of the tooth, or the distal phalanges of the fingers and the toes.

Pupillary (**PEW**-pih-lair-ee) pertaining to the pupil of the eye.

Purging (**PERJ**-ing) the means of ridding the body of what has been consumed; that is, the individual may induce vomiting or use laxatives to rid the body of food that has just been eaten.

Purpura (**PURR**-pew-rah) a collection of blood beneath the skin in the form of pinpoint hemorrhages appearing as red-purple skin discolorations.

Purulent (**PEWR**-yoo-lent) containing pus.

Pustule (**PUS**-tyool) a small elevation of the skin filled with pus; a small abscess on the skin.

Pyelitis (pye-eh-**LYE**-tis) inflammation of the renal pelvis.

Pyelography (**pie**-eh-**LOG**-rah-fee) technique in radiology for examining the structures and evaluating the function of the urinary system.

Pyloric sphincter (pye-**LOR**-ik **SFINGK**-ter) a thickened muscular ring in the stomach that regulates the passage of food from the pylorus of the stomach into the duodenum.

Pyorrhea (pye-oh-**REE**-ah) discharge or flow of pus.

Pyrexia (pie-**REK**-see-ah) fever.

Pyrosis (pye-**ROH**-sis) heartburn; indigestion.

Q

Quadriplegia (**kwad**-rih-**PLEE**-jee-ah) follows severe trauma to the spinal cord between the fifth and seventh cervical vertebrae, generally resulting in loss of motor and sensory function below the level of injury.

Quickening (**KWIK**-en-ing) the first feeling of movement of the fetus felt by the expectant mother; usually occurs at about 16 to 20 weeks' gestation.

R

Rad (**RAD**) abbreviation for *radiation absorbed dose*; the basic unit of absorbed dose of ionizing radiation.

Radiation (ray-dee-**AY**-shun) the emission of energy, rays, or waves.

Radiation therapy (ray-dee-**AY**-shun **THAIR**-ah-pee) the treatment of neoplastic disease by using X-rays or gamma rays, usually from a cobalt source, to deter the growth of malignant cells by decreasing the rate of cell division or impairing DNA synthesis. Also called radiotherapy.

Radical prostatectomy (**RAD**-ih-kal **pross**-tah-**TEK**-toh-mee) the surgical removal of the entire prostate gland as a treatment for cancer.

Radiculotomy (rah-dick-yoo-**LOT**-oh-mee) the surgical resection of a spinal nerve root (a procedure performed to relieve pain); also called a rhizotomy.

Radioactive iodine uptake (RAIU) (ray-dee-o-**AK**-tiv **EYE**-oh-dine **UP**-tayk) a thyroid function test that evaluates the function of the thyroid test gland by administering a known amount of radioactive iodine and later placing a gamma ray detector over the thyroid gland to determine the percentage or quantity of radioactive iodine absorbed by the gland over specific time periods. It is used in the diagnosis of thyroid problems, particularly hyperthyroidism.

Radioactivity (ray-dee-oh-**ak-TIV**-ih-tee) ability of a substance to emit rays or particles (alpha, beta, or gamma) from its nucleus.

Radiocurable tumor (ray-dee-oh-**KYOOR**-ah-bul **TOO**-mor) pertaining to the susceptibility of tumor cells to destruction by ionizing radiation.

Radioresistant tumor (ray-dee-oh-ree-SIS-tant TOO-mor) a tumor that resists the effects of radiation.

Radioresponsive tumor (**ray**-dee-oh-ree-**SPON**-siv **TOO**-mor) a tumor that reacts favorably to radiation.

Radiosensitive tumor (ray-dee-oh-**SEN**-sih-tiv **TOO**-mor) a tumor capable of being changed by or reacting to radioactive emissions such as X-rays, alpha particles, or gamma rays.

Radiographer (ray-dee-**OG**-rah-fer) an allied health professional trained to use X-ray machines and other imaging equipment to produce images of the internal structures of the body; also known as a radiologic technologist.

Radioimmunoassay (ray-dee-oh-**im**-yoo-noh-**ASS**-ay) a technique in radiology used to determine the concentration of an antigen, antibody, or other protein in the serum.

Radioisotope (ray-dee-oh-**EYE**-soh-tohp) a radioactive isotope (of an element) used for therapeutic and diagnostic purposes.

Radiologist (ray-dee-**OL**-oh-jist) a physician who specializes in radiology.

Radiology (ray-dee-**OL**-oh-jee) the study of the diagnostic and therapeutic uses of X-rays; also known as roentgenology.

Radiolucent (ray-dee-oh-**LOO**-sent) pertaining to materials that allow X-rays to penetrate with a minimum of absorption.

Radionuclide (radioisotope) (ray-dee-oh-**NOO**-kleed) (**ray**-dee-oh-**EYE**-soh-tohp) an isotope (or nuclide) that undergoes radioactive decay.

Radiopaque (ray-dee-oh-**PAYK**) not permitting the passage of X-rays or other radiant energy. Radiopaque areas appear white on an exposed X-ray film.

Radiopharmaceutical (ray-dee-oh-farm-ah-**SOO**-tih-kal) a drug that contains radioactive atoms.

Radiotherapy (ray-dee-oh-**THAIR**-ah-pee) the treatment of disease by using X-rays or gamma rays.

Random specimen (**RAN**-dom **SPEH**-sih-men) a urine specimen that is collected at any time.

Rationalization (rash-un-al-ih-**ZAY**-shun) attempting to make excuses or invent logical reasons to justify unacceptable feelings or behaviors; most commonly used defense mechanism.

Rebound tenderness a sensation of severe pain experienced by the patient when the doctor applies deep pressure to the abdomen and releases it quickly. When this deep pressure is applied to the lower right quadrant of the abdomen at McBurney's point, and this type of pain is experienced, it is a strong indicator of appendicitis.

Receptor (ree-**SEP**-tor) a sensory nerve ending (i.e., a nerve ending that receives impulses and responds to various types of stimulation).

Rectal medication (**REK**-tal) medication inserted into the rectum and slowly absorbed into the mucous membrane lining of the rectum. It is in the form of a suppository, which melts as the body temperature warms it, or a retention enema.

Rectal temperature temperature as measured in the rectum.

Rectoscope (**REK**-toh-skohp) an instrument used to view the rectum that has a cutting and cauterizing (burning) loop. Also known as proctoscope.

Rectum (REK-tum) the portion of the large intestine, about 4.7 inches long, continuous with the descending sigmoid colon (just proximal to the anal canal).

Recumbent (ree-KUM-bent) lying down.

Red blood cell count (RBC) the measurement of the circulating number of RBCs in 1 mm³ of peripheral blood.

Red blood cell morphology (mor-FOL-oh-jee) an examination of the RBC on a stained blood smear that enables the examiner to identify the form and shape of the RBCs.

Red bone marrow the soft, semifluid substance located in the small spaces of cancellous bone that is the source of blood cell production.

Regression (rih-GRESH-un) a response to stress in which the individual reverts to an earlier level of development and the comfort measures associated with that level of functioning.

Relapse (ree-LAPS) to exhibit again the symptoms of a disease from which a patient appears to have recovered.

Remission (rih-MISH-un) the partial or complete disappearance of the symptoms of a chronic or malignant disease.

Renal angiography (REE-nal an-jee-OG-rah-fee) X-ray visualization of the internal anatomy of the renal blood vessels after injection of a contrast medium.

Renal artery (REE-nal AR-teh-ree) one of a pair of large arteries, branching from the abdominal aorta, that supplies blood to the kidneys, adrenal glands, and ureters.

Renal calculus a stone formation in the kidney (plural: *renal calculi*); also called a nephrolith.

Renal cell carcinoma (REE-nal SELL kar-sih-NOH-mah) a malignant tumor of the kidney occurring in adulthood.

Renal failure, chronic (REE-nal FAIL-yoor, KRON-ik) **(uremia)** (yoo-REE-mee-ah) progressively slow development of kidney failure occurring over a period of years. The late stages of chronic renal failure are known as end-stage renal disease (ESRD).

Renal pelvis (REE-nal PELL-viss) the central collecting part of the kidney that narrows into the large upper end of the ureter. It receives urine through the calyces and drains it into the ureters.

Renal scan (REE-nal scan) a procedure in which a radioactive isotope (tracer) is injected intravenously, and the radioactivity over each kidney is measured as the tracer passes through the kidney.

Renal tubule (REE-nal TOOB-yool) a long, twisted tube that leads away from the glomerulus of the kidney to the collecting tubules. As the glomerular filtrate passes through the renal tubules, the water, sugar, and salts are reabsorbed into the bloodstream through the network of capillaries that surround them.

Renal vein (REE-nal VAYN) one of two vessels that carries blood away from the kidney.

Repression (rih-PRESH-un) involuntary blocking of unpleasant feelings and experiences from one's conscious mind.

Resectoscope (ree-SEK-toh-skohp) instrument used to remove tissue surgically from the body. It has a light source and lens attached for viewing the area.

Residual urine (rih-ZID-yoo-al YOO-rin) urine that remains in the bladder after urination.

Residual urine specimen obtained by catheterization after the patient empties the bladder by voiding. The amount of urine remaining in the bladder after voiding is noted as the residual amount.

Resistance the body's ability to counteract the effects of pathogens and other harmful agents.

Resorption (ree-SORP-shun) the process of removing or digesting old bone tissue.

Restless legs syndrome (RLS) condition of the legs involving annoying sensations of uneasiness, tiredness, itching, or tingling of the leg muscles while resting. The individual feels an overwhelming desire to get up and move around due to the jerking sensation and painful twitching of the muscles. It is sometimes referred to as Ekbom's syndrome, after the doctor who first recognized it.

Reticulocyte (reh-TIK-yoo-loh-sight) an immature erythrocyte characterized by a meshlike pattern of threads and particles at the former site of the nucleus.

Reticulocyte count (reh-TIK-yoo-loh-sight) a measurement of the number of circulating reticulocytes, immature erythrocytes, in a blood specimen.

Retinal detachment (RET-in-al detachment) the partial or complete splitting away of the retina from the pigmented vascular layer called the choroid, interrupting vascular supply to the retina and thus creating a medical emergency.

Retinal photocoagulation (RET-in-al foh-toh-coh-ag-yoo-LAY-shun) surgical procedure that uses an argon laser to treat conditions such as glaucoma, retinal detachment, and diabetic retinopathy.

Retinal tear (RET-in-al tear) an opening in the retina that allows leakage of vitreous humor under the retina.

Retinopathy (ret-in-OP-ah-thee) any disease of the retina.

Retractions (rih-TRAK-shun) displacement of tissues to expose a part or structure of the body; retractions may be seen around the ribs in a child or infant with respiratory distress.

Retrograde pyelogram (RP) (RET-roh-grayd PYE-eh-loh-gram) a radiographic procedure in which small-caliber catheters are passed through a cystoscope into the ureters to visualize the ureters and the renal pelvis.

Reye's syndrome (RISE SIN-drom) acute brain encephalopathy along with fatty infiltration of the internal organs that may follow acute viral infections; occurs in children between 5 and 11, often with a fatal result. There are confirmed studies linking the onset of Reye's syndrome to aspirin administration during a viral illness.

Rh incompatibility incompatibility between an Rh negative mother's blood with her Rh positive baby's blood, causing the mother's body to develop antibodies that will destroy the Rh positive blood.

Rheumatic fever (roo-**MAT**-ic fever) an inflammatory disease that may develop as a delayed reaction to insufficiently treated group A beta-hemolytic streptococcal infection of the upper respiratory tract.

Rheumatoid arthritis (**ROO**-mah-toyd ar-**THRY**-tis) chronic, systemic, inflammatory disease that affects multiple joints of the body, mainly the small peripheral joints such as in those of the hands and feet.

Rheumatoid factor (**ROO**-mah-toyd factor) blood test that measures the presence of unusual antibodies that develop in a number of connective tissue diseases, such as rheumatoid arthritis.

Rhinitis (rye-**NYE**-tis) inflammation of the mucous membranes of the nose, usually resulting in obstruction of the nasal passages, rhinorrhea, sneezing, and facial pressure or pain, also known as coryza.

Rhizotomy (rye-**ZOT**-oh-mee) surgical resection of a spinal nerve root (a procedure performed to relieve pain); also called a radiculotomy.

Ribonucleic acid (RNA) (**rye**-boh-**new**-**KLEE**-ik **ASS**-id) a nucleic acid found in both the nucleus and cytoplasm of cells that transmits genetic instructions from the nucleus to the cytoplasm.

Ribosomes (**RYE**-boh-sohmz) cell organs (or organelles) that synthesize proteins; often called the cell's "protein factories."

Roentgenology (**rent**-jen-**OL**-oh-jee) see *radiology*.

Rorschach inkblot test (**ROR**-shak) personality test that involves the use of 10 inkblot cards, half black-and-white and half in color. The cards are shown to the individual one at a time. The person is shown a card and asked to describe what he or she sees in the card.

Romberg test (**ROM**-berg test) test used to evaluate cerebellar function and balance.

Rosacea (roh-**ZAY**-she-ah) chronic inflammatory skin disease that mainly affects the skin of the middle third of the face. The individual has persistent redness over the areas of the face, nose, and cheeks.

Roseola infantum (**roh**-zee-**OH**-lah in-**FAN**-tum) viral disease with a sudden onset of a high fever for three to four days, during which time the child may experience mild cold-like symptoms and slight irritability. Febrile seizures may occur.

Rotation (roh-**TAY**-shun) movement that involves the turning of a bone on its own axis.

Rotator cuff tear tear in the muscles that form a "cuff" over the upper end of the arm (head of the humerus). The rotator cuff helps lift and rotate the arm and hold the head of the humerus in place during abduction of the arm.

Rouleaux (roo-**LOH**) aggregation of RBCs viewed through the microscope that may be an artifact or may occur with persons with multiple myeloma as a result of abnormal proteins.

Route of administration method of introducing a medication into the body.

Rubella (German measles; 3-day measles) (roo-**BELL**-lah) mild febrile (fever-causing) infectious disease resembling both scarlet fever and measles but differing from these in its short course; characterized by a rash of both macules and papules that fades and disappears in three days.

Rubeola ("red measles," 7-day measles) (roo-bee-**OH**-lah) acute, highly communicable viral disease that begins as an upper respiratory disorder with fever, sore throat, cough, runny nose, sensitivity to light, and possible conjunctivitis. Typical red, blotchy rash appears four to five days after onset of symptoms, beginning behind the ears, on the forehead, or on the cheeks and progressing to extremities and trunk and lasting about five days.

Rugae (**ROO**-gay) a ridge or fold (such as the rugae of the stomach) that presents large folds in the mucous membrane of that organ.

Rupture of the amniotic sac may occur prior to the onset of labor, may occur during labor, or may not occur without assistance. Expectant mothers are usually advised to report to the hospital or birthing center for evaluation if the membranes rupture prior to the onset of labor. This is important because the amniotic sac serves as a barrier between the baby and the unsterile outside environment, and when broken the chance for infection is increased. Women often refer to the rupture of the amniotic sac by saying their "water broke," because there may be a sudden gush of amniotic fluid as the membranes rupture.

S

SA node sinoatrial node; pacemaker of the heart. See also *pacemaker*.

Sacrum (**SAY**-krum) singular triangular-shaped bone that results from the fusion of the five individual sacral bones of the child.

Saliva (sah-**LYE**-vah) the clear, viscous fluid secreted by the salivary and mucous glands in the mouth.

Salivary glands (**SAL**-ih-vair-ee glands) one of the three pairs of glands secreting into the mouth, thus aiding the digestive process.

Salpingectomy (sal-pin-**JEK**-toh-mee) surgical removal of a fallopian tube.

Salpingitis (sal-pin-**JYE**-tis) inflammation of the fallopian tubes; also known as pelvic inflammatory disease (included in this section because it is associated with sexually transmitted diseases).

Sarcoidosis (**sar**-koyd-**OH**-sis) systemic inflammatory disease resulting in the formation of multiple small, rounded lesions (granulomas) in the lungs (comprising 90%), lymph nodes, eyes, liver, and other organs.

Sarcoma (sar-**KOH**-mah) malignant neoplasm of the connective and supportive tissues of the body, usually first presenting as a painless swelling.

Scabies (**SKAY**-beez) a highly contagious parasitic infestation caused by the "human itch mite," resulting in a rash, pruritus, and slightly raised thread-like skin lines.

Scales thin flakes of hardened epithelium shed from the epidermis.

Scanning (bone, brain, liver, lungs) process of recording the emission of radioactive waves using a gamma camera (scanner) after an intravenous injection of a radionuclide material (tracer) into the particular part of the body being studied. The tracer doesn't remain active for long, with radioactivity being completely eliminated by two days.

Scarlet fever (scarlatina) (**SCAR**-let **FEE**-ver) (scar-lah-**TEE**-nah) an acute, contagious disease characterized by sore throat, abrupt high fever, increased pulse, strawberry tongue (red and swollen), and punctiform (pointlike) bright red rash on the body.

Schilling test a diagnostic analysis for pernicious anemia.

Schizophrenia (skiz-oh-**FREN**-ee-ah) any of a large group of psychotic disorders characterized by gross distortion of reality, disturbances of language and communication, withdrawal from social interaction, and the disorganization and fragmentation of thought, perception, and emotional reaction.

Sciatica (sigh-**AT**-ih-kah) inflammation of the sciatic nerve; characterized by pain along the course of the nerve, radiating through the thigh and down the back of the leg.

Scirrhous (**SKIR**-us) pertaining to a carcinoma with a hard structure.

Sclerectomy (skleh-**REK**-toh-mee) excision, or removal, of a portion of the sclera of the eye.

Scleritis (skleh-**RYE**-tis) the presence of inflammation in the white, outside covering of the eyeball (the sclera).

Scleroderma (sklehr-oh-**DER**-mah) gradual thickening of the dermis and swelling of the hands and feet to a state in which the skin is anchored to the underlying tissue.

Scotoma (skoh-**TOH**-mah) area of depressed vision (blindness) within the usual visual field, surrounded by an area of normal vision; an abnormal "blind spot."

Scrotum (**SKROH**-tum) external sac that houses the testicles. It is located posterior to the penis and is suspended from the perineum.

Sebaceous cyst (see-**BAY**-shus **SIST**) cyst filled with a cheesy material consisting of sebum and epithelial debris that has formed in the duct of a sebaceous gland; also known as an epidermoid cyst.

Sebaceous gland (see-**BAY**-shus) oil gland located in the dermis; its secretions provide oil to the hair and surrounding skin.

Seborrhea (seb-or-**EE**-ah) excessive secretion of sebum, resulting in excessive oiliness or dry scales.

Seborrheic keratosis (seb-oh-**REE**-ik kair-ah-**TOH**-sis) appears as brown or waxy yellow wartlike lesion(s) 5 to 20 mm in diameter, loosely attached to the skin surface.

Sebum (**SEE**-bum) the oily secretions of the sebaceous glands.

Secondary teeth see *permanent teeth.*

Sedative agent that decreases functional activity and has a calming effect on the body.

Semen (**SEE**-men) combination of sperm and various secretions that is expelled from the body through the urethra during sexual intercourse.

Semen analysis (**SEE**-men ah-**NAL**-ih-sis) assessment of a sample of semen for volume, viscosity, sperm count, sperm motility, and percentage of any abnormal sperm.

Seminal vesicles (**SEM**-ih-nal **VESS**-ih-kulz) glands that secrete a thick, yellowish fluid (known as seminal fluid) into the vas deferens.

Seminiferous tubules (**SEM**-in-**IF**-er-us **TOO**-byools) specialized coils of tiny tubules responsible for production of sperm; located in the testes.

Senescence (seh-**NESS**-ens) the process of growing old.

Senile dementia (**SEE**-nile dee-**MEN**-shee-ah) an organic mental disorder of the aged, resulting from the generalized atrophy (wasting) of the brain with no evidence of cerebrovascular disease. This condition is characterized by loss of memory, impaired judgment, decreased moral and ethical values, inability to think abstractly, and periods of confusion and irritability. These symptoms may range from mild to severe.

Senile lentigines (**SEE**-nyle lin-**TIH**-jeh-nez) age spots; brown macules found on areas of the skin that are frequently exposed to the sun such as the face, neck, or back of the hands of many older people. The singular form of the word is *lentigo.*

Sensory (**SEN**-soh-ree) pertaining to sensation.

Sensory nerves (**SEN**-soh-ree nerves) transmitters of nerve impulses toward the CNS; also known as afferent nerves.

Septicemia (sep-tih-**SEE**-mee-ah) systemic infection in which pathogens are present in the circulating bloodstream, having spread from an infection in any part of the body.

Septum (**SEP**-tum) a wall, or partition, that divides or separates two cavities. The interatrial septum separates the right and left atria, the atrioventricular septum separates the atria and the ventricles, and the interventricular septum separates the right and left ventricles.

Seroconversion (see-roh-con-**VER**-zhun) a change in serologic tests from negative to positive as antibodies develop in reaction to an infection or vaccine.

Serology (see-**ROL**-oh-jee) branch of laboratory medicine that studies blood serum for evidence of infection by evaluating antigen–antibody reactions.

Serous (**SEER**-us) pertaining to producing serum.

Serous otitis media (SOM) (**SEER**-us oh-**TYE**-tis **MEE**-dee-ah) a collection of clear fluid in the middle ear that may follow acute otitis media or be due to an obstruction of the eustachian tube.

Serum (**SEE**-rum) also called blood serum. The clear, thin, and sticky fluid portion of the blood that remains after coagulation. Serum contains no blood cells, platelets, or fibrinogen.

Serum bilirubin (SEE-rum bill-ih-**ROO**-bin) measurement of the bilirubin level in the serum. Serum bilirubin levels are a result of the breakdown of red blood cells.

Serum glucose test (SEE-rum **GLOO**-kohs) measures the amount of glucose in the blood at the time the sample was drawn.

Serum glutamic-oxaloacetic transaminase (SGOT) (SEE-rum **TAM**-ik **oks**-ah-loh-ah-**SEE**-tik trans-**AM**-in-ays) enzyme that has very high concentrations in liver cells; (also known as ASPT: aspartate aminotransferase)

Serum lipid test (SEE-rum **LIP**-id test) measures the amount of fatty substances (cholesterol, triglycerides, and lipoproteins) in a sample of blood obtained by venipuncture.

Serum sickness (SEE-rum) hypersensitivity reaction that may occur two to three weeks after administration of an antiserum. Symptoms include fever, enlargement of the spleen (splenomegaly), swollen lymph nodes, joint pain, and skin rash.

Sesamoid bones (SES-a-moyd bones) irregular bones imbedded in tendons near a joint, as in the kneecap.

Sessile (SESS-il) attached by a base rather than by a stalk or a peduncle.

Sexual intercourse the sexual union of two people of the opposite sex in which the penis is introduced into the vagina; also known as copulation or coitus.

Sexual sadism/sexual masochism a sexual disorder that involves the act (real, not simulated) of being humiliated, beaten, bound, or otherwise made to suffer; or the act of inflicting psychological or physical suffering on the victim.

Shaken baby syndrome (SBS) serious form of child abuse that describes a group of unique symptoms resulting from repetitive, violent shaking. The violent shaking (forward and backward shaking) produces acceleration–deceleration forces within the head of the child that can cause brain injury. This whiplash-type injury is not caused by playful bouncing of the child and is not an accidental injury.

Shingles (herpes zoster) (SHING-ulz) (HER-peez ZOSS-ter) acute viral infection seen mainly in adults who have had chicken pox, characterized by inflammation of the underlying spinal or cranial nerve pathway (producing painful vesicular eruptions on the skin along these nerve pathways).

Short bones bones that are about as long as they are wide and somewhat box-shaped, such as the wrist bone.

Shunt a tube or passage that diverts or redirects body fluid from one cavity or vessel to another; may be a congenital defect or artificially constructed for the purpose of redirecting fluid, as a shunt used in hydrocephalus.

Side effect an additional effect on the body by a drug that was not part of the goal for that medication. Nausea is a common side effect of many drugs.

Sigmoid colon (SIG-moyd colon) the portion of the colon that extends from the end of the descending colon in the pelvis to the juncture of the rectum.

Signs objective findings as perceived by an examiner, such as the measurement of a fever on the thermometer, the observation of a rash on the skin, or the observation of a bluish-violet color of the cervix.

Silicosis (sill-ih-**KOH**-sis) a lung disease resulting from inhalation of silica (quartz) dust, characterized by formation of small nodules.

Simple to complex language, for example, develops from simple to complex.

Single-photon emission computed tomography (SPECT) (single-**FOH**-ton ee-**MISH**-un kom-**PEW**-ted toh-**MOG**-rah-fee) nuclear imaging procedure that shows how blood flows to tissues and organs.

Sinus (SIGH-nuss) an opening or hollow space in a bone; a cavity within a bone.

Sinusitis (sigh-nus-**EYE**-tis) inflammation of a sinus, especially a paranasal sinus.

Skeletal muscle (SKELL-eh-tal) muscle that is attached to bone and is responsible for the movement of the skeleton.

Skin biopsy (BYE-op-see) the removal of a small piece of tissue from a skin lesion for the purpose of examining it under a microscope to confirm or establish a diagnosis.

Skin graft process of placing tissue on a recipient site, taken from a donor site, to provide the protective mechanisms of skin to an area unable to regenerate skin (as in third-degree burns).

Skin tags small brownish or flesh-colored outgrowth of skin occurring frequently on the neck; also known as a cutaneous papilloma.

Skull fracture (depressed) (SKULL FRAK-chur) (deh-**PREST**) a broken segment of the skull bone thrust into the brain as a result of a direct force, usually a blunt object.

Slit-lamp exam the examination of the external and internal structures of the eye, using a low-power microscope combined with a high-intensity light source that can be focused to shine as a slit beam; also known as biomicroscopy.

Small bowel follow-through oral administration of a radiopaque contrast medium, barium sulfate, which flows through the GI system. X-ray films are obtained at timed intervals to observe the progression of the barium through the small intestine.

Smooth muscle muscle found in the walls of the hollow internal organs of the body such as the stomach and intestines.

Solute (SOL-yoot) a substance dissolved in a solution, as in the waste products filtered out of the kidney into the urine.

Somatic nervous system (soh-**MAT**-ik nervous system) the part of the PNS that provides voluntary control over skeletal muscle contractions.

Somatic symptom disorders (soh-**MAT**-ik **SIM**-tohm dis-**OR**-ders) any group of neurotic disorders characterized by symptoms suggesting physical illness or disease for which there are no demonstrable organic causes or physiologic dysfunctions.

Somatotropic hormone (soh-mat-oh-**TROH**-pik) a hormone secreted by the anterior pituitary gland that regulates the cellular processes necessary for normal body growth; also called the growth hormone.

Specific gravity (speh-**SIH**-fik **GRAV**-ih-tee) weight of a substance compared with an equal volume of water, which is considered to be the standard. Water is considered to have a specific gravity of 1.000 (one). Therefore, a substance with a specific gravity of 2.000 would be twice as dense as water.

Sperm a mature male germ cell; spermatozoon.

Spermatozoan (**sper**-mat-oh-**ZOH**-ahn) a mature male germ cell; also known as spermatozoon (plural: *spermatozoa*).

Spermatozoon (**sper**-mat-oh-**ZOH**-on) see *spermatozoan*.

Sphincter (**SFINGK**-ter) a circular band of muscle fibers that constricts a passage or closes a natural opening in the body, such as the hepatic sphincter in the muscular coat of the hepatic veins near their union with the superior vena cava (and the external anal sphincter, which closes the anus).

Spina bifida cystica (**SPY**-nah **BIFF**-ih-dah **SISS**-tih-kah) congenital defect of the CNS in which the back portion of one or more vertebrae is not closed normally and a cyst protrudes through the opening in the back, usually at the level of the fifth lumbar or first sacral vertebrae.

Spina bifida occulta (**SPY**-nah **BIFF**-ih-dah oh-KULL-tah) congenital defect of the CNS in which the back portion of one or more vertebrae is not closed. A dimpling over the area may occur.

Spinal cavity cavity that contains the nerves of the spinal cord; also known as the spinal canal.

Spinal cord injuries severe injuries to the spinal cord, such as vertebral (paraplegia and dislocation or vertebral fractures, resulting in impairment of spinal quadriplegia) cord function below the level of the injury.

Spinal stenosis narrowing of the vertebral canal, nerve root canals, or intervertebral foramini (openings) of the lumbar spinal canal. The narrowing causes pressure on the nerve roots prior to their exit from the foramini.

Spine a sharp projection from the surface of a bone, similar to a crest.

Splenomegaly (**splee**-noh-**MEG**-ah-lee) an abnormal enlargement of the spleen.

Sprains injury involving the ligaments that surround and support a joint, caused by a wrenching or twisting motion.

Sputum (**SPEW**-tum) substance coughed up from the lungs, bronchi, and trachea that is expelled through the mouth; sputum is not the same as saliva, which is secreted by the salivary glands.

Sputum specimen (**SPEW**-tum specimen) a specimen of material expectorated from the mouth. If produced after a cough, it may contain (in addition to saliva) material from the throat and bronchi.

Squamous epithelial cells (**SKWAY**-mus ep-ih-**THEE**-lee-ul) flat scalelike cells arranged in layers (strata).

Squamous epithelium (**SKWAY**-mus ep-ih-**THEE**-lee-um) single layer of flattened platelike cells that cover internal and external body surfaces.

Staging (**STAY**-jing) the determination of distinct phases or periods in the course of a disease.

Standards rules that have been established to control the strength, quality, and purity of medications prepared by various manufacturers.

Stapedectomy (stay-pee-**DEK**-toh-mee) microsurgical removal of the stapes diseased by otosclerosis, typically under local anesthesia.

Stature (**STAT**-yoor) natural height of a person in an upright position.

Stem cell formative cell; a cell whose daughter cells may give rise to other cell types.

Stenosis (stin-**OH**-sis) an abnormal condition characterized by a narrowing or restriction of an opening or passageway in a body structure.

Stereotaxic neurosurgery (**ster**-eh-oh-**TAK**-sik **noo**-roh-**SER**-jer-ee) performed on a precise location of an area within the brain that controls specific function(s) and may involve destruction of brain tissue with various agents such as heat, cold, and sclerosing or corrosive fluids.

Stimulus (**STIM**-yoo-lus) any agent or factor capable of initiating a nerve impulse.

Stomach (**STUM**-ak) the major organ of digestion located in the left upper quadrant of the abdomen and divided into a body and pylorus.

Stool analysis for occult blood (stool analysis for uh-**CULT** blood) analysis of a stool sample to determine the presence of blood not visible to the naked eye (i.e., hidden or occult blood).

Stool culture (**STOOL KULL**-chir) involves collection of a stool specimen placed on one or more culture mediums and allowed to grow colonies of microorganisms to identify specific pathogen(s).

Stool guaiac (**STOOL GWEE**-ak *or* **GWY**-ak) test on a stool specimen using guaiac as a reagent, which identifies the presence of blood in the stool.

Strabismus (strah-**BIZ**-mus) failure of the eyes to gaze in the same direction due to weakness in the muscles controlling the position of one eye. The most common type of strabismus is nonparalytic strabismus, an inherited defect in which the eye position of the two eyes has no relationship.

Strains injury to the body of the muscle or attachment of the tendon, resulting from overstretching, overextension, or misuse (i.e., a "muscle pull").

Stratified (**STRAT**-ih-fyd) layered; arranged in layers.

Stratum (**STRAT**-um) a uniformly thick sheet or layer of cells.

Stratum basale (**STRAT**-um **BAY**-sil) the layer of skin where new cells are continually being reproduced, pushing older cells toward the outermost surface of the skin.

Stratum corneum (**STRAT**-um **COR**-nee-um) the outermost layer of the epidermis (consisting of dead cells that have converted to keratin), which continually sloughs off or flakes away; known as the keratinized (or "horny") cell layer (*kerat/o* = horn).

Stress incontinence, urinary (**STRESS** in-**CON**-tin-ens, **YOO**-rih-**nair**-ee) the inability to hold urine when the bladder is stressed by sneezing, coughing, laughing, or lifting.

Stretch marks linear tears in the dermis that result from overstretching from rapid growth. They begin as pinkish-blue streaks with jagged edges and may be accompanied by itching. As they heal and lose their color, they remain as silvery-white scar lines, also known as striae.

Striae gravidarum (**STRIGH**-ay grav-ih-**DAR**-um) stretch marks that occur during pregnancy due to the great amount of stretching that occurs. They appear as slightly depressed, pinkish-purple streaks in the areas of greatest stretch (which are the abdomen, the breasts and the thighs).

Striated muscle (**STRY**-ay-ted muscle) muscles that have a striped appearance when viewed under a microscope. Skeletal and cardiac muscles are examples.

Stridor (**STRYE**-dor) abnormal, high-pitched, musical sound caused by an obstruction in the trachea or larynx.

Stupor (**STOO**-per) a state of lethargy. The person is unresponsive and seems unaware of his or her surroundings.

Subarachnoid space (sub-ah-**RAK**-noyd space) the space located just under the arachnoid membrane that contains cerebrospinal fluid.

Subcutaneous medication (**sub**-kyoo-**TAY**-nee-us) medication injected into the subcutaneous layer, or fatty tissue, of the skin.

Subcutaneous tissue (**sub**-kyoo-**TAY**-nee-us) the fatty layer of tissue located beneath the dermis.

Subdural space (**sub**-**DOO**-ral space) the space located just beneath the dura mater that contains serous fluid.

Sublimation (sub-lih-**MAY**-shun) rechanneling or redirecting one's unacceptable impulses and drives into constructive activities.

Sublingual medication (sub-**LING**-gwal) medication placed under the tongue, where it dissolves in the patient's saliva and is quickly absorbed through the mucous membrane lining of the mouth.

Subluxation (**sub**-luks-**AY**-shun) an incomplete dislocation.

Subungual hematoma (sub-**UNG**-gwall heemah-**TOH**-ma) a collection of blood beneath a nail bed, usually the result of trauma (injury).

Sudden burst of energy occurs in some women shortly before the onset of labor. These women may suddenly have the energy to do major housecleaning duties—things they have not had the energy to do previously.

Sudden infant death syndrome completely unexpected and unexplained death of an apparently well, or virtually well, infant. SIDS, also known as crib death, is the most common cause of death between the second week and first year of life.

Sudoriferous gland (soo-door-**IF**-er-us) a sweat gland.

Sulcus (**SULL**-kus) depression or shallow groove on the surface of an organ; as a sulcus that separates any of the convolutions of the cerebral hemispheres (plural: *sulci*).

Superficial pertaining to the surface of the body or near the surface.

Superior (soo-**PEE**-ree-or) above or upward toward the head.

Supination (soo-pin-**AY**-shun) the act of turning the palm up or forward.

Supine (soo-**PINE**) lying horizontally on the back, faceup.

Supine hypotension (soo-**PINE high**-poh-**TEN**-shen) low blood pressure that occurs in a pregnant woman when she is lying on her back. It is caused by the pressure of the pregnant uterus on the vena cava; also known as supine hypotension syndrome or vena cava syndrome.

Suppression (suh-**PRESH**-un) voluntary blocking of unpleasant feelings and experiences from one's mind.

Suppurative otitis media (**SOO**-per-ah-tiv oh-**TYE**-tis **MEE**-dee-ah) purulent collection of fluid in the middle ear, causing the person to experience pain (possibly severe), an elevation in temperature, dizziness, decreased hearing, vertigo, and tinnitus; also called acute otitis media.

Suprapubic prostatectomy (**soo**-prah-**PEW**-bik **pross**-tah-**TEK**-toh-mee) surgical removal of the prostate gland by making an incision into the abdominal wall, just above the pubic bone.

Susceptible (suh-**SEP**-tih-bul) a state of having a lack of resistance to pathogens and other harmful agents. For example, the individual is said to be "susceptible."

Sutures (**SOO**-chers) immovable joints, such as those of the cranium.

Sweat the clear, watery fluid produced by the sweat glands; also known as perspiration.

Sweat gland one of the tiny structures within the dermis that produces sweat, which carries waste products to the surface of the skin for excretion; also known as a sudoriferous gland.

Sydenham's chorea (**SID**-en-hamz koh-**REE**-ah) a form of chorea (involuntary muscle twitching) associated with rheumatic fever, usually occurring in childhood.

Sympathectomy (**sim**-pah-**THEK**-toh-mee) surgical procedure used to interrupt a portion of the sympathetic nerve pathway for the purpose of relieving chronic pain.

Sympathetic nerves (sim-pah-**THET**-ik) nerves of the ANS that regulate essential involuntary body functions such as increasing the heart rate, constricting blood vessels, and raising the blood pressure.

Sympathomimetic (sim-pah-thoh-mim-**ET**-ik) copying or producing the same effects as those of the sympathetic nerves; "to mimic" the sympathetic nerves.

Symptoms (**SIM**-toms) subjective indication of a disease or a change in condition as perceived by the patient; something experienced or felt by the patient.

Synapse (**SIN**-aps) the space between the end of one nerve and the beginning of another, through which nerve impulses are transmitted.

Syncope (**SIN**-koh-pee) fainting.

Syndrome (**SIN**-drohm) a group of symptoms occurring together, indicative of a particular disease or abnormality.

Synechia (sin-**ECK**-ee-ah) an adhesion in the eye that develops as a complication of trauma, inflammation, or surgery or as a secondary condition of one of the following pathological conditions: cataracts, glaucoma, keratitis, or uveitis.

Synovial fluid (sin-**OH**-vee-al) a thick lubricating fluid located in synovial joints.

Synovial joint (sin-**OH**-vee-al) in a synovial joint, the bones have a space between them called the joint cavity. The joint cavity is lined with a synovial membrane, which secretes a thick lubricating fluid called the synovial fluid. The bones of the synovial joint are held together by ligaments. The surfaces of the connecting bones are protected by a thin layer of cartilage called the articular cartilage. A synovial joint allows free movement.

Synovial membrane (sin-**OH**-vee-al **MEM**-brayn) the lining of a synovial joint cavity.

Syphilis (**SIF**-ih-lis) a sexually transmitted disease characterized by lesions that may involve any organ or tissue. It is spread by sexual intercourse with an infected partner and can also be passed through the placenta from an infected mother to her unborn infant. The spirochete *Treponema pallidum* is the causative organism of this highly contagious disease. If left untreated, this disease progresses through three stages (each with characteristic signs and symptoms): primary syphilis, secondary syphilis, and tertiary syphilis.

System organs that work together to perform the many functions of the body as a whole.

Systemic circulation (sis-**TEM**-ik ser-kew-**LAY**-shun) circulation of blood from the left ventricle of the heart, throughout the body, and back to the right atrium of the heart. Oxygenated blood leaves the left ventricle of the heart and is distributed to the capillaries. Deoxygenated blood is picked up from the capillaries and is transported back to the right atrium of the heart.

Systemic effect (sis-**TEM**-ik effect) a generalized response to a drug by the body. The drug has a widespread influence on the body because it is absorbed into the bloodstream.

Systemic lupus erythematosus (sis-**TEM**-ik **LOO**-pus er-rih-them-ah-**TOH**-sus) a chronic inflammatory connective-tissue disease affecting the skin, joints, nervous system, kidneys, lungs, and other organs. The most striking symptom of the disease is the "butterfly rash" that appears on both cheeks, joined by a narrow band of rash across the nose.

T

T cells Specialized lymphocytes that are involved in the immune response.

Tachycardia (tak-eh-**CAR**-dee-ah) rapid heartbeat, consistently over 100 beats per minute.

Talipes equinovarus clubfoot.

Tay-Sachs disease (**TAY**-**SACKS** dih-**ZEEZ**) congenital disorder caused by altered lipid metabolism, resulting from an enzyme deficiency.

Telangiectasia (tell-**an**-jee-ek-**TAY**-zee-ah) permanent dilation of groups of superficial capillaries and venules. These dilated vessels may be visible through the skin as tiny red lines. Common causes include but are not limited to rosacea, elevated estrogen levels, and actinic damage.

Teletherapy (tell-eh-**THAIR**-ah-pee) Radiation therapy administered by a machine positioned at some distance from the patient.

Tendon (**TEN**-dun) a strong fibrous band of tissue that extends from a muscle, attaching it to the bone by becoming continuous with the periosteum of the bone.

Tension headache (**TEN**-shun headache) occurs from long, endured contraction of the skeletal muscles around the face, scalp, upper back, and neck.

Testes (**TESS**-teez) the paired male gonads that produce sperm. They are suspended in the scrotal sac in the adult male. See also *testicles*.

Testicles (**TESS**-tih-kuls) the male gonads, or male sex glands, responsible for production of spermatozoa (the male germ cell) and for the secretion of the male hormone testosterone.

Testosterone (tess-**TOSS**-ter-own) a male hormone secreted by the testes, responsible for the secondary sex characteristic changes that occur in the male with the onset of puberty. These changes include growth of facial hair (beard), growth of pubic hair, and deepening of the voice.

Tetany (**TET**-ah-nee) a condition characterized by severe cramping and twitching of the muscles and sharp flexion of the wrist and ankle joints; a complication of hypocalcemia.

Tetralogy of Fallot (teh-**TROL**-oh-jee of fal-**LOH**) congenital heart anomaly that consists of four defects: pulmonary stenosis, interventricular septal defect, dextroposition (shifting to the right) of the aorta so that it receives blood from both ventricles, and hypertrophy of the right ventricle; named for the French physician, Etienne Fallot, who first described the condition.

Thalamus (**THAL**-ah-mus) the part of the brain located between the cerebral hemispheres and the midbrain. The thalamus receives all sensory stimuli, except those of smell, and relays them to the cerebral cortex.

Thalassemia (thal-ah-**SEE**-mee-ah) hereditary form of hemolytic anemia in which the alpha or beta hemoglobin chains are defective and the production of hemoglobin is deficient, creating hypochromic microcytic RBCs.

Thallium stress test (**THAL**-ee-um stress test) one of several nuclear stress tests. It is a combination of exercise stress testing with thallium imaging (myocardial perfusion scan) to assess changes in coronary blood flow during exercise.

Thematic apperception test (TAT) (thee-**MAT**-ik **ap**-er-**SEP**-shun) designed to elicit stories that reveal something about an individual's personality. This test consists of a series of 30 black-and-white pictures, each on an individual card.

Therapeutic dose (thair-ah-**PEW**-tik) dose of a medication that achieves the desired effect.

Thoracentesis (thoh-rah-sen-**TEE**-sis) use of a needle to collect pleural fluid for laboratory analysis or to remove excess pleural fluid or air from the pleural space.

Thoracic cavity (thoh-**RASS**-ik) the chest cavity, which contains the lungs, heart, aorta, esophagus, and trachea.

Thoracic vertebrae (thoh-**RASS**-ik) the second segment of 12 vertebrae that make up the vertebral bones of the chest; identified as T1 through T12.

Thorax (**THOH**-raks) the chest; that part of the body between the base of the neck and the diaphragm.

Thrombin (**THROM**-bin) enzyme formed from prothrombin, calcium, and thromboplastin in plasma during the clotting process. It causes fibrinogen to change to fibrin, which is essential in the formation of a clot.

Thrombocyte (**THROM**-boh-sight) a clotting cell; a platelet.

Thrombocytopenia (**throm**-boh-**sigh**-toh-**PEE**-nee-ah) an abnormal hematologic condition in which the number of platelets is reduced.

Thrombophlebitis (**throm**-boh-fleh-**BY**-tis) inflammation of a vein associated with the formation of a thrombus (clot); usually occurs in an extremity, most frequently a leg.

Thromboplastin (throm-boh-**PLAST**-in) a complex substance that initiates the clotting process by converting prothrombin into thrombin in the presence of calcium ion.

Thrombosis (throm-**BOH**-sis) the formation or existence of a blood clot.

Thrombus (**THROM**-bus) a clot.

Thrush (**THRUSH**) a fungal infection in the mouth and throat, producing sore, creamy white, slightly raised curdlike patches on the tongue and other oral mucosal surfaces. Thrush is caused by *Candida albicans*.

Thymopoietin (thigh-moh-**POY**-eh-tin) a hormone secreted by the thymus, thought to stimulate the production of T cells (which are involved in the immune response).

Thymosin (thigh-**MOH**-sin) a hormone secreted by the thymus. This hormone is thought to stimulate the production of specialized lymphocytes, called T cells, which are involved in the immune response.

Thyroid cancer (cancer of the thyroid gland) (**THIGH**-royd gland **CAN**-sir) malignant tumor of the thyroid gland that leads to dysfunction of the gland and thus inadequate or excessive secretion of the thyroid hormone.

Thyroid echogram (**THIGH**-royd **EK**-oh-gram) **(ultrasound)** an ultrasound examination important in distinguishing solid thyroid nodules from cystic nodules.

Thyroid function tests (**THIGH**-royd) laboratory tests that measure the blood levels of the T_3, T_4, and TSH hormones. These blood tests indicate how well the thyroid gland is working.

Thyroiditis, chronic (thigh-royd-**EYE**-tis) **(Hashimoto's)** (**HASH**-ee-moh-**TOZ**) chronic inflammation of the thyroid gland, leading to enlargement of the thyroid gland.

Thyroid panel (**THIGH**-royd) a laboratory blood test that produces an enhanced thyroid profile.

Thyroid scan (**THIGH**-royd) a test that determines the position, size, shape, and physiological function of the thyroid gland through the use of radionuclear scanning.

Thyroid-stimulating hormone (TSH) blood test a test that measures the concentration of TSH in the blood.

Thyroid storm thyrotoxicosis (thyroid storm) (**THIGH**-royd storm) (**thigh**-roh-toks-ih-**KOH**-sis) an acute, sometimes fatal, incident of overactivity of the thyroid gland resulting in excessive secretion of thyroid hormone.

Thyroxine (thigh-**ROKS**-in) a hormone secreted by the thyroid gland. This hormone helps maintain normal body metabolism (abbreviated as T_4).

Tinea (**TIN**-ee-ah) more commonly known as ringworm, a chronic fungal infection of the skin that is characterized by scaling, itching, and sometimes painful lesions. The lesions are named according to the body part affected.

Tinea capitis (**TIN**-ee-ah **CAP**-ih-tis) ringworm of the scalp is more common in children.

Tinea corporis (**TIN**-ee-ah **COR**-poh-ris) ringworm of the body is characterized by round patches with elevated red borders of pustules, papules, or vesicles that affect the nonhairy skin of the body. The lesion actually looks like a circle and is raised.

Tinea cruris (**TIN**-ee-ah **KROO**-ris) ringworm of the groin is also known as jock itch.

Tinea pedis (**TIN**-ee-ah **PED**-is) ringworm of the foot is also known as athlete's foot.

Tinnitus (tin-**EYE**-tus) a ringing or tinkling noise heard in the ears; may be a sign of injury to the ear, some disease process, or toxic levels of some medications from prolonged use (such as aspirin).

Tissue a group of cells that performs specialized functions.

Tolerance (**TAHL**-er-ans) the body's decreased response to the effect of a drug after repeated dosages.

Tomography (toh-**MOG**-rah-fee) X-ray technique used to construct a detailed cross section, at a predetermined depth, of a tissue structure.

Tonic-clonic seizure (**TON**-ik-**KLON**-ik **SEE**-zhur) a seizure characterized by the presence of muscle contraction or tension followed by relaxation, creating a "jerking" movement of the body.

Tonometry (tohn-**OM**-eh-tree) process of determining the intraocular pressure by calculating the resistance of the eyeball to an applied force causing indentation.

Tonsillectomy (ton-sill-**ECK**-toh-mee) surgical removal of the palatine tonsils.

Tonsillitis (ton-sill-**EYE**-tis) inflammation of the palatine tonsils, located in the area of the oropharynx.

Tonsils (**TON**-sills) masses of lymphatic tissue located in a protective ring, just under the mucous membrane, surrounding the mouth and back of the throat.

Topical medication (**TOP**-ih-kal) medication applied directly to the skin or mucous membrane for a local effect to the area.

Torso (**TOR**-soh) see *trunk*.

Toxic (**TOKS**-ik) poisonous.

Toxicology (**tocks**-ih-**KOL**-oh-jee) the study of poisons, their detection, and their effects and establishing antidotes and methods of treatment for conditions they produce and prevention of poisoning.

Toxoid (**TOKS**-oyd) toxin that has been treated with chemicals or with heat to decrease its toxic effect but that retains its ability to cause the production of antibodies.

Trabeculae (trah-**BEK**-yoo-lay) needlelike bony spicules within cancellous bone that contribute to the spongy appearance. Their distribution along lines of stress adds to the strength of the bone.

Trabeculectomy (trah-bek-yool-**EK**-toh-mee) the surgical excision of a portion of corneoscleral tissue to decrease the intraocular pressure in persons with severe glaucoma.

Trabeculoplasty (trah-**BEK**-yoo-loh-plass-tee) the surgical creation of a permanent fistula used to drain fluid (aqueous humor) from the eye's anterior chamber, usually performed under general anesthesia.

Trachea (**TRAY**-kee-ah) a cylinder-shaped tube lined with rings of cartilage (to keep it open) that is 4.5 inches long, from the larynx to the bronchial tubes; the windpipe.

Trachoma (tray-**KOH**-mah) an infectious eye disease caused by *Chlamydia trachomatis*, which is chronic and will lead to blindness without effective treatment.

Tractotomy (trak-**TOT**-oh-mee) a tractotomy involves a craniotomy, through which the anterolateral pathway in the brain stem is surgically divided in an attempt to relieve pain.

Trade name brand name copyrighted by a pharmaceutical company.

Transcutaneous electrical nerve stimulation (TENS) (tranz-kyoo-**TAY**-nee-us ee-**LEK**-trih-kul nerve **stim**-yoo-**LAY**-shun) a form of cutaneous stimulation for pain relief that supplies electrical impulses to the nerve endings of a nerve close to the pain site.

Transdermal (tranz-**DER**-mal) method of applying a drug to unbroken skin using an adhesive patch. The drug is absorbed continuously and produces a systemic effect.

Transducer (trans-**DOO**-sir) handheld device that sends and receives a sound-wave signal.

Transposition of the great vessels (tranz-poh-**ZIH**-shun) a condition in which the two major arteries of the heart are reversed in position, which results in two noncommunicating circulatory systems.

Transurethral resection of the prostate (TUR or TURP) (**trans**-yoo-**REE**-thral) the surgical removal of a portion of the prostate gland by inserting a resectoscope (an instrument used to remove tissue from the body) through the urethra and into the bladder to remove small pieces of tissue from the prostate gland.

Transvaginal ultrasonography (trans-**VAJ**-in-al **ull**-trah-son-**OG**-rah-fee) an ultrasound image that is produced by inserting a transvaginal probe into the vagina. The probe is encased in a disposable cover and is coated with a gel for easy insertion. The gel also promotes conductivity. This procedure allows clear visualization of the uterus, gestational sac, and embryo in the early stages of pregnancy. It also allows the examiner to visualize deeper pelvic structures such as the ovaries and fallopian tubes.

Transverse plane (trans-**VERS**) any of the planes cutting across the body perpendicular to the sagittal and the frontal planes, dividing the body into superior (upper) and inferior (lower) portions.

Trichomoniasis (**trik**-oh-moh-**NYE**-ah-sis) a sexually transmitted protozoal infection of the vagina, urethra, or prostate. It is usually spread by sexual intercourse and affects approximately 15% of all sexually active people. The causative organism is *Trichomonas vaginalis*.

Trigeminal neuralgia (*tic douloureux*) (try-**JEM**-ih-nal noo-**RAL**-jee-ah) (tik **DOO**-loh-roo) short periods of severe unilateral pain, which radiates along (*tic douloureux*) the fifth cranial nerve.

Triglycerides (try-**GLISS**-er-eyeds) a compound consisting of a fatty acid (oleic, palmitic, or stearic) and glycerol.

Triiodothyronine (**try**-eye-oh-doh-**THIGH**-roh-neen) a hormone secreted by the thyroid gland. This hormone helps regulate growth and development of the body and control metabolism and body temperature (abbreviated as T_3).

Trimester (**TRY**-mes-ter) one of the three periods of approximately three months into which pregnancy is divided. The first trimester consists of weeks 1 to 12, the second trimester consists of weeks 13 to 27, and the third trimester consists of weeks 28 to 40.

Trochanter (tro-**CAN**-ter) large bony process located below the neck of the femur.

True ribs the first seven pairs of ribs, which connect to the vertebrae in the back and to the sternum in the front.

Trunk the main part of the body, to which the head and the extremities are attached; also called the torso.

Truss an apparatus worn to prevent or block the herniation of the intestines or other organ through an opening in the abdominal wall.

Tubal ligation (**TOO**-bal lye-**GAY**-shun) surgically cutting and tying the fallopian tubes to prevent passage of ova or sperm through the tubes, consequently preventing pregnancy; female sterilization.

Tubercle (**TOO**-ber-kul) a small rounded process of a bone.

Tuberculin skin test (TST) (too-**BER**-kew-lin skin test) used to determine past or present tuberculosis infection present in the body. This is based on a positive skin reaction to the introduction of a purified protein derivative (PPD) of the tubercle bacilli, called tuberculin, into the skin.

Tuberculosis (too-**ber**-kyoo-**LOH**-sis) an infectious disease caused by the *Mycobacterium tuberculosis* tubercle bacillus and characterized by inflammatory infiltrations, formation of tubercles, and caseous (cheeselike) necrosis in the tissues of the lungs. Other organ systems may also be infected.

Tuberosity (too-ber-**OSS**-ih-tee) an elevated, broad, rounded process of a bone.

Tumor (**TOO**-mor) a new growth of tissue characterized by progressive, uncontrolled proliferation (growth) of cells. The tumor may be localized or invasive, benign or malignant.

Tumors, intracranial (**TOO**-mors, in-trah-**KRAY**-nee-al) occur in any structural region of the brain and may be malignant or benign. They are classified as primary or secondary and are named according to the tissue from which they originate.

Tumors, metastatic intracranial (**TOO**-mors, **met**-ah-**STAT**-ik in-trah-**KRAY**-nee-al) occur as a result of metastasis from a primary site such as the lung or breast.

Tumors, primary intracranial (**TOO**-mors, primary in-trah-**KRAY**nee-al) arise from gliomas (malignant glial cells that are a support for nerve tissue) or from the meninges are known as primary intracranial tumors.

Tuning fork test (Rinne test) (**RIN**-nee test) examination that compares bone conduction and air conduction.

Tuning fork test (Weber test) examination used to evaluate auditory acuity and to discover whether a hearing deficit is a conductive loss or a sensorineural loss.

Turbid (**TER**-bid) cloudy.

Tympanic temperature (tim-**PAN**-ik **TEM**-per-ah-chur) the body temperature as measured electronically at the tympanic membrane.

Tympanoplasty (tim-pan-oh-**PLASS**-tee) see *myringoplasty*. A tympanoplasty may also involve surgical repair of the bones in the middle ear (ossicles).

Tympanotomy (tim-pan-**OT**-oh-mee) see *myringotomy*.

U

Ulcer (**ULL**-ser) a circumscribed, open sore or lesion of the skin that is accompanied by inflammation.

Ulcerative colitis (**ULL**-sir-ah-tiv koh-**LYE**-tis) a chronic inflammatory condition resulting in a break in the continuity of the mucous membrane lining of the colon in the form of ulcers. Ulcerative colitis is characterized by large watery diarrheal stools containing mucus, pus, or blood.

Ultrasonography (**ull**-trah-son-**OG**-rah-fee) also called ultrasound. This is a procedure in which sound waves are transmitted into the body structures as a small transducer is passed over the patient's skin.

Ultrasound (**ULL**-trah-sound) sound waves at the very high frequency of more than 20,000 kHz (vibrations per second).

Umbilical cord (um-**BILL**-ih-kal cord) flexible structure connecting the umbilicus (navel) of the fetus with the placenta in the pregnant uterus. It serves as passage for the umbilical arteries and vein.

Umbilical hernia (um-**BILL**-ih-kahl **HER**-nee-ah) outward protrusion of the intestine through a weakness in the abdominal wall around the umbilicus (navel, or "belly button").

Umbilical region the region of the abdomen located in the middle section of the abdomen, between the right and left lumbar regions and directly beneath the epigastric region.

Umbilicus the navel; also called the belly button.

United States Pharmacopeia (**far**-mah-koh-**PEE**-ah) an authorized publication of the United States Pharmacopeial Convention that contains formulas and information that provide a standard for preparation and dispensation of drugs. Recognized by the U.S. government as the official listing of standardized drugs.

Upper GI tract the upper part of the gastrointestinal tract consisting of the mouth, pharynx, esophagus, and stomach.

Uptake (**UP**-tayk) the drawing up or absorption of a substance.

Uremia (yoo-**REE**-mee-ah) the presence of excessive amounts of urea and other nitrogenous waste products in the blood; also called *azotemia*.

Ureter (**YOO**-reh-ter) one of a pair of tubes that carries urine from the kidney to the bladder.

Urethra (yoo-**REE**-thrah) a small tubular structure that drains urine from the bladder to the outside of the body.

Urethritis (yoo-ree-**THRYE**-tis) inflammation of the urethra. Urethritis, characterized by dysuria, is usually the result of an infection of the bladder or kidneys.

Urinalysis (**yoo**-rih-**NAL**-ih-sis) physical, chemical, or microscopic examination of urine.

Urinary bilirubin (**YOO**-rih-nair-ee bill-ih-**ROO**-bin) a test performed on urine to check for conjugated or direct bilirubin in a urine specimen.

Urinary incontinence (**YOO**-rih-**nair**-ee in-**CON**-tin-ens) inability to control urination; the inability to retain urine in the bladder.

Urinary retention (**YOO**-rih-**nair**-ee ree-**TEN**-shun) an abnormal involuntary accumulation of urine in the bladder; the inability to empty the bladder.

Urination (**YOO**-rih-**NAY**-shun) the act of eliminating urine from the body; also called *micturition* or *voiding*.

Urine (**YOO**-rin) the fluid released by the kidneys, transported by the ureters, retained in the bladder, and eliminated through the urethra. Normal urine is clear, straw colored, and slightly acid.

Urine culture (**YOO**-rin) a procedure used to cultivate the growth of bacteria present in a urine specimen for proper microscopic identification of the specific pathogen (disease-producing microorganism).

Urticaria (**ur**-tih-**KARE**-ree-ah) a reaction of the skin in which there is an appearance of smooth, slightly elevated patches (wheals) that are redder or paler than the surrounding skin and often accompanied by severe itching (pruritus).

Uterus (**YOO**-ter-us) the hollow, pear-shaped organ of the female reproductive system that houses the fertilized, implanted ovum as it develops throughout pregnancy; also the source of the monthly menstrual flow from the nonpregnant uterus.

Uveitis (yoo-vee-**EYE**-tis) inflammation of all or part of the middle vascular layer of the eye made up of the iris, the ciliary body, and the choroid.

Uvula (**YOO**-vyoo-lah) the small, cone-shaped process suspended in the mouth from the middle of the posterior border of the soft palate.

V

Vaccine (**VAK**-seen; vak-**SEEN**) a suspension of attenuated or killed microorganisms administered intradermally, intramuscularly, orally, or subcutaneously to induce active immunity to infectious disease.

Vagina (vah-**JEYE**-nah) the muscular tube that connects the uterus with the vulva. It is approximately 3 inches long and rests between the bladder (anteriorly) and the rectum (posteriorly).

Vaginal medication (**VAJ**-in-al) medication inserted into the vagina; may be in the form of a suppository, cream, foam, or tablet.

Vaginitis (vaj-in-**EYE**-tis) inflammation of the vagina and the vulva.

Varicocele (**VAIR**-ih-koh-seel) an abnormal dilation of the veins of the spermatic cord leading to the testicle.

Varicose veins (**VAIR**-ih-kohs veins) enlarged, superficial veins; a twisted, dilated vein with incompetent valves.

Vas deferens (vas **DEF**-er-enz) the narrow, straight tube that transports sperm from the epididymis to the ejaculatory duct.

Vasectomy (vas-**EK**-toh-mee) a surgical cutting and tying of the vas deferens to prevent the passage of sperm, consequently preventing pregnancy; male sterilization.

Vasoconstriction (**vaz**-oh-con-**STRIK**-shun) narrowing of the lumen of a blood vessel.

VDRL test a serological test for syphilis (test performed on blood serum); widely used to test for primary and secondary syphilis. The acronym stands for Venereal Disease Research Laboratory test.

Vegetation (vej-eh-**TAY**-shun) an abnormal growth of tissue around a valve.

Venography (vee-**NOG**-rah-fee) also called phlebography, venography is a technique used to prepare an X-ray image of veins that have been injected with a contrast medium that is radiopaque.

Venous insufficiency (**VEE**-nuss in-syoo-**FISH**-in-see) an abnormal circulatory condition characterized by decreased return of venous blood from the legs to the trunk of the body. Venous insufficiency occurs as a result of prolonged venous hypertension, which stretches the veins and damages the valves. Standing or sitting in one position for long periods of time, pregnancy, and obesity may cause chronically distended veins, which leads to damaged valves.

Ventral pertaining to the front; belly side.

Ventricle, brain (**VEN**-trih-kul) a small hollow within the brain that is filled with cerebrospinal fluid.

Ventricular tachycardia (ven-**TRIK**-yoo-lar **TAK**-ee-**CAR**-dee-ah) ventricular tachycardia is a condition in which the ventricles of the heart beat at a rate greater than 100 beats per minute; characterized by three or more consecutive premature ventricular contractions (PVCs). It is also known as "V-tach" (VT).

Verruca (veh-**ROO**-kah) wart; *see verrucae.*

Verrucae (veh-**ROO**-kee) small, hard skin lesions caused by the human papillomavirus; warts (plural form).

Verrucous (veh-**ROO**-kus) rough; warty.

Vertebral foramen (**VER**-teh-bral for-**AY**-men) a large opening in the center of each vertebra that serves as a passageway for the spinal cord.

Vertex (**VER**-teks) the top of the head; crown.

Vertigo (**VER**-tih-goh) a sensation of spinning around or of having things in the room or area spinning around the person; a result of disturbance of the equilibrium.

Vesicle (**VESS**-ih-kul) a small thin-walled skin lesion containing clear fluid; a blister.

Vesicocele (**VESS**-ih-koh-**seel**) herniation or downward protrusion of the urinary bladder through the wall of the vagina; also called a *cystocele.*

Vesicoureteral reflux (vess-ih-koh-yoo-**REE**-ter-al **REE**-fluks) an abnormal backflow (reflux) of urine from the bladder to the ureter.

Villi (**VIL**-eye) one of the many tiny projections barely visible to the naked eye clustered over the entire mucous surface of the small intestine.

Virilism (**VEER**-il-izm) the development of masculine physical traits in the female (such as growth of facial and body hair, increased secretion of the sebaceous glands, deepening of the voice, and enlargement of the clitoris); also called masculinization. This condition may be due to an abnormality or dysfunction of the adrenal gland, as in adrenal virilism.

Visceral pertaining to the internal organs.

Visceral muscle see *smooth muscle.*

Visceral pleura (VISS-er-al PLOO-rah) portion of the pleura that is closest to the internal organs.

Viscous (VISS-kus) sticky; gelatinous.

Vitiligo (vit-ih-LYE-goh) a skin disorder characterized by nonpigmented white patches of skin of varying sizes that are surrounded by skin with normal pigmentation.

Vitreous (VIT-ree-us) pertaining to the vitreous body of the eye.

Voiding (VOYD-ing) the act of eliminating urine from the body; also called *micturition* or *urination.*

Voiding cystourethrography (VOY-ding sis-toh-yoo-ree-THROG-rah-fee) X-ray visualization of the bladder and urethra during the voiding process, after the bladder has been filled with a contrast material.

Volvulus (VOL-vyoo-lus) a rotation of loops of bowel, causing a twisting on itself that results in an intestinal obstruction. See also *intestinal obstruction.*

Vomiting (VOM-it-ing) ejection through the mouth of the gastric content. The forcible expulsion of the content of the stomach through the mouth; also called emesis.

Vulva (VULL-vah) the external genitalia that consists of the mons pubis, labia majora, clitoris, labia minora, vestibule, urinary meatus, vaginal orifice, Bartholin's glands, and the perineum; also known as the pudendum.

W

Waddling gait (WOD-ling gait) a manner of walking in which the feet are wide apart and the walk resembles that of a duck.

Wart (verruca) (ver-ROO-kah) a benign, circumscribed, elevated skin lesion that results from hypertrophy of the epidermis; caused by the human papilloma virus.

Weakness (WEEK-ness) lacking physical strength or vigor (energy).

Well-child visit routine health visit in which health professionals assess the current health status of the child, the progression of growth and development, and the need for immunizations.

Western blot a test that detects the presence of the antibodies to HIV, the virus that causes AIDS, used to confirm validity of ELISA tests.

Wet mount; wet prep the microscopic examination of fresh vaginal or male urethral secretions to test for the presence of living organisms.

Wheal (WHEEL) a circumscribed, slightly elevated lesion of the skin that is paler in the center than its surrounding edges; hives.

Wheezing (HWEEZ-ing) a breath sound, characterized by a high-pitched musical quality heard on both inspiration and expiration. Wheezes may be associated with asthma and chronic bronchitis as well as with other illnesses.

Whiplash an injury to the cervical vertebrae and their supporting structures due to a sudden back-and-forth jerking movement of the head and neck. Whiplash may occur as a result of an automobile being struck suddenly from the rear.

White blood cell (WBC) count the measurement of the circulating number of WBCs in 1 mm^3 of peripheral blood.

White blood cell differential (diff-er-EN-shal) measurement of the percentage of each specific type of circulating WBCs present in 1 mm^3 of peripheral blood drawn for the WBC count.

Whitehead a closed comedo caused by accumulation of keratin and sebum within the opening of a hair follicle; the content within is not easily expressed.

White matter the part of the nervous system consisting of axons covered with myelin sheath, giving a white appearance.

Wilms tumor a malignant tumor of the kidney occurring predominantly in childhood.

Wood's lamp an ultraviolet light used to examine the scalp and skin for the purpose of observing fungal spores.

X

Xanthoderma (zan-thoh-DER-mah) any yellow coloration of the skin.

Xeroderma (zee-roh-DER-mah) a chronic skin condition characterized by roughness and dryness.

X-rays the use of high-energy electromagnetic waves, passing through the body onto a photographic film, to produce a picture of the internal structures of the body for diagnosis and therapy. A chest X-ray is a visualization of the interior of the chest; critical in the complete evaluation of the cardiac and pulmonary systems.

Y

Yellow marrow located in the diaphysis of long bones, yellow marrow consists of fatty tissue and is inactive in the formation of blood cells.